Quick Reference to Standard Protocols for All Nursing Interventions

All nursing skills must include certain basic steps for the safety and well-being of the client and the nurse. To prevent repetition, these steps are not included in each skill unless it is necessary to clarify them as applied in that skill. *Remember that these steps are essential and must be consistently followed.*

HAND HYGIENE

The Centers for Disease Control and Prevention have issued guidelines for Hand Hygiene in Health Care settings (Boyce & Pittet, 2002). The published guidelines provide health care workers with specific recommendations to promote improved hand hygiene practices and reduce transmission of pathogenic microorganisms to clients and health care personnel. *Hand hygiene* is the new general term that applies to handwashing, antiseptic hand wash, antiseptic hand rub, and surgical hand antisepsis. Traditional handwashing refers to washing hands with plain, nonantimicrobial soap and water, which may not effectively remove pathogens. An antiseptic hand wash involves washing hands with water and soap containing an antimicrobial agent. An antiseptic hand rub involves use of an alcohol-based hand rub that reduces bacteria on the hands without causing irritation to the skin. Alcohol-based hand rubs are now recommended by the CDC for hand antisepsis in most clinical situations. However, when hands are visibly dirty or contaminated with proteinaceous material or are visibly soiled with blood or other body fluids, handwashing or antiseptic handwashing is recommended. For more information about hand hygiene see Chapter 3.

GLOVE LOGO

A logo is used in this text. The logo identifies circumstances in which the use of clean gloves is recommended because of increased probability of contact with mucous membranes, nonintact skin, or moist body substances. The Occupational Safety and Health Administration (OSHA) mandates that gloves be worn during all client care activities that may involve exposure to blood or body fluids that may be contami-

nated with blood (Occupational Safety and Health Administration. 29 CFR Part 1910.1030). Clean gloves are used to protect both caregivers and the clients. By wearing clean, disposable gloves before client contact, most microorganisms are kept off the caregiver's hands. However, gloves are not 100% effective and can have invisible small holes or tears. Gloves must not be washed or reused. **Effective hand hygiene and changing clean gloves is required between clients and between activities with the same client or when gloves become excessively soiled** (Murray, 2002).

Synthetic vinyl gloves may be effective; however, the barrier integrity varies based on intensity of use and length of time used. Because of increased concerns with latex allergies of both clients and health care workers, having more than one type of glove available is desirable in order to select the type that best suits the necessary activity. If latex products are used, use powder-free gloves with reduced protein content. Clients need to be questioned regarding latex allergies so that exposure can be avoided (DHHS [NIOSH] Publication No. 98-113).

Some skills require the use of **sterile gloves** for certain steps to protect the client from infection. Color print is used in this text to emphasize when sterile gloves are used.

Equipment   This includes standard equipment for all nursing procedures.

Armband for client identification

Consent Form if required by agency policy (see Chapter 1)

Clean disposable gloves (if contact with mucous membranes, nonintact skin, or moist body substances is anticipated)

BEFORE THE SKILL

1. Verify physician's orders if skill is a dependent or collaborative nursing intervention. Independent nursing interventions may be verified with the nursing care plan or primary nurse.
2. Identify the client by checking armband and having the client state name (if able to do so). In many long-term care settings, armbands are not used; however, pictures are available for identification.

To my children and grandchildren
whose love constantly reminds me of the most important things in life,
To my partner, Mary Ann,
whose love, patience, and encouragement empowered me
throughout the many long hours of manuscript preparation,
and
To the many nursing students
who have provided valuable input into this book
from the unique viewpoint of learners.
Martha Keene Elkin

To professional nurses
who accept the challenges of nursing and today's health care environment
and consistently incorporate care, compassion, scientific knowledge,
and standards of excellence into their nursing practices.
Anne Griffin Perry

To Kathy Teal
whose resolve to produce an accurate and
well-organized text is greatly appreciated.
We wish her a quick recovery.
Patricia Potter

3RD EDITION

NURSING INTERVENTIONS & CLINICAL SKILLS

Martha Keene Elkin, RN, MSN, IBCLC
Nursing Educator for Associate Degree Nursing
Private Practice Lactation Consultant
MotherCare of Maine, Comprehensive Breastfeeding Services
Sumner, Maine

Anne Griffin Perry, RN, MSN, EdD, FAAN
Professor and Coordinator, Adult Health Specialty
Saint Louis University School of Nursing
Saint Louis University Health Sciences Center
St. Louis, Missouri

Patricia A. Potter, RN, MSN, PhD
Research Scientist
Barnes-Jewish Hospital
St. Louis, Missouri

With over 900 illustrations

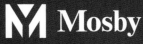
Mosby
An Affiliate of Elsevier

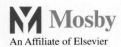

Mosby

An Affiliate of Elsevier

11830 Westline Industrial Drive
St. Louis, Missouri 63146

NURSING INTERVENTIONS AND CLINICAL SKILLS   ISBN 0-323-02201-4

Copyright © 2004, Mosby, Inc. All rights reserved.

NOTICE

Nursing is an ever-changing field. Standard safety precautions must be followed, but as new research and clinical experience broaden our knowledge, changes in treatment and drug therapy may become necessary or appropriate. Readers are advised to check the most current product information provided by the manufacturer of each drug to be administered to verify the recommended dose, the method and duration of administration, and contraindications. It is the responsibility of the licensed prescriber, relying on experience and knowledge of the patient, to determine dosages and the best treatment for each individual patient. Neither the publisher nor the authors assume any liability for any injury and/or damage to persons or property arising from this publication.

Previous editions copyrighted 2000, 1996

International Standard Book Number 0-323-02201-4

Executive Editor: Susan R. Epstein
Developmental Editor: Robyn L. Brinks
Publishing Services Manager: John Rogers
Senior Project Manager: Kathleen L. Teal
Senior Project Manager: Beth Hayes
Senior Designer: Kathi Gosche
Photography: Rick Brady
Design: Rokusek Design

Printed in China

Last digit is the print number: 9   8   7   6   5   4   3   2

Contributors

Margaret R. Benz, RN, MSN(R), BC, APN
Adjunct Assistant Professor
St. Louis University School of Nursing
St. Louis, Missouri

V. Christine Champagne, APRN, BC
Adult Nurse Practitioner
Midwest Chest Consultants
St. Charles, Missouri

Janice C. Colwell, RN, MS, CWOCN
Clinical Nurse Specialist, Wound, Ostomy & Skin Care
University of Chicago Hospitals
Chicago, Illinois

Eileen Costantinou, MSN, RN
Practice Consultant
Barnes-Jewish Hosptial
St. Louis, Missouri

Deborah Crump, RN, MS, CHPN
Hospice/Palliative Care Nurse
Androscoggin Home Care and Hospice
Oxford, Maine

Wanda Cleveland Dubuisson, RN, MSN
Assistant Professor of Nursing
College of Nursing
The University of Southern Mississippi
Hattiesburg, Mississippi

Susan Jane Fetzer, RN, BA, BSN, MBA, MSN, PhD
Associate Professor
University of New Hampshire
Durham, New Hampshire

Amy M. Hall, RN, BSN, MS, PhD
Assistant Professor
Saint Francis Medical Center College of Nursing
Peoria, Illinois

Mimi Hirshberg, RN, MSN
Barnes College of Nursing and Health Studies
University of Missouri   St. Louis
St. Louis, Missouri
IV Therapist
Vascular Access Service
Barnes-Jewish Hospital
St. Louis, Missouri

Meredith Hunt, MSN, RNC, NP
Nurse Practitioner
TriCounty Health Services
Norway, Maine

Kristine M. L'Ecuyer, RN, MSN
Adjunct Assistant Professor
Saint Louis University School of Nursing
St. Louis, Missouri

Cynthia L. Maskey, RN, MS
Professor, Associate Degree Nursing
Lincoln Land Community College
Springfield, Illinois

Peter R. Miller, RN, MSN, ONC
Faculty
Central Maine Medical Center School of Nursing
Lewiston, Maine

Jacqueline Raybuck Saleeby, PhD, RN, CS
Associate Professor
Jewish Hospital College of Nursing and Allied Health
St. Louis, Missouri

Lynn Schallom, RN, MSN, CCNS
Surgical Critical Care Clinical Nurse Specialist
Barnes-Jewish Hospital
St. Louis, Missouri

Kelly M. Schwartz, BSN, RN
Professional Practice Consultant
Barnes-Jewish Hospital
St. Louis, Missouri

Julie S. Snyder, MSN, RN, C
Adjunct Faculty
Old Dominion University
Norfolk, Virginia

Patricia A. Stockert, RN, BSN, MS, PhD
Associate Professor, Senior Coordinator
Saint Francis Medical Center College of Nursing
Peoria, Illinois

Contributors

Nancy Tomaselli, RN, MSN, CS, CRNP, CWOCN, CLNC
President and CEO
Premier Health Solutions LLC
Cherry Hill, New Jersey

Paula J. Vehlow, RN, MS
Professor
Lincoln Land Community College
Springfield, Illinois

Joan Domigan Wentz, MSN, RN
Assistant Professor
Jewish Hospital College of Nursing and Allied Health
St. Louis, Missouri

Terry L. Wood, PhD(c), RN
Assistant Professor
Jewish Hospital College of Nursing and Allied Health
St. Louis, Missouri

Rita J. Wunderlich, RN, MSN PhD
Nurse Manager Medicine, St. Louis University Hospital
Clinical Instructor, St. Louis University School of
   Nursing
St. Louis, Missouri

Reviewers

Marianne Adam, MSN, RN, CRNP
Assistant Professor
St. Luke's School of Nursing
Moravian College
Bethlehem, Pennsylvania

Marie H. Ahrens, MS, RN
Clinical Instructor
The University of Tulsa School of Nursing
Tulsa, Oklahoma

Tracy C. Babcock, RN, MSN
Adjunct Assistant Professor
Montana State University College of Nursing
Bozeman, Montana

Sylvia K. Baird, RN, BSN, MM
Manager of Patient Safety
Spectrum Health
Grand Rapids, Michigan

Martha C. Baker, PhD, RN, CS, CCRN
Associate Professor of Nursing
Missouri Southern State College
Joplin, Missouri

Doris Bartlett, RN, BSN, MS
Assistant Professor
Bethel College
Mishawaka, Indiana

Julie Baylor, RN, MSN, PhD(c)
Assistant Professor
Bradley University
Peoria, Illinois

Margaret W. Bellak, MN, RN
Associate Professor
Indiana University of Pennsylvania
Indiana, Pennsylvania

Teri Boese, MSN, BSN
Assistant Professor (Clinical)
Learning Resource Services Coordinator
The University of Iowa
College of Nursing
Iowa City, Iowa

Janice Boundy, RN, PhD
Professor, Director of Graduate Program
Saint Francis College of Nursing
Peoria, Illinois

Therese M. Bower, EdD, RN, CNS
Nursing Instructor
Firelands Regional Medical Center School of Nursing
Sandusky, Ohio

Margie E. Brown, RNC, MS, ANP
Staff Nurse, Surgery
St. Mary's Medical Center
Long Beach, California

Susan M. Burchiel, MSN, RN, C
Instructor, Nursing
Cuesta College
San Luis Obispo, California

Susan Burkett, RN, MSN, CPNP, CPN
Chief Administrative Officer T.C. Thompson
    Children's Hospital
Erlanger Health System
Chattanooga, Tennessee

Jeanie Burt, MSN, MA, RN
Assistant Professor
Harding University College of Nursing
Searcy, Arkansas

Darlene Nebel Cantu, RNC, MSN
Director
Baptist Health System
School of Professional Nursing
San Antonio, Texas
Faculty at San Antonio College in Nursing
San Antonio, Texas

Kathlyn Carlson, RN, MA, CPAN
Clinical Staff Nurse
Post Anesthesia Care Unit (PACU)
Abbott Northwestern Hospital
Minneapolis, Minnesota

Reviewers

Elaine M. Caron, MS, RN, C
Patient Educator
Diabetes Center
St. Mary's Regional Medical Center
Lewiston, Maine

Patricia A. Castaldi, RN, BSN, MSN
Director, Practical Nursing Program
Union County College
Plainfield, New Jersey

Barbara A. Caton, RN, MSN
Assistant Professor
Southwest Missouri State University   W est Plains
West Plains, Missouri

Laura H. Clayton, RN, MSN
Assistant Professor of Nursing
Department of Nursing Education
Shepherd College
Shepherdstown, West Virginia

Janice C. Colwell, RN, MS, CWOCN
Clinical Nurse Specialist, Wound, Ostomy & Skin Care
University of Chicago Hospitals
Chicago, Illinois

Barbara P. Daniel, CRNP, MEd, MS
Professor of Nursing
Cecil Community College
North East, Maryland

Karen Delrue, RN, MSN, CEN
Clinical Nurse Specialist Emergency Services
Spectrum Health
Grand Rapids, Michigan

Michael Dreher, DNSc, RN
Associate Director of Undergraduate Nursing Programs
College of Nursing & Health Professions
Drexel University
Philadelphia, Pennsylvania

Linda Evans, RN, MSN
Instructor of Clinical Nursing
University of Missouri Sinclair School of Nursing
Columbia, Missouri

Susan Jane Fetzer, RN, BSN, BA, MSN, MBA, PhD
Associate Professor
University of New Hampshire
Durham, New Hampshire

Margaret S. (Peg) Freel, RN, MSN, CNRN, APN/CNS
Instructor A cute, Chronic and Long-Term Care Nursing
Coordinator C linical Stimulation and Learning
    Laboratory
Niehoff School of Nursing
Loyola University   C hicago
Chicago, Illinois

Lois C. Hamel, PhD, RN, CS
Adult Nurse Practitioner
University of Southern Maine
Portland, Maine

Adrienne Hentemann, BSN, MS
Administrative Associate
Spectrum Health   Butterworth Campus
Grand Rapids, Michigan

Monica M. Hentemann, BSN
Nursing
Spectrum Health
Grand Rapids, Michigan

Mary A. Herring, MSN, BSN, COHN-S
Nursing Faculty
University of Phoenix
Phoenix, Arizona

Janice Hoffman, MSN, RN, CCRN
SPRING Program Director
Department of Nursing
The Johns Hopkins Hospital
Baltimore, Maryland

Beth Hogan Quigley, RN, MSN, CRNP
Clinical Faculty and Lecturer
University of Pennsylvania School of Nursing
Philadelphia, Pennsylvania

Christine A. Hudak, RN, MEd, PhD
Assistant Professor of Nursing
Case Western Reserve University
Frances Payne Bolton School of Nursing
Cleveland, Ohio

Patricia Jacobson, BSN, MSN
Nursing Instructor
Bullard Havens Regional Vocational Technical School
Bridgeport, Connecticut

Susan Junaid, MSN, ARNP, WHNP
Assistant Professor
Allen College
Waterloo, Iowa

Linda L. Kerby, RNC, BSN, MA
Educational Consultant
Leawood, Kansas

Stephen P. Kilkus, RN, MSN
Consultant
Heartspace Coaching
Madison, Wisconsin

Deborah Klaas Kindy, RN, PhD
Associate Professor
Department of Nursing
Sonoma State University
Rohnert Park, California

Maryanne F. Lachat, RNC, PhD
Associate Professor
School of Nursing and Health Studies
Georgetown University
Washington, DC

Virginia D. Lester, RN, BSN, MSN
Clinical Nurse Specialist (Inactive Status)
Assistant Professor of Nursing
Angelo State University
San Angelo, Texas

Suzanne Lockwood-Rayermann, RN, PhD
Assistant Professor
Texas Christian University
Harris School of Nursing
Fort Worth, Texas

Rosemary Macy, RN, MS
Assistant Professor
Boise State University
Boise, Idaho

Mary Jo Mattocks, RN, MN, PhD
Nurse Clinician
Benefits Health Care
Great Falls, Montana

Claudia Louth Mitchell, RN, MS, Certificate in Gerontology
Professor of Nursing
Santa Barbara City College
Santa Barbara, California

Mary E. Newell, RN, MSN
Director of Nursing
Highline Community College
Des Moines, Washington

Kathleen Ahern Nieubuurt, RN, MS
Nursing Instructor
Chemeketa Community College
Salem, Oregon

Patricia K. O'Brien, RN, MSN
Instructor
Penn Valley Community College
Kansas City, Missouri

Gay Oyco-Divinagracia, MA, RN, BC, CNA
Associate Professor, Nursing Department
Indian River Community College
Fort Pierce, Florida

Melissa L. Powell, MSN
Assistant Professor
Eastern Kentucky University
Richmond, Kentucky

Elaine T. Princevalli, RN, BSN, MS
Instructor, Practical Nurse Education Program
State of Connecticut Department of Education
Hamden, Connecticut

Sharon Halloran Proctor, RN, BSN, WOCN
Wound Ostomy Continence Nurse
Manager, Stephens Memorial Wound Program
Infection Control Coordinator
Stephens Memorial Hospital
Norway, Maine

Anita K. Reed, MSN, RN
Instructor of Nursing
St. Elizabeth School of Nursing
Lafayette, Indiana

Kevin J. Ribby, BSN, MSN, GCNS, APRN, BC
Clinical Nurse Specialist Medicine/Surgery
North Mississippi Medical Center
Tupelo, Mississippi

Jane Ruhland, RN, MSN, BSN, C
Education Coordinator
Barnes-Jewish St. Peter's Hospital
St. Peters, Missouri

Susan T. Sanders, MSN, RN, CNAA
Director of Nursing Education
Motlow State Community College
Lynchburg, Tennessee

Alwilda Scholler-Jaquish, PhD, APRN, BC
Assistant Professor
School of Nursing
Texas Tech University Health Sciences Center
Lubbock, Texas

Susan Parnell Scholtz, RN, DNSc
Associate Professor of Nursing
St. Luke's School of Nursing
Moravian College
Bethlehem, Pennsylvania

Ellen Shannon, RN, MSN, PhD(c)
Assistant Professor
East Stroudsburg University
East Stroudsburg, Pennsylvania

Tracy Sheffield-Lindsay, BSN, RNC
Instructor
Mississippi College School of Nursing
Clinton, Mississippi

Sharon Souter, RN, PhD
Director of Nursing Programs
New Mexico State University   Carlsbad
Carlsbad, New Mexico

Rowena Tessmann, PhD, RN-CS
Executive Director
PROTEA Behavioral Health Services
Bangor, Maine

Peggy Lea Thweatt, RN, MSN
Assistant Professor of Nursing
Faculty Development Coordinator
Coppin State College, School of Nursing
Baltimore, Maryland

Heidi Hahn Tymkew, PT, MHS, CCS
Physcial Therapist
Barnes-Jewish Hospital
St. Louis, Missouri

Anne Falsone Vaughan, MSN, RN
Clinical Instructor, Medical-Surgical and Critical Care
Bellarmine University
Louisville, Kentucky

Debra J. Walden, MNSc, RNP
Assistant Professor of Nursing
Arkansas State University
Jonesboro, Arkansas

Jennifer Whitley, RN, MSN, CNOR
Instructor, Associate Degree Nursing Program
Calhoun Community College
Decatur, Alabama

Kevin Wilson, EdS, MSN, RN, C, CNRN
Nursing Department Chairperson
St. Louis Community College at Forest Park
St. Louis, Missouri

Rosemary H. Wittstadt, EdD, RN
Assistant Professor
Towson University
Department of Nursing
Towson, Maryland

Contributors to Previous Editions

Elizabeth A. Ayello, RN, BSN, MS, PhD, CS, CETN
Clinical Assistant Professor of Nursing
New York University
New York, New York

Sheila A. Cunningham, BSN, MSN
Assistant Professor
Neumann College
Aston, Pennsylvania

Julie Eddins, RN, BSN, MSN, CRNI
Staff Nurse, IV Therapy
Barnes Hospital   Christian Health Services
Faculty
The Jewish College of Nursing and Allied Health
St. Louis, Missouri

Deborah Oldenburg Erickson, RN, BSN, MSN
Instructor, School of Nursing
Methodist Medical Center of Illinois
Peoria, Illinois

Joan O. Ervin, RN, BSN, MN, CCRN
Adjunct Faculty
Florence Darlington Technical College
Florence, South Carolina

Melba J. Figgins, MSN, BSN
Associate Professor
The University of Tennessee at Martin
Martin, Tennessee

Janet B. Fox-Moatz, RN, BSN, MSN
Assistant Professor
Neumann College
Aston, Pennsylvania

Lynn C. Hadaway, MEd, RNC, CRNI
Principal
Hadaway and Associates
Milner, Georgia

Susan A. Hauser, RN, BSN, BA, MS
Instructor
Mansfield General Hospital School of Nursing,
Mansfield, Ohio

Carolyn Chaney Hoskins, RN, BSN, MSN
Clinical Instructor
Rockingham Community College
Wentworth, North Carolina

Nancy Jackson, RN, BSn, MSN(R), CCRN
Pulmonary Clinical Nurse Specialist
St. Mary's Health Center
St. Louis, Missouri

Linda L. Kerby, RNC, BSN, MA, BA
Educational Consultant
Leawood, Kansas

Marilee Kuhrik, BSN, MSN, PhD
Associate Professor
Colorado Mountain College
Glenwood Springs, Colorado

Nancy Kuhrik, BSN, MSN, PhD
Associate Professor
Colorado Mountain College
Glenwood Springs, Colorado

Amy Lawn, BSN, MS, CIC
Infection Control Coordinator
Spectrum Health
Grand Rapids, Michigan

Antoinette Kanne Ledbetter, RN, BSN, MS, TNS
Clinical Education Coordinator
Missouri Baptist Medical Center
St. Louis, Missouri

Mary MacDonald, RN, MSN
Staff Educator
Spectrum Health
Grand Rapids, Michigan

Mary Kay Knight Macheca, MSN(R), RN, CS, ANP, CDE
Adult Nurse Practitioner/Certified Diabetes Educator
The Bortz Diabetes Control Center
Richmond Heights, Missouri

Barbara McGeever, RN, RSM, BSN, MSN, DNS(c)
Assistant Professor
Neumann College
Aston, Pennsylvania

Mary "Dee" Miller, RN, BSN, MS, CIC
Clinical Nursing Specialist/Infection Control and
  Epidemiology
St. Joseph's Hospital and Medical Center
Faculty, BSN and MSN Nursing and Business
University of Phoenix
Phoenix, Arizona

Rose M. Miller, RN, BSN, MSN, MPA, ACLS
Instructor
Wallace College
Dothan, Alabama

Kathleen Mulryan, RN, BSN, MSN
Professor
LaGuardia Community College
Long Island, New York

Elaine K. Neel, RN, BSN, MSN
Instructor, School of Nursing
Methodist Medical Center of Illinois
Peoria, Illinois

Marsha Evans Orr, RN, MS
Owner
CreativEngergy, LLC Healthcare Consultants
Mesa, Arizona

Deborah Paul-Cheadle, RN
Registered Nurse, Infection Control
Spectrum Health
Grand Rapids, Michigan

Roberta J. Richmond, MSN, RN, CCRN
Cardiac Case Manager
Central Maine Medical Center
Lewiston, Maine

Paulette D. Rollant, RN, BSN, MSN, PhD, CCRN
Consultant and President
Adult Health Clinical Specialist
Multi-Resources, Inc.
Grantville, Georgia

Linette M. Sarti, RN, BSN, CNOR
Senior Coordinator
University Community Hospital
Tampa, Florida

Phyllis G. Stallard, BSN, MSN, ACCE
Assistant Professor
Neumann College
Aston, Pennsylvania

Victoria Steelman, PhD, RN, CNOR
Advanced Practice Nurse, Intensive and Surgical Services
University of Iowa Hospitals and Clinics
Iowa City, Iowa

Sue G. Thacker, RNC, BSN, MS, PhD
Professor
Wytheville Community College
Wytheville, Virginia

Stephanie Trinkl, BSN, MSN
Instructor, Department of Nursing
Immaculata College
Immaculata, Pennsylvania

Kathryn Tripp, BSN
Nursing Instructor
Southeastern Community College
Keokuk, Iowa

Pamela Becker Weilitz, MSN(R), RN, CN, ANP
Board Certified Adult Nurse Practitioner and Medical-
  Surgical Clinical Nurse Specialist
Private Practice
St. Louis, Missouri
Assistant Clinical Professor
St. Louis University School of Nursing
St. Louis, Missouri

Jana L. Weindel-Dees, RN, BSN, MSN
Registered Nurse
Barnes Hospital
St. Louis, Missouri

Trudie Wierda, RN, MSN
Staff Educator
Spectrum Health
Grand Rapids, Michigan

Laurel A. Wiersema-Bryant, MSN, RN, CS
Clinical Nurse Specialist, Adult Nurse Practitioner
Barnes-Jewish Hospital
St. Louis, Missouri

Clinical Consultants

Mimi Hirshberg, RN, MSN
Barnes College of Nursing and Health Studies
University of Missouri   St. Louis
St. Louis, Missouri
IV Therapist
Vascular Access Service
Barnes-Jewish Hospital
St. Louis, Missouri

Leah Frederick, MS, RN, CIC
Consultant
Infection Control Consultants
Phoenix, Arizona

Preface to the Student

This text was designed to be clear and easy to follow. The five-step nursing process provides the overall framework that is also used in most nursing textbooks. Each section and every feature was carefully developed to describe how to perform the skills and how to effectively provide nursing care. We've developed checklists to enable self-evaluation of your performance for each of the skills in the text. These checklists can be purchased separately (ISBN 0-323-02200-6) or packaged with the text (ISBN 0-323-02202-2).

Quick Reference to Standard Protocols for all Nursing Skills highlights basic essential steps required for every nursing skill. Placing this information inside the front cover and including a reminder at the beginning of each skill reduces repetition and directs you quickly to the essential steps of the individual skill.

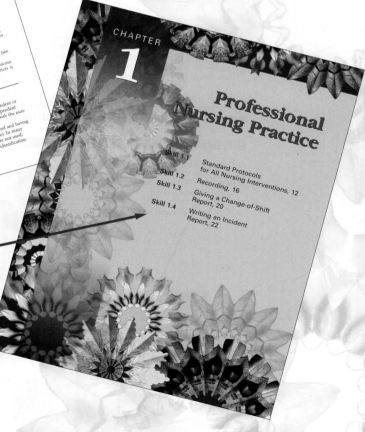

Chapter Format: Chapters open with a list of skills and pages for ease in location. Introductory information relating to these skills includes purposes, influencing factors, and principles. Each skill opens with a brief introduction, focusing on the importance and clinical use of the skills.

Delegation Considerations provide students with guidelines for assigning a skill to assistive personnel.

Chapter 18   Administration of Injections

Skill 18.3

Intradermal Injections

Intradermal injections are used for administering small amounts of local anesthetic and skin testing, such as in TB screening and allergy tests. Because these medications are potent, they are injected in small amounts into the dermis where blood supply is reduced and drug absorption occurs slowly. A client may have an anaphylactic reaction if the medication enters the circulation too rapidly. For clients with a history of numerous allergies, the physician may perform skin testing.

Skin testing requires the identification of changes in color and tissue integrity. Therefore intradermal sites should be lightly pigmented, free of lesions, and relatively hairless. The inner forearm and upper back are ideal locations.

A TB or 1-ml syringe with a short ($\frac{1}{4}$- to $\frac{1}{2}$-inch), fine-gauge (26 or 27) needle is used for intradermal injections. Very small amounts of medication (0.01 to 0.1 ml) are injected. If a bleb does not appear or if the site bleeds after needle withdrawal, the medication may enter SQ tissues. In this case, skin test results will not be valid.

ASSESSMENT

1. Review physician's medication order for client's name, drug name, dose, time, and route of administration.
2. Know information regarding drug action, purpose, normal route, dosage, and expected reaction when testing skin with specific allergen or medication.
3. Assess client's history of allergies, substance to which client is allergic, and normal allergic reaction.
4. Determine if client has had previous reaction to skin testing. *Rationale: Can prevent a major allergic response.*
5. Check date of expiration for medication vial or ampule.
6. Assess client's knowledge of purpose and reactions of skin testing. *Rationale: Reveals need for client education.*

PLANNING

Expected outcomes focus on safe administration and the identification of allergies or exposure to tuberculosis.

Expected Outcomes

1. Desired effect of medication is achieved.
2. Client experiences very mild burning sensation during injection but no discomfort or adverse effects from the medication after the injection.
3. Small, light-colored bleb, approximately 6 mm ($\frac{1}{4}$ inch) in diameter, forms at site and gradually disappears.
4. Client verbalizes and identifies signs of a skin reaction.

Equipment

- 1-ml TB syringe with 26- or 27-gauge ($\frac{1}{4}$- to $\frac{1}{2}$-inch) needle
- Alcohol swab
- Dry sterile gauze pad
- Vial or ampule of skin test solution
- Disposable gloves
- Skin pencil (optional)
- MAR or computer printout

Delegation Considerations

The skill of administering intradermal injections requires problem-solving and critical-thinking skills unique to a professional nurse. Delegation is inappropriate. Inform AP of possible allergic reactions to report immediately to the RN.

IMPLEMENTATION FOR INTRADERMAL INJECTIONS

Steps	Rationale
1. See Standard Protocol (inside front cover).	

NURSE ALERT *Review the five rights for administration of medications.*

2. Check expiration date of test solution, and prepare in syringe.

Nurse Alerts help you remember important safety issues.

Each skill is presented in an easy-to-follow two-column format with *Rationales for key steps* that explain why specific techniques are used.

Skill 18.3   **Intradermal Injections**

Steps	Rationale
3. Select appropriate injection site. Inspect skin surface for bruises, inflammation, or edema. If possible, select site three to four fingerwidths below antecubital space and one hand above wrist. If forearm cannot be used, inspect the upper back. If necessary, sites appropriate for SQ injections (see Figure 18-11) can be used (Workman, 1999).	Injection sites should be free of abnormalities that may interfere with drug absorption. An intradermal site should be clear so results of skin test can be seen and read correctly.
4. Assist client to comfortable position with elbow and forearm extended and supported on flat surface.	Stabilizes injection site for easiest accessibility.
5. Cleanse site with an antiseptic swab, beginning at center of the site and rotating outward in a circular direction for about 5 cm (2 inches). Allow to dry.	Mechanical action of swab removes secretions containing microorganisms. Drying prevents antiseptic from affecting test results.
6. Hold swab or square of sterile gauze between fingers of nondominant hand.	Swab or gauze remains readily accessible when needle is withdrawn.
7. Remove needle cap or sheath from needle by pulling it straight off.	Preventing needle from touching sides of cap prevents contamination.
8. Hold syringe between thumb and forefinger of dominant hand with bevel of needle pointing up.	Bevel up facilitates correct needle placement.
9. With nondominant hand, stretch skin over site with forefinger or thumb.	Needle pierces tight skin more easily.
10. With needle almost against client's skin, insert it carefully at a 5- to 15-degree angle until resistance is felt (see illustration), and advance needle through epidermis to approximately 3 mm ($\frac{1}{8}$ inch) below skin surface. Needle tip can be seen through skin.	
11. Inject medication slowly. It is not necessary to aspirate, because dermis is relatively avascular. Normally resistance is felt. If not, needle is too deep; remove and begin again.	Slow injection minimizes discomfort at site. Dermal layer is tight and does not expand easily when solution is injected.
12. While injecting medication, a bleb resembling a mosquito bite approximately 6 mm ($\frac{1}{4}$ inch) in diameter forms at site (see illustration).	Ble

Communication Tips guide you in preparing clients for what they will experience, see, hear, or feel as the skill is performed.

COMMUNICATION TIP *During this time, explain to client what the skin will look like: Normally the skin will remain clear, or you might notice a needle mark. If the test is positive, you will notice redness and a lump at the site.*

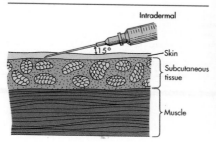

Step 10 Inject intradermal needle at a 5- to 15-degree angle.

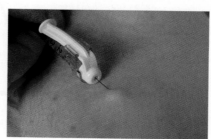

Step 12 Injection creates a small bleb.

A special *Glove Logo* reminds you when to apply clean gloves.

More than 900 *full-color photographs and drawings* with legends clearly show how steps are performed.

Sample Documentation shows you how to record a narrative note with proper terminology and phrasing.

Chapter 18   **Administration of Injections**

Steps	Rationale

13. Withdraw needle while applying alcohol swab or gauze gently over site.
14. Do not massage site.
15. Discard uncapped needle and syringe in appropriately labeled receptacle. Discard gloves, and wash hands.
16. If skin testing, read site within appropriate amount of time, designated by type of medication or skin test given. If client is tested in a clinic or other outpatient setting, have client call in results to health care provider's office.
17. See Completion Protocol (inside front cover).

Support of tissue around injection site minimizes discomfort during needle withdrawal.
Massage may disperse medication into underlying tissue layers and alter test results.
Prevents injury to client and health care personnel.

There is a prescribed wait of 20 minutes to several days (depending on the antigen) before the local reaction should be evaluated for positive test. TB tests should be read in 48 to 72 hours (McKenry and Salerno, 2001).

· · · · · · · · · · ·

EVALUATION
1. Evaluate for desired effect of medication. If medication is for skin testing, assess site at appropriate time for erythema and induration.
2. Assess for pain and any allergic reactions.
3. Inspect bleb. Optional: Use skin pencil and draw circle around perimeter of injection site. Tell client not to wash off markings around injection site.
4. Ask client to describe implications of skin testing and signs of expected skin reaction or hypersensitivity.

Unexpected Outcomes and Related Interventions
1. Erythema or induration appears around injection site, indicating sensitivity to injected allergen or positive test for tuberculin skin testing.
   a. Document results, and notify client's health care provider.

b. Notify client's health care provider immediately.
c. Anticipate administration of epinephrine and need for respiratory and circulatory support (McKenry and Salerno, 2001).

Recording and Reporting
Record amount, type of medication, site of injection, and date and time on medication record.
Record results of skin testing in client's record.

Sample Documentation
1000 PPD injection site in left lower forearm read at 72 hours; test site without redness or induration.

Unexpected Outcomes and Related Interventions describe how to assess for complications related to each skill and take the appropriate action.

...ration 9 mm ...m is a question ...gated further ...hat a positive ...ctive disease ...dividual with ...nduration) is more than 5 mm should have a chest x-ray film and be considered for preventive therapy. Contacts who initially have negative skin test results should receive a repeat skin test 10 to 12 weeks after the initial test.
2. Onset of anaphylactic response occurs within minutes.
   a. Follow institutional policy or guidelines for appropriate response to allergic reactions.

✪ SPECIAL CONSIDERATIONS ✪

Pediatric Considerations
• Only amounts up to 0.5 ml can be administered intradermally to small children (Wong and others, 1999).

Geriatric Considerations
• TB skin testing in older adults is an unreliable indicator of TB. Older adults often display a false-negative skin test as a result of reduced immune system activity.
• The skin becomes less elastic during physiological changes in the older adult. Therefore the skin must be held taut to ensure the intradermal injection is administered correctly.

Special Considerations highlight specific needs for children and older adults and help you to work in home care and long-term care settings.

Preface to the Instructor

We are grateful for the enthusiastic responses to *Nursing Interventions and Clinical Skills* and have carefully preserved the features that made it unique: its streamlined and concise approach, language, and format easily understood by beginning and advanced nursing students. Generous use of color photographs illustrates skills, and the way they are best learned and performed.

This third edition builds on the basic organization and format of the previous editions. Early chapters include basic skills typically introduced before or during initial clinical experiences, such as infection control, safety, hygiene, and vital signs. Later chapters focus on more complex skills often encountered in medical-surgical nursing, such as gastric intubation and enteral nutrition. All chapters include a brief introduction including a unique segment that describes related nursing diagnoses in a way that helps students identify their potential application. Skills are presented in the nursing process format. Steps of the skills include parallel rationales to explain underlying scientific principles and research-based best practice techniques. Hundreds of close-up, full-color photographs facilitate learning. Delegation considerations, communication tips, and pediatric, geriatric, home care, and long-term care considerations help students adapt skills into the context of clinical care.

We have enlisted contributors and clinical consultants throughout the country who have provided their expertise in revising and updating each chapter. We carefully reviewed and refined the contributors' material ourselves to maintain a consistent organization and writing level to help beginning nursing students effectively grasp essential information.

KEY FEATURES

- Comprehensive coverage of nursing skills from beginning, basic skills to the complex advanced skills of central lines, parenteral nutrition, mechanical ventilation, and dialysis.
- Nearly 1000 full-color photographs are conveniently placed near the accompanying text.
- Standard Protocols for beginning and completion of each skill emphasize safety and infection control practices.
- The new 2002 CDC hand hygiene guidelines are incorporated.
- A Glove Logo is used to visually highlight the circumstances when the use of clean gloves is recommended.

- Delegation Considerations are included in the planning section for each skill to help the learner identify when delegation to assistive personnel is appropriate and what to include to clarify expectations regarding performance of the task.
- Communication Tips provide guidelines on how to prepare, support, and instruct clients during a skill. In addition, there are tips that help students know when to offer valuable instruction.
- Recording and Reporting provides a concise, bulleted list of information to be documented and reported.
- Sample Documentation provides examples of clear, concise variance notes or narrative documentation.
- Special Considerations include guidelines for adaptation of skills in various settings, including home care and long-term care, and highlight specific needs for children and older adults.

NEW FEATURES

- Sterile Gloving is visually highlighted in skills to emphasize the importance of this essential action.
- Expanded Client Teaching is incorporated into Communication Tips to assist students to more effectively prepare clients for self-care.
- Legends for Illustrations allow for quick identification of figures and skill steps.
- Updated infection control content includes brushless surgical scrubbing, hand hygiene guidelines, and new needleless systems for blood draws, injections, and IV therapy.

NEW CONTENT

- A Wound Care unit has been organized to include surgical wounds, pressure ulcers, dressings, and hot and cold therapy, covered comprehensively and logically in one convenient unit.
- Six new skills better prepare students for practice
  - Wound Vacuum Assisted Closure
  - Verifying Tube Placement for a Large-Bore or Small-Bore Feeding Tube
  - Removal of an Indwelling Catheter
  - Adapting the Home Setting for Clients With Cognitive Deficits
  - Medication and Medication Device Safety

- Local Anesthetic Infusion Pump for Management of Postoperative Pain
- A chapter on Palliative Care includes Care of the Dying Client

TEACHING-LEARNING PACKAGE

The comprehensive teaching and learning package includes the following:

- *Instructor's Resource With Test Bank* (available online or as a CD) includes a list of skills, teaching strategies, and student activities; answers to critical thinking exercises; skills checklists for each skill; and a revised/updated test bank with over 600 questions in NCLE format.
- *Skills Checklists Booklet* is sold separately or packaged with the text.
- *Mosby's Nursing Skills Video Series* provides valuable visual reinforcement for learning. Also available in CD-ROM format.

- *Skills Exercises* accompany the innovative series of engaging, action-packed videos that provide clear demonstrations of how to perform key nursing procedures in real-life clinical situations. Actual nurses perform each skill, incorporating contemporary concepts such as delegation, critical thinking, standard CDC precautions, and communication techniques.
- *EVOLVE* course management system provides Internet-based course content that reinforces and expands on the concepts delivered in class. EVOLVE can also be used to publish your class syllabus, outline, and lecture notes; set up "virtual office hours" and e-mail communication; share important dates and information through the online class *Calendar;* and encourage student participation through Chat Rooms and Discussion *Boards.*

We hope that each chapter will help students develop a solid base on which to build the knowledge and ability to use critical thinking and the nursing process to provide nursing care for clients safely, effectively, and with an awareness of why, as well as how, the steps of each skill are performed.

Acknowledgments

We are especially grateful to the students who have provided valuable input into the revision of this book from the unique viewpoint of the learner; the many nursing faculty members and practitioners who have offered their comments, recommendations, and suggestions; the contributors who revised selected chapters of this edition; and the reviewers for their insightful feedback.

Thanks to Rick Brady for the expert color photography and to John and Kim Rokusek of Rokusek Designs for the creative design that provides attractive and unique visual appeal. These contributions significantly enhance the process of learning.

Thanks also to the talented and dedicated professionals at Mosby: Suzi Epstein, Executive Editor, who provided leadership, energy, and enthusiasm for the revision process; Robyn Brinks and Shari Malchow, Developmental Editors, who greatly enhanced the quality of this book by their organizational skills, persistent and courteous communications, and dedication to accuracy and quality; Lisa Kopp, Editorial Assistant, who cheerfully assisted with a myriad of details; Kathy Teal and Beth Hayes, Senior Project Managers, whose careful editing and thoughtful handling of the production process ensured an accurate, consistent book.

Finally, thanks to our friends and families for their understanding, patience, and encouragement.

Martha "Marty" Keene Elkin
Anne Griffin Perry
Patricia A. Potter

Contents

Contents

Nursing Interventions & Clinical Skills

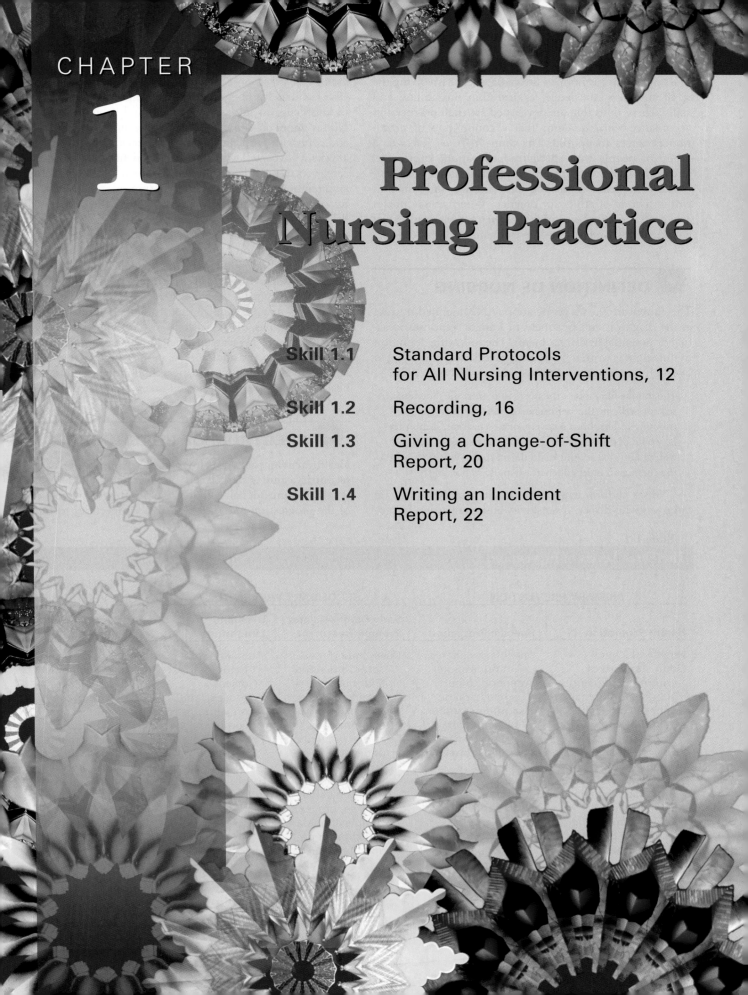

Professional Nursing Practice

Nursing practice is both an art and a science involving the application of knowledge, critical thinking ability, and skills. These skills that are developed are then practiced in accordance with standards that a community of practitioners agrees to uphold. The term *profession* refers to a group of people with specialized education, knowledge, and skills that serve a specific need. Professionals have autonomy in decision making and practice and function within a code of ethics for practice. When we say nurses act "professionally," we imply that they are knowledgeable, conscientious, and responsible to themselves and others.

DEFINITION OF NURSING

The American Nurses Association (ANA) defined nursing as the diagnosis and treatment of human responses to actual or potential health problems. The following definition of nursing was written by Virginia Henderson and adopted by the International Council of Nurses (ICN) in 1973:

> The unique function of the nurse is to assist the individual, sick or well, in the performance of those activities contributing to health, its recovery, or to a peaceful death that he would perform unaided if he had the necessary strength, will, or knowledge. And to do this in such a way as to help the client gain independence as rapidly as possible.

Nurses perform many roles simultaneously. Nurses are caregivers who display a sensitivity and compassion in providing care in response to clients' needs. Nurses are teachers, who facilitate learning as an interactive process that results in knowledge to improve, maintain, and promote health. Nurses are counselors, who help individuals to recognize and cope with problems and improve relationships. Nurses are client advocates, who defend client rights and encourage caregivers to provide what is best for them. Nurses are leaders attempting to influence others to improve the health status of individuals and groups and improve the systems of delivery of health care in a variety of settings. Nurses are managers, responsible for planning, providing adequate staffing patterns, problem solving to achieve established standards, and developing health care policies. They coordinate and supervise the delivery of nursing care, including delegation of nursing tasks to others.

Nurses may become generalists, able to function in a variety of settings, or specialize in medical-surgical nursing, gerontologic nursing (care of older adults), pediatric nursing (care of children and adolescents), perinatal nursing (care of families before, during, or after childbirth), community health nursing, or psychiatric and mental health nursing.

SPECTRUM OF HEALTH CARE

Health activities and nursing care occur at the primary, secondary, and tertiary levels of prevention (Table 1-1). Prevention includes all activities that limit either the onset or the progression of a disease. Primary prevention is true

Table 1-1
The Three Levels of Prevention

PRIMARY PREVENTION		SECONDARY PREVENTION		TERTIARY PREVENTION
Health Promotion	**Specific Protection**	**Early Diagnosis and Prompt Treatment**	**Disability Limitations**	**Restoration and Rehabilitation**
Health education Good standard of nutrition adjusted to developmental phases of life Attention to personality development Provision of adequate housing and recreation and agreeable working conditions Marriage counseling and sex education Genetic screening Periodic selective examinations	Use of specific immunizations Attention to personal hygiene Use of environmental sanitation Protection against occupational hazards Protection from accidents Use of specific nutrients Protection from carcinogens Avoidance of allergens	Case-finding measures: individual and mass Screening surveys Selective examinations Cure and prevention of disease process to prevent spread of communicable disease, prevent complications, and shorten period of disability	Adequate treatment to arrest disease process and prevent further complications Provision of facilities to limit disability and prevent death	Provision of hospital and community facilities for training and education to maximize use of remaining capacities Education of the public and industries to use rehabilitated persons to the fullest possible extent Selective placement Work therapy in hospitals

Modified from Leavell HR, Clark AE: *Preventive medicine for doctors in the community*, ed 3, New York, 1965, McGraw-Hill.

prevention. The focus of primary prevention is the promotion of health, a positive, dynamic state that is more than merely the absence of disease. Primary prevention precedes disease or dysfunction and is applied to clients considered physically and emotionally healthy (Edelman and Mandle, 1998). It is not a therapeutic level of care. Primary prevention can be delivered to an individual or to a general population. The United States Department of Health and Human Services (USDHHS) has developed a national strategy to promote health called *Healthy People 2010* (USDHHS, 2000). The objectives of this program include continuing the objectives identified for *Healthy People 2000* to increase the span of healthy life by risk reduction, health services and protection, and research.

Secondary prevention focuses on persons who are experiencing health problems or illnesses and who are at risk for developing complications or worsening conditions. Activities are directed at diagnosis and prompt intervention, reducing the severity of disease, and enabling a client to return to a normal level of health as soon as possible (Edelman and Mandle, 1998). Tertiary prevention occurs when a defect or disability is permanent and irreversible. It involves minimizing the effects of long-term disease or disability by interventions directed at preventing complications or deterioration (Edelman and Mandle, 1998). Activities are directed at rehabilitation.

The health care system provides levels of care: preventive, primary, secondary, tertiary, restorative, and continuing care (Figure 1-1). Levels of care describe the scope of services and settings where health care is offered to clients in all stages of health and illness. For example, preventive care settings focus on education and prevention (e.g., care activities in the physician's office or the home), whereas tertiary care settings focus on highly technical care (e.g., care delivered in the intensive care unit setting). Levels of care are not the same as levels of prevention. Levels of prevention describe the focus of health-related activities. At any level of care, nurses and other health care providers offer a variety of levels of prevention. The nurse working in an acute care, tertiary setting, for example, monitors the recovery of a postoperative open heart surgery client while also providing health promotion information to the client and family concerning healthy diet and exercise.

CARE MANAGEMENT

Care management is a health care delivery system that coordinates health care services during hospitalization, to home, to the clinic, and when possible extending into wellness. In care management, the health professionals who care for clients are held accountable to some standard of cost management and quality. Nurses and other health care professionals work together as an interdisciplinary team focusing on daily evaluation of client progress toward specific outcomes. The care provided is modified as needed based on the evaluation of client progress. Preparing clients for timely discharge or transition to other care areas is an important part of the planning process (Lynn and Kelley, 1997).

In some settings, care management includes the use of multidisciplinary plans that include established interventions, timelines, and anticipated outcomes for clients with a specific illness or surgery. These plans are called critical pathways. Critical pathways are multidisciplinary plans, developed in collaboration by all members of the health care team who care for a specific type of client. The pathways map out anticipated interventions and expected outcomes each day over a projected length of stay or series of visits to a health care setting. Each day or visit includes clinical assessments, treatments, dietary interventions, activity and exercise, client education, and other plans that promote a normal recovery process.

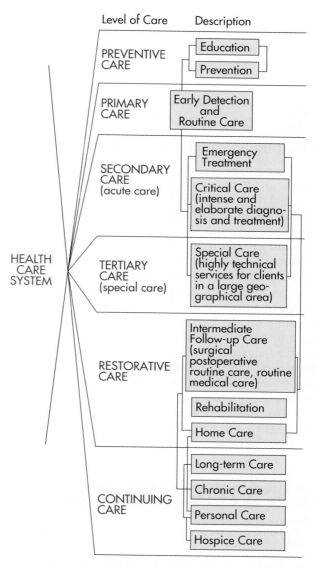

Figure 1-1 Spectrum of health services delivery. (Modified from Cambridge Research Institute: *Trends affecting the U.S. health care system,* 262, Health Planning Information Series, Human Resources Administration, Public Health Service, Department of Health, Education, and Welfare, Washington, DC, 1976, revised and updated 1992, U.S. Government Printing Office.)

Care management is just one model of care approach designed to promote a client's timely recovery. One of the most significant factors influencing how health care institutions manage client care is prospective reimbursement. The prospective payment system was established by Congress in 1983 and eliminated cost-based reimbursement. This means hospitals serving Medicare clients were no longer paid for all costs incurred to deliver care to a client. Instead, inpatient hospital services were bundled into 468 diagnosis-related groups (DRGs). Each group has a fixed reimbursement amount based upon a client's diagnosis or type of surgery. Prospective reimbursement now applies to Medicare clients and clients in managed care plans. In addition, home health settings are now reimbursed on the basis of a prospective payment plan. With hospitals now financially responsible if clients exceed the allotted DRG hospital stay, more clients are discharged at earlier stages of recovery. This has increased the need for home care and increased the need for skilled care in long-term care settings.

 ## LEGAL CONCEPTS

Client Rights and Responsibilities

The Patient Care Partnership: Understanding Expectations, Rights, and Responsibilities was adopted by the American Hospital Association (AHA) in 2003 (Box 1-1). Health care institutions are encouraged to adapt and simplify the language to promote client and family understanding. According to this document, effective health care requires collaboration between clients and physicians and other health care professionals. Open and honest communication, respect for personal and professional values, and sensitivity to differences are integral to optimal client care. As a setting for the provision of health services, a hospital must provide a foundation for understanding and respecting the rights and responsibilities of clients, their families, physicians, and other caregivers. Hospitals must ensure a health care ethic that respects the role of clients in decision making about treatment choices and other aspects of their care. Hospitals must be sensitive to cultural, racial, linguistic, religious, age, gender, and other differences, as well as the needs of persons with disabilities (Dunn, 1999).

The collaborative nature of health care requires that clients, or their families, participate in their care and recognizes that "family is defined by the client" (Dudley, 2001). The effectiveness of care and client satisfaction with the course of treatment depend to a large extent on the client fulfilling certain responsibilities. Clients are responsible for providing information about past illnesses, hospitalizations, medications, and other matters related to health status. To participate effectively in decision making, clients must be encouraged to take responsibility for requesting additional information or clarification about their health status or treatment when they do not fully understand information and instructions. Clients are responsible for informing their physicians and other caregivers if they anticipate problems in following prescribed treatment (AHA, 1992).

A client may choose to implement an advance directive, which documents the client's wishes in the event that the client becomes incapacitated and unable to speak for himself or herself. This requires that the client, family, and health care providers grapple with issues related to quality of life and end-of-life care. Clients are also responsible for ensuring that the health care institution has a copy of their written advance directive if they have one.

Clients should also be aware of the hospital's obligation to be reasonably efficient and equitable in providing care to other clients and the community. The hospital's rules and regulations are designed to help the hospital meet this obligation. Clients and their families are responsible for making reasonable accommodations to the needs of the hospital, other clients, medical staff, and hospital employees. Clients are responsible for providing necessary information for insurance claims and for working with the hospital to make payment arrangements, when necessary.

Informed Consent

The law requires the person who will be performing an invasive procedure to discuss it with the client to obtain informed consent. This involves explaining treatments and alternatives in terms the client understands, and the person must invite and answer all questions. The nurse is responsible for assessment of the level of comprehension and ability to make an informed decision. The role of the professional nurse is to be an advocate for the client and

Box 1-1

The Patient Care Partnership: Understanding Expectations, Rights, and Responsibilities

When you need hospital care, your doctor and the nurses and other professionals at our hospital are committed to working with you and your family to meet your health care needs. Our dedicated doctors and staff serve the community in all its ethnic, religious, and economic diversity. Our goal is for you and your family to have the same care and attention we would want for our families and ourselves.

The sections below explain some of the basics of how you can expect to be treated during your hospital

stay. They also cover what we will need from you to care for you better. If you have questions at any time, please ask them. Unasked or unanswered questions can add to the stress of being in the hospital. Your comfort and confidence in your care are very important to us.

WHAT TO EXPECT DURING YOUR HOSPITAL STAY
• **High quality hospital care.** Our first priority is to provide you the care you need, when you need it, with skill,

Box 1-1

The Patient Care Partnership: Understanding Expectations, Rights, and Responsibilities—cont'd

compassion, and respect. Tell your caregivers if you have concerns about your care or if you have pain. You have the right to know the identity of doctors, nurses, and others involved in your care, as well as when they are students, residents, or other trainees.

- **A clean and safe environment.** Our hospital works hard to keep you safe. We use special policies and procedures to avoid mistakes in your care and keep you free from abuse or neglect. If anything unexpected and significant happens during your hospital stay, you will be told what happened and any resulting changes in your care will be discussed with you.

- **Involvement in your care.** You and your doctor often make decisions about your care before you go to the hospital. Other times, especially in emergencies, those decisions are made during your hospital stay. When they take place, making decisions should include:

  ? *Discussing your medical condition and information about medically appropriate information about medically appropriate treatment choices.* To make informed decisions with your doctor, you need to understand several things:
  — The benefits and risks of each treatment.
  — Whether it is experimental or part of a research study.
  — What you can reasonably expect from your treatment and any long-term effects it might have on your quality of life.
  — What you and your family will need to do after you leave the hospital.
  — The financial consequences of using uncovered services or out-of-network providers.
  Please tell your caregivers if you need more information about treatment choices.

  ? *Discussing your treatment plan.* When you enter the hospital, you sign a general consent to treatment. In some cases, such as surgery or experimental treatment, you may be asked to confirm in writing that you understand what is planned and agree to it. This process protects your right to consent to or refuse a treatment. Your doctor will explain the medical consequences of refusing recommended treatment. It also protects your right to decide if you want to participate in a research study.

  ? *Getting information from you.* Your caregivers need complete and correct information about your health and coverage so that they can make good decisions about your care. That includes:
  — Past illnesses, surgeries, or hospital stays.
  — Past allergic reactions.
  — Any medications or diet supplements (such as vitamins or herbs) that you are taking.
  — Any network or admission requirements under your health plan.

  ? *Understanding your health care goals and values.* You may have health care goals and values or spiritual beliefs that are important to your well-being. They will be taken into account as much as possible throughout

your hospital stay. Make sure your doctor, your family, and your care team know your wishes.

  ? *Understanding who should make decisions when you cannot.* If you have signed a health care power of attorney stating who should speak for you if you become unable to make health care decisions for yourself, or a "living will" or "advance directive" that states your wishes about end-of-life care, give copies to your doctor, your family and your care team. If you or your family need help making difficult decisions, counselors, chaplains and others are available to help.

- **Protection of your privacy.** We respect the confidentiality of your relationship with your doctor and other caregivers, and the sensitive information about your health and health care that are part of that relationship. State and federal laws and hospital operating policies protect the privacy of your medical information. You will receive a Notice of Privacy Practices that describes the ways we use, disclose, and safeguard patient information and that explains how you can obtain a copy of information form our records about your care.

- **Help preparing you and your family for when you leave the hospital.** Your doctor works with the hospital staff and professionals in your community. You and your family also play an important role. The success of your treatment often depends on your efforts to follow medication, diet, and therapy plans. Your family may need to help care for you at home.

  You can expect us to help you identify sources of follow-up care and to let you know of our hospital has a financial interest in any referrals. As long as you agree we can share information about your care with them, we will coordinate our activities with your caregivers outside the hospital. You can also expect to receive information and, where possible, training about the self-care you will need when you go home.

- **Help with your bill and filing insurance claims.** Our staff will file claims for you with health care insurers or other programs such as Medicare and Medicaid. They will also help your doctor with needed documentation. Hospital bills and insurance coverage are often confusing. If you have questions about your bill, contact our business office. If you need help understanding your insurance coverage or health plan, start with your insurance company or health benefits manager. If you do not have health coverage, we will try to help you and your family find financial help or make other arrangements. We need your help with collecting needed information and other requirements to obtain coverage or assistance.

While you are here, you will receive more detailed notices about some of the rights you have as a hospital patient and how ot exercise them. We are always interested in improving. If you have questions, comments, or concerns, please contact _____.

serve as a witness to the client's signature on the agency form. This includes protecting the client's rights, identifying related fears, and determining the client's level of understanding and approval of the procedure. It is effective to ask the client to state in his or her own words what information was conveyed by the physician or provider. If there is any doubt about understanding or the client's decision, the nurse notifies the provider (Dunn, 1999).

Nurse Practice Acts

Nurse Practice Acts, laws which define nursing practice for each state, specify those actions that a nurse can perform independently and those that require a physician's order. The authorization to practice nursing requires becoming licensed by the State Board of Nursing. The applicant for registered nurse (RN) licensure must graduate from an accredited school of nursing and be successful in completing a state board examination.

STANDARDS OF CARE

Standards of care are guidelines that establish expectations for the provision of safe and appropriate nursing care. Standards of care in each state are represented in the form of Nurse Practice Acts, the State Board of Nursing rules and regulations in each state, by federal and state laws regulating hospitals and other health care institutions, by professional and specialty nursing organizations, and by the written policies and procedures of employing institutions (Potter and Perry, 2001).

The ANA has established standards of nursing practice and policy statements that delineate the scope, function, and role of the nurse and establish clinical practice standards. These standards serve as guidelines and correlate to the nursing process (Figure 1-2). It is important for professional nurses to be involved in establishing and maintaining standards of practice, because these standards define the responsibility and accountability for the profession. In addition, professional and government organizations have developed clinical practice guidelines for management of certain symptoms of diseases. These guidelines reflect current research that supports changes in practice. For example, the Agency for Healthcare Research and Quality (AHRQ) has evidence-based guidelines in the areas of pain management and pressure ulcer prevention and treatment.

CRITICAL THINKING IN NURSING PRACTICE

Critical Thinking Defined

Nurses have the responsibility of making accurate and appropriate clinical decisions using knowledge and experience. Critical thinking is a process used to carefully examine the thought process in an organized way. A critical thinker identifies and challenges assumptions, considers what is important in a situation, explores alternatives, sets priorities, draws conclusions, and thus makes informed decisions. When a nurse directs thinking toward understanding and assisting clients in finding solutions to their health problems, the process becomes purposeful and goal oriented. Critical thinking also involves reflection. Reflection is a process of thinking about an experience and factors that influenced it. This promotes self-evaluation and facilitates the incorporation of the learning experience into future decisions.

Delegation

As a result of the changing demands in health care systems and increasing need for accessible, affordable, quality health care, there is a trend toward use of a variety of health care workers with different levels of education and training. In addition, professional nurses are finding themselves in situations that require more support to perform the daily, repetitive tasks of care. The RN is needed to assess, diagnose, plan, and evaluate client needs and responses to care; coordinate care delivery for groups of clients; make the professional judgments necessary to adjust therapies and deliver care; deliver complex therapies; and provide client education and counseling. The best use of the RN's time requires wise and efficient use of ancillary personnel.

Ancillary staff include both licensed and unlicensed personnel. The licensed practical or vocational nurse (LPN/LVN), who works under the supervision of a professional nurse, has 12 to 18 months of basic nursing education. Although the LPN/LVN uses the nursing process under the direction of the RN, there are some limitations based on the scope of practice determined by the Nurse Practice Acts in each state (Box 1-2). In many states the

---

Box 1-2

Role of the LPN/LVN in the Nursing Process

Assessment: Observe and report significant cues (e.g., signs, symptoms) to RN or physician.
Diagnosis: Assist in validating current nursing diagnoses.
Planning: Assist with goal identification and priority setting; suggest nursing interventions.
Implementation: Carry out physician and nursing orders.
Evaluation: Assist with evaluation of progress toward goals and suggest alternative nursing interventions when necessary.

Modified from Christensen B, Kockrow E: *Foundations of nursing,* ed 4, St Louis, 2002, Mosby.

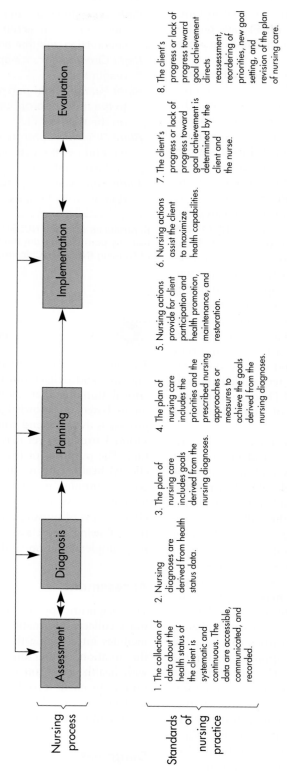

Figure 1-2 Nursing process compared with standards of nursing practice. (Modified from American Nurses Association: *Nursing's social policy statement*, Washington, DC, 1995, American Nurses Foundation/American Nurses Association. Reprinted with permission.)

LPN administers medications and with additional education may initiate intravenous (IV) therapy. Certified nursing assistants have 2 to 3 months of basic nursing care training with a focus on basic skills administered in long-term care facilities. Assistive personnel (AP) have on-the-job training of specific, usually noninvasive tasks in a particular health care setting.

Delegation is entrusting the performance of selected nursing tasks to an individual who is qualified, competent, and able to perform such tasks. The RN retains the accountability for the total nursing care of the individual (ANA, 1999). In delegating there is a decision-making process that must take into account which tasks can be delegated and in what situations, according to the Nurse Practice Act of each state. RNs delegate tasks to LPNs and AP, whereas LPNs delegate tasks to AP. The nurse needs to know the qualifications of the caregiver, including the caregiver's education, skills, and experience, as well as the caregiver's demonstrated and documented evidence of current competency. Delegation requires assessment of each client situation and effective prioritization of client needs and therapies. In addition, the professional nurse must provide direction and clear expectations regarding performance of the task and evaluate the effectiveness of the performance in relation to established standards. Ancillary staff are important members of the health care team and can be very productive when their contributions are recognized and valued. Box 1-3 lists the Five Rights of Delegation recommended by the National Council of State Boards of Nursing (Habgood, 2000).

Throughout this text, boxes are included to assist learners in identifying delegation considerations that should be taken into account as RNs, and in many cases LPNs, decide which tasks can be delegated and how to safely delegate tasks to others. The RN is responsible for assessing the needs of the client and the skills of the caregivers to determine if the two match. Part of delegation includes specific instructions regarding how tasks are to be adapted to client needs and under what circumstances the caregiver should communicate with the licensed nurse. Delegation of any given task may be appropriate in some situations and inappropriate in others. For example, AP routinely provide baths for assigned clients. However, if the professional nurse wishes to assess the client more thoroughly, it may be appropriate for the professional nurse to give the bath. The licensed nurse must decide whether the client's response to the performance of the task is reasonably predictable and whether the caregiver will achieve results similar to those the licensed nurse will achieve in performing that task. When the RN determines that someone who is not licensed to practice nursing can safely provide a selected nursing task for a client and delegates that task, the nurse remains responsible and accountable for the care provided (Wong and Perry, 2002).

Box 1-3
Five Rights of Delegation

Right Task: One that can safely be delegated for a specific client, such as repetitive tasks that require little supervision and that are relatively noninvasive.

Right Circumstances: Appropriate client, setting, and resources.

Right Person: Right person delegates the right task to the most appropriate person, to be performed on the right client.

Right Direction/Communication: Clear, concise description of the task, including its objective, limits, and expectations.

Right Supervision: Appropriate monitoring, evaluation, intervention, as needed, and feedback.

Reproduced from the NCSBN website (www.ncsbn.org) and used by permission from the National Council of State Boards of Nursing (NCSBN), Chicago, IL, copyright May, 2000.

NURSING PROCESS

The nursing process is an approach that enables a nurse to organize and deliver nursing care. This process involves critical thinking that allows decision making and judgments based on knowledge and experience. The nursing process is dynamic and continuous. It is a creative organizational structure, yet it is flexible and useful in any setting. The purposes of the nursing process are to identify clients' health care needs, determine priorities, establish goals, communicate the plan of care, provide nursing interventions designed to meet client needs, and evaluate the effectiveness of nursing care. The nursing process includes the following steps: assessment, nursing diagnosis, planning, implementation, and evaluation (Table 1-2).

Assessment

The diagnostic process begins with assessment, as the nurse collects information about the client (Box 1-4). This includes interviewing the client and others significant to the situation, conducting a physical assessment, conferring with health care team members, and reviewing information in the client record. Assessment is an ongoing process of data collection beginning with the first contact with a client and continuing with each additional contact.

Diagnosis

A nursing diagnosis is a clinical judgment about individual, family, or community responses to actual or potential health problems (Potter and Perry, 2001). To identify

Table 1-2

Summary of the Nursing Process

Component	Purpose	Steps
Assessment	To gather, verify, and communicate data about a client so that a database is established	1. Collecting nursing health history 2. Performing physical examination 3. Collecting laboratory data 4. Validating data 5. Clustering data 6. Documenting data
Nursing diagnosis	To identify health care needs of a client, to formulate nursing diagnoses	1. Analyzing and interpreting data 2. Identifying client problems 3. Formulating nursing diagnoses 4. Documenting nursing diagnosis
Planning	To identify a client's goals; to determine priorities of care, to determine expected outcomes, to design nursing strategies to achieve goals of care	1. Identifying client goals 2. Establishing expected outcomes 3. Selecting nursing actions 4. Delegating actions 5. Writing nursing care plan 6. Consulting
Implementation	To administer nursing actions necessary for accomplishing the care plan	1. Reassessing client 2. Reviewing and modifying existing care plan 3. Performing nursing actions
Evaluation	To determine the extent to which goals of care have been achieved	1. Comparing client response to criteria 2. Analyzing reasons for results and conclusions 3. Modifying care plan

Box 1-4

Creating a Nursing Diagnosis

STEP 1
Start with information from a client assessment.
a. Make a comprehensive list of all significant cues, such as symptoms, laboratory data, subjective data, and other information. This would not include medical diagnosis, physician orders, treatments, or interventions.
b. Group cues according to ways that make sense to you.
c. Each group of cues then provides supporting defining characteristics for a nursing diagnosis label.

STEP 2
Determine the etiology or contributing factors for the diagnosis. (This becomes the "related to" part of the statement.)
a. "What makes or maintains the client's unhealthy response?"
b. The related factor should clearly indicate what nurses can independently do to help alleviate the problem.

c. Compare with contributing factors or related factors as listed in references. NOTE: Watch out for medical diagnoses that may be there and may not be used in this step except by using the phrase ". . . secondary to. . . ."
d. The related factor directs the nursing interventions and becomes the second part of the diagnostic statement.
e. In some cases the contributing factors are "unknown."

STEP 3
Identify the client problem or response from the NANDA listing.
a. This becomes the stem or label and the first part of the diagnostic statement.
b. For this part you must use the exact NANDA words.

a nursing diagnosis, client data are analyzed and organized into clusters of related cues, which then lead to the formulation of a nursing diagnosis. Clusters of subjective and objective cues support the selection of the nursing diagnosis (Table 1-3). Numerous resources are available to assist nurses in identifying characteristics that may be included in cue clusters for a given nursing diagnosis. Many agencies have initial nursing assessment forms that facilitate identification of nursing diagnoses (see Appendix A).

A nursing diagnosis is composed of a problem and an etiology statement:

- The problem statement describes a physiological or psychological response to a health problem, for example, "Impaired Skin Integrity."
- The etiology statement describes contributing factors that influence development of the response, for example, "immobility."

Identifying the First Part of the Diagnostic Statement. The list of accepted nursing diagnoses of the North American Nursing Diagnosis Association (NANDA) can also be categorized into the 11 functional patterns listed in Appendix C. For each of the 11 patterns, the nurse assesses clients by organizing patterns of behavior and physiological responses that pertain to a functional pattern category. The assessment of each of the 11 patterns represents the interaction of the client and the environment, and each pattern interacts with other patterns (Gordon, 2002).

The first part of the diagnostic statement, the problem or stem, may be an actual or high-risk nursing diagnosis. The "actual" nursing diagnosis has data that support the presence of the problem. A high-risk nursing diagnosis indicates the client is at risk for this response, although it is not yet present. Most nursing diagnosis labels can be used as either actual or high-risk nursing diagnoses. For example, a client may have a nursing diagnosis of actual **Impaired Physical Mobility** or **High Risk for Impaired Physical Mobility.**

Identifying the Second Part of the Diagnostic Statement. Etiology or contributing factors for a nursing diagnosis are the second part of the statement and are linked with the connecting phrase "related to." It is essential that the related factor communicate something that nurses can address within the domain of nursing practice. Interventions are selected based primarily on this part of the nursing diagnosis. The contributing factors are validated with the client when possible. For example, the diagnosis of Impaired Physical Mobility could be related to "pain, weakness, or lack of balance." One can understand that interventions for pain are very different from those for weakness or lack of balance. In some cases the contributing factors are unknown. The statement could read, ". . . related to unknown factors," and interventions involve assessment for contributing factors. More than one contributing factor may be identified for a single nursing diagnosis.

When the primary nursing focus needs to be client teaching, the second part of the nursing diagnosis is "lack of knowledge of (specific topic)"; for example, **High Risk for Injury** related to lack of knowledge of safe transfer and crutch-walking techniques.

When assessment reveals that a client has significant risk factors that could contribute to a nursing diagnosis, the second part of the statement includes identified risk factors, and the focus becomes prevention; for example, **High Risk for Impaired Skin Integrity** related to immobility and diaphoresis. In this case, interventions are directed toward promoting mobility, positioning, and dry skin, all of which prevent skin breakdown.

Because physicians are responsible for the treatment of medical diagnoses, it is not appropriate to use a medical diagnosis in a nursing diagnosis statement. When it is difficult to identify an etiology or contributing factor different from the medical diagnosis, the client's response to the medical problem may be the contributing factor. For example, **Impaired Mobility** related to fractured femur would be incorrect. However, the nurse might ask, "What is this client's response to the fracture?" **Impaired Mobility** related to pain secondary to fracture would be accurate.

Table 1-3

Example of the Diagnostic Process

Assessment	Data Clusters	Analysis	Nursing Diagnosis
Inspection of skin	Open lesion on sacrum 1 × 1 cm Red area 33 cm around coccyx	Pressure on coccyx	
Palpation of skin	Skin moist from diaphoresis Tenderness noted around lesion	Skin moisture promotes breakdown	**Impaired Skin Integrity** related to immobility secondary to traction
Historical data	Fractured left leg on 5/3 Positioned on back for traction to leg for 2 weeks; anticipate 4 more weeks minimum	Immobility	

It is also incorrect to repeat the same concept in different words for the first and second parts of the nursing diagnosis; for example, **Deficient Fluid Volume** related to dehydration. This statement does not identify contributing factors, which could include either increased losses or decreased intake. Knowing the contributing factors directs the nurse toward identifying appropriate interventions.

This text includes information in each chapter that identifies nursing diagnoses that are related to the interventions and skills for that chapter. This information includes a description of the diagnostic statement, related factors that may be pertinent, and the focus for related nursing care. By reviewing this information, the reader is able to compare applicable data and determine which diagnosis would best communicate a particular client's needs.

Planning

Planning includes identifying goals and expected outcomes derived from the nursing diagnosis, determining priorities, and selecting nursing actions that will facilitate goal achievement. Planning also involves selecting the appropriate equipment.

Goals and expected outcomes are statements of client behaviors or responses that the nurse anticipates from nursing care. Goals tend to be more general and reflect the client's highest level of wellness, for example, client practices self-management techniques for diabetes.

Expected outcomes are specific, step-by-step achievements that help the client achieve the goals of care and resolution of the etiology for the nursing diagnosis. To be effective, expected outcomes must fit the following criteria:

1. Client centered (states what the client will do)
2. Realistic
3. Observable (e.g., lungs will be clear to auscultation)
4. Measurable (e.g., apical pulse will be between 60 and 100 beats per minute)
5. Time designated (e.g., by the end of the shift, by discharge, in 1 month)
6. Mutually set with the client (something the client agrees with)

An example of an expected outcome is as follows: Client will demonstrate insulin self-injection by 3/20. At the time specified, progress toward achievement is evaluated, and if necessary, the plan of care is revised.

Setting priorities involves critical thinking to determine the urgency of intervention needed. The first priority is for life-threatening problems involving airway, breathing, or circulation. Maslow's hierarchy of needs can act as a useful guide in setting priorities. These needs include, in the order of priority, physical safety, love and belonging, esteem, and self-actualization.

Another way to determine priorities for a client involves the client's perception of what is important. When the client is not aware of the significance of a particular intervention, explanations and teaching can help the client understand why one aspect of care is more important than another. Often it is appropriate to address the client's priorities before working with other areas of concern. In some situations it is possible to deal with more than one priority simultaneously. For example, the nurse may promote the client's independence and mobility while bathing the client. Such an approach increases the effectiveness and efficiency of each client contact.

Implementation

Implementation involves putting the plan into action. To be most effective, the care plan will include nursing interventions that are individualized to the client's needs. These include what, when, how much, how far, how long, how often, where, by whom, and with what. For example, in the case of a client with impaired physical mobility, "Encourage ambulation" is not adequate. Acceptable nursing interventions may include "Assist with walking to bathroom 2 times on 5/9"; "Assist with ambulating in hall at least 20 feet 2 times on 5/9"; and "Assist with ambulating 50 feet 3 times on 5/10." There are a variety of nursing interventions from which to choose, such as the following:

1. Performing an activity completely for a client (administering pain medication)
2. Assisting the client (helping bathe the areas the client cannot manage independently)
3. Teaching (explaining the rationale for the treatment plan)
4. Monitoring (laboratory test results)

Evaluation

The nursing process is dynamic and continuous, and evaluation is an ongoing process. As a nurse assesses a client's status and plans and implements interventions directed at a specific area of concern, the nurse continuously observes the effectiveness of the intervention and the client's response and progress. Whether or not outcomes were achieved by the target date must be clearly documented. When expected outcomes are not being met, evaluation reveals the need to revise approaches to care, introduce different interventions, or continue current interventions for a longer time. When expected outcomes are achieved, the nursing diagnosis can be documented as "resolved." Keeping focus on *evaluation of the client's progress* lessens the chances of becoming distracted by the tasks of care. Evidence of systematic evaluation of the nursing process is one of the standards of the Joint Commission on Accreditation of Healthcare Organizations (JCAHO) (2001).

NURSING PRACTICE AND SKILLS

The practice of professional nursing includes the performance of skills requiring substantial critical thinking and specialized judgment with knowledge of biological, physical, and social sciences (ANA, 1955). Essential components of professional nursing include care and coordination. The caring is more than "to take care of"; it is also "caring for" and "caring about" the client. Caring involves listening, evaluating, and intervening appropriately. The clinical area of practice determines the skills and knowledge needed to practice. Advances in technology have required the nurse to be able to operate complex equipment while remaining client focused.

Nursing practice includes cognitive, psychomotor (technical), and interpersonal skills. Each type of skill is needed to implement care. The nurse is responsible for knowing when one of these methods is preferred over another and for having the necessary theoretical knowledge and psychomotor skills to implement them.

Cognitive skills involve the application of nursing knowledge. The nurse must continually think and anticipate so that each client contact is individualized and appropriate. The nurse needs to know the rationale for each intervention and recognize normal and abnormal physiological and psychological responses. Psychomotor skills involve providing direct care to clients, such as changing a dressing, giving an injection, or bathing. With practice, the nurse learns to perform skills smoothly, confidently, and efficiently. Interpersonal skills include clear, open, and honest communication and teaching and counseling at the client's level of understanding. The nurse must be sensitive to the client's emotional response to illness and treatment.

Skill 1.1

Standard Protocols for All Nursing Interventions

All nursing skills must include certain basic steps for the safety and well-being of the client and the nurse. To save space and prevent repetition, in this text the steps typically performed before and after a skill are not included in each skill unless it is necessary to clarify them as applied for that skill. Remember that these steps are essential and must be followed to deliver appropriate and responsible nursing care.

This logo is used in this text to identify circumstances when the use of clean gloves is recommended. Clean gloves are used to protect both caregivers and clients. By wearing clean, disposable gloves before contact with mucous membranes, nonintact skin, or moist body substances, most microorganisms are kept off the caregiver's hands. However, gloves are not 100% effective and can have invisible small holes or tears. Hand hygiene or the use of antiseptic hand disinfectant after removing the gloves effectively prevents transfer of microorganisms to other clients. The logo is used to indicate situations in which the probability of contact with mucous membranes, nonintact skin, or moist body substances is increased. Hand hygiene refers to either handwashing (use of soap and water), antiseptic handwashing (use of alcohol-based product), and surgical antisepsis (Boyce & Pittet, 2002).

Effective hand hygiene, as well as changing clean gloves, is required between clients and between activities with the same client when gloves become excessively soiled (Centers for Disease Control and Prevention [CDC], 1992). Antiseptic disinfectant can now be used in select situations instead of handwashing, but handwashing is always required when hands are visibly soiled (see Chapter 3). Refer to agency policy for hand hygiene guidelines.

Equipment

- Arm band for client identification
- Consent form (if required by agency policy)
- Clean disposable gloves (if contact with body secretions or excretions is anticipated)

IMPLEMENTATION FOR STANDARD PROTOCOLS FOR ALL NURSING INTERVENTIONS

Steps	Rationale
Standard protocol (before each skill)	
1. Verify physician's orders if skill is a dependent or collaborative nursing intervention. Independent nursing interventions may be verified with the nursing care plan, Kardex, or primary nurse.	Dependent and collaborative interventions include most invasive procedures, such as medications and urinary catheterization. Check agency policy.

Steps	**Rationale**
2. Identify client by checking arm band and having client state name (if able to do so).	Arm bands are standard for client identification in most agencies. Clients who have difficulty hearing or have an altered level of consciousness may answer to a name other than their own. Some agencies use arm bands to communicate special safety concerns, such as allergies.
3. Introduce yourself to client, including your name and title or role, and explain what you plan to do.	Clients have the right to know what will be done and by whom and when those involved are students.
4. Explain the procedure and the reason it is to be done in terms client can understand.	Understanding what is being done enhances client's ability and willingness to cooperate. Client has the right to relevant, current, and understandable information.
5. Assess client to determine that the intervention is still appropriate. (Each skill in the text has an assessment section that includes appropriate specific findings.)	Clients have the right to make decisions about the plan of care before and during the course of treatment.
6. Gather equipment, and complete necessary charges.	Some equipment is reusable and is kept at the bedside. Some equipment is disposable and charged to the client as used. Check agency policy.
7. Perform hand hygiene for at least 10 to 15 seconds before each new client contact (see Skill 3.1, p. 52).	Handwashing is the most important technique in prevention and control of the transmission of microorganisms.

NURSE ALERT *Manufacturers of various antiseptic hand disinfectants may include recommended duration for hand hygiene.*

---

8. Adjust the bed to appropriate height, and lower side rail (if raised) on the side nearest you.	This minimizes muscle strain on caregivers and helps prevent injury and fatigue.
9. Provide privacy for client. Position and drape client as needed.	Respect for privacy is basic for preserving human dignity. Clients have the right to privacy

During each skill

10. Promote client involvement if possible.	Participation enhances client motivation and cooperation.
11. Assess client tolerance, being alert for signs of discomfort and fatigue. Inability to tolerate a procedure is described in the nurses' notes.	Clients' ability to tolerate interventions varies depending on severity of illness and disability. Nurses need to use judgment in providing the opportunity for rest and comfort measures.

Completion protocol (end of skill)

12. Assist client to a position of comfort, and place needed items within reach. Be certain client has a way to call for help and knows how to use it.	Clients may attempt to reach items and risk falling or injury.
13. Raise the side rails, and lower the bed to the lowest position.	This minimizes the risk of clients getting out of bed unattended. Nursing judgment may allow alert, cooperative clients to have side rails down during the day without risking injury (see Chapter 5).
14. Store or remove and dispose of soiled supplies and equipment.	See Centers for Disease Control and Prevention (CDC) guidelines for handling and disposal of contaminated supplies/equipment (see Chapter 3).
15. Perform hand hygiene for at least 10 to 15 seconds after client contact.	Wearing gloves does not eliminate the need to perform hand hygiene. Handwashing and disinfection are effective in preventing and controlling the transmission of microorganisms.
16. Document client's response and expected or unexpected outcomes.	Quality documentation enhances continuity of nursing care.

COMMUNICATION WITHIN THE HEALTH CARE TEAM

Records and reports communicate specific information about a client's health care. Reports include oral and written information shared between caregivers in several ways. Nurses give a verbal or taped report when responsibility for care is being transferred (Figure 1-3). A physician may call a nursing unit to receive a verbal report on a client's progress. The laboratory provides written reports or results of diagnostic tests.

Confidentiality

Nurses are legally and ethically obligated to keep information about clients confidential. Recently the United States Department of Health and Human Services (USDHHS) finalized regulations through the Health Information and Privacy Act (HIPA), which protects the privacy of health information. Under this legislation clients have access to their medical records and consent must be received from the client before information is released for health-related purposes (USDHHS, 2000). When health care professionals have reason to use records for data gathering, research, or education, records may be used with permission and according to established agency, state, and federal guidelines. Many states require reporting of certain infectious or communicable diseases through the public health department, which must be done through proper channels.

Nurses may not disclose a client's status, including diagnosis, laboratory results, and prognosis, to other clients or staff not involved in the client's care. Nurses must be aware of confidentiality issues in elevators, waiting areas, and during lunch and coffee breaks. It is essential that protection be provided for the privacy and rights of clients who do not want information about their health information disseminated to others. For example, a nurse is responsible for respecting a client's wishes with regard to informing family members of a terminal illness. Further, a nurse cannot assume that a client's family members know all of the client's history, particularly with respect to private issues such as mental illness, medications, pregnancy, abortion, birth control, or sexually transmitted diseases.

The Medical Record

The medical record is a legal document. Through accurate documentation the record serves as a description of exactly what happened in the health care system. The purpose of the record is to provide information for communication, education, assessment, research, financial billing, auditing, and legal accountability. Nursing care actually provided may have been excellent; however, in a court of law, "care not documented is care not done." The nursing process shapes a nurse's approach and direction of care, and good reporting and recording reflects the nursing process.

- Assessment results are recorded to offer to all health care team members a database from which to draw conclusions about the client's problems.
- Information describing the client's concerns or condition assists caregivers in planning and setting priorities.
- Description of details of care given reflects implementation of the plan.
- Evaluation of client responses to nursing care determines the client's success in achieving expected outcomes of care.

Nurses involved in the direct care of clients are responsible for recording thorough assessments of a client's condition, descriptions of changes in a client's condition, a detailed accounting of nursing interventions, and an evaluation of the client's response to care.

Care Management and Critical Pathways. The care management model of delivering care may use its own documentation format. This model uses a multidisciplinary plan of care that is often summarized into critical pathways. These are usually one- to two-page formats that include key interventions and expected outcomes that allow the health care team to follow integrated care plans for client problems specific to a medical condition or surgical procedure (see Appendix A).

The critical paths are used to direct and monitor the flow of client care. Because of the nature of human responses, there are variances in outcomes as the client deviates from the critical path plan. These variances refer to either the positive or negative changes in a client's progression toward expected outcomes.

Guidelines for Effective Recording and Reporting

Various methods are used for nursing progress notes. Regardless of the method, certain basic guidelines must be followed.

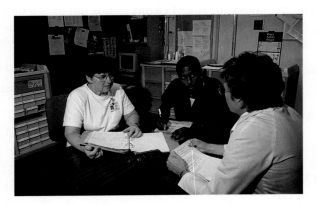

Figure 1-3 Nurses collaborate with the health care team.

Factual. A factual record or report contains descriptive objective information about what a nurse sees, hears, feels, or smells. An objective description (e.g., pulse 54, strong, and irregular) is the result of physical assessment skills. Words such as *good, adequate, fair,* or *poor* are subject to interpretation and should be avoided. Inferences are conclusions based on factual data. For example, an inference might be "The client has a poor appetite." The factual data is "The client ate only two bites of toast for breakfast." Suppose that in one case the client was nauseated, whereas in another case the client was hungry but did not like the food on the tray. If nurses document inferences or conclusions without supportive factual data, misinterpretations about the client's health status occur.

Subjective data include clients' perceptions about their health problems. Documentation using the client's words in quotes, for example: The client states she is "nauseated" or the client states she "does not like the food choices," is factual and acceptable. In both cases, it would be helpful to document the actual food intake, as well as the subjective data.

Accurate. Accurate documentation uses reliable, precise measurements as a means to make comparisons and to determine when a client's condition has changed. Charting that "abdominal wound is 5 cm in length, without redness or edema" is more accurate and descriptive than "large abdominal wound is healing well." To avoid misunderstandings, use only approved agency abbreviations and write out all terms that may be confusing. For example, o.d. (once daily) could be misinterpreted to mean OD (right eye). Correct spelling is essential, because terms can easily be misinterpreted (e.g., *accept* or *except, dysphagia* or *dysphasia*). When observations are reported to another caregiver and interventions are performed by someone else, clearly indicate that fact (e.g., "Surgical dressings removed by Dr. Kline. Pulse of 104 reported to J. Kemp, RN"). End each entry with first name or first initial, last name, and title. Nursing students include the approved abbreviation for the school and level.

Complete. Complete and concise information is essential to describe a client's clinical progress. Consider the following example of what may occur when a note has not been recorded completely.

A nurse does not document or report the teaching session about giving insulin injections. During the next shift, another nurse spends time assessing Mrs. Blake's learning needs because the previous teaching was not communicated. Time is wasted, and Mrs. Blake becomes frustrated with the unnecessary repetition.

A comparison of a concise and lengthy note follows:

Concise, Factual Entry
0900 L toes cool and pale; capillary return >5 sec;

Lengthy Entry Using Vague Terms
0900 The client's left toes are cool, with pale color. There

L pedal pulse 1++; R pedal pulse 4+. Describes pain in L foot as dull, aching 4 (scale 0-10).

is no inflammation. There is slow capillary return present exceeding 5 seconds. Dorsalis pedis pulse in left foot is weak, and the client complains of some discomfort. The pain in left foot is described as aching at a level of 4 on a scale of 0-10.

Current. To be current, the following activities or findings need to be communicated at the time of occurrence:

1. Critical changes in vital signs
2. Administration of medications and treatments
3. Preparation for diagnostic tests or surgery
4. Critical change in status
5. Admission, transfer, discharge, or death of a client

Refer to the client's concern, nursing interventions provided, and client response as soon as possible after the occurrence. Writing scratch notes on a work pad at the time of the event helps ensure accuracy when completing formal documentation. Many agencies use military time, a 24-hour system that uses digit numbers to indicate morning, afternoon, and evening times (Figure 1-4).

Organized. The following compares a well-organized note with a disorganized note:

Organized Note
7/17 0630 Client reports sharp pain 9 (scale 0-10)

Disorganized Note
7/17 0630 Client experiencing sharp pain in

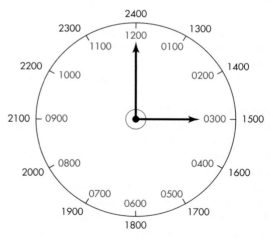

Figure 1-4 Comparison of military time and standard time.

Organized Note

in left lower quadrant
of abdomen, worsened
by turning onto right side.
Positioning on left side
decreases pain to 8
(scale 0-10). Abdomen
is tender to touch
and rigid. Bowel sounds
are absent. Dr. Phillips
notified. To x-ray for
CT scan of abdomen.
T. Reis, RN

Disorganized Note

lower quadrant of abdomen.
MD notified. Abdomen
tender to touch, rigid,
with bowel sounds absent.
Positioning on left side
offers minimal relief of
pain. CT scan ordered
of the abdomen.
J. Adams, RN

Computerized Records. Computers are used in health care facilities in a variety of ways, including computerized documentation systems. There are many benefits to computerized documentation, such as reduction of transcription errors, standardization of nursing care, increasing nursing efficiency, and easier monitoring of quality improvement. Computerization of data results in complete legibility and offers a structure through software design that reinforces standards of nursing care.

Computerized documentation continues to change drastically with the increased use of new technological interfaces. Notebook-size computers with pen-based reading functions, handwriting recognition capabilities, and automated speech recognition systems are examples of technology that is influencing nursing documentation.

Skill 1.2

Recording

Nurses practice in a variety of settings, and a variety of forms and formats are used to communicate specific information about a client's health care. Documentation is a major indicator of quality and an important means of communication of the nursing care provided. Accreditation agencies such as the JCAHO establish standards for the quality of documentation.

Agencies use a variety of forms to make documentation of medical and nursing interventions easy, quick, and comprehensive. Ideally, forms are designed to make data

easy to find and interpret and to avoid unnecessary duplication. Most of the forms have a place for client identification, date and times, and a key to indicate the meaning of abbreviations/entries used and the type of information required. Because of legal requirements, certain requirements for correct recording must be followed (Box 1-5). Medical record forms that nurses have traditionally used for documentation include nursing admission history, physical assessment and vital signs graphic, medication administration records, nurses' notes, and nursing care flow sheets (see Appendix A).

In addition, many agencies have a variety of worksheets that are useful for routine client care and that are not a permanent part of the record (Box 1-6). One example includes a computerized care summary printed as updated each shift, which includes current orders for activities of daily living (ADLs), diagnostic tests ordered, and in some cases standard or individualized nursing care plans. In some long-term care agencies where information is not computerized a "Kardex" is handwritten in pencil to serve this purpose.

Because the nursing process shapes a nurse's approach to client care, good documentation reflects the nursing process. Assessment data are recorded to provide all health care team members with a database from which to make decisions about the client's needs and problems. After a plan of care is developed, with goals and expected outcomes established, documentation needs to include a description of nursing care provided. Evaluation of care communicates the client's degree of progress toward wellness and success in meeting expected outcomes of care. One of the major challenges of effective documentation is to complete it in a timely fashion. Prompt documenta-

---

Box 1-5

Legal Requirements for Recording

- Draw a single line through the error, write the word "error" above it, and sign your name or initials. Then record the note correctly. Do not erase, apply correction fluid, or scratch out errors made while recording.
- To avoid blank spaces in nurses' notes draw a line horizontally through the space and sign your name at its end.
- Record all entries legibly and permanently. Use black or blue ink for all entries (check agency policy for type of ink preferred). Never use pencil, which can be erased.
- Sign using first initial, complete last name, and title (C. Robinson, RN or T. Wallace, SN, U of I). Begin each entry with the time, and end with your signature and title (students may be required to sign an abbreviation of their school).

tion increases accuracy and promotes effective communication to other members of the health care team. Prompt documentation also provides an accurate record of client status and prevents omissions resulting from unexpected events.

NURSING HISTORY FORMS

Completed when a client is admitted to a nursing unit. Includes basic biographical data (e.g., age, method of admission, physician), admitting medical diagnosis or chief complaint, a brief medical-surgical history (e.g., previous surgeries or illnesses, allergies, medication history, client's perceptions about illness or hospitalization, physical assessment of all body systems). Encourages a systematic complete assessment and identification of relevant nursing diagnoses. Provides baseline data to compare with changes in the client's condition. The JCAHO (2001) requires a nursing assessment be completed for each client at the time of admission to a health care agency.

GRAPHIC SHEETS AND FLOW SHEETS

Include routine observations on a repeated basis using a check mark (e.g., when bath is given, client is turned). When completing a flow sheet, the nurse should review previous entries to identify changes.

COMPUTERIZED PATIENT CARE SUMMARY

Includes pertinent information about clients and their ongoing care plans, such as the following:
1. Basic demographical data (e.g., age, religion, physician's name)
2. Primary medical diagnosis
3. Current physician's orders to be carried out routinely
4. Nursing orders or interventions
5. Scheduled tests or procedures
6. Safety precautions to be used in the client's care
7. Factors related to ADLs

NURSING KARDEX (WORKSHEET)

Includes information needed for daily care on a flip card or in a notebook. Usually kept at the nurses' station. Information can be used for change-of-shift report and facilitates access to information without referring to the client record. Includes demographical data, tests ordered, therapies, and information related to ADLs. May include standardized or individualized nursing care plans.

Progress notes are a form of recording that document a client's progress. A variety of formats may be used for progress notes, including SOAP (acronym for Subjective data, Objective data, Assessment or Analysis, and Plan); SOAPE (which adds Evaluation to the previous acronym); PIE (acronym for Problem, Intervention, and Evaluation); APIE (acronym for Assessment, Plan, Intervention, and Evaluation); and DAR (Data, Action, and Response), used in focus charting (Box 1-7). Any caregiver needs to be able to read a progress note and understand what type of problem a client has, the level of care provided, and the results of the interventions. The nurse who is responsible for the client care provided signs each entry. The signature includes the full name and title.

CHARTING BY EXCEPTION

Charting by exception is an innovative approach to streamline documentation by reducing repetition and time spent in charting (Iyer and Camp, 1999). It is a shorthand method for documenting normal findings and routine care based on clearly defined standards of practice and predetermined criteria for nursing assessments and interventions. With standards integrated into documentation forms, such as predefined normal assessment findings or predetermined interventions, a nurse needs to document only significant findings or exceptions to the predefined norms. In other words, the nurse writes a variance note only when the standardized statement on the form is not met. Assessments are standardized on forms so that all caregivers evaluate and document findings consistently.

Because the standard assessments are located in the chart, client data are already present on the permanent record, so nurses do not have to keep temporary notes for later transcription. In addition, caregivers have easy access to current data. The assumption with charting by exception is that all standards are met with a normal or expected response unless otherwise documented. When nurses see entries in the chart, they know that something out of the ordinary has been observed or has occurred.

ASSESSMENT

1. Review assessments, goals and expected outcomes, interventions, and client responses as soon as possible after contact with each client. *Rationale: This facilitates use of documentation as a method of reviewing and evaluating the effectiveness of the nursing care provided and the need for a change in the plan.*

PLANNING

Planning documentation includes reviewing the nursing process as it has been utilized and clarifying pertinent subjective and objective data that communicate progress toward goals.

Box 1-7

Formats for Recording

PIE: Acronym for Problem, Intervention, and Evaluation. Problem-oriented system in which progress notes are written based on a list of numbered or labeled according to the client's problems. For example:

P: Problem—Preoperative anxiety: Client stated, "I am dreading this surgery because last time I had a terrible reaction to the anesthesia and had such terrible pain when they made me get out of bed." Noted muscle tension and loud, agitated voice.

I: Intervention—Notified anesthesiologist, Dr. Moore, of experience. Discussed alternatives for anesthesia and pain-control options. Stressed importance of activity for circulation and healing. Encouraged to keep nurses informed of pain level and need for medication and told client that pain usually is present, but manageable.

E: Evaluation—Client stated she was "very relieved." Stated she would tell the nurses about pain.

SOAP: Acronym for Subjective data, Objective data, Assessment or Analysis, and Plan. Usually based on a numbered list of problems or nursing diagnoses. For example:

1. Anxiety related to preparation for surgery

   S: Subjective data—The client's statements regarding the problem (e.g., Client stated, "I am dreading this surgery because last time I had a terrible reaction to the anesthesia and had such terrible pain when they made me get out of bed.")

   O: Objective data—Observations that support or are related to subjective data (e.g., Noted muscle tension and loud, agitated voice.)

   A: Assessment/Analysis—Conclusions reached based on data. Intense fear related to pain/anesthesia.

   P: Plan—The plan for dealing with the situation (e.g., Notified anesthesiologist, Dr. Moore, of experience. Discussed alternatives for anesthesia and pain-control options. Stressed importance of activity for circulation and healing. Encouraged to keep nurses informed of pain level and need for medication and told client that pain usually is present, but manageable.)

Focus Charting: A way to organize progress notes to make them more clear and organized. For example:

D: Data—Client states, "I am dreading this surgery because last time I had a terrible reaction to the anesthesia and had such terrible pain when they made me get out of bed." Noted muscle tension and loud, agitated voice.

A: Action—Notified anesthesiologist, Dr. Moore, of experience. Discussed alternatives for anesthesia and pain-control options. Stressed importance of activity for circulation and healing. Encouraged to keep nurses informed of pain level and need for medication and told client that pain usually is present, but manageable.

R: Response—Client stated she was "very relieved." Stated she would tell the nurses about pain.

Narrative Note: Describes client data in a narrative paragraph. For example:

Client states, "I am dreading this surgery because last time I had a terrible reaction to the anesthesia and had such terrible pain when they made me get out of bed." Noted muscle tension and loud, agitated voice. Notified anesthesiologist, Dr. Moore, of experience. Discussed alternatives for anesthesia and pain-control options. Stressed importance of activity for circulation and healing. Encouraged to keep nurses informed of pain level and need for medication and told client that pain usually is present, but manageable.

Delegation Considerations

Charting progress notes requires the critical thinking and knowledge application unique to a nurse. Delegation to assistive personnel (AP) is inappropriate. Some documentation may be delegated, including vital signs, intake and output (I&O), and routine care related to ADLs. It is essential to give clear information regarding what should be reported for appropriate follow-up.

IMPLEMENTATION FOR RECORDING

Steps	Rationale
1. Identify the forms you are expected to maintain and where they are located.	

2. After each client contact, identify information that needs to be documented. Consider:
  a. Abnormal findings
  b. Changes in status
  c. New problems identified
	Improves quality and accuracy of documentation and promotes effective communication to other members of the health care team.

3. Document in a timely fashion, without leaving open spaces between notes, and include date and time.	Increases accuracy and helps prevent omission of significant information.

4. Using agency format, determine the most effective way to include significant changes, including:
  a. Pertinent, factual, objective data
  b. Selected subjective data that validates or clarifies
  c. Nursing actions taken
  d. Client responses to actions taken
  e. Additional plans that should be implemented
  f. To whom the information has been reported, including name and status
	When follow-up is needed, documenting to whom information was reported shares responsibility with that individual.

5. Sign progress note with full name or first initial and last name and status according to agency policy. Students are usually required to indicate their level of education and school affiliation.	Identifies person legally responsible for client care provided.

• • • • • • • • • •

 ## SPECIAL CONSIDERATIONS

Home Care Considerations

For continuity of nursing care, documentation provides evidence of achieving nursing standards and is the basis for reimbursement for home health care services. Both quality of care and justification for financial reimbursement depend on effective documentation. Because Medicare has specific guidelines for eligibility for reimbursement, documentation that fulfills these guidelines is essential. Some parts of the record are needed in the home, and other parts are needed in the agency office, which is being addressed by development of new methods using modems and laptop computers.

Long-Term Care Considerations

For stable long-term care residents, certain documentation entries may be made weekly or monthly. Outside agencies such as the state department of health determine the standards and policies for long-term care documentation. The RN is responsible for identifying and documenting episodic changes that may require more intensive nursing intervention and pertinent data for residents who become ill.

Skill 1.3

Giving a Change-of-Shift Report

In addition to written documentation, nurses report information about their assigned clients to the nurses working on the next shift. The purpose of the report is to provide continuity of care for the client. A change-of-shift report may be given in a report room orally in person, by audiotape recording, or during walking rounds from client to client (Figure 1-5). Oral reports are given in a conference room with nurses from both shifts participating. When an audiotape is used, the report is recorded before the end of the shift. This allows the nurses who are preparing to leave to finish last-minute tasks while the oncoming staff listens to the report. It is beneficial to allow time for clarification or updates before the previous nurses leave the unit. Reports given in person or on rounds allow immediate feedback when questions are raised. Confidentiality must be maintained.

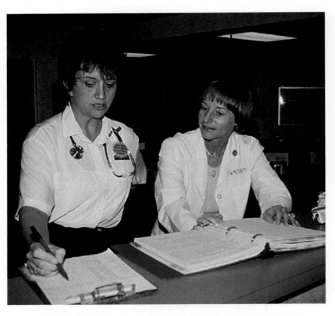

Figure 1-5   Giving a change-of-shift report.

ASSESSMENT

1. Review information on worksheets, get report from co-workers to whom care has been delegated, and gather other relevant information (e.g., pertinent assessment data, laboratory reports, physicians' orders). *Rationale: Data reported needs to reflect changes during the shift and be pertinent, specific, and accurate. Preparation enhances a clear, well-organized report with fewer pauses.*

PLANNING

Expected outcomes focus on identifying appropriate information to report to the nurses on the next shift.

Equipment

- Worksheets, nursing Kardex or client care profile, nursing care plan, critical pathway, or multidisciplinary treatment plan
- Tape recorder (according to agency policy)

Delegation Considerations

The skill of change-of-shift report requires the critical thinking and knowledge application unique to a nurse. For this skill, delegation is inappropriate. However, assistive personnel (AP) should know what to report to a nurse (e.g., apparent change in client's level of pain, reduction in level of consciousness, or change in vital signs) so that the nurse may include any pertinent information (after validation) in the report.

IMPLEMENTATION FOR GIVING A CHANGE-OF-SHIFT REPORT

Steps	Rationale
1. Develop an organized format for delivering report that provides a description of the client's needs and concerns.	Organizes data based on priorities and individualized by the reporting nurse.

Steps	**Rationale**
2. For each client, include:	
a. *Background information*—Include client's name, gender, age, and current primary reason for hospitalization. Also include any known allergies, code status (i.e., do not resuscitate), and special needs as related to any physical challenges (e.g., blind, hearing deficit, amputee).	A more in-depth background report may be needed if a nurse new to a unit or an inexperienced nurse will be working the next shift.
b. *Assessment data*—Provide objective observations and measurements made by the nurse during the shift. Describe client's condition, and emphasize any recent changes. Include any relevant information reported by client, family, or health care team members, such as laboratory data and diagnostic test results.	Oncoming nurse will use data as a baseline for comparison during next shift.
c. *Nursing diagnoses*—If appropriate, state the nursing diagnoses appropriate for client. (Some agencies do not use nursing diagnosis in report.)	Clarifies the type of problems client is experiencing.
d. *Interventions and evaluation*—(steps can be combined in a report).	Clarifies client's current responses to health problems.
(1) Describe therapies or treatments administered during shift and expected outcomes (e.g., medication changes, laboratory results, consultation visits). Specify how interventions are uniquely given for this client. Explain client's response and whether outcomes are met. Do not explain basic steps of procedure.	Staff learn the effect interventions are having on client's recovery and progress.
(2) Describe instructions given in teaching plan and client's ability to demonstrate learning.	Ensures continuity of teaching, minimizing repetition, but communicating any needs for reinforcement.
e. *Family information*—Report on family visitation or involvement, specifically as it influenced client. Explain if family members were included in care procedures or instruction.	Informs staff of level of involvement family members have assumed in client's care.
f. *Discharge plan*—The client's progress in reaching discharge is reviewed on an ongoing basis during each change-of-shift report. Discuss status of educational progress, communication with referral agencies, and preparation of family members for clients who are being discharged. This plan also identifies the roles and responsibilities of the multidisciplinary team and their follow-up visits.	All team members need to collaborate to follow the plan of care that promotes discharge each day to facilitate a smooth transition from hospital or health care facility to home.
g. *Current priorities*—Explain clearly the priorities to which oncoming nurse must attend.	
(1) Report on the immediate treatment planned for a newly admitted client.	
(2) Explain the status of specific preparatory activities for clients who are going for diagnostic or treatment procedures.	
(3) Describe current physical status of clients returning from diagnostic or operative procedures.	

• • • • • • • • •

EVALUATION

1. Ask staff from the oncoming shift if they have questions regarding information reported.

2. When using a tape recorder, periodically self-evaluate for clarity, organization, rate of speaking, and volume level.

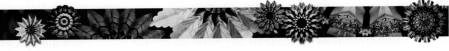

Skill 1.4

Writing an Incident Report

An incident is defined as any event that is not consistent with the routine operation of the health care unit or routine care of a client. Clients, visitors, and employees are at risk when unusual occurrences take place. Examples of incidents include falls, needle-stick injuries, and medication errors. Incidents may involve both actual and potential injuries. When an incident occurs, the nurse involved completes an incident report, which helps identify circumstances or system problems that may be correctable. The first priority is the safety and well-being of the client. Assess the need to notify the physician immediately.

Because an incident can result in a lawsuit, accuracy in reporting is essential. The incident report is essential even when no injury is apparent and establishes a factual basis for comparison with later developments. Incident reports provide a mechanism for keeping all appropriate persons informed. Client's medical records are legally recoverable and can be used in court through a subpoena if information in the medical record validates that a report was completed; therefore no reference to completing the report may appear in the nurses' progress notes.

The incident reporting process may identify actions that could help prevent similar occurrences. The professional nurse can then collaborate with the appropriate persons to institute new or revised policies. Risk management programs and quality improvement programs are enhanced by involvement of professional nursing staff.

ASSESSMENT

1. Use critical-thinking skills to systematically and carefully determine exactly what was involved in the incident and factors that may have contributed to the situation. *Rationale: The best reporting includes objective, accurate, and detailed information in chronological order.*

2. Assess injury and potential risk to the client, and determine the need to notify the physician immediately. *Rationale: The first priority is the safety and well-being of the client.*

PLANNING

Planning includes a thorough review of the details involved in the incident, clarifying contributing factors, and identifying potential outcomes.

Delegation Considerations

Incident reporting may involve assistive personnel (AP) who actually find the client situation requiring the report. Caregivers need to know what immediate actions to take and the importance of observing specific details when reporting to the nurse. Writing the incident report requires the critical thinking and knowledge application unique to a nurse. Therefore delegation is inappropriate.

IMPLEMENTATION FOR WRITING AN INCIDENT REPORT

Steps	Rationale
1. Complete the incident report form as promptly as possible, completely, and accurately, within time required by agency policy (usually 8 to 24 hours).	An incident can result in a lawsuit. Prompt documentation enhances accuracy.
2. Describe objectively what was observed when the incident was discovered, taking care to avoid personal opinions and feelings. Include times, witnesses (names and status), condition of individual, and who was notified at what time (Table 1-4).	

Table 1-4

Comparison of Correct and Incorrect Incident Report Entries

Correct Entry	Incorrect Entry
1800 Client found on floor at foot of bed; able to respond to name when called. 2-cm abrasion noted across left forehead. Vital signs stable. Dr. Smith notified and arrived on floor at 1825. Placed client on fall-prevention protocol.	Client found on floor at foot of bed, probably fell on way to bathroom. Small abrasion over left forehead. Dr. Smith notified. Client instructed to use call light when needing to go to bathroom.
1600 Morphine 10 mg given IM. Dr. Jones notified. 1615 Vital signs stable. Will monitor q15 min for 4 hr.	Administered 10 mg morphine sulfate at 1600. When 6 mg was ordered because order on medication record was unclear. Client resting quietly.
2000 Vital signs stable. Client alert and oriented. Right index finger punctured by 18-gauge angiocath while turning client. Minimal bleeding. Reported to employee health department for follow-up.	Needle-stick injury to right index finger caused by RN who left 18-gauge needle in bed after starting IV 1 hour earlier.

Steps	Rationale
3. Describe measures taken by any caregivers at the time of the incident, including assessment of body systems.	
4. Sign the report and obtain additional signatures (e.g., physician, nursing supervisor) as required by agency.	Provides a mechanisms for keeping all appropriate persons informed.
5. Document factual data on the client's medical record, including the incident and related assessments and interventions. Do not include details contrary to agency policy, and do not include any reference to having completed an incident report.	Client's medical records are legally recoverable and can be used in court. Incident reports are the property of the institution. If the medical record indicates a report was completed, a subpoena can make the incident report admissible in court.

• • • • • • • • • • •

EVALUATION

Seek to identify actions that could help prevent similar occurrences, and collaborate with the appropriate persons to institute new or revised policies. Risk management programs and quality improvement programs are enhanced by involvement of professional nursing staff.

CRITICAL THINKING EXERCISES

1. The nurse checks the client, Mr. Rawls, a 62-year-old man who was admitted to the hospital with pneumonia. Mr. Rawls has been coughing profusely and has required nasotracheal suctioning. He also has an IV infusion of antibiotics. Mr. Rawls is febrile with a temperature of 101° F (38.3° C). Mr. Rawls asks the nurse if he can perhaps have a bed bath because he has been perspiring profusely. The most appropriate task for the nurse to delegate to the nurse assistant working with her today is:
   a. Temperature measurement
   b. Changing IV dressing
   c. Nasotracheal suctioning
   d. Administering a bed bath
2. A professional nurse is responsible for the following two clients. What factors need to be considered in deciding how to prioritize care?
   Client 1: First postoperative day after major surgery with difficulty with pain control.
   Client 2: Recovering from knee surgery and anticipating discharge tomorrow.
3. A nursing diagnosis of Anxiety related to unknown factors manifested by restlessness, shakiness, hyperventilation (rapid breathing), and withdrawal is established for a 72-year-old female client who has never been hospitalized before. When planning nursing interventions, what would be the priority for dealing with the anxiety?

REFERENCES

American Hospital Association: *The patient care partnership: understanding expectations, rights, and responsibilities,* Chicago, 2003, The Association.

American Nurses Association: ANA news, *Am J Nurs* 55:1474, 1955.

American Nurses Association: *Nursing's social policy statement,* Washington, DC, 1999, American Nurses Foundation/American Nurses Association.

Boyce JM, Pittet D: *Guidelines for hand hygiene in health care settings. Am J Infect Control* 30(8):S1, 2002.

Cambridge Research Institute: Trends affecting the US health care system, 262, Health Planning Information Series, Human Resources Administration, Public Health Service, Department of Health, Education, and Welfare, Washington, DC, 1976. Revised and updated 1992, US Government Printing Office.

Centers for Disease Control and Prevention: Universal precautions for prevention of human immunodeficiency virus, hepatitis B virus, and other blood-borne pathogens in health care settings, *MMWR Morb Mortal Wkly Rep* 37:377, 1992.

Centers for Disease Control and Prevention: Surveillance, prevention and control of nosocomial infections, *MMWR Morb Mortal Wkly Rep* 41:783, 1992.

Christensen B, Kockrow E: *Foundations of nursing,* ed 4, St Louis, 2002, Mosby.

Dudley A: Journey toward family-centered care, *Advance for Nurses,* New England, 1(6):10, Oct 8, 2001.

Duffy ME: Determinants of health-promoting lifestyles in older persons, *Image J Nurs Sch* 25(1): 23-28, 1993.

Dunn D: Exploring the gray areas of informed consent, *Nursing,* July 1999, p. 44.

Edelman CL, Mandle CL: *Health promotion through the life span,* ed 4, St Louis, 1998, Mosby.

Gordon M: *Manual of nursing diagnosis,* ed 10, St Louis, 2002, Mosby.

Habgood, CM: Ensuring proper delegation to unlicensed assistive personnel, *AORN J* 71(5):1058, 2000.

International Council of Nurses: *The 1973 code for nurses,* Geneva, 1973, Impimeries Populaires.

Iyer PW, Camp NH: *Nursing documentation: a nursing process approach,* ed 3, St Louis, 1999, Mosby.

Joint Commission on Accreditation of Healthcare Organizations: *Accreditation manual for hospitals,* Chicago, 2001, The Commission.

Leavell HR, Clark AE: *Preventive medicine for doctors in the community,* ed 3, New York, 1965, McGraw-Hill.

Lynn MR, Kelley B: Effects of case management on the nursing context: perceived quality of care, work satisfaction, and control over practice, *Image J Nurs Sch* 29(3):237-241, 1997.

National Council of State Boards of Nursing: *Delegation: concepts and decision making process,* Chicago, 1995, The Association.

National Council of State Boards of Nursing (NCSBN), Five rights of delegation, Chicago, 2000, The Council.

Potter PA, Perry AG: *Fundamentals of nursing,* ed 5, St Louis, 2001, Mosby.

U.S. Department of Health and Human Services: *Healthy people 2010: national health promotion and disease prevention objectives,* Washington, DC, 2000, US Government Printing Office.

Wong DL, Perry SE: *Maternal child nursing care,* ed 2, St Louis, 2002, Mosby.

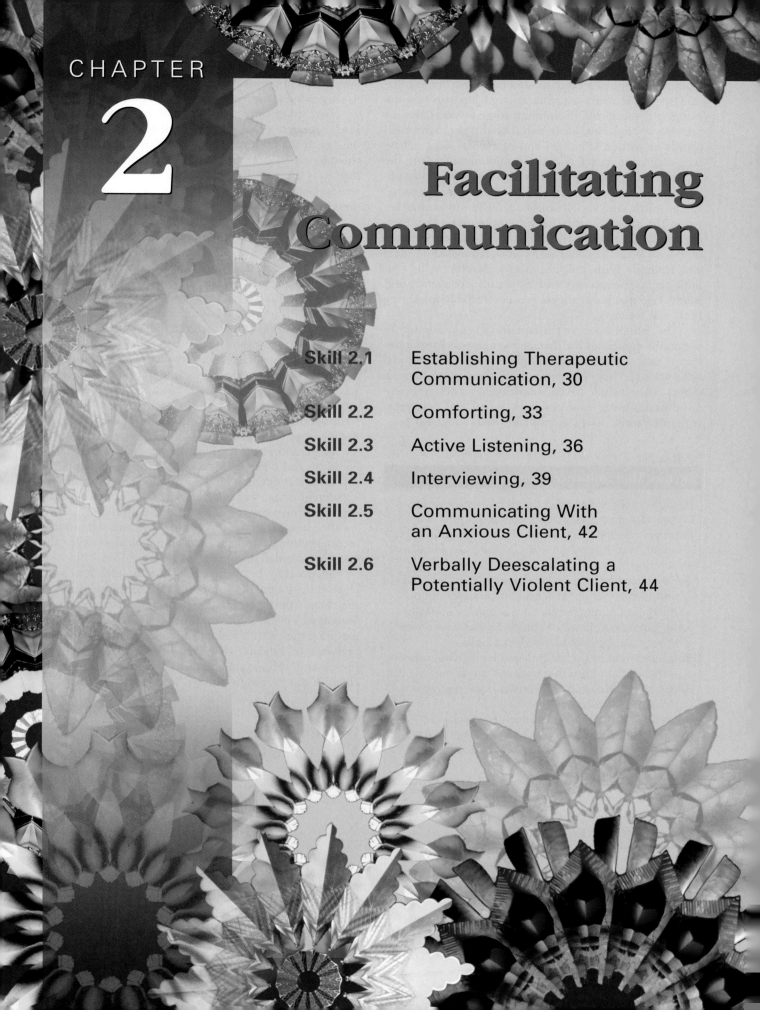

CHAPTER 2

Facilitating Communication

Communication is a basic human need and the foundation for establishing a caring relationship between the nurse and the client. Communication involves the expression of emotions, ideas, and thoughts through verbal (words or written language) and nonverbal (e.g., behaviors) exchanges. Verbal communication includes both the spoken and written word. Nonverbal communication includes body movement, physical appearance, personal space, touch, and facial expression. The interaction between the nurse and the client then progresses to a therapeutic level in which the nurse offers goal-directed activities to help the client feel comfortable sharing ideas and feelings. With practice, nurses develop skills that limit social interactions and maintain a congenial and warm style that helps clients feel comfortable in sharing ideas and feelings.

The importance of interpersonal communication within the context of the therapeutic nurse-client relationship is well documented. Multiple essential interpersonal skills are necessary to communicate therapeutically with clients. They include having empathy and a nonjudgmental attitude, being aware of both verbal and nonverbal communication; using appropriate body language (e.g.,

eye contact or personal space), being patient and sensitive to client's cues, and giving feedback appropriately.

The basic elements of communication include a message, a sender, a receiver, and feedback (Figure 2-1). The message is the information expressed, which can be motivated by experience, emotions, ideas, or actions. The message may be sent through visual, auditory, and tactile senses. Generally, the more channels used, the better the message is understood.

For communication to be effective, the receiver must be aware of the sender's message. The message received is understood as filtered through perceptions shaped from previous experiences. People tend to interpret life experiences through general assumptions and values they hold; in essence, this is the concept of filtering. The more aware people are of how these assumptions influence how they perceive the world and others, the more open they can be when interacting with others.

Feedback, verbal or nonverbal, is a response to the sender that can indicate the meaning of the message that was received. Because communication is a two-way process, the nurse must give feedback to clients and seek feedback from clients to validate clients' understanding of the messages conveyed.

Communication is a complex process that is influenced by many factors (Box 2-1). Each person is unique and associates different ideas with a message and interprets it differently than any other person. For example, a facial expression may convey anger to one person and pain to another. It is essential for nurses to clarify messages so that incorrect inferences and miscommunication with the client are avoided (Figure 2-2).

Silence can be therapeutic. It gives the nurse and client time to think. It is important for the nurse to notice the client's inner feelings. It is also important to pay attention to a client's nonverbal behavior for cues that suggest what the client is feeling and to reflect the nurse's impressions to validate what the client is experiencing. If silence lasts too long or becomes uncomfortable for the client, it can be helpful to say, "You seem very quiet," or

---

Box 2-1

Factors That Influence Communication

Perceptions: Personal views based on past experiences.

Values: Beliefs a person considers important in life.

Emotions: Subjective feelings about a situation (e.g., anger, fear, frustration, pain, anxiety, personal appearance).

Sociocultural background: Language, gestures, and attitudes common for a specific group of people relating to family origin, occupation, or lifestyle.

Knowledge level: Level of education and experience influences a person's knowledge base.

Roles and relationships: Conversation between two nurses differs from that between nurse and client.

Environment: Noise, lack of privacy, and distractions influence effectiveness.

Space and territoriality: Distance of 18 inches to 4 feet is ideal for sitting with a client for an interaction. Clients may have different needs for personal space.

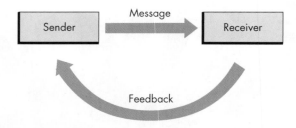

Figure 2-1 Communication is a two-way process.

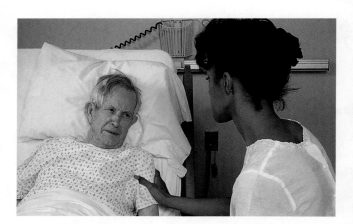

Figure 2-2 Clarify nonverbal language.

"Could you tell me what you need right now?" or "How are you feeling?"

Barriers to effective therapeutic communication techniques exist in the form of ineffective responses and behaviors (Box 2-2). The use of these nontherapeutic techniques can hinder the therapeutic relationship between the client and the nurse.

Preoccupation with the techniques of communication can interfere with rather than enhance the process; however, effective communication can be learned and requires practice, as does any other skill. An attitude of acceptance is helpful to promote open communication. to listen effectively, it helps to face clients, maintain eye contact, pay attention to what is being conveyed, and give feedback to verify accurate understanding. Even though the nurse may not agree with clients, the nurse can accept clients' rights to their opinions. It is best to avoid arguing with clients. The nurse simply reflects an understanding of what clients are communicating without agreeing or disagreeing. Ineffective communication may not halt conversation, but it tends to inhibit clients' willingness to express concerns openly. the nurse needs to find an appropriate place, allow sufficient time, and facilitate communication according to clients' circumstances and needs. Table 2-1 summarizes techniques that facilitate and inhibit communication.

Cultural Considerations Relating to Communication

It is important to recognize cultural diversity and to demonstrate respect for people as unique individuals. Culture is just one factor that influences communication

Box 2-2
Ineffective Responses and Behaviors

Not listening	Talking too much
Looking too busy	Not paying attention
Seeming uncomfortable with silence	Laughing nervously
	Smiling inappropriately
Being opinionated	Showing disapproval
Avoiding sensitive topics	Belittling feelings
Arguing	Minimizing problems
Changing the subject	Being defensive
Being superficial	Focusing on personal problems of the nurse
Having a closed posture	
Ignoring the client	
Making false promises	Using cliches
Making sarcastic remarks	Making flippant remarks
	Lying/being insincere

From Keltner N, Schwecke L, Bostrom C: *Psychiatric nursing: a psychotherapeutic management approach,* ed 4, St Louis, 2002, Mosby.

Table 2-1
Facilitating and Inhibiting Communication

Technique	Examples	Rationale
Initiating and Encouraging Interaction		
Giving information	"It is time for me to . . ."	Informs client of facts needed to understand situation.
	"I will be here until . . ."	Provides a means to build trust and develop a knowledge base for clients to make decisions.
Stating observations	"You are smiling." "I see you are up already."	By calling client's attention to what is observed, nurse encourages client to be aware of behavior.
Open questions/ comments	"What is your biggest concern?" "Tell me about your health."	Allows client to choose the topic of discussion according to circumstances and needs.
General leads	"And then?" "Go on . . ." "Say more . . ."	Encourages client to continue talking.
Focused questions/ comments	"Tell me about your pain or comfort." "What did your doctor say?" "How has your family reacted?" "What is your biggest fear?"	Encourages client to give more information about specific topic of concern.
Helping Client Identify and Express Feelings		
Sharing observations	"You look tense." "You seem uncomfortable when . . ."	Promotes client's awareness of nonverbal behavior and feelings underlying the behavior. Helps clarify meaning of the behavior.

Continued

Table 2-1

Facilitating and Inhibiting Communication—cont'd

Technique	Examples	Rationale
Helping Client Identify and Express Feelings—cont'd		
Paraphrasing	Client: "I could not sleep last night." Nurse: "You've had trouble sleeping?"	Encourages client to describe the situation more fully. Demonstrates that nurse is listening and concerned.
Reflecting feelings	"You were angry when that happened?" "You seem upset . . ."	Focuses client on identified feelings based on verbal or nonverbal cues.
Focused comments	"That seems worth talking about more." "Tell me more about . . ."	Encourages client to think about and describe a particular concern in more detail.
Ensuring Mutual Understanding		
Seeking clarification	"I don't quite follow you . . ." "Do you mean . . ?" "Are you saying that . . ?"	Encourages client to expand on a topic that is not yet clear or that seems contradictory.
Summarizing	"So there are three things you are upset about, your family being too busy, your diet, and being in the hospital so long."	Reduces the interaction to three or four points identified by nurse as significant. Allows client to agree or add other concerns.
Validation	"Did I understand you correctly that . . ?" "Why did you eat that when you know it gives you stomach pain?"	Allows clarification of ideas that nurse may have interpreted differently than intended by client.
Inhibiting Communication		
"Why" questions	"Why did you go back to bed?"	Asks client to justify reasons. Implies criticism and makes client feel defensive. Better to focus on what happened and encourage telling the whole story.
Sidestepping or changing subject	Client: "I'm having a hard time with my family." Nurse: "Do you have any grandchildren?"	This eases nurse's own discomfort. It avoids exploring topic identified by client.
False reassurance	"Everything will be okay." "Surgery is no big deal."	This is vague and simplistic and tends to belittle client's concerns. It does not invite a response.
Giving advice	"You really should exercise more." "You shouldn't eat fast food every day."	This keeps client from actively engaging in finding a solution. Often client knows what should/should not be done and needs to explore alternative ways of dealing with issue.
Stereotyped responses	"You have the best doctor in town." "All clients with cancer worry about that."	This does not invite client to respond.
Defensiveness	"The nurses here work very hard." "Your doctor is extremely busy."	Moves focus away from client's feelings without acknowledging concerns.

between two persons. It is imperative that nurses be aware of cultural norms or values to enhance understanding of nonverbal cues. The nurse must consider any potential communication differences to effectively communicate with persons from other cultures.

- Who is the nurse from a cultural perspective?
- Who is the client from a cultural perspective?
- What is the nurse's heritage?
- What is the client's heritage?

- What are the health traditions of the nurse's heritage?
- What are the health traditions of the client's heritage?

Transcultural communication is most effective when each person attempts to understand the other's point of view from that person's cultural heritage.

Use of language, gestures, and vocal emphasis of words: Take care to determine if understanding was achieved. Avoid overly technical jargon, or terms unique to a culture.

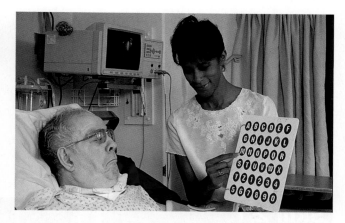

Figure 2-3   Tracheostomy interferes with speech.

Box 2-4

Communication Aids

Pad and felt-tipped pen or magic slate

Board with words, letters, or pictures denoting basic needs (e.g., water, bedpan, pain medication)

Call bells or alarms

Sign language

Use of eye blinks or movement of fingers for simple responses (e.g., "yes" or "no")

Flash cards with pictures rather than words

Eye contact: Direct eye contact is valued in some cultures, whereas other cultures find it improper and intrusive; it may be improper to make eye contact with authority figure.

Use of touch/personal space: Some cultures are "noncontact" cultures and have needs for clear boundaries; other cultures value close contact, handshakes, and embracing.

Time orientation: Many cultures are oriented to the present; some cultures value planning for the future.

Nonverbal behaviors: Use gestures with shared meaning.

Nurses need to adopt an attitude of flexibility, respect, and interest to bridge any communication barriers imposed by cultural differences.

If a client does not speak the nurse's language, a translator is needed. Often, however, the client speaks the nurse's language with limited ability or uses language with meaning different from the nurse's meaning. For example, the client may know customary greetings such as "How are you?" but not understand "pain" or "nausea." However, the client may understand "Are you comfortable?" or "Do you feel ill?" When communication fails, nurses tend to speak louder, stop talking and concentrate on the tasks, or begin doing things for, rather than with, the client. This can result in painful isolation, anger, or misunderstanding for the client and inability of the client to cooperate. Special approaches that can help avoid these outcomes are described in Box 2-3.

Gerontologic Considerations

Older adults with sensory losses require communication techniques that maximize existing sensory and motor functions (see Chapter 36). Some clients are unable to

speak because of physical or neurological alterations, such as paralysis, a tube in the trachea to facilitate breathing (Figure 2-3), or a stroke resulting in receptive or expressive aphasia. When a client experiences receptive aphasia, there is impaired comprehension of both written and spoken language. Expressive aphasia affects the motor function of speech so that the client has difficulty speaking and writing; however, the client can hear and understand. Hearing loss affects one's quality of life and may be easily overlooked by health care providers. Older adults are at higher risk for hearing impairments than the younger population. Communication is impaired when a message is lost or misinterpreted because the message is not heard due to the client's hearing loss (Lindblade and McDonald, 1995). Communication aids can facilitate communication (Box 2-4).

 NURSING DIAGNOSES

Communication, involving an exchange of information, is a basic human need. **Impaired Verbal Communication** is the state in which an individual experiences a decreased or absent ability to use or understand language in human interaction. If a client has difficulty communicating, either sending or receiving information, several factors should be considered. Perhaps there are language barriers; sensory/perceptual deficits; or psychological barriers such as **Anxiety, Fear,** or **Fear of loneliness** that are interfering with the communication process. **Anxiety, Ineffective Coping,** or **Risk for Other-Directed Violence** may be an appropriate nursing diagnosis when the focus is to help the client deal with a crisis, facilitating the expression of

anxiety or anger. **Disturbed Sensory Perception** or **Disturbed Thought Processes** may be an appropriate nursing diagnosis when the focus is to help enhance the client's altered communication patterns. **Social Isolation** or **Impaired Social Interaction** may be an appropriate nursing diagnosis when the client experiences loneliness or has an insufficient quantity or ineffective quality of social exchange.

Skill 2.1

Establishing Therapeutic Communication

The primary goal of effective therapeutic communication for the nurse is to promote wellness and growth in clients (see Table 2-1). Therapeutic communication empowers clients to make decisions. Therapeutic communication differs from social communication in that it is client centered and goal directed with limited disclosure from the professional. However, an important aspect of therapeutic communication is the nurse's ability to show caring for the client. Caring establishes trust and creates an openness on the part of the client to communicate.

Usually nurses should avoid sharing intimate details of their personal lives with clients. This personal self-disclosure by the nurse (e.g., if they have any children or what nursing school they attended) may occur if it may be of help to the client, such as helping the client focus on key issues. The nurse should answer questions and return the focus to the client. This may assist the nurse in establishing a professional relationship with the client. Social communication that involves equal opportunity for personal disclosure and in which both participants seek to have personal needs met is not appropriate between nurses and clients (Keltner, Schwecke, and Bostrom, 1999). Factors that influence communication include the client's perceptions, values, sociocultural background, and knowledge level.

ASSESSMENT

1. Determine client's need to communicate (e.g., client who constantly uses call light, client who is crying, client who does not understand an illness, client who has just been admitted to the hospital or nursing home).
2. Assess reason client needs health care.
3. Assess factors about self and client that normally influence communication: perceptions, values and beliefs, emotions, sociocultural background, severity of illness, knowledge, age level, verbal ability, roles and relationships, environmental setting, physical com-

fort, and discomfort. *Rationale: Communication is a dynamic process influenced by interpersonal and intrapersonal processes. By assessing factors that influence communication, the nurse can more accurately assess the experiences of the client.*

4. Assess client's language and ability to speak. Does the client have difficulty finding words or associating ideas with accurate word symbols? Does the client have difficulty with expression of language and/or reception of messages? What is the client's primary language? *Rationale: A determination must be made as to why the client cannot speak so the appropriate communication aids can be used (e.g., use of a translator, use of communication board).*
5. Observe client's pattern of communication and verbal or nonverbal behavior (e.g., gestures, tone of voice, eye contact). *Rationale: Client's patterns of communication may determine the type and manner of communication used by the nurse.*
6. Encourage the client to ask for clarification at any time during the communication. *Rationale: This gives the client a sense of control and keeps the channels of communication open.*

PLANNING

Expected outcomes focus on using therapeutic communication skills to obtain information about the client's ideas, fears, and concerns.

Expected Outcomes

1. Client expresses ability to communicate with the nurse without feeling threatened or defensive.
2. Client expresses thoughts and feelings to the nurse through verbal and nonverbal communication.

Delegation Considerations

Effective communication is a goal of all client interactions. Although establishing therapeutic communication is a professional nursing skill, often assistive personnel (AP) are able to facilitate effective communication because of the extended length of time they are with the client. It is essential for AP to be aware of the following guidelines:

*   All information discussed must be considered confidential.
*   Client concerns, including anger and anxiety, should be communicated to the nurse to determine if additional nursing interventions are needed.
*   All interactions need to be respectful and kind, including special considerations for clients who have cognitive or sensory impairment.

IMPLEMENTATION FOR ESTABLISHING THERAPEUTIC COMMUNICATION

Steps	Rationale
1. See Standard Protocol (inside front cover).	
2. Create a climate of warmth and acceptance. Consider the need to alter the environment by lowering noise level and providing privacy and comfort. Also consider timing in relation to visitors or personal routines.	Environmental factors can promote open communication.
3. Provide an introduction by addressing the client by name and introducing self and role. For example: "Hello, my name is Jane, and I am the nurse who will take care of you today."	
4. Be aware of nonverbal cues that are both sent and received (e.g., eye contact, facial expression, posture, body language). Be particularly alert to behaviors that are incongruent with the client's verbal message.	Incongruence is an indication that something may be interfering with open communication. Behaviors are often more accurate than words, and clarification may be indicated before proceeding.
5. Explain purpose of the interaction when information is to be shared.	Confidentiality is maintained whereby client information is shared only with members of the health care team. Confidentiality is respected outside the treatment setting.
6. Encourage the client to ask for clarification at any time during the communication.	
7. Use questions carefully and appropriately. Ask one question at a time, and allow sufficient time to answer. Use direct questions. Avoid asking questions about information that may not have yet been disclosed to the client (e.g., medical diagnosis). Avoid asking "why" questions.	"Why" questions may cause increased defensiveness in the client and may hinder communication.
8. Use clear and concise statements with a client who experiences altered levels of consciousness and cognition; repeat information, orient to surroundings, and offer reassurance.	

Steps	Rationale
9. Focus on understanding the client, providing feedback and assisting in problem solving, and providing an atmosphere of warmth and acceptance.	Need to clarify clients' misinterpretations because clients experiencing emotionally charged situations may not comprehend the message (Keltner, Schwecke, and Bostrom, 1999).
10. Adjust the amount and quality of time for communicating depending on clients' needs.	Flexibility and adaptation of techniques may be necessary to encourage client's self-expression.
11. Be aware of cultural and gender differences when interacting with clients. Plan for identified communication difficulties associated with culture, language, age, and gender. Be alert to literacy status, such as the inability to read or write English.	The nurse needs to be aware of any nonverbal cures that may indicate discomfort, confusion, or anxiety and to determine if these cues are related to cultural differences or illness experience.
12. Summarize with clients what was discussed during the interaction. Ask clients to state their understanding of the information shared or conclusion reached if the nurse suspects clients may in any way have misunderstood the communication.	Encourages the client to compare perceptions with the nurse and to determine if clarifications need to be made.
13. See Completion Protocol (inside front cover).	

• • • • • • • • • • •

Evaluation

1. Observe client's verbal and nonverbal responses toward your communication.
2. Ask client for feedback regarding message communicated.
3. Verify if information obtained from client is accurate regarding client's ideas, fears, and concerns.

Unexpected Outcomes and Related Interventions

1. Client continues to verbally and nonverbally express feelings of anxiety, fear, anger, confusion, distrust, and helplessness.
   a. Assess client's level of anxiety, fear, and distrust.
   b. Come back at another time to repeat the message.
   c. Determine cultural, literacy influences affecting clear communication.
2. Feedback between nurse and client reveals a lack of understanding.
   a. Assess for and remove barriers to communication.
   b. Repeat the message.
3. Nurse is unable to acquire information about client's ideas, fears, and concerns.
   a. Use alternative communication techniques to promote the client's willingness to communicate openly.
   b. Offer another professional for the client to talk with to obtain the necessary information.
   c. Rephrase question after time for understanding and response.

Recording and Reporting

- Report pertinent information, subjective data, and nonverbal cues, including:
  Response to illness
  Response to therapy
  Questions
  Concerns
- Record information interventions, and client responses.

Sample Documentation

1345 Client continues to be anxious and fearful about current hospitalization. Client appears to be fidgeting in the bed, wringing his hands, and is expressing much concern about the outcomes of recent diagnostic tests. He uses the call light frequently, asking the same questions repeatedly to the nurse. Client seems to focus only on his illness and cannot be redirected.

SPECIAL CONSIDERATIONS

Pediatric Considerations

- Use vocabulary that is familiar to the child, based on the child's level of understanding.
- Evaluate the child's usual patterns of communication.
- Consider the child's developmental level to select the most appropriate communication techniques (e.g., storytelling and drawing). Be sure to include parent and child (Wong and others, 1999).

Geriatric Considerations

- Be aware of any cognitive or sensory impairment.
- Each client needs to be assessed individually. Avoid stereotyping older adults as having cognitive or sensory impairments.
- Speak face-to-face with the hard-of-hearing client, articulate clearly in a moderate tone of voice, and assess whether the client hears and understands the words.
- Encourage clients with visual impairments to use assistive devices such as eyeglasses and large-print read

ing material to aid in communication (Smith, Buckwalter, and Maxson, 2002).

Home Care Considerations

- Identify a primary caregiver for the client. This individual may be a family member, friend, or neighbor.
- Assess level of understanding of the client and primary caregiver regarding the client's condition.
- Incorporate the client's usual daily habits and routines into the communication event (e.g., bathing and dressing client).

Long-Term Care Considerations

- Assess for cognitive impairment or physical difficulty that may impair the client's communication.
- Assess level of understanding of the client regarding the health condition.
- Incorporate the client's usual daily habits and routines into the communication event (e.g., bathing and dressing client).

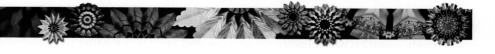

Skill 2.2

Comforting

It is quite common for a nurse to encounter a client who needs comfort and support while experiencing threatening situations. A newly diagnosed illness, separation from family, the discomfort of surgery or diagnostic and treatment procedures, grief, and loss are just a few examples of health-related situations that may require this skill.

ASSESSMENT

1. Observe interactions between client and others in the environment, including family or persons who provide the support system.
2. Identify medications that may alter speech. *Rationale: Medications such as antidepressants, antipsychotics, or sedatives may cause a client to slur words or use incomplete sentences.*
3. Identify body language that conveys positive or negative responses. *Rationale: A person's body language communicates messages about an individual's feelings such as self-esteem and comfort level. Evaluating body language may clarify inconsistent/confusing verbal messages.*

PLANNING

Expected outcomes focus on helping clients and families communicate effectively.

Expected Outcomes

1. Client verbalizes feelings regarding identified threat or concern.
2. Client identifies factors that provide support and comfort.
3. Client contacts one or more support systems.

Delegation Considerations

Effective communication is a goal of all client interactions. Although comforting is a nursing skill, often assistive personnel (AP) are able to provide comfort to clients because of the extended length of time they are with the client. It is essential for assistive personnel to be aware of the following guidelines:

- Client concerns, including anger and anxiety, should be communicated to the nurse to determine if additional nursing interventions are needed.
- Be aware of nonverbal behaviors, both of self and of client.

IMPLEMENTATION FOR COMFORTING

Steps	Rationale
1. See Standard Protocol (inside from cover).	
2. Provide a private, quiet, and calm environment.	Environmental factors can promote open communication.
3. Acknowledge and respond to physical discomfort by positioning, medication, or other comfort measures. Consider individual preferences and expressed needs.	Physical discomfort, difficulty breathing, or pain interferes with communication.
4. Convey interest by maintaining eye contact and using open, relaxed posture (see illustration).	
5. Convey acceptance without judgment. Avoid facial expressions or gestures that suggest disapproval.	Acceptance is not the same as agreement but is a willingness to hear the person without conveying doubt or disagreement.
6. Provide empathy, which involves a sensitive and accurate awareness of client's feelings.	Empathy helps clients explain and explore their feelings so that problem solving might occur.
7. Remain centered on the current concern. Avoid introducing new information.	Clients may be overwhelmed by additional information. Talking about self, other people, or events shifts the focus away from clients (Fortinash and Holoday-Worret, 2000).

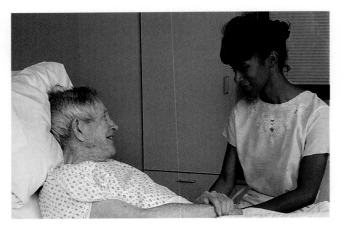

Step 4 The nurse talks with the client.

Steps	Rationale
8. Guide client's description of the situation to include what happened, thoughts about the experience, and feelings about the experience (e.g., "What happened then?" "How did you feel after that?").	This assists the process of clarifying the experience.
9. Communicate understanding by repeating what you understand the message to be (e.g., "I understand you . . . ," "I hear you saying . . . ," "I sense that . . . ").	Communicating understanding tends to decrease the intensity of feelings and conveys empathy (Keltner, Schwecke, and Bostrom, 1999).
10. Use open questions to explore possible alternatives.	Open questions cannot be answered by "yes" or "no" and encourage expression of ideas or thoughts.
11. Offer honest reassurance to the extent possible (e.g., that someone cares, that there is hope, that client is not alone).	Offering of self by the nurse shows interest and concern for the client (Keltner, Schwecke, and Bostrom, 1999).
12. Explore support services available and what services client has previously used. Refer as appropriate.	
13. See Completion Protocol (inside front cover).	

• • • • • • • • • •

EVALUATION

1. Ask for feedback about effectiveness of support and comfort provided.
2. Observe client's response (e.g., body language, verbal statements) after discussion of feelings and circumstances that have been identified.
3. Ask in what way support systems are expected to become available and helpful.

Unexpected Outcomes and Related Interventions

1. Client is unable or unwilling to express feelings or circumstances.
   a. Consider the level of trust that has been established. If appropriate, facilitate greater level of trust in relation to other matters, such as providing for physical needs.
   b. Respect client's need, and offer opportunity to discuss the situation at another time or with another person.
2. Client expresses continued anger of discontent with alternatives available.
   a. Suggest taking more time to explore possibilities.
   b. Avoid telling client how to feel or what to think.
   c. Acknowledge and name the expressed feelings.

3. Client is unable to identify family or friends that can provide support. Family is too far away or estranged and unwilling to become involved.
   a. Identify community resources that may be helpful (e.g., church, neighbors, support groups).
   b. Facilitate a telephone support system.

Recording and Reporting

• Document summary of client concerns. Include the following:
   Subjective data (e.g., significant quote)
   Objective data (e.g., body language)

Sample Documentation

1900 Client states, "I am having major surgery tomorrow and I feel so alone and scared." Client reports that her family lives out of town and she has felt increasingly isolated since a recent move to an assisted living facility. Client is unable to identify any other people or community agencies that she considers part of her support system.

SPECIAL CONSIDERATIONS

Pediatric Considerations
- Evaluate the child's usual pattern of communication, including use of age-appropriate language.
- Consider the child's developmental level when providing comfort to the child.
- Include parents in the comforting process when appropriate.

Geriatric Considerations
- Be aware of any cognitive or sensory impairment
- Encourage clients with auditory and/or visual impairments to use assistive devices to aid in communication.

Home Care Considerations
- Assess for the presence of any cognitive and/or physical impairments that may hinder communication.
- Identify who constitutes client's support and caregiver systems.
- Assess level of understanding of client and caregiver regarding the client's condition.

Long-Term Care Considerations
- Assess for cognitive impairment and/or physical difficulties that may impair the client's communication.
- Identify who constitutes the client's support system.
- Assess level of understanding of the client and support system regarding the client's condition.

Skill 2.3

Active Listening

Active listening is one of the most effective ways to facilitate communication. It conveys interest in the client's needs, concerns, and problems and requires complete attention to understand the entire verbal and nonverbal message. A synonym for active listening is empathy. Empathy is the act of communicating to other persons that we have understood their feelings and what makes them feel that way. This requires acceptance of the individual in need of help. Once people know they have been understood and accepted, they do not have to struggle to explain or justify their reactions (Fortinash and Holoday-Worret, 2000).

Listening techniques are learned behaviors. At first they seem awkward and time consuming, and, as with any skill, they become more comfortable with practice. It is essential that the nurse appear natural, relaxed, and at ease while listening.

ASSESSMENT

1. Assess patterns of communication with caregivers:
   a. Does client initiate conversation and ask appropriate questions?
   b. Does body language support and complement the verbal message?
   c. Does client talk excessively and control the topic of conversation?
   d. Does client avoid expressing feelings or thoughts and confine conversation to necessary facts? *Rationale: Awareness of communication patterns facilitates planning for the interaction.*

2. Identify sensory and neurological factors that affect the client's ability to communicate. *Rationale: Altered vision or hearing or expressive aphasia (in which words cannot be formed or expressed) or receptive aphasia (in which language is not understood) interferes with communication (Fortinash and Holoday-Worret, 2000).*

3. Identify cultural influences that affect communication (Giger, 1999). What language does client predominantly use in thinking? Does client need an interpreter? Is client able to read and/or write in English? What verbal or nonverbal communication shows respect (e.g., tempo, eye/body contact, topic restrictions)? *Rationale: Respecting and allowing a free exchange of the client's thoughts and feelings can facilitate effective communication (Giger, 1999).*

PLANNING

Expected outcomes focus on achieving clear understanding of client's communication.

Expected Outcomes

1. Client demonstrates comfort and willingness to communicate, stating that the nurse is listening to identified needs.
2. Client verbalizes a sense of feeling understood.

Delegation Considerations

Effective communication is a goal of all client interactions. The nurse can encourage assistive personnel (AP) to improve listening skills, using these guidelines:
- When performing procedures, pay attention to what client has to say and do not ignore questions or concerns that may cause a temporary delay.
- Eye contact is critical in showing interest in the client.
- Do not anticipate what the client wants to say. Let him or her finish.
- Report client concerns to the nurse.

IMPLEMENTATION FOR ACTIVE LISTENING

Steps	Rationale
1. See Standard Protocol (inside front cover).	
2. Use physical attending to convey interest by sitting within 4 feet of client, maintaining eye contact, and using open, relaxed posture (arms and legs not crossed).	This nonverbal language conveys interest and concern. The nurse makes self available to client (Keltner, Schwecke, and Bostrom, 1999).
3. Ask one related open-ended question at a time following a logical sequence that encourages client to tell the whole story.	Open questions encourage client to elaborate and provide more accurate and detailed descriptions.
4. Listen without interrupting until a natural break occurs.	This avoids interference with client's flow of thoughts.
5. Offer feedback that lets client know what you understood. Paraphrase by restating client's message using fewer words.	
6. If the message is unclear, back up the conversation and clarify. Admit confusion and ask for more information.	Without clarification, valuable information is lost.
7. Focus questions on one area at a time. Avoid numerous direct questions and "why" questions that may result in defensiveness.	Focusing eliminates vagueness in communication by limiting the area of discussion. The use of "why" questions may place client in defensive position and may block further communication (Fortinash and Holoday-Worret, 2000).
8. Identify when a verbal message conflicts with nonverbal cues. Stating observations gives feedback that helps increase awareness of whether client communicated the intended message.	People may be unaware of the way the message was received unless the impressions created by the nonverbal cues are described. This also encourages further discussion (Keltner, Schwecke, and Bostrom, 1999).
9. Allow silence, which can be an effective means of allowing the organization of thoughts and processing of information. When client becomes emotionally upset or cries, a quiet period can be helpful.	Silence shows that nurse is accepting and willing to wait for client to be ready to continue.
10. At the conclusion of the interaction, summarize by giving a concise review of the key aspects of the main ideas.	Client is able to review information and make additions or corrections.
11. See Completion Protocol (inside front cover).	

• • • • • • • • • •

EVALUATION

1. Ask client what facilitates or interferes with communication of needs.
2. Ask if the communication was accurately interpreted by caregivers.

Unexpected Outcomes and Related Interventions

1. Client shifts conversation back to the nurse rather than discussing own issues.
   a. Answer questions briefly if appropriate, then state your need to focus on client issues.
   b. Ask what client is most concerned about at this time.
2. Client has difficulty hearing the questions.
   a. Reduce or remove background noise.
   b. If client has a hearing aid, be sure it is clean, is inserted properly, and has a functioning battery.
   c. Adjust volume of hearing aid to a comfortable level.
   d. Speak slowly and articulate clearly.
   e. Face client to provide opportunity for lip reading.
   f. Talk toward client's best ear.
3. Client has dysarthria (difficult, poorly articulated speech from interference in control of muscles of speech) or expressive aphasia.
   a. Ask simple, closed questions. Client can answer "yes" or "no" or nod or shake head in response.
   b. Allow time for understanding and a response.
   c. Use visual cues (pictures, objects, gestures).
   d. Encourage continued efforts to speak.
   e. Allow time, and demonstrate an interested and patient attitude.
   f. Refer to speech therapist as needed.

Recording and Reporting

- Document summary of client concerns. Include the following:
  Subjective data (e.g., significant quote)
  Objective data (e.g., body language)

Sample Documentation

1500 Client has spent much of the conversations during this shift focusing on the nurse rather than his own issues with prostrate cancer. He has been unable to redirect back to the reasons for his hospitalization. He appears uncomfortable and tense (by assessing his nonverbal cues and body language) when discussing his health issues.

SPECIAL CONSIDERATIONS

Pediatric Considerations

- The nurse must adapt own communication level to the developmental age of the child to match the client's ability to comprehend.
- The nurse needs to present a verbal and nonverbal environment in which the child feels comfortable.
- The nurse should include parents during interactions with the client when appropriate.

Geriatric Considerations

- Be aware of any cognitive or sensory impairment.
- Encourage clients with auditory and/or visual impairments to use assistive devices to aid in communication.

Home Care Considerations

- Assess for the presence of any cognitive and/or physical impairments that may hinder communication.
- Assess level of understanding of the client and identified caregiver/support system regarding the client's condition.

Long-Term Care Considerations

- Assess for cognitive impairment and/or physical difficulties that may impair the client's communication.
- Assess level of understanding of the client regarding health condition.

Skill 2.4

Interviewing

The interview involves communication initiated for a specific purpose and focused on a specific content area, such as the initial assessment of newly admitted clients or obtaining a health history in a health care provider's office. In nursing, the interviewer obtains information about the client's health state, lifestyle, support systems, patterns of illness, patterns of adaptation, strengths and limitations, and resources. This information can be used for an admission database or health history and provides data for identifying the client's expectations and for responding appropriately to individualized client needs (Box 2-5).

The interview can facilitate a positive nurse-client relationship, which makes it easier for clients to ask questions about the health care environment and expectations regarding daily routines and procedures. It is important to indicate to clients that they may ask questions at any time. They also have the right not to answer questions. Indicating the purpose of the interview helps to establish trust and to put the client at ease.

The interview involves phases of orientation, working, and termination. The interview may be scheduled at a time when interruptions will be minimal and visitors are not present. In some cases it is possible to include family members in the interview while the focus is clearly kept with identifying the client's needs.

ORIENTATION PHASE

Before beginning, the nurse tells the client the purpose of the interview and the types of data to be obtained. Then time is spent becoming acquainted with the client. Establish a time frame for the interview, and honor this commitment to the client.

WORKING PHASE

The nurse asks questions to form a database from which a care plan can be developed (See Box 2-5). The nurse observes for evidence of discomfort and is willing to stop the interview when appropriate.

A direct-question technique is a structured format requiring one- or two-word answers and is frequently used to clarify previous information or obtain basic routine information (e.g., allergies, marital status). The open-question technique is used to promote a more complete description of identified areas of concern. Examples of open questions/comments include "What are your health concerns?" "How have you been feeling?" and "Tell me about your problem."

TERMINATION PHASE

The client is given an indication that the interview is coming to an end a few minutes before conclusion is anticipated. This allows the client to ask questions and keeps the client aware of what to expect. The interview is terminated in a friendly manner, indicating specifically if there will be further contact. It is helpful to ask if anything else is needed before leaving the client's bedside.

ASSESSMENT

1. Review available information, which may include admission information such as name, address, age, marital status, employment, and reason for admission or reason for office visit.
2. Consider factors that may influence ability or willingness of client or significant other to respond to the questions, such as physical pain, discomfort, or anxiety. *Rationale: These factors may need to be alleviated before the interview. Intellectual level affects the choice of words used in the questions.*
3. Determine if client is alert and oriented. Assess for hearing and speech difficulties (see Chapter 36). *Rationale: These factors may interfere with the interview, and another source of information will be needed.*

PLANNING

Expected outcomes focus on gathering information for a database to develop an appropriate plan of care.

Expected Outcomes

1. Client (or significant other) is able to describe health concerns.
2. Verbal and nonverbal messages are congruent.

Box 2-5

Interview Database

- Health-related concerns
- Perception of health status
- Past health problems and therapies
- Effect of health status on role; influence on relationship with members of household
- Influence on occupation
- Ability to complete activities of daily living (ADLs)

Delegation Considerations

This skill requires the critical thinking and knowledge application unique to a nurse. Delegation is inappropriate.

IMPLEMENTATION FOR INTERVIEWING

Steps	Rationale

Orientation phase

1. Greet client and significant others and introduce yourself by name and job title. Tell client why the interview is being done. Tell client you need to ask some questions that will require about 15 to 20 minutes. Assure client that this information will be kept confidential.

This allays anxiety about divulging information to a stranger and encourages participation.

2. Provide privacy and eliminate distractions, unnecessary noise, and interruptions by going to a quiet unoccupied room and/or closing the door. If others are present, ask client if they should stay.

Distractions and interruptions may interfere with therapeutic interactions between nurse and client.

3. Sit facing client at approximately the same eye level.

This facilitates active listening and places client more at ease.

4. If client is alert enough to state name, where he or she is, and what day it is, proceed with the interview.

Confirm information obtained from client with other caregivers or family members if client is disoriented or confused or does not seem reliable.

Working phase

5. If client is talkative, refocus the interview when client strays from the topic.

6. Ask what led client to seek health care. Attempt to obtain a descriptive account of all the events in the order in which they occurred.

Active listening encourages the exchange of information (see Skill 2.3, p. 36). Conducting an interview by only asking questions may make client feel like a subject of interrogation.

7. Observe and clarify nonverbal behaviors. Listen to client responses.

This provides a focus for collecting more specific data related to the primary areas of concern.

8. For each symptom, determine when, where, and under what circumstances it occurred. Also determine location; quality; quantity; duration; and aggravating, alleviating, and associated factors (Table 2-2).

9. Within each symptom, also clarify the absence of other symptoms that are generally associated with the problem.

10. Identify past hospitalizations, past surgical procedures and complications, and previous major health problems.

11. Determine whether client regularly takes medications and, if so, for what period of time. Ask the name, reason for taking, dosage, and frequency. Specifically ask about dietary supplements or over-the-counter (OTC) medications such as aspirin, acetaminophen, ibuprofen, laxatives, sleeping pills, diet pills, herbal supplements/remedies, or other types of alternative therapies.

Clients may not think of dietary supplements or over-the-counter (OTC) medications, because these do not require prescriptions. However, both of these classifications of medications may have interactive effects with current or future prescribed medications.

Table 2-2

Dimensions of a Symptom			
Dimensions	**Questions to Ask**	**Dimensions**	**Questions to Ask**
Location	"Where do you feel it?" "Does it move around?" "Show me where."	Timing	"When did you first notice it?" "How long does it last?" "How often does it happen?"
Quality or character	"What is it like? Sharp, dull, stabbing, aching?"	Setting	"Does it occur in a particular place or under certain circumstances?"
Severity	"On a scale of 0 to 10, with 10 the worst, how would you rate what you feel right now?" "What is the worst it has been?" "In what ways does this interfere with your usual activities?"	Aggravating or alleviating factors	"What makes it better?" "What makes it worse?" "When does it change?" "Have you noticed other changes associated with this?"

Steps	**Rationale**
12. Also ask if client takes narcotics, insulin, digitalis, contraceptives, steroids, or hormone replacements.	Clients may not mention these if such drugs seem unrelated to the reason for admission or when they think that the physician would have previously conveyed this information.
13. Identify risk factors related to lifestyle that influence the client's health, knowledge level, and awareness of the risk.	Risk factors include smoking, alcohol use, drug abuse, lack of exercise, stress, nutritional factors (e.g., fluids, cholesterol, carbohydrates, fiber, salt), exposure to violence, and sexual activity that is unprotected.
14. Continue with additional areas of interest or concern according to the focus of the interview.	

Termination phase

15. Give information that tells clients you are nearly finished.	This offers client a chance to ask final questions before nurse is finished.
16. Summarize your understanding of client's health concerns.	
17. Completion Protocol (inside front cover).	

• • • • • • • • • •

EVALUATION

1. Ask if client or significant other has had an adequate opportunity to describe health concerns.
2. Observe client's nonverbal expressions during interview. Do they match verbal statements?

Unexpected Outcomes and Related Interventions

1. Family or significant other answers for client, even when client is capable of answering.
   a. Direct the question to client, using client's name.
   b. Avoid giving eye contact to family member.
   c. Acknowledge the answer given by a family member, then state you are interested specifically in what client has to say about it.

   d. Conclude the interview, and resume again after the family members are gone. If necessary, you may suggest that family take a break for a while, get coffee or a meal, or walk outside briefly for some fresh air.
2. Client is unable to communicate, and family members are present.
   a. Interview family member as you would client.
   b. Explore the needs of family and client.

Recording and Reporting

• List what is to be included in the admission profile:
  Reason for admission
  Medical-surgical history, family history

Allergies
Health habits
Current prescribed therapies (include all OTC medications and supplements)
Current nonprescribed therapies/alternative treatments

Sample Documentation

Documentation involves use of a standard format for a database (see Admission Patient Profile, Appendix A).

SPECIAL CONSIDERATIONS

Pediatric Considerations
- Evaluate the child's usual pattern of communication, including use of age-appropriate language.
- Consider the child's developmental level when interviewing the child.
- Include parents in the interviewing process when appropriate.

Geriatric Considerations
- Be aware of any cognitive or sensory impairment.
- Encourage clients with auditory and/or visual impairments to use assistive devices to aid in communication.

Home Care Considerations
- Assess for the presence of any cognitive and/or physical impairments that may hinder communication.
- Identify the client's primary caregiver and include in interviewing process.
- Assess level of understanding of the client and caregiving regarding client's condition.

Long-Term Care Considerations
- Assess for cognitive impairment and/or physical difficulties that may impair the client's communication.
- Identify who constitutes the client's support system, and include in interviewing process when appropriate.
- Assess level of understanding of the client regarding health condition.

Skill 2.5

Communicating With an Anxious Client

Clients in the health care setting may experience anxiety for a variety of reasons. A newly diagnosed illness, separation from loved ones, threat associated with diagnostic tests or surgical procedures, a language barrier, and expectations of life changes are just a few factors that can cause anxiety. How successfully a client copes with anxiety depends in part on previous experiences, the presence of other stressors, the significance of the event causing anxiety, and the availability of supportive resources. The nurse can be a support to the client. The nurse can help to decrease anxiety through effective communication. Communication methods reviewed in this skill assist the nurse in helping the anxious client clarify factors causing anxiety and cope more effectively. There are stages of anxiety with corresponding behavioral manifestations: mild, moderate, severe, and panic (Box 2-6).

ASSESSMENT

1. Observe for physical, behavioral, and verbal cues that indicate the client is anxious, such as dry mouth, sweaty palms, tone of voice, frequent use of call light, difficulty concentrating, wringing of hands, and statements such as "I am scared." *Rationale: Anxiety can interfere with usual manner of communication and thus interfere with client's care and treatment. Extreme anxiety can interfere with comprehension, attention, and problem-solving abilities.*
2. Assess for possible factors causing client anxiety (e.g., hospitalization, fatigue, fear, pain).
3. Assess factors influencing communication with the client (e.g., environment, timing, presence of others, values, experiences, need for personal space because of heightened anxiety).

Box 2-6

Behavioral Manifestations of Anxiety: Stages of Anxiety

MILD ANXIETY
- Increased auditory and visual perception
- Increased awareness of relationships
- Increased alertness
- Able to problem solve

MODERATE ANXIETY
- Selective inattention
- Decreased perceptual field
- Focus only on relevant information
- Muscle tension; diaphoresis

SEVERE ANXIETY
- Focus on fragmented details
- Headache, nausea, dizziness
- Unable to see connections between details
- Poor recall

PANIC STATE OF ANXIETY
- Does not notice surroundings
- Feeling of terror
- Unable to cope with any problem

4. Assess own level of anxiety as nurse, and make a conscious effort to remain calm. *Rationale: Anxiety is highly contagious, and one's own anxiety can exacerbate the client's anxiety.*

PLANNING

Expected outcomes focus on reducing the client's anxiety through the use of effective communication techniques.

Expected Outcomes

1. Client establishes rapport, achieves a sense of calm, and discusses coping and decision making about current situation.
2. Client's physical and emotional discomforts are acknowledged.
3. Client discusses factors causing anxiety.

Delegation Considerations

Therapeutic communication is a goal of all client interactions, delegated or not. Communicating effectively with an anxious client is a skill that can be delegated to assistive personnel (AP). However, before delegation of this skill, the nurse should adhere to the following guidelines:
- Inform assistive care provider in proper way to interact verbally and nonverbally with the client.
- Review skills with AP for communicating with the anxious client.

IMPLEMENTATION FOR COMMUNICATING WITH AN ANXIOUS CLIENT

Steps	Rationale
1. See Standard Protocol (inside front cover).	
2. Provide brief, simple introduction; introduce yourself and explain purpose of interaction.	Anxiety may limit amount of information client may understand.
3. Use appropriate nonverbal behaviors (e.g., relaxed posture, eye contact) and active listening skills, such as staying with the client at the bedside.	Clients experiencing emotionally charged situations may not comprehend the delivered message. Focus on understanding the client, providing feedback and assisting in problem solving, and providing an atmosphere of warmth and acceptance.
4. Use appropriate verbal techniques that are clear and concise to respond to the anxious client.	Coping mechanisms provide the foundation for effective communication so that the client can explore causes of anxiety and steps to alleviate anxious feelings.
5. Help client acquire alternative coping strategies, such as progressive relaxation, slow deep-breathing exercises, and visual imagery (see Chapter 10).	Stress-reduction techniques are nonpharmacologic strategies that client can use to reduce anxiety, pain, and/or discomfort.
6. Minimize noise in physical setting.	Decreasing environmental stimuli may reduce client's anxiety.

Steps	**Rationale**
7. Adjust the amount and quality of time for communicating depending on client's needs.	Flexibility and adaptation of techniques may be necessary based on client's ability to communicate, level of anxiety, and need for more time to establish trust.
8. See Completion Protocol (inside front cover).	

• • • • • • • • • •

EVALUATION

1. Have client discuss ways to cope with anxiety in the future and make decisions about current situation.
2. Observe for continuing presence of physical signs and symptoms or behaviors reflecting anxiety.
3. Ask client to discuss factors causing anxiety.

Unexpected Outcomes and Related Interventions

1. Physical signs and symptoms of anxiety continue.
   a. Utilize refocusing or distraction skills, such as relaxation and imagery, to reduce anxiety (see Skill 10.2, p. 228).
   b. Be direct and clear when communicating with client, to avoid misunderstanding.
   c. Touch, when used appropriately, may help control feelings of panic.
   d. Administering an antianxiety medication may be necessary.

Recording and Reporting

• Record in nurses' notes the following:
  Cause of anxiety
  Nonverbal behaviors
  Methods used to relieve anxiety (pharmacologic and nonpharmacologic methods)
  Client response (verbal and nonverbal)

Sample Documentation

1130 Client appears to be severely anxious and repeatedly approached the nurses' station with complaints of headaches and dizziness. He does not recall that the doctor is coming to see him to discuss the upcoming surgery. He seems easily agitated by the noise around the nurses' station and in the halls. He responds poorly to redirection by the nurse and is unable to follow directions for using progressive relaxation techniques.

SPECIAL CONSIDERATIONS

Pediatric Considerations
• The nurse must evaluate the child's usual pattern of communication, including use of age-appropriate language.
• Children may express anxiety through restless behavior, physical complaints, or behavioral regression.

Geriatric Considerations
• Be aware of any cognitive or sensory impairment.
• Anxiety is often seen among the older adult population, resulting from change in usual patterns.

Home Care Considerations
• Assess for the presence of any cognitive and/or physical impairments that may hinder communication.
• Antianxiety should be managed based on client's presenting behavior.
• Determine community resources to assist client and caregiver.

Long-Term Care Considerations
• Assess for cognitive impairment and/or physical difficulties that may impair client's communication and cause social isolation.
• Anxiety should be managed based on client's presenting behaviors.

Skill 2.6

Verbally Deescalating a Potentially Violent Client

Anger is the common underlying factor associated with a potential for violence. The degree and frequency of anger ranges from everyday mild annoyance, to anger related to feelings of helplessness and powerlessness, and ultimately to rage when usual coping methods are no longer effective to manage the situation. There are positive functions of anger, including anger as an energizing behavior, anger to protect positive image, and anger to give a person greater control over a situation. A client can become angry for a variety of reasons. Anger may be directly related to a client's experience with illness, or it can be associated with problems that existed before the client entered the health care system.

In the health care setting, the nurse has frequent contact with a client and thus may become the target of the client's anger when the client cannot express it toward a significant other. It is important for the nurse to understand that in many cases the client's ability to express anger is important to recovery. For example, when a client has experienced a significant loss, anger becomes a means to help cope with grief. A client may express anger toward the nurse, but the anger often hides a specific problem or concern. For example, a client diagnosed as having cancer may voice displeasure with the nurse's care instead of expressing a fear of dying.

It can be stressful for a nurse to deal with an angry client. Anger can represent rejection or disapproval of the nurse's care. A nurse's efforts at satisfying the needs of one angry client can result in a failure to meet the priorities of other clients. The nurse needs to allow the client to express anger openly and not feel threatened by the client's words (Adams and Murray, 1998).

The client's anger cannot be allowed to compromise care. Skills for communicating with an angry client or a potentially violent client will allow a nurse to assist the client in dealing with anger constructively and in refocusing emotional energy toward effective problem solving. Deescalation skills are useful techniques that can be used to manage the potentially violent client; these skills range from using nonthreatening verbal and nonverbal messages to safely disengaging and controlling the aggressor physically (Fortinash and Holoday-Worret, 2000).

ASSESSMENT

1. Observe for behaviors that indicate the client is angry (e.g., pacing, clenched fist, loud voice, throwing objects) and/or expression that indicate anger (e.g., repeated questioning of the nurse, irrational complaints about care, nonadherence to requests, belligerent outbursts, threats). *Rationale: Anger is a normal expression of frustration or a response to feeling threatened. However, the expression can interfere with or block communication and interactions.*
2. Assess factors that influence communication of the angry client, such as refusal to comply with treatment goals, use of sarcasm or hostile behavior, having a low frustration level, or being emotionally immature.
3. Consider resources available to assist in communicating with the potentially violent client, such as members of the health care team and family members.

PLANNING

Expected outcomes focus on promoting effective and socially appropriate verbal and nonverbal expressions of anger.
1. Client's feelings of anger subside without harm to self or others.
2. Client's anger is diffused, and problem solving is initiated.

 Delegation Considerations

Therapeutic communication is a goal of all client interactions. Communicating effectively with the potentially violent client is a skill that should be taught to all assistive personnel (AP) who may need to use it (e.g., security personnel, AP who work in psychiatric units).

IMPLEMENTATION FOR VERBALLY DEESCALATING A POTENTIALLY VIOLENT CLIENT

Steps	Rationale
1. See Standard Protocol (inside front cover).	
2. Create a climate of client acceptance. Maintain nonthreatening verbal and nonverbal communication skills when interacting with the angry or potentially violent client.	A relaxed atmosphere may prevent further escalation (Ross, Gwyther, and Kahn, 1999).
3. Respond to the potentially violent client with therapeutic silence, and allow client to ventilate feelings.	These techniques often deescalate anger, because anger expends emotional and physical energy; client runs out of momentum and energy to maintain anger at a high level.

Steps	Rationale
4. Answer questions; if client presents a power-struggle type of question (e.g., "Who said you were in charge; I don't have to listen to you"), redirect and set limits by giving clear, concise expectations. Inform client of potential consequences, and follow through with consequences if behaviors are not altered. Do not argue with client, because arguing will escalate anger. Do not get defensive with client.	By setting limits on power-struggle questions, structure is provided and anger is diffused (Fortinash and Holoday-Worret, 2000).
5. Encourage client to write about negative thoughts.	
6. Encourage physical exercise as a means of directing energy in an acceptable way.	
7. If the client is making verbal threats to harm others, remain calm yet professional and continue to set limits with inappropriate behavior. If a strong likelihood of imminent harm to others is present, the nurse should notify the proper authorities (e.g., nurse manager, security).	Angry clients lose the ability to process information rationally and therefore may impulsively express themselves through intimidation.
8. Maintain personal space and safety with the client who is making verbal threats of violence directed at others. It may be necessary to have someone with you and to keep the door open. Maintain nonthreatening nonverbal behaviors, including body language (e.g., relaxed posture, arms open and hands not in pockets, not invading the client's personal space).	Clients experiencing emotionally charged situations may not comprehend the message. Focus on understanding the client, providing feedback and assisting in problem solving, and providing an atmosphere of warmth and acceptance.

NURSE ALERT *The potentially violent client can be impulsive and explosive, and therefore it is imperative the nurse keep personal safety skills in mind. In this case, avoid touch.*

Steps	Rationale
9. Adjust the amount and quality of time for communicating depending on the client's needs. Try to deescalate the client's anger first, then return later to deliver the message.	It is futile to try to communicate a complicated message to a client in the height of anger.
10. If the client appears to be calm and anger is diffused, explore alternatives to the situation or feelings of anger.	May prevent future explosive outbursts and teach the client effective ways of dealing with anger.
11. See Completion Protocol (inside front cover).	

· · · · · · · · · · ·

EVALUATION

1. Ask client if feelings of anger have subsided.
2. Determine client's ability to answer questions and solve problems.

Unexpected Outcomes and Related Interventions

1. Client continues to demonstrate behaviors or verbal expression of anger or violence. Nurse is unable to assist the client in relieving source of anger or in expressing anger openly without violent acts.
   a. If anger continues to escalate, reassess factors contributing to anger.
   b. Remove or alter factors contributing to anger.

Recording and Reporting

• Record interaction, including: observations related to factors precipitating anger
Use exact quotes
Threats of violence made and who was notified
Nursing action for deescalation and limit setting
Response

Sample Documentation

1800 Despite limit setting measures used by staff, client continues to be verbally assaultive to staff and other clients on the hospital division. He has made verbal threats to harm his doctor: "Just wait until my doctor comes to see me, he is really going to get it bad." The nurse manager and the client's doctor were notified of client's threats.

SPECIAL CONSIDERATIONS

Pediatric Considerations

Immediately setting limits for inappropriate behaviors exhibited by child are effective, because children tend to have less internal control over their behaviors (Wong and others, 1999).

Geriatric Considerations

Clients who have cognitive impairments may exhibit tantrum-like behaviors in response to real or perceived frustration. The nurse can use distraction techniques to remove the cognitively impaired adult client from the disturbing stimuli, or the nurse can use redirection to an activity that is pleasurable to the client.

Home Care Considerations

- Personal safety for the nurse against potentially violent client or family member extends to all health care settings, including the client's home. The nurse may be in potentially dangerous situation while giving care to the client at home; the nurse may give care to the client without support from other staff members.
- Be aware of physical surroundings, including possible exits. Maintain nonthreatening position, including body language, position, and rate of speech, when interacting with an angry or potentially violent client. The nurse should attempt to deescalate the client. If deescalation does not occur and the nurse feels safety may be threatened, the nurse should call for assistance or remove staff from situation.
- Have posted near phone, numbers for emergency use (e.g., mental health provider, emergency response units, neighbors).

Long-Term Care Considerations

- Personal safety is a major concern in settings in which there is no access to additional support from other health care personnel. The nurse should not enter an unsafe environment. In all settings, the nurse needs to be aware of both verbal and nonverbal cues that indicate escalating anger. In settings in which additional support is not readily available, it is also important to be aware of physical surroundings, possible exits, and communication systems to call for assistance (e.g., telephone, emergency call system). A quick exit is appropriate if efforts to deescalate are not successful.
- Allow adequate personal space, and use a firm and calm tone of voice at a moderate pace. The level of speech should be clearly audible, avoiding both shouting and timid tones.
- Use a nonthreatening posture (e.g., avoid standing over the individual, shaking a finger, putting hands on hips).

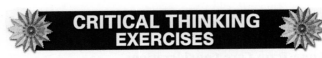

CRITICAL THINKING EXERCISES

1. Mr. Jones was recently admitted for complications from diabetes mellitus. He was diagnosed 10 years ago, and in the past few weeks he has experienced numbness and tingling in both legs. The nurse attempts to gather information to develop an appropriate plan of care. He is very anxious about his condition, is fearful about the hospitalization, and suffers from a hearing loss. Identify possible barriers to effective communication, and state the techniques to be used during the client interview to initiate interaction and facilitate communication.

2. A 78-year-old woman was admitted with an exacerbation of diverticulitis. She appears moderately anxious, with complaints of muscle tensions and sweating. She focuses on only parts of the conversation with the nurse. The nurse needs to attend to other clients, so she delegates communicating with the anxious client to the AP. Discuss how the nurse will delegate this skill and how the AP will communicate with the client.

3. The nurse is involved in a pediatric interview. The client is a 9-year-old boy admitted with complaints of abdominal pain. He has a history of gastrointestinal problems. Discuss strategies for interviewing a pediatric client.

REFERENCES

Adams J, Murray R III: The general approach to the difficult patient, *Emerg Med Clin North Am* 689, 1998.

Erber NP, Scherer SC: Sensory loss and communication difficulties in the elderly, *Australas J Ageing* 4, 1999.

Fortinash K, Holoday-Worret P: *Psychiatric-mental health nursing,* ed 2, St Louis, 2000, Mosby.

Giger J: *Transcultural nursing: assessment and intervention,* ed 3, St Louis, 1999, Mosby.

Keltner N, Schwecke L, Bostrom C: *Psychiatric nursing: a psychotherapeutic management approach,* ed 3, St Louis, 1999, Mosby.

Ross R, Gwyther L, Kahn D: Treatment of agitation in older persons with dementia, *Health Care Consultant* 19, 1999.

Smith M, Buckwalter KC, Maxson E: Psychiatric and geriatric nurses together at the table: evaluation of a combined conference, *J Am Psychiatr Nurses Assoc* 3, 2002.

Wong DL and others: *Whaley and Wong's nursing care of infants and children,* ed 6, St Louis, 1999, Mosby.

CHAPTER

3

Medical Aseptic Techniques

Infections present a significant hazard in all health care settings. Infection-control practices that reduce and/or eliminate sources and transmission of infection help to protect clients and health care providers from disease. Knowledge of the infectious process and disease transmission and critical thinking associated with how and when to use infection-control practices cannot be overemphasized. Today's nurse plays a vital role in the prevention and control of infection.

Nosocomial infections are those that develop as a result of a stay or visit in a health care facility and that were not present or incubating at the time of admission (Bobo, 1994). Risk factors for nosocomial infection include crowding within a health care facility and the client's length of stay (Rubino, 2001). In addition, infection is more likely to develop in persons with chronic illnesses or compromised immunity. Stress related to the uncertainty of diagnosis or the implications of an illness causes susceptibility because of circulating infectious agents (Rubino, 2001). In acute care or ambulatory care facilities, clients can be exposed to new or different microorganisms. Some of these microorganisms may be resistant to most antibiotics. In all settings, clients may have procedures or treatments that lower their resistance to infections. For example, clients' immune systems may be altered after receiving radiation or chemotherapy; therefore they are more susceptible to infections, even from their own normal flora. In addition, invasive procedures, such as the insertion of intravenous (IV) or urinary catheters, disrupt the body's natural defense barriers. In all health care settings the nurse is responsible for teaching clients and their families about the source and transmission of infections, reason for susceptibility, and infection-control principles.

The mere presence of a pathogen does not mean that an infection will begin. Development of an infection occurs in a cyclical process, described as the chain of infection, that depends on the presence of six elements: (1) an infectious agent or pathogen, (2) a reservoir or source for pathogen growth, (3) a portal of exit from the reservoir, (4) a method or mode of transmission, (5) a portal of entrance into the host, and (6) a susceptible host. An infection develops if the chain remains intact (Figure 3-1). However, a nurse who uses infection-control practices can break an element of the chain so that infection will not be transmitted. For example, cleansing contaminated objects, washing or disinfecting hands, changing soiled dressings, keeping work surfaces clean and dry, and wearing gloves when handling blood or body fluids are just a few ways to break the infection chain. Asepsis is defined as the absence of disease-producing (pathogenic) organisms (DeCastro, Fauerback, and Masters, 1996). Aseptic technique involves the purposeful prevention of transfer of microorganisms (DeCastro, 2000). The two types of aseptic technique a nurse practices are medical and surgical asepsis.

Medical asepsis, or clean technique, includes procedures used to reduce the number of and prevent the spread of microorganisms. Handwashing and use of disposable gloves and masks (barrier techniques) are examples of medical asepsis. Surgical asepsis, or sterile technique, includes procedures used to eliminate all microorganisms from an area. For example, sterilization destroys all microorganisms and their spores (Rutala, 1996). Use of sterile instruments and gloves in the operating room and special procedural areas are additional examples of surgical aseptic technique. Surgical aseptic techniques are more rigid than those performed under medical asepsis. Chapter 4 discusses sterile techniques.

Barrier protection protects the health care worker from the client's blood and body fluids and helps prevent the transfer of organisms to other clients, health care workers, and the environment. It is also an important technique for protecting those clients who are immunosuppressed (e.g., clients with cancer who are receiving chemotherapy). Barrier protection includes use of

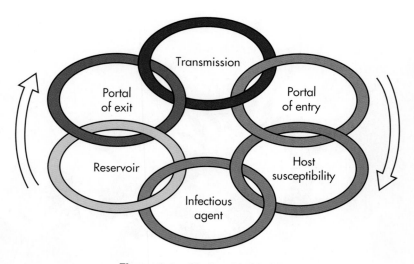

Figure 3-1 Chain of infection.

gowns, masks, protective eyewear, and gloves. Some form of personal protective equipment (PPE) is indicated for all clients who potentially have an infection that can be transmitted to others. Because of the increased attention to the prevention of certain diseases, such as hepatitis B, acquired immunodeficiency syndrome (AIDS), and tuberculosis (TB), the Centers for Disease Control and Prevention (CDC) and the U.S. Occupational Safety and Health Administration (OSHA) have stressed the importance of the use of barriers and precautions (Garner, 1996a; OSHA, 1991, 1994).

In 1996 the CDC published guidelines for the set of precautions known as standard precautions (Garner, 1996a). Part of the rationale for the development of standard precautions is the fact that any client may be a source for infection, requiring health care workers to use PPE to prevent exposure. Table 3-1 describes standard precautions, the primary strategies for reducing the risk of transmission of blood-borne and other pathogens. Standard precautions should become a routine part of a nurse's practice and thus be observed in every client encounter. Increased knowledge of and adherence to standard precautions have been associated with decreased skin and mucous membrane exposures and percutaneous injuries (e.g., needlestick injuries) (McCoy and others, 2001).

In addition to standard precautions, the Hospital Infection Control Practice Advisory Committee (HICPAC) of the CDC published revised guidelines for isolation precautions. Isolation precautions are based upon the assumption that microorganisms are transmitted by several routes;

Table 3-1

Centers for Disease Control and Prevention Isolation Guidelines

Standard Precautions (Tier One)

Standard precautions apply to blood, all body fluids, secretions, excretions (except sweat), nonintact skin, and mucous membranes.

Hands are washed between client contacts; after contact with blood, body fluids, secretions, and excretions and after contact with equipment or articles contaminated by them; and immediately after gloves are removed.

Gloves are worn when touching blood, body fluids, secretions, excretions, nonintact skin, mucous membranes, or contaminated items. Gloves should be removed and hand hygiene performed between client care.

Masks, eye protection, or face shields are worn if client care activities may generate splashes or sprays of blood or body fluid.

Gowns are worn if soiling of clothing is likely from blood or body fluid. Perform hand hygiene after removing gown.

Client care equipment is properly cleaned and reprocessed, and single-use items are discarded.

Contaminated linen is placed in leakproof bag and handled so as to prevent skin and mucous membrane exposure.

All sharp instruments and needles are discarded in a puncture-resistant container. CDC recommends that needles be disposed of uncapped or that a mechanical device be used for recapping.

A private room is unnecessary unless the client's hygiene is unacceptable. Check with an infection-control professional.

Transmission Categories (Tier Two)

Category	Disease	Barrier Protection
Airborne precautions	Droplet nuclei smaller than 5 μm; measles; chickenpox (varicella); disseminated varicella zoster; pulmonary or laryngeal TB	Private room, negative-pressure airflow of at least six exchanges per hour, mask or respiratory protection device
Droplet precautions	Droplets larger than 5 μm; diphtheria (pharyngeal); rubella; streptococcal pharyngitis, pneumonia, or scarlet fever in infants and young children; pertussis; mumps; mycoplasmal pneumonia; meningococcal pneumonia or sepsis; pneumonic plague	Private room or cohort clients; mask
Contact precautions	Direct client or environmental contact; colonization or infection with multidrug-resistant organism; respiratory syncytial virus; shigella and other enteric pathogens; major wound infections; herpes simplex; scabies, varicella zoster (disseminated)	Private room or cohort clients; gloves, gowns

Modified from Garner JS: Guidelines for isolation precautions in hospitals, *Infect Control Hosp Epidemiol* 17(1):54, 1996b.

the five main routes are contact, droplet, airborne, common vehicle, and vectorborne. The developed guidelines are aimed at using barrier precautions to interrupt the mode of transmission (see Procedural Guideline 3-1, p. 57, and Skill 3-2, p. 56).

In 1994 the CDC issued guidelines for the prevention of transmission of tuberculosis in health care facilities. The guidelines include medical screening and require that all health care workers be fit-tested and trained in the wearing and storage of a high-efficiency particulate air (HEPA) respirator or N95 mask that meets or exceeds the standard. Other requirements include annual TB skin testing for health care workers and the isolation of clients suspected of having TB (see Skill 3-3, p. 58).

Nurses can play a very important role in the prevention of infection. As advocates, nurses can help to ensure that all health care providers (e.g., respiratory therapists, physicians, and other nurses) working with clients and support staff (e.g., housekeepers) maintain infection-control practices at all times. This applies also to family members. When a hospitalized client has an infection, the nurse can play a role in deciding the optimal room placement to minimize the chances of infection spreading to other clients. In addition, two clients with "like" infections can be placed in the same room together. The knowledgeable

and judicious use of infection-control practices can make a difference as to whether a client recovers from an illness or develops serious or even fatal complications.

NURSING DIAGNOSES

Several nursing diagnoses may be appropriate when using infection-control measures. **Risk for Infection** relates to clients who may have specific risk factors that may increase their potential for acquiring an infection. These include pathological conditions (immunosuppression, chronic disease, or obesity), treatments (surgery, invasive procedures, or steroids), situational factors (disease exposure, inadequate immunizations, or lack of handwashing by caregiver), or maturation (the very young and very old).

A diagnosis of **Deficient Knowledge** regarding infection prevention is appropriate when the nurse teaches individuals, families, or groups information about infection-control measures. Clients can experience **Fear** or a feeling of **Powerlessness** when restricted to a respiratory isolation type of environment or when required to use protective barriers. **Social Isolation** may also be appropriate when use of protective barriers and environmental restrictions are required.

Skill 3.1

Handwashing and Disinfection

Handwashing has been considered the most important measure for controlling and preventing the spread of infection in health care facilities. Handwashing is a vigorous, brief rubbing together of all surfaces of the hands lathered in soap, followed by rinsing under a stream of water. The purpose is to remove soil and transient microorganisms from the hands and areas around the nails, to reduce total microbial counts over time (Larson, 1996).

Research has shown that most health care workers fail to wash their hands thoroughly as recommended (Boyce & Pittet, 2002). The recommended duration for lathering hands is *at least 15 seconds* and preferably 30 seconds. However, hospital personnel typically wash their hands for less than 15 seconds. Contaminated hands are a prime cause of transmission of infection. Health care workers function in a busy environment. Client care activities are fast paced. With a busy workload, frequent interruptions in client care activities, inaccessible sinks or supplies, and irritating hand-washing agents, handwashing adherence can be a problem. Nishimura and others (1999) have found that hand-washing adherence among intensive care unit (ICU) personnel is low. After videotaping staff as they entered the ICU, the researchers found only 71% of ICU

personnel washed their hands before beginning client care. *Handwashing is not optional, it is a critical responsibility of all health care workers.*

The Healthcare Infection Control Practices Advisory Committee as part of the Centers for Disease Control and Prevention (CDC) recently released new guidelines for *hand hygiene* in health care settings (Boyce & Pittet, 2002). The development of alcohol-based hand antiseptics in reducing bacterial counts on the hands, offers an alternative to traditional handwashing that is highly effective. Hand hygiene refers to either handwashing (use of soap and water), antiseptic handwashing (use of antiseptic soap), antiseptic hand rub (use of alcohol based product) and surgical hand antisepsis (Chapters 4 and 20).

Hand hygiene can effectively reduce health care–acquired infection, when performed correctly. The decision to perform hand hygiene depends on three factors: (1) the intensity or degree of contact with clients or contaminated objects, (2) the amount of contamination that may occur with the contact, (3) the client's or health care worker's susceptibility to infection, and the procedure or activity to be performed (Larson, 2000). For example, if a nurse touches an object that is not visibly soiled, hand-

Table 3-2

Guidelines for Hand Hygiene Based on Degree of Antisepsis

Type of Hand Care	Purpose	Method
Hand wash	Remove soil and transient microorganisms.	Soap or detergent for at least 10-15 seconds.
Hand antisepsis	Remove or destroy transient microorganisms.	Antimicrobial soap or detergent or alcohol-based hand rub for at least 10-15 seconds.
Surgical hand scrub	Reduce, remove, or destroy transient microorganisms and reduce resident flora.	Antimicrobial soap or detergent preparation and brushing to create friction for at least 120 seconds, or alcohol-based preparation for at least 120 seconds.

Modified from Larson EL: APIC guideline for handwashing and hand antisepsis in health care settings, *Am J Infect ControL* 23(4):251, 1995.

washing may not be required. In contrast, prolonged contact with a soiled dressing from a client's wound would require thorough handwashing (Table 3-2). The CDC hand hygiene guidelines suggest the following:

1. When hands are visibly dirty or contaminated with proteinaceous material or are visibly soiled with blood or other body fluids, wash hands with either a nonantimicrobial soap and water or an antimicrobial soap and water.
2. If hands are nor visibly soiled, use and alcohol-based hand rub for routinely decontaminating the hands in all of the following clinical situations:

Ba. Before having direct contact with clients.
   b. Before donning sterile gloves when inserting a central IV catheter.
   c. Before inserting indwelling urinary catheters, peripheral vascular catheters, or other invasive devices that do not require a surgical procedure.
   d. After contact with a client's intact skin (e.g. after taking a pulse or blood pressure, and lifting a client).
   e. After contact with body fluids or excretions, mucous membranes, nonintact skin, and wound dressings *if hands are not visibly soiled.*
   f. If moving from a contaminated-body site to a clean-body site during client care.
   g. After contact with inanimate objects (e.g. medical equipment) in the immediate vicinity of the client.
   h. After removing gloves.

Routine handwashing may be performed with soap in any convenient form (bar, leaflets, liquid, or powder). Nonantimicrobial soaps have cleaning activity because of their detergent properties, which results in removal of soil, dirt, and organic substances from the hands. The soaps contain little if any antimicrobial activity. Bar soap that remains wet or in pooled water may harbor microorganisms. The use of antimicrobial soap (antiseptic) is encouraged in health care settings. Antimicrobials are effective in reducing bacte-

rial counts on the hands and often have residual antimicrobial effects for several hours. There are a number of effective antimicrobial soaps that contain alcohols, chlorhexidine gluconate (CHG), triclosan, and iodophors. Certain antimicrobial soaps can irritate the skin, and their use must be weighed against the potential for skin irritation.

Decontamination of the hands by a hand rub involves the use of alcohol-based, waterless products. The products have low irritancy potential, particularly when staff decontaminate their hands multiple times a shift (Larson and others, 2001). Typically the product solutions contain alcohol in addition to products that prevent skin dryness. When hands are vigorously cleansed with the alcohol solution, a significantly greater reduction in the number of microbial counts on the hands results, when compared with traditional handwashing (Zaragoza and others, 1999).

ASSESSMENT

1. Assess client's risk for or extent of infection (e.g., elevated white blood cell [WBC] count, open wound, known medical diagnosis).
2. Inspect surface of nurse's hands for breaks or cuts in skin or cuticles. Note condition of nails. Report and cover any skin lesions before providing client care. Avoid wearing artificial nails or extenders when having direct contact with clients at high risk (e.g. ICU). *Rationale: Chipped nail polish may support growth of larger numbers of organisms on fingernails (Baumgardner, Maragos, and Larson, 1993). Health care workers who wear artificial nails are more likely to harbor gram-negative pathogens on their fingertips than are those who have natural nails (Boyce and Pittet, 2002)*
3. Keep natural nails less than $\frac{1}{4}$ inch long (Boyce and Pittet, 2002). *Rationale: Enhances ability to clean subungual area of nail.*
4. Consider the type of nursing activity being performed. *Rationale: Determines need for antiseptic hand rub.*
5. Inspect hands for visible soiling. *Rationale: Determines the need for hand wash.*

PLANNING

Expected outcomes focus on preventing the transmission of infection.

Expected Outcomes

1. Hands and areas under fingernails are clean and free of debris.

Equipment

Handwashing
- Easy-to-reach sink with warm running water
- Antimicrobial or regular soap
- Paper towels

Antiseptic hand rub
- Waterless alcohol-based product

Delegation Considerations

Hand hygiene or antisepsis involves a set of basic procedures that should be performed correctly by all caregivers. If you observe other caregivers or family caregivers incorrectly cleanse their hands, reinforce the importance of the technique and correct procedural steps.
- Observe the consistency and thoroughness of staff in washing or disinfecting hands.

IMPLEMENTATION FOR HANDWASHING AND DISINFECTION

Steps	Rationale
1. Handwashing a. Push wristwatch and long uniform sleeves above wrists. Avoid wearing rings.	Studies have shown that skin underneath rings is more heavily colonized than comparable areas of skin on fingers without rings. Gram-negative bacilli and *Staphylococcus aureus* are commonly found under rings (Boyce and Pittet, 2001)
b. Stand in front of sink, keeping hands and uniform away from sink surface. (If hands touch sink during handwashing, repeat.)	Inside of sink is a contaminated area. Reaching over sink increases risk of touching edge, which is contaminated.
c. Turn on water. Turn faucet on (see illustration) or push knee pedals laterally or press pedals with foot to regulate flow and temperature.	
d. Avoid splashing water against uniform.	Microorganisms travel and grow in moisture.
e. Regulate flow of water so that temperature is warm.	Hands are the most contaminated parts to be washed.
f. Wet hands and wrists thoroughly under running water. Keep hands and forearms lower than elbows during washing.	Water flows from least to most contaminated area, rinsing microorganisms into sink.

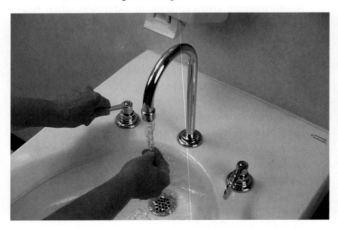

Step 1c   Turning on water.

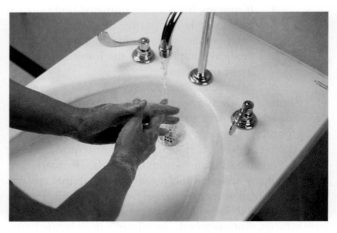

Step 1g   Lathering hands thoroughly.

Steps	Rationale
g. Apply 3 to 5 ml of detergent (see product recommendation) and rub hands together vigorously, lathering thoroughly (see illustration). Soap granules and leaflet preparations may be used instead.	Necessary to ensure that all surfaces of hands and fingers are covered and cleansed.
h. Perform hand hygiene using plenty of lather and friction for *at least* 15 seconds. Interlace fingers and rub palms and back of hands with circular motion at least 5 times each. Keep fingertips down to facilitate removal of microorganisms.	Friction and rubbing mechanically loosen and remove dirt and transient bacteria. Adequate time is needed to expose skin surfaces to antimicrobial agent.
i. Areas underlying fingernails are often soiled. Clean with fingernails of other hand and additional soap or clean orangewood stick *(optional).*	Area under nails can be highly contaminated, which will increase the risk of infections for the nurse or client.

NURSE ALERT *Do not tear or cut skin under or around nail.*

Steps	Rationale
j. Rinse hands and wrists thoroughly, keeping hands down and elbows up (see illustration).	Rinsing mechanically washes away dirt and microorganisms.
k. *Optional:* Repeat Steps 1 through 9, and extend period of washing if hands are heavily soiled.	
l. Dry hands thoroughly from fingers to wrists and forearms with paper towel.	Drying from cleanest (fingertips) to least clean (forearms) area avoids contamination. Drying hands prevents chapping and roughened skin.
m. Use towel to turn off hand faucet. Avoiding touching handles with hands (see illustration). Turn off water with foot or knee pedals (if applicable).	Prevents transfer of pathogens from faucet to hands.
n. If hands are dry or chapped, use a small amount of lotion or barrier cream dispensed from an individual-use container.	Large, refillable containers of lotion have been associated with nosocomial infections.

2. **Antiseptic hand rub**

Steps	Rationale
a. Apply adequate amount of product to cover all surfaces of hands and fingers during rubbing (follow manufacturer's directions for volume to use).	
b. Rub hands together, covering all surfaces of the hands and fingers, until hands are dry (see illustrations on p. 56).	If an adequate volume of an alcohol-based hand rub is used, it should take 15 to 25 seconds for hands to dry (Boyce and Pittet, 2001).

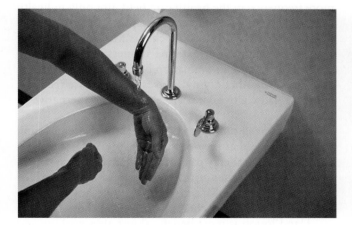

Step 1j Rinsing hands.

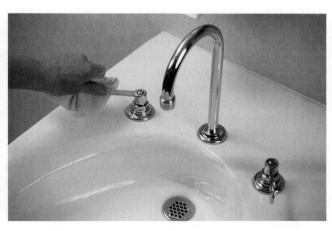

Step 1m Turning off faucet.

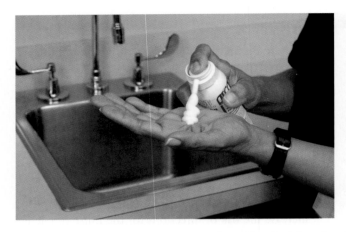 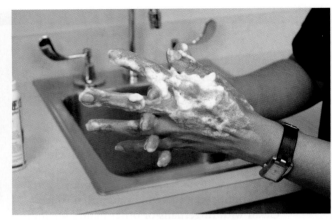

Step 2b   Rub hands with antiseptic hand rub.

• • • • • • • • • •

EVALUATION

1. Inspect surfaces of hands for obvious signs of soil or other contaminants.
2. Inspect hands for dermatitis or cracked skin.

Unexpected Outcomes and Related Interventions

1. Hands or areas under fingernails remain soiled.
   a. Repeat handwashing
2. Repeated use of soaps/antiseptics may cause dermatitis or cracked skin.
   a. Rinse and dry hands thoroughly, avoid excessive amounts of soap/antiseptic, try various products, use hand lotions or barrier creams, or wear gloves. (This should be temporary because glove wearing can increase bacterial growth and may increase incidence of latex allergies.)

Recording and Reporting

- It is unnecessary to document handwashing.
- Report dermatitis to employee health and/or infection-control department of agency.

Skill 3.2

Using Disposable Clean Gloves

Disposable gloves must be worn before coming in contact with mucous membranes, nonintact skin, blood, body fluids, or other infectious material. Nurses wear gloves routinely when performing a variety of procedures (e.g., nasogastric tube insertion, enema administration, perineal hygiene, and removal of soiled dressings). In addition, gloves are indicated when there are cuts; abrasions; or oozing, draining wounds on the caregiver's hands (Larson, 1996). Gloves should be inspected before use for cuts, tears, or holes. Gloves found with any of these deficiencies will not provide proper barrier protection. Disposable gloves are easy to apply (Procedural Guideline 3-1). Remove gloves after caring for a client. Also, change gloves during client care if moving from a contaminated site to a clean body site.

There are many types of gloves available to the health care worker. It is important that individuals choose gloves that suit their needs. Latex allergies are occurring with more frequency in the health care field, not only in health care workers but also in clients. Chapter 4 describes in detail the approach for assessing clients for latex allergies. If redness, inflammation, extreme dryness, or vesicles appear on the hands, an evaluation by a physician should be performed. Synthetic vinyl gloves are just as effective a barrier as latex gloves and are an excellent alternative to latex.

Clients need to be questioned regarding allergies, and it is imperative that they be specifically asked about latex allergies. A latex allergy can precipitate a respiratory arrest, which is a life-threatening event, and must not be ignored or forgotten. The health care worker should not wear latex gloves when caring for clients with latex allergies.

Hand lotion is most beneficial just after washing and lightly drying your hands. Avoid using lotions that contain mineral oil or petroleum as their main ingredients, because these impair the integrity of latex and the effectiveness of gloves. Use the facility-provided lotion, which should be compatible with antimicrobial soaps. Lotion is a culture media for organisms. Do not share a lotion bottle or buy large economy jugs and refill a small portable container.

Delegation Considerations

Applying disposable gloves is a basic procedure that should be performed correctly by assistive personnel (AP). If you observe AP failing to use gloves when necessary, reinforce the importance of the procedure.

Procedural Guideline 3-1

Using Disposable Clean Gloves

Equipment: 1 pair of disposable gloves (latex or latex-free)

1. Application
   a. Inspect hands for cuts, abrasions, or wounds that indicate need for gloves.
   b. Inspect skin for redness, inflammation, extreme dryness, or vesicles that may indicate latex allergy.
   c. Select appropriate glove size, and apply gloves (no special technique required). If wearing an isolation gown, pull cuffs of gloves over cuffs of gown. If not wearing a gown, pull up the gloves to cover the wrist (see illustration).
   d. Interlink fingers to adjust glove fit.
2. Removal
   a. Remove first glove by grasping outer surface of lower cuff, taking care to touch only glove to glove (see illustration).
   b. Pull glove inside out over hand, taking care to touch only inside of glove with hand.
   c. Grasp soiled glove in remaining gloved hand.
   d. With ungloved hand, tuck finger inside cuff of remaining glove and pull it off, inside out, enclosing both soiled gloves. Discard in receptacle (see illustration).
3. Perform hand hygiene when washing hands, do so thoroughly for at least 10 to 15 seconds. Decreases exposure to latex residue on hands.

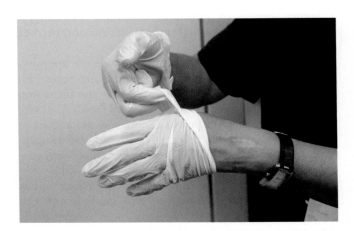

Step 2a   Remove first glove.

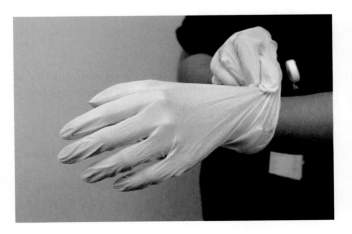

Step 1c   Pull glove cuff up over wrist.

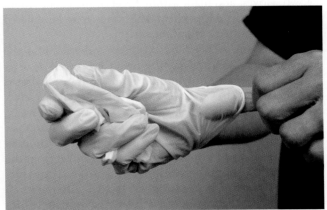

Step 2d   Remove second glove while holding soiled glove.

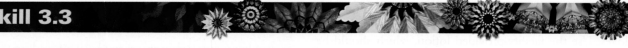

Skill 3.3

Caring for Clients Under Isolation Precautions

Standard precautions are always used as a basic form of clinical practice for all clients. The majority of organisms causing nosocomial infections are found in the colonized body substances of clients, regardless of whether or not a culture has confirmed infection and a diagnosis has been made (Jackson and Lynch, 1992). Body substances such as feces, urine, mucus, and wound drainage can contain potentially infectious organisms. However, when a client has a known source of infection, additional precautions, above and beyond those of standard precautions, become necessary.

Isolation or barrier precautions include the appropriate use of gloves, gowns, masks, eyewear, and other PPE when a client is infected or colonized with specific organisms. The revised guidelines developed by the CDC (1996) include special precautions for clients who are known or suspected to be infected or colonized with microorganisms transmitted by airborne, droplet, or contact with contaminated surfaces or dry skin (see Table 3-1, p. 51).

The three types of transmission-based precautions may be combined for diseases that have multiple routes of transmission. When used singularly or in combination, they are to be used in addition to standard precautions when required by the specific infection. When a client requires isolation, determine the reason and the mode of transmission. Evaluate the task to be performed to identify the barrier equipment that will be needed. For example, a client in respiratory isolation for measles or pertussis has an organism that can be carried on droplets. A mask is necessary when entering the room for any reason. To hold and feed an infant, it would be appropriate to wear both a mask and gown, to protect clothing from secretions from the infant's nose or mouth. It would be appropriate to add gloves to assist in intubating the infant. When a client is in contact isolation for a resistant organism in sputum, wear a gown, gloves, and mask within 3 feet of the client. To introduce yourself to the client, the room may be entered without any protective equipment.

Taking care of a client requires understanding the chain of infection and how the organism travels to a receptive host. The most common mode of transmission is your hands. *Wash or decontaminate your hands after every client contact,* even when gloves have been worn. Be aware of unconscious actions such as rubbing your eyes or nose, picking teeth, or biting fingernails. For respiratory/droplet-spread organisms, a safe zone beyond 3 to 5 feet from the client can be assumed, unless a client is on airborne precautions. Therefore it is appropriate to walk into the room of a client in isolation, without barrier equipment, to introduce yourself and be seen without your face covered. This is a good opportunity to inform the client why it is necessary to wear masks, gowns, or gloves while doing certain tasks.

When a client requires isolation in a private room, the nurse must remember that loneliness can develop. Isolation disrupts normal social relationships with visitors and caregivers. A client who suffers from an infectious disease may also experience self-concept or body image changes. Unless the nurse acts to reduce feelings of psychological and physical isolation, the client's emotional state can interfere with recovery. Clients and families need to be reassured with appropriate education regarding the infectious agent, its mode of transmission, and the purpose of isolation. This education helps maintain the client's self-concept or body image, minimizes feelings of isolation, and facilitates recovery.

ASSESSMENT

1. Assess client's medical history and possible indications for isolation (e.g., purulent productive cough, major draining wound). Review the precautions necessary for the specific isolation system.
2. Review laboratory test results (e.g., wound culture, acid-fast bacillus [AFB] smears, serology testing, and changes in WBC count). *Rationale: Reveals type of organism infecting a client.*
3. Consider types of care measures to be performed while in client's room. *Rationale: Allows nurse to organize all equipment needed in room.*
4. Determine from nursing care plan, nursing colleagues, or family members the client's emotional state and reaction to isolation. Also assess client's understanding of purpose of isolation.
5. Before applying gloves, assess if the client has a known latex allergy. *Rationale: Allows nurse to select nonlatex gloves for use.*

PLANNING

Expected outcomes focus on preventing transmission of infection to nurse and other clients and improving client's knowledge of the purpose of isolation.

Expected Outcomes

1. Client and/or family verbalizes purpose of isolation and treatment plan.
2. Infection does not develop in neighboring clients.

Equipment

- Disposable gloves
- Mask

- Eyewear, protective goggles or glasses, face shield
- Fluid-resistant gown
- Medication
- Hygiene items

Delegation Considerations

Basic care procedures (e.g., bathing and feeding) performed under isolation can be delegated to assistive personnel (AP). The RN is responsible for assessing whether it is more effective to provide direct care or delegate care activities, depending on the client's clinical status. Procedures such as medication administration and IV care require the critical thinking and knowledge application unique to an RN.

- Clarify for assistive personnel the type of isolation precautions to use.

IMPLEMENTATION FOR CARING FOR CLIENTS UNDER ISOLATION PRECAUTIONS

Steps	Rationale

1. See Standard Protocol (inside front cover).
2. Enter the client's room, and remain by the door. Introduce yourself, and explain the care you are to provide and the purpose of isolation precautions before applying protective equipment.

    Allows client to sense the nurse's caring without exposing nurse to risk of infection transmission.

3. Prepare for entrance into isolation room. Choice of barrier protection depends on type of isolation and facility policy (see Table 3-1, p. 51).

  a. Apply either surgical mask or respirator around mouth and nose (type depends on type of isolation and facility policy). Tie or attach a mask securely to make sure it fits snugly. (see illustration).

    Prevents exposure to airborne microorganisms or exposure to microorganisms from splashing of fluids.

  b. Apply eyewear or goggles snugly around face and eyes (when needed) (see illustration).

    Protects nurse from exposure to microorganisms that may occur during splashing of contaminated fluids.

  c. Apply gown, being sure it covers all outer garments; pull sleeves down to wrist. Tie securely at neck and waist (see illustration).

    Prevents transmission of infection when client has excessive drainage or discharge. Also reduces contamination of clothing from splashes or splatters.

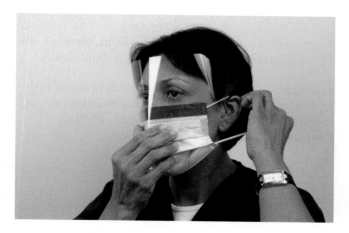

Step 3a   Mask snugly in place.

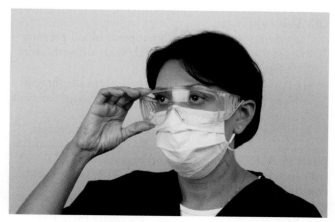

Step 3b   Eye goggles in place.

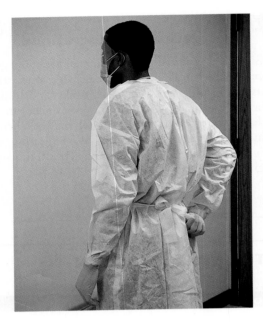

Step 3c   Nurse tying gown.

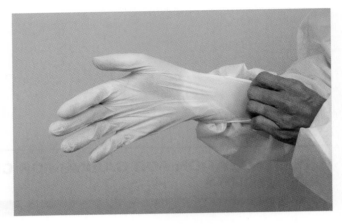

Step 3d   Application of disposable glove over edge of gown sleeve.

Steps	Rationale
d. Apply disposable gloves. (NOTE: Unpowdered latex-free gloves should be worn if the client or the health care worker has a latex allergy.) If worn with gown, bring cuffs over edge of gown sleeves (see illustration).	Gloves are applied last so that they can be placed over the cuffs of the gown.

COMMUNICATION TIP   *Reassure clients and families that isolation is used for diseases that are easily spread, not for diseases that are "extra terrible." It protects other clients in the facility from exposure to the microorganism. Be positive, and focus on what they can do (e.g., receive/send mail, watch TV, use the phone, receive visitors). Assure them that the goal is for isolation to be as short and pleasant as possible.*

---

4. Enter client's room. Arrange supplies and equipment. (If equipment will be removed from room for reuse, place on clean paper towel.)	Minimizes contamination of care items.
5. Assess vital signs.	
a. Avoid contact of stethoscope or blood pressure cuff with infective material. Wipe off with disinfectant as needed.	If stethoscope is used later on other clients, there is a risk of transmitting infection unless it is disinfected.
b. If stethoscope is to be reused, clean diaphragm or bell with 70% alcohol or liquid soap. Set aside on clean surface.	Systematic disinfection with 70% alcohol or liquid soap will minimize chance of spreading infectious agents between clients (Bernard and others, 1999).
c. Use an individual or disposable thermometer.	Prevents cross contamination.

NURSE ALERT   *If a resistant organism (e.g., vancomycin-resistant Enterococcus [VCE]) is present, equipment remains in room.*

---

6. Administer medications (see Chapters 17 and 18).
    a.   Give oral medication in wrapper or cup.
    b.   Dispose of wrapper or cup in plastic-lined receptacle.

Steps	Rationale

c. Administer injection, being sure gloves are worn.

d. Discard disposable syringe (with protective shield) or syringe with uncapped needle (if applicable) into designated sharps container (see illustration).

Reduces risk of needle-stick injury.

NURSE ALERT *Hepatitis B virus and Hepatitis C virus are the most prevalent blood-borne pathogens. Spread occurs mainly through direct parenteral or percutaneous exposure to tainted blood (Sattar and others, 2001).*

---

e. Place reusable plastic syringe (e.g., Carpuject) on clean towel for eventual removal and disinfection.

7. Administer hygiene, encouraging the client to verbalize any questions or concerns regarding isolation.

COMMUNICATION TIP *This is an excellent time to provide informal teaching.*

---

a. Avoid allowing isolation gown to become wet: carry washbasin outward away from gown; avoid leaning against wet tabletop.

b. Assist client in removing own gown; discard in impervious linen bag.

c. Remove linen from bed; avoid contact with isolation gown. Place in impervious linen bag.

d. Provide clean bed linen and set of towels.

e. Change gloves and perform hand hygiene if hands become excessively soiled and further care is necessary.

8. Collect specimens (see Chapter 14).

a. Place specimen container on clean paper towel in client's bathroom, and follow procedure for collecting specimen.

b. Transfer specimen to container without soiling outside of container. After gloves are removed, place container in plastic bag and label correctly for transport to laboratory.

Moisture allows organisms to travel through gown to uniform.

Reduces transfer of microorganisms.

Linen soiled by client's body fluids is handled so as to prevent contact with clean gown.

Container will be taken out of client's room, thus outer surface must not be contaminated.

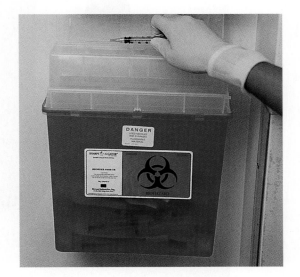

Step 6d Dispose of uncapped needle and syringe in sharps receptacle.

Steps	**Rationale**

9. Dispose of linen, trash, and disposable items.
   a. Use single bags that are impervious to moisture and sturdy to contain soiled articles. Use double bag if necessary for heavily soiled linen or heavy wet trash.
   b. Tie bags securely at top in knot.

Linen or refuse should be totally contained to prevent exposure of personnel to infective material.

10. Remove all reusable pieces of equipment. Clean any contaminated surfaces with disinfectant (see agency policy).

Items must be properly cleaned, disinfected, or sterilized for reuse.

11. Resupply room as needed. Have staff hand new supplies to you.

Limiting trips into and out of room reduces nurse's and client's exposure to microorganisms.

12. Leave isolation room. Order of removal of protective equipment depends on what is worn in room. This sequence describes steps to take if all barriers were required to be worn.
   a. Remove gloves (see Procedural Guideline 3-1, p. 57).

Prevents nurse from contacting contaminated glove's outer surface.

   b. Untie *top* mask string and then bottom strings, pull mask away from face and drop into trash receptacle (Do not touch outer surface of mask).

Ungloved hands will not be contaminated by touching only mask strings.

   c. Untie neck strings, then back strings of gown. Allow gown to fall from shoulders. Remove hands from sleeves without touching outside of gown (see illustration). Hold gown inside at shoulder seams and fold inside out. Discard in laundry bag (see illustration).

Hands do not come in contact with soiled front of gown. Hands have not been soiled.

   d. Remove eyewear or goggles.
   e. Perform handwashing or antisepsis a minimum of 10 to 15 seconds.

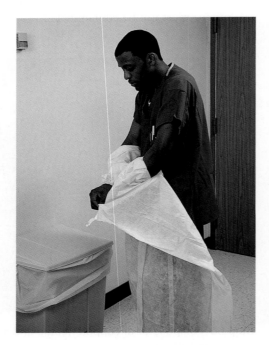
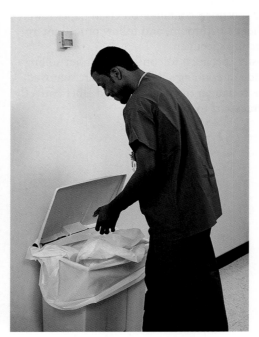

Step 12c Turn gown inside out and discard.

Steps	Rationale

f. Retrieve wristwatch and stethoscope (unless remains in room), and record vital signs on notepaper or clean paper towel.

Clean hands can contact clean items.

g. Explain to client when you plan to return to room. Ask if client has any requests or needs.

h. Leave room, and close door.

Keeping door open too long equalizes pressure in room and allows organisms to flow out.

13. See Completion Protocol (inside front cover).

• • • • • • • • • • •

EVALUATION

1. Ask client and family member to explain purpose of isolation in relation to diagnosed condition.
2. Monitor clinical status of neighboring clients.

Recording and Reporting

- Procedures performed (including education) and client's response
- Type of isolation in use and the microorganism (if known)
- Client's response to social isolation

Sample Documentation

1320 Contact isolation in place for salmonella in stool. Client incontinent of liquid stool. Wife at bedside, asking questions about barrier equipment. Discussed the method by which salmonella is transmitted and explained the purpose of gown and gloves. Wife verbalized good understanding when she requested gloves and gown to assist in cleanup.

SPECIAL CONSIDERATIONS

Pediatric Considerations

Strange environment of isolation confuses a child. Preschoolers are unable to understand cause-effect relationship for isolation. School-agers may understand cause but still fantasize. Offer children simple explanations, "You need to be in this room to help you get better." Show all barrier equipment to a child. Toys and games that are brought into the room should be ones that can be effectively cleaned with an approved germicide. Parents must be actively involved in any explanations. Nurse lets child see face before applying mask so child does not become frightened.

Geriatric Considerations

Isolation can increase confusion in older adults who have already demonstrated signs of confusion or depression. Many times clients become more confused when confronted by a nurse wearing a mask or gown or when they are left in a room with the door closed. Assess need for closing door along with safety of client and additional safety measures required. Assess older adult for signs of depression: loss of appetite, decrease in verbal communications, or inability to sleep.

Home Care Considerations

- If client returns home with draining wound or productive cough, educate family on potential sources of contamination in the home and techniques for disposing of any biological wastes.
- Encourage clients to use vigilant handwashing and to avoid sharing personal care items with other family members.
- Have clients store contaminated linens in plastic bags and then launder them in hot soapy water with a bleach solution (e.g., Clorox). It is also important for clients to wear gloves when handling blood- or body fluid–soiled linens.
- Have clients use a 10% bleach solution when performing household kitchen/bathroom cleaning of spills containing blood or other body fluids.

Long-Term Care Considerations

Protective isolation is typically not used in long-term care settings.

Skill 3.4

Special Tuberculosis Precautions

The dramatic upsurge of TB, some cases involving drug-resistant strains of the microorganism, has increased concern regarding nosocomial transfer. Guidelines for preventing TB in health care settings stress the importance of early identification and treatment of persons with known or suspected TB and proper isolation in the health care setting. In 1994 the CDC released guidelines for stricter adherence to infection-control measures (CDC, 1994). A nurse should suspect TB in any client with respiratory symptoms lasting longer than 3 weeks. It is essential that nurses have good assessment skills, because the risk of exposure is greatest before a diagnosis is made and isolation precautions are implemented. Suspicious symptoms include fatigue, unexplained weight loss, dyspnea, fever and night sweats, and a cough that can sometimes be productive of blood. Isolation for clients with known or suspected TB includes a special, private AFB isolation room (Box 3-1). Such rooms in existing facilities have negative

Box 3-1
TB Isolation

- TB isolation should be practiced for all clients with known or suspected TB. (Suspected TB is defined by agency policy and generally means any client with a positive AFB smear, a cavitating lesion seen on chest x-ray study, or identified as high risk by a screening tool.)
- Isolation must be in a single-client room designated as negative airflow and having at least six air exchanges per hour. Room air must be vented to the outside. The door must be closed to maintain negative pressure.
- Health care workers must wear an N95 particulate respirator mask or HEPA respirator when entering an AFB isolation room. (Check agency's policy for type of mask.)
- Workers must be fit-tested* before using a respirator for the first time. This ensures type and size of respirator appropriate for an individual.
- Workers must fit-check† the respirator's fit before each use.
- Respirator may be reused and stored according to agency policy.

AFB, Acid-fast bacillus.
Fit test: Procedure to determine adequate fit of respirator, usually by qualitative measure (wearers are exposed to a concentrated saccharin solution and asked if they can detect taste wearing respirator).
†*Fit check:* Procedure in which worker uses negative pressure to see if mask is properly sealed to face.

pressure in relation to surrounding areas so that room air is exhausted directly to the outside or through special HEPA filters if recirculation is unavoidable. High-hazard procedures on clients with suspected or confirmed infectious TB must be performed in AFB treatment rooms.

OSHA and CDC guidelines require health care workers who care for active or suspected TB clients to wear HEPA respirators. The respirators are high-efficiency particulate masks that have the ability to filter particles 1 μm in size with a filter efficiency of 95% or higher. Health care employees who work in the rooms of TB clients must be fit-tested in a reliable way to obtain a face-seal leakage of 10% or less (CDC, 1994). Under National Institute for Occupational Safety and Health (NIOSH) criteria the minimally acceptable level of respiratory protection for TB is the Type 95 Respirator. Hospital staff must be trained in the wearing and storage of the HEPA respirator. OSHA also requires employers to provide training concerning transmission of TB, especially in areas where risk of exposure is high, such as in bronchoscopy procedural areas. Other requirements include annual TB skin testing for health care workers and appropriate follow-up when previously negative skin tests become positive (OSHA, 1993).

ASSESSMENT

1. Assess client's potential for infectious pulmonary or laryngeal TB (e.g., documentation of positive AFB smear or culture, signs or symptoms of TB, cavitation on chest x-ray study, history of a recent exposure, physician progress notes indicating plan to rule out TB).
2. Assess effectiveness of isolation room (e.g., check negative airflow using flutter strip or smoke stick, or consult with institution's plant engineering department).
3. Consider type of care measures to be performed while in client's room. *Rationale: Allows nurse to organize all necessary equipment.*

PLANNING

Expected outcomes focus on prevention of transmission of TB and client understanding of TB transmission.

Expected Outcomes

1. Client describes how TB may be transmitted.
2. Neighboring clients or staff do not develop TB.

Equipment

- TB isolation room
- Respiratory protective device (check agency policy)
- Disposable gloves, gown, protective eyewear (based on client's clinical condition)
- Basic care items (e.g., medication equipment, hygiene items)

Delegation Considerations

Basic care procedures (e.g., bathing and feeding) performed under TB isolation can be delegated to assistive personnel (AP). The nurse is responsible for assessing whether it is more effective to provide direct care or delegate care activities, depending on the client's clinical status. Procedures such as medication administration and IV care require the critical thinking and knowledge application unique to a nurse.

- Clarify for assistive personnel special precautions in use of a fitted respirator.

IMPLEMENTATION FOR SPECIAL TUBERCULOSIS PRECAUTIONS

Steps	Rationale
1. See Standard Protocol (inside front cover).	
2. Before entering room, apply recommended mask. Be sure it fits snugly.	Reduces transmission of airborne droplet nuclei.
3. Explain purpose of AFB isolation to client, family, and others.	Improves ability of client to participate in care. TB cannot be transmitted through contact with clothing, bedding, food, or eating utensils.

COMMUNICATION TIP *TB is transmitted by inhalation of droplets that remain suspended in the air when client coughs, sneezes, speaks, or sings (CDC, 1994). Offer opportunity for questions.*

4. Instruct client to cover mouth with tissue when coughing and to wear disposable surgical mask when leaving the room.	Reduces spread of droplet nuclei.

NURSE ALERT *The particulate respirator that the health care worker wears is not to be placed on the client. The added work of breathing through the respirator is an added stress on an already compromised pulmonary system. Simply apply a regular surgical mask.*

5. Provide care (see Skill 3-3, p. 58).	
6. Leave the room, and close the door.	Maintains negative pressure in room.
7. Remove respiratory protective device.	Most fitted respiratory devices are reusable.
8. Place reusable device in labeled paper bag for storage, being careful not to crush device. (Check agency policy for number of times it can be reused.)	Plastic bags seal in moisture.
9. See Completion Protocol (inside front cover).	

• • • • • • • • • •

EVALUATION

1. Assess client's laboratory data for repeated AFB smears that may be negative.
2. Ask client and/or family to identify method of transmission for TB.
3. Be alert, and assess any suspected respiratory symptoms in neighboring clients.

Unexpected Outcomes and Related Interventions

1. Client fails to follow precautions for preventing transmission (e.g., fails to cover mouth when coughing, improperly disposes of soiled tissue).
   a. Reexplain significant risk to family and friends.
   b. Discuss client's concerns/feelings about the disease.

Recording and Reporting

- Procedures performed in isolation room and client's response
- Type of isolation precaution system
- Education given to client/family and their response to instruction
- Response of client/family to isolation

Sample Documentation

0800 Client on TB isolation, coughing productively blood-tinged sputum. Client having difficulty in disposing of soiled tissues, explained nature of how TB can be transmitted to family members and other nurses. Client able to explain importance of disposing of soiled tissues in a receptacle, verbalized concern about family exposure.

 SPECIAL CONSIDERATIONS

Pediatric Considerations

Strange environment of isolation confuses a child. Preschoolers are unable to understand cause-effect relationship for isolation. School-agers may understand cause but still fantasize. Offer children simple explanations, "You need to be in this room to help you get better." Show all barrier equipment to a child. Toys and games that are brought into the room should be ones that can be effectively cleaned with an approved germicide. Parents must be actively involved in any explanations. Nurse lets child see face before applying mask so child does not become frightened.

Geriatric Considerations

Isolation can increase confusion in older adults who have already demonstrated signs of confusion or depression. Many times clients become more confused when confronted by a nurse wearing a mask or gown or when they are left in a room with the door closed. Assess need for closing door along with safety of client and additional safety measures required. Assess older adult for signs of depression: loss of appetite, decrease in verbal communications, or inability to sleep.

CRITICAL THINKING EXERCISES

1. When Sally enters Mrs. Lyon's room, she begins to conduct a physical assessment. As she turns Mrs. Lyon to check the condition of her skin, she notices moisture on her hand. Close inspection reveals the moisture is from an open, oozing lesion of Mrs. Lyon's sacral area. After assessing the wound, Sally quickly checks the condition of Mrs. Lyon's IV site and then washes her hands before leaving Mrs. Lyon's room. What elements of the infection chain were intact or broken as a result of Sally's care?

2. Joseph is caring for two clients in the same room, Mr. Isadore and Mr. Lee. Joseph enters the room and begins by repositioning Mr. Isadore and making him more comfortable. He inspects Mr. Isadore's abdominal dressing and adds a gauze bandage for reinforcement. Next, he checks the rate of Mr. Isadore's IV and examines the IV site. Mr. Lee calls for assistance because of discomfort from his nasogastric tube. Joseph checks the tube, retapes it at the nose, and irrigates the tube for patency. At what point should Joseph have performed hand hygiene? At what point should Joseph have worn gloves?

3. Last month you were working in an acute care facility and were caring for a client with MRSA (a resistant staphylococcal blood infection) in the sputum and blood. This client was in contact isolation, and you wore a mask, gown, and gloves when you gave personal care. Today you are working at a nursing home and have the same client. You are surprised that there is no sign on the door designating that this is a client in contact isolation. The client's wife recognizes you and asks you to tell the nurses that her husband must be in isolation as he was at the hospital. How would you handle this situation?

4. Cyndi is caring for a client who requires an irrigation of a deep abdominal wound. A wound irrigation involves the instillation of a sterile solution such as saline into a cavity that usually contains infectious drainage. What type of barrier protection should Cyndi wear?

REFERENCES

Baumgardner CA, Maragos CS, Larson EL: Effects of nail polish on microbial growth of fingernails, *AORN J* 58:84, 1993.

Bernard L and others: Bacterial contamination of hospital physicians' stethoscopes, *Infect Control Hosp Epidemiol* 20(9):626, 1999.

Bobo L: The microbiologic environment. In Soule B, Larson E, Preson G, editors: *Infection and nursing practice: prevention and control*, St Louis, 1994, Mosby.

Boyce JM, Pittet D: *HICPAC/SHEA/APIC/IDSA Hand Hygiene Task Force and the CDC Healthcare Infection Control Practices Advisory Board draft guideline for hand hygiene in healthcare settings*, 2001.

Boyce JM, Pittet D: Guidelines for Hand Hygiene in Health-Care Settings, *Am J Infect Control* 30(8):S1, 2002.

Centers for Disease Control and Prevention: Guidelines for preventing the transmission of *mycobacterium tuberculosis* in health-care facilities, *MMWR Morb Mortal Wkly Rep* 43(RR-13), 1994.

Centers for Disease Control and Prevention, Hospital Infection Control Practice Advisory Committee: Guidelines for isolation precautions in hospitals, *Am J Infect Control* 24:24, 1996.

DeCastro M, Fauerback L, Masters L: Aseptic technique. In Olmsted R, editor: *APIC infection control and applied epidemiology,* St Louis, 1996, Mosby.

DeCastro MG: Aseptic technique. In *APIC Text of Infection control and Epidemiology,* Washington, DC, 2000, Association for Professionals in Infection Control and Epidemiology.

Garner JS: Guidelines for isolation precautions in hospitals, *Am J Infect Control* 24:24, 1996a.

Garner JS: Guidelines for isolation precautions in hospitals, *Infect Control Hosp Epidemiol* 17(1):54, 1996b.

Jackson M, Lynch P: Body substance isolation, *Infect Control Hosp Epidemiol* 13(14):191, 1992.

Larson E: APIC guideline for the use of topical antimicrobial agents, *Am J Infect Control* 16(6):253, 1996.

Larson E: Antiseptic. In Olmsted R, editor: *APIC infection control and applied epidemiology,* St Louis, 2000, Mosby.

Larson E and others. Assessment of two hand hygiene regimens for intensive care unit personnel, *Crit Care Med* 29:944, 2001.

Larson EL: APIC guideline for handwashing and hand antisepsis in health care settings, *Am J Infect Control* 23(4):251, 1995.

McCoy KD and others: Monitoring adherence to standard precautions, *Am J Infect Control* 29:24, 2001.

Nishimura S and others: Handwashing before entering the intensive care unit: what we learned from continuous video camera surveillance, *Am J Infect Control* 27(4):367, 1999.

Occupational Safety and Health Administration: Occupational exposure to bloodborne pathogens: final rule, 29 CFR 1919:1030, *Federal Register* 56:64003, 1991.

Occupational Safety and Health Administration: Enforcement policies on procedures for occupational exposure to tuberculosis, Washington, DC, 1993, OSHA.

Occupational Safety and Health Administration: Respiratory protection, *Federal Register* 59(219):58884, 1994.

Rubino JR: Infection control practices in institutional settings, *Am J Infect Control* 29:241, 2001.

Rutala W: Disinfection and sterilization of patient-care items, *Infect Control Hosp Epidemiol* 17(6):377, 1996.

Sattar SA and others: Preventing the spread of hepatitis B and C viruses: where are germicides relevant? *Am J Infect Control* 29:187, 2001.

Zaragoza M and others: Handwashing with soap or alcoholic solutions? A randomized clinical trial of its effectiveness, *Am J Infect Control* 27:258, 1999.

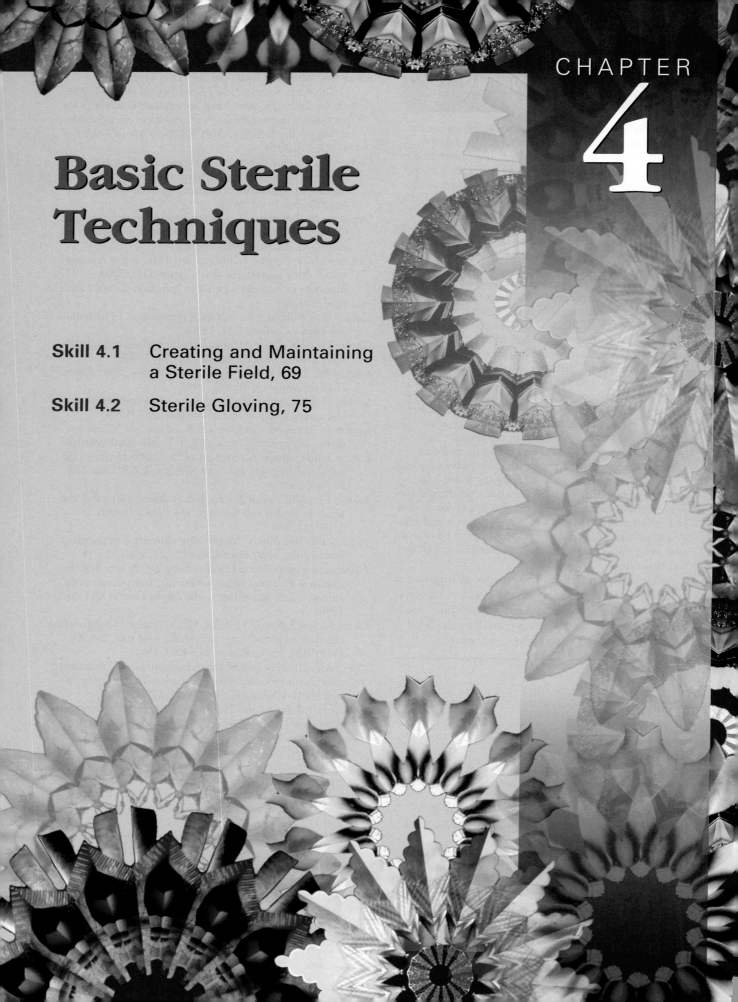

Basic Sterile Techniques

Sterile technique, or surgical asepsis, is designed to render and maintain objects and areas free from pathogenic microorganisms (Crow and others, 1995). As in medical asepsis, hand hygiene with an appropriate soap or antiseptic is essential before the initiation of an aseptic procedure. Surgical asepsis does require more precautions than medical asepsis (see Chapter 3). Strict adherence to the principles of sterile technique limits a client's risk for infection during invasive procedures, although infection can occur because of the presence of endogenous organisms on the skin and mucous membranes.

Surgical asepsis is routine in the operating room, labor and delivery areas, and some procedural areas (e.g., cardiac catheterization laboratory and gastrointestinal endoscopy). However, the skills presented in this chapter can also be performed at a client's bedside. Nurses use principles of sterile technique (Box 4-1) at the client's bedside in the following three types of situations:

- During procedures that require intentional perforation of a client's skin, such as insertion of an intravenous (IV) catheter
- When the skin's integrity is broken, such as with a surgical incision, burn, or pressure ulcer
- During procedures requiring insertion of devices or instruments into a sterile body cavity, such as urinary catheterization

Principles of sterile technique are used for certain procedures, such as parenteral injections, although open gloving and use of a sterile field are not needed because of the use of sterile barriers to cover the needle. Nurses must recognize the importance of strict adherence to aseptic principles. All individuals involved in surgical asepsis have a responsibility to provide and maintain a safe environment by following aseptic principles (Association of Operating Room Nurses [AORN], 2001). In a treatment area and at the bedside, it is important to have clients positioned properly and to gain their full cooperation to minimize contamination of a work area. The nurse prepares a client before a procedure, explaining how a procedure is to be performed and what a client can do to avoid contaminating sterile items (e.g., maintain position, avoid sudden body movements, refrain from touching sterile supplies, and avoid coughing or talking over a sterile area). The nurse serves as an excellent role model and client advocate, reinforcing principles when another caregiver breaks technique.

Box 4-1

Principles of Surgical Asepsis

1. All items used within a sterile field must be sterile.
2. A sterile barrier that has been permeated by moisture must be considered contaminated.
3. Once a sterile package is opened, the edges are considered unsterile.
4. Gowns, once put on, are considered sterile in front from chest to waist or table level; sleeves are considered sterile from 5 cm (2 inches) above elbows to fingertips of gloved hand. (NOTE: Cuffs are not considered sterile once glove has been removed.)
5. Tables draped as part of sterile field are considered sterile only at table level.
6. If there is any question or doubt of an item's sterility, the item is considered to be unsterile.
7. Persons with sterile barriers (gloves) or sterile items contact only sterile areas/items. Persons without sterile barriers contact only unsterile items.
8. Movement around and in the sterile field must not compromise or contaminate the sterile field.

The use of sterile technique is intended to protect the client from exogenous infections. However, there are situations in which this technique is expanded to include the use of standard precautions to protect the nurse from potential contact with blood and body fluids. Standard precautions include the use of masks, eye protection, and gowns when there is risk of being splattered with infectious materials (see Chapter 3).

NURSING DIAGNOSES

The nursing diagnosis most directly related to clients requiring procedures involving sterile technique is **Risk for Infection.** Use of meticulous sterile technique has substantially reduced the incidence of wound infections in surgical clients. However, endogenous microorganisms can cause infections even when the principles of surgical asepsis have been carefully followed.

Skill 4.1

Creating and Maintaining a Sterile Field

A sterile field is an area that provides a sterile surface for placement of sterile equipment. For minor procedures, a sterile kit or container of supplies (e.g., a urinary catheterization or tracheal suction kit) can be opened on a clean surface and used as the sterile field (Figure 4-1). Some institutions wrap and process their own bundles of equipment for

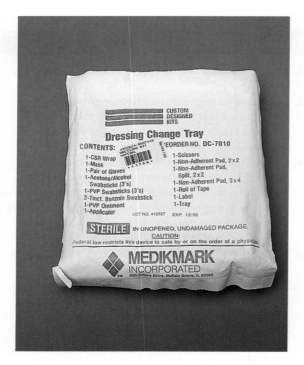

Figure 4-1 Sterile dressing changing kit.

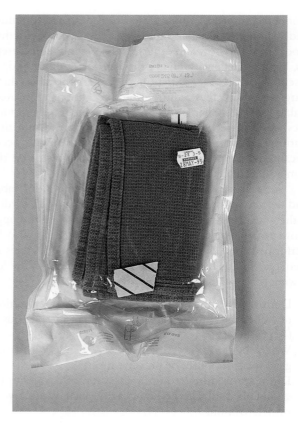

Figure 4-2 Tape with stripes changes color after sterilization.

procedures such as lumbar punctures or thoracentesis trays. Bundles packaged by the institution generally contain external and internal sterile (chemical) indicators that indicate the item has completed a sterilization process (Figure 4-2). Once the bundle is opened, the inside surface of the linen cover can be used as a sterile field. For more complicated procedures or those requiring several supplies, a table can be covered with a sterile, water-repellent drape. Sterile drapes can be linen, paper, or plastic but must be water repellent. Sterile supplies and solutions can then be placed on the sterile field.

The following basic rules are essential for creating and maintaining a sterile field (AORN, 2001):

- A sterile field is established immediately before the procedure, because there is a direct relationship between the time the sterile field is open and the presence of airborne contaminants.
- The sterile field must always be within view of the nurse, to prevent unobserved contamination.
- The sterile field is not covered, because it is too difficult to uncover without contaminating the field.

ASSESSMENT

1. Verify that procedure requires surgical aseptic technique.
2. Assess client's comfort, oxygen requirements, and elimination needs before procedure. *Rationale: Certain sterile procedures may last a long time. Nurse anticipates client's needs so that client can relax and avoid any unnecessary movement that might disrupt the procedure.*

3. Assess for latex allergies (see Skill 4-2, p. 75). *Rationale: A focused review may reveal latex allergies even when no known allergies are indicated during the chart review.*
4. Check sterile package integrity for punctures, tears, discoloration, or moisture. If using commercially packaged supplies or those prepared by agency, check sterilization indicator. *Rationale: Inspection of packaging ensures that only sterile items are presented to the sterile field (AORN, 1998).*
5. Anticipate number and variety of supplies needed for procedure.

PLANNING

Expected outcomes focus on prevention of localized or systemic infection.

Expected Outcomes

1. Client remains afebrile 24 to 48 hours after the procedure or during course of repeated procedures.
2. Client displays no signs of localized infection (e.g., redness, tenderness, edema, drainage) or systemic infection (e.g., fever, change in white blood cell count) 24 hours after the procedure.

Equipment

- Sterile gloves
- Sterile, water-repellent drapes (often included within a kit)
- Sterile equipment and solutions (as appropriate)
- Sterile gown, cap, mask, and protective eyewear (if required based on type of procedure and agency policy)
- Waist-high table/countertop surface

Delegation Considerations

Procedures requiring sterile technique are generally performed by nurses and should not be delegated. In some settings, assistive personnel (AP) (e.g., surgical technicians) are specifically trained to perform sterile technique under the supervision of a nurse.

IMPLEMENTATION FOR CREATING AND MAINTAINING A STERILE FIELD

Steps	Rationale
1. See Standard Protocol (inside front cover).	
2. Apply cap, mask, protective eyewear, and/or gown as needed (consult agency policy) (see Chapter 3).	
3. Select a clean, dry work surface at or above waist level.	

COMMUNICATION TIP *Now is a good time to instruct the client not to touch the work surface or equipment during the procedure, and to remain still.*

Steps	Rationale
4. **Preparing a sterile commercial kit or tray containing sterile items**	
a. Place sterile kit or package containing sterile items on the work surface.	Once created, sterile field is sterile only at table level.
b. Open outside cover of kit. Remove kit from dust cover and place on work surface (see illustration).	Inner kit remains sterile.
c. Grasp outer surface of tip of outermost flap.	Outer surface of package is considered unsterile. There is a 2.5-cm (1 inch) border around any sterile drape or wrap that is considered contaminated.
d. Open outermost flap away from body, keeping arm outstretched and away from sterile field (see illustration).	Reaching over sterile field contaminates it.

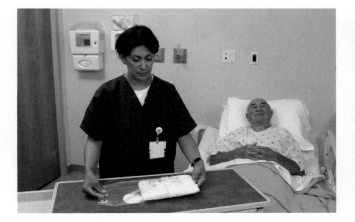

Step 4b Opening sterile kit.

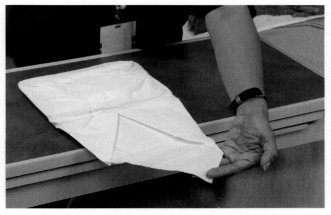

Step 4d Open outermost flap of sterile kit away from body.

Steps	**Rationale**
e. Grasp outside surface of edge of first side flap. Open side flap, pulling to side and allowing it to lie flat on table surface. Keep arm to the side and not extended over the sterile surface (see illustration).	Outer border is cosidered unsterile. Flap should lie flat so it will not accidentally rise up and contaminate inner surface or the sterile items placed on its surface.
f. Repeat steps for second side flap (see illustration).	
g. Grasp outside border of last and innermost flap (see illustration). Stand away from sterile package and pull flap back, allowing it to fall flat on work surface.	Reaching over sterile field contaminates it.
5. Preparing a paper supply bundle processed by agency	
a. Place package on work surface. Remove outer plastic wrap if present. Remove sterile (chemical) indicator tape from outside of package and discard.	Paper-wrapped items have one or two layers and may be enclosed in plastic. The first is a dust cover, and the second layer must be opened to view the sterile (chemical) indicator.
b. Open outer wrapper layer and each successive layer as seen in Steps 4c-g above. Use opened paper wrapper as sterile field.	

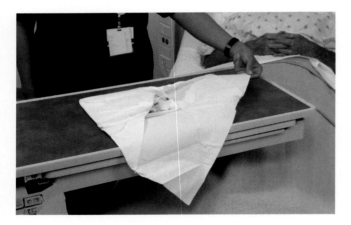

Step 4e   Open first side flap, pulling to side.

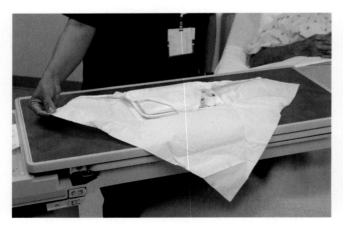

Step 4f   Open second side flap, pulling to side.

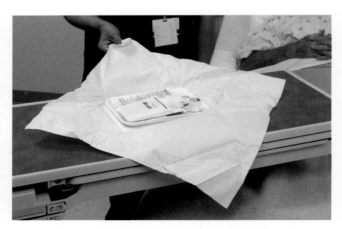

Step 4g   Open last and innermost flap standing away from sterile field.

Steps	**Rationale**

6. **Preparing a sterile drape**
   a. Place pack containing the sterile drape on the work surface. **Apply sterile gloves.** (NOTE: This is an option depending on agency policy. Nurse may touch outer 1-inch border of drape without wearing gloves.)

   b. Grasp folded top edge of drape with fingertips of one hand. Gently lift drape up from its wrapper without touching any object.

   c. Allow drape to unfold, keeping it above waist and the work surface and away from the body. (Carefully discard outer wrapper with other hand.)

   d. With other hand, grasp the adjacent corner of drape. Hold drape straight over work surface.

   e. Holding drape, first position the bottom half over top half of the intended work surface. Then allow top half of drape to be placed over bottom half of work surface. A sterile surface is now available for placement of sterile items.

7. **Adding sterile items to a sterile field**
   a. Open sterile item (following package directions) by carefully peeling back the outer wrapper over the nondominant hand (see illustration).

   b. Being sure wrapper does not fall down on sterile field, place item onto field at an angle so that arm does not reach over field (see illustration). Continue to add items as needed.

   c. Dispose of outer wrapper.

8. **Pouring sterile solutions**
   a. Verify contents and expiration date of solution.
   b. Be sure receptacle for solution is located near or on sterile surface. Sterile kits have cups or plastic molded sections into which fluids can be poured. Remove sterile seal and cap from bottle in an upward motion. If cap is to be reused, place on a clean surface in an inverted position.

Rationale column:

Sterile on sterile remains sterile.
Outer 1-inch border is always considered contaminated.

If a sterile object touches any nonsterile object, it becomes contaminated.

Object held below person's waist, and above chest is contaminated.

Drape cannot be properly placed with two hands.

Creates flat, sterile work surface

If outer wrap flips back against item, it could cause contamination. Inner surface of wrapper is considered sterile.
Reaching over or touching sterile field contaminates field.
Sterile items may be arranged later on field after all supplies are assembled following sterile gloving.

Ensures proper solution and sterility of contents.
Prevents reaching over sterile field.

Prevents contamination of bottle lip.
Maintains sterility of inside of cap.

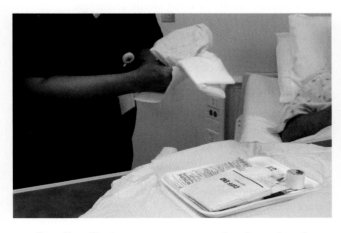

Step 7a   Peel wrapper over nondominant hand.

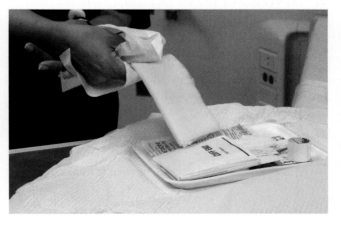

Step 7b   Place sterile item on field.

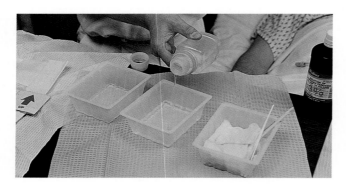

Step 8c Pour water into sterile container.

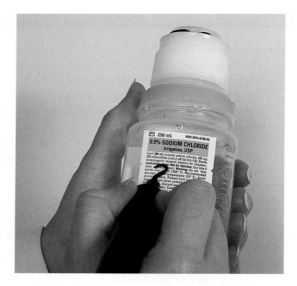

Step 8e Label date bottle is opened.

Steps	Rationale
c. With solution bottle held away from sterile field, and bottle lip above inside of sterile receiving container, slowly pour necessary amount of solution without splashing (see illustration).	Edge and outside of bottle are considered contaminated. Slow pouring prevents splashing liquids, which causes fluid permeation of the sterile barrier, called strike through, resulting in contamination.
d. If pouring solution from container previously opened, pour a small amount of fluid into a nonsterile container before pouring into sterile receptacle.	Lipping of previously used container is believed to remove any microorganisms that might be present on edge of bottle.
e. Label container with expiration date and time (see illustration).	Solution is considered contaminated 24 hours after opening (check agency policy).
9. Proceed with intended sterile procedure.	

• • • • • • • • • • •

EVALUATION

1. Evaluate client for fever for 48 hours after procedure.
2. Inspect treated area for localized signs of infection (e.g., redness, tenderness, edema, warmth, odor, drainage).

Unexpected Outcomes and Related Interventions

1. Client develops signs of infection.
   a. Notify physician of findings.
   b. Continue strict aseptic technique and hand hygiene.
   c. Monitor temperature every 4 hours and as needed (prn).
   d. Encourage and document client's intake of fluids.

Recording and Reporting

- Depending on the procedure, include the following:
  Procedure performed using sterile technique
  Proper position
  Client's understanding/knowledge of the procedure
  Client's response
  Number and type of supplies used

Sample Documentation

1400 Abdominal dressing changed using sterile technique with client supine. Client able to state steps of procedure and keep hands away from sterile supplies. Wound well approximated except for small 2-cm separation at top end of incision. Draining small amount of serous drainage. Used four 4 × 3's and ABD. Secured dressing with paper tape. Client denies discomfort.

SPECIAL CONSIDERATIONS

Pediatric Considerations

Children may not be able to cooperate during a sterile procedure depending on level of developmental maturity. Instruct family members in how they may assist so that child does not contaminate sterile field.

Geriatric Considerations

- Older adults may be at greater risk for infection because of compromised circulation, inadequate nutrition, or decreased body defenses caused by chronic illness.
- Memory and sensory deficits may impair client's ability to understand and cooperate with the procedure.

Home Care and Long-Term Care Considerations

- Adaptations may be made for some procedures, such as self-catheterization and home tracheostomy care. In some cases clients use medical asepsis rather than surgical technique (see Chapters 3 and 35).
- If possible, the client/family learns to perform sterile procedures well before discharge from acute care so that skill and adaptations can be worked out with professional assistance.
- Home visits should include assessing cleanliness of the environment, as well as the understanding and ability of client and family to perform procedure safely.

Skill 4.2

Sterile Gloving

Sterile gloves act as a barrier against the transmission of pathogenic microorganisms and are applied before performing any sterile procedure, such as a sterile dressing change or urinary catheter insertion. The nurse must remember that sterile gloves do not replace hand hygiene.

The open glove application method is used for most sterile procedures not requiring a sterile gown. The nurse must take care not to contaminate the gloved hands by touching clean, contaminated, or possibly contaminated items or areas. If a glove becomes contaminated or torn, it must be changed immediately. The hands should remain clasped about 12 inches in front of the body, above waist level, and below the shoulders until the nurse is ready to perform a procedure.

It is important to select the correct size and type of gloves. Gloves should not stretch so tightly over the fingers that they can easily tear, yet they should be tight enough that objects can be picked up easily. Sterile gloves are available in sizes (6, 6½, 7, and so on). There are also sterile gloves available in a "one size fits all" style. It is also important to choose gloves made from appropriate material. Many clients and health care workers have developed allergies to latex, the natural rubber used in most gloves and medical products (Allen-Bridson and Olmstead, 2000). Latex proteins can enter the body through skin or mucous membranes, intravascularly, or by inhalation. The cornstarch powder used to make latex gloves slip on easily is a carrier of latex proteins (Burt, 1998). This is one reason why vigorous hand hygiene is necessary following glove removal. Studies have shown that individuals who are highly sensitive to latex develop local and systemic reactions when latex gloves are removed and the latex glove powder particles are suspended in the air, often for hours (Fleishman and Olmstead, 2000). Reactions to latex can be mild to severe (Box 4-2). For individuals at high risk or with suspected sensitivity to latex, it is important to choose latex-free or synthetic gloves and to inspect the contents of all sterile kits for items that contain latex. Institutions have latex-free procedure kits available for use.

ASSESSMENT

1. Verify that the procedure to be performed requires sterile gloves. *Rationale: Some sterile procedures can use a "no-touch" technique without gloves.*
2. Determine if the client has a history of spina bifida, congenital or urogenital defects, indwelling catheter placement or repeated catheterizations, adverse reactions during surgery or dental procedures, using condom catheters, multiple childhood surgeries, food allergies (papaya, avocado, banana, peach, kiwi, tomato), and high latex exposure (e.g., housekeepers, food handlers, health care workers). *Rationale: High risk factors for latex allergy (Gritter, 1998; Kim and others, 1998).*
3. Inspect condition of hands for cuts, open lesions, or abrasions. *Rationale: Presence of such lesions may contraindicate nurse's participation in procedure.*

PLANNING

Expected outcomes focus on prevention of localized or systemic infection.

Box 4-2
Levels of Latex Reactions

Contact dermatitis—a nonallergic response characterized by skin redness and itching.

Type IV hypersensitivity—cell-mediated allergic reaction to chemicals used in latex processing. Reaction can be delayed up to 48 hours, including redness, itching, and hives. Localized swelling, red and itchy or runny eyes and nose, and coughing may develop.

Type I hypersensitivity—a true latex allergy that can be life threatening. Reactions vary based on type of latex protein and degree of individual sensitivity, including local and systemic. Symptoms include hives, generalized edema, itching, rash, wheezing, bronchospasm, difficulty breathing, laryngeal edema, diarrhea, nausea, hypotension, tachycardia, and respiratory or cardiac arrest.

Modified from Gritter M: The latex threat, *Am J Nurs* 98(9):26, 1998.

Expected Outcomes

1. Client remains afebrile 24 to 48 hours after the procedure or during the course of repeated procedures.
2. Client displays no signs of localized infection (e.g., redness, tenderness, edema, drainage) 72 hours after the procedure.

Equipment

- Package of correct-size sterile gloves: latex or synthetic nonlatex. (NOTE: Hypoallergenic, low-powder, or low-protein gloves may contain enough protein to cause an allergic reaction [Burt, 1998].)

Delegation Considerations

Procedures requiring sterile technique are generally performed by nurses and should not be delegated. In some settings, assistive personnel (AP) (e.g., surgical technicians) are specifically trained to perform sterile technique under the supervision of a nurse. Check agency policy.

IMPLEMENTATION FOR STERILE GLOVING

Steps	Rationale
1. See Standard Protocol (inside front cover).	
2. Examine glove package to determine if it is dry and intact	Torn or wet package is contaminated.
3. Open sterile gloves by carefully separating and peeling open adhered package edges (see illustration).	Prevents inner glove package from accidentally opening and touching contaminated objects.
4. Grasp inner glove package, and lay it on a clean, dry, flat surface at waist level. Open package, keeping gloves on wrapper's inside surface (see illustration).	Inner surface of glove package is sterile. Sterile object held below waist level is contaminated.
5. Identify right and left glove. Each glove has a cuff approximately 5 cm (2 inches) wide. Glove dominant hand first.	Eases glove application and dexterity.
6. With thumb and first two fingers of nondominant hand, grasp edge of cuff of glove for dominant hand. Touch only glove's inside surface and pull glove over dominant hand, carefully working thumb and fingers into correct spaces (see illustrations). Gently let go of cuff while preventing it from rolling up wrist.	Inner edge of cuff will touch skin and is no longer considered sterile.
7. Slide fingers of gloved hand underneath second glove's cuff (see illustration). Pull glove over fingers of nondominant hand. Do not touch exposed areas with gloved hands; keep thumb of dominant hand abducted back (see illustrations).	Cuff protects gloved fingers; abducting thumb prevents contamination from contact with unsterile surface.
8. Interlock fingers of gloved hands and hold away from body, above waist level, until beginning procedure (see illustration on p. 78).	Prevents accidental contamination from hand movement.
9. Proceed with intended procedure.	

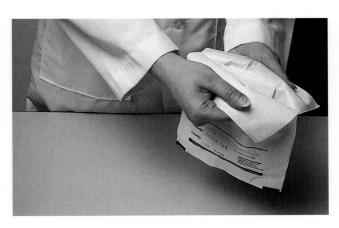

Step 3   Open outer glove package wrapper.

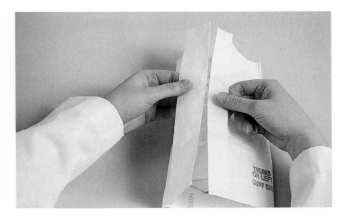

Step 4   Open inner glove package on clean, uncluttered work surface.

A

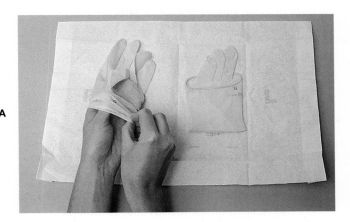

B

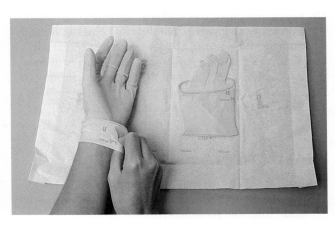

Step 6   **A,** Grasp cuff and insert fingers of dominant hand into glove. **B,** Pull glove over dominant hand.

A

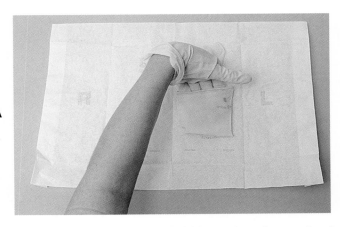

B

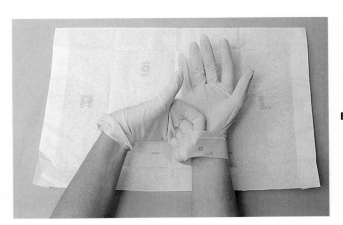

Step 7   **A,** Pick up glove for nondominant hand. **B,** Pull second glove over nondominant hand.

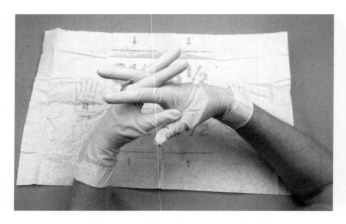

Step 8 Interlock gloved hands.

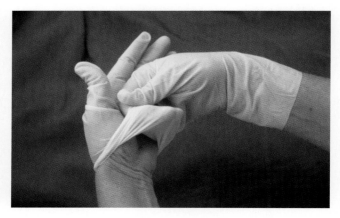

Step 10 Remove first glove by turning it inside out.

Steps	Rationale

Glove removal

10. Grasp outside of one cuff with other gloved hand; avoid touching wrist. Pull glove off, turning it inside out (see illustration). Discard in proper receptacle.

Outside of glove should not touch skin surface.

11. Remove remaining glove by placing fingers of bare hand under cuff, and pull off by turning inside out. Discard in proper receptacle.

Fingers do not touch contaminated glove surface.

12. See Completion Protocol (inside front cover).

• • • • • • • • • •

EVALUATION

1. Evaluate client for signs and symptoms of infection (e.g., fever, development of wound drainage) for 48 hours after the procedure.
2. Inspect treated area for localized signs of infection (e.g., redness, tenderness, edema, warmth, odor, drainage).

Unexpected Outcomes and Related Interventions

1. Client develops signs of infection.
   a. Notify physician of findings. Cultures (see Chapter 14) and antibiotic therapy may be needed.
   b. Apply standard precautions (see Chapter 3) and sterile technique (as appropriate).
   c. Monitor temperature every 4 hours or per orders.

CRITICAL THINKING EXERCISES

1. Dr. Johnson has requested that you assist him in performing a lumbar puncture on Mr. Smith, who has agreed to the procedure. It takes several minutes to position the client, prepare the area, and inject the local anesthetic. Mr. Smith becomes very restless and complains about feeling very uncomfortable in the required position. Dr. Johnson reaches for the spinal needle but does not notice that it is touching the edge of the sterile field. Is this a problem? If so, why? How would you handle the situation?

2. Which of the following procedures require sterile (aseptic) technique? Which require only clean technique?
   a. Urinary catheterization
   b. Tracheal suctioning
   c. Insertion of rectal suppository
   d. Insertion of a feeding tube
   e. Lumbar puncture
   f. Sitz bath

3. You have several dressing changes to perform this morning and have just spent an hour with another client that had to be transferred to the intensive care unit. After first checking on all your clients, you start with Mrs. Martinez, a pleasant but confused lady with an abdominal wound infection. Trying to make up for lost time, you start opening supplies and preparing Mrs. Martinez for the dressing change. You realize you do not have everything you need for the dressing change. As you turn around to look for the missing supplies, Mrs. Martinez sits up in bed, contaminating the sterile field. What preparations could you make ahead of time to avoid this situation?

4. You have applied the first sterile glove on your right hand. You take your gloved right hand and pick up the remaining glove at the top of the cuff and slip it over your left hand. Is this correct? Explain.

REFERENCES

Allen-Bridson K, Olmstead RM: Surgical services. In *APIC text of infection control and applied epidemiology,* Washington, DC, 2000, Association for Professionals in Infection Control and Epidemiology.

Association of Operating Room Nurses: Recommended practices for aseptic technique. In *AORN standards and recommended practices for perioperative nursing,* Denver, 2001, The Association.

Beezold D, Kostyol D, Wiseman J: The transfer of protein allergens from latex gloves, *AORN J* 59:30, 1994.

Burt S: What you need to know about latex allergy, *Nursing* 28(10):33, 1998.

Crow S and others: Antisepsis: disinfection and sterilization. In Soule B, Larson E, Preston G, editors: *Infection and nursing practice: prevention and control,* St Louis, 1995, Mosby.

Fleischman CA, Olmstead RM: Ask APIC: a comprehensive reference anthology. In *APIC Text of Infection Control and Epidemiology,* Washington, DC, 2000, Association for Professionals in Infection Control and Epidemiology.

Gritter M: The latex threat, *Am J Nurs* 98(9):26, 1998.

Kim KT and others: Implementation recommendations for making health care facilities latex safe, *AORN J* 67:615, 1998.

Promoting a Safe Environment

Safety is a basic human need often defined as freedom from psychological and physical injury. Nurses in any setting are responsible for identifying and eliminating safety hazards and providing communication and support that promote a feeling of security and allow clients to focus on recovery. Client safety is a priority in health care agencies, in long-term care facilities, and in the home.

Promoting client safety in the acute care setting reduces the length and cost of treatment, the frequency of treatment-related accidents, the potential for lawsuits, and the number of work-related injuries to personnel. There are many safety features that are part of the structure and design of a health care environment, such as specialized equipment, including beds, handrails, call bells, and alarm systems.

Promoting client safety in the home and community helps enhance confidence and maximize self-care and provides freedom to interact with the environment. In many communities special programs such as escort services, crime prevention education, and safety information have been initiated. Nurses working in the community can contact the local law enforcement agency or AARP (formerly known as the American Association for Retired Persons) to familiarize themselves with programs in crime protection and prevention and how to obtain assistance.

 ## ACCIDENTS

Beginning at about age 70, the death rate from falls increases dramatically and continues to increase with age. Accidental falls in the home are the cause of most deaths in the older population (Ebersole and Hess, 2001). The National Center for Injury Prevention and Control (2000) estimates that falls were the leading cause of accidental death among people 65 years of age and older in 1999. Falls are also a leading cause of injury in older adult clients. Factors that contribute to the risk of falls include being in an unfamiliar environment; difficulty communicating because of impaired vision, hearing, or speech; and impaired cognition. In many agencies a falls risk assessment is routinely completed on admission and may be repeated at specified intervals (Box 5-1). Signs, special arm bands, or color-coded footwear may be used to identify clients at risk for falls.

 ## FIRE SAFETY

Fire prevention in health care agencies is a basic responsibility of all health care workers. Fires in health care agencies are most often related to electrical safety and anesthesia (Potter and Perry, 2001). Because smoking is both a health hazard and a safety hazard, it is not permitted in the hospital setting without a physician's order. Some clients need supervision while smoking. Fires in health

care agencies may result from malfunction or damage to electrical equipment or from anesthetic gases. Electrical equipment must be maintained in good condition and must be grounded. All health care workers are responsible for inspecting electrical cords and reporting damaged equipment to the maintenance department.

If a fire occurs in a health care agency, the nurse protects clients from injury, reports the location of the fire, and contains the fire. One helpful acronym in the event of a fire is RACE: *rescue* or *remove* the client from immediate danger (Box 5-2); pull the *alarm; confine* the fire by closing all doors and windows; and *extinguish* the fire if manageable by using a blanket, sheet, or water pitcher.

Fire extinguishers are available in specified locations. They are to be used by persons who have been trained and have had the opportunity to practice. The three basic types of fires for which extinguishers are used are paper, wood, and rubbish (type A); grease and anesthetic gas (type B); and electrical (type C). The appropriate extinguisher should be used for each type of fire (Table 5-1). A portable dry chemical fire extinguisher is also available for general use and can be used on type A, B, and C fires.

 ## PHYSICAL RESTRAINTS

The optimal goal for all clients is a restraint-free environment. Adults who have altered cognitive ability often are at risk for injury from wandering, falls, and disruptive or agitated behavior and may need restraints temporarily. Restraints do not necessarily prevent injuries. In fact, it has been shown that clients may suffer fewer injuries if left unrestrained (Capezuti and others, 1998; Strumpf and others, 1998). Growing research findings indicate that the hazards of restraints outweigh the apparent benefits. Regulatory agencies such as the Joint Commission on Accreditation of Healthcare Organizations (JCAHO, 2001) and the Centers for Medicare and Medicaid Services (CMS, 2000) promote limiting the use of restraint devices and enforce standards for safe use of such devices. When restraints are needed, the least restrictive type of restraint should be used and a physician's order must specify time limitations, type of restraint, and the client's behavior requiring the restraint. Some medications, such as those given to calm an agitated patient, can be considered a chemical restraint when they are not a standard part of the client's treatment plan.

A wide variety of electronic options (e.g., bed alarms) are available to alert staff when clients under supervision need assistance. Nurses are responsible for identifying and using all other alternatives before using physical restraints. Sometimes having someone sit and spend time talking with clients helps to reorient them and reduces wandering. When restraints are necessary, documentation must show the reason for restraint and that the restraint is the only appropriate intervention that will maintain a client's safety.

Box 5-1
Risk for Falls Assessment Tools

TOOL 1: RISK ASSESSMENT TOOL FOR FALLS

Directions: Place a check mark in front of elements that apply to your client. The decision of whether a client is at risk for falls is based on your nursing judgment. *Guideline:* A client who has a check mark in front of an element with an asterisk (*) or four or more of the other elements would be identified as at risk for falls.

General Data
___ Age over 60
___ History of falls before admission*
___ Postoperative/admitted for surgery
___ Smoker

Physical Condition
___ Dizziness/imbalance
___ Unsteady gait
___ Diseases/other problems affecting weight-bearing joints
___ Weakness
___ Paresis
___ Seizure disorder
___ Impairment of vision
___ Impairment of hearing
___ Diarrhea
___ Urinary frequency

Mental Status
___ Confusion/disorientation*
___ Impaired memory or judgment
___ Inability to understand or follow directions

Medications
___ Diuretics or diuretic effects
___ Hypotensive or central nervous system suppressants (e.g., narcotic, sedative, psychotropic, hypnotic, tranquilizer, antihypertensive, antidepressant)
___ Medication that increases gastrointestinal motility (e.g., laxative, enema)

Ambulatory Devices Used
___ Cane
___ Crutches
___ Walker
___ Wheelchair
___ Geriatric (Geri) chair
___ Braces

TOOL 2: REASSESSMENT IS SAFE "KARE" (RISK) TOOL

Directions: Place a check mark in front of any element that applies to your client. A client who has a check mark in front of any of the first four elements would be identified as at risk for falls. In addition, when a high-risk client has a check mark in front of the element "Use of a wheelchair," the client is considered to be at greater risk for falls.
___ Unsteady gait/dizziness/imbalance
___ Impaired memory or judgment
___ Weakness
___ History of falls
___ Use of a wheelchair

Data from Brians LK and others: Development of the RISK tool for fall prevention, *Rehabil Nurs* 16(2):67, 1991.

Table 5-1
Fire Extinguishers and Their Uses

Class of Fire	Fire Extinguisher
Class A: Paper, wood, rubbish	Contains water or a solution with a large percentage of water; quenches and cools
Class B: Flammable liquids (gasoline, oil, grease, or solvents)	Dry chemical, carbon dioxide, foam, and halogenated hydrocarbons cut off oxygen supply
Class C: Electrical	Carbon dioxide or dry chemical cuts off oxygen supply

Both the client and family need to be informed that the restraint is temporary and protective. Measures to prevent the hazards of immobility and other complications must be initiated.

 SEIZURE PRECAUTIONS

Clients who are at risk for seizure activity need to have seizure precautions instituted to protect them from injury during a seizure. Seizures may occur in several forms and result from a variety of conditions. The most alarming form of seizure activity is called a grand mal seizure, which is characterized by loss of consciousness and alternating rigid and jerking movements. Clients may also have altered breathing and loss of bowel and bladder control. Objects are not to be placed in the client's mouth during

---

Box 5-2

Client Removal Methods

INFANT AND CHILD REMOVAL

1. Place a blanket or sheet on the floor.
2. Place two infants in each bassinet, using diapers or small blankets for padding.
3. Place the bassinet in the middle of the blanket.
4. Use the baby vest if available or fold the blanket over one end, fold the corners in, then roll the sides in to form a pocket.
5. Grasp the folded corners of the blanket and pull the infants to safety. Two persons (or, if necessary, one person) can drag eight babies to the prescribed area.
6. Alternatively, place as many children as possible in one crib and pull the crib to the prescribed area.

UNIVERSAL CARRY

The universal carry is a method of removing a client from a bed to the floor. It is a quick and effective method for removing a client who is in immediate danger. This carry can be used by anyone, regardless of client size.

1. Spread a blanket, sheet, or bedspread on the floor alongside the bed, placing one third of it under the bed and leaving about 8 inches to extend beyond the client's head.
2. Grasp the client's ankles, and move the client's legs until they fall at the knee over the edge of the bed.
3. Grasp each shoulder, slowly pulling the client to a sitting position.
4. From the back, encircle the client with your arms, place your arms under the client's armpits, and lock your hands over the client's chest.
5. Slide the client slowly to the edge of the bed, and lower the client to the blanket. If the bed is high, instruct the client to slide down one of your legs.

6. Taking care to protect the client's head, gently lower the head and upper torso to the blanket and wrap the blanket around the client.
7. At the client's head, grip the blanket with both hands, one above each shoulder, holding the client's head firmly in the 8 inches of blanket. Do not let the client's head snap back.
8. Lift the client to a half-sitting position, and pull the blanketed client to safety.

BLANKET DRAG

If vertical or downward evacuation by an interior stairway is necessary, in many cases one person can handle a helpless client by using the blanket drag.

1. Double a blanket lengthwise, and place it on the floor parallel and next to the bed, leaving 8 inches to extend above the client's head.
2. Using cradle drop, kneel drop, or other suitable means, remove the client from the bed to the folded blanket on the floor alongside the bed.
3. Grasping the blanket above the client's head with both hands, drag the client headfirst to the stairway.
4. Position yourself one, two, or three steps lower than the client, depending on your height and the client's height. The client's lower body inclines upward.
5. Place your arms under the client's arms, and clasp your hands over the client's chest.
6. Back slowly down the stairs, constantly maintaining close contact with the client, keeping one leg against the client's back.

---

a seizure, because this practice may result in injury to the oral cavity or aspiration. Clients experiencing a seizure should not be restrained but do need to be observed closely and protected from injury. The client should be assisted to the bed or floor, equipment and furniture moved aside, and side rails padded to prevent injury to the client's head or extremities.

 ## RADIATION SAFETY

Another source of environmental hazard in health care settings is use of radioactive materials that may be present in radiology departments, nuclear medicine, clinical laboratories, and client care areas. The safe handling, use, and dis-

posal of radioactive materials is under the management of the Nuclear Regulatory Commission (NRC). Regulations require limiting the exposure of employees to radiation. Reduction to exposure can be achieved by including use of caution signs, personal radiation dose meters, and actions to be taken after accidental exposure.

 ## CHEMICAL SAFETY

Various forms of chemicals used in health care settings are an additional source of an environmental hazard. Chemicals such as mercury (Box 5-3) and those found in some medications, anesthetic gases, cleaning solutions, and disinfectants can be potentially toxic. These chemicals

Box 5-3

Steps to Take in the Event of Mercury Spill

1. Do NOT touch spilled mercury droplets. If skin contact has occurred, immediately flush the area with water for 15 minutes.
2. If possible, remove client from immediate contaminated environment.
3. Change any clothing or linen that has been contaminated with mercury. Wash hands thoroughly after changing. Wash clothing before reuse.
4. Notify the Environmental Services Department, or obtain a mercury spill kit if available.
5. Follow procedures for mercury removal as directed by Material Safety Data Sheet (MSDS). Spills are removed using special absorbent materials, filtered vacuum equipment, and protective clothing.
6. Promote exhaust ventilation to reduce concentration of mercury vapors.
7. Complete occurrence report as directed by institution procedure.

can cause damage or irritation to the body after skin contact, if ingested, or when vapors are inhaled. Health care facilities are required to provide employees access to a Material Safety Data Sheet (MSDS) for each hazardous chemical used. These sheets provide detailed information about the chemical, any health hazards imposed, precautions for safe handling and use, and steps to take in case the material is released or spilled.

NURSING DIAGNOSES

Risk for Injury (trauma) is appropriate for clients with safety issues for a variety of reasons. Risk factors may include altered cognitive ability (e.g., disorientation, impaired judgment); unfamiliar setting or inability to use call system; impaired mobility resulting from weakness, paralysis, balance and coordination problems, or dizziness; and sensory/perceptual alterations including vision, hearing, or touch. **Deficient Knowledge** due to a lack of knowledge of safety precautions is appropriate when teaching the client and family about home safety, fire safety, and radiation safety.

Skill 5.1

Safety Equipment and Fall Prevention

It is important for nurses and other health care workers to be acutely aware of potential safety hazards in acute care and long-term care settings. Confusion, multiple medical problems, sedating medications, generalized weakness, postural instability, and an unfamiliar environment are major contributors to falling when a client is hospitalized (Ebersole and Hess, 2001). Among older adults, most falls occur in the home; however, 10% of the falls occur in health care facilities. In addition, hip fractures result in more hospital admissions than any other injury (National Center for Injury Prevention and Control, 2000). Clients at risk for falling need to be identified by a visual system (e.g., sign on the door or bedside or color-coded arm band). These clients need to be watched closely under all circumstances.

For clients who need assistance to get out of bed and do not remember to call for assistance, electronic monitoring devices can be used (see Skill 5.2, p. 92). Hospital units are designed with safety as a major concern. Floor surfaces must be kept dry and free of clutter. Spills of water, food, or urine must be immediately wiped up from the floor or a safety cone placed to alert staff and clients of the hazard. One side of the hallways is to be kept free of equipment and clutter to provide a clear pathway for safe ambulation. Lighting must be adequate, without glare.

Adequate ventilation and stable room temperature and humidity provide both comfort and safety.

Hospital beds have a frame that can raise or lower the entire bed. To promote good body mechanics for caregivers the bed is raised when care is being provided. The bed is kept in low position at all other times. Be sure side rails are used appropriately. A full set of raised side rails may be considered a restraint when used to prevent the client from getting out of bed (CMS, 2000). Raising the two upper side rails gives the client room to exit a bed safely and to maneuver within the bed.

Every client must have a call light or signaling device easily accessible and must be given instructions on its use. Call bells or intercom systems at each bedside and in bathrooms and treatment rooms facilitate emergency calls for assistance. Safety features in bathrooms include shower chairs that allow clients to sit safely during the shower. Safety grips and nonskid surfaces are provided in bathrooms and shower areas (Figure 5-1). A raised toilet seat with arms may be used for clients who have difficulty sitting down and standing after having been seated.

Most hospital rooms have a straight-back chair and a lounge chair to be used by the client and visitors. Reclining chairs with elevated foot support and an at-

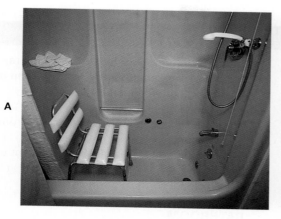
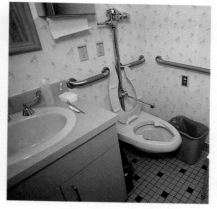

Figure 5-1   A, Nonslip surface in tub prevents falls. Shower chair allows clients to sit while in the shower. **B,** Safety features in bathrooms include safety grip bar and emergency call bell.

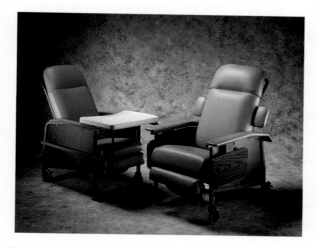

Figure 5-2   A Geri chair with attached tray and elevated foot support may be used for nonambulatory clients. (Courtesy Invacare Corporation, Elyria, Ohio.)

tached tray are often used for older clients who are not ambulatory (Figure 5-2).

At home or in the health care setting, it is important that clients have adequate footwear when ambulating. Clients should have well-fitting sturdy shoes or slippers with nonskid rubber soles. A walking shoe or sneaker is recommended. In addition, cotton socks absorb moisture and prevent friction.

When preparing clients for discharge to home and when making home care visits, assessment of safety hazards in the home environment is essential. Assessment should include access to the home, such as sidewalks, railings, and stairs; general safety concerns (e.g., lighting, floors, furniture, and electrical and fire safety); and specific concerns relating to the kitchen, bedroom, and bathroom (see Chapter 40). Adequate lighting, removal of clutter and throw rugs, and installation of safety features, such as grip

bars, nonslip floor surfaces, and smoke and carbon monoxide detectors, can minimize many physical hazards.

ASSESSMENT

1. Assess the client's motor, sensory, balance, and cognitive status, including ability to follow directions and cooperate. *Rationale: Physiologic alterations increase client's physical risk factors for falls.*
2. Assess client's medical history and medications. *Rationale: Antihypertensives, diuretics may cause hypotension; narcotics, antihistamines may cause drowsiness.*
3. Assess the environment for potential threats to client's safety (e.g., poor lighting, cluttered pathways, wet floors). *Rationale: Reveals client's environmental risk factors for falls.*
4. Assess the degree of assistance client needs by observing client ambulate. Look for signs of grabbing for support, swaying, stumbling, hesitancy, and dizziness while pivoting. *Rationale: Promotes client independence and determines whether client needs assistance to ambulate.*

PLANNING

Expected outcomes focus on preventing client injury and appropriate use of safety equipment.

Expected Outcomes

1. Client does not fall or suffer injury while in the health care agency.
2. Client and family demonstrate use of the call bell to obtain assistance.
3. Client and family state reasons why safety devices are used.

Box 5-4

Home Hazard Assessment

HOME EXTERIOR
Are sidewalks uneven?
Are steps in good repair?
Is ice and snow removal adequate?
Do steps have securely fastened handrails?
Is there adequate lighting?
Is outdoor furniture sturdy?

HOME INTERIOR
Do all rooms, stairways, and halls have adequate
  lighting?
Are night-lights available?
Are area rugs secured?
Are wooden floors nonslippery?
Is furniture placed appropriately to permit mobility?
Is furniture sturdy enough to provide support for get-
  ting up and down?
Are temperature and humidity within normal range?
Are there any steps or thresholds that may pose a
  hazard?
Are step edges clearly marked with colored tape?
Are handrails available and secure?
Are extension cords used appropriately?
Are smoke, fire, and carbon monoxide detectors
  installed?

KITCHEN
Are hand-washing facilities available?
Is the pilot light on for the gas stove?
Are the dials on the stove readable?
Are storage areas within easy reach?
Are cleaning fluids, bleach, etc., in original containers
  and stored properly?

Is the water temperature within normal range?
Are there clean areas for food storage and preparation?
Is refrigeration adequate?
Are appliances in good working order?
Are electrical appliances located away from water
  sources?
ABC fire extinguisher available and client understands
  how to use?
Are electrical cords in good condition?

BATHROOM
Are hand-washing facilities available?
Are there skidproof strips or surfaces in the tub or
  shower?
Are bath mats secured?
Does the client need grip bars near the bathtub and
  toilet?
Does the client need an elevated toilet seat?
Is the medicine cabinet well lighted?
Are medications in their original containers?
Have outdated medications been discarded?

BEDROOM
Are beds of adequate height to allow getting on and
  off easily?
Is day and night lighting adequate?
Are floor coverings nonskid?
Is nonskid footwear available?
Does the client have a telephone nearby?
Are emergency numbers visible near the phone?

Modified from Tideiksaar R: Home safe home: practical tips for fall-proofing, *Geriatr Nurs* 11(6):284, 1989; and Ebersole P, Hess P: *Toward healthy aging: human needs and nursing process,* ed 5, St Louis, 1998, Mosby.

Equipment

- Home Hazard Assessment
- Risk for Falls Assessment Tool
- Hospital bed with side rails
- Call bell/intercom system
- Wheelchair (for transport of clients too unsteady or weak to walk)
- Wedge cushion (if available)
- Stretcher (for transport of clients unable to safely sit upright)

Delegation Considerations

Fall prevention is the responsibility of all caregivers, including assistive personnel (AP). However, assessment for risk of fall or injury requires the critical thinking and knowledge application unique to the nurse and is not delegated. When delegating safety measures, the nurse needs to stress the importance of the following:

- The client's mobility limitations and any specific measures to minimize risks
- Environmental safety precautions (e.g., bed locked and in low position, call bell and personal items within reach, clear pathway, nonskid footwear)
- What to do when a client starts to fall while being assisted with ambulation (i.e., ease client into a sitting position in a chair or on the floor, and alert the nurse)

IMPLEMENTATION FOR SAFETY EQUIPMENT AND FALL PREVENTION

Steps	Rationale

1. See Standard Protocol (inside front cover).

NURSE ALERT   *Before using any equipment for the first time, make sure you understand the safety features and proper method of operation.*

2. Explain the use of the call bell or intercom (see illustration).
  - a. Provide client with hearing aid and glasses if used.
  - b. Demonstrate to both client and family how to turn the call bell on and off at bedside and in the bathroom.
  - c. Have client/family return demonstration.

Reinforces understanding and evaluates ability to manipulate controls.

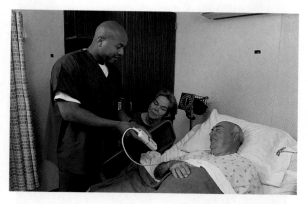

Step 2   Nurse demonstrates the use of the call light and secures it in an accessible location.

Steps	Rationale

d. Inform client and family of expectations for when the call bell/intercom is to be used (e.g., to use the bathroom, to get out of bed).

e. Secure call bell in an accessible location, such as on the side rails or clipped to bedding. Make sure client can reach the device easily and is aware of its location.

Prevents client from searching for device, overreaching and possibly falling out of bed.

3. **Use of hospital bed and side rails**

a. Keep bed in low position with wheels locked whenever care is not being provided (see illustration).

Minimizes risks if client attempts to get out of bed without help.

b. Teach the client/family that the purpose of side rails is to remind the client to call for assistance before getting out of bed and to assist with moving and turning in bed.

Client and family understanding promote cooperation.

c. Check agency policies regarding side rail use.

Side rails may be considered a restraint device when used to prevent the ambulatory client from getting out of bed (CMS, 2000).

Reminds client upon awakening of unfamiliar environment and to call for assistance.

d. Keep side rails up if client is weak, sedated, or confused.

e. Leave one side rail up and one down (on side where oriented and ambulatory client gets out of bed).

Can be used to enhance transfer ability and as a proprioceptive cue (Hammond and Levine, 1999).

4. Arrange necessary items (e.g., water pitcher, telephone, reading materials) within the client's easy reach.

Facilitates independence and self-care and prevents falls from attempts to reach too far.

5. Provide adequate, nonglare lighting throughout care area.

Reduces likelihood of falling over objects or bumping into them. Glare is a major problem for older adults (Ebersole and Hess, 2001).

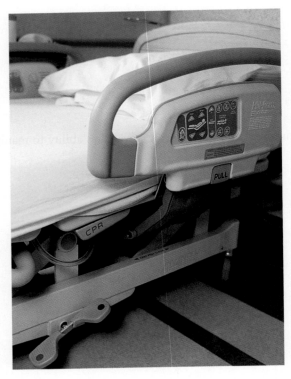

Step 3a The hospital bed should be kept in low position with wheels locked and side rails up (when appropriate).

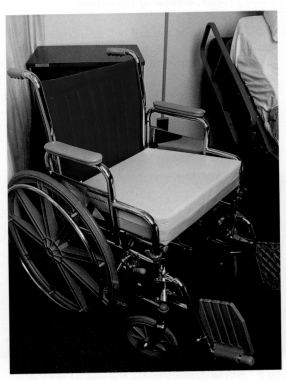

Step 7 Wheelchair with brakes locked, raised foot plates, and wedge cushion in place.

Steps	Rationale
6. Remove unnecessary objects from room, hallway and stairs. Pay particular attention to items outside client's field of vision, and ensure that pathway to bathroom facilities is clear.	Eliminates potential hazards.
7. Safe transport using a wheelchair (see illustration)	
a. The brakes on both wheels must be locked securely when a client is transferred into or out of a wheelchair (see Chapter 6).	Keeps chair steady and secure.
b. Raise the foot plates before the transfer; lower them, placing the client's feet on them, after the client is seated.	Promotes client's stability during transfer.
c. Make sure the client is seated with buttocks well back in the seat. Use a seat belt or wedge cushion if available.	Protects client from sliding out of the chair.
d. Back the wheelchair into and out of an elevator, rear large wheels first.	Makes a smoother ride and prevents smaller wheels from catching in the crack between the elevator and the floor.
e. When navigating on a ramp or incline, turn so that the chair pushes against your body, which is between the chair and the bottom of the ramp.	Prevents a runaway wheelchair that can pull away and roll faster down ramp than intended.
8. Safe transport using a stretcher	

NURSE ALERT *Clients are not to be left on a stretcher unattended, especially when medicated or confused.*

Steps	Rationale
a. Lock the wheels during transfer from bed to stretcher or stretcher to bed.	Prevents bed or stretcher from moving apart.
b. Use a safety belt across the client's upper thighs, or raise side rails (see illustration).	Reduces risk of falling from stretcher.
c. Push the stretcher from the end where the client's head rests. Some stretchers may have the head raised for comfort. For stretchers with stationary wheels on one end and swivel wheels on the other, the head of the stretcher has the stationary wheels.	Protects the client's head in case of a collision.
d. Maneuver the stretcher into an elevator head first.	Facilitates entry without bumping the sides.

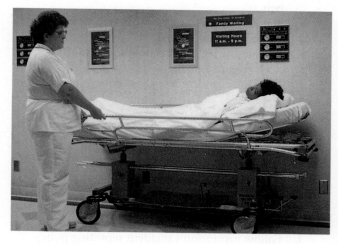

Step 8b   Side rails are raised to prevent client from rolling or falling off the stretcher.

Steps	Rationale
9. **Assisting the client with ambulation**	
a. Explain to client specific safety measures to prevent falls (e.g., dangle feet for a few minutes before standing, walk slowly, call for help if dizzy or weak).	Promotes client understanding and cooperation. Dangling allows blood pressure to stabilize before ambulating.
b. While standing next to the client's stronger side, have the client take a few steps. If using an assistive device, stand next to client's weak side.	Position of health care professional in such a manner provides for immediate assistance if needed.
c. Support client by placing arm closest to client on gait belt or around client's waist and other arm.	Providing constant contact by nurse reduces the risk of falls or injury.
d. Take a few steps forward with client, assessing client's strength and balance.	Ensures client has satisfactory strength and balance to continue.
e. If client becomes weak or dizzy, return the client to bed or chair, whichever is closer.	Prevents fall to floor.

COMMUNICATION TIP *At this time, talk to the client about risks for falls: "Some medications, tests, or procedures and long periods of immobility may make you feel dizzy or weak. Always ask for assistance before trying to walk under these conditions." "Falls can be prevented if safety measures are instituted." Also let the client who has a fear of falling know that confidence can be regained with continued practice.*

10. See Completion Protocol (inside front cover).

• • • • • • • • • •

EVALUATION

1. Determine client's response to safety modifications and that no falls or injuries have occurred.
2. Observe appropriate use of the call bell to obtain assistance.
3. Ask client and family to explain reasons for safety devices.

Unexpected Outcomes and Related Interventions

1. Client starts to fall while ambulating with a caregiver.
   a. Put both arms around client's waist or grasp gait belt.
   b. Stand with feet apart to provide broad base of support (Figure 5-3, *A*).
   c. Extend one leg and let client slide against it to the floor (Figure 5-3, *B*).
   d. Bend knees to lower body as client slides to floor (Figure 5-3, *C*).
2. Client suffers a fall.
   a. Call for assistance.
   b. Assess client for injury.
   c. Stay with the client until assistance arrives to help lift client to bed or to a wheelchair.
   d. Notify physician.
   e. Note pertinent events related to fall and resultant treatment in medical record.
   f. Follow institution's incident reporting policy.
   g. Reassess client and environment to determine if fall could have been prevented.

h. Reinforce identified risks with client, and review safety measures needed to prevent a fall.

Recording and Reporting

- Record in progress notes specific interventions to prevent falls and promote safety.
- Report to all health care personnel specific risks to client's safety and measures taken to reduce risks.
- Report immediately if the client sustains a fall or an injury.
- Document instructions given to client and any information related to the use of side rails or call bell.

Sample Documentation

0900 Risk for Falls Assessment Tool completed. Client placed on fall precautions due to history of falls, weakness, urinary frequency, and use of diuretics. Call bell within reach, side rails up × 2, hourly room checks, night-light on at all times, bedside commode in place. Instructed in safety measures and instructed to call for help when ambulating. Client voiced understanding.

1615 Found client on floor in bathroom after responding to emergency call light. Client stated, "I slipped on the wet floor." Alert and oriented × 3. Assisted back to bed and assessed for injury. No apparent injury noted from fall. BP 110/74, P 82 and regular, R 20. Instructed to call for help before getting out of bed. Call bell placed within client's reach. Side rails up × 3. Physician notified of client's fall.

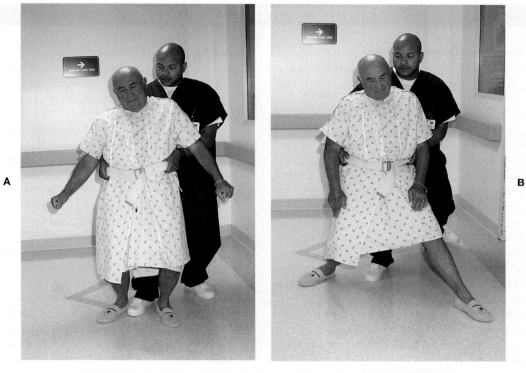

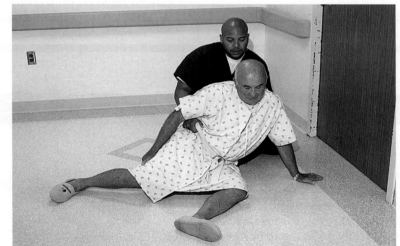

Figure 5-3 **A,** Stand with feet apart to provide broad base of support. **B,** Extend one leg and let client slide against it to the floor. **C,** Bend knees to lower body as client slides to floor.

SPECIAL CONSIDERATIONS

Pediatric Considerations
- Never leave a child of any age unattended or unrestrained on a raised surface (Hockenberry and others, 2003).
- Hoods or tents may be placed over the infant or child's crib to prevent accidental falls.
- Falling from stairs is a major cause of injury in the toddler. Gates should be placed at both ends of the stairs.
- Toddlers and children should wear helmets to protect the head from injury due to a fall sustained while bicycling, skateboarding, or riding a scooter.

Geriatric Considerations
- Older clients with short-term memory loss or cognitive dysfunction may be unable to follow directions and may attempt to climb out of bed or get up from a chair unassisted.
- Older adults, especially postmenopausal women, are at risk for fractured hips. Fractures can cause independent clients to become more dependent or immobilized (Lueckenotte, 2000).

Home Care Considerations
- The home environment should be assessed carefully.
- Night-lights, grip bars, handrails, raised toilet seats, and skid-proof strips or surfaces for tub or shower should be used.
- Items should be kept in their familiar positions and within easy reach.
- Client should have well-fitting, flat footwear with non-skid soles.
- Carpeting, mats, and tile should be secured, and non-skid backing placed under area rugs.
- If client has a history of falls and lives alone, recommend an electronic safety alert device that is turned on by the wearer to alert a monitoring site to call emergency services for help.

Long-Term Care Considerations
- Clients who wander from a facility are at risk for injury. Specific interventions such as electronic wandering devices can be used to reduce this risk.
- Make sure assistive devices (e.g., canes, handrails, walkers) are in proper working order.

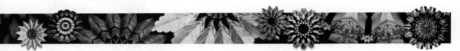

Skill 5.2

Designing a Restraint-Free Environment

The standard of care for institutionalized older adults is avoidance of mechanical restraints, except as needed under exceptional circumstances, and only after all other reasonable alternatives have been tried. Physical restraints are devices that limit a client's movement. The immobility resulting from physical restraints can result in serious complications, including death (see Skill 5.3, p. 96). Care of the person who may be prone to threats to safety and security requires a creative, systematic, and attentive approach to care.

A wide variety of electronic devices are available to alert staff to a client's need for assistance. One type is a battery-operated alarm attached to the client's leg. When the client changes position to get out of bed, the alarm sounds and alerts staff to provide assistance. A tether alarm is a device that can be attached to a chair, bed, or doorway and clipped to the client's garment. When a magnet connection is disrupted, the alarm sounds. A weight-sensitive alarm can be placed under the client in bed or in a chair. When the person tries to get up, an audible alarm sounds (Figure 5-4).

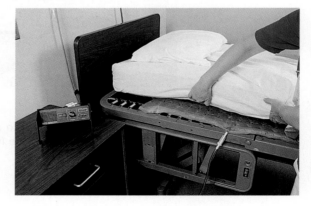

Figure 5-4 Weight-sensitive alarm. (From Sorrentino SA: *Assisting with patient care,* St Louis, 1999, Mosby.)

ASSESSMENT

1. Identify factors that place the client at an increased risk for injury, such as a history of falls, impaired cognition, poor balance, altered gait, impaired vision and hearing, urinary frequency, and orthostatic hy-

potension (dizziness upon arising quickly, because of a fall in blood pressure). *Rationale: Presence of these risk factors increase the likelihood of restraint use.*

2. Review prescribed medications (e.g., sedatives, hypnotics) for interactions and untoward effects. *Rationale: Medications may be the cause for client's altered mental status or increased risk for falling.*

3. Assess orientation to time, place, and person.

4. Use one-on-one observation or behavior-monitoring logs to document specific risks related to inability to understand, remember, and follow directions. *Rationale: Helps identify client's behavior patterns.*

PLANNING

Expected outcomes focus on maintaining client safety while avoiding the need for physical restraints.

Expected Outcomes

1. The client will remain free of injury without the use of restraints.
2. The client will not exhibit violence toward others.

Equipment

- Visual or auditory stimuli (e.g., calendar, clock, radio, television)
- Diversional activities (e.g., puzzles, games, audio books, music, videotapes)
- Wedge pillow
- Ambularm or pressure-sensitive bed or chair alarm

Delegation Considerations

Monitoring client behavior for risk of injury and promoting a safe environment may be delegated to assistive personnel (AP). Assessment of client behaviors and decisions about less restrictive interventions require the critical thinking and knowledge application unique to the nurse.

IMPLEMENTATION FOR DESIGNING A RESTRAINT-FREE ENVIRONMENT

Steps	Rationale
1. See Standard Protocol (inside front cover).	
2. Orient client and family to surroundings, introduce to staff, and explain all treatments and procedures.	Promotes client understanding and cooperation.

COMMUNICATION TIP   *When orienting client, approach client in a calm, nonthreatening, professional manner. Orientation information may need to be repeated often, especially when the environment has changed from what the client is accustomed to.*

3. Encourage family and friends to stay with the client. Sitters and companions can be helpful.	Presence of a consistent companion reduces client anxiety and increases feelings of security.
4. Place the client in a room close to the nurses' station.	Facilitates close observation. Watching the unit's activities distracts client (Rogers and Bocchino, 1999).
5. Provide visual and auditory stimuli, including a clock, radio, television, and calendar with large print (see illustration).	Assists with orientation to day, time, and physical surroundings.

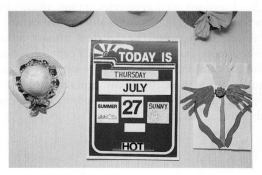

Step 5   Calendar with large print orients client to physical surroundings. (From Sorrentino SA: *Assisting with patient care,* St Louis, 1999, Mosby.)

Steps	Rationale
6. Encourage family to supply family pictures and personal belongings of sentimental value.	Promotes orientation to person and provides psychological comfort.
7. Provide the same caregivers to the extent possible.	Provides stability of routine care and consistency in approach.
8. Respond promptly to client's needs for toileting, relief of pain, and requests for activity.	Promotes comfort, minimizes anxiety, and reduces risk of falls from client attempts to get out of bed unassisted.

NURSE ALERT　*Getting out of bed for toileting purposes is one of the most common events leading to a client's fall.*

Steps	Rationale
9. Organize a predictable daily routine that provides opportunity for stimulation alternated with sleep and rest.	Routine facilitates psychological security and avoids overstimulation.
10. Use a wedge pillow on chair, with the thickest part toward the front of the chair.	Prevents clients with limited mobility from being able to rise to a standing position.
11. Use a pressure-sensitive bed or chair pad with alarms for alerting staff to an unsteady client who is standing without help. To use Ambularm monitoring device: 　a. Explain the use of the device to the client and family. 　b. Measure the client's thigh circumference just above the knee to determine appropriate size (see illustration). For a leg circumference less than 18 inches, use the regular size; use a large size for 18 inches or greater.	A band that is too loose may slip off; a band that is too tight may interfere with circulation or cause skin irritation.

NURSE ALERT　*Use of Ambularm is contraindicated in the presence of impaired circulation, swelling, skin irritation, or breaks in the skin.*

　c. Test battery and alarm by touching snaps to corresponding snaps on leg band.
　d. Apply the leg band just above the knee and snap battery securely in place (see illustration).
　e. Instruct client that alarm will sound unless the leg is kept in a horizontal position (see illustration).
　f. To assist client to ambulate, deactivate the alarm by unsnapping the device from the leg band.
12. Use stress reduction techniques such as massage and guided imagery (see Chapter 10).
13. Use diversions such as puzzles, games, music, books, or videotapes chosen specifically for the client.
14. Position intravenous (IV) catheters, urinary catheters, tubes/drains out of client view, or camouflage an IV site by wrapping with bandage or stockinet, place undergarments on client with urinary catheters, or cover abdominal feeding tubes/drains with loose abdominal binder.

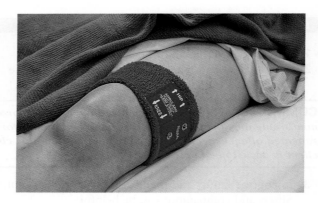

Step 11b　Client's thigh circumference is measured to determine appropriate size. (Courtesy AlertCare, Mill Valley, California.)

Diversional activities assist client's orientation and may reduce wandering and confusion.
Facilitates medical treatment and reduces client access to tubes/lines.

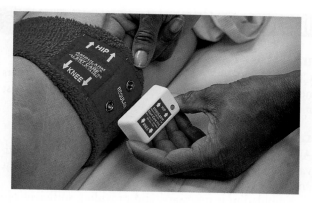

Step 11d Snap battery in place to activate alarm. (Courtesy AlertCare, Mill Valley, California.)

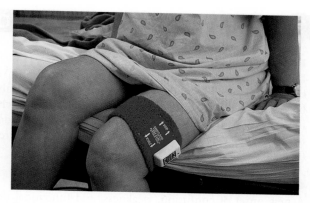

Step 11e Audio alarm will sound when client approaches a near vertical position. (Courtesy AlertCare, Mill Valley, California.)

Steps	Rationale

15. Consult with physical therapy, speech therapy, and occupational therapy for appropriate activities to provide stimulation and exercise.
16. See Completion Protocol (inside front cover).

• • • • • • • • • •

EVALUATION

1. Review incidence of behaviors that increase risk for injury without the use of restraints.
2. Verify absence of violence toward others.

Unexpected Outcomes and Related Interventions

1. Client displays behaviors that substantially increase risk for injury to self or others.
   a. Intensify supervision of client, and notify physician.
   b. Review episodes for a pattern (e.g., activity, time of day) that indicate alternatives that could eliminate the behavior.
   c. Engage in creative thinking with all caregivers and support service personnel for alternative interventions that promote safe, consistent care.
2. The client sustains an injury or is out of control, placing others at risk for injury.
   a. Notify physician, and complete an incident report according to agency policy.
   b. Identify alternative measures to promote safety without a restraint. As a last resort, identify appropriate restraint to use (see Skill 5.3, p. 96).

Recording and Reporting

Document all behaviors that relate to cognitive status and ability to maintain safety:
- Orientation to time, place, and person
- Ability to follow directions
- Mood and emotional status
- Understanding of condition and treatment plan
- Medication effects related to behaviors
- Interventions used and client response

Sample Documentation

0900 Up and dressed, oriented to person but not time or place. Upset and crying when unable to call wife on the telephone. Pacing in room.

1000 Participated for 15 minutes with ball toss to music at O.T.; then resting in rocking chair, smiling, and interacting socially with roommate.

SPECIAL CONSIDERATIONS

Pediatric Considerations

Distraction techniques, such as having a child hold a stuffed animal while an IV is being inserted, blowing bubbles while tubes or drains are being removed, and watching television during a dressing change or burn debridement, can decrease the need for restraining measures (Selekman and Snyder, 1996).

Geriatric Considerations

A new onset of confusion, weakness, and functional decline may indicate the presence of an underlying illness in the older client. It is important to assess for physical causes of behavior changes such as urinary or respiratory infection, hypoxia, fluid and electrolyte imbalance, side effects of multiple drug administration, depression, anemia, hypothyroidism, or fecal impaction (Ebersole and Hess, 2001).

Home Care Considerations

Clients at risk for self-injury or violence toward others need intensive supervision. Family and/or caregiver must recognize this and be able to provide it.

Long-Term Care Considerations

Allow the client to reminisce about past events to cultivate a sense of security, to enhance the client's identity, and to help maintain orientation.

Ambulation is necessary, and providing sufficient opportunities to ambulate in areas that are not hazardous is important. Interruption of wandering behaviors may cause more distress for the client; it is more productive to identify the stimulus for wandering and modify the environment so that wandering is not likely to be hazardous (Ebersole and Hess, 2001).

Skill 5.3

Applying Physical Restraints

Although the goal in health care settings today is a restraint-free environment, there are some extreme circumstances in which clients need to be temporarily restrained when other measures have failed (see Skill 5.2, p. 92). Physical restraint involves the use of any physical or mechanical device that the person cannot remove, that restricts the person's physical activity or normal access to the body, and that is not a usual part of treatment plans indicated by the person's condition or symptoms. Clients needing temporary restraints include those at risk for falls and confused or combative clients at risk for self-injury or violence to self or others. In addition, restraints are used to prevent interruption of therapy such as an IV catheter, urinary or surgical drains, nasogastric tube, traction, or life support equipment.

Restraints are not a solution to a client problem, but rather a temporary means to maintain client safety. The use of restraints is associated with serious complications, including pressure ulcers, constipation, urinary and fecal incontinence, and urinary retention. In some cases restricted breathing or circulation has resulted in death. Loss of self-esteem, humiliation, fear, and anger are additional serious concerns. The Food and Drug Administration (FDA), which regulates restraints as medical devices, requires manufacturers to label restraints as "prescription only." In most agencies a specific physician's order is required for their use. Orders may not be on an as-needed

(prn) basis and must specify the type of behavior requiring restraint, the type of restraint, and time limitations (JCAHO, 2001). Orders should be renewed according to agency policy and based upon reassessment and reevaluation of the restrained client. When restraints are required, both the client and family should be informed that the restraint is temporary and protective.

ASSESSMENT

1. Assess the need for restraint when all other measures have failed to prevent interruption of therapy or injury to self or others. *Rationale: Using a restraint may place the client at greater risk for injury.*

2. Review agency policies regarding restraints. Check physician's order for purpose, type, location, and duration. Determine if a signed consent is needed. *Rationale: Physician's order is required for physical restraints.*

3. Review manufacturer's instructions for restraint application and determine the most appropriate size restraint. *Rationale: Incorrect application and size may result in client injury or death.*

4. Inspect the area where the restraint is to be placed, including the condition of the skin and the adequacy of circulation. *Rationale: Provides baseline to evaluate onset of injury.*

NURSE ALERT   *The least restrictive type of restraint should be used, avoiding interference with therapeutic equipment, such as IV access devices, arteriovenous (AV) shunt used for dialysis, and drainage tubes.*

PLANNING

Expected outcomes focus on protecting the client from injury and maintaining prescribed therapy.

Expected Outcomes

1. The client will be free of injury.
2. The prescribed therapies will be continued without interruption.
3. The client's self-esteem and dignity will be maintained.

Equipment

*   Appropriate restraint and padding if needed. Restraint options include the following:
    Jacket restraint (vest or Posey)
    Belt restraint
    Extremity (ankle or wrist) restraint
    Mitten restraint

Delegation Considerations

Application of restraints may be delegated to assistive personnel (AP). However, assessment of when restraints are needed and the appropriate type to use requires the critical thinking and knowledge application unique to the nurse and should not be delegated. Stress the importance of the following:
*   Correct placement of the restraint
*   Observing for constriction of circulation, skin integrity, and adequate breathing
*   When and how to change position, provide range of motion, skin care, toileting, and opportunities for socialization

IMPLEMENTATION FOR APPLYING PHYSICAL RESTRAINTS

Steps	Rationale
1. See Standard Protocol (inside front cover).	
COMMUNICATION TIP *Explain to both the client and family the reason for the restraint, and stress that it is temporary and protective. Explain other measures that have been taken to avoid the restraint and that they have failed.*	
2. Place the client in proper body alignment.	Promotes comfort, prevents contractures, and prevents neurovascular injury.
3. If necessary, pad bony prominences where restraints will be placed.	Protects the skin from irritation.
4. Apply the proper-size restraint according to manufacturer's directions.	
a. *Jacket restraint:* Vestlike garment applied over clothing or hospital gown; used when client is in bed or chair. The front and back of the garment are labeled to facilitate correct application (see illustration). Straps are placed at client's hips.	Proper application prevents suffocation or choking. Clothing or gown prevents friction against the skin.
b. *Belt restraint:* Secures client in bed or stretcher. Make sure it is placed at the waist, not the chest. Remove wrinkles while placing around the waist, and avoid excessive tightness (see illustration).	Tight application or misplacement can interfere with ventilation.

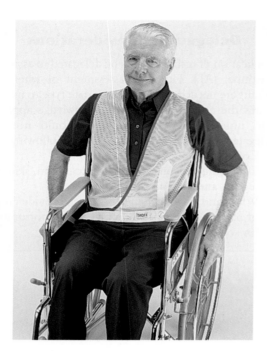

Step 4a Jacket (vest or Posey) restraint. (Courtesy JT Posey Co., Arcadia, California.)

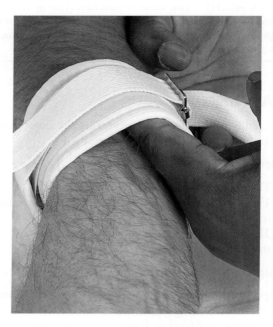

Step 4c Two fingers are placed under the limb restraint to check for constriction. (Courtesy JT Posey Co., Arcadia, California.)

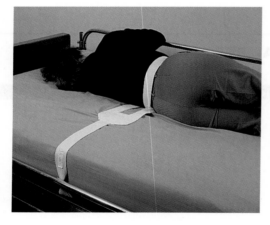

Step 4b Belt restraint placed around the waist. (Courtesy JT Posey Co., Arcadia, California.)

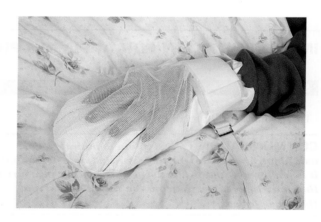

Step 4d Mitten restraint. (From Sorrentino SA: *Assisting with patient care,* St Louis, 1999, Mosby.)

Steps	Rationale
c. *Extremity/limb restraint (wrist or ankle):* With client in the lateral position, may be used to immobilize one or all extremities. Commercial restraints have sheepskin or foam padding. Check that two fingers can be inserted under the restraint (see illustration).	The lateral position helps prevent aspiration if the client vomits. Tight restraints may constrict circulation or ventilation and cause neurovascular injury or cause therapeutic devices to become occluded.
d. *Mitten restraint:* A thumbless mitten device to restrain client's hands (see illustration).	Prevents use of fingers to scratch skin, remove dressings, or dislodge equipment, yet allows more movement than a wrist restraint.
5. Attach restraints to the moveable part of bed frame, which moves when the head of the bed is raised or lowered (see illustration).	When the bed is raised/lowered, the strap will not tighten and restrict circulation.

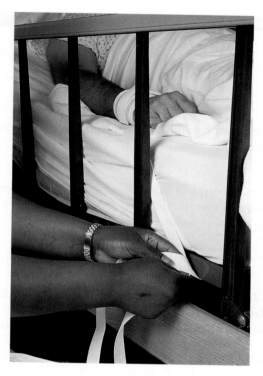

Step 5 Restraints are attached to the bed frame and to an area that does not cause the restraint to tighten when bed frame is raised or lowered.

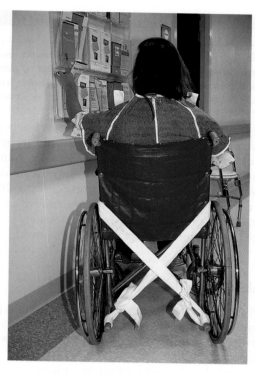

Step 6 Jacket restraint secured under the armrests and to the back of the wheelchair.

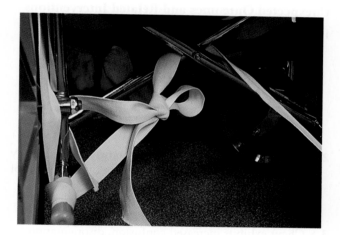

Step 7 Quick-release tie.

Steps	Rationale

NURSE ALERT *Do not attach restraints to side rails, which could cause injury when side rail is lowered.*

6. When the client is in a wheelchair, the jacket restraint should be secured with the ties under the armrests and tied at the back of the chair (see illustration).
7. Secure restraint with a quick-release tie (see illustration).
8. Before leaving client, make sure call bell is within reach and tell the client when you will return.

When ties are not under the armrests, clients may be able to slide the ties up the back of the chair and free themselves.

Allows for quick release in an emergency.

Steps	Rationale

9. At least every hour or according to agency policy, the restraint should be checked for proper placement and the client evaluated for pulses, temperature, color, and sensation of the distal part of the extremities.

Prevents complications from constriction and impaired circulation.

10. Every 2 hours, release the restraints (Zusman, 2001). If client is violent or noncompliant, remove one restraint at a time and/or have staff assistance.

Provides opportunity to change client's position, perform range of motion, toileting, and exercise and to provide food or fluids.

11. See Completion Protocol (inside front cover).

• • • • • • • • • •

EVALUATION

1. Observe for effectiveness of chosen restraint in preventing harm to the client.
2. Verify that prescribed therapies are continued without interruption.
3. Reassess client's need for restraint at least every 24 hours with the intent of discontinuing restraint at the earliest possible time (JCAHO, 2001).

Unexpected Outcomes and Related Interventions

1. Client experiences impaired skin integrity.
   a. Assess skin, and provide appropriate therapy.
   b. Notify the physician, and reassess the need for continued use of restraint.
   c. Consider if alternatives to restraint can be used.
   d. Ensure correct application of restraint, pad skin under restraints, and remove restraints more frequently.
2. Client has altered neurovascular status to an extremity (cyanosis, pallor, coldness of the skin or complaints of tingling, pain, or numbness)
   a. Remove restraint immediately, stay with the client, and notify the physician.
3. Client exhibits increased confusion, disorientation, or agitation.
   a. Identify reason for change in behavior, and attempt to eliminate cause.
   b. Attempt restraint alternatives.

4. Client escapes from the restraint device and suffers a fall or injury.
   a. Attend to client's immediate physical needs, and inform the physician.
   b. Reassess type of restraint used, correct application, and if alternatives can be used.

Recording and Reporting

• Document evidence that client's safety was at risk and specific restraint was warranted, including the following:
   Behavior before restraints were applied
   Level of orientation
   Client/family understanding and consent for application
   Type and location of restraint used and time applied
   Client behavior after restraint was applied and during attempts to use restraint alternatives
   Assessments related to oxygenation, circulation, and skin integrity
   Times of each subsequent assessment and release, range of motion, turning, and position
   Time restraints were removed and client response
Also see behavioral restraint flow sheet (Figure 5-5).

Holy Family Hospital and Medical Center
70 East Street, Methuen, MA 01844

RESTRAINT FLOW SHEET

Less Restrictive
Alternative Measures Attempted
(check all that apply)
- ☐ Pain/comfort measures
- ☐ Position changes
- ☐ Place near nurse's station
- ☐ Schedule toileting
- ☐ Attempt to reorient
- ☐ Alternatives discussed w/family
- ☐ Encourage family to visit
- ☐ Provide 1:1 observation
- ☐ Other:

Justification/Rationale for Restraints
(circle all that apply)

A. Harm to self
B. Harm to others
C. Removing medical devices
D. Confusion
E. Combative
F. Other:

ALL PATIENTS THAT NEED RESTRAINT MUST ALSO HAVE:

- A *Computer order* for the *"Restraint"*
- *MD order* with *"date and time"* noted by an RN – *No PRN orders!*
- *All* of the items on this flow sheet must be *__completed__*
- *Face-to-face* observation of the pt. by an RN or designated person *Q 15 minute –behavioral/safety check – and documented Q 2 hours*
- *Documented* assessment by RN Q 2 hours
- *A Problem/Progress note* regarding notification of patient/family and response to Less Restrictive Measures
- *Documented* restraint renewal every 24 hours by the physician

Was the Patient/Family Notified?
☐ yes; ☐ no; ☐ Brochure given
Who was notified?

Date/Time:
If not notified, why?

Type of Restraint Used
(check all that apply)
- ■ Right wrist; ☐ Left wrist
- ■ Right leg; ☐ Left leg
- ■ Jacket
- ■ 4 side rails up
- ■ Other:

Date/Time that the restraint was first applied:
(the first date and time that the order was obtained)

_____/_____/_____ @ _____ am/pm

Date/Time that the restraint order was discontinued:
(the last date and time that the order was valid)

_____/_____/_____ @ _____ am/pm

KEY: NN = Nurses Notes; X = Patient off Unit; R = Removed; ✓ = Observation; S = Sleeping

	Date:										
	Time:										
Document Every 2 Hours											
• Reason for restraint (A-F above)											
• Assess for early release (N/A = still required)											
• Hydration / Nutrition / Elimination											
• Condition of skin/CSM											
• ROM / Reposition											
• Neurovascular changes											
• Restraint reduced / released q2 hours											
• Vital signs taken if applicable											
• Behavioral / Safety check q15 minutes											
Initials of Observer:											

Comments:

Renewal Date:	**Date:**										
Renewal Time:	**Time:**										
Document Every 2 Hours											
• Reason for restraint (A-F above)											
• Assess for early release (N/A = still required)											
• Hydration / Nutrition / Elimination											
• Condition of skin/ CSM											
• ROM / Reposition											
• Neurovascular changes											
• Restraint reduced / released q2 hours											
• Vital signs taken if applicable											
• Behavioral / Safety check q15 minutes											
Initials of Observer:											

Comments:

Renewal Date:	**Date:**										
Renewal Time:	**Time:**										
Document Every 2 Hours											
• Reason for restraint (A-F above)											
• Assess for early release (N/A = still required)											
• Hydration / Nutrition / Elimination											
• Condition of skin/ CSM											
• ROM / Reposition											
• Neurovascular changes											
• Restraint reduced / released q2 hours											
• Vital signs taken if applicable											
• Behavioral / Safety check q15 minutes											
Initials of Observer:											

Comments:

Initials	Signature	Initials	Signature	Initials	Signature	Initials	Signature	Initials	Signature

Revised: 3/01; 5/02; 9/02

MF683A

Figure 5-5   Behavioral restraint flow sheet. (Courtesy Holy Family Hospital and Medical Center, Methuen, Massachusetts.)

SPECIAL CONSIDERATIONS

Pediatric Considerations

- When a child needs to be restrained for a procedure, it is best that the person applying the restraint not be the child's parent or guardian.
- A mummy restraint is a safe, efficient, short-term method to restrain a small child or infant for examination or treatment.
  - Open a blanket, and fold one corner toward the center. Place the infant on the blanket with shoulders at the fold and feet toward the opposite corner (Figure 5-6, *A*).
  - With infant's right arm straight down against body, pull the right side of the blanket firmly across the right shoulder and chest, and secure beneath the left side of body (Figure 5-6, *B*).
  - Place the left arm straight against the body, bring the left side of the blanket across the shoulder and chest, and lock beneath the infant's body on the right side (Figure 5-6, *C*).
  - Align the infant's legs, pull the corner of the blanket near the feet up toward the body, and tuck snugly in place or fasten securely with safety pins (Figure 5-6, *D*) (Wong and others, 1999).
- Remain with the infant while restrained, and remove the restraint immediately after treatment is complete. If restraint is required for an extended period of time, remove it at least every 2 hours and perform range-of-motion exercises on all extremities.

Geriatric Considerations

Advanced age alone is not an indication for use of restraints. The need for restraints and the risk of injury can be reduced by individual assessment of risk factors, creative planning, modifying the environment, and promoting functional restoration (Ebersole and Hess, 2001).

Home Care Considerations

A physical restraint should not be sent home with family unless the device is needed to protect the client or others from injury. If a restraint is needed for use at home, a physician's order is required and clear instructions should be given to the caregiver regarding proper application, care needed while in restraint, and potential complications.

Long-Term Care Considerations

- Unnecessary restraint is a violation of the client's right to freedom of movement. The client and family must understand the reason for the restraint, how the restraint will help planned medical treatment, and the risks associated with the use of restraint (Perry and Potter, 2002).
- Restraints are never used to discipline a person or for staff convenience (Sorrentino, 2000).

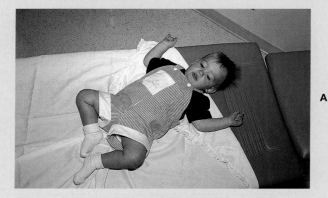

A

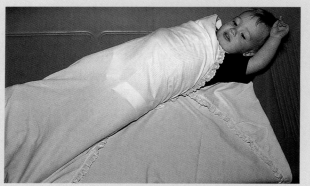

B

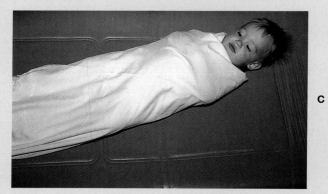

C

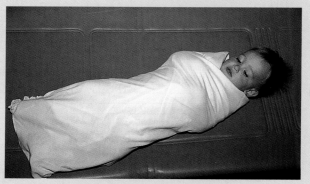

D

Figure 5-6   Mummy restraint.

Skill 5.4

Seizure Precautions

A seizure involves sudden, violent, involuntary muscle contractions that occur rhythmically, such as during acute or chronic seizure disorders, febrile episodes (especially in children), and after a head injury. Status epilepticus, generalized tonic-clonic seizures that last longer than 5 minutes or are followed quickly by subsequent seizures, is a medical emergency and requires intensive monitoring and treatment. Seizure precautions include nursing interventions to protect the client from traumatic injury, positioning for adequate ventilation and drainage of secretions, providing privacy, and support after the seizure. It is important for the nurse to observe and accurately document the sequence of events before, during, and after the seizure, including the duration of the seizure.

ASSESSMENT

1. Assess seizure history, noting frequency and presence of a visual, auditory, or other type of aura before a seizure. *Rationale: Provides a baseline to evaluate onset of seizure activity.*
2. Assess for factors that may precipitate a client's seizure (e.g., nonadherence to seizure medication, surgery, stress, infection). *Rationale: These factors place the client at greater risk for seizure activity.*
3. Inspect the client's environment for potential safety hazards if a seizure occurs. *Rationale: Prevents client from injury sustained by striking the head or body on furniture or equipment.*

PLANNING

Expected outcomes should focus on safety, prevention of airway obstruction and aspiration, and maintenance of self-esteem.

Expected Outcomes

1. Client does not suffer traumatic physical injury during a seizure episode.
2. Client's airway is maintained, and secretions are not aspirated during a seizure episode.
3. Client verbalizes positive self-feelings after a seizure episode.

Equipment

- Padded side rails and headboard
- Suction machine and oral airway
- Clean, disposable gloves

Delegation Considerations

Setting up seizure precautions and protection for clients at risk for seizures may be delegated to assistive personnel (AP). Stress the importance of protection from falls, avoiding attempts to restrain, and not placing anything in the client's mouth. Interventions for a client experiencing a seizure may not be delegated. Assessment of the client's airway patency, breathing, and circulatory status requires the critical thinking and knowledge application unique to the nurse and may not be delegated.

IMPLEMENTATION FOR SEIZURE PRECAUTIONS

Steps	Rationale
1. See Standard Protocol (inside front cover).	
2. Prepare bed with padded side rails and headboard and bed in lowest position. Provide equipment for oral suction (see illustration).	Modifications to the environment minimize risks associated with seizure activity. Oral suctioning may be required after a seizure to prevent aspiration of secretions.
3. Provide or encourage use of bracelet or identification card noting seizure disorder and medications taken.	Communicates client's risk for seizure activity to emergency health care providers.

COMMUNICATION TIP *Explain to the client and family what to expect during a seizure and the safety measures that are in place to protect the client from injury.*

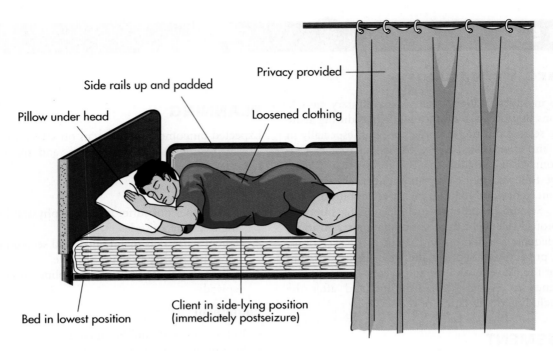

Privacy provided

Side rails up and padded

Loosened clothing

Pillow under head

Client in side-lying position
(immediately postseizure)

Bed in lowest position

Step 2 Seizure precautions.

Steps	**Rationale**

4. **If a seizure occurs (see illustration)**
    a.   Stay with the client. Protect head from injury, loosen clothing, and turn client on side, with head flexed slightly forward (see illustration).

Position protects the client from injury and reduces the risk of aspiration.

NURSE ALERT *Injury may result from forcible insertion of a hard object. Soft objects may break or come apart and be aspirated. Do not place fingers near or in the client's mouth, because this could result in a bite injury. If the client has dentures, do not try to remove them during the seizure. If loosened, remove after the seizure (Lannon, 1995).*

---

b. Provide client privacy if possible.
c. Observe the sequence and timing of seizure activity and client's skin color and respirations.
d. If a client is experiencing status epilepticus, an oral airway (see illustration) may need to be inserted when the jaw is relaxed between seizures. Hold airway with curved side up, insert downward until airway reaches back of throat, then rotate downward and follow natural curve of the tongue.
e. After the seizure, assess airway status, identify possible precipitating factors, and assess for bruising or injury. Remove gloves.
f. Explain what happened, and provide a quiet, nonstimulating environment.
5. See Completion Protocol (inside front cover).

Embarrassment is common after a seizure.
Accurate observations will assist in diagnosis and treatment of the seizure disorder.
Airway occlusion and aspiration are potential complications of this medical emergency.

Client may be confused and experience postictal drowsiness.

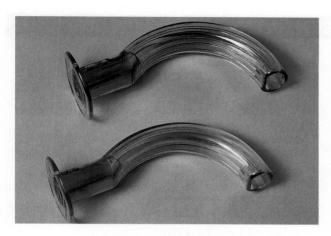

Step 4d Oral airways.

• • • • • • • • • •

EVALUATION

1. Assess client for traumatic injury during and after the seizure episode.
2. Observe client's color and respiratory rate and pattern during and after the seizure.
3. Ask client to verbalize feelings after the seizure.
4. Ensure a quiet, nonstimulating environment after the seizure.

Unexpected Outcomes and Related Interventions

1. Client suffers traumatic injury.
   a. Continue to protect client from further injury.
   b. Notify the physician immediately.
   c. Ensure environment is free of safety hazards.
2. Client verbalizes feelings of embarrassment and humiliation.
   a. Offer support and allow client to verbalize feelings.
   b. Encourage client and family to participate in decision making and planning care.

Recording and Reporting

- Document events before, during, and after the seizure, including the following:
  Presence/absence of aura
  Level of consciousness
  Posture
  Color
  Sequence and movements of extremities
  Presence/absence of incontinence
  Objective and subjective data immediately afterward
Notify physician immediately when seizure begins because status epilepticus requires immediate medical therapy.

Sample Documentation

1000 Observed client sitting in chair in room. Cry heard, client observed sliding to floor, not responding to verbal stimuli. Client assisted to floor with head supported. Pillow placed under head. Tonic and clonic movements of all four extremities noted, lasting 2 minutes. Color remained good, respiratory pattern slightly irregular. No incontinence noted. At conclusion of tonic and clonic movements, client slept for 20 minutes, during which time respirations were 16 per minute and regular.

  1020 Client awake and alert. Requested nurse to describe sequence of events. Stated that this was his "usual type of seizure."

SPECIAL CONSIDERATIONS

Pediatric Considerations

Benign febrile seizures occur in 3% to 5% of children under the age of 5 years with no cause for the seizure other than a high fever. It is important, however, that benign febrile convulsions be differentiated from epilepsy (Rolak, 1998).

Geriatric Considerations

- Older adults metabolize anticonvulsants more slowly; therefore drugs may accumulate, resulting in toxicity. Therapeutic blood levels should be monitored carefully (McKenry and Salerno, 1999).
- Older adults may have symptoms that impede the recognition of a seizure disorder such as confusion lasting several days, unusual behaviors, or receptive and expressive language problems (Lannon, 1995).

Home Care Considerations

- Discuss with the client and family precipitating factors and care of the client experiencing a seizure.
- The client's home should be assessed for environmental hazards.
- Unless seizure activity is well controlled, instruct client to avoid swimming activities or taking a tub bath unless a knowledgeable family member is present. Driving may also be restricted until seizures are controlled for at least 1 year.
- Refer client and family to the Epilepsy Foundation to improve coping ability.

Skill 5.5

Safety Measures for Radioactive Materials

Radiation and radioactive materials are used in the diagnosis and treatment of clients. Nurses may be exposed to radiation when assisting clients who are undergoing x-ray examinations. Clients with some forms of cancer may be treated with internal radioactive implants placed in a body cavity, using sealed tubes, ribbons, wires, seeds, capsules, or needles. Nurses need to be familiar with agency policies for the care of clients who are receiving radiation and radioactive materials. Nurses who are or may be pregnant are not to be involved in the care of clients with radiation therapy. Nurses need to reduce the exposure to radiation by applying the principles of time, distance, and shielding. The time near the source is limited (a dosimeter badge may be worn to measure exposure), distance from the source is maximized, and shielding devices (e.g., lead shields or aprons) are used. Lead-shielded containers are used for storage of radioactive materials. Nurses need to check with agency policy or safety office regarding specific information about safe times and distances to ensure that their occupational exposure is as low as reasonably achievable.

ASSESSMENT

1. Consult with radiation protection officer to identify the type and amount of radiation to be used and its side effects and hazards. *Rationale: Minimizes risk of overexposure to client, visitors, and staff.*
2. Identify the restrictions related to time and distance.

PLANNING

Expected outcome focuses on minimizing exposure to radiation.

Expected Outcome

1. The client will be diagnosed or treated using radiation with the least exposure possible for client, visitors, and staff.

Equipment

- Protective lead shields
- Dosimeter badge
- Sign for door: "Caution—Radioactive Material" (Figure 5-7)
- Bright-colored tape for floor
- Lead or disposable rubber gloves

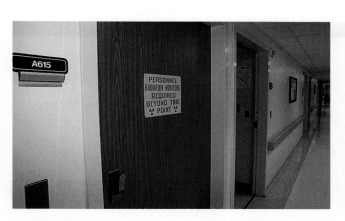

Figure 5-7 Signage indicates materials are in room.

Delegation Considerations

Care of the client receiving radiation therapy may be delegated to assistive personnel (AP). Stress the importance of the following:

- Client's activity limitations
- Safety regulations (e.g., dosimeter, time and distance limits)
- Use of protective equipment (shields, gloves)
- Visitor restrictions (no one under 18 years of age or who is or may be pregnant)
- Care and handling of patient care related items (e.g., linen, trash, dietary tray, specimens, urine, feces)

IMPLEMENTATION FOR SAFETY MEASURES FOR RADIOACTIVE MATERIALS

Steps	Rationale
1. See Standard Protocol (inside front cover).	
2. Explain the treatment plan to the client and family, including activity limitations and expected side effects.	

NURSE ALERT *Rotate care providers to provide nursing care needed while keeping staff exposure to radiation within safe limits. Avoid exposure to persons in early pregnancy to prevent risks related to fetal development.*

COMMUNICATION TIP *Radiation therapy can sound frightening. Allow the client and family to verbalize their fears and concerns. Describe to the client and family what procedures are involved and what they will experience.*

Steps	Rationale
3. Prepare the room with a sign on the door and yellow tape on the floor to mark the distance from the bed required for safety. A private room is required.	Provides a visual alert to visitors and staff to minimize exposure to radiation (Otto, 1997).
4. Provide client with diversional activities such as watching television, reading a book, listening to music, or playing cards.	Helps relieve boredom imposed by the physical and psychosocial limitations of radiation therapy.
5. Explain safety regulations, time limits, and distance limits to client and visitors.	
6. Wear a badge or dosimeter that indicates extent of radiation exposure.	Protects staff from overexposure to radioactive materials.
7. Wear appropriate shield (e.g., lead apron or gloves, rubber gloves) when providing care. Wash gloves before removal, and dispose of in designated waste container. Wash hands thoroughly after removing gloves.	Provides protection to care providers during patient care activities such as collecting or transferring urine, feces, or other contaminated items.
8. Leave nondisposable items (e.g., equipment) and soiled items (e.g., linen) sealed in a plastic bag in the client's room.	Items must stay in client's room until checked for radioactivity (Otto, 1997).

Steps	Rationale
9. Identify special requirements relating to laboratory specimens, dietary tray, secretions and excretions, dressings, linens, and trash.	
10. Request a discharge survey by radiation protection officer.	Client's room and all items in it are surveyed for any residual radioactivity (Otto, 1997).
11. See Completion Protocol (inside front cover).	

· · · · · · · · · · ·

EVALUATION

Determine the amount of radiation exposure to client, visitors, and staff.

Unexpected Outcome and Related Interventions

1. Questions arise about radiation exposure, spillage, dislodged implant, or systemic treatment.
   a. Notify radiation protection officer immediately.
   b. Avoid direct contact with source of radiation.
   c. Wash with soap and water if skin becomes contaminated.

Recording and Reporting

Document radiation therapy and related safety measures used, including the following:
- Length of exposure
- Apparent side effects if noted
- Teaching provided to client and family

Sample Documentation

1300 Admitted for radiation treatments. Client and family instructed on expectations relating to side effects of therapy and routines for minimizing unnecessary exposure by limiting time, maintaining appropriate distance, and use of protective equipment.

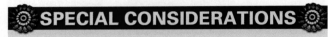

SPECIAL CONSIDERATIONS

Pediatric Considerations

Boredom is a common problem for children receiving internal radiation therapy. Play therapy can help relieve the boredom. A family-centered approach works best where children, parents, and staff work together toward planning for and coping with such procedures (McKay and Hirano, 1998).

Geriatric Considerations

When providing radiation therapy to older clients, it is important to maintain psychological well-being. Many geriatric clients are used to a daily routine. Physical and psychosocial limitations imposed by radiation therapy may contribute to frustration and confusion.

CRITICAL THINKING EXERCISES

1. An 88-year-old woman is admitted to a long-term care facility after having had several falls resulting from weakness and loss of balance. The most recent fall resulted in a fractured hip, which was surgically treated. She is being given Tylenol with codeine every 4 hours as needed for pain. She tells you she is accustomed to being very independent, having lived alone for several years since her husband died. She appears alert and oriented on arrival at the facility. However, during the first night she is found wandering in the hall, looking for the bathroom. What can be done to avoid restraining this client?

2. A client is admitted for surgery. She has a history of grand mal seizures for which she is taking medication. She has been ill for several days and has been unable to take the medication. When delegating the care of the client to AP, what information should you communicate about initiating seizure precautions and caring for the client if a seizure occurs?

3. While moving a client in the bed, you accidentally knock over the portable blood pressure apparatus. The mercury contained in the manometer spills on the floor. What would be your priority actions in this situation?

REFERENCES

Brians LK and others: Development of the RISK tool for fall prevention, *Rehabil Nurs* 16(2):67, 1991.

Capezuti E and others: The relationship between physical restraint removal and falls and injuries among nursing home residents, *J Gerontol A Biol Sci Med Sci* 53A: M47, 1998.

Centers for Medicare and Medicaid Services: *Conditions of participation: interpretive guidelines,* 2000, US Department of Health and Human Services, Bethesda, Maryland.

Ebersole P, Hess P: *Toward healthy aging: human needs and nursing process,* ed 5, St Louis, 1998, Mosby.

Ebersole P, Hess P: *Geriatric nursing and healthy aging,* St Louis, 2001, Mosby.

Hammond M, Levine J: Bedrails: choosing the best alternative, *Geriatr Nurs* 20(6):297, 1999.

Hockenberry MJ and others: *Wong's nursing care of infants and children,* ed 7, St Louis, 2003, Mosby.

Joint Commission on Accreditation of Healthcare Organizations: *Comprehensive Accreditation Manual for Hospitals,* 2001, Chicago, The Association.

Lannon S: Epilepsy in the elderly, *Clin Nurs Pract Epilepsy* 2(2):5, 1995.

Lueckenotte AG: *Gerontologic nursing,* St Louis, 2000, Mosby.

McKay J, Hirano N: *The chemotherapy and radiation survival guide,* Oakland, Calif, 1998, New Harbinger.

McKenry L, Salerno E: *Mosby's pharmacology in nursing,* ed 20, St Louis, 1999, Mosby.

National Center for Injury Prevention and Control: *Fact book for the year 2000,* 2000, Centers for Disease Control and Prevention, Atlanta, Georgia.

Otto SE: *Oncology Nursing,* ed 3, St Louis, 1997, Mosby.

Perry A, Potter P: *Clinical nursing skills and techniques,* ed 5, St. Louis, 2002, Mosby.

Potter PA and Perry AG: *Fundamentals of nursing,* ed 5, St Louis, 2001, Mosby.

Rogers P, Bocchino N: Restraint free care: is it possible? *Am J Nurs* 99(10):26, 1999.

Rolak LA: *Neurology secrets,* ed 2, Philadelphia, 1998, Hanley & Belfus.

Selekman J, Snyder B: Uses of and alternatives to restraints in pediatric settings, *AACN Clin Issues* 7(4):603, 1996.

Sorrentino SA: *Assisting with patient care,* St Louis, 1999, Mosby.

Sorrentino SA: *Mosby's textbook for nursing assistants,* ed 5, St Louis, 2000, Mosby.

Strumpf N and others: *Restraint free care: individualized approaches for frail elders,* New York, 1998, Springer.

Tideiksaar R: Home safe home: practical tips for fall-proofing, *Geriatr Nurs* 11(6):284, 1989.

Wong DL and others: *Whaley and Wong's nursing care of infants and children,* ed 6, St Louis, 1999, Mosby.

Zusman J: *Restraint and seclusion: understanding the JCAHO standards and federal regulations,* ed 3, Marblehead, Mass, 2001, Opus Communications.

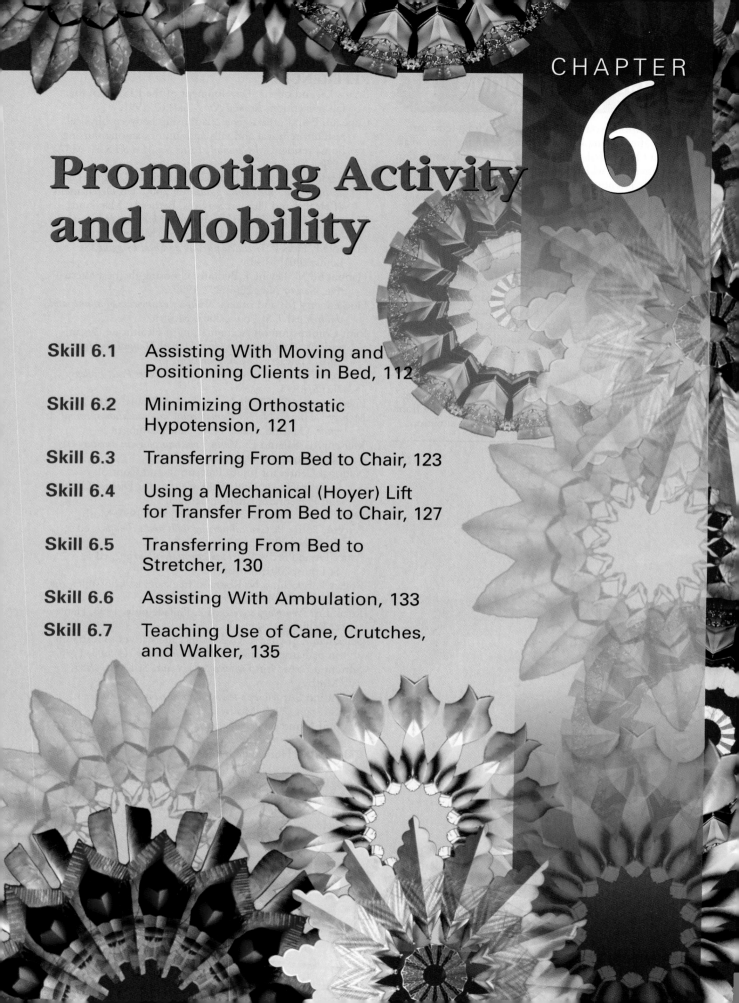

Promoting Activity and Mobility

Regular physical activity and exercise contributes to both physical and emotional well-being (Huddleston, 1998; Konradi and Anglin, 2001). The benefits of physical activity include increased energy, improved sleep, better appetite, less pain, and improved self-esteem. It is useful to incorporate active exercises into activities of daily living (ADLs) (Box 6-1). Every effort must be made to promote and maintain functional mobility. Physical activities that clients are able to perform indicate their physical capacity, functional ability, and personal desires.

Three elements essential for mobility include (1) ability to move based on adequate muscle strength, control, coordination, and range of motion (ROM); (2) motivation to move; and (3) absence of barriers in the environment. To prevent injury to both client and caregiver, use of good body mechanics is essential (Table 6-1). For information about range of motion, see Chapter 27.

Immobilized clients, clients with chronic illnesses, and older adults are at a greater risk of developing complications that affect all body systems very quickly. These complications include muscle atrophy, loss of bone mass, contractures of joints, pressure ulcers, cardiovascular and respiratory problems, constipation, urinary stasis, mental confusion, and depression (Jitramontree, 2001; McCance and Huether, 2002).

Bed rest is a medical intervention in which the client is restricted to bed for one of the following purposes: (1) decreasing oxygen requirements of the body, (2) reducing pain, and (3) allowing rest and recovery.

NURSING DIAGNOSES

Activity Intolerance and **Risk for Activity Intolerance** are situations in which clients experience altered vital signs (pulse, respiration, or blood pressure) in response to activity. **Impaired Physical Mobility** is associated with pain or discomfort resulting from trauma or surgery, decreased strength and endurance, prolonged bed rest, or restrictive

---

Box 6-1

Examples of Incorporating Exercise Into Activities of Daily Living

UPPER BODY

Nodding head "yes": neck flexion

Shaking head "no": neck rotation

Reaching to bedside stand for book: shoulder extension

Scratching back: shoulder hyperextension

Brushing or combing hair: shoulder hyperextension

Eating, bathing, and shaving: elbow flexion and extension

Writing and eating: fingers and thumb flexion, extension, and opposition

LOWER BODY

Walking: hip flexion, extension, and hyperextension; knee flexion and extension; ankle dorsiflexion; plantar flexion

Moving to side-lying position: hip flexion, extension, and abduction; knee flexion and extension

Moving from side-lying position: hip extension and adduction; knee flexion and extension

While sitting, lifting knees up and straightening legs: strengthens muscles used for walking

---

Table 6-1

Body Mechanics for Health Care Workers

Action	Rationale
1. When planning to move a client, arrange for adequate help. Use mechanical aids if help is unavailable.	Two workers lifting together divide the workload by 50%.
2. Encourage client to assist as much as possible.	This promotes client's abilities and strength while minimizing workload.
3. Keep back, neck, pelvis, and feet aligned. Avoid twisting.	Twisting increases risk of injury.
4. Flex knees, keep feet wide apart.	A broad base of support increases stability.
5. Position self close to client (or object being lifted).	The force is minimized.
6. Use arms and legs (not back).	The leg muscles are stronger, larger muscles capable of greater work without injury.
7. Slide client toward yourself using a pull sheet. When transferring a client onto a stretcher, a slide-board is more appropriate.	Sliding requires less effort than lifting. Pull sheet minimizes shearing forces, which can damage client's skin.
8. Set (tighten) abdominal and gluteal muscles in preparation for move.	Preparing muscles for the load minimizes strain.
9. Person with the heaviest load coordinates efforts of team involved by counting to three.	Simultaneous lifting minimizes the load for any one lifter.

external devices such as casts, splints, braces, or drainage and intravenous (IV) tubing. Psychological factors such as **Fear** relating to a history of falling results in a client's refusal to ambulate. **Risk for Disuse Syndrome** is a diagnosis that applies when inactivity is desired or unavoidable, increasing the risk for deterioration of cardiovascular, respiratory, musculoskeletal, and psychosocial body systems.

In this case, maintenance of the client's present abilities is the primary focus of activity. When a client has mental confusion, weakness, or orthostatic hypotension, the diagnosis of **Risk for Injury** should be considered. Finally, a client with a nursing diagnosis of **Acute Pain** or **Chronic Pain** is susceptible to developing impaired mobility resulting from the nature and extent of discomfort.

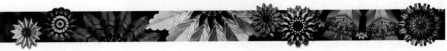

Skill 6.1

Assisting With Moving and Positioning Clients in Bed

This skill includes moving dependent clients up in bed with one or more nurses with or without a pull sheet and positioning clients in the Fowler's, supine, prone, lateral, and semiprone (Sims') positions. Each position offers advantages and limitations. When moving and positioning clients, it is important to be aware of potential pressure points (Figure 6-1).

Correct body alignment involves positioning so that no excessive strain is put on joints, tendons, ligaments, and muscles. Clients with impaired nervous or musculoskeletal system functioning, with increased weakness, or those restricted to bed rest benefit from repositioning (Hoeman, 2001). In general, clients should be repositioned as needed and at least every 2 hours if they are in bed and every 20 to 30 minutes if they are sitting in a chair. Additional variables influencing frequency of position changes include level of comfort, amount of spontaneous movement, presence of edema, loss of sensation, and overall physical and mental status (Hoeman, 2001). Dependent clients need a regularly scheduled program of assisted ROM exercises (see Chapter 27).

Care must be taken to protect the skin from damage caused by shearing forces resulting from sliding rather than lifting the client (Figure 6-2). Shear injury occurs when the skin remains stationary and the underlying tissue shifts, resulting in tissue damage. This is especially important when the client is thin, has fragile skin, is nutritionally compromised, or is unable to move independently.

For immobilized clients, pillows or foam wedges should be used to keep bony prominences such as heels and ankles from excessive or extended pressure. The use of air or water mattresses is also recommended (see Chapter 26).

ASSESSMENT

1. Assess client's weight, age, level of consciousness, disease process, and ability to cooperate. *Rationale: Determines how much assistance will be needed.*
2. Assess strength of muscles and mobility of joints to be used by observing client movement in bed and by applying gradual pressure to a muscle group (e.g., attempting to extend client's elbow). Compare strength in muscle groups, including arms and legs. *Rationale: Provides a baseline to determine ability to assist caregivers and to assess the client's progress toward improved activity tolerance and muscle endurance. The plan of care should be adjusted if the client is losing or gaining muscle strength and joint mobility over time.*
3. Assess need for analgesic medication 30 to 60 minutes before position changes. *Rationale: Analgesics enhance client's ability to tolerate movement. Peak levels vary according to the specific analgesic and route of administration.*
4. Assess for tubes, incisions, and equipment. *Rationale: Will alter positioning procedure.*

PLANNING

Expected outcomes focus on mobility, self-care, interaction, and prevention of complications within the confines of the prescribed activity.

Expected Outcomes

1. Client's skin remains intact without redness.
2. Client verbalizes a sense of comfort after each repositioning.
3. Client maintains assisted changes in position in bed for at least 1 hour.
4. Client lists two benefits of position changes and good body alignment:
   a. Improved circulation
   b. Reduced skin breakdown

Equipment

- Pillows
- Footboard (optional)
- High-top sneakers
- Trochanter roll (optional)
- Sandbag (optional)
- Hand rolls
- Side rails
- Trapeze bar (optional)
- Pull sheet

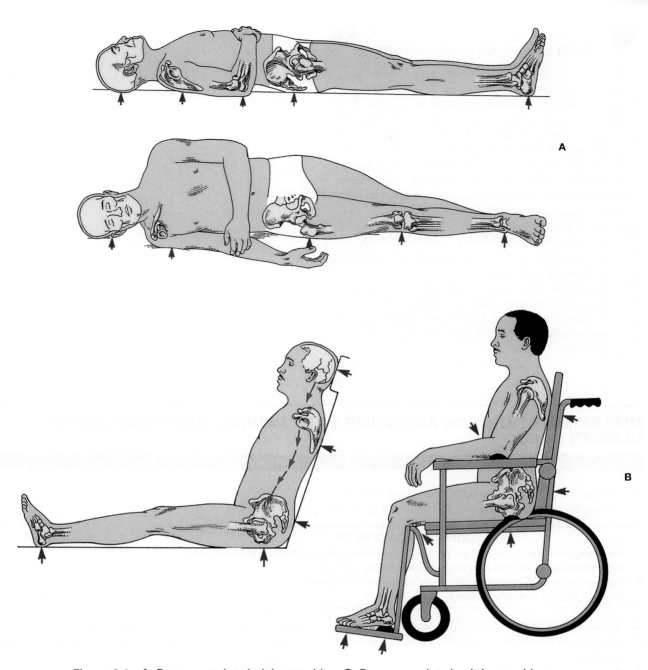

Figure 6-1   **A,** Pressure points in lying position. **B,** Pressure points in sitting position.

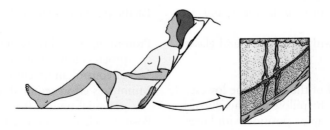

Figure 6-2   Shearing forces against sacrum cause tissue damage.

Delegation Considerations

The skill of moving and positioning clients with acute spinal cord trauma requires critical thinking and knowledge application unique to a nurse. The skills of moving and positioning clients without neurological trauma in bed can be delegated to assistive personnel (AP). When delegating these skills, it is important for caregivers to know how to protect themselves from injury and to report changes in the client condition that indicate problems requiring the assessment and intervention of the nurse.

- Identify ability to maintain personal safety by use of correct body mechanics, including height of bed, broad base of support, use of large muscles, and coordinated team effort.
- Encourage caregivers to have the client participate as much as possible in the process.
- Evaluate the client's comfort and alignment after repositioning, and assess pressure points for skin integrity.

IMPLEMENTATION FOR ASSISTING WITH MOVING AND POSITIONING CLIENTS IN BED

Steps	Rationale
1. See Standard Protocol (inside front cover). Review principles of body mechanics (see Table 6-1, p. 111).	

COMMUNICATION TIP

- *Encourage clients to assist as much as possible, discuss steps involved, and determine ways clients can assist while being moved.*
- *Review each step again as the move is about to be made.*
- *Include family in explanations.*

Steps	Rationale
2. Raise level of bed to comfortable working height.	Raises level of work toward nurse's center of gravity.
3. Remove all pillows and devices used in previous position.	Reduces interference from bedding during positioning procedure.
4. Get extra help as needed.	Provides for client and nurse safety.
5. Position client.	
a. **Moving a dependent client up in bed with one nurse and client assistance**	
(1) Adjust position of IV pole, tubes, and catheters.	Facilitates movement without tension and disruption.
(2) Provide client with hearing aid and glasses if used.	Promoting client involvement motivates and speeds progress toward independence and provides a sense of control and security.
(3) Lower the head of the bed to the lowest position. Place the pillow near headboard.	Minimizes effort required to move client and minimizes potential trauma from head contacting headboard.
(4) Assist client to supine position with knees flexed so that soles of one or both feet are flat on the bed.	Positions client to exert effort when moving up in bed.

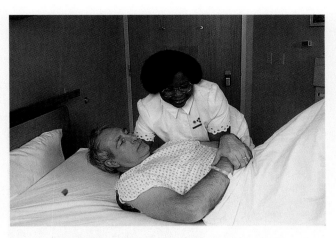

Step 5a(5) Moving client with one nurse.

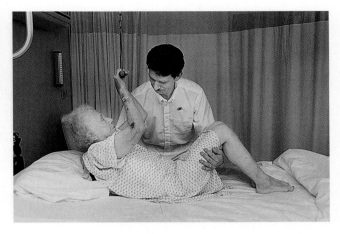

Step 5a(6) Moving client with aid of trapeze.

Steps	Rationale
(5) If there is no trapeze, slide arm nearest the head of the bed under client's shoulders, reaching under and supporting client's opposite shoulder. Place other arm under client's upper back (see illustration). Have client push with feet as you lift on the count of three.	
(6) If there is a trapeze, assist client with grasping it. Slide one arm under thighs and one arm under trunk (see illustration).	
(7) Have client lift with trapeze and/or push with feet on the count of three. Repeat if needed to move up farther in the bed.	Coordinates client's movement with nurse's lifting action.
(8) Ask client about level of comfort, and adjust as necessary.	

b. Assisting client to move up in bed when client cannot assist

(1) Remove pillow, lower the head of the bed to the lowest position client can tolerate, and lower side rails. Place pillow at head of bed.	Minimizes effort required to move client and minimizes potential trauma from head contact on headboard. Clients with hypoxia may not tolerate lying flat.
(2) Roll client side to side, placing a pull sheet that extends from shoulders to thighs. A pull sheet can be made using a small sheet folded in half.	
(3) With one nurse on each side of client, grasp pull sheet firmly with hands near client's upper arms and hips, rolling sheet material until hands are close to client.	The closer nurses are to client, the less height of lifting is required to clear the bed during the move.

NURSE ALERT *Review principles of body mechanics (see Table 6-1, p. 111). This move requires at least two nurses and pull sheet when client is unable to assist. If client is very heavy, consider using more personnel.*

(4) Nurses' knees are flexed with body facing the direction of the move. The foot away from the bed faces forward for a broader base of support (see illustration on p. 116).

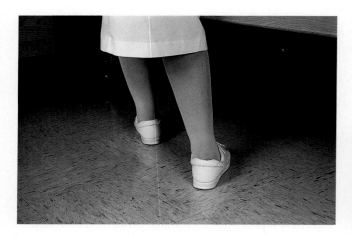

Step 5b(4)   Nurse flexes knees with wide base of support.

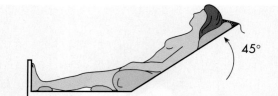

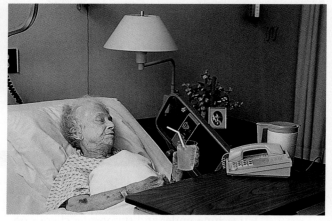

Step 5c(1)   Raise head of bed to appropriate level.

Steps	Rationale

(5)   Instruct client to rest arms on body and to lift head on the count of three.

(6)   Lift client toward the head of the bed on the count of three. Repeat the move if necessary.

(7)   Assist client as needed in shifting to attain position of comfort.

c.   **Positioning in semi-Fowler's and Fowler's position.** For the semi-Fowler's position the head of the bed is raised 45 to 60 degrees. The high-Fowler's position, with the head of the bed raised 90 degrees, is recommended for eating.

   Both positions improve breathing by decreasing pressure on the diaphragm as gravity pulls abdominal contents downward. These positions also facilitate visiting and diversional activities. In this position clients tend to slide toward the foot of the bed.

(1)   With client in supine position, raise the head of the bed to the appropriate level (45 to 90 degrees) (see illustrations).

(2)   Use pillows to support client's arms and hands if upper body is immobilized.

   Minimizes development of dependent edema and prevents shoulder dislocation if client has upper extremity impairment.

(3)   Position a pillow under client's head if desired, and raise the knee break of the bed slightly. Avoid pressure under the popliteal space (back of the knee).

   Pressure under the popliteal space can interfere with circulation and contribute to thromboemboli (blood clots) (Brough, 1998).

(4)   Change the degree of elevation of the head of bed 5 to 10 degrees frequently.

   Alters the pressure points slightly and promotes comfort.

(5)   Identify potential pressure points, including scapulae, elbows, sacrum or coccyx, and heels (see Figure 6-1, p. 113) (implement pressure ulcer prevention, Chapter 23).

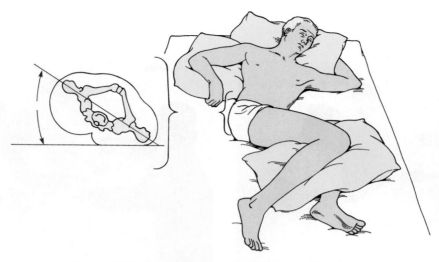

Step 5d(8)   Side-lying position with pillow placement.

Steps	Rationale
d. Moving dependent client to 30-degree lateral (side-lying) position. This move removes pressure from bony prominences of entire back.	If client can move freely, a side-lying position with upper and lower shoulders aligned is acceptable.
(1) Lower the head of the bed as much as client can tolerate, keeping head of bed below 30-degree angle. Lower side rail.	Reduces shear. Avoids working against gravity. Ensures that client will be in center of the bed when turned.
(2) Using a pull sheet, move client to the side of the bed opposite to the one toward which client will be turned. Raise side rail. Go to opposite side of the bed, and lower side rail.	
(3) Prepare to turn client onto side. Flex client's knee that will not be next to mattress once turned. Assist client with raising arm nearest you above head, adjusting pillow if needed.	
(4) Place one hand on client's hip and one hand on client's shoulder and hip, and assist client with rolling toward you onto side.	Turning client toward you promotes client's sense of security
(5) Flex both client's knees after the turn, and support upper leg from knee to foot using a pillow or folded blanket.	Keeps spine in good alignment.
(6) Ease lower shoulder forward, and bring upper shoulder back slightly. Check client's comfort.	Prevents excessive pressure directly on shoulder.
(7) Support upper arm with pillows so that arm is level with shoulder.	Improves ventilation by minimizing pressure on chest.
(8) *Optional:* Place pillow behind client's back and under so that it is tucked smoothly against back (see illustration).	Provides support and prevents client from rolling onto back.
(9) Make sure client's back is straight without evidence of twisting. Adjust as needed for comfort.	
(10) Pressure points to check include the ear, shoulder, anterior iliac spine, trochanter, lateral side of the knee, malleolus, and foot (see Figure 6-1, p. 113).	

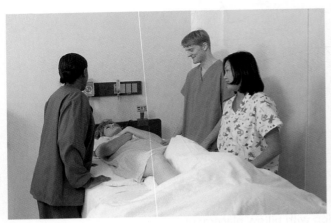 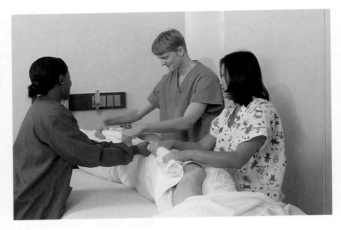

Step 5e(5) Logrolling a client. (From Sorrentino SA: *Assisting with patient care,* St. Louis, 1999, Mosby.)

Steps	Rationale
e. Logrolling to maintain neck and spinal alignment following injury or surgery	
(1) Determine number of staff required to logroll client.	To prevent injury to client and/or caregivers a minimum of three or four staff is recommended (Groeneveld, McKenzie, and Williams, 2001).
(2) Lower the head of the bed as much as client can tolerate.	Maintains alignment of the spinal column.
(3) Place a pillow between the legs. Use of a pull sheet placed between shoulders and knees can facilitate turning.	Maintains position of the lower extremities.
(4) Cross client's arms on chest.	Prevents injury to arms during turning.
(5) Position two nurses on side of bed to which the client will be turned. Position third nurse on the other side of bed (see illustration).	Distributes weight equally between nurses.
(6) Fanfold or roll the drawsheet or pullsheet.	Provides strong handles in order to grip the drawsheet or pull the sheet without slipping.
(7) Using the count of three, turn client as one unit with a continuous, smooth, and coordinated effort.	Maintains body in alignment, preventing stress on any part of the body.
(8) Support client with pillows along the length of the client. Gently lean client as a unit back towards the pillows for support.	
f. Moving dependent client to Sims' (semiprone) position. For this alternative to the lateral position, client lies somewhat forward onto abdomen.	This position is useful to discourage clients from rolling back to the supine position.
(1) With client in the lateral position, arm against mattress is externally rotated with elbow extended. Prevent internal rotation of hip and adduction of leg by extending the lowermost leg and supporting the other leg level with the hip (see illustration).	Minimizes pressure on the hip and shoulder.
(2) Support client's uppermost arm in flexed position level with shoulder.	Decreases internal rotation and adduction of shoulder and protects joint. Allows better chest expansion and improves ventilation.

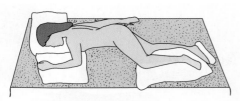

Step 5f(1)   Sims' (semiprone) position.

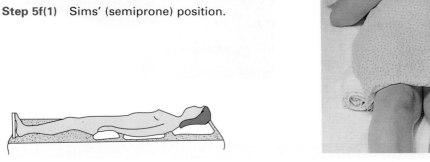

Step 5g(2)   Pillow placement for supine position.

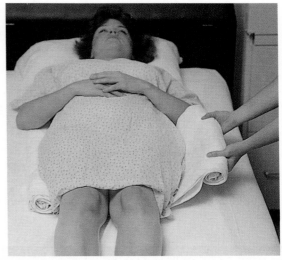

Step 5g(3)   Positioning of trochanter roll.

Steps	Rationale
(3) Pressure points include ear, front of shoulder, iliac crest, lateral knee, malleolus, and side of foot of lower leg, as well as medial knee and malleolus of upper leg (see Figure 6-1, p. 113).	
g. Positioning dependent client in supine position	
(1) Place client on back with head of bed flat.	Supports normal curvature of lumbar spine.
(2) Place pillow under upper shoulders, neck, and head (see illustration).	Prevents excessive flexion of cervical spine.
(3) To position trochanter roll at client's hips, place a folded bath blanket under hips and roll ends under until toes point directly up (see illustration)	Prevents external rotation of hips and may be bilateral or unilateral depending on extent and location of muscle weakness.
(4) Place small support under ankles to minimize pressure on heels. A footboard or use of high top tennis shoes may be used to prevent footdrop. Shoes should be removed at least 3 times a day for ROM exercises to prevent contractures.	Footboard or tennis shoes keep ankles in flexed position.
(5) Place small supports under forearms with hand-wrist splints or small rolls to support fingers and thumb in a functional position.	A functional position allows the fingers to be flexed and the thumb to touch the fingertips.
(6) Pressure areas to check include the back of the head, scapulae, elbows, posterior iliac spine, sacrum or coccyx, ischium, Achilles tendons, and heels (see Figure 6-1, p. 113).	
h. Positioning client in prone position	Prone positioning improves oxygenation in clients with severe pulmonary problems, such as adult respiratory distress syndrome (ARDS). This position is contraindicated in clients with spinal cord or facial trauma or surgery, obese clients, and those with increased intracranial pressure (Marion, 2001).
(1) Roll client to one side.	
(2) Roll client over arm positioned close to body, with elbow straight and hand under hip. Position client on abdomen in center of bed.	Positions client correctly so alignment can be maintained.

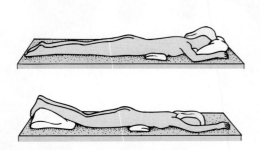

Steps 5h(3) and 5h(4) Prone position with pillows in place.

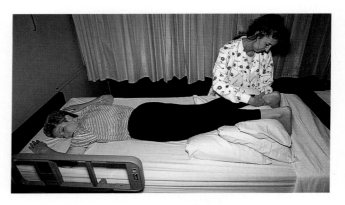

Step 5h(6) Prone position with pillows supporting lower legs.

Steps	Rationale
(3) Turn client's head to one side, and support head with small pillow (see illustration).	Reduces flexion or hyperextension of cervical vertebrae.
(4) Place small pillow under client's abdomen below level of diaphragm (see illustration).	Reduces pressure on breasts of some female clients and decreases hyperextension of lumbar vertebrae and strain on lower back. Improves breathing by reducing mattress pressure on diaphragm.
(5) Support arms in flexed position level at shoulders.	Maintains proper body alignment. Support reduces risk of joint dislocation.
(6) Support lower legs with pillow to elevate toes (see illustration).	Prevents footdrop. Reduces external rotation of legs. Reduces mattress pressure on toes.
6. See Completion Protocol (inside front cover).	

• • • • • • • • • •

EVALUATION

1. Inspect skin overlying pressure areas for erythema (redness) and blanching. Observe again in 60 minutes.
2. Ask client if position is comfortable.
3. Observe client's body alignment and position.
4. Ask client to identify two benefits of position changes and correct body alignment.

Unexpected Outcomes and Related Interventions

1. Client develops areas of abnormal reactive hyperemia, blistering, or skin irritation.
   a. Change client's position more frequently.
   b. Avoid prolonged pressure on any one pressure area.
2. Client complains of discomfort from stretching because of altered alignment.
   a. Readjust position according to client's comfort level.
   b. Readjust supportive pillows to maintain alignment.
3. Client turns back to same position frequently and expresses discomfort with alternate positions.
   a. Reinforce the rationale for position changes.
   b. Provide diversional activities in various positions.
   c. Identify client's perception of position preference and attempt to create incentive for compliance with alternate positions.

4. Client complains of respiratory distress.
   a. Readjust client's position. Underlying respiratory and/or cardiac diseases may limit the client's tolerance to certain positions.

Recording and Reporting

- Position client was moved from
- Position client was moved to
- Supportive devices used
- Condition of skin on pressure points
- Instructions given to client and/or family
- Client's tolerance of change in position

Sample Documentation

0800 Turned from back to left lateral position. Area of erythema approximately 3 cm in diameter noted over coccyx. Blanches easily. Urged client not to lie on back.

1000 Found client lying on back. Turned to right side and supported with pillows. Coccyx remains reddened, blanches to fingertip pressure.

1100 Continues on right side watching television. Denies discomfort.

SPECIAL CONSIDERATIONS

Pediatric Considerations

- Children should be encouraged to be as active as their condition and restrictive devices allow. Opportunity, materials, or objects to stimulate activity and encouragement and participation of others must be available (Hockenberry and others, 2003).
- Children not able to move will need passive exercise and movement (see Chapter 27).

Geriatric Considerations

- Immobilized older adult clients are at higher risk of developing complications that affect all body systems. These complications include muscle atrophy, contractures, pressure ulcers, blood clots, pneumonia, constipation, urinary stasis, depression, and mental confusion (Jitramontree, 2001).
- Activity is especially important in older adults to maintain functional status (Lueckenotte, 2000).
- Provide support to avoid strain on joints, tendons, ligaments, and muscles.
- Frequent repositioning (see Chapter 23) and a regular program of ROM exercises are essential.
- Physical therapy or occupational therapy consultation is appropriate.
- In the presence of thin, fragile skin and/or nutritionally compromised state, lubricants or protective films or padding can reduce friction injury (see Chapter 23).
- Use a pull sheet to avoid shearing forces that damage client tissues.

Home Care Considerations

- Teach family members body mechanics.
- In the absence of a hospital bed and equipment, creative adaptation will be required.
- Consider the need for a bed that places the bedridden client at caregiver's waist level.
- Teach caregivers to change client's position every 1 to 2 hours if possible, to maintain musculoskeletal alignment, and to reduce pressure on bony prominences. Develop a realistic turning schedule that is posted.

Long-Term Care Considerations

- Clients who have maintained bed rest for a long period of time may revert back to a favorite position. Frequently assess these clients, and turn more often as needed.
- Use lift (draw) sheet as often as possible to prevent shearing force on fragile skin.
- Allow client to assist with moving and positioning whenever possible to promote independence.

Skill 6.2

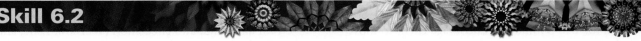

Minimizing Orthostatic Hypotension

Orthostatic or postural hypotension involves a drop in blood pressure when changing from the horizontal to a sitting or standing position (McCance and Huether, 2002; Phipps, Sands, and Marek, 1999). A drop in blood pressure of approximately 15 mm Hg in systolic pressure and 10 mm Hg in diastolic pressure with symptoms of dizziness, pallor, or fainting indicates orthostatic hypotension (Winslow, Lane, and Woods, 1995). Orthostatic hypotension may be related to bed rest, hypovolemia (decreased circulating blood volume), hypokalemia (low serum potassium level), and certain medications, including sedatives, hypnotics, analgesics, antihypertensives, antiemetics, antihistamines, diuretics, and antianxiety agents (McFarland and McFarlane, 1997).

ASSESSMENT

1. Assess blood pressure, pulse readings, and client's current activity level. *Rationale: Provides a baseline to determine if client tolerates position change.*
2. Identify factors that may precipitate orthostatic hypotension, including decreased intravascular volume, hypokalemia, prolonged immobility, and medications. *Rationale: Alerts the caregiver to potential preexisting medical conditions that contribute to orthostatic hypotension.*

PLANNING

Expected outcomes focus on preventing hypotension and increasing tolerance of activity with minimal risk of falls.

Expected Outcomes

1. Client demonstrates no evidence of weakness, light-headedness, diaphoresis, dizziness, or decrease in blood pressure greater than 15 mm Hg (systolic) to 10 mm Hg (diastolic) in response to sitting or standing.
2. Client describes interventions to minimize orthostatic hypotension and prevent injury.
3. Client ambulates 10 feet while maintaining blood pressure within systolic baseline.

Equipment

- Blood pressure equipment
- Stethoscope

Delegation Considerations

The following information is needed when delegating the skill of position changes to minimize orthostatic hypotension to nursing staff or family members:
- Have client wear shoes with a nonslip surface during transfer or ambulation.
- Make slow, gradual position changes.
- Observe client for nausea, pallor, and dizziness.
- Have client sit in chair or return to bed if client has symptoms of orthostatic hypotension.

When assisting with ambulation:
- Do not try to hold clients if they become dizzy or faint. Ease them into a sitting position in a chair or onto the floor (Skill 5-1, p. 84).
- Use assistive devices such as walkers, crutches, or cane when appropriate.
- Be sure the area is free of clutter, wet areas, and rugs that may slide.

IMPLEMENTATION FOR MINIMIZING ORTHOSTATIC HYPOTENSION

Steps	Rationale

1. See Standard Protocol (inside front cover).
2. Explain reason for gradual position change.

COMMUNICATION TIP *Include family in explanation. Explain to client the importance of slow, gradual position change to minimize dizziness, light-headedness.*

3. Raise head of bed slowly to semi-Fowler's and then to high-Fowler's position and reassess blood pressure, pulse, and respirations. Instruct client to report any dizziness or light-headedness during position change.

   Raising slowly allows body to adjust to change in position. If client has a drop in blood pressure when upright, orthostatic hypotension is evident and risk of falls significant (Winslow, Lane, and Woods, 1995).

4. If no evidence of hypotension occurs, proceed to dangle client (allow feet to hang over the side of the bed for 1 to 3 minutes). Encourage client to move shoulders in circles and flex and extend ankles and knees. Reassess blood pressure.

   Allows autonomic nervous system to adapt to postural changes. Movement of muscles increases venous return and stimulates circulation (Winslow, Lane, and Woods, 1995).

5. If there are no signs of orthostatic hypotension, proceed with planned activity.

NURSE ALERT *DO NOT attempt to ambulate if client reports dizziness, nausea, or appears pale. Lower head and allow client to rest for a few minutes, and try again more gradually.*

6. See Completion Protocol (inside front cover).

• • • • • • • • • •

EVALUATION

1. Observe client for signs of weakness, dizziness, and pallor.
2. Obtain blood pressure, pulse, and respirations if client experiences weakness or dizziness at any point and on completion of activity. Normally blood pressure, pulse, and respirations increase slightly in response to exercise and return to baseline within 5 minutes of resting.

3. Ask client to describe interventions to minimize orthostatic hypotension and prevent injury (e.g., slow, gradual position changes; remain in bed/chair if dizzy or light-headed; do not attempt to ambulate without assistance).

Unexpected Outcomes and Related Interventions

1. Client becomes light-headed and dizzy when upright.
   a. Return client to supine position.
   b. If client faints, lower to floor safely.
   c. Take blood pressure immediately.
   d. After 3 to 5 minutes, attempt the same procedure. If unsuccessful, wait 1 to 2 hours before attempting again.

Recording and Reporting

- Resting pulse and blood pressure
- Type of exercise/exertion
- Pulse and blood pressure after activity
- Subjective response (dizziness, weakness)

Sample Documentation

0900 BP 110/70, pulse 86, respirations 18 in supine position. Assisted to sitting position over 1 minute. Complained of dizziness. BP 90/50, pulse 102, respirations 22. Assisted back to supine position.

0905 Assisted to upright position over 3 minutes without dizziness. BP 104/72, pulse 90, respirations 20.

0908 Ambulated to bathroom slowly with steady gait. Stated, "I feel weak, but not dizzy."

0930 Sitting in chair; BP 112/70, pulse 88, respirations 20.

SPECIAL CONSIDERATIONS

Pediatric Considerations

- Children who have volume losses resulting in dehydration have an increased potential for orthostatic hypotension (Hockenberry and others, 2003).
- Maintain hydration status and provide safety precautions to prevent falls or injuries.

Geriatric Considerations

- Older adults who have volume losses or have undergone prolonged bed rest have greater risk for hypotension with postural change (Lueckenotte, 2000).
- Clients using medications to reduce blood pressure are at greater risk for orthostatic hypotension.

Home Care Considerations

- Instruct family or caregiver in the rationale for slow, gradual position change.
- Instruct family or caregiver in the use of a gait belt and correct body mechanics for transfer of client.
- Instruct family or caregiver to not attempt ambulation if client complains of dizziness or light-headedness.

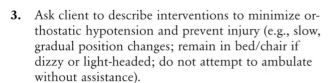

Skill 6.3

Transferring From Bed to Chair

Moving clients to a chair after bed rest stimulates them physically and mentally and promotes involvement in self-care activities. It is important to allow clients to proceed at their own pace, encouraging as much independence as possible. Transfers may be from bed to chair, wheelchair, or bedside commode.

ASSESSMENT

1. Assess muscle strength of legs and upper arms, comparing right with left. *Rationale: Clients with hemiplegia have weakness on one side. Clients with paraplegia may have spastic or flaccid paralysis.*
2. Assess joint mobility and limitations caused by contractures or discomfort. Assess for history of osteoporosis. *Rationale: Osteoporosis increases risk of pathological fractures with minimal stress.*
3. Assess vision, hearing, and altered sensation. Assess ability to follow verbal instructions and appropriateness of response to simple commands. *Rationale: Determines the extent to which the client is able to assist during a transfer.*
4. Assess client's level of motivation. *Rationale: Clients who fear falling may avoid activity or make excuses.*
5. Determine the position and functioning of IV tubing and poles, need for oxygen therapy, Foley catheter, surgical drains, and other drains or tubes. *Rationale: Prevents accidental removal of client's tubes and drains.*
6. Assess the need for prescribed analgesic medication before transfer. Plan activity for the period in which adequate pain relief is apparent without dizziness or excessive sedation. *Rationale: Analgesics enhance client's ability to tolerate movement. Peak levels vary according to the specific analgesic and route of administration.*

PLANNING

Expected outcomes focus on improving the client's functional abilities and strength. It is also essential to promote body alignment and safety.

Expected Outcomes

1. Client assists with transfer to chair by standing erect, pivoting, and grasping arm of chair to sit.
2. Client tolerates sitting in chair 30 to 40 minutes and is able to shift weight independently, at least every 15 minutes.
3. Client expresses benefit from change of environment while in the chair.

Equipment

- Gait belt/transfer belt
- Nonskid footwear
- Bath blanket
- Pillows
- Wheelchair: position chair close to bed, lock brakes, and remove or fold footrests out of the way.
- Bedside commode or supportive chair

Delegation Considerations

The skills of safe and effective transfer from bed to chair can be delegated to assistive personnel (AP) who have successfully demonstrated good body mechanics and safe transfer techniques for clients involved.

IMPLEMENTATION FOR TRANSFERRING FROM BED TO CHAIR

Steps	Rationale
1. See Standard Protocol (inside front cover).	
2. Position the chair or wheelchair so that the move will be toward client's stronger side. Chair should be at an appropriate distance to allow client participation and safety.	Facilitates balance and movement.
3. Lower bed to lowest position. Lower side rails, and turn client to one side with knees flexed.	

NURSE ALERT *When in doubt about the ability to transfer a client safely, nurses should request assistance. It is advisable to use a gait (transfer) belt.*

NURSE ALERT *Check the equipment to be used, and familiarize yourself with safety factors involved, such as wheelchair brakes, removable arm, adjustable footrest or leg rest, and reclining features.*

Steps	Rationale
4. Raise the head of the bed to the highest position. Wait a minute and ask if client feels dizzy.	Minimizes onset of orthostatic hypotension (see Skill 6.2, p. 121).
5. Face client with feet comfortably apart and a broad base of support.	Maximizes nurse's stability and balance and prevents twisting that could result in muscle strain.
6. Assist client to the sitting position by lifting upper body as the legs swing over edge of the bed (see illustrations).	Client should be able to place feet flat on floor for balance and stability.

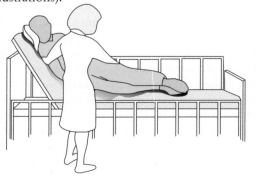

Step 6 Assisting client to sitting position.

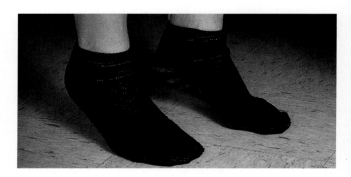

Step 9 Nonskid slippers.

7. Encourage client to assist as much as possible as legs and feet are assisted over side of bed and client's shoulders are raised.

8. Instruct client to take a deep breath and sit upright for 1 to 2 minutes. Encourage movement of shoulders, legs, feet, and toes. Apply gait belt around client's waist.

    Muscle activity promotes venous circulation and allows adjustment to the sitting position. Gait belt offers means to transfer client safely.

9. Assist client with putting on nonskid slippers or shoes and placing feet flat on the floor (see illustration).

10. Spread feet apart. Flex hips and knees, aligning knees with client's knees (see illustration).

    Flexion of knees and hips lowers nurse's center of gravity to object to be raised; aligning knees with client's allows for stabilization of knees when client stands.

COMMUNICATION TIP *Psychological support and encouragement during transfer is important.*

---

11. Apply a sling if client has flaccid arm.
12. Grasp gait belt from underneath.

    Supports arm and prevents stress or injury.
    Gait belt is grasped at client's side to provide movement of client at center of gravity. Client with upper extremity paralysis or paresis should never be lifted by or under arms.

NURSE ALERT *A gait belt or walking belt with handles should be used in place of the under-axilla technique. The under-axilla technique has been found to be physically stressful for nurses and uncomfortable for clients (Owens, Welden, and Kane, 1999).*

---

13. Rock client up to standing position on count of three while straightening hips and legs and keeping knees slightly flexed (see illustration). Unless contraindicated, client may be instructed to use hands to push up if applicable.

    Rocking motion gives client's body momentum and requires less muscular effort to lift client.

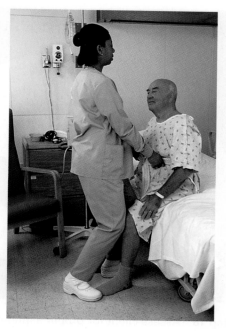

Step 10 Nurse flexes hips and knees, aligning with client's knees.

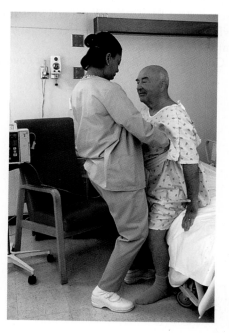

Step 13 Nurse rocks client to standing position.

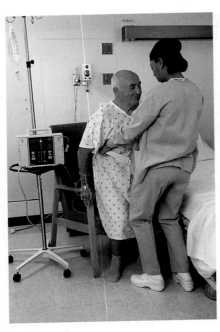

Step 16   Client uses armrest for support.

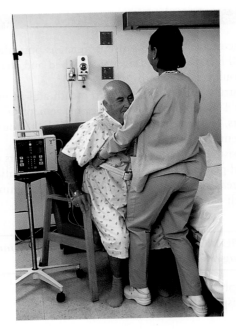

Step 17   Nurse eases client into chair.

Steps	Rationale
14. Maintain stability of client's weak or paralyzed leg with your knee.	Ability to stand can often be maintained in paralyzed or weak limb with support of knee to stabilize.
15. Once standing, pivot client toward seat of chair. Client should then reach for arm of chair and assist with easing self into chair.	
16. Instruct client to use armrests on chair for support and ease into chair (see illustration).	Increases client's stability.
17. Flex hips and knees while lowering client into chair (see illustration).	
18. Observe client for proper alignment for sitting. Provide pillows to support affected (paralyzed) extremities (see illustration).	
19. See Completion Protocol (inside front cover).	

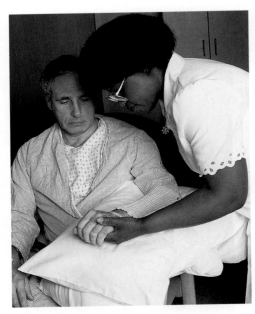

Step 18   Assess client for proper alignment.

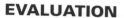
EVALUATION

1. Observe client's ability to bear weight (or avoid bearing weight if prescribed), ability to pivot, and number of personnel needed. Ask client to describe level of strength and control.
2. Monitor length of time client sits in chair and ability to shift weight every 15 minutes.
3. Ask client to describe response to environmental and positional changes.

Unexpected Outcomes and Related Interventions

1. Client does not follow directions for transfer.
   a. Identify interfering factors (e.g., anxiety) and provide positive reinforcement for effort and achievement.
   b. Demonstrate the procedure for the client in a step-by-step manner.
2. Client's weakness of lower extremities does not permit active transfer.
   a. Consider physical therapy consultation.
   b. Develop a plan for isotonic or isometric leg-strengthening exercises to be done while lying in bed or sitting in chair.
   c. Use a gait belt for balance and support.
3. Client tends to bear weight on non–weight-bearing leg.
   a. Have another caregiver support affected leg as a reminder.
   b. Use a gait belt to facilitate balance and control.

Recording and Reporting

- Ability to bear weight and pivot
- Length of time in chair
- Subjective response

Sample Documentation

0800 Transferred client from bed to chair with gait belt and assistance of one. Cooperative and able to stand erect with encouragement.

0815 Requested to return to bed. Stated, "I'm so tired, I just can't sit up any longer." Needed assistance of two with transfer back to bed. Knees buckled and legs were shaking during attempt to stand.

SPECIAL CONSIDERATIONS

Pediatric Considerations
- Children should be encouraged to be as active as their condition and restrictive devices allow. Opportunity, materials, or objects to stimulate activity and encouragement and participation of others must be available.
- Children's activities always require special safety precautions.

Geriatric Considerations
- Older persons who fear falling may be reluctant to move from bed to chair.
- Older adult clients who are depressed often prefer to stay in bed, especially when accustomed to being very independent and active and now need assistance.

Home Care Considerations
- Transfer ability at home is greatly enhanced by prior teaching of family, assessment of home for safety risks and functionality, and provision of applicable aids.
- Family should practice transfer in hospital to achieve success before taking client home.
- Alternatively, client (if living alone) should practice activities as they will be used at home, commode, and shower. Clients should be taught to transfer to armchairs for ease of rising and sitting.
- Home should be free of risks (i.e., throw rugs, electric cords, slippery floors). If wheelchair is used, access must be possible through all doors, and space for transfer must be available in bedroom and bathroom.

Long-Term Considerations
Allow client to assist with moving and positioning whenever possible to promote independence.

Skill 6.4

Using a Mechanical (Hoyer) Lift for Transfer From Bed to Chair

Mechanical lifts are used to transfer large, dependent clients who do not have spinal cord injury. Use of a lift does not require assistance from the client and should be used only when required.

NURSE ALERT *Before using the device, practice using controls that spread the base to provide stability, the lever that raises the sling, and the release that lowers the sling.*

ASSESSMENT

1. Compare the weight limit for the lift with the client's current weight. *Rationale: Mechanical (Hoyer) lifts have a maximum weight-carrying capacity.*
2. Assess client's muscle strength of legs and upper arms, joint mobility, and limitations from contractures or discomfort. *Rationale: Overextension of contracted joints can cause the client pain or discomfort.*
3. Assess client's heart rate and blood pressure. *Rationale: Provides baseline to determine if client's cardiovascular status changes during transfer.*
4. Assess client's level of motivation. *Rationale: Clients who fear falling may avoid being transferred.*

PLANNING

Expected outcomes focus on promoting safety and comfort during the transfer.

Expected Outcomes

1. Client verbalizes feeling secure and comfortable during transfer.
2. Client transfers safely.
3. Client maintains correct body alignment after transfer.
4. Client maintains heart rate and systolic blood pressure within 10% of resting baseline during transfer.

Equipment

* Mechanical (Hoyer) lift: hydraulic lift frame with supporting boom and attached chains, canvas sling (Figure 6-3).
* Pillows
* Chair/Wheelchair

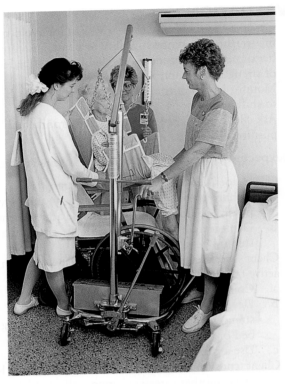

Figure 6-3   Mechanical (Hoyer) lift.

Delegation Considerations

The skill of safe and effective transfer using a Hoyer lift can be delegated to assistive personnel (AP) who have demonstrated ability to use good body mechanics and safe transfer techniques, as well as equipment (Hoyer lift).

IMPLEMENTATION FOR USING A MECHANICAL (HOYER) LIFT FOR TRANSFERRING FROM BED TO CHAIR

Steps	Rationale

1. See Standard Protocol (inside front cover).
2. Ask another caregiver to assist. Move the lift to the bedside. Place a comfortable chair with supportive arms in a convenient location.

COMMUNICATION TIP *A mechanical lift may frighten the client. Reassurance and ability to convey knowledge of procedure by caregivers will decrease anxiety.*

3. Raise the bed to a comfortable height. Turn client to side, and place the canvas sling under the client, extending from popliteal space of the knees to beneath the head. The hole of the canvas is placed under the buttocks. Turn client to opposite side to center sling placement.

Raises bed to accommodate nurses' center of gravity and thus maintains proper body mechanics.

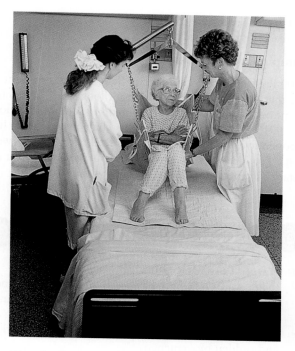

Step 8   Proper placement of sling under client.

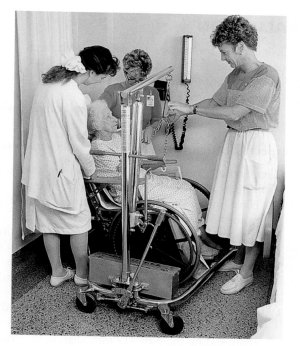

Step 11   Removal of hydraulic lift.

Steps	Rationale
4. With the client lying supine and arms crossed over the body, position the lift with the base under the bed and spread the base of the lift.	A broad base of support enhances stability and prevents tipping.
5. Attach the shorter chains to the section of the sling (may be narrower) that supports the upper body.	
6. Raise the boom slightly, and attach the longer chains to the (wider) sling that supports the hips and thighs.	It may help if one caregiver supports and flexes the client's knees as another attaches the chains to the sling.
7. Adjust the sling as necessary so that the client's weight is evenly distributed.	Promotes stability and security during the move.
8. Pump the lift to elevate it just enough to clear the bed, and guide client's legs over the side (see illustration).	
9. Instruct client to keep arms folded during the transfer.	Keeps the device balanced and prevents injury from bumping against objects.
10. Check the chair's position and stability before the move. While supporting the client, guide the lift to-ward the chair, commode, or wheelchair so that when the boom is lowered, client will be centered in the chair.	

NURSE ALERT   *Apply brakes on wheelchair. If transferring to a chair or com-mode, have another caregiver hold on to the chair or commode to prevent move-ment or slippage while client is lowered.*

---

11. Release valve slowly, and lower client into the chair. Protect client's head from striking the equipment. Once client is securely seated, remove the chains and store the lift nearby (see illustration).	Leaving the sling under client facilitates transfer back to bed.
12. See Completion Protocol (inside front cover).	

• • • • • • • • • •

EVALUATION

1. Ask client if the transfer felt safe, smooth, and comfortable.
2. Observe client transfers.
3. Observe for correct body alignment.
4. Measure heart rate and blood pressure, compare with baseline.

Unexpected Outcomes and Related Interventions

1. Client's buttocks are too far forward in the chair seat, resulting in a slouched position.
   a. Have one caregiver stand in front of client to push the pelvis back into the chair.
   b. A second caregiver stands behind client, placing arms under client's axillae and grasping client's wrists, which places the force on client's arms rather than at axillae and prevents injury from pressure on axillae.
   c. As caregiver behind client lifts upward, second caregiver pushes the knees toward back of the chair, sliding the buttocks into alignment. Avoid shearing forces.
2. Client develops orthostatic BP changes (Skill 6-2).
   a. Have client extend and flex knees and ankles to encourage venous blood flow.
   b. If dizziness increases, have client lower head and close eyes, and encourage deep breaths.
   c. Reassess blood pressure in 5 minutes.

Recording and Reporting

- Type of equipment and number of caregivers
- Client's subjective response
- Teaching performed

Sample Documentation

0900 Refuses to transfer to chair. Stated, "I do not want to use that thing (Hoyer lift); it doesn't look safe." Instructed client on use of Hoyer lift; provided mock demonstration.

0915 Transferred from bed to chair using Hoyer lift. Cooperative with move. Stated, "I felt very secure with that." Propped with pillows and encouraged to call for assistance if uncomfortable. Call light within reach.

SPECIAL CONSIDERATIONS

Geriatric Considerations

- Older clients may have fragile skin that tears easily and tissues that bruise easily. Take care to provide padding and prevent pinching of tissues during the transfer.
- Explain each step in simple language, and avoid jerky and sudden movements

Home Care Considerations

- Transfer ability at home is greatly enhanced by prior teaching of family and support persons, assessment of home for safety risks and functionality, and provision of applicable aids.
- Family or support person should practice transfer in hospital to achieve success before taking client home. Arrangements must be made for home health nurse to continue to assist family or support person at home.

Skill 6.5

Transferring From Bed to Stretcher

This transfer involves movement from the bed to a stretcher for client transport from one department to another, to surgery, or for diagnostic tests when the client is too ill to tolerate sitting, client is sedated, or diagnostic equipment requires a supine position.

ASSESSMENT

1. Assess client's level of consciousness and ability to cooperate with the move. *Rationale: Determine client's ability to assist as much as possible to promote independence and a sense of control over situation.*
2. Assess client's joint mobility and limitations. *Rationale: Overextension of contracted or arthritic joints can cause the client extreme pain or discomfort.*
3. Assess client's pain, including location and severity. When appropriate, offer prescribed analgesic medication before transfer. *Rationale: Analgesics enhance client's ability to tolerate movement. Peak levels vary according to the specific analgesic and route of administration.*

PLANNING

Expected outcomes focus on comfort and safety.

Expected Outcomes

1. Client follows instructions for transfer to stretcher.
2. Client is transferred safely.
3. Client verbalizes feeling comfortable and secure during transfer.

Equipment

- Stretcher with side rails or safety straps and brake locks
- IV pole (if needed and not attached to stretcher)
- Roller device or plastic slider board (heavy plastic to minimize shearing forces while sliding client)
- Bath blanket or sheet
- Pillow

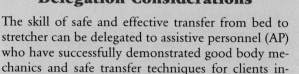

Delegation Considerations

The skill of safe and effective transfer from bed to stretcher can be delegated to assistive personnel (AP) who have successfully demonstrated good body mechanics and safe transfer techniques for clients involved. Clients who have acute spinal trauma or multiple acute injuries may require transfer and moving by nurses.

IMPLEMENTATION FOR TRANSFERRING FROM BED TO STRETCHER

Steps	Rationale

1. See Standard Protocol (inside front cover).

COMMUNICATION TIP
- *Caution client not to move until all caregivers are in position. Explain to client to fold arms over chest to facilitate transfer.*
- *Reassure client that move will be made slowly and gently according to client's level of tolerance.*

2. Position the bed flat, and raise to the same height as the stretcher. Lower side rails.

3. Cover client with a sheet or bath blanket, and remove top covers of the bed without exposing client.

4. Check for IV line, Foley catheter, tubes, or surgical drains, and position them to avoid tension during the move.

5. Position the stretcher as close to the bed as possible, and lock the wheels of the bed and stretcher. Side rails should be lowered (see illustration).   Aligns stretcher and bed for safe transfer.

6. Transfer when client can assist

  a. Stand near the side of the stretcher, and instruct client to move feet, then buttocks, and finally upper body to the stretcher, bringing cover along.   Promotes safety and security.

  b. After moving, check to be sure client's body is centered on the stretcher.

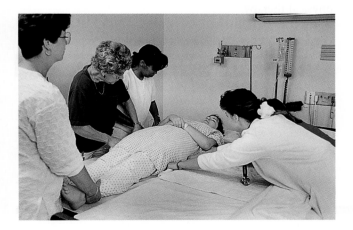

Step 5   Proper placement of stretcher and personnel.

Steps	Rationale

7. Client is unable to assist

NURSE ALERT *As many as five caregivers may be required for a safe transfer of a heavy client who cannot assist.*

---

a. Place a folded sheet or bath blanket under the client so that it supports client's head and extends to midthighs.

b. Roll the ends of the sheet or bath blanket close to client's body. Assist client with crossing arms over chest.

c. Two caregivers reach over the bed to client, and two caregivers stand as close as possible to the stretcher. A fifth caregiver stands at the foot of the bed to lift the feet (see illustration).

d. Using a coordinating count of three, all five caregivers simultaneously lift client to edge of the bed.

e. With another coordinated lift, move client from edge of the bed to the stretcher.

8. Raise both side rails and head of the stretcher if desired.

9. Instruct client to keep hands inside while moving and to avoid grasping side rail, which could bump against door frames during transport.

10. See Completion Protocol (inside front cover).

Pull sheet will be used to transfer client.

Being closer to weight being lifted reduces risk of back injury to caregiver.

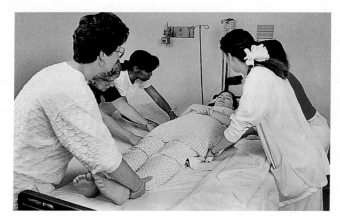

Step 7c   Transfer of client unable to assist.

• • • • • • • • • • •

EVALUATION

1. Observe client's ability to follow instructions and assist with transfer.
2. Ask client if the transfer felt safe, smooth, and comfortable.
3. Ask client if change in environment was positive.

Unexpected Outcomes and Related Interventions

1. Client resists transfer and interferes with move by grasping bed or caregivers.
    a. Explain reason for transfer to encourage client's cooperation.
    b. Identify client's reasons for resisting transfer.
    c. Assess for the possibility of premedication for pain before transfer.

Recording and Reporting

• Equipment used and number of caregivers
• Subjective response of client
• Destination for transport

Sample Documentation

1030 Attempt transfer to stretcher with assistance of staff. Client reports incisional pain and refuses transfer at this time. States that pain is at a 7 on a scale of 1 to 10 (10 being the worst). Tylenol #3 given.

1100 States pain is subsiding.

1115 Rates pain at level 2 and is ready to transfer to stretcher. Reports comfortable transfer. Transported to physical therapy.

❂ SPECIAL CONSIDERATIONS ❂

Pediatric Considerations
Whenever possible, transporting child by stretcher, stroller, or wheelchair outside confines of room will increase environmental stimuli and provide social contact with others.

Skill 6.6

Assisting With Ambulation

In the normal walking posture, the head is erect; the cervical, thoracic, and lumbar vertebrae are aligned; the hips and knees have slight flexion; and the arms swing freely. Illness, surgery, injury, and prolonged bed rest can reduce activity tolerance so that assistance is required. Clients with hemiparesis (one-sided weakness) have difficulty with balance. Temporary or permanent damage to the musculoskeletal or nervous system may necessitate use of an assistive device such as a cane, crutches, or walker (see Skill 6-7, p. 135). Clients with altered cardiovascular or respiratory function may experience difficulty with ambulation, evidenced by chest pain, altered vital signs, dyspnea, or fatigue.

ASSESSMENT

1. Assess client's most recent activity experience, including distance ambulated and tolerance of activity. *Rationale: This facilitates realistic planning and identifies degree of assistance needed.*
2. Determine the best time to ambulate, considering other scheduled activities such as bathing and physical therapy. *Rationale: Rest is needed after activities requiring exertion and after meals. Energy is needed to digest food.*
3. Check the availability of handrails on the walls. Consider whether the assistance of one or two caregivers is required, and determine the need for an assistive device.
4. Observe the environment, and remove obstacles such as chairs, tables, and equipment. If client has an IV line, a rolling IV pole is needed. *Rationale: Provides a safe, clutter-free environment.*
5. Assess client's motivation and ability to cooperate. *Rationale: Comparing this activity with client plans for the home environment often enhances motivation.*
6. Assess for medications that may alter stability, including antihypertensive or narcotic medications. *Rationale: These drugs may cause hypotension, dizziness, or instability.*

7. Before beginning ambulation assess baseline vital signs. *Rationale: Postambulation vital signs can be compared to baseline to determine client's activity tolerance.*

PLANNING

Expected outcomes focus on developing activity and rest patterns that support increased tolerance of activity. It is essential that these are tailored to each client's needs and abilities.

Expected Outcomes

1. Client will ambulate without episode of injury.
2. Client is able to ambulate without excessive fatigue or dizziness.
3. Client maintains respirations, pulse, and blood pressure within 10% of resting values.
4. Client maintains erect posture while standing and walking.

Equipment

- Robe
- Nonskid footwear
- Portable IV pole
- Gait belt (required for clients with unsteady gait or balance)

Delegation Considerations

The skill of assisting the client with ambulation may be delegated to assistive personnel (AP). The following information is needed when delegating this skill to nursing staff or family members:
- Have client wear shoes with a nonskid surface during ambulation.
- Do not try to hold clients if they become dizzy or faint. Ease them into a sitting position in a chair or on the floor (Skill 5-1, p. 84).
- Be sure the area is free of clutter, wet areas, and rugs that may slide or buckle.

IMPLEMENTATION FOR ASSISTING WITH AMBULATION

Steps	Rationale
1. See Standard Protocol (inside front cover)	

COMMUNICATION TIP
- *Explain importance of nonskid shoes or slippers.*
- *Encourage client to move slowly at own pace, maintain erect posture, and look straight ahead.*

Steps	Rationale
2. Assist the client with putting on shoes or slippers with nonslip soles.	Provides stable walking support.
3. Assist client to stand at the bedside. Encourage to stand fully erect with shoulders back and looking ahead (not at the floor).	Standing at bedside allows client opportunity to stabilize before ambulating.
4. If client is unstable, seat client and apply safety belt before proceeding. Consider need for additional help. If client is very heavy, unstable, or fearful, a second person is needed.	Provides added stability.
5. If client has an IV line, place the IV pole on the same side as the site of infusion, and instruct client to hold and push the pole while ambulating (see illustration).	
6. If a Foley catheter is present, client or caregiver carries the bag below the level of the bladder and prevents tension on the tubing.	Prevents reflux of urine from the bag back into bladder.
7. Take a few steps supporting client with one arm around the waist and the other under the elbow of the flexed arm. Grasp gait belt in the middle of client's waist.	This provides balance and facilitates lowering client to the floor if client is unable to continue because of weakness or dizziness.
8. When ambulating in a hallway, position client between yourself and the wall. Encourage client to use handrails if available.	The wall provides stable support for clients who start to fall away from nurse.
9. See Completion Protocol (inside front cover).	

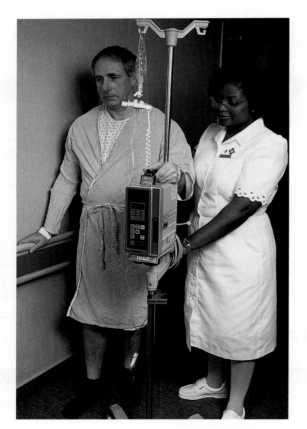

Step 5   Assisting a client with ambulation.

• • • • • • • • • •

EVALUATION

1. Observe client ambulating.
2. Observe tolerance of the activity by noting the frequency of rest periods.
3. Compare client's heart rate, respiratory rate, and blood pressure with baseline values immediately after ambulation and again after 5 minutes of rest.
4. Observe client's body alignment and balance while standing and walking.

Unexpected Outcomes and Related Interventions

1. Vital signs are altered: pulse more than 10% to 20% over resting rate or greater than 120 beats per minute; systolic blood pressure shows orthostatic changes; or dyspnea, labored breathing, and wheezing present. Client reports feelings of excessive fatigue or weakness.
    a. Plan activity after adequate rest period.
    b. Pace activity to proceed more slowly, and allow time to stop and rest at regular intervals. Sitting periodically may be helpful.
    c. Provide a wheelchair to be pushed by the client to provide balance and support.
    d. Assistive devices such as a cane or walker may decrease energy required (see Skill 6.7).
2. Client starts to fall.
    a. Call for help.
    b. Put both arms around client's waist from behind and spread feet apart for a broad base of support.
    c. If necessary, ease client slowly to the floor, bending knees to prevent strain on back muscles.
    d. Stay with client until assistance arrives to help lift client to wheelchair.

Recording and Reporting

*   Distance ambulated
*   Client's subjective response
*   Changes in vital signs

Sample Documentation

1300 Ambulated client 100 feet in hall with assistance of one. Gait steady. States, "I am so tired, I don't know if I can make it back to my room." Gait steady. B/P 160/82, heart rate 120. Placed in wheelchair.

1305 Back in bed with assistance. B/P 145/78, heart rate 92. Denies dizziness.

1315 Resting comfortably at this time. No complaints voiced. States, "I think I overdid it." B/P 130/70, heart rate 80.

SPECIAL CONSIDERATIONS

Geriatric Considerations
*   Older clients are often fearful of falling when ambulatory. Encouragement, reassurance, and assistance from family or caregiver decreases anxiety.
*   Older adults may need more time in the morning to resume activity.

Skill 6.7

Teaching Use of Cane, Crutches, and Walker

Assistive devices (i.e., canes, crutches, and walkers) are usually recommended for clients who cannot bear full weight on one or more joints of the lower extremities. Other indications for their use are instability, poor balance, or pain in weight bearing. Nurses are expected to supervise clients in using their assistive devices correctly (Phipps, Sands, and Marek, 1999). It is important for the nurse to know the client's weight-bearing status and any specific movement precautions ordered by the physician. The wrong weight-bearing status or improper movement can cause further damage to the injured extremity.

Non–weight-bearing status requires the client to support weight on the assistive device and the unaffected limb. The affected leg is kept off the floor at all times. Partial or touch-down weight bearing is similar to that for non–weight bearing, but either limb can be advanced initially. Partial weight bearing more closely approximates normal walking except that less weight is placed on the affected limb. Total weight bearing allows the client to distribute equal weight between each limb with minimal weight on the assistive device. Muscle-strengthening exercises such as knee-and-foot extension (kicking leg straight out while sitting in a chair) or hip flexion (marching while sitting in a chair) and walking in parallel bars help the client increase strength and confidence before using an assistive device.

Rubber tips on the ends of assistive devices prevent slipping when using any of the aids. Teaching to lift rather than slide the device lessens the possibility of catching the tips, which could cause the user to lose balance, trip, or fall. Personnel should attend to clients when using an assistive device until they are assured that the client's understanding and strength are sufficient for safe solo ambulation. Observing unaccompanied clients on their walks may reveal a need for attendance and/or additional or continued reminding about the amount of weight permitted or the distance covered.

CANES

Canes primarily increase the person's security and balance by broadening the base of support. Canes also absorb or take the body weight when necessary for mobility during partial weight-bearing periods. Instruction for use of cane-assisted ambulation is required to assess the client's balance, strength, and confidence. When canes are unilaterally used, they are most often used opposite the weak or injured side and are advanced forward with the injured or affected limb.

CRUTCHES

Persons using one or two crutches as aids for ambulation are frequently seen. The user's proficiency varies with age, condition, degree or extent of injury, musculoskeletal functions, and so on. Use of crutches may be a temporary aid for persons with sprains, in a cast, or following surgical treatments; crutches may be routinely and continuously used for those with congenital or acquired musculoskeletal anomalies, neuromuscular weakness, or paralysis; or they may be used after amputations.

Placing the crutches in an easily accessible and safe location is the first requirement when crutches are used to rise to a standing position. Accessible sites are on the back or side of the chair or upright against a near cabinet or wall. The hand rests of the crutches may be used for bracing while rising if the chair is solid and heavy enough to preclude tipping, and if only one arm is to be used with the crutches for bracing while rising. If the chair is lightweight, both armrests should be used for even bracing while rising, and then the crutches placed for ambulating. When sitting down or rising, the client should be instructed to use either both armrests, or one armrest and both crutches together, to maintain balance. Balance can be lost or chairs can be tipped from uneven or one-sided pressure.

WALKERS

Constructed of aluminum or metallic alloys, walkers are lightweight aids strong enough to withstand prolonged use. Heights are adjustable for individual needs. The use of a walker facilitates partial, full, or non–weight bearing. Before using a walker, the client should understand the specific amount of weight bearing permitted or non–weight

bearing to be maintained and how to use and care for the walker. Demonstrating the technique to be used for a particular client is beneficial, because techniques vary for non–weight bearing on one extremity versus partial weight bearing. For both walking activities, the assistant supports the client to prevent loss of balance, tipping, or uneven balance on the walker.

ASSESSMENT

1. Review client's chart, including medical history, previous activity level, and current activity order. *Rationale: Reveals client's current and previous health status.*
2. Assess client's physical readiness: vital signs; presence of confusion; and orientation to time, place, and person. *Rationale: Baseline vital signs offer a means of comparison after exercise. Level of orientation or confusion may reveal risk for fall.*
3. Assess ROM and muscle strength or the presence of foot deformities. *Rationale: Determines if assistance is needed for client to ambulate safely.*
4. Assess client for any visual, perceptual, or sensory deficits. *Rationale: Determines if client can use assistive device safely.*
5. Assess environment for potential threats to client safety (e.g., bed brake, bed position, objects in pathway). Make sure floor is dry and area is well lighted. *Rationale: Provides for a safe, clutter-free environment.*
6. Assess client for discomfort. *Rationale: Determines if client needs prescribed analgesic before exercise.*
7. Assess client's understanding of technique of ambulation to be used. *Rationale: Allows client to verbalize concerns.*

PLANNING

Expected outcomes focus on improving mobility, minimizing activity intolerance, preventing risk for injury, minimizing fatigue, and improving client's knowledge.

Expected Outcomes

1. Client demonstrates correct use of assistive device.
2. Client demonstrates correct gait pattern and weight-bearing status.
3. Client rates pain/discomfort as 4 or less on a scale of 0 to 10 during ambulation.
4. Client performs activities with return of vital signs to baseline 3 to 5 minutes after rest.
5. Client independently performs all ADLs using assistive device safely.

Equipment

- Ambulation device (cane, crutches, walker)
- Well-fitting, flat shoes or slippers with nonskid soles
- Robe; well-fitting pants or dress
- Gait belt

Delegation Considerations

Teaching the client the use of assistive devices requires critical thinking and knowledge application unique to a nurse. However, assistive personnel (AP) may assist clients who ambulate with assistive devices.

- Have client wear shoes with a nonskid surface during ambulation.
- Be sure the area is free of clutter, wet areas, and rugs that may slide or buckle.
- Make sure client uses the correct gait and weight bearing during ambulation.
- Ease client to a sitting position in a chair or on the floor if he or she becomes dizzy or faint.
- Alert the nurse if client becomes dizzy or light-headed or suffers a fall.

IMPLEMENTATION FOR TEACHING USE OF CANE, CRUTCHES, AND WALKER

Steps	Rationale
1. See Standard Protocol (inside front cover).	

NURSE ALERT *Make sure that surface client will walk on is clean, dry, and well lighted. Remove objects that might obstruct the pathway.*

Steps	Rationale
2. Prepare client for procedure.	
a. Explain reasons for exercise and demonstrate specific gait technique to client or caregiver.	Teaching and demonstration enhance learning, reduce anxiety, and encourage cooperation.
b. Decide with client how far to ambulate.	Determines mutual goal.
c. Schedule ambulation around client's other activities.	Avoids client fatigue.
d. Place bed in low position.	Reduces risk of injury.
e. Help client put on well-fitting, flat shoes or non-skid slippers.	
f. Slowly assist client from a lying to a sitting or standing position. Assist client with standing stationary until balance is maintained. Check blood pressure as appropriate.	Prevents orthostatic hypotension.
3. Make sure that the assistive device is the appropriate height.	Wrong height causes client to expend more energy, experience greater discomfort, and feel unable to achieve adequate weight transmission through the arms (Borgman-Gainer, 1996).
4. Make sure assistive device has rubber tips.	Rubber tips increase surface tension and reduce the risk of the assistive device slipping.
5. Apply safety belt if unsure of client's stability. Gait belt encircles client's waist and has space for nurse to hold while client walks. Assist client to standing position and observe balance. If client appears weak or unsteady, return client to bed. Grasp safety belt in middle of client's back, or place hands at client's waist if safety belt is not available.	Providing constant contact by nurse reduces risk of fall or injury.

Steps	Rationale

COMMUNICATION TIP

- *Let the client know that use of the ambulation device may seem awkward at first. Independence will be gained after practice.*
- *Instruct the client to use good posture and always look ahead while using the ambulation device.*

---

6. **Cane**

a. Client should hold cane on uninvolved side 4 to 6 inches (10 to 15 cm) to side of foot. Cane should extend from greater trochanter to floor. Allow approximately 15 to 30 degrees elbow flexion.

Offers most support when on stronger side of body. Cane and weaker leg work together with each step. If cane is too short, client will have difficulty supporting weight and be bent over and uncomfortable. As weight is taken on by hands and affected leg is lifted off floor, complete extension of elbow is necessary.

b. Assist client in ambulating with cane. (Same steps are taught whether standard or quad canes are used.)

c. Begin by placing cane on the side opposite the involved leg.

Provides added support for the weak or impaired side.

d. Place cane forward 6 to 10 inches (15 to 25 cm), keeping body weight on both legs.

Distributes body weight equally.

e. Move involved leg forward, even with the cane (see illustration).

Body weight is supported by cane and uninvolved leg.

f. Advance uninvolved leg past cane.

Aligns client's center of gravity. Returns client body weight to equal distribution.

g. Move involved leg forward, even with uninvolved leg.

h. Repeat these steps.

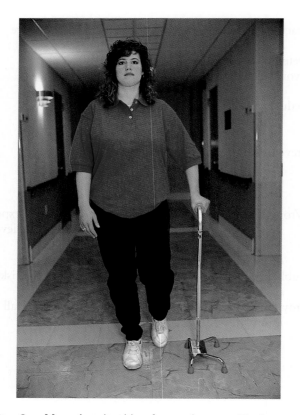

Step 6e   Move involved leg forward even with the cane.

Steps	Rationale

7. Crutches

a. Crutch measurement includes three areas: client's height, distance between crutch pad and axilla, and angle of elbow flexion. Measurements may be taken with client standing or lying down. Make sure shoes are on before performing measurements.

Measurement promotes optimal support and stability. Radial nerves that pass under axilla are superficial. If crutch is too long, it can cause pressure on axilla. Injury to nerve causes paralysis of elbow and wrist extensors, commonly called crutch palsy (Borgman-Gainer, 1996). If crutch is too long, shoulders are forced upward and client cannot push body off the ground. If ambulation device is too short, client will be bent over and uncomfortable.

NURSE ALERT *Instruct client to report any tingling or numbness in upper torso. This may mean crutches are being used incorrectly or that they are wrong size.*

---

(1) *Standing:* Position crutches with crutch tips at point 4 to 6 inches (10 to 15 cm) to side and 4 to 6 inches in front of client's feet. Position crutch pads 1½ to 2 inches (4 to 5 cm) below axilla. Two or three fingers should fit between top of crutch and axilla (see illustration).

(2) *Supine:* Crutch pad should be 3 to 4 finger-widths under axilla, with crutch tips positioned 6 inches (15 cm) lateral to client's heel (see illustration).

(3) Elbow flexion is verified with goniometer (see illustration). Handgrip should be adjusted so that client's elbow is flexed 15 to 20 degrees.

Low handgrips cause radial nerve damage. High handgrips cause client's elbow to be sharply flexed, and strength and stability of arms are decreased.

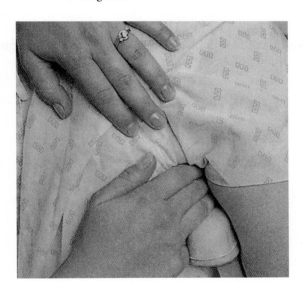

Step 7a(1)   Top of crutch.

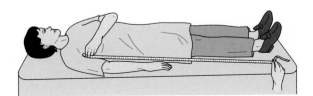

Step 7a(2)   Measuring length of crutch.

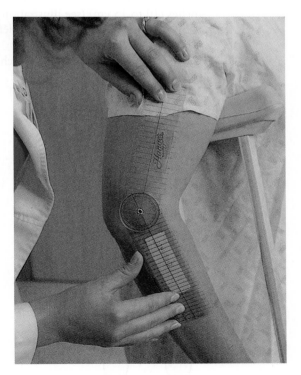

Step 7a(3)   Goniometer determines elbow flexion.

Steps	Rationale

b. To use crutches, client supports self with hands and arms. Therefore strength in arm and shoulder muscles, ability to balance body in upright position, and stamina are necessary. Type of gait client uses in crutch walking depends on amount of weight client is able to support with one or both legs.

c. Have client stand up from a sitting position.
   (1) Move to the edge of the chair, with the strong leg slightly under chair seat.
   (2) Place both of the crutches in the hand on the affected side. If chair has armrests and is heavy and solid enough to avoid tipping, one armrest and both crutches may be used for bracing while rising. If the chair is lightweight, both armrests should be used for even bracing.

   Balance can be lost or chairs tipped with uneven or one-sided pressure.

   (3) Push down on the crutch hand rests while raising the body to a standing position.

d. Choose appropriate crutch gait (darkened areas in illustrations indicate movement).
   (1) *Four-point gait*
      (a) Begin in tripod position (see illustration). Crutches are placed 6 inches (15 cm) in front and 6 inches to side of each foot. Posture should be erect head and neck, straight vertebrae, and extended hips and knees.

      Most stable of crutch gaits because it provides at least three points of support at all times. Requires weight bearing on both legs. Often used when client has paralysis, as in spastic children with cerebral palsy (Wong and others, 1999). May also be used for arthritic clients. Improves client's balance by providing wider base of support.

      (b) Move right crutch forward 4 to 6 inches (10 to 15 cm) (see illustration).

      Crutch and foot position are similar to arm and foot position during normal walking.

      (c) Move left foot forward to level of left crutch (see illustration).
      (d) Move left crutch forward 4 to 6 inches (see illustration).
      (e) Move right foot forward to level of right crutch (see illustration).
      (f) Repeat sequence.

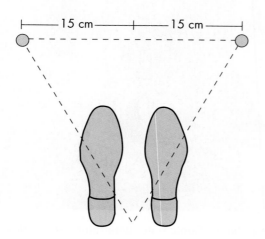

Step 7d(1a) Tripod position.

Steps	**Rationale**

(2) *Three-point gait:* Requires client to bear all weight on one foot. Weight is borne on un-involved leg, then on both crutches. Affected leg does not touch ground during early phase of three-point gait. May be useful for client with broken leg or sprained ankle.

   (a) Begin in tripod position.

                                             Improves client's balance by providing wide base of support.

   (b) Advance both crutches and affected leg (see illustration).

   (c) Move stronger leg forward.

   (d) Repeat sequence.

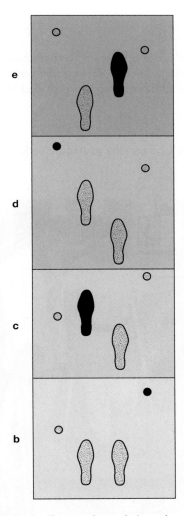

Step 7d(1b-e) Four-point gait (starting at bottom).

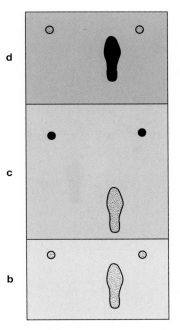

Step 7d(2b-d) Three-point gait.

Steps	Rationale
(3) *Two-point gait:* Requires at least partial weight bearing on each foot. Is faster than the four-point gait. Requires more balance because only two points support body at one time.	
(a) Begin in tripod position.	Improves client's balance by providing wider base of support.
(b) Move left crutch and right foot forward (see illustration).	Crutch movements are similar to arm movement during normal walking.
(c) Move right crutch and left foot forward.	
(d) Repeat sequence.	
(4) *Swing-to gait*	Frequently used by clients whose lower extremities are paralyzed or who wear weight-supporting braces on their legs. This is the easier of the two swinging gaits. It requires the ability to bear body weight partially on both legs.
(a) Move both crutches forward.	
(b) Lift and swing legs to crutches, letting crutches support body weight.	
(c) Repeat two previous steps.	
(5) *Swing-through gait:* Requires that client have the ability to sustain partial weight bearing on both feet.	
(a) Move both crutches forward.	Increases client's base of support so that when the body swings forward, client is moving the center of gravity toward the additional support provided by crutches.
(b) Lift and swing legs through and beyond crutches.	
(6) *Climbing stairs with crutches*	
(a) Begin in tripod position.	Improves client's balance by providing wider base of support.

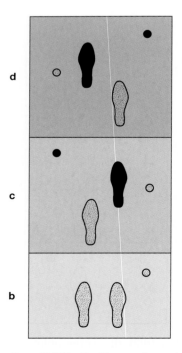

Step 7d(3b-d) Two-point gait.

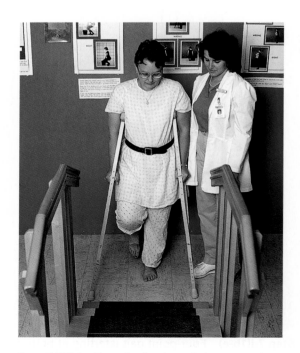

Step 7d(6b) Transfer body weight to crutches.

Steps	Rationale
(b) Client transfers body weight to crutches (see illustration).	Prepares client to transfer weight to unaffected leg when ascending first stair.
(c) Advance unaffected leg onto the step (see illustration).	Crutch adds support to affected leg. Client then shifts weight from crutches to unaffected leg.
(d) Align both crutches with the unaffected leg on the step (see illustration).	Maintains balance and provides wide base of support.
(e) Repeat sequence until client reaches top of stairs.	Improves client's balance by providing wider base of support.
(7) *Descending stairs with crutches*	
(a) Begin in tripod position.	Prepares client to release support of body weight maintained by crutches.
(b) Transfer body weight to unaffected leg.	Maintains client's balance and base of support.
(c) Move crutches to stair below, and instruct client to transfer body weight to crutches and move affected leg forward.	Maintains balance and provides base of support.
(d) Move unaffected leg to stair below and align with crutches.	
(e) Repeat sequence until client reaches bottom step.	The non–weight-bearing client should be able to balance on one leg before transferring both crutches to the same hand.
e. *Teach client to sit in a chair*	
(1) Transfer both crutches to the same hand and transfer weight to crutches and unaffected leg.	
(2) Grasp arm of chair with free hand and extend the affected leg out while lowering into chair (see illustration).	

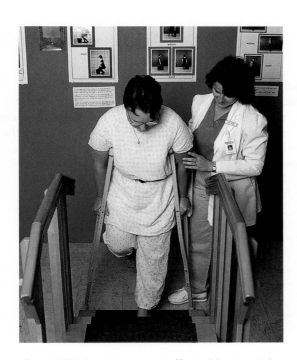

Step 7d(6c)   Advance unaffected leg to stair.

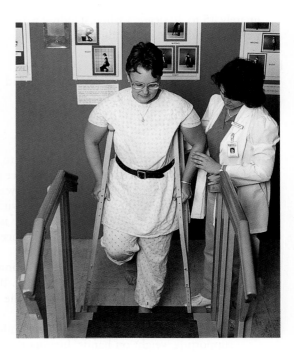

Step 7d(6d)   Align crutches with unaffected leg.

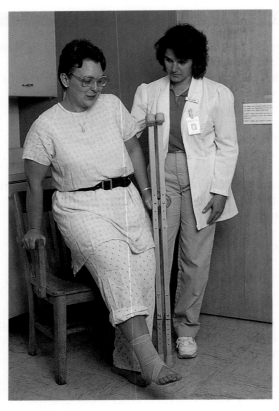

Step 7e(2) Grasp arm of chair with free hand.

Steps	Rationale

8. Walker

a. Upper bar of walker should be slightly below client's waist. Elbows should be flexed at approximately 15 to 30 degrees when standing with walker, with hands on handgrips.

Walkers without wheels must be picked up and moved forward. Client must have sufficient strength to be able to move walker. A four-wheeled walker, which does not have to be picked up, is not as stable and may cause injury.

b. Assist client in ambulating.

(1) Have client stand in center of walker and grasp handgrips on upper bars.

Client balances self before attempting to walk.

Position provides broad base of support between walker and client. Client then moves center of gravity toward the walker. Keeping all four feet of the walker on the floor is necessary to prevent tipping of the walker.

(2) Lift walker, moving it 6 to 8 inches (15 to 20 cm) forward, making sure all four feet of walker stay on the floor. Take a step forward with either foot. Then follow through with the other foot (see illustrations). If there is unilateral weakness after walker is advanced, instruct client to step forward with the weaker leg, support self with the arms, and follow through with the uninvolved leg. If client is unable to bear full weight on the weaker leg after advancing walker, have client swing the stronger leg through while supporting weight on hands. Instruct the client not to advance the lower extremity past the front bar of the walker.

Moving 6-8 inches stimulates normal distance of steps. Providing constant contact of all four walker feet with the floor reduces the risk of injury or fall. Advancing with weaker extremity allows client to have maximal support of walker.

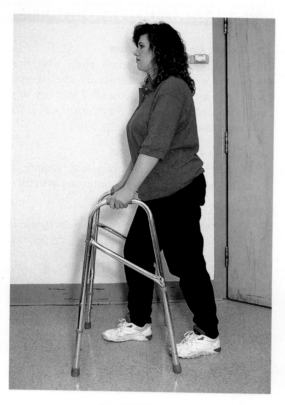 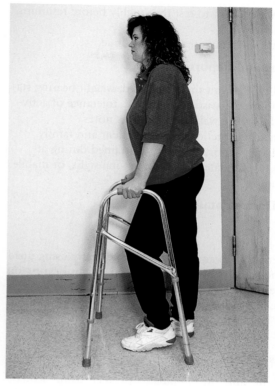

Step 8b(2)   Lift walker, move it 6 to 8 inches, take step forward.

Steps	Rationale
9. Have client take a few steps with the assistive device being used. If client is hemiplegic (one-sided paralysis) or has hemiparesis (one-sided weakness), stand next to client's unaffected side. Then support client by placing arm closest to client on gait belt.	Ensures client has satisfactory strength and balance to continue.
10. Take a few steps forward with client. Then assess for strength and balance.	Allows client to rest.
11. If client becomes weak or dizzy, return to bed or chair, whichever is closer.	
12. See Completion Protocol (inside front cover).	

· · · · · · · · · · ·

EVALUATION

1. Observe client using assistive device.
2. Inspect hands and axillae for redness, swelling, or skin irritation caused by using assistive device.
3. Ask client to rate level of pain or discomfort if present after ambulating.
4. Monitor client for postural hypotension; increased heart rate, decreased blood pressure, increased respirations or shortness of breath during and after ambulation.
5. Ask client/family about the ease with which ADLs are performed using assistive device.

Unexpected Outcomes and Related Interventions

1. Client is unable to ambulate correctly.
   a. Reassess client for correct fit of assistive device.
   b. Have added assistance nearby to ensure safety.
   c. Reassess comfort level.
   d. Reassess muscle strength in uninvolved extremities. Alternative device may be needed.
   e. Obtain referral for physical therapy to assist with gait training.
2. Client becomes dizzy and light-headed.
   a. Call for assistance.
   b. Have client sit or lie down on nearest chair or bed.

c. Assess client's vital signs.

   d. Allow client to rest thoroughly before resuming activity.

   e. Ask if client is ready to continue.

Recording and Reporting

- Record type of gait the client used, weight-bearing status, amount of assistance required, tolerance of activity, and distance walked in progress notes.
- Document instructions given to client and family.
- Immediately report any injury sustained during attempts to ambulate, alteration in vital signs, or inability to ambulate.

Sample Documentation

Cane

0900 Client able to ambulate 20 feet correctly using quad cane, standby assist of one, and partial weight bearing on right lower extremity. Requested pain pills. Rates pain in right knee at 6 (scale 0 to 10). Returned to bed.

    0910 Prescribed analgesic given.

    0930 Resting quietly in bed. Denies discomfort.

Crutches

0900 Client able to ambulate 40 feet using axillary crutches and standby assist of one. Gait slow and steady, maintaining non–weight-bearing status on right leg. Able to ambulate up and down stairs correctly using axillary crutches; standby assistance of two needed to steady gait. Voiced no complaints of pain. Returned to bed. Client instructed not to get out of bed without assistance of health care personnel. Voiced understanding.

Walker

0900 Client able to ambulate 20 feet correctly using walker, with full weight-bearing status. Became dizzy and light-headed. Assisted to chair with assistance of two personnel. Vital signs: BP 126/70, pulse 78, respirations 18. Client rested 5 minutes and then continued ambulating back to bed. Vital signs: BP 124/80, pulse 72, respirations 16. Denies dizziness or discomfort.

SPECIAL CONSIDERATIONS

Pediatric Considerations

For rehabilitation of a small child who has not yet learned to walk or who is unsteady, special crutches with three or four legs provide needed stability to allow the child to maintain an upright posture and learn to walk (Wong and others, 1999).

Geriatric Considerations

The older adult with arthritis may require additional time in the morning before resuming activities.

Home Care Considerations

- Client should be instructed in how to use the ambulation aid on various terrains (e.g., carpet, stairs, rough ground, inclines).
- Client should be instructed in how to maneuver around obstacles such as doors and how to use the aid when transferring, such as to and from a chair, toilet, tub, and car (Borgman-Gainer, 1996).
- Attach a "saddle bag" to client's walker to carry objects; caution client not to overfill to prevent forward tipping of walker.

Long-Term Care Considerations

- Safety and maintenance checks of ambulation devices should be done on a routine basis.
- Periodic assessments should be performed to ensure that the client is using ambulation device properly.

CRITICAL THINKING EXERCISES

1. Mrs. Smith has had a cerebral infarct (stroke), and her left side is paralyzed. The plan is to discharge her in 1 week. Her twin daughters, age 24, are anxious to care for her at home. Mrs. Smith lives with her 64-year-old husband in a one-story town house in a senior community. Her daughters live together 1 mile from their parents. Coordinate plan of home care for this family related to her activity, mobility, and normal daily routines.

2. Mrs. George is on bed rest at home. Develop a plan of care for the family to prevent pressure sores.

3. Safety is an important issue for all hospitalized clients. What important safety measure(s) was (were) overlooked in each of the following situations, and what consequence could have occurred to the clients as a result of the oversight?
   a. Sarah was transferring Martha from her bed to a stretcher. Sarah positioned the bed flat and placed a bath blanket beneath Martha from her shoulders to her hips. Sarah then moved the stretcher as close to the bed as possible and locked the wheels of the stretcher in place.
   b. Jim is in the process of transferring Mr. Blue from his bed to a chair using a mechanical lift. Jim has prepared the chair and placed it near the bed. Jim turns Mr. Blue to his side, places the sling under Mr. Blue to ensure adequate support of Mr. Blue's head, returns Mr. Blue to his back, and slowly begins to lift Mr. Blue from his bed.
   c. Tom has an order to ambulate Mrs. Rucker twice daily in her room. On entering Mrs. Rucker's room, Tom notes that she is lying in bed. He explains that she needs to take a short walk, assists her to a standing position, and encourages her to walk toward the door. Mrs. Rucker states that she is dizzy.

4. You observe an AP using the under-axilla method to assist a client out of bed and into a chair. Instruct in the importance of using a gait belt.

5. Mrs. Orbe has undergone extensive abdominal surgery. This is her first time out of bed. What assessment parameters need to be considered before transferring her to the chair?

REFERENCES

Borgman-Gainer M. Independent function: movement and mobility. In Hoeman S, editor: *Rehabilitation nursing: process and application,* ed 2, St Louis, 1996, Mosby.

Brough E: Deep vein thrombosis, *Prof Nurs* 13(10):687, 1998.

Groeneveld A, McKenzie ML, Williams D: Logrolling: establishing consistent practice, *Orthop Nurs* 20(2):45, 2001.

Hockenberry MJ and others: *Wong's nursing care of infants and children,* ed 7, St Louis, 2003, Mosby.

Hoeman SP: *Rehabilitation nursing: process and application,* ed 3, St Louis, 2001, Mosby.

Huddleston JS: Exercise. In Edelman C, Mandle C, editors: *Health promotion throughout the lifespan,* ed 4, St Louis, 1998, Mosby.

Jitramontree N: Evidence-based protocol: exercise promotion, *J Gerontol Nurs* 27(10):7, 2001.

Konradi DB, Anglin LT: Moderate-intensity exercise: for our patients, for ourselves, *Orthop Nurs* 20(1):47, 2001.

Lueckenotte AG: *Gerontologic nursing,* ed 2, St Louis, 2000, Mosby.

Marion BS: A turn for the better: prone positioning of patients with ARDS, *Am J Nurs* 101(5):26, 2001.

McCance K, Huether S: *Pathophysiology: the biologic basis for disease in adults and children,* ed 4, St Louis, 2002, Mosby.

McFarland G, McFarlane E: *Nursing diagnosis and intervention,* ed 3, St Louis, 1997, Mosby.

Owens B, Welden N, Kane J: What are we teaching about lifting and transferring patients? *Res Nurs Health* 22:3, 1999.

Phipps W, Sands JK, Marek JF: *Medical-surgical nursing: concepts and clinical practice,* ed 6, St Louis, 1999, Mosby.

Winslow EH, Lane L, Woods R: Dangling: a review of relevant physiology, research, and practice. *Heart Lung* 24(2):263, 1995.

Wong D and others: *Whaley and Wong's nursing care of infants and children,* ed 6, St Louis, 1999, Mosby.

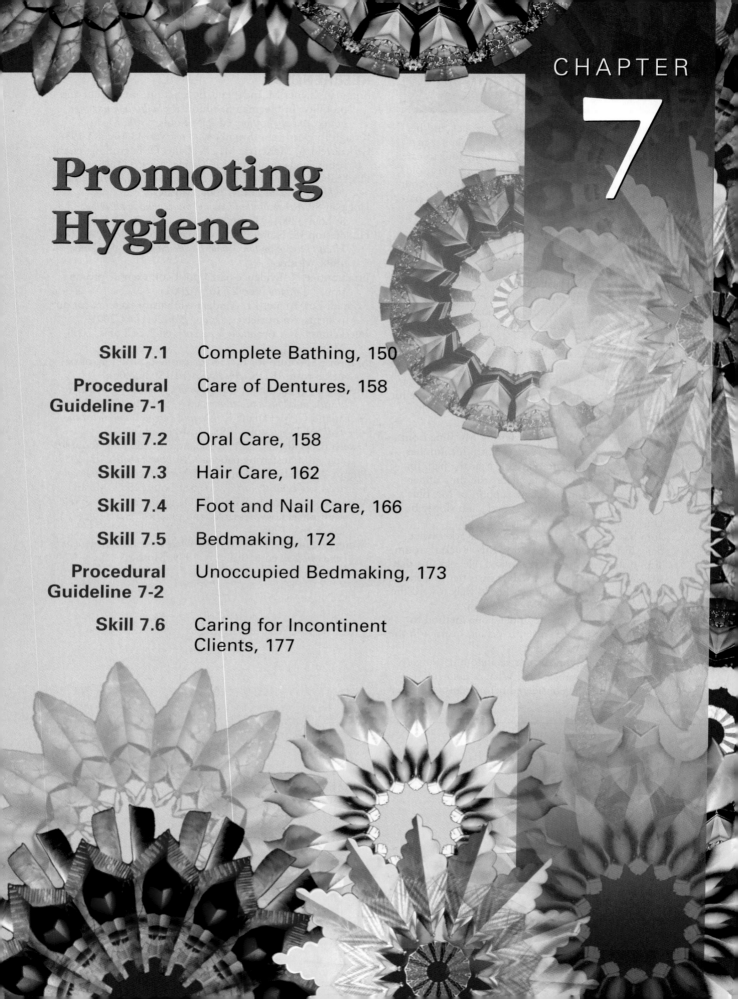

CHAPTER

7

Promoting Hygiene

Many clients require assistance with personal hygiene during illness or recovery. Maintenance of personal hygiene is necessary for comfort and a sense of well-being. Because personal hygiene requires close contact with the client, it provides an opportunity for interactions that focus on immediate and future emotional, social, and health-related concerns.

Box 7-1

Benefits of Bathing

Cleansing the skin: removal of perspiration, some bacteria, sebum, and dead skin cells minimizes skin irritation and reduces the chance of infection.

Stimulating circulation: muscle activity, warm water, and stroking extremities enhance circulation.

Promoting range of motion (ROM): movement of extremities assists in maintaining joint function.

Reducing body odors: secretions and excretions from axillae and perineal areas result in body odors that are eliminated by bathing.

Improving self-image: promotes relaxation and feeling clean and comfortable. Care of hair and teeth enhances appearance and sense of well-being.

The nurse needs to convey sensitivity and respect for personal beliefs and habits and to ensure as much privacy as possible. Bathing should be done according to the client's usual routines and preferences. Some clients need encouragement to be independent and to participate in self-care. If the client cannot participate, the family or significant other may be encouraged to assist when possible. Some clients lack the physical energy to perform self-care and need to be temporarily dependent on others to enhance the healing and recovery process.

Personal hygiene is essential to maintain skin integrity by promoting adequate circulation and hydration. Intact skin functions include (1) defense against infection; (2) awareness of touch, pain, heat, cold, and pressure; and (3) control of body temperature. Bathing should be done when any body part becomes soiled. Linen changes are usually required as well. Problems such as incontinence, wound drainage, or diaphoresis may require frequent bathing. In addition to cleansing the skin, bathing a client has several benefits (Box 7-1).

Age influences the skin's condition. Normally the skin is elastic, well hydrated, firm, and smooth. With age the skin becomes thinner, dry, less vascular, more fragile, and prone to bruising and tears. Bathing is an excellent opportunity to assess the skin for common skin problems that may require special interventions (Table 7-1). Bathing

Table 7-1

Common Skin Problems and Related Interventions

Problem	Interventions
Dry skin: flaky, rough texture to skin, which may crack and become infected.	Bathe less frequently; rinse away all soap or use a waterless cleanser rather than soap; increase fluid intake; use moisturizing lotion.
Acne: inflammatory papulopustular skin eruption, usually involving bacterial breakdown of sebum, typically on face, neck, shoulders, and back.	Wash hair daily. Wash skin twice daily with warm water and soap to remove oils and cosmetics (if used); cosmetics that can accumulate in pores should be used sparingly. Topical antibiotics, if prescribed, may minimize problems.
Hirsutism: excessive growth of body and facial hair, especially in women; may cause negative body image by giving women a male appearance.	Shaving is safest method; electrolysis and laser permanently remove hair by destroying hair follicles; tweezing and bleaching are temporary measures; depilatories may remove unwanted hair but may cause infection, rashes, or dermatitis.
Skin rashes: skin eruption from overexposure to sun or moisture or from allergic reaction; may be flat, raised, localized, or systemic; may be associated with pruritus (itching).	Wash thoroughly; apply antiseptic spray or lotion to prevent further itching and aid in healing process; warm or cold soaks relieve inflammation.
Contact dermatitis: inflammation of skin characterized by abrupt onset with erythema, pruritus, pain, and scaly, oozing lesions; usually results from contact with substance difficult to identify and eliminate.	Identify and avoid contributing agents; provide linens rinsed and sterilized to minimize irritation.
Abrasion: scraping or rubbing away of epidermis that results in localized bleeding and later weeping of serous fluid; easily infected.	Wash with mild soap and water; observe dressings for retained moisture, which can increase risk of infection.

older clients too frequently may contribute to dry skin and should be avoided. A full bath 3 times a week may be adequate for many older clients; however, optimal frequency depends on individual needs.

There are prepackaged, disposable bathing systems available over the counter for use in the home and in health care agencies. Each bath kit contains 8 to 10 disposable cloths premoistened with a cleansing solution that does not require rinsing or towel drying. Time to complete the bath is decreased, and the products are meant to be gentle to the skin. These systems are easier to use, take less time, and save money on linens and other supplies.

NURSING DIAGNOSES

Bathing/Hygiene Self-Care Deficit is appropriate when the focus of care is helping the client move toward independence in bathing. The client may be unable to wash body parts, to obtain or have access to a water source, or to regulate water temperature or flow (Kim, McFarland, and McLane, 1997). Contributing factors may include impaired physical mobility in which range of motion (ROM) or muscle strength is limited or an alteration in mental state. Shortness of breath with activity or excessive fatigue when bathing may also be contributing factors. **Risk for Impaired Skin Integrity** should be considered when the client has re-

duced sensation, immobility, impaired circulation, incontinence, inadequate nutrition, or fragile skin associated with advancing age. **Impaired Skin Integrity** is an appropriate diagnosis for the client who has actually experienced a loss in skin integrity. Pressure ulcers, vascular ulcerations, and blistering are examples of impaired skin integrity.

Impaired Oral Mucous Membrane is appropriate when mucous membranes are damaged, such as by ulcerations, erythema, and irritation. Contributing factors may include sensory changes (pain, burning, or numbness), decreased level of consciousness, medication side effects, or altered oral intake for any reason. **Imbalanced Nutrition: Less Than Body Requirements** should be considered when a client's appetite and intake are diminished because of altered mucous membranes, and the aim is to increase oral intake by improving oral hygiene. **Dressing/ Grooming Self-Care Deficit** is appropriate when the focus is to improve a client's ability to provide self-care with oral hygiene or hair care.

Disturbed Body Image is often appropriate when the client loses interest in grooming or experiences hair loss. This should also be considered when the client displays a lack of interest in appearance, especially when medical treatment alters body appearance or function.

Ineffective Health Maintenance is appropriate when client teaching related to foot care is the focus of care for a diabetic.

Skill 7.1

Complete Bathing

The extent of the bath and the methods used depend on the client's ability to participate, the condition of the client's skin, and in some settings, time of day (Box 7-2). A partial bath consists of bathing only body parts that would cause discomfort or odor if left unbathed, such as hands, face, breasts, perineal area, and axillae. Clients who cannot tolerate a complete bath and self-sufficient clients unable to reach all body parts may be given a partial bed bath. A tub bath or shower can be used to give a more thorough bath. In the tub or shower, washing and rinsing all body parts is easier; however, safety is of primary concern, and clients must have adequate strength, mobility, and mental capacity.

ASSESSMENT

1. Assess degree of assistance needed for bathing. Factors may include vision, ability to sit without support, hand grasp, ROM of extremities, and cognitive ability.
2. Assess client's tolerance of activity, level of discomfort with movement, and presence of shortness of breath or chest pain with exertion. *Rationale:*

Determines what type of cleansing bath is appropriate for the client.

3. Assess client's preferences for time of day, products used, and frequency of bathing.
4. Identify any problems related to condition of the skin:
    a. Excessive moisture from diaphoresis or incontinence
    b. Drainage or excretions from lesions or body cavities
    c. External devices (catheters, drains, dressings, restraints)
    d. Rashes or skin damage related to pruritus and scratching
    Rationale: Determines what toiletry items and/or other equipment to have available for the client.
5. Identify any prescribed limitations of activity or positioning required by client's illness or treatment plan. This information is available from the primary caregiver's report or information from a nursing care plan. *Rationale: Determines safety needs of the client to prevent injury.*

Box 7-2

AM and PM Care

In the morning when the client wakes and prior to breakfast:
- Assist the client with toileting.
- Assist the client with washing hands and face and oral care.
- Make sure the client's environment is neat and set up for breakfast.

In the evening before the client goes to sleep:
- Assist the client with toileting.
- Assist the client with washing hands and face and oral care.
- Make sure that the client's bed is clean, dry, and wrinkle free with adequate blankets for warmth.
- Offer the client a back massage to promote comfort and relaxation.
- Make sure client's environment is neat and free of hazards and that call button is within reach.

Equipment

- Washcloths and towels
- Bath blanket
- Soap and soap dish
- Warm water
- Toiletry items (deodorant, powder, lotion)
- Clean hospital gown or client's own pajamas
- Laundry bag
- Disposable gloves (when body secretions are present)
- Washbasin

PLANNING

Expected outcomes focus on promoting comfort, mobility, and self-care abilities.

Expected Outcomes

1. Client's skin is clean and free of excretions, drainage, or odor.
2. Client demonstrates functional ROM of hands and shoulders.
3. Client demonstrates ability to wash face, hands, and chest independently.
4. Client expresses comfort and relaxation.

NOTE: This procedure assumes client is totally dependent. When client is able to assist, encourage and allow as much involvement as possible.

Delegation Considerations

Skills of bathing are often delegated to assistive personnel (AP); however, skin and ROM assessment require the critical thinking and knowledge application unique to the nurse. The nurse should:
- Instruct the care provider in what type of bath (complete, partial assist, tub, shower) is appropriate to the client's diagnosis and needs
- Remind the care provider to notify the nurse of any skin integrity problems so the nurse can inspect areas of breakdown or potential breakdown
- Remind the care provider to use an organized approach and reassuring tone of voice so the client feels safe and comfortable during bathing
- Instruct the care provider to encourage the client to report any concerns or discomfort during the bath
- Instruct the care provider to encourage as much independence in the client's self-care skills as appropriate and to provide positive feedback

IMPLEMENTATION FOR COMPLETE BATHING

Steps	Rationale
1. See Standard Protocol (inside front cover).	

COMMUNICATION TIP
- *Use an organized approach and reassuring tone of voice so the client feels safe and comfortable during bathing.*
- *Encourage the client to report any concerns or discomfort.*

Steps	Rationale
2. Promote independence and participation as much as possible during bath. If appropriate, involve the family or significant other.	Increases client's cooperation and comfort.

Steps	Rationale
3. Provide privacy. Close the door and/or pull the curtains around the area. Expose only the areas being bathed.	Promotes client's emotional and physical comfort.
4. Provide safety. If it is necessary to leave the room, be sure the call light is within reach. Provide assistance according to client's needs.	
5. The room should be comfortably warm. Protect the client from injury by assessing and controlling bath water temperature.	Avoids chilling the client and promotes safety.
6. Consider the client's cultural preferences in regard to grooming techniques and products. However, the nurse may have opportunities to caution against the use of products that can damage or injure skin, hair, or nails.	
7. With client supine, place bath blanket over client and remove top covers without exposing client. Place soiled linen in laundry bag.	Prevents chilling and provides privacy.
8. Remove client's gown or pajamas.	
a. If an extremity is injured or has limited mobility, begin removal from unaffected side first.	Removing gown from unaffected side or arm without an IV reduces risk of injury or accidental dislodgement of IV.
b. If client has an intravenous (IV) line, remove gown from arm without IV first, then slide IV container and tubing through sleeve and rehang. Check flow rate, and regulate if necessary (see illustration). Gowns with sleeves that snap may also be available for clients with IVs.	
c. If IV pump is in use, turn pump off, clamp tubing, remove tubing from pump, and proceed as in Step b. Insert tubing into pump, unclamp tubing, and turn pump on at correct rate. Observe flow rate, and regulate if necessary.	Sterility and patency of IV infusion must be maintained.
9. Remove pillow. Place one bath towel under client's head and another over chest.	Removing pillow facilitates bathing ears and neck. Towels absorb moisture.
10. Wash face.	
a. Form mitt with washcloth (see illustration), and wash client's eyes with plain warm water using a clean area of cloth for each eye, bathing from inner to outer canthus (see illustration on p. 153). Dry around eyes gently and thoroughly.	Mitt prevents loose ends from dripping or annoying client. Bathing inner to outer canthus prevents secretions from entering nasolacrimal duct. Soap irritates eyes. Using a clean area of the cloth reduces the possibility of infection transmission.

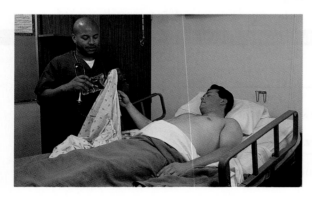

Step 8b Slide IV container and tubing through sleeve and rehang.

Steps	**Rationale**

b. Wash, rinse, and dry forehead, cheeks, nose, neck, and ears without using soap. Ask men if they want to be shaved (see Skill 7.3, p. 162).

Soap tends to dry face, which is exposed to air more than other body parts. If client has a preferred face wash, it should be used.

11. Provide eye care for the unconscious client.

a. Cleanse the eyelids with a washcloth from the inner to outer canthus using plain warm water.

Clients who are unconscious have lost the normal protective actions of the eye, which increases their risk for corneal drying, corneal abrasions, and eye infections.

b. Instill prescribed eye drops or ointment as per physician's order or agency policy. Reassess eyes every 2 to 4 hours or as ordered for dryness.

Lubricants will help keep the client's eyes moist in the absence of tearing and/or blinking.

c. In the absence of a blink reflex the eyelids should be kept closed and covered with an eye patch or shield. Do not tape the eyelid.

Eyelids should be kept closed to keep eyes moist and prevent injury. Taping can injure the eyelid (American Society of Health-Systems Pharmacists, 2002).

12. Wash the trunk and upper extremities.

a. Remove bath blanket from over client's arm. Place bath towel lengthwise under arm. Bathe with minimal soap and water using long, firm strokes from distal to proximal (fingers to axilla).

Promotes circulatory return to heart.

b. Raise and support arm above head (if possible) to wash, rinse, and dry axilla thoroughly.

Raising arm promotes ROM and facilitates thorough cleansing.

c. Repeat Steps a and b with other arm (see illustration). Apply deodorant or powder to underarms, if needed.

d. Cover client's chest with bath towel, and fold bath blanket down to umbilicus. Bathe chest using long, firm strokes. Take special care with skin under female clients' breasts, lifting breast upward if necessary. Rinse and dry well.

Skin under breasts is vulnerable to excoriation if not kept clean and dry.

13. Wash the abdomen and lower extremities.

a. Place bath towel over chest and abdomen, and fold bath blanket down to just above pubic region. Bathe, rinse, and dry abdomen with special attention to umbilicus and skinfolds of abdomen and groin.

Keeping skinfolds clean and dry helps prevent odor and skin irritation.

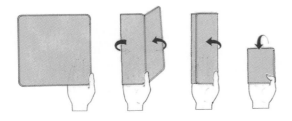

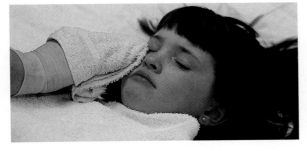

Step 10a   Wash eye from inner to outer canthus.

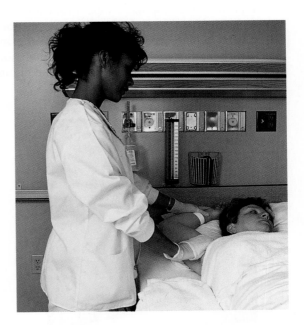

Step 12c   Positioning the arm to wash axilla.

Steps	Rationale
b. Expose client's leg nearest to you, leaving perineum covered. Place bath towel under leg, supporting leg at knee and with foot flat on bed. If desired, place client's foot in a basin to soak while washing and rinsing. If client is unable to support leg, assistance will be needed or soaking omitted. Wash and dry leg using long, firm strokes from ankle to knee, then knee to thigh (see illustration). Wash between toes of the foot. Rinse and dry thoroughly.	Soaking softens calluses and rough skin.

NURSE ALERT *It is not recommended to soak the feet of clients with diabetes mellitus or peripheral vascular disease. This may lead to maceration (excessive softening of the skin) and infection (American Diabetes Association, 2001).*

Avoid long, firm strokes when washing the legs of a client at risk of deep vein thrombosis (blood clots) or emboli. Use short, light strokes (Perry and Potter, 2002).

c. Raise side rail, move to opposite side, lower the side rail, and repeat Step b with other leg and foot. If skin is dry, apply lotion.	Promotes good body mechanics for the nurse.
d. Cover with bath blanket, and raise side rail. Change bath water. Remove contaminated gloves.	Provides client warmth and safety.

14. Wash perineum.

NURSE ALERT *Along with care of the perineum, be sure to provide care of any indwelling urinary catheter according to agency policy.*

a. Assist client in assuming side-lying position, placing towel lengthwise along client's side and keeping client covered with bath blanket as much as possible.	If client is totally dependent, assistance is necessary to support client in side-lying position and to raise leg as perineum is bathed.
b. If fecal material is present, enclose it in a fold of underpad and remove as much as possible with disposable wipes first. Cleanse anal area from front to back with special attention to folds of buttocks (see illustration). Use as many washcloths as necessary to cleanse and rinse thoroughly. Dry area completely. Remove and discard underpad, and replace with a clean one.	Washing from front to back or side to side prevents transmission of microorganisms from anus to urethra or genitalia.

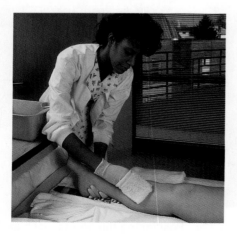

Step 13b Washing the leg.

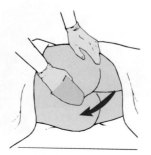

Step 14b Cleanse anal area from front to back.

Steps	Rationale

15. Provide perineal care.
 a.   Female
  (1)   Position waterproof pad under client's buttocks with client supine. Drape client with bath blanket placed in the shape of a diamond. Lift lower edge of bath blanket to expose perineum (see illustration). Wash labia majora using washcloth, soap, and warm water. Then gently retract labia from thigh, and wash groin from perineum toward rectum.

Washing from front to back prevents contamination of urethral meatus with fecal matter.

  (2)   Gently separate labia, and expose urethra and vagina. Wash from pubic area toward rectum, cleansing thoroughly. Avoid tension on indwelling catheter if present, and clean area around it thoroughly.

Minimizes risk for developing infection because of presence of indwelling catheter or fecal incontinence.

  (3)   Rinse and dry area thoroughly. Assess for redness, swelling, discharge, irritation, or skin breakdown. Make sure catheter is secure and positioned over (not under) the thigh.

Prevents pulling of catheter on urethral canal and promotes urinary drainage.

 b.   Male
  (1)   Gently grasp shaft of penis, and if client is not circumcised, retract foreskin.

Gentle handling reduces risk of having an erection. Secretions and microorganisms tend to collect under foreskin.

  (2)   Wash tip of penis at urethral meatus first. Using circular motion, cleanse away from meatus (see illustration). Replace foreskin to its natural position.

Discharge may indicate presence of infection or inflammation. Replacing foreskin prevents constriction of the penis, which may result in edema.

  (3)   Gently cleanse shaft of penis and scrotum, washing underlying skinfolds. Rinse and dry.

Minimizes risk of discomfort from secretions or moisture.

16. Cover client with bath blanket, change bath water, remove and discard contaminated gloves, and apply clean gloves.

17. Wash back.
 a.   Assist client to side-lying position, and place towel lengthwise along the back. Wash, rinse, and dry back from neck to buttocks using long, firm strokes.
 b.   Remove gloves, and dispose of them properly.

18. Apply body lotion to skin as needed and topical moisturizing agents to dry, flaky, or scaling areas. Replace gown.

Dry skin results in reduced pliability and cracking. Moisturizers may help prevent skin breakdown (Agency for Health Care Policy and Research [AHCPR], 1992).

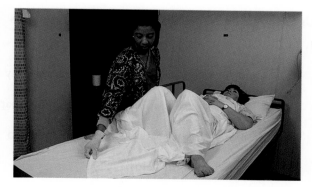

Step 15a(1)   Drape the client for perineal care.

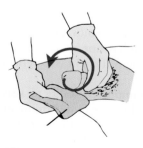

Step 15b(2)   Wash the penis in a circular motion.

Steps	**Rationale**

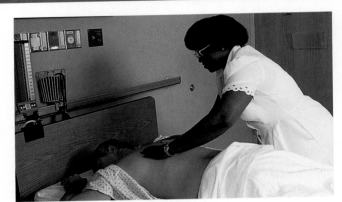

A

19. Massage back

NURSE ALERT *Massaging over bony prominences is no longer recommended. Evidence suggests that massage may result in decreased blood flow and tissue damage in some clients (AHCPR, 1992).*

a. Position client prone (on abdomen) if possible. Side-lying position is also frequently used.

b. Provide back massage using lotion to stimulate circulation (see illustration). Begin at sacral area. Massaging in circular motion, stroke upward from buttocks to shoulders and upper arms and over scapulae with smooth, firm strokes (see illustration). Keep hands on skin, and continue massage pattern for 3 to 4 minutes.

c. Knead skin by grasping tissue between thumb and fingers. Knead upward along each side of spine and around muscles of neck, avoiding bony prominences.

d. End massage with long stroking movements, and tell client you are ending massage.

e. Observe skin for redness and skin breakdown, paying particular attention to any bony prominences. Remove excess lotion from back with bath towel.

f. Apply clean gown or pajamas, dressing affected side first.

20. See Completion Protocol (inside front cover).

B

Step 19b A, Massage the back. **B,** Massage in circular motion upwards from buttocks.

Long strokes promote comfort and relaxation.

Excess lotion could promote maceration of skin.

Allows easier manipulation of gown over restricted body part.

• • • • • • • • • •

EVALUATION

1. Observe areas on skin for erythema, exudate, drainage, or breakdown.
2. Measure ROM in hands, arms, and shoulders, and compare with baseline.
3. Assess vital signs if client is experiencing distress or restlessness.
4. Observe for improved ability to assist with self-bathing and hygiene to determine progress.
5. Ask client to view self in mirror and comment on appearance and comfort.

Unexpected Outcomes and Related Interventions

1. Client's skin on lower extremities is dry and flaky and itches.
   a. Limit the frequency of baths to every other day or less.
   b. Use antibacterial soap sparingly. Use a mild soap that is nondrying.
   c. Blot skin dry after bathing, and apply lotion to skin.
   d. Increase hydration status.

e. Administer antipruritics as ordered to control itching.

f. Use distraction techniques to remove focus from itching.

2. The client has evidence of rashes, redness, scaling, or cracking.

a. Evaluate the need for a change in frequency of bathing and soap product used.

b. Collaborate with the physician regarding application of ointments or creams to provide a protective barrier and help maintain moisture within the skin.

3. The rectum, perineum, or genital region is inflamed, is swollen, or has foul-smelling discharge.

a. Bathe area frequently enough to keep clean and dry.

b. Apply protective barrier or antiinflammatory cream.

c. Report to physician.

Recording and Reporting

- Routine documentation may include check marks on a flow sheet. Observations made during the bath that should be charted may include:
Type of bath given
Client's ability to assist or cooperate
Condition of client's skin and any nursing interventions related to skin integrity
Client's response to bathing and any concerns voiced by client regarding self-care needs

Sample Documentation

0900 Complete bed bath given. Client unable to assist but cooperative with turning. Skin on both legs dry and flaking, complains of severe itching. Bath oil added to bath water. Emollient lotion applied after bath. States itching is less now.

 ## SPECIAL CONSIDERATIONS

Pediatric Considerations

- Infants may chill easily.
- Use only mild soap for bathing infants and children (Wong, Perry, and Hockenberry-Eaton, 2002).
- Safety is always the major concern in caring for children. Attempts should also be made to maintain a child's bathing routine (Wong, Perry, and Hockenberry-Eaton, 2002).

Geriatric Considerations

- Consider conditions of older adult's skin when planning hygiene routine. Older adults may require less frequent bathing. Because of the aging process, more moisture is needed; client's skin can be rehydrated with lotions and fluids (Lueckenotte, 2000).
- Older adults may chill easily.
- Older adults with limited mobility need assistance in perineal care. Using a side-lying position increases client's comfort and provides nurse with opportunity to provide perineal care and inspect surrounding skin as well.
- Older adults with urinary incontinence need meticulous skin care to reduce skin irritation from urine and feces (see Skill 7.6, p. 177).

Home Care Considerations

- Type of bath chosen depends on assessment of the home, availability of running water, and condition of bathing facilities.
- In home setting, set up equipment according to established routines. Client is best resource for what works in terms of convenience and saving time.
- The three types of bath for the homebound client are the complete bed bath; the abbreviated bed bath, during which only parts of the body are washed that, if neglected, might cause illness, odor, or discomfort; and the partial bath, which may take place at the sink, in the tub, or in the shower.
- Never leave bathing client unattended. Adhesive strips on bottom of tub or shower, handrails, chairs, or stools in tub or shower will further protect client.
- Clients at risk for falls may wish to have grab bars installed around tub and have bathroom floor carpeted. Client also may use portable shower seat.

Long-Term Care Considerations

- Skin-related problems in long-term care may include methicillin-resistant *Staphylococcus aureus* (MRSA) infections, pressure ulcers, and dermatitis (Lueckenotte, 2000).
- Residents in long-term care facilities should be encouraged to do as much of their own personal care as able and to wear their own clothes (Sorrentino, 1999).

Skill 7.2

Oral Care

Oral hygiene helps maintain healthy structures of the oral cavity and comfort of the mouth, teeth, gums, and lips. Brushing cleanses the teeth of food particles, plaque, and bacteria; massages the gums; and relieves discomfort resulting from unpleasant odors and tastes. Many factors can influence oral hygiene (Box 7-3). Inadequate oral hygiene can create a general sense of discomfort and also diminish appetite.

Clients may experience altered oral mucous membranes when they are dehydrated; have inadequate nutrition, particularly vitamin B deficiency; or are unable to take food or fluids orally (NPO). Mouth breathing may result in dry mucous membranes. Trauma to oral mucous membranes may also occur from oral tubes, oxygen therapy, suctioning, hot foods, or trauma from broken teeth or ill-fitting dentures. Chemical injury may result from irritating substances such as alcohol, tobacco, acidic foods, or side effects of medications, including chemotherapy, antibiotics, steroids, and antidepressants. Chronic inflammatory disease may be caused by bacteria, viral or fungal infections, or ineffective oral hygiene.

Dentures should be cleaned as regularly as natural teeth to prevent gingival infection and irritation (Procedural Guideline 7-1). Loose dentures can cause discomfort and make it difficult for clients to chew food and speak clearly. Loose dentures may result from weight loss.

Box 7-3

Factors Influencing Oral Hygiene

- Client lacks upper-extremity strength or dexterity to perform oral hygiene (e.g., is paralyzed or has limited ROM).
- Client unable or unwilling to attend to personal hygiene needs (e.g., is unconscious, depressed, or confused).
- Client is diabetic and prone to dryness of mouth, gingivitis, periodontal disease, and loss of teeth.
- Client is prone to dehydration or has a fever. Thick secretions develop on tongue and gums. Lips become cracked and reddened.
- Radiation therapy causes soreness, mild erythema, swollen mucosa, dysphagia, dryness, taste changes, and possible oral infection.
- Chemotherapy causes ulcerations and inflammation of mucosa and possible oral infection.
- Tissues in oral cavity become traumatized with swelling, ulcerations, inflammation, and possible bleeding.

Procedural Guideline 7-1
Care of Dentures

Equipment: Soft-bristled toothbrush or denture toothbrush, denture cleaning agent or toothpaste, denture adhesive (optional), glass of water, emesis basin or sink, washcloth, disposable gloves, denture cup (if dentures are to be stored after cleaning).

1. Clean dentures for client during routine mouth care.
2. Fill emesis basin with tepid water or if using sink, place washcloth in bottom of sink and fill sink with an inch of water (see illustration).
3. Remove dentures: If client is unable to do this independently, apply gloves, grasp upper plate at front with thumb and index finger wrapped in gauze, and pull downward. Gently lift lower denture from jaw, and rotate one side downward to remove from client's mouth. Place dentures in emesis basin or sink.
4. Apply cleaning agent to brush, and brush surfaces of dentures (see illustration). Hold dentures close to water. Hold brush horizontally, and use back-and-forth motion to cleanse biting surfaces. Use short strokes from top of denture to biting surfaces to clean outer and inner teeth surfaces. Hold brush vertically, and use short strokes to clean inner tooth surfaces. Hold brush horizontally, and use back-and-forth motion to clean undersurface of dentures.
5. Rinse thoroughly in tepid water.
6. Some clients use an adhesive to seal dentures in place. Apply a thin layer to undersurface before inserting.
7. If client needs assistance with insertion of dentures, moisten upper denture and press firmly to seal it in place. Then insert moistened lower denture. Ask if dentures feel comfortable.
8. Some clients prefer to have their dentures stored to give the gums a rest and to reduce risk of infection. Keeping dentures moist will prevent warping and facilitate easier insertion. Store in a secure place to prevent loss.
9. Remove and discard gloves.

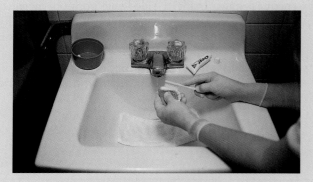

Step 2 Washcloth in bottom of basin with one inch of water.

Dentures can be easily lost or broken. They are stored in an enclosed, labeled cup and should be soaking when not worn (e.g., during surgery or a diagnostic procedure). They should be reinserted as soon as possible. The change in appearance when they are not worn may be of major concern to the client.

ASSESSMENT

1.   Determine presence or absence of gag reflex by placing tongue blade or suction tip on back of tongue. *Rationale: Clients with no gag reflex are at risk for aspiration. Suction equipment must be available.*
2. Inspect lips, teeth, gums, buccal mucosa, palate, and tongue, using tongue depressor and penlight if necessary (see Chapter 13). Observe for color, texture, moisture, lesions or ulcers, and condition of teeth (or dentures). Ask if areas of tenderness exist. *Rationale: Every effort should be made to prevent or minimize oral problems.*
3. Identify presence of oral problems, and remove gloves.
    a. Dental caries: discoloration of tooth enamel
    b. Gingivitis: inflammation of gums
    c. Periodontitis: receding gum lines, inflammation, gaps between teeth, rough or jagged teeth
    d. Halitosis: bad breath
    e. Cracked lips
    f. Dry, cracked, coated tongue
    Rationale: Any oral problems put clients at risk for infection or nutritional deficiencies.

For Denture Care

1. Ask client if dentures fit and if there is any gum or mucous membrane tenderness or irritation.

2. Ask client about preferences for denture care and products used. If client is unable to care for own dentures, the nurse must provide this care (see Procedural Guideline 7-1).

PLANNING

Expected outcomes focus on promoting comfort, preventing aspiration, and promoting integrity of oral mucous membranes.

Expected Outcomes

1. Client's oral mucous membranes are smooth, moist, pink, and without lesions.
2. Client maintains clean dental surfaces.
3. Client verbalizes comfort and displays no restlessness or facial grimacing during oral care.
4. The client, spouse, or significant other demonstrates proper oral hygiene regimen.

Equipment (Figure 7-1)

*   Soft-bristled toothbrush or sponge toothettes (if toothbrush is contraindicated)
*   Antiinfective oral cleaning solution or normal saline to loosen crusts (check agency policy)
*   Glass of water
*   Padded tongue blade
*   Emesis basin
*   Face towel
*   Paper towels
*   Suction equipment (optional): suction machine or small bulb syringe
*   Disposable gloves
*   Water-soluble lubricant

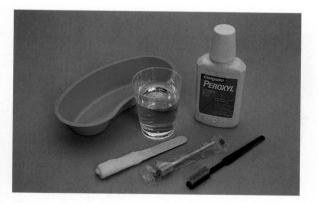

Figure 7-1   Oral hygiene equipment. *Clockwise from left:* Emesis basin, water, mouthwash, toothbrush, sponge toothette, and a padded tongue blade.

Delegation Considerations

Skills of oral care, toothbrushing, and denture care can be delegated to assistive personnel (AP). The nurse must first assess the client's gag reflex.
*   Instruct the care provider in the proper way to position client if client is unconscious or debilitated.
*   Remind the care provider to report any changes in oral mucosa.
*   Review the use of oral suction for cleansing oral secretions with the care provider if the client may require it.

IMPLEMENTATION FOR ORAL CARE

Steps	Rationale

1. See Standard Protocol (inside front cover).

2. Position unconscious client in side-lying position with bed flat and towel placed under chin. Have emesis basin available.

Side-lying position minimizes risk of aspiration. Debilitated client may be positioned with head of bed elevated if not in danger of aspirating.

Some clients tend to bite on any object placed in mouth.

3. Separate upper and lower teeth gently with padded tongue blade between back molars (see illustration). Client needs to be relaxed. Wait until client is relaxed with mouth open, then insert blade with smooth, quick motion and without using force.

4. Suction should be on and ready for use if gag reflex is absent (see Chapter 31).

Some clients who are unconscious do not have a gag reflex and so are at increased risk of aspiration. Suctioning of excess oral secretions reduces this risk.

Brushing action removes food particles between teeth and along chewing surfaces.

5. Clean mouth using brush or sponge toothettes moistened with normal saline, water, or antiinfective oral cleaning solution. Clean tooth surfaces, roof of mouth, inside cheeks, and tongue. Swab roof of mouth, gums, and inside cheek. Rinse with clean toothette and water. Avoid stimulating gag reflex (if present), and use as little fluid as possible to prevent aspiration.

Swabbing helps remove secretions and crusts from mucosa and moistens mucosa.

6. Suction secretions as they accumulate.

Suction removes secretions that collect in posterior pharynx.

7. Apply water-soluble jelly to lips (see illustration).

8. Remove gloves and inform client that you are finished.

Lubricates lips and prevents drying and cracking.

Provides meaningful stimulation and reality orientation.

9. Provide oral care to prevent or minimize mucositis.

Mucositis (inflammation of the mucous membranes in the mouth) is a common complication in hospitalized clients, especially those receiving radiation or chemotherapy (Lecours, 2001).

  a. Provide mouth care at least 4 times per day and often enough to keep the mouth clean and moist.

  b. Clean the mouth by brushing the teeth with a soft-bristled toothbrush angled at 45 degrees or a sponge toothette and rinsing well with normal saline. Avoid the use of lemon and glycerine swabs.

Angling the toothbrush or using the toothette avoids injury to the oral mucosa. Lemon and glycerine swabs are drying to the oral mucosa and should not be used (Lecours, 2001).

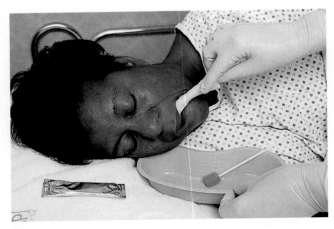

Step 3 Gently separate the teeth with a padded tongue blade.

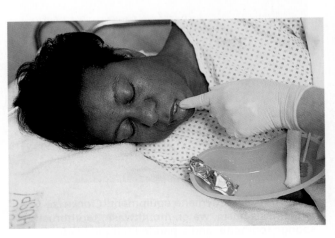

Step 7 Apply water-soluble jelly to lips.

Steps	Rationale

c. Rinse the mouth and carefully remove secretions (check agency policy or specific order) and remove gloves.

10. See Completion Protocol (inside front cover).

Agencies and physicians have different protocols for oral rinses. These mouth rinse mixtures will generally include some combination of alcohol-free antifungals, a commercial oral rinse or normal saline for cleaning, a topical anesthetic such as lidocaine for pain, and ice chips (Lecours, 2001).

• • • • • • • • • •

EVALUATION

1. Inspect oral mucous membranes for moistness, color, smoothness, and intact appearance.
2. Inspect dental surfaces for cleanliness.
3. Observe for restlessness or grimace during care. Ask client if mouth feels more comfortable.
4. Observe client, spouse, or significant other providing oral hygiene regimen.

Unexpected Outcomes and Related Interventions

1. Mucosa, tongue, or gums remain coated with thick secretions.
   a. Provide mouth care more frequently if secretions are thick or if oral ulcers are present (Lecours, 2001).
   b. To loosen and remove thick mucus, use toothette or soft toothbrush for cleaning and rinse with normal saline or a solution of tepid water.
2. Lips are cracked or inflamed.
   a. Lubricate lips more frequently with water-soluble lubricant.
3. Client has gurgles in back of throat from accumulation of liquid and is unable to clear throat or cough.
   a. Suction back of throat to clear airway and prevent aspiration.

Recording and Reporting

• Routine documentation may include check marks on a flow sheet. Observations made during oral care that should be charted include:
   Condition of mucous membranes and lips
   Client's level of consciousness and ability to cooperate and/or swallow
   Whether suction is necessary for oral care and if the client's gag reflex is present
   How the client tolerated the procedure

Sample Documentation

0800 Mouth care given. Mucous membranes are moist and pink, with no inflammation. Lips are dry and cracked. Moisturizing gel applied to lips. Client unresponsive. No gag reflex elicited. Oral pharynx suctioned frequently during oral care.

❋ SPECIAL CONSIDERATIONS ❋

Pediatric Considerations

• Infants will need the nurse to perform mouth care.
• Children will need reminders that oral care is needed and usually also need some supervision and/or assistance (Wong, Perry, and Hockenberry-Eaton, 2002).
• Proper oral hygiene and the importance of regular dental care should be taught to parents and care providers (Wong, Perry, and Hockenberry-Eaton, 2002).

Geriatric Considerations

• Older adults are more prone to oral injury and periodontal disease. Good oral hygiene practices can help older adults preserve their ability to eat.
• Clients unable to grasp a toothbrush can have an enlarged handle placed on toothbrush (e.g., push handle through center of a plastic ball).
• Clients with diabetes will require visits to the dentist a minimum every 6 months.
• Older adults, especially those at risk for oral problems, should avoid spicy, coarse, acidic, and sugary foods, which can irritate the mouth and cause dental caries (Kim, McFarland, and McLane, 1997).

Home Care Considerations

• During the initial admission visit, document the condition of the client's mouth, teeth, and gums, thus providing a baseline for assessment of the client's ability to comply with special diets and fluid intake and to carry out oral hygiene practices.
• On regular visits, assess for signs and symptoms of infection or irritation, including reddened, bleeding oral lesions.
• Provide special care to clients undergoing head and neck radiation, because gums may be dry and swollen and may interfere with proper denture fit.

Long-Term Care Considerations

Residents of long-term care facilities continue to require regular dental care and examinations and need to have their dentures evaluated for proper fit.

Skill 7.3

Hair Care

A person's appearance and feeling of well-being are influenced by how the hair looks and feels. Brushing, combing, and shampooing are basic measures for all clients unable to provide self-care. Male clients should be offered the opportunity to shave or be shaved when their condition allows. Some hospitals have a beauty shop where clients can go for professional hair care.

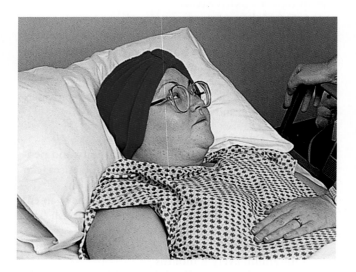

Figure 7-2 Clients may choose to wear a turban because of hair loss.

Fever, malnutrition, emotional stress, and depression affect the condition of hair. Diaphoresis leaves hair oily and unmanageable. Excessively dry or oily hair may be associated with hormone changes. Dry, brittle hair occurs with aging and excessive use of shampoo.

Certain chemotherapy agents and radiation therapy may cause alopecia (hair loss). Many clients choose to wear a wig; however, some choose to wear head scarves or turbans (Figure 7-2). The average growth of healthy hair is ½ inch per month. Table 7-2 describes common hair and scalp conditions and nursing interventions.

When caring for clients from different cultures, it is important to learn as much as possible about the client's cultural customs and beliefs and to be sensitive to the uniqueness of each client; preferred hair care methods. For example, African-Americans' hair is quite dry. Special lanolin conditioners may be used to maintain conditioning. The neglect of hair care may be interpreted by the client or family as rejection.

Frequency of shampooing depends on the hair's condition and the person's personal preferences. Dry hair, which often results from aging and protein deficiency, requires less frequent shampooing than oily hair or hair of people who exercise actively. Hospitalized clients who have excess perspiration or treatments that leave blood or solutions in the hair may need a shampoo.

Some clients are able to sit in a chair in front of a sink, positioned facing away from the sink with the head and

Table 7-2

Common Hair and Scalp Conditions and Related Interventions

Problem	Interventions
Alopecia (hair loss): chemotherapeutic agents kill cells that rapidly multiply, including both tumor and normal cells.	Some clients wear scarves. Some clients prefer hairpieces. Referral may be needed for professional consultation for long-term interventions.
Dandruff: scaling of scalp accompanied by itching; if severe, may involve eyebrows.	Shampoo regularly with medicated shampoo.
Pediculosis	
Head lice: parasites attached to hair strands. Eggs look like oval particles. Bites or pustules may be found behind ears and at hairline. May spread to furniture and other people.	Shampoo with a medicated shampoo or conditioner for lice, and repeat 12 to 24 hours later. Change bed linens, and follow isolation precautions for pediculosis according to agency policy.
Body lice: parasites tend to cling to clothing. Client itches. Hemorrhagic spots may appear on skin where lice are sucking blood. Lice may lay eggs on clothing and furniture.	For body lice, apply a medicated lotion for lice, and repeat according to instructions on product. Follow appropriate agency isolation precautions.
Crab lice: found in pubic hair, are grayish white with red legs, and may spread via sexual contact.	For pubic lice, shave hair off affected area, use medicated product for lice, and notify sexual partner of proper treatment.

neck hyperextended over the sink's edge. This is contraindicated for clients who have had neck injuries or back pain.

Some clients may be placed on a stretcher with head extended over a sink. A plastic shampoo trough or board facilitates a shampoo in bed. Water is poured over the client's head and allowed to drain into a container on the side of the bed.

Dependent clients with beards or mustaches need to have assistance keeping the facial hair clean, especially after eating. A brush or comb may be used. Shaving of facial hair is a task most men prefer to do for themselves. Men without beards usually shave daily. A beard or mustache should be combed or washed as needed. Food particles easily collect in the hair. Some religions and cultures forbid cutting or shaving any body hair (Galanti, 1997); therefore nurses should not shave or cut the hair of a client without consent.

ASSESSMENT

1. Determine any restrictions that may be necessary. Often a physician's order is required to wash a client's hair. If exposure to moisture is contraindicated, dry shampoo may be used. *Rationale: Shampoo may be contraindicated if client has increased intracranial pressure; cerebrospinal fluid leaks; open incisions of face, head, or neck; cervical neck injuries; tracheostomy; facial edema; or respiratory distress.*

2. Assess condition of hair and scalp. Note distribution of hair, oiliness, and texture. Inspect scalp for abrasions, lacerations, lesions, inflammation, and infestation. *Rationale: Determines the need for further interventions, such as conditioner or medicated shampoo.*

3. Before shaving client, assess for bleeding tendency. Review medical history, and check laboratory values, including platelet count, prothrombin time (PT), and activated partial thromboplastin time (aPTT). *Rationale: Clients with leukemia, hemophilia, or disseminated intravascular coagulation and clients receiving anticoagulant therapy (heparin or coumadin) or taking high doses of aspirin may have abnormally long clotting times. An electric razor is generally recommended for these clients. Electric razors may be a safety hazard in the presence of oxygen therapy.*

4. If client wants to shave himself, assess ability to manipulate razor to determine how much assistance will be needed.

PLANNING

Expected outcomes should focus on comfort and promoting self-concept.

Expected Outcomes

1. Client expresses increased sense of comfort.
2. Client verbalizes improved self-image.
3. Skin remains free of cuts.

Equipment

- Brush
- Comb
- Shampoo board
- Shampoo
- Conditioner (optional)
- Towels (two or more)
- Razor
- Shaving cream
- Basin of very warm water

Delegation Considerations

The skills of shampooing and shaving can be delegated to assistive personnel (AP) unless the client has a trauma or injury of the cervical spine. The nurse should:

- Instruct the care provider how to properly position individual clients and any special products indicated
- Make sure the care provider knows how to correctly use medicated shampoos for lice or other conditions and the appropriate steps to prevent transmission to other clients
- Remind the care provider to report how the client tolerated the procedure and any changes that may indicate inflammation or injury

IMPLEMENTATION FOR HAIR CARE

Steps	Rationale
1. See Standard Protocol (inside front cover).	
2. **Shampoo for client confined to bed**	

NURSE ALERT *Caution is needed in providing hair care if clients have neck pain or neck or back injury.*

Steps	**Rationale**

a. Place a towel under head. Brush and comb client's hair by separating hair into small sections, releasing tangles with fingers.

b. Place a waterproof pad under client's shoulders, neck, and head. Position client supine with plastic trough under head and spout extending beyond edge of mattress. Position container under spout to collect water (see illustration).

c. Pour warm water over hair until it is completely wet (see illustration). The client or another caregiver can protect client's face with towel or washcloth over eyes, as needed.

d. Apply small amount of shampoo, and work up a lather with both hands. Start at hairline, and work toward back of neck. Lift head slightly to wash back of head. Massage scalp gently. Rinse thoroughly, and repeat if necessary. Dry using a second towel if needed.

e. Assist client to a comfortable position, and complete styling of hair. Braids may be helpful for clients with very long hair.

Moistening with water or mineral oil may help free tangles. Anchoring tangled hair at scalp prevents painful pulling of scalp.

3. **Caring for coarse, curly hair**

a. Shampooing of coarse, curly hair is identical to shampooing wavy or straight hair, but the hair should be conditioned after washing. Ask clients if they use a particular product.

b. To untangle wet coarse, curly hair use the wide teeth of a comb. Beginning at the nape of the neck, comb small subsections of the hair starting at the hair ends. Continue to work through small sections until hair is free of tangles.

c. To comb through dry hair it is best to lubricate the hair by applying a conditioner and loosening any tangles with your fingers. Then, using a wide-tooth comb, start on either side of the head, insert the comb with the teeth upward to the hair near the scalp. Comb through the hair in a circular motion by turning the wrist while lifting up and out. Continue until the hair is combed through, and then comb into place using hands to shape.

Coarse, curly hair, seen, for example, in African-American clients, does not retain moisture as other types of hair do. Shampooing may be necessary only once a week (Crute, 1997).

Working on small sections of the hair keeps fragile hair from becoming entangled.

Coarse, curly hair can be very dry and fragile and will be damaged if not combed carefully. Dry areas of the hair may require further lubrication with a leave-in conditioner and/or styling lotion (Crute, 1997).

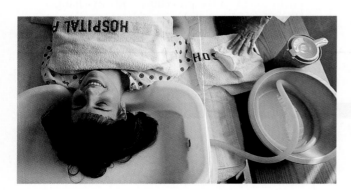

Step 2b Position client with plastic trough under head.

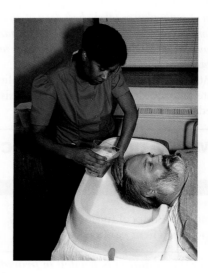

Step 2c Pour warm water over hair.

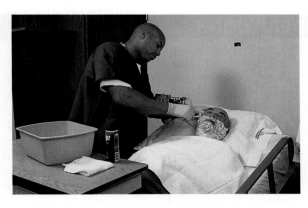

Step 4c   Shaving a client.

Steps	Rationale

4. **Shave beard**
   a. Assist client to sitting position if possible, and place towel over chest and shoulders.
   b. Place a warm, moist washcloth over client's face for several seconds. Apply shaving cream, using product client prefers. — Softens beard. Skin sensitivity can occur with some products.
   c. With the razor at a 45-degree angle, shave in direction of hair growth using short strokes. Hold skin taut with nondominant hand. Remind client to tell you if it becomes uncomfortable (see illustration). — Holding skin taut helps prevent razor cuts and discomfort during shaving.
   d. Dip razor blade in water as shaving cream accumulates on blade's edge. — Keeps cutting surface of razor blade clean.
   e. Rinse and dry face. Remove gloves. Apply aftershave if desired. — Provides a positive effect for comfort and self-esteem.
5. See Completion Protocol (inside front cover).

• • • • • • • • • •

EVALUATION

1. Offer a mirror, and ask how client feels and looks.
2. Inspect condition of shaved area of skin for nicks, cuts, or areas of dryness.

Unexpected Outcomes and Related Interventions

1. Client has small nicks or cuts on skin.
   a. Apply pressure and if necessary a small dressing or Band-Aid.
2. Client has areas of skin surface that appear dry.
   a. Use moisturizing shaving foam next time, and apply moisturizing lotion to skin.

Recording and Reporting

Routine documentation may include check marks on a flow sheet. It is usually not necessary to document hair care unless it is included on the agency's checklist.

SPECIAL CONSIDERATIONS

Pediatric Considerations

African-American children will require special hair care, including some type of hair dressing specified by their parents. Do not use petroleum jelly (Wong, Perry, and Hockenberry-Eaton, 2002).

Geriatric Considerations

- Hair growth declines sharply between 50 and 60 years.
- Usually the facial hair of older clients does not grow quickly. Thus a shave might not be necessary each day.

Home Care Considerations

- Assess room temperature, availability of water, and most satisfactory position for the client.
- Provide extra protection from wetness for clients with casts.
- Obtain dry shampoo preparations when a wet shampoo is contraindicated.

- Construct a trough by arranging a plastic shower curtain or tablecloth under the client's head and then tapering the cloth to form a narrow end that can drain into a bucket or basin next to the client's bed.
- In the home setting, one of the nurse's greatest challenges is to find ways the client can shampoo the hair without causing injury. For example, a client with a long leg cast may need to wash the hair at a sink until it is safe to shower or until the cast is removed and tub baths can be resumed.
- Caution clients about using chemicals and hot combs for straightening hair. Such practices can cause considerable damage to the hair. Misuse can result in scalp burns, hair loss, and allergic reactions that can cause severe skin rashes, urticaria, and conjunctivitis (Crute, 1997).

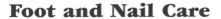

Skill 7.4

Foot and Nail Care

Most people are required to walk or stand to perform their jobs, and foot pain can cause strain on muscle groups. Often people are unaware of foot or nail problems until pain occurs. Various skin problems involving the feet are the result of improperly fitted shoes. Tight shoes, socks, garters, or knee-high hose may interfere with circulation. Foot pain may cause a person to change gait, resulting in strain on different muscle groups. If job performance requires a person to walk or stand comfortably, a foot disorder can become a serious problem.

Nail and foot care should be included in a client's daily hygiene; the best time is during the client's bath. Feet and nails often require special care to prevent infection, odors, and injury to soft tissues. Many conditions often result from inadequate care of the feet and hands, such as biting nails or trimming them improperly, exposure to harsh chemicals, or wearing ill-fitting shoes (American Diabetes Association, 2001). Changes also occur in the shape, color, and texture of nails that may result from various nutritional, infectious, and circulatory disorders (Table 7-3).

Many older clients may have poor vision, hand tremors, obesity, or limited joint mobility that contribute to difficulties with foot and nail care (Lueckenotte, 2000). Older clients may also have excessive dryness of the skin and poor circulation.

Circulation is assessed by palpation of the pedal and posterior tibial pulses. The nurse also palpates the skin for edema, texture, and coolness. Changes in skin color may be noted. Clients with peripheral vascular disease, such as diabetes, may have inadequate arterial or venous circulation or both. These clients are at high risk for neuropathy, a degeneration of peripheral nerves with loss of sensation. Sensation can be checked by light touch, use of a pinprick, or asking client to discriminate hot and cold temperatures. These clients need to inspect their feet daily, because injuries may not be felt. These injuries are easily infected and heal slowly because of inadequate circulation (American Diabetes Association, 2001).

ASSESSMENT

1. Identify client's risk for foot or nail problems.
   a. Poor vision, lack of coordination, and inability to bend over contribute to older adults' difficulty in performing foot and nail care. *Rationale: Normal physiological changes of aging also result in nail and foot problems.*
   b. Vascular changes associated with diabetes reduce blood flow to peripheral tissues. *Rationale: Break in skin integrity places diabetic clients at high risk for skin infection (American Diabetes Association, 2001).*

Table 7-3

Common Foot and Nail Problems and Related Interventions

Problem	Prevention	Interventions
Callus: thickened epidermis, usually flat, painless, and on underside of foot or palm; caused by friction or pressure.	Wear gloves when working with hands. Wear proper footwear, and always wear clean socks/stockings.	Soak callus in warm water to soften. Creams or lotions can help prevent reformation. Refer diabetic client to a podiatrist.
Corns: caused by friction and pressure from shoes, mainly on toes, over bony prominence; usually cone shaped, round, raised, and tender; may affect gait (Figure 7-3).	Wear proper footwear; pain is aggravated by tight shoes. Always wear clean socks or stockings.	Surgical removal may be necessary. Use oval corn pads carefully, because they increase pressure on toes and reduce circulation.
Plantar warts: fungating lesions on sole of foot caused by papillomavirus (Figure 7-4).	Warts are contagious. Avoid going barefoot, especially in public places.	Treatment ordered by physician may include applications of acid, burning, or freezing for removal.
Athlete's foot: fungal infection of foot; scaling and cracking of skin occur between toes and on soles of feet; may have small blisters containing fluid. Apparently induced by tight footwear (Figure 7-5).	Feet should be well ventilated. Avoid tight footwear. Dry feet well after bathing; apply powder. Wear clean socks.	May be treated with medicated powder or cream. Refer to physician if condition does not improve with medicated products.
Ingrown nails: toenail or fingernail grows inward into soft tissue around nail; may be painful (Figure 7-6).	Cut with a nail clipper and file toenails straight across after bathing when they are soft. If nails are thick or vision is poor, have toenails trimmed by a podiatrist.	Frequent warm soaks in antiseptic solution and surgical removal of portion of nail that has grown into skin. Diabetic clients need to be referred to a podiatrist.
Fungus infection: thick, discolored nails with yellow streaks.	Keep feet and nails clean and dry. Check feet and nails daily.	Refer to podiatrist.

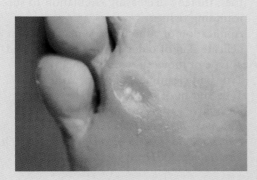

Figure 7-3   Corn. (From Weston WL, Lane AT: Color textbook of pediatric dermatology, ed 3, St Louis, 2002, Mosby.)

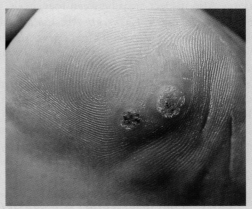

Figure 7-4   Plantar warts. (From Zitelli BJ, Davis HW: *Atlas of pediatric physical diagnosis*, ed 3, St Louis, 1997, Mosby.)

Continued

Table 7-3

Common Foot and Nail Problems and Related Interventions—cont'd

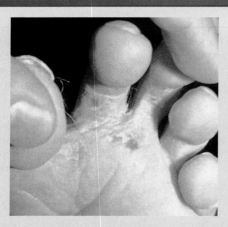

Figure 7-5 Athlete's foot, tinea pedis. (From Greenberger NJ, Hinthorn DR: *History taking and physical examination: essentials and clinical correlates,* St Louis, 1993, Mosby. Courtesy Dr. Loren Amundson, University of South Dakota, Sioux Falls, SD.)

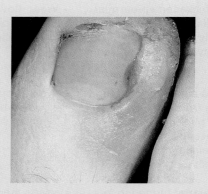

Figure 7-6 Ingrown toenail. (From Habif TP: *Clinical dermatology: a color guide to diagnosis and therapy,* ed 2, St Louis, 1990, Mosby.)

c. Edema associated with cardiac or renal conditions can have symptoms of increased tissue edema, particularly in dependent areas (e.g., feet). *Rationale: Edema reduces blood flow to neighboring tissues.*

d. Presence of muscle weakness or paralysis of one lower extremity after a stroke is a risk factor. *Rationale: May result in altered walking patterns, which increase friction and pressure on the affected foot.*

2. Inspect all surfaces of toes, feet, and nails. Pay particular attention to areas of dryness, inflammation, or cracking. Also inspect areas between toes, heels, and soles of feet. *Rationale: Changes in skin associated with aging include thinning of epidermis and dryness. The nails may become opaque, tough, scaly, brittle, and hypertrophied (Lueckenotte, 2000).*

3. Assess color and warmth of toes and feet. Assess capillary refill of nails. Palpate the dorsalis pedis pulse of both feet simultaneously, comparing the strength of pulses. *Rationale: Circulatory alterations may change integrity of nails and increase client's chance of localized infection when a break in skin integrity occurs (Armstrong and Lavery, 1998).*

NURSE ALERT *A physician's order is required for trimming nails, especially when impaired circulation is suspected (e.g., diabetes mellitus, peripheral vascular disease, leg ulcers).*

---

4. Determine client's ability to perform self-care. *Rationale: Limited vision, lack of coordination, and inability to reach feet influence degree of assistance required.*

5. Assess client's knowledge of foot and nail care practices and type of home remedies client uses for existing foot problems. *Rationale: Over-the-counter liquid preparations to remove corns may cause burns and ulcerations.*

a. Cutting of corns or calluses with razor blade or scissors may result in infections. *Rationale: Proper foot care is essential if the client is to avoid foot ulcers, infections, and complications (American Diabetes Association, 2001).*

b. Use of oval corn pads may exert pressure on toes, thereby decreasing circulation to surrounding tissues.

c. Application of adhesive tape may tear thin and delicate skin of older adults when removed.

6. Assess type of footwear worn by clients.

a. Type and cleanliness of socks worn?

b. Type and fit of shoes?

c. Restrictive garters or knee-high hose worn? *Rationale: Improper footwear and constrictive clothing contribute to foot problems (American Diabetes Association, 2001).*

PLANNING

Expected outcomes focus on self-care practices that maintain healthy nails and feet and promote circulation and comfort.

Expected Outcomes

1. Client maintains nail integrity and cleanliness.
2. Client correctly demonstrates nail care.
3. Client walks steadily in appropriate footwear.
4. Client identifies ways to minimize sources of pressure or irritation when walking.

Equipment

- Basin (appropriate size for soaking)
- Washcloth
- Bath or face towel
- Nail clippers
- Orange stick (optional)
- Emery board or nail file

Delegation Considerations

The skill of care of the fingernails and foot care for the nondiabetic clients and clients without any circulatory compromise can be delegated to assistive personnel (AP). The nurse should:

- Instruct care provider in the proper way to use nail files and clippers (check agency policy on whether AP may use nail clipper on clients)
- Caution care provider to use warm water
- Remind care provider to report any changes that may indicate inflammation or injury

---

IMPLEMENTATION FOR FOOT AND NAIL CARE

Steps	Rationale

1. See Standard Protocol (inside front cover).
2. **Soak feet**
   a. Explain that soaking requires 10 to 20 minutes.
   b. Assist ambulatory client to sit in chair with disposable bath mat under feet. If confined to bed, assist to a semi-Fowler's position with a waterproof pad and bath towel under feet.

COMMUNICATION TIP   *Now is the time to stress to the client the importance of foot care routine. Nurse may say, "Now let's look at your feet together to see if there are any problem areas."*

NURSE ALERT   *It is not recommended to soak the feet of clients with diabetes mellitus or peripheral vascular disease. Soaking may lead to maceration (excessive softening of the skin), ulceration, or infection (American Diabetes Association, 2001).*

---

   c. Fill washbasin with warm water. Test temperature of water with back of hand.
   d. Place basin on bath mat or towel, and help client place one foot in basin. Place call light within client's reach and position over-bed table in front of client. Offer diversional activity.

Clients with decreased sensation to feet are unable to detect temperature of water.
Clients with muscular weakness or tremors may have difficulty positioning feet.

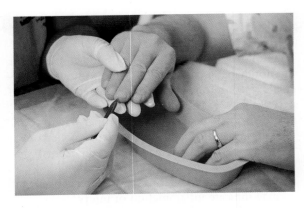

Step 2e Soaking fingers in basin.

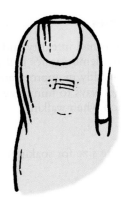

Step 3a Shape and trim nails straight across and even with digit.

Steps	Rationale
e. If desired, allow client to soak fingers in a small basin on over-bed table with arms in a comfortable position (see illustration).	Prolonged positioning can cause discomfort unless alignment is maintained.
f. Allow client's feet and nails to soak for 10 to 20 minutes. If necessary, rewarm water after 10 minutes. Begin care on foot that has soaked, and place other foot in basin.	Softening of corns, calluses, and cuticles ensures easy removal of dead cells and easy manipulation of cuticle (Armstrong and Lavery, 1998).
g. ✋ Using an orange stick, clean gently under nails while they are immersed in water. Remove from basin and dry thoroughly.	Thorough drying slows fungal growth and prevents maceration of tissues. Friction removes dead skin layers (Perry and Potter, 2002)
3. Trim nails	
a. With nail clippers, clip nails straight across and even with ends of digits. Shape nails with emery board or file (see illustration).	Cutting straight across prevents splitting of nail margins and formation of sharp nail spikes that can irritate lateral nail margins (Strauss, Hart, and Winant, 1998).

NURSE ALERT *Clients with severe hypertrophy of nails or diabetes should be referred to podiatrist for care to avoid risk of additional tissue injury.*

---

b. If client has circulatory problems, file the nails only.	Filing prevents cutting soft tissues, which could become infected and heal slowly.
c. Push cuticle back gently with orange stick, apply lotion to hands and feet, and remove gloves.	Reduces incidence of inflamed cuticles. Lotion lubricates dry skin by helping to retain moisture.
4. Teach foot care	
a. Instruct client to inspect feet daily: tops and soles, heels, and area between toes. Use a mirror to check soles and heels.	Irritated areas may not be painful initially, so are noted only by observation.
b. Instruct nondiabetic client to wash and soak feet daily using lukewarm water and to dry thoroughly, especially between toes.	Warm water softens nails and thickened epidermal cells, reduces inflammation of skin, and promotes local circulation (Armstrong and Lavery, 1998).
c. Instruct to consult a physician or podiatrist rather than cutting corns or calluses or using commercial removers.	
d. If feet tend to perspire, instruct client to use a mild foot powder.	
e. Instruct client to wear clean socks or stockings daily (change twice a day if feet perspire heavily). Check for holes or roughness that might cause pressure. Wearing absorbent liners also helps reduce perspiration and foot odors.	Light-colored or white cotton socks do not contain dyes and are more absorbent (Strauss, Hart, and Winant, 1998).

Steps	Rationale
f. If dryness is noted along the feet or between the toes, instruct or assist the client in applying lotion.	Lotion lubricates dry skin by helping to retain moisture (Perry and Potter, 2002).
g. Instruct client to avoid wearing elastic stockings, knee-high hose, or constricting garters and to avoid crossing legs at knees and ankles.	Impairs circulation to the lower extremities.
h. Instruct client with impaired sensation to wear protective footwear at all times and to check inside of shoes daily for pebbles, foreign objects, and roughness or tears in the inner liners.	Reduced circulation is often accompanied by reduced sensation, allowing injuries to go untreated unless detected by inspection. Foreign objects may cause sores that go unnoticed (Slovenkai, 1998).
i. Instruct client to wear shoes with flexible nonslip soles, sturdy porous uppers, and closed-in toes. Fit should not be restrictive to the feet.	
j. Any minor cuts should be washed immediately and dried thoroughly. Only mild antiseptics (e.g., Neosporin ointment) should be applied to the skin. Avoid iodine or merbromin (Perry and Potter, 2002). Notify a physician.	With reduced circulation, infections are more likely and heal more slowly.

5. See Completion Protocol (inside front cover).

• • • • • • • • • •

EVALUATION

1. Inspect nails and surrounding skin surfaces after soaking and nail trimming. Note any remaining rough areas.
2. Ask client to explain and demonstrate nail care.
3. Observe client's walk after toenail care using appropriate footwear.

Unexpected Outcomes and Related Interventions

1. Nails are discolored, rough, and concave or irregular in shape. Cuticles and surrounding tissues may be inflamed and tender to touch. Localized areas of tenderness are present on feet, with calluses or corns at points of friction.
   a. Repeated nail and foot care is necessary to help relieve inflammation and remove layers of cells from calluses or corns. Referral to a podiatrist may be needed.
   b. Change in footwear or corrective foot surgery may be needed for permanent improvement in corns or calluses.
2. Client unable to explain or perform foot care.
   a. Provide repeated opportunities for practice in controlled setting.
   b. Refer to podiatrist for regular follow-up care.

3. Client complains of pain while walking and has unsteady gait.
   a. Special footwear may be required, or client may need referral to a podiatrist.

Recording and Reporting

- Foot care and condition of the feet and nails should be documented, including:
  Condition of feet and nails
  Clients' ability to care for their own feet
  Any apparent area of inflammation, infection, ulceration, or injury with any interventions provided
  All teaching given to clients about foot care and their comprehension of information

Sample Documentation

0900 Right great toe red, inflamed, and tender. Client states this was first noted before admission 1 week ago. Feet soaked for 10 minutes in warm water and dried thoroughly. Lotion applied. Client instructed on necessity of cutting nails straight across to avoid this problem. Stated, "This is so sore, I'll be careful how I trim my nails now." Toe inflammation reported to physician.

SPECIAL CONSIDERATIONS

Pediatric Considerations

- The nails of infants and children should be kept short and clean (Wong, Perry, and Hockenberry-Eaton, 2002).
- It is best to cut an infant's nails with manicure scissors with rounded tips while the infant is sleeping (Wong, Perry, and Hockenberry-Eaton, 2002).

Geriatric Considerations

- Changes in aging skin include thinning of epidermis and subcutaneous fat and dryness because of decreased activity of oil and sweat glands. These changes can be seen in the feet. In addition, nails become opaque, tough, scaly, brittle, and hypertrophied.
- A lifetime of limited exercise can result in laxity of foot ligaments and musculature and lead to instability and impaired mobility.
- Common foot problems of older adults include heel pain caused by tearing of plantar fascia and foot musculature, metatarsalgia (pain beneath metatarsal head), hammer toes and claw toes, corns and calluses, pathological nail conditions (e.g., ingrown toenails, fungal infections), arthritis, and neuropathies that cause diminished sensation in foot (Lueckenotte, 2000).

- Older persons are also more vulnerable to bunions because feet tend to spread with aging (Lueckenotte, 2000).

Home Care Considerations

- Alternative therapies: moleskin applied to areas of feet that are under friction is less likely to cause local pressure than corn pads; spot adhesive bandages can guard corns against friction, but do not have padding to protect against pressure; wrapping small pieces of lamb's wool around toes reduces irritation of soft corns between toes (Beuscher, 1998).
- Assess use of bathroom sink for soaking client's hands and tub for soaking feet.
- Financial constraints may contribute to clients' wearing poorly fitted shoes, which can cause foot problems.

Skill 7.5

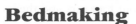

Bedmaking

The nurse makes a client's bed with safety and comfort in mind. The sheets must be clean, dry, and wrinkle free. Whenever a client's bed is soiled, it must be changed. The sheets should be straightened out and tightened periodically throughout the day to keep them wrinkle free.

Within Skill 7.5 there are three bedmaking procedures:

1. Unoccupied bed, used when the client is able to get out of bed, is left open with the top sheets folded down (Procedural Guideline 7-2).
2. Postoperative (postop) or surgical bed, used when clients have left for the operating room or procedural area, is left with the top sheets fanfolded lengthwise and not tucked in to facilitate the client's return to bed.
3. Occupied bed, used when the client is not allowed out of bed.

When a client is discharged and housekeeping cleans the unit, the bed is made with the top sheets left up. This is known as a closed bed.

ASSESSMENT

1. Check the activity order, and assess the client's ability to get out of bed. *Rationale: This determines whether an unoccupied or occupied bed should be made.*
2. Assess the client's self-toileting ability; note the presence of any wounds, drainage tubes. *Rationale: This determines if placement of waterproof pads should be on the bed.*

PLANNING

Expected outcomes focus on the client's safety and comfort.

Expected Outcomes

1. Client has a clean, safe environment throughout hospitalization.
2. Client verbalizes a sense of comfort while in bed.
3. Client's skin remains free of irritation throughout hospitalization.

Procedural Guideline 7-2

Unoccupied Bedmaking

Equipment: Linen bag, mattress pad (change only when soiled), bottom sheet (flat or fitted), drawsheet (optional), top sheet, blanket, bedspread, waterproof pads (optional), pillowcases, bedside chair or table, disposable gloves (if linen is soiled), washcloth, and antiseptic cleanser.

1. Determine if client has been incontinent or if excess drainage is on linen. Gloves will be necessary.
2. Assess activity orders or restrictions in mobility in planning if client can get out of bed for procedure. Assist to bedside chair or recliner.
3. Lower side rails on both sides of bed, and raise bed to comfortable working position.
4. Remove soiled linen, and place in laundry bag. Avoid shaking or fanning linen.
5. Reposition mattress, and wipe off any moisture using a washcloth moistened in antiseptic solution. Dry thoroughly.
6. Apply all bottom linen on one side of bed before moving to opposite side.
7. Be sure fitted sheet is placed smoothly over mattress. To apply a flat unfitted sheet, allow about 25 cm (10 inches) to hang over mattress edge. Lower hem of sheet should lie seam down, even with bottom edge of mattress. Pull remaining top portion of sheet over top edge of mattress.
8. While standing at head of bed, miter top corner of bottom sheet (see Skill 7-5, Step 3g, p. 172).
9. Tuck remaining portion of unfitted sheet under mattress.
10. Optional: Apply drawsheet, laying center fold along middle of bed lengthwise. Smooth drawsheet over mattress, and tuck excess edge under mattress, keeping palms down.
11. Move to opposite side of bed, and spread bottom sheet smoothly over edge of mattress from head to foot of bed.
12. Apply fitted sheet smoothly over each mattress corner. For an unfitted sheet, miter top corner of bottom sheet (see Step 8), making sure corner is taut.
13. Grasp remaining edge of unfitted bottom sheet, and tuck tightly under mattress while moving from head to foot of bed. Smooth folded drawsheet over bottom sheet, and tuck under mattress, first at middle, then at top, and then at bottom.
14. If needed, apply waterproof pad over bottom sheet or draw sheet.
15. Place top sheet over bed with vertical center fold lengthwise down middle of bed. Open sheet out from head to foot, being sure top edge of sheet is even with top edge of mattress.

16. Make horizontal toe pleat; stand at foot of bed and fan fold in sheet 5 to 10 cm (2 to 4 inches) across bed. Pull sheet up from bottom to make fold approximately 15 cm (6 inches) from bottom edge of mattress.
17. Tuck in remaining portion of sheet under foot of mattress. Then place blanket over bed with top edge parallel to top edge of sheet and 15 to 20 cm (6 to 8 inches) down from edge of sheet. (Optional: Apply additional spread over bed.)
18. Make cuff by turning edge of top sheet down over top edge of blanket and spread.
19. Standing on one side at foot of bed, lift mattress corner slightly with one hand, and with other hand tuck top sheet, blanket, and spread under mattress. Be sure toe pleats are not pulled out.
20. Make modified mitered corner with top sheet, blanket, and spread. After triangular fold is made, do not tuck tip of triangle (see illustration).
21. Go to other side of bed. Spread sheet, blanket, and spread over evenly. Make cuff with top sheet and blanket. Make modified corner at foot of bed.
22. Apply clean pillowcase.
23. Place call light within client's reach on bed rail or pillow, and return bed to height allowing for client transfer. Assist client to bed.
24. Arrange client's room. Remove and discard supplies. Perform hand hygiene.

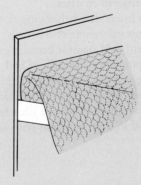

Step 20   Modified mitered corner.

Equipment

- Linen bag or hamper
- Bath blanket (if available)
- Bottom sheet (flat or fitted)
- Drawsheet (optional)
- Waterproof pads (optional)
- Top sheet
- Blanket
- Mattress pad (needs to be changed only when soiled)
- Spread
- Pillowcase
- Disposable gloves

COMMUNICATION TIP

- *Use an organized approach and reassuring tone of voice so the client feels safe and comfortable during bedmaking.*
- *Encourage the client to report any discomfort or special requests while the bed is being made.*
- *When making an occupied bed, ask the client to assist as able and to report any discomfort or the need to rest.*
- *Interact throughout the entire procedure, even if client is not responsive.*

Delegation Considerations

Bedmaking is usually delegated to assistive personnel (AP). The nurse should:

- Instruct care provider on whether an unoccupied or occupied bed is to be made
- Review safety precautions or activity restrictions for client with care provider; stress the use of side rails and the call system in the event that staff assistance is needed
- Tell care provider what to do if wound drainage, dressing material, drainage tubes, or IV tubing becomes dislodged or is found in the linen
- Instruct care provider on what to do if the client becomes fatigued

---

IMPLEMENTATION FOR BEDMAKING—OCCUPIED BED

Steps	Rationale

1. See Standard Protocol (inside front cover).
2. **Postoperative (postop) or surgical bed.** Begin with clean unoccupied bed (see Procedural Guideline 7-2, p. 173).   *Facilitates transfer of postoperative client from stretcher to bed.*
   a. Fold all top linen from foot of bed toward center of mattress. Linen fold should be flush with bottom edge of mattress.
   b. Fold top linen that is hanging down over sides of bed toward center of mattress. Face one side of bed and fold nearest bottom corner back and over toward opposite side of bed, forming a triangle. Repeat for top corner (see illustration).
   c. Grasp apex of triangle and fanfold top linen over to far side of bed (see illustration).
   d. Leave bed in high position with side rails down.   *Matches height of stretcher and facilitates client transfer.*

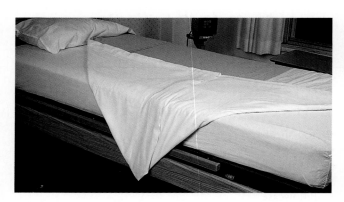

Step 2b   Fold top linen to form a triangle.

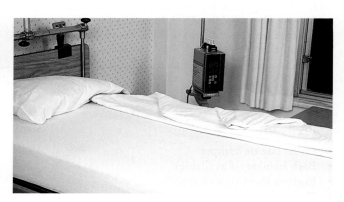

Step 2c   Fanfold linen over to far side of bed.

Steps	Rationale

3. Occupied bed

a. Raise entire bed to comfortable working height. Lower head of bed, if tolerated by client. Lower side rail on nurse's side; leave far side rail up.

It is easier to apply wrinkle-free, tight linens if bed is in the flat position.

b. 🖐 Loosen all top linens. Remove spread and blanket, leaving client covered with top sheet or bath blanket. Fold spread and blanket in quarters, and place over bottom of bed or on back of chair if they are clean and are to be reused.

Gloves are worn to remove linen only if it is soiled with body secretions.

c. Assist client to a side-lying position on far side of bed. Slide pillow over so it remains under client's head. Check that any tubing is not being pulled.

Provides privacy and warmth.

d. Roll bottom sheet, drawsheet, and any pads as far as possible toward client. Clean and dry mattress if necessary.

Reduces transmission of organisms and keeps new linen dry.

e. Place clean bottom sheet on bed with seam side down.
   (1) Bottom sheets may be fitted.
   (2) If flat, center sheet on bed and pull bottom hem to foot end of mattress. Open sheet toward client (see illustration).

f. Unfold flat bottom sheet lengthwise to cover mattress. Tuck top of sheet under head end of mattress.

g. Miter top corner of a flat bottom sheet, and tuck in side of sheet under mattress (see illustration).

Mitered corners do not loosen easily.

h. Place folded drawsheet and/or waterproof pads on center of bed with seam side down. Fanfold toward client.

Provides additional protection to bed linen.

i. Cover unoccupied portion of bed with half the material, tucking drawsheet under mattress. Place remaining materials as close to client as possible. Keep clean linen and soiled linen separate.

j. Place waterproof pads with absorbent side up and plastic side down. Some pads go under cloth drawsheet. Newer, larger absorbent pads go on top of drawsheet or replace it (check agency policy).

Waterproof absorbent pads protect bedding and keep moisture away from client's skin.

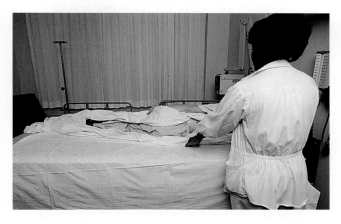

Step 3e(2)   Open clean flat bottom sheet toward client.

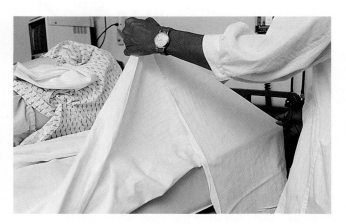

Step 3g   Miter the top corner of flat bottom sheet.

Steps	**Rationale**
k. Assist client with logrolling over all linen and facing you. Keep client covered with top sheet or bath blanket. Raise side rail on the side client is facing. Go to other side of bed, and lower side rail.	
l. Remove soiled linens. Hold them away from uniform. Place on chair seat or in disposable bag or hamper if it is close by. Do not leave client alone with side rail down, even for a moment. Remove gloves if worn, and dispose of them properly.	Reduces transmission of microorganisms.
m. Gently slide clean linen toward you, and straighten the clean linen out.	Avoids friction of linen being pulled across skin.
n. Miter the top corner of bottom sheet as before.	
o. Grasp side of flat bottom sheet tightly. Keeping it taut, tuck it under mattress. Proceed from head to foot.	
p. Repeat by tucking drawsheet, proceeding from middle to top to bottom.	
q. Straighten out waterproof pads that are on top of drawsheet.	
r. Assist client into a supine position; place a clean top sheet, blanket, and spread over client, leaving several inches of sheet at top to be folded down.	
s. With client grasping clean top linens, slide out used top sheet or bath blanket (see illustration). Cuff top sheet over blanket and spread.	Prevents exposure of client. Gives a neat appearance to bed and keeps client's face off blanket.
t. Make a modified miter corner with top linens at foot of bed. Miter the corner as before, but do not tuck in lower edge of triangle (see illustration).	
u. Loosen linen at client's feet to client's comfort.	Allows for movement of client's feet, prevents top linen from forcing feet into plantar flexion, and prevents pressure ulcers from developing.
v. Supporting client's head, remove pillow and change pillowcase.	

4. See Completion Protocol (inside front cover).

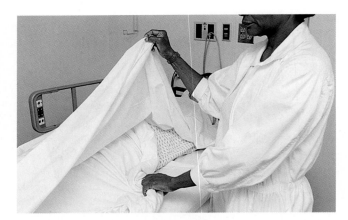

Step 3s Slide out used top sheet while keeping client covered.

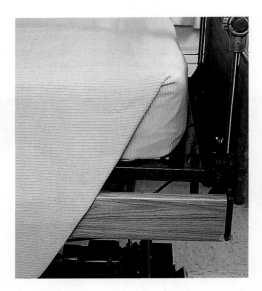

Step 3t Modified miter corner with top linens.

EVALUATION

1. Observe client's linens for cleanliness and tightness.
2. Ask if client is comfortable after bed is made.
3. Observe client's skin for signs of irritation.

Unexpected Outcomes and Related Interventions

1. Client is not comfortable in bed.
   a. Check that linens are clean and dry. Tighten them.
   b. Assist client with changing position in bed.

2. Client's skin appears red and irritated.
   a. Reposition client frequently. Consider use of pressure-relieving mattress (see Chapter 23).
   b. Keep client's bedding clean and dry.

Recording and Reporting

Bedmaking is usually not documented. Some agencies require the nurse to check off this activity on a flow sheet.

SPECIAL CONSIDERATIONS

Pediatric Considerations

Infants and children must be kept in cribs and with bedding that has met the safety guidelines from the U.S. Consumer Product Safety Commission (Wong, Perry, and Hockenberry-Eaton, 2002).

Geriatric Considerations

- Older adults have fragile skin and require more protection. Be sure bed linens are clean, dry, and free of wrinkles.
- Encourage older adults to spend as much time out of bed as possible.
- Use drawsheets and waterproof pads with caution. Accumulation of moisture creates a risk for skin maceration and breakdown.

Home Care Considerations

- Assess the primary caregiver's ability and willingness to maintain a clean environment for the client.
- Assess home laundry facilities to plan with the primary caregiver the frequency with which linens could reasonably be laundered.
- Assess the amount of linen in the home to establish with the primary caregiver the number of changes of sheets that could be reserved for the client's use.

Skill 7.6

Caring for Incontinent Clients

Incontinence is a very common problem, especially among older adults. Regardless of the cause, incontinence is a psychologically distressing and socially disruptive problem.

Urinary incontinence occurs because pressure in the bladder is too great, because the sphincters are weak, or because the innervation has been compromised due to illness or injury. The nurse can collaborate with other members of the health care team to assess the cause and extent of incontinence and to assist in the management of the problem. The physical therapist, for example, can assess the extent of musculoskeletal involvement and determine methods of treatment (Frahm 1997).

Incontinence may involve a small leakage of urine when the person laughs, coughs, or lifts something heavy. The client can be taught exercises to strengthen muscles around the external sphincters to help manage this type of incontinence. Pelvic floor exercises (Kegel exercises) involve tightening of the ring of muscle around the vagina and anus and holding them for several seconds. This should be done a minimum of 10 times, 3 times a day.

Alert clients need an incontinence product that is discreet and promotes self-care. Some incontinence products are designed for small amounts of leakage. Persistent urge, stress, or overflow incontinence may need referral for urological evaluation (Lewis, Collier, and Heitkemper, 2000).

Incontinence characterized by urine or fecal flow at unpredictable times requires the use of disposable adult undergarments or underpads as the primary means of management (Box 7-4). Urine and feces are very irritating to the skin. Skin that is continuously exposed quickly becomes in-

Box 7-4

Containment Devices

Diapers can hold large amounts of urinary leakage. They are large and bulky and best used for clients with total incontinence and confined to bed or wheelchair.

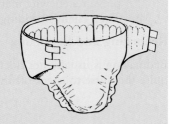

Adult undergarments can hold relatively large amounts of urinary leakage and are best for ambulatory clients.

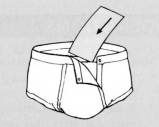

Underpants with absorbent pads can hold relatively large amounts of urinary leakage.

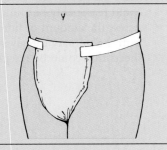

Sanitary pads can hold small amounts of urinary leakage. They are constructed for menstrual flow and are not as absorbent as incontinent pads.

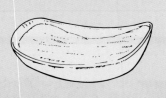

Male drip collectors can absorb small amounts of urine and fit comfortably over the penis.

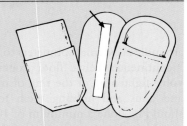

Modified from Gray M: *Genitourinary disorders,* Mosby's Clinical Nursing Series, St Louis, 1992, Mosby.

flamed and irritated. Cleansing the skin thoroughly after each episode of incontinence with warm soapy water and drying it thoroughly help prevent skin breakdown.

When urinary incontinence results from decreased perception of bladder fullness or impaired voluntary motor control, bladder training can be helpful. Bladder train-

ing provides cooperative clients with opportunity to void at regular intervals (every 1½ to 2 hours) to achieve continence. On such a schedule, clients need to be asked if they are wet or dry, checked for wetness, reminded or assisted to the toilet, and praised for appropriate toileting. Limiting fluids after the evening meal minimizes the need for voiding during the night.

When paralyzed clients have overflow incontinence, Credé's method may be used. This involves manual pressure over the lower abdomen to express urine from the bladder at regular intervals. Credé's method requires a measure of expertise to prevent injury to the bladder (Lewis, Collier, and Heitkemper, 2000).

The first step in care of the client with fecal incontinence is to assess if fecal impaction is the cause and to remove the impaction (see Skill 34.1, p. 821). Management of fecal incontinence includes educating the client about dietary measures, abdominal exercises, and physical activity (Lewis, Collier, and Heitkemper, 2000).

ASSESSMENT

1. Assess the frequency of episodes of incontinence. *Rationale: Determine if there is a pattern.*
2. Assess the amount of leakage experienced. Determine if it is frequent dribbling of small amounts or unpredictable loss of large amounts of urine and stool. *Rationale: Determines type of incontinence and appropriate choice of therapies.*
3. Assess episodes related to specific events such as coughing, sneezing, or exercise.
4. Assess the condition of client's skin in the perineal area. *Rationale: Identifies the need for special skin care products, barrier films, or creams.*
5. Assess fluid intake and the color, odor, and appearance of urine. *Rationale: Some clients drink less to minimize incontinence, resulting in dark, concentrated urine and increased risk for infection.*

PLANNING

Expected outcomes focus on promoting continence.

Expected Outcomes

1. Client achieves continence 75% of the time.
2. Client remains clean and dry 90% of the time.
3. Client maintains skin integrity without redness or irritation of the perineum.

Equipment

- Disposable gloves
- Washcloths and towels
- Soap
- Warm water
- Absorbent pad
- Skin barrier or sealant
- Incontinence briefs or sanitary pads if needed

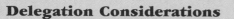

Delegation Considerations

The skill of providing care for incontinent clients can be delegated to assistive personnel (AP).

- Caution personnel to be aware of the client's dignity and self-esteem needs and to take measures to avoid violating these needs.
- Ensure personnel know standard precautions guidelines related to handling of body fluids.
- Be sure personnel report information to the nurse such as abdominal pain, increased episodes of incontinence, changes in appearance of urine or stool, and evidence of skin breakdown.
- Credé's maneuver is to be done by the nurse.

IMPLEMENTATION FOR CARING FOR INCONTINENT CLIENTS

Steps	Rationale
1. See Standard Protocol (inside front cover).	
2. Provide client with opportunity to use the bathroom, bedpan, or commode to void and defecate at appropriate regular times.	Promotes episodes of continence.
3. Keep a record of episodes of continence and incontinence for 48 hours.	Record allows identification of patterns of elimination.
4. Turn client to the supine position with legs abducted (see Skill 6.1, p. 112).	
a. *Female:* Wash labia using a washcloth, soap, and warm water. Then gently retract labia from thigh, and wash groin from perineum toward rectum (front to back).	Cleansing from front to back prevents transmission of microorganisms from anus to urethra.
b. *Male:* Wash the penis beginning with the urinary meatus, retracting the foreskin if client is uncircumcised. Gently cleanse shaft of penis and scrotum, taking care to thoroughly reach all skinfolds. Return foreskin to its natural position.	

COMMUNICATION TIP *Avoid all negative verbal and nonverbal expressions. Cleanse the perineum in a professional, caring, and matter-of-fact manner. Under no circumstances should client be reprimanded or humiliated for having "accidents."*

Steps	Rationale
5. Turn client to side, and continue cleansing, using as many washcloths as necessary and drying thoroughly.	
6. Place absorbent underpad from waist to knees with absorbent side toward client; or use other appropriate incontinent product if absolutely necessary.	Use of these products emphasizes the incontinence and affects the client's dignity and self-esteem.
7. If skin is red or irritated, exposure to air whenever possible is beneficial. A vitamin-enriched cream may promote healing. Apply a skin barrier or sealant to protect the skin from moisture (see Chapter 23).	Reduces risk of further skin breakdown.
8. Ambulatory clients may wear briefs with pads to absorb urine (see Box 7-4, p. 166).	Sanitary pads can hold small amounts of urinary leakage but are not intended for this purpose.
9. Discard gloves.	
10. See Completion Protocol (inside front cover).	

• • • • • • • • •

EVALUATION

1. Determine percentage of continent episodes in relation to total number of events of elimination in specified time.
2. Observe effectiveness of absorbent pads or garments used to contain incontinent episodes.
3. Observe the perineum for evidence of redness or irritation.

Unexpected Outcomes and Related Interventions

1. Client describes episodes of incontinence as urgency associated with frequency and burning with voiding.
   a. Increase fluid intake, and encourage cranberry juice, if appropriate.
   b. Consider the possibility of urinary tract infection. Report to physician for evaluation and treatment.
2. Client experiences overflow incontinence associated with urinary retention and bladder distention.
   a. Teach and encourage voiding according to a planned schedule.

   b. Notify physician if prescribed drugs may be contributing to urinary retention (e.g., anticholinergics, antispasmodics, antidepressants, seizure medications). Dosage or schedule of administration may be adjusted.
   c. Consult with physician regarding catheterization for residual urine (see Chapter 35).

Recording and Reporting

- Document each episode of incontinence.
- Include appearance and amount of stool or urine.
- Include appearance of skin.
- Document interventions that are carried out.

Sample Documentation

0800 C/O urgency and frequency of urination that started 24 hours ago; now C/O burning when urinating. Voided 50 ml concentrated urine every 1 to 2 hours in the last 24 hours. Reddened area around urinary meatus and labia. Perineal area cleansed with warm soapy water and dried thoroughly. Increased fluid intake encouraged, 200 ml of water intake now. Physician notified. Urine culture sent to lab as ordered.

 SPECIAL CONSIDERATIONS

Geriatric Considerations

- The aging process contributes to changes in voiding and defecating. The aging client may require immediate response to a request for the bedpan or urinal or a trip to the toilet.
- Incontinence of urine or stool is NOT an expected result of the aging process.

Home Care Considerations

- Assess the client before determining a treatment program; include health history, voiding diary, cognitive ability, physical functions, urinalysis, and environment (Colling, 1996).
- Teach the primary home caregiver methods of assisting the client to manage incontinence, such as prompted voiding or a voiding schedule.

Long-Term Care Considerations

- Personnel in long-term care facilities need to emphasize methods to manage incontinence, instead of emphasizing custodial care.
- Long-term use of incontinence products can lead to skin breakdown, although this can be minimized with conscientious care.
- Personnel in long-term care facilities must maintain professional, respectful attitudes toward both cognitively impaired and alert clients experiencing repeated, continuing problems.

Chapter 7

CRITICAL THINKING EXERCISES

1. The AP is getting ready to assist a client on heparin therapy with his bath, oral hygiene, and shaving. What instructions will you give the AP regarding equipment and safety needs?
2. A 70-year-old client with a history of breast cancer is being discharged following a course of chemotherapy. What instructions would you include regarding oral care, nutrition, and when to contact the health care provider?

REFERENCES

Agency for Health Care Policy and Research: *Pressure ulcers in adults: prediction and prevention*, Clinical practice guideline, Rockville, Md, 1992, U.S. Department of Health and Human Services.

American Diabetes Association: Preventive foot care in people with diabetes, *Diabetes Care* 21(Suppl 1):S56, 2001.

American Society of Health-Systems Pharmacists: Clinical practice guidelines for sustained neuromuscular blockade in the adult critically ill patient, *Am J Health Syst Pharm* 59(2):179, 2002.

Armstrong DG, Lavery LA: Diabetic foot ulcers: prevention, diagnosis, and classification, *Am Fam Physician* 57(6): 1325, 1998.

Buescher TL: Community outreach foot care for the elderly: a winning proposition, *Home Healthc Nurse* 16(1):37, 1998.

Colling J: Noninvasive techniques to manage urinary incontinence among care-dependent persons, *J Wound Ostomy Continence Nurs* 23(6):302, 1996.

Crute S, editor: *Health and healing for African-Americans*, Emmaus, Pa, 1997, Rodale Press.

Frahm J: The role of the PT in incontinence innovation and communication to improve patient care, *Ostomy/Wound Manage* (43):42, 1997.

Galanti G: *Caring for patients from different cultures*, ed 2, Philadelphia, 1997, University of Pennsylvania Press.

Gray M: *Genitourinary disorders*, Mosby's clinical nursing series, St Louis, 1992, Mosby.

Greenberger NJ and others: *History taking and physical examination: essentials and clinical correlates*, St Louis, 1993, Mosby.

Habif TP: *Clinical dermatology: a color guide to diagnosis and therapy*, ed 1, St Louis, 1994, Mosby.

Kim MJ, McFarland GK, McLane AM: *Pocket guide to nursing diagnoses*, ed 7, St Louis, 1997, Mosby.

Lecours AD: Understanding common oral lesions associated with HIV, *Clin Rev* 11(6):96, 2001.

Lewis SM, Collier IC, Heitkemper MM: *Medical surgical nursing: assessment and management of clinical problems*, ed 5, St Louis, 2000, Mosby.

Lueckenotte AG: *Gerontologic nursing*, ed 2, St Louis, 2000, Mosby.

Perry AG, Potter PA: *Clinical nursing skills and techniques*, ed 5, St Louis, 2002, Mosby.

Slovenkai NP: Getting and keeping a leg up on diabetes-related foot problems, *J Musculoskeletal Med* 15(12):46, 1998.

Sorrentino SA: *Assisting with patient care*, St Louis, 1999, Mosby.

Strauss MB, Hart JD, Winant DM: Preventive foot care: a user friendly system for patients and physicians, *Postgrad Med* 103(5):233, 1998.

Weston WL, Lane AT: *Color textbook of pediatric dermatology*, ed 2, St Louis, 1996, Mosby.

Wong DL, Perry SC, Hockenberry-Eaton M: *Maternal-child nursing care*, ed 2, St Louis, 2002, Mosby.

Zitelli BJ, Davis HW: *Atlas of pediatric physical diagnosis*, ed 3, St Louis, 1997, Mosby.

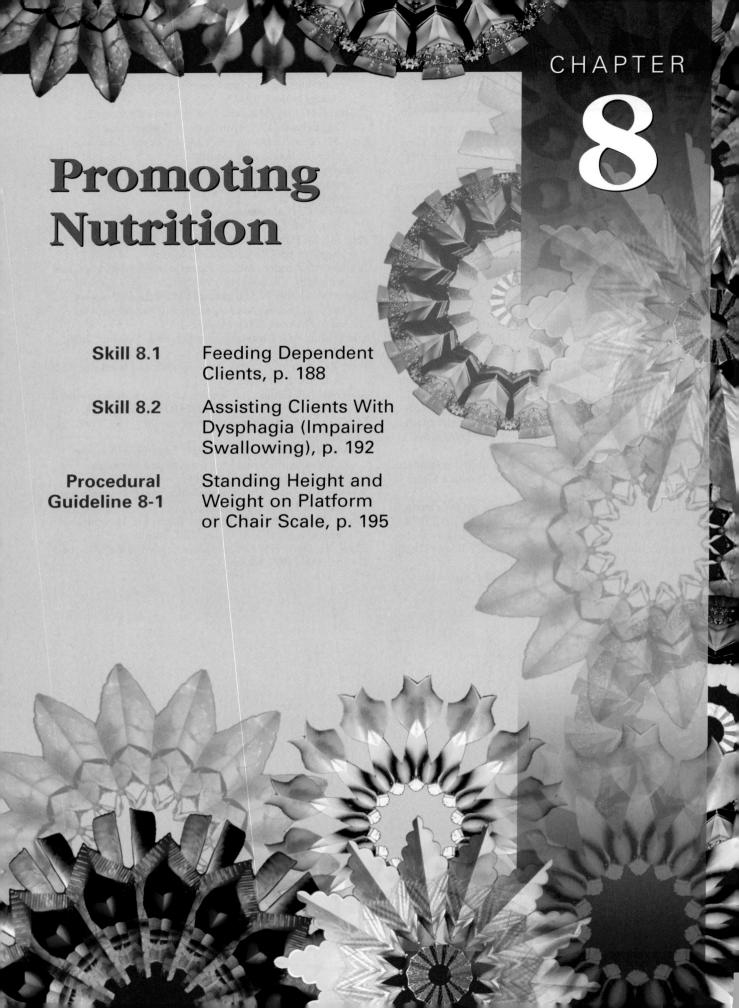

Promoting Nutrition

Nutrition is considered one of the foundations for life and health. It involves the process of ingesting food and using it to maintain body tissue and provide energy. Nutrients needed include water, carbohydrates, fats, proteins, lipids, vitamins, and minerals. Digestion is the mechanical and chemical processes by which food is broken down into its simplest form for absorption. The body needs to absorb nutrients in various combinations to continue daily activities, provide energy, heal, resist infection, grow, and survive.

The U.S. Department of Agriculture has recommended the Food Guide Pyramid (Figure 8-1) to emphasize the grain and cereal group as the basic food in the diet, with progression of intake of other food groups in smaller quantities toward the top. In the United States current dietary guidelines advocate reduced intake of fat, saturated fat, salt, refined sugar, and cholesterol and increased intake of complex carbohydrates and fiber (Potter and Perry, 2001).

The vegetarian pyramid differs in its emphasis on plant sources of nutrients most likely to be missed when animal foods are not included. This includes soy milk with added calcium, vitamin B$_{12}$, vitamin D, and at least 3 teaspoons of added vegetable oil each day. Variety in food choices is the key to a nutritious vegetarian diet. More Americans are choosing vegetarian diets for health reasons or because of their beliefs (Morgan and Weinsier, 1998).

The U.S. Department of Health and Human Services (USDHHS) developed recommendations in the form of an official strategy for improving our nation's health, published as *Healthy People 2000: National Health Promotion and Disease Prevention Objectives*. These recommendations focus on achieving a healthy weight and reducing disease risks through reducing fat and cholesterol, increasing carbohydrate and fiber, limiting sodium and sugar, and consuming alcohol only in moderation, while maintaining adequate intake of calcium and fluoride (Healthy People 2000, 1990). Many nutrition-related goals from *Healthy People 2000* indicated progress, including an increase in overall life expectancy, decreasing fat consumption, and lowered death rates from coronary heart disease. Obesity remains problematic. The challenge for nutrition-related goals remains to motivate consumers to put dietary recommendations into practice. These goals are continued as *Healthy People 2010* (USDHHS, 2000).

Early recognition of malnourished or at-risk clients can have a strong positive influence on health outcomes (Covinsky and others, 1999). Studies have identified that a large proportion of adult hospitalized clients are either malnourished or at risk (Bickford and others, 1999). Clients who receive nothing by mouth (NPO) and receive only intravenous (IV) fluids for more than 7 days are at nutritional risk. In addition, nutritional problems often occur in chronic disease, eating disorders, critical illness, metabolic diseases, and obesity. Box 8-1 lists some diagnoses, procedures, and therapies that place clients at nutritional risk or indicate malnutrition is present (Bankhead, 1999).

Nutritional assessment can be performed by a dietitian, nurse, or physician. A nutritional assessment has five com-

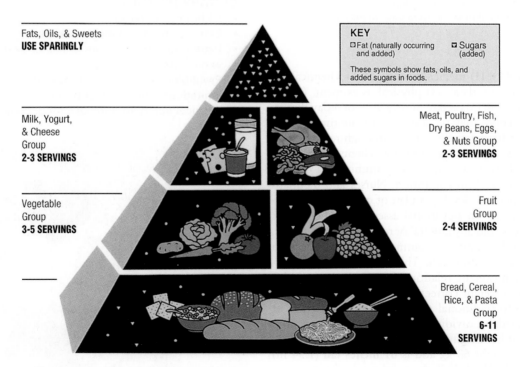

Figure 8-1 Food Guide Pyramid. (From U.S. Department of Agriculture: USDA's food guide pyramid, USDA Human Nutrition Information Pub No. 249, Washington, DC, 1992, U.S. Government Printing Office.)

Box 8-1
Clients at High Nutritional Risk

DIAGNOSIS/CONDITIONS
Cancer
HIV
Malabsorption syndromes
Sepsis
Inflammatory bowel disease
Trauma
Burns
Alcoholism
Anorexia
Dysphagia
Metabolic disorders
Cognitive dysfunction
Renal/hepatic/pancreatic dysfunction
Psychosocial disorders
Loss of independence

SURGERIES/THERAPIES
Head and neck resection
Bowel resection
Gastric surgery
Liver or bile duct surgery
Chemotherapy
Radiation therapy
Multiple medications

Modified from Bankhead RR: Integration of nutrition screening into case management practice, *Nurs Case Manag* 4(3):122, 1999.

Box 8-2
Components of a Nutritional Assessment

MEDICAL HISTORY
- Illnesses, conditions, or medications that required a change in the kind and/or amount of food eaten

PHYSICAL ASSESSMENT
- Height and usual weight
- Dentition status
- Weight gain or loss of 10 pounds in the last 6 months
- Ideal body weight
- Frame size

ANTHROPOMETRICS
- Triceps skinfold (TSF) (see illustration)
- Midarm circumference (MAC)
- Midarm muscle circumference (MAMC) or estimated skeletal muscle mass
  $MAMC = MAC \text{ (cm)} - [TSF \text{ (cm)} \times 3.14]$

LABORATORY TESTS
- Serum albumin (measures protein stores)
- CBC (nutrition-related anemia)
- Electrolytes and liver panel (for clotting issues with alcoholic clients)
- Cholesterol

DIETARY HISTORY
- 24-hour food recall
- Eats less than two meals per day
- Pattern of three or more drinks of beer, liquor, or wine almost every day
- Psychological status, religious beliefs, economic limitations, and social support
- Physical ability to purchase food, cook, and feed self

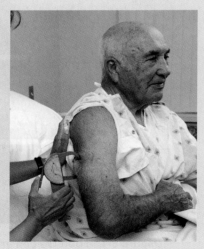

Box 8-1 Measuring triceps skinfold.

ponents (Box 8-2): (1) medical history, (2) biochemical parameters (laboratory data), (3) physical assessment, (4) anthropometrics, and (5) dietary history. A 2- or 3-day diet recall or calorie count may be done to estimate the quantity and content of food actually eaten. Although registered dietitians possess expertise in assessing clients' nutritional needs, nurses have very frequent opportunities to observe many aspects of a client's nutrition. Nurses and dietitians working together can develop a plan of care to meet nutritional needs based on nutritional assessment, the client's food preferences, and any cultural or religious requirements.

Height and weight are routinely obtained for each client on hospital admission. This is compared to standards for height-weight relationships. Body mass index (BMI) measures weight corrected for height and serves as an alternative to traditional weight charts. Calculation of BMI is achieved by dividing the client's weight in kilograms by his or her height in meters squared. For example, a person who weighs 68 kg and is 61 inches tall (1.54 m) would have a BMI of 28.7. A useful guide for assessing health risk according to BMI is given in Table 8-1. A BMI of less than 20 or greater than 35 places a client at high risk of illness (Grodner, Anderson, and DeYoung, 2000).

Table 8-1

Body Mass Index	
BMI	Health Risks
<20	Increased risk of respiratory disease, tuberculosis, digestive disease, and some cancers
20-35	Within normal limits
>35	Increased risk of coronary heart disease, some cancers, diabetes mellitus, and hypertension

Box 8-3

Selected Examples of Cultural or Religious Beliefs Related to Food

- The theory of hot and cold foods predominates in many cultures. Filipinos, Caribbean Islanders, Mexicans, and Latinos may plan their meals based on these beliefs. Food classification as hot or cold varies slightly from culture to culture.
- Mexicans believe hot is warmth, strength, and reassurance, whereas cold is menacing and weak. Classification has nothing to do with spiciness. Hot foods include rice, grains, alcohol, beef, lamb, chili peppers, chocolate, cheese. By contrast, cold foods include beans, citrus fruits, dairy products, most vegetables, honey, raisins, chicken, fish, and goat. Foods can be made hot or cold through methods of preparation.
- Orthodox Judaism requires adherence to kosher food preparation methods and prohibits eating pork, predatory fowl, shellfish, blood, and mixing of milk or dairy products with meat dishes. No cooking is done on the Sabbath (Saturday). For all Jewish sects no leavened bread is eaten during Passover.
- The Church of Jesus Christ of Latter-Day Saints (Mormons) prohibits the use of alcohol, tobacco, and caffeine.
- Seventh-Day Adventists encourage a vegetarian diet and prohibit intake of pork, shellfish, or alcohol.

Modified from Potter P, Perry A: *Fundamentals of nursing,* ed 5, St Louis, 2001, Mosby.

Another method of weight assessment is ideal body weight (IBW). This can be calculated as follows: for women IBW equals 100 pounds plus 5 additional pounds for each inch of height over 60 inches (5 feet); for men IBW can be estimated with a baseline of 106 pounds plus 6 additional pounds for each inch of height over 60 inches.

Bioelectrical impedance analysis (BIA) is noninvasive and is increasingly replacing traditional methods, but it is not available at all health care settings. An innocuous electrical current travels from one externally attached pole to another (one on each distal arm and leg). The speed of current is different for lean versus fat tissue. BIA is considered a more direct and immediate measure of lean body mass (Bioelectrical impedance analysis, 1996).

Laboratory and biochemical tests also assist in nutritional assessment; however, there is no one test that is diagnostic for malnutrition. Some of the basic laboratory tests to study nutritional status include plasma protein values such as serum albumin. Serum albumin value is the best-studied indicator of protein stores, but it is not specific for malnutrition and is affected by many factors, for example, hydration, hemorrhage, steroids, and surgery. However, hypoalbuminemia (less than 3.5 g/dl) is very suggestive of protein malnutrition and has been associated with subsequent morbidity and mortality in older populations. Cholesterol level is also helpful. A cholesterol level less than 160 may indicate malnutrition. A complete blood count (CBC) is useful for nutritionally related anemias. Low values for hemoglobin and hematocrit may indicate nutritional deficiency. Further testing is indicated to determine if anemia is related to nutritional intake. A total lymphocyte count less than 1500 mm^3 is suggestive of protein malnutrition (Morgan and Weinsier, 1998).

Dietary history and health history focus on the client's usual intake of foods and liquids and information about preferences, allergies, and food availability. Illness and activity levels affect energy needs. Assessment includes age; socioeconomic status; personal preference; psychological factors; use of alcohol or illegal drugs; vitamin, mineral, or herbal supplements; prescription or over-the-counter (OTC) drugs, and knowledge level. Eating patterns and food choices are also significantly affected by ethnicity, culture, and religious influences. Cultural awareness helps in incorporating preferences into dietary recommendations (Box 8-3).

Clinical observation involves physical assessment of body systems for signs of nutritional status (Table 8-2). Most nutritional problems develop insidiously over weeks and months. Because improper nutrition affects all body systems, clues to malnutrition require careful analysis of data from the physical assessment.

Clients rely on health care professionals to identify problems. A firm knowledge base of nutrition requirements and food sources of specific nutrients is important to help identify potential problems. In many cases a 24-hour or 3- to 7-day food diary may be kept to allow the nurse to calculate nutritional intake and compare it with daily requirements to see what dietary concerns need to be addressed. Nurses are in a key position to educate clients about good nutrition. Early identification of potential problems helps to avoid more serious problems. The nurse's role as educator often involves providing information about community resources, referral to a dietitian, supporting healthy changes, and monitoring progress.

Table 8-2

Clinical Signs of Nutritional Status

Body Area	Signs of Good Nutrition	Signs of Poor Nutrition
General appearance	Alert, responsive	Listless, apathetic, cachectic
Weight	Normal for height, age, body build	Overweight or underweight (special concern for underweight)
Posture	Erect, arms and legs straight	Sagging shoulders, sunken chest, humped back
Muscles	Well-developed, firm, good tone, some fat under skin	Flaccid, poor tone, undeveloped, tender, "wasted" appearance, cannot walk properly
Nervous control	Good attention span, not irritable or restless, normal reflexes, psychologic stability	Inattentive, irritable, confused, burning and tingling of hands and feet (paresthesia), loss of position and vibratory sense, weakness and tenderness of muscles (may result in inability to walk), decrease or loss of ankle and knee reflexes
Gastrointestinal function	Good appetite and digestion, normal regular elimination, no palpable (perceptible to touch) organs or masses	Anorexia, indigestion, constipation or diarrhea, liver or spleen enlargement
Cardiovascular function	Normal heart rate and rhythm, no murmurs, normal blood pressure for age	Rapid heart rate (above 100 beats per minute, tachycardia), enlarged heart, abnormal rhythm, elevated blood pressure
General vitality	Endurance, energetic, sleeps well, vigorous	Easily fatigued, no energy, falls asleep easily, looks tired, apathetic
Hair	Shiny, lustrous, firm, not easily plucked, healthy scalp	Stringy, dull, brittle, dry, thin and sparse, depigmented, can be easily plucked
Skin (general)	Smooth, slightly moist, good color	Rough, dry, scaly, pale, pigmented, irritated, bruises, petechiae
Face and neck	Skin color uniform, smooth, healthy appearance, not swollen	Greasy, discolored, scaly, swollen, skin dark over cheeks and under eyes, lumpiness or flakiness of skin around nose and mouth
Lips	Smooth, good color, moist, not chapped or swollen	Dry, scaly, swollen, redness and swelling (chiolosis), or angular lesions at corners of the mouth or fissures or scars (stomatitis)
Mouth, oral membranes	Reddish pink mucous membranes in oral cavity	Swollen, boggy oral mucous membranes
Gums	Good pink color, healthy, red, no swelling or bleeding	Spongy, bleed easily, marginal redness, inflamed, gums receding
Tongue	Good pink color or deep reddish in appearance, not swollen or smooth, surface papillae present, no lesions	Swelling, scarlet and raw, magenta color, beefy (glossitis), hyperemic and hypertrophic papillae, atrophic papillae
Teeth	No cavities, no pain, bright, straight, no crowding, well-shaped jaw, clean, no discoloration	Unfilled caries, absent teeth, worn surfaces mottled (fluoresis), malpositioned
Eyes	Bright, clear, shiny, no sores at corner of eyelids, membranes moist and healthy pink color, no prominent blood vessels or mound of tissue or sclera, no fatigue circles beneath	Eye membranes pale (pale conjunctivae), redness of membrane (conjunctival injection), dryness of infection, Bitot's spots, redness and fissuring of eyelid corners (angular palpebritis), dryness of eye membrane (conjunctival xerosis), dull appearance of cornea (corneal xerosis), soft cornea (keratomalacia)
Neck (glands)	No enlargement	Thyroid enlarged
Nails	Firm, pink	Spoon-shaped (koilonychia), brittle, ridged
Legs and feet	No tenderness, weakness, or swelling; good color	Edema, tender calf, tingling, weakness
Skeleton	No malformation	Bowlegs, knock-knees, chest deformity at diaphragm, beaded ribs, prominent scapulae

Data from Williams SR: Nutritional guidance in prenatal care. In Worthington-Roberts BS and others: *Nutrition in pregnancy and lactation,* St Louis, 1985, Mosby.

Table 8-3

Diets of Modified Consistency

Diet	Description
Clear-liquid	Allows clear, bland liquids, such as chicken broth, gelatin, and apple juice, which leave little residue and are easily absorbed. Is commonly ordered for short-term use (24 to 48 hours) after episodes of vomiting, diarrhea, or surgery.
Full-liquid	Consists of foods that liquefy at room or body temperature and are easily digested and absorbed. Includes foods allowed on clear-liquid diet plus milk and some milk-containing foods, such as creamed, strained soups. Is commonly ordered before or after surgery for clients who are acutely ill from infection or for clients who cannot chew or tolerate solid foods.
Pureed	Includes easily swallowed foods that do not require chewing. May be ordered for clients with head and neck abnormalities or who have had surgery.
Mechanical or dental-soft	Consists of foods that do not need chewing, such as chopped or ground foods. Avoids tough meats, nuts, bacon, and fruits with tough skins or membranes. May be ordered for clients who have chewing problems caused by lack of teeth or sore gums.
Soft	Includes foods that are low in fiber, easily digested, easy to chew, and simply cooked. Does not permit fatty, rich, and fried foods. Is sometimes referred to as low-fiber diet.
High-fiber	Includes sufficient amounts of indigestible carbohydrate to relieve constipation, increase gastrointestinal motility, and increase stool weight. May be ordered for clients with diverticulosis or irritable bowel syndrome.
Therapeutic Diets	
Restricted fluid intake	Required in severe heart failure and kidney failure.
Sodium-restricted	Allows low levels of sodium and may include a 4-g (no added salt), 2-g (moderate), 1-g (strict), or 500-mg (very strict) diet. May be ordered for clients with congestive heart failure, renal failure, cirrhosis, or hypertension.
Fat-modified	Low total and saturated fat and low cholesterol. Cholesterol intake less than 300 mg daily and fat intake to 30% to 35% by eliminating or reducing fatty foods for hypercholesterolemia.
Diabetic	Ordered as essential treatment for clients with diabetes mellitus. Provides clients with a diet recommended by American Diabetes Association, which allows for clients to select set amount of food from basic food groups.

Modified from Morgan SL, Weisner RL: *Fundamentals of clinical nutrition,* ed 2, St Louis, 1998, Mosby.

THERAPEUTIC DIETS

Food provided to hospitalized clients requires a physician's order. Diet therapy can be used for many disease states, complementing and at times even replacing drug therapy. A useful way to understand therapeutic diets breaks the general diet into its basic components: water, carbohydrate, protein, fat, vitamins, and minerals. Modifications of the amounts of these components may form a therapeutic diet. For example, clients with diabetes mellitus have inadequate production or effectiveness of insulin, resulting in high levels of plasma glucose. Type 2 diabetes mellitus, also called non–insulin dependent diabetes mellitus (NIDDM), accounts for 90% to 95% of individuals with diabetes. This type of diabetes is often managed with diet and exercise. The diet is individualized according to the client's age, build, weight, and activity level. Protein constitutes 10% to 20% of daily intake. Fats are moderately controlled (30% or less), complex carbohydrates make up the majority (50% to 60%) of the diet rather than simple carbohydrates, and a daily intake of 40 g of fiber is recommended. If diet and exercise are inadequate to control glucose levels, drug therapy such as oral hypoglycemic agents or insulin may be necessary.

Therapeutic diets may also be modified in consistency or texture. After surgery clients may initially require a liquid diet. A dental-soft diet is for clients without teeth, and a high-fiber, high-residue diet is for clients with constipation. When there are no restrictions, the order may be diet as tolerated (DAT) or regular diet. Other examples of therapeutic diets include diets low in fat or cholesterol, low in protein, and low in sodium. For specific information about special diets see the agency dietary manual or contact a dietitian. Table 8-3 has a summary of several common hospital therapeutic diets.

Several related topics are beyond the scope of this chapter and are included in other chapters. Enteral nutrition (EN), including feeding tubes, is discussed in Chapter

33, and total parenteral nutrition (TPN), administration of nutrients via IV access, is included in Chapter 38.

NURSING DIAGNOSES

Imbalanced Nutrition: Less Than Body Requirements is the general nursing diagnosis for clients when the focus is increasing the quantity or quality of nutritional intake. **Feeding Self-Care Deficit** may be related to inability of clients to prepare food or feed themselves because of mobility or coordination problems, visual problems, or mental problems. **Impaired Swallowing** may be related to an altered gag reflex or inability to cough, weakened muscles of chewing, or mechanical alterations such as cancer of the upper airway, an obstructing tumor, or a fistula (abnormal opening between the esophagus and adjacent body cavity). Nausea may be an appropriate diagnosis for clients who have gastric irritation or distention, or psychosocial disorders. **Risk for Aspiration** may also be appropriate for clients who have difficulty swallowing or who are relearning to swallow after neurological damage or surgery. **Imbalanced Nutrition: More Than Body Requirements** is appropriate when clients are more than 10% to 20% over the desired weight range for their height.

Skill 8.1

Feeding Dependent Clients

Hospitalized clients may be unable to feed themselves adequately because of the severity of their illness or the fatigue and debilitation associated with their disease. Others are limited by loss of arm or hand movement, by impaired vision, by brain injury, or by the need to remain in a flat or prone position. When assisting the client with feeding, the nurse encourages the client to ingest an adequate volume of food at a comfortable pace. It is important to facilitate independence when possible with the use of adaptive devices or finger foods and with comfortable and safe positioning for swallowing. Because mealtime is often viewed as a social time for clients, sitting and talking during mealtime is important.

ASSESSMENT

1. Assess level of consciousness, ability to cooperate, mobility/activity orders, and physical limitations. *Rationale: Determines appropriate positioning for meals and level of assistance required.*
2. Assess need for toileting, handwashing, and oral care before feeding. *Rationale: Reduces interruptions and improves appetite during the meal.*
3. Assess food tolerance, cultural and religious preferences, and food likes and dislikes. *Rationale: Determines if certain foods will improve appetite and desire to feed independently.*
4. Measure client's weight, and determine whether the client requires a diet that has been altered in nutrients (low protein, low fat), flavoring (low salt, nonspicy), or consistency (pureed, liquid). Routine diets used in the hospital and sometimes in the home care or long-term care setting are shown in Table 8-3 on p. 187. *Rationale: Weight provides a baseline. Clients with chronic diseases, such as cardiac or renal disease, may need alterations in nutrient content or flavoring. After surgical procedures the client may progress from a clear liquid diet to a regular diet as the client's ability to digest or tolerance of more complex nutrients returns.*
5. Assess pertinent laboratory values indicative of nutritional balance

PLANNING

Expected outcomes focus on increased independence with eating, improved nutritional intake, and safe intake of food.

Expected Outcomes

1. Client's body weight remains stable or trends toward the normal level.
2. Client's nutrition-related laboratory values trend toward normal. (Note serum albumin and hemoglobin values.)
3. Client demonstrates increased ability to feed self or open items on tray.
4. Client coughs appropriately when eating with no new signs of respiratory compromise.
5. Client demonstrates use of adaptive utensils as appropriate.
6. Client's intake improves in the quality of nutrients ingested.

Equipment

- Meal tray
- Over-bed table
- Adaptive utensils if appropriate (Figure 8-2)
- Damp washcloth (optional)
- Oral hygiene supplies (optional)

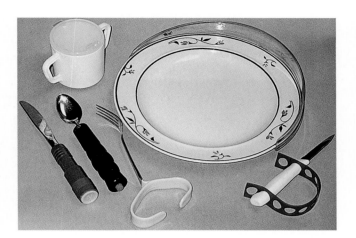

Figure 8-2 Adaptive equipment. *Clockwise from upper left:* Two-handled cup with lid, plate with plate guard, utensils with splints, and utensils with enlarged handles.

 Delegation Considerations

The skill of assisting the client with oral nutrition can be delegated to assistive personnel (AP) who have demonstrated ability to feed clients safely. Instruct care provider to observe for any swallowing problems and to notify nurse immediately. Clients with swallowing difficulty require the problem-solving and critical-thinking skills unique to a nurse. Delegation is inappropriate.

IMPLEMENTATION FOR FEEDING DEPENDENT CLIENTS

Steps	Rationale
1. See Standard Protocol (inside front cover).	
2. Offer toileting and handwashing before meal.	Increases level of comfort.
3. Offer toothbrush or mouthwash before meal.	May improve appetite in client with stomatitis or other oral hygiene problems
4. Check the environment for distractions. Reduce the noise level if possible.	

5. Position client appropriately for safe eating within limitations of ability.
  a. Up in chair
  b. High-Fowler's position in bed (see illustration)
  c. Side-lying position if flat in bed
	Positioning helps to improve swallowing and digestion and to avoid aspiration.

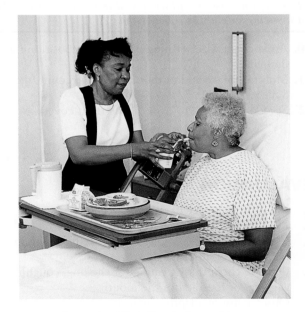

Step 5b High-Fowler's position.

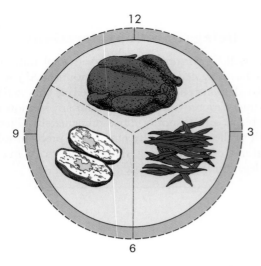

Step 8   Location of food using clock.

Steps	Rationale
6. Assist client with setting up meal tray if able: open packages, cut up food, apply seasonings/condiments, butter bread, and place napkin.	
7. Place adaptive utensils on tray if indicated, and instruct in their use.	
8. If client is visually impaired, identify food location on plate as if it were a clock (e.g., the chicken is at 12 o'clock) (see illustration).	Visually impaired client may feed self when given adequate information about tray.
9. Pace feeding to avoid client fatigue. Ask client the order in which he or she wishes to eat food. Interact with client during mealtime. Verbally encourage self-feeding attempts.	Gives client some control of situation and avoids embarrassment of limitations. Social interaction may improve appetite.

COMMUNICATION TIP   *Use simple verbal prompts and touch: for example, "Here is your bread" (place bread in the client's hand). Pantomime desired behaviors, such as drinking a beverage.*

---

10. Assist client with washing hands and repositioning as desired.	
11. Monitor intake and output and calorie count (see Skill 9.1, p 200).	
12. See Completion Protocol (inside front cover).	Physician's orders may require identifying the specific number of calories consumed.

• • • • • • • • • •

EVALUATION

1. Monitor body weight daily or weekly.
2. Monitor laboratory values as ordered.
3. Observe client's technique for self-feeding: certain items, part or all of meal.
4. Observe client during eating for choking, coughing, gagging, or food left in the mouth.
5. Observe use of adaptive utensils.
6. Observe amount of food on tray after meal.

Unexpected Outcomes and Related Interventions

1. Client refuses to eat food offered.
   a. Try to identify and resolve possible interferences.
      (1) Determine if client has other food preferences, cultural influences, or religious restrictions.
      (2) Determine if different times of the day are better.
      (3) Determine if discomfort or anxiety should be treated before eating.

(4) Determine if client is mentally incapable of cooperating.

2. Client chokes on food.
  a. Use suction equipment if necessary to clear food from airway.
  b. If choking occurs repeatedly, stop feeding and notify physician.

3. Food sits on side or back of mouth (see Skill 8.2, p. 192).
  a. Initiate interventions designed to assist dysphagic clients with eating (see Skill 8.2, p. 192).

Recording and Reporting

- Food and fluids actually consumed (for calorie count and intake and output)

- Degree of participation/independence
- Client response
- Description of the swallowing
- Description of choking or possible aspiration
- Report food tolerance/intolerance and significant changes to the dietitian

Sample Documentation

0800 Client able to feed self 5 bites with encouragement. Reported "that is all I can do." Remaining breakfast fed to client. No difficulty swallowing or coughing noted.

SPECIAL CONSIDERATIONS

Pediatric Considerations

- Females of childbearing age anticipating pregnancy need folic acid to prevent neural tube birth defects. It is most easily obtained from a daily multivitamin supplement.
- Food allergies are common in infancy because the immature intestinal tract is more permeable to proteins. Severe reactions can be minimized by prenatal precautions, including avoiding known food allergens, milk and dairy products, peanuts, and eggs during the last trimester of pregnancy. Food allergies may be prevented by feeding breast milk exclusively for at least 6 months, avoiding solid foods for the first 6 months, and avoiding eggs, fish, corn, citrus, peanuts, nuts, or chocolate for 12 months.
- Age affects the requirements for essential nutrients. Periods of rapid growth increase the need for protein, vitamins, and minerals.
- Eating habits established in toddler years tend to have lasting effects in subsequent years.

Geriatric Considerations

- Changes in taste perception, oral mucus production, and dentition with aging may affect the client's food choices and ability to chew or swallow. The nurse needs to assess the client's food patterns for nutrient, calorie, and fluid adequacy.

- Adequate calcium intake is essential for older men and women to prevent the development of osteoporosis.
- Older adults may have difficulty eating because of physical symptoms or lack of teeth or dentures.
- Thirst sensation may diminish in older adults, leading to inadequate fluid intake or dehydration.
- An estimated 2.5 million community-dwelling older adults suffer from food inadequacies within any 6-month period, and 40% to 50% of this group have a moderate to high risk of malnutrition.

Home Care Considerations

- Homebound older adults may benefit from Meals on Wheels, which recently instituted a program to provide breakfast as a second meal (USDHHS, 1997).
- Clients who are unable to feed themselves independently may eat better if other family members participate at mealtimes to avoid social isolation.

Long-Term Care Considerations

Institutionalized older adults often have nutrition issues related to poor appetite, infections, weight loss, pressure ulcers, and polypharmacy. In 1997 the American Dietetic Association (ADA) published a position statement endorsing liberalized diets for older adults in long-term care (ADA, 1997).

Skill 8.2

Assisting Clients With Dysphagia (Impaired Swallowing)

Dysphagia is a decreased ability to voluntarily pass fluids and/or solids from the mouth to the stomach. Swallowing is a complex event, requiring both voluntary and involuntary movements. It requires the coordination of cranial nerves and the muscles of the tongue, pharynx, larynx, and jaw. Clients with neuromuscular diseases involving the brain, brain stem, cranial nerves, or muscles of swallowing should be assessed for swallowing difficulties before feeding. Speech pathologists are trained to perform evaluation of swallowing and to recommend appropriate interventions.

A speech therapist or radiologist may conduct swallowing assessments. A videofluoroscopic swallowing study (VFSS) may be performed in the fluoroscopy room with a radiologist and speech pathologist present. The client is given puree-, liquid-, and solid-consistency barium in varied amounts while visualizing the swallowing mechanism (Bastian, 1998).

Maintaining an upright position to enhance the effects of gravity is important. When feeding the client, the nurse places food on the unaffected side of the mouth (as in clients with hemiparesis) and observes the swallowing event closely for delays. Providing verbal coaching throughout the swallowing process can greatly help the client swallow more effectively. Food that is the consistency of mashed potatoes is easiest for dysphagic clients to swallow. Liquids and solids are more likely to pose a threat. In some cases, thickeners may be added to food or fluids to increase the consistency and thus allow the client more control of the volume in the mouth.

ASSESSMENT

1. Assess client's level of alertness; drooling; problems with speech; and wet, gurgly voice. *Rationale: Indicates difficulty with muscle control and may put the client at risk for aspiration.*
2. Assess client's lung sounds, ability to cough on request, and the presence of gagging or involuntary coughing when back of the throat is tickled with a tongue depressor or wet cotton swab. *Rationale: Assessment of lung sounds provides a baseline.*

Absence of gag or cough reflexes indicates that client is at high risk for aspiration with swallowing.

3. Assess client's swallowing reflex before feeding by placing fingers on client's throat at level of the larynx, then asking client to swallow saliva. *Rationale: Movement of the larynx normally can be palpated.*
4. Assess client's body weight and nutrition-related laboratory values. *Rationale: Provide objective baseline measures for nutrition status.*

PLANNING

Expected outcomes focus on adequate food and fluid intake to prevent malnutrition and dehydration while avoiding aspiration.

Expected Outcomes

1. Client swallows without retaining food in mouth.
2. Client demonstrates a complete, effective swallowing event.
3. Client exhibits no symptoms of aspiration or new respiratory distress.
4. Oral intake is adequate for nutrition and fluids.
5. Client's body weight trends toward IBW.
6. Nutrition-related laboratory values all trend toward normal.

Equipment

- Meal tray
- Thickener (if ordered)
- Suction equipment
- Oxygen

Delegation Considerations

The skill of assisting clients with impaired swallowing requires the critical thinking and knowledge application unique to a nurse and based on the evaluation and recommendations of a speech pathologist.

IMPLEMENTATION FOR ASSISTING CLIENTS WITH DYSPHAGIA

Steps	Rationale
1. See Standard Protocol (inside front cover).	
2. Position client upright in bed or chair with head slightly flexed forward.	This position reduces risk of aspiration.
3. Reduce distractions in the room	Helps to keep client focused on swallowing.

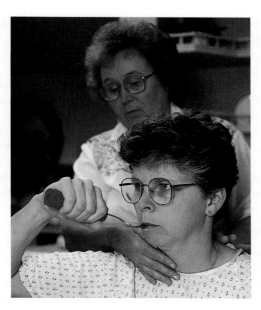

Step 6 Palpate swallowing.

Steps	Rationale
4. Add thickener to thin liquids to create the consistency of mashed potatoes, or serve client pureed foods.	Thin liquids such as water and fruit juice are difficult to control in the mouth and are more easily aspirated (Goulding and Bakheit, 2000).
5. Place ½ to 1 teaspoon of food on unaffected side of the mouth, allowing utensil to touch the mouth or tongue.	
6. Place hand on throat as shown to gently palpate swallowing event as it occurs (see illustration). Swallowing twice is often necessary to clear the pharynx.	
7. Provide verbal coaching while feeding client and positive reinforcement to client.	Verbal cueing keeps client focused on swallowing. Positive reinforcement enhances client's confidence in ability to swallow.

   a.   Open your mouth.
   b.   Feel the food in your mouth.
   c.   Chew and taste the food.
   d.   Raise your tongue to roof of your mouth.
   e.   Think about swallowing.
   f.   Close your mouth and swallow.
   g.   Swallow again.
   h.   Cough to clear airway.

Steps	Rationale
8. Observe for coughing, choking, gagging, and drooling of food; suction airway as necessary.	These are indications that suggest dysphagia and risk for aspiration (Dangerfield and Sullivan, 1999).
9. Provide rest periods as necessary during meal.	Avoiding fatigue decreases the risk of aspiration.
10. Maintain upright position for 15 to 30 minutes after eating.	Helps avoid aspiration or regurgitation.
11. Provide mouth care after meals.	This dislodges any food or fluids that may have accumulated inside client's cheeks.
12. Advance diet to thicker foods that require more chewing and finally to thin liquids as tolerated.	Dietitian and/or speech pathologist can direct safest advancement of diet.
13. See Completion Protocol (inside front cover).	

• • • • • • • • • •

EVALUATION

1. Observe contents of client's mouth during meal for food pocketing.
2. Observe client for a continuous (not prolonged or delayed) swallowing event.
3. Observe client for coughing or choking during meal.
4. Monitor intake and output (see Skill 9.1, p. 200), calorie count, and food eaten from tray.
5. Monitory daily or weekly weight (see Procedural Guideline 8.1, p. 195)
6. Monitor nutrition-related laboratory values as ordered.

Unexpected Outcomes and Related Interventions

1. Client begins coughing, choking, or turning blue.
   a. Stop feeding client.
   b. Position client in high-Fowler's position or, if unable, position on side.
   c. Suction airway until clear (see Skill 31.3, p. 760).
   d. Provide oxygen if color has not returned to normal.
2. Food and/or fluids drain out of client's nose during the meal.
   a. Stop feeding client.
   b. Suction nasopharyngeal area.
   c. Resume feeding with increased head flexion.
3. On inspection, food is found pocketed in client's cheeks.
   a. Teach client to use the tongue or to massage the cheek externally to move food to a more functional area of the mouth.
4. A registered dietitian may calculate calorie count, which requires an accurate recording of the amount or percentage of food eaten in 24 hours.

Recording and Reporting

- Time of meal
- Amount of food and fluid ingested
- Any symptoms of intolerance to foods or fluids or symptoms of difficulty chewing, swallowing, or ingesting

Sample Documentation

1200 Client fed ½ of pureed diet and 4 oz juice with 1 teaspoon of thickener added with much encouragement. Client refused additional food. No coughing or aspiration noted.

 ## SPECIAL CONSIDERATIONS

Pediatric Considerations

Swallowing is an automatic reflex for the first 3 months of life, and the infant has no voluntary control until approximately 6 weeks of age. Coordinated muscle action typical of the adult type of swallowing gradually develops with neural and muscular development. By 6 months of age the infant is capable of swallowing, holding food in the mouth, or spitting it out at will (Wong and others, 1999).

Geriatric Considerations

Degenerative changes in the esophagus result in a decline in its motility, leading to dysphagia, heartburn, or vomiting and decreased food intake from fear of a recurrence of symptoms (Lueckenotte, 2000).

Home Care Considerations

Consultation with a speech therapist for recommendations about how to assist the client with impaired swallowing may be indicated.

Long-Term Care Considerations

It is estimated that 40% to 60% of nursing home residents have some degree of dysphagia, which can lead to aspiration pneumonia, chronic malnutrition, decreased quality of life, and frustration for residents, family, and staff (Shanley and Loughlin, 2000).

OBTAINING BODY WEIGHTS

A person's general level of health is reflected in the ratio of height to weight. Standardized tables can help reveal the normal expected weight for a client at a given height. Rapid weight gain of 5 pounds in a day can indicate fluid retention problems. A loss of 5% in a month or 10% in 6 months is significant. The Joint Commission for the Accreditation of Healthcare Organizations (JCAHO) requires all hospitalized and home care clients to have height-weight measurement.

Obtaining a body weight must be done accurately because it is one of the important parameters used to evaluate and treat many diseases, including congestive heart failure, fluid overload, and renal failure. When monitoring weight for therapeutic purposes, care must be taken in using the same scale at or near the same time of the day, weighing the same amount of clothing or linen, and weighing client after emptying drainage bags (e.g., colostomy or catheter bag). Weight of drainage alters body weight (500 ml equals 1 pound). A chair scale should be used if client cannot stand independently. A bed scale should be used if client is unable to bear weight. Some of the newer models of beds have scales built into their structures. Obtaining a client's weight on this type of scale requires following the manufacturer's instructions.

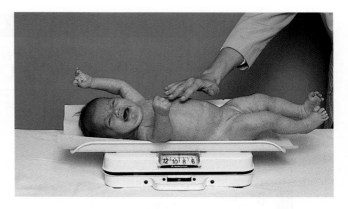

Figure 8-3 Weighing an infant. (From Wong DL: *Whaley & Wong's nursing care of infants and children,* ed 6, 1999, Mosby.)

Infants may be weighed on a calibrated beam balance scale (Figure 8-3) or electronic scale. The infant is best weighed unclothed.

Weights for ambulatory home care clients may be obtained using a good-quality standard bathroom scale; however, the scale should be tested periodically for accuracy with a known weight. The scale should be disinfected if it is taken from one client to another.

Procedural Guideline 8-1

Standing Height and Weight on Platform or Chair Scale

Equipment: Appropriate scale: standing, chair, or stretcher/bed scale

1. See Standard Protocol (inside front cover).
2. Determine client's ability to bear weight and safely stand on a scale. If your client is alert but unable to stand, a chair scale may be used. If the client is not alert or is critically ill, a bed scale is the safest means to obtain a weight.
3. 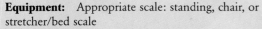 Empty any pouches or drainage devices attached to client that contain drainage.
4. Weigh client
    a. Platform or chair scale
        (1) Place platform or chair scale at client's bedside.
        (2) Balance and calibrate scale to 0 pounds/kilograms. Balance beam should be in the middle of mark; digital scale should read 0.
        (3) Ask client to step up onto platform scale and stand still (see illustration), or assist client with sitting on chair scale (see illustration).
        (4) Adjust balance on scale until it is in middle of mark or until digital scale displays a reading (see illustration).

    (5) With the client standing erect with good posture and without shoes, swing the metal rod attached to the back of the scale over the crown of the head (see illustration).
    (6) With the rod horizontal to the measuring stick, measure height in inches or centimeters.
    b. Bed scale
        (1) Place sling with same type and amount of linen and a client gown on arms of scale.
        (2) Calibrate scale to 0 with linens and gown.
        (3) With nurse on each side of the bed, roll client onto side. Place sling under client (see illustration) using good body mechanics (see Chapter 6).
        (4) Attach scale, and elevate until clear of bed (see illustration).
        (5) Instruct client to remain still, if possible.
        (6) Read digital weight on scale (see illustration).
        (7) Lower client onto bed, roll over stretcher, then remove stretcher and scale from client's bed.
5. Compare weight obtained with previous weight.
6. Record weight on appropriate form (see agency policy).
7. See Completion Protocol (inside front cover).

Continued

Procedural Guideline 8-1

Standing Height and Weight
on Platform or Chair Scale–cont'd

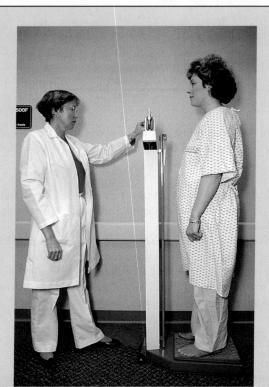

Step 4a(3)   Standing weight.

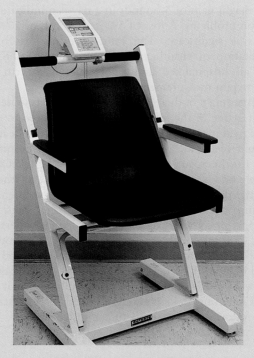

Step 4a(3)   Using chair scale.

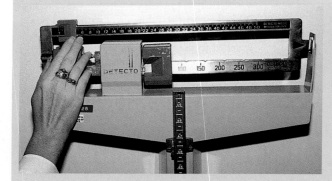

Step 4a(4)   Balance the scale by moving the weight.

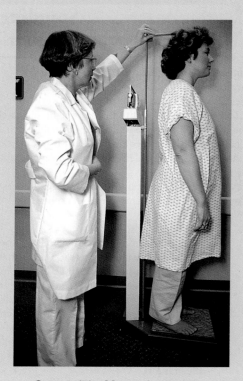

Step 4a(5)   Measuring height.

Procedural Guideline 8-1

Standing Height and Weight
on Platform or Chair Scale—cont'd

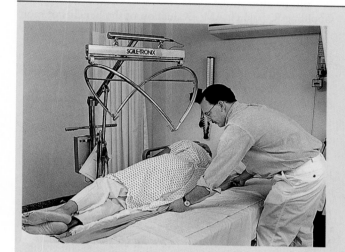

Step 4b(3)   Place sling under client.

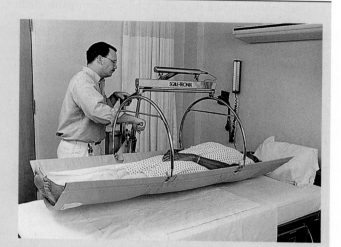

Step 4b(4)   Elevate sling.

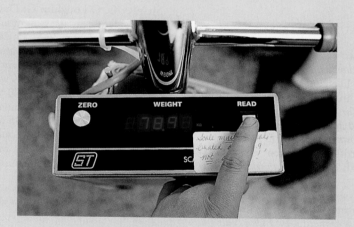

Step 4b(6)   Read digital weight.

CRITICAL THINKING EXERCISES

1. Mr. Littlefeather has a progressive neuromuscular disease, which affects his speech and throat muscles. What precautions should the nurse take in assisting this client with meals?

2. Identify the type of scale that is appropriate and precautions that should be taken for each of the following clients to obtain a weight safely and accurately:
   a. A 25-year-old client who has an ileostomy and is able to stand without assistance
   b. A 75-year-old client who has had a recent amputation of his left leg and is able to get up in a chair
   c. A 15-year-old client with cerebral palsy who needs the assistance of two people to get out of bed

3. Ms. Garrett is an 80-year-old who is below her estimated calorie requirement by 800 kcal/day. She tries to eat three meals a day, but because of feeling full, she cannot. She is 20% below her IBW. She is asking for help to gain weight. What is your first priority in this situation? What would be an appropriate goal for her? How would you evaluate achievement of this goal?

REFERENCES

American Dietetic Association: *Position of the American Dietetic Association: nutrition, aging, and the continuum of care,* Chicago, American Dietetic Association, 1997.

Bankhead RR: Integration of nutrition screening into case management practice, *Nurs Case Manag* 4(3):122, 1999.

Bastian RW: Contemporary diagnosis of the dysphagic patient, *Otolaryngol Clin North Am* 31(3):489, 1998.

Bickford GR and others: Nutrition assessment outcomes: a strategy to improve health care, *Clin Lab Manage Rev* 13(6):357, 1999.

Bioelectrical impedance analysis in body composition measurement: National Institutes of Health Technology Assessment Conference statement, *Am J Clin Nutr* 64 (suppl 3):524s, 1996.

Covinsky EK and others: The relationship between clinical assessments of nutritional status and adverse outcomes in older hospitalized medical patients, *J Am Geriatr Soc* 47(5):532, 1999.

Dangerfield L, Sullivan R: Screening for and managing dysphagia after stroke, *Nurs Times* 95(19):44, 1999.

Goulding R, Bakheit AM: Evaluation of the benefits of monitoring fluid thickness in the dietary management of dysphagic stroke patients, *Clin Rehabil* 14(2):119, 2000.

Grodner M, Anderson S, DeYoung S: *Foundations and clinical applications of nutrition: a nursing approach,* ed 2, St Louis, 2000, Mosby.

Healthy People 2000: national health promotion and disease prevention objectives, U.S. Department of Health and Human Services, Public Health Service, DHHS Pub No. (PHS) 91-50213, Washington, DC, 1990, U.S. Government Printing Office.

Joint Commission on Accreditation of Healthcare Organizations: *Accreditation manual for hospitals,* Chicago, 2000, The Commission.

Lueckenotte A: *Gerontologic nursing,* ed 2, St Louis, 2000, Mosby.

Morgan SL, Weinsier RL: *Fundamentals of clinical nutrition,* ed 2, St Louis, 1998, Mosby.

Potter P, Perry A: *Fundamentals of nursing,* ed 5, St Louis, 2001, Mosby.

Shanley C, O'Loughlin G: Dysphagia among nursing home residents: an assessment and management protocol, *J Gerontol Nurs* 26(8):35, 2000.

U.S. Department of Health and Human Services, 1997.

U.S. Department of Health and Human Services: *Healthy people 2010 objectives,* http://web.health.gov./healthypeople, 2000.

Williams SR: Nutritional guidance in prenatal care. In Worthington-Roberts BS and others: *Nutrition in pregnancy and lactation,* St Louis, 1985, Mosby.

Wong D and others: *Whaley and Wong's nursing care of infants and children,* ed 6, St Louis, 1999, Mosby.

CHAPTER

9

Assisting With Elimination

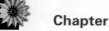

To promote normal elimination, nurses determine a client's normal pattern of elimination and attempt to accommodate that pattern. Elimination patterns are often disturbed by physiological and psychological factors during illness. Most people have been culturally indoctrinated to believe elimination is a very private activity. In a hospital or long-term care setting, bathroom facilities may be shared with a roommate. The sights, sounds, and odors associated with elimination may be embarrassing, which may prompt the client to decrease fluid intake to minimize the need to void or to ignore the urge to defecate for as long as possible. Clients who have difficulty lowering to and rising from a sitting position may need assistance with an elevated toilet seat. Those having difficulty ambulating may need assistance using a bedside commode, bedpan, or urinal. A young child recently toilet trained may have difficulty in unfamiliar circumstances.

Emotional factors often affect elimination. Anxiety may result in urinary frequency and urgency or urinary retention. Anxiety, fear, and anger may also accelerate peristalsis, resulting in diarrhea and gaseous distention. Depressed persons may have decreased peristalsis, resulting in reabsorption of water from the stool and constipation.

During illness fluid and electrolyte balance is often altered; therefore intake and output (I&O) are monitored. Intake to be measured and recorded includes liquids taken orally, intravenous (IV) solutions (see Chapter 29), and tube feedings. Output to be measured and recorded includes urine, vomitus, liquid stool, nasogastric drainage, and wound drainage (see Chapter 22). Excessive fluid losses resulting from diarrhea, which also results in losses of sodium, potassium, chloride, and bicarbonate, contribute to fluid and electrolyte imbalance (see Chapter 30).

NURSING DIAGNOSES

Many different nursing diagnoses pertain to clients with altered elimination. **Toileting Self-Care Deficit** is appropriate for clients when the focus is to promote independence with toileting activities. **Constipation** refers to decreased frequency of stool passage and/or passage of hard, dry stool related to inadequate dietary fiber, limited physical activity, altered routines, or chronic use of laxatives. **Perceived Constipation** results when a client expects a daily bowel movement at the same time and uses laxatives, enemas, or suppositories to achieve this.

Diarrhea is characterized by frequent loose, liquid, and unformed stools associated with abdominal pain, cramping, and urgency or loss of control. **Bowel Incontinence** involves weakness of the rectal sphincter or inability to know when a bowel movement occurs, which may occur following anal surgery, cerebrovascular accident (CVA), dementia, spinal cord injury, or ulcerative colitis. Numerous nursing diagnoses relate to urinary incontinence (see Chapter 7). The nursing diagnoses of **Impaired Skin Integrity** and **Impaired Tissue Integrity** may be appropriate for incontinent clients.

The client may also develop or be at risk for **Deficient Fluid Volume** or **Excess Fluid Volume** depending on disease process or fluid intake. Additional diagnoses associated with the care of indwelling catheters may be **Deficient Knowledge** and **Risk for Infection.**

Skill 9.1

Monitoring Intake and Output

Measuring and recording I&O may be a dependent or independent nursing intervention. Physicians often order I&O as a routine practice following surgery or for select medical conditions (e.g., congestive heart failure [CHF] or renal disease). Nurses can initiate I&O when they assess a client having problems in maintaining an adequate fluid balance (e.g., change in drinking habits or increased urinary output). The measuring and recording of I&O is appropriate if a client has a fever, has edema, is receiving IV or diuretic therapy, or is placed on restricted fluids. It is also important when a client has excessive fluid or electrolyte loss, as associated with vomiting, diarrhea, gastrointestinal drainage, or extensive open wounds. At specified times, usually every 8 hours, I&O is totaled and evaluated. Significant alterations are apparent by comparing 24-hour totals over several days.

Intake and output should be recorded as soon as they are measured to maintain accuracy. If more than one client is in the same room, each must have measuring receptacles labeled with name and bed location. Liquid intake includes all liquids taken orally, by feeding tube, and parenterally. Liquids include any substance that becomes liquid at room temperature, such as gelatin and ice cream. Liquid output includes urine, diarrhea, vomitus, gastric suction, and contents of drainage devices. When possible, assistance from the alert client or family facilitates accuracy, independence, and a sense of accomplishment.

ASSESSMENT

1. Identify medications that may alter urine output.
   Rationale: Diuretics cause water, sodium, and potassium excretion, resulting in an increased output; steroids (e.g., prednisone, cortisone) cause sodium and water retention and potassium excretion, resulting in a decreased output (Lewis, Heitkemper, and Dirkson, 2000).

2. Monitor hematocrit (Hct). *Rationale: Increased Hct value suggests fluid volume deficit (FVD); decreased Hct value suggests fluid volume excess (FVE) (Ignatavicius and Workman, 2002).*

3. Weigh the client daily at the same time, on the same scale, in the same clothes. Weight loss greater than 2% suggests FVD, whereas sudden weight gain greater than 2% may indicate FVE (see Procedural Guideline 8-1, p. 195). *Rationale: Fluid retention is demonstrated by differences in weight before changes in edema appear.*

4. Assess signs and symptoms of dehydration and fluid overload (see Chapter 30).

5. Assess the client's and family's knowledge of the purpose of I&O measurement and ability to participate actively in measurement. *Rationale: Identifying the gap between the known and unknown helps to focus the teaching process (Lewis, Heitkemper, and Dirkson, 2000).*

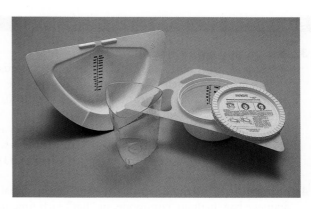

Figure 9-1 Graduated measuring containers. *Clockwise from left to right:* "Hat" receptacle, specipan, and graduated measuring container.

PLANNING

Expected outcomes focus on maintaining fluid balance, encouraging adequate fluid intake, and achieving normal laboratory values and body weight.

Expected Outcomes

1. Client's urine is neither concentrated or dilute.
2. Client maintains fluid balance, as evidenced by intake approximately 600 ml greater than output, with total 24-hour output of at least 1500 ml.
3. Client's Hct level is within a range of 40% to 54% for males or 38% to 47% for females.
4. Client's weight remains within 2% of baseline.

Equipment

- Graduated measuring containers (Figure 9-1)
  - 180- to 240-ml container for intake
  - 1000-ml container or smaller for output
- Bedpan, urinal, or bedside commode
- Specipan or "hat" (a receptacle that fits inside the commode)
- Disposable gloves

Delegation Considerations

The skills of evaluating I&O totals at the end of the shift, assessing trends in 24-hour totals over several days, monitoring and recording of IV therapy, wound or chest tube drainage, and tube feedings require the critical thinking and knowledge application of the nurse. The skill of measuring and recording I&O can be delegated to assistive personnel (AP).

- Stress the importance of accuracy in measuring and recording I&O.
- Ensure that personnel use standard precautions relating to body fluids.
- Verify that personnel can use the metric system to measure with standard containers.
- Have personnel report changes in color, amount, and odor of stool and urine and episodes of incontinence.
- Emphasize the importance of maintaining privacy for the client.

IMPLEMENTATION FOR MONITORING INTAKE AND OUTPUT

Steps	Rationale
1. See Standard Protocol (inside front cover).	
2. Explain to client and family that accurate I&O measurements are important to identify potential fluid overload or excessive losses.	Information presented must be perceived as important for the individual to learn effectively (Fox, 1998).

COMMUNICATION TIP *Tell client or family exactly what is to be measured and where to record it. Have client or family demonstrate ability to measure and record accurately.*

Steps	**Rationale**

3. Measure and record all fluid intake.

   a. Liquids with meals may include gelatin, custards, ice cream, popsicles, and sherbets. Ice chips are recorded as 50% of measured volume (e.g., 100 ml ice equals 50 ml water).

   b. Liquid medicines such as antacids are counted as fluid intake, as are liquids taken with medicines.

   c. Enteral nutrition (tube feedings) (see Chapter 33).

   d. IV fluids (see Chapter 29).

4. Instruct client and family to call nurse to empty urinal, drainage bag, bedpan, commode, or "hat" each time it is used (see illustration). Observe color and characteristics of urine. Alert, cooperative clients may keep own tally using scratch paper or a copy of facility's I&O chart. Report urine output less than 30 ml/hr.

   Promotes accurate method for recording output. Urine output less than 30 ml/hr may indicate decreased renal perfusion (Lewis, Heitkemper, and Dirkson, 2000). Dark, concentrated urine suggests dehydration; colorless urine may indicate overhydration (Lewis, Heitkemper, and Dirkson, 2000).

5. Empty and record urine output from Foley catheter into clean, graduated container at end of each shift (see illustration). Do not touch edge of graduated container or floor with tip of port while draining and before recapping. If tip of port becomes contaminated, cleanse with antiseptic swab.

   Contamination of port can create source for infection that could spread up urine drainage system to client.

6. Observe color and characteristics of urine in Foley tubing. Some clients may have a special device that is emptied into the larger container hourly. Report urine output less than 30 ml/hr.

   Dark, concentrated urine suggests dehydration. Colorless urine may indicate overhydration (Lewis, Heitkemper, and Dirkson, 2000).

COMMUNICATION TIP *Tell client or family member exactly what is to be measured and where to record it. Have client and family demonstrate ability to measure output and record volume.*

---

7. Measure and record all output from all other sources, including emesis, nasogastric suction (see Chapter 32), and all measurable wound drainage (see illustration *A*), or measure chest tube drainage by marking and recording the time on the collection chamber (see illustration *B*) (see Chapter 31).

8. Remove gloves.

9. See Completion Protocol (inside front cover).

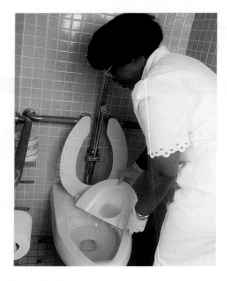

Step 4 Emptying specipan or "hat."

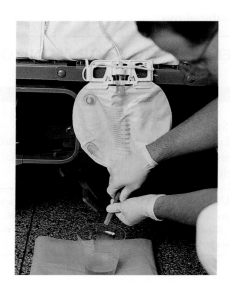

Step 5 Emptying a Foley bag.

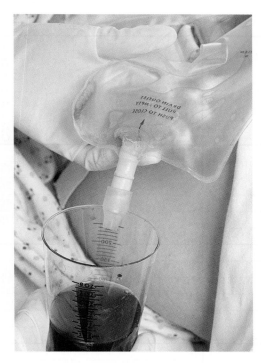

Step 7 (A)   Measuring wound drainage.

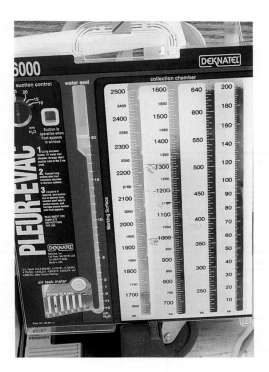

Step 7 (B)   Measuring chest tube drainage.

• • • • • • • • • •

EVALUATION

1. Observe amount and characteristics of urine such as color.
2. Calculate total I&O at the end of each shift and for 24 hours.
3. Monitor laboratory test reports for serum Hct values. The Hct is an indication of hydration status (Ignatavicius and Workman, 2002)
4. Compare daily weights, noting increase or decrease greater than 2% within 48 hours.

Unexpected Outcomes and Related Interventions

1. Client develops FVE or fluid overload (see Chapter 30), as evidenced by intake greater than output and weight gain greater than 2% over 24 to 48 hours and a low Hct value.
   a. Assess other signs and symptoms of fluid excess.
   b. In collaboration with other health care team members, administer diuretics and carefully regulate IV and oral intake.
   c. Reeducate client and family regarding fluid intake and medications.
2. Client develops FVD (see Chapter 30), as evidenced by output greater than intake, weight loss greater than 2% in 24 to 48 hours, and a high Hct value.
   a. Assess other signs and symptoms for FVD.

   b. In collaboration with other health care team members, administer oral and IV fluids consistently (see Chapter 29).
   c. Reeducate client and family regarding fluid intake.

Recording and Reporting

- Collect I&O data from client's bedside at specified time, usually every 8 hours, and document it on the specified intake and output summary in the client's chart (Figure 9-2).
- Document any changes or clinical signs in nursing note.

Sample Documentation

1500 States feels as though she cannot eat or drink anything, refused lunch. 300 ml PO fluid intake in 8 hours, temperature 38.5° C. Over 8 hours 250 ml dark, concentrated urine drained per Foley. Physician notified.

1515 1000 ml lactated Ringer's solution started IV in back of right hand with #18 angiocath. Infusing per pump at 125 ml/hr without signs of swelling or redness. Client denies discomfort at site.

Intake and Output Summary

Patient Label	P.O. Intake	Tube Feedings	Hyperalimentation	I.V. Primary	I.V.P.B.	Blood/Blood Products	Other:	Urine	Emesis	G.I. Suction	Drainage	Other: Chest tube
Date: 6-10-XX												
2200–0600	120				50			325			50	75
0600–1400	800							700			75	50
1400–2200	650				50			500			30	50
24Hr. Subtotal	1570				100			1525			155	175
Total Intake/Output	1670							1855				
Date:												
2200–0600												
0600–1400												
1400–2200												
24Hr. Subtotal												
Total Intake/Output												
Date:												
2200–0600												
0600–1400												
1400–2200												
24Hr. Subtotal												
Total Intake/Output												
Date:												
2200–0600												
0600–1400												
1400–2200												
24Hr. Subtotal												
Total Intake/Output												
Date:												
2200–0600												
0600–1400												
1400–2200												
24Hr. Subtotal												
Total Intake/ Output												
Date:												
2200–0600												
0600–1400												
1400–2200												
24Hr. Subtotals												
Total Intake/Output												
Date:												
2200–0600												
0600–1400												
1400–2200												
24Hr. Subtotals												
Total Intake/Output												

Figure 9-2　Intake and output summary.

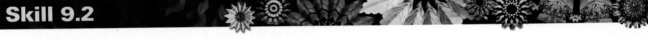

SPECIAL CONSIDERATIONS

Pediatric Considerations
- Infants and young children have a greater need for water and are more vulnerable to alterations in fluid and electrolyte balance than other age group (Wong and others, 1999).
- Infants ingest and excrete a greater amount of fluid per kilogram of body weight than do older children (Wong and others, 1999).
- Accurate I&O for infants and young children is obtained by weighing diapers (1 g weight equals 1 ml urine) or by using urine collection bags (Wong and others, 1999).

Geriatric Considerations
- Older adults are more susceptible to fluid imbalances with fever, chronic illness, gastroenteritis, or trauma.

- Incontinence may be discovered when I&O is monitored; however, incontinence is not a function of age (Lueckenotte, 2000).

Home Care Considerations
- Assess client's or primary caregiver's ability to maintain accurate I&O at home.
- Demonstrate measuring, recording, and weighing, and request return demonstration from client or home caregiver.

Long-Term Care Considerations
- Promote continuity between acute care and long-term care facilities.
- Clients in long-term care facilities can take an active part in their care if they are taught to measure and record I&O.

Skill 9.2

Providing a Bedpan and Urinal

In many cultures squatting is the usual position for defecation and urination for females. For males, squatting is the usual position during defecation and standing is the custom for voiding. For the client confined to bed, it is impossible to assume the customary positions for normal elimination, and the upright position needs to be facilitated to the extent possible. Adults may resist using a bedpan or urinal because of the emphasis on privacy. Children may find the equipment unfamiliar and threatening.

ASSESSMENT

1. Check physicians' orders for prescribed bed rest. When determining the need for a bedpan or urinal, consider factors that limit mobility (e.g., fractures, pain, surgery, postcardiac catheterization, arteriogram with potential for bleeding). Unless contraindicated, it is generally beneficial for clients to get up from bed to use the bathroom.
2. Discuss client's elimination needs in a professional, open manner using common language familiar to client. *Rationale: Language and facial expressions that indicate disapproval or revulsion contribute to embarrassment and create communication barriers.*
3. Assess elimination pattern. When does client normally defecate (e.g., after breakfast)? Are laxatives

or stool softeners routinely used? *Rationale: The normal patterns of elimination establishes a baseline for comparison.*

4. Assess the length and extent of immobility. *Rationale: Decreased mobility slows peristalsis of intestines and ureters, increasing risk for alterations such as constipation.*
5. Assess client's ability to assist, including ability to lift hips or turn. *Rationale: Determines the type of assistance needed to assist client on and off bedpan.*
6. Determine if a urine or stool specimen is to be collected. *Rationale: Ensures nurse gathers necessary supplies.*
7. Assess patterns of fluid intake. Adequate hydration (1200 to 1500 ml water daily) facilitates normal bowel elimination by keeping stools soft. Hot fluids are especially effective in softening stool and increasing peristalsis. *Rationale: Decreased fluid intake slows the passage of food through the intestines, peristalsis slows, and there is increased absorption of fluid and hardening of feces.*
8. Assess dietary intake, including high-fiber foods such as raw fruit, whole grains, bran, and green leafy vegetables. *Rationale: High-fiber foods increase bulk, which helps increase fluid content in stool, normalize consistency, and decrease transit time in the colon.*
9. Assess extent and location of pain that may influence ability to void, defecate, or position on a bed-

pan. It may be advisable to administer a prescribed analgesic about a half hour before the normal time of elimination.

10. Assess bowel sounds, and palpate abdomen and bladder for distention. Ask client if flatus is being passed. *Rationale: Abnormal bowel sounds or a distended bladder are indicative of urinary or bowel elimination problems.*

PLANNING

Expected outcomes focus on the management of bowel and urinary elimination.

Expected Outcomes

1. Client assists with movement onto bedpan and self-cleaning.
2. Client successfully defecates soft stool while on the bedpan.
3. Client uses the bedpan or urinal to void at least 1500 ml in 24 hours.
4. Client's skin integrity in perineal and perianal area remains intact without redness or irritation.

Equipment

- Bedpan (regular or fracture) (Figure 9-3)
- Urinal
- Specipan
- Toilet paper
- Underpads
- Disposable gloves

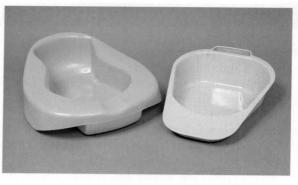

Figure 9-3   Type of bedpans. *Left,* Regular bedpan; *right,* fracture bedpan. (From Sorrentino A: *Assisting with patient care.* St Louis, 1999, Mosby.)

Delegation Considerations

The skill of assisting a client with using a bedpan or urinal can be delegated to assistive personnel (AP).

- Ensure that personnel are aware of standard precautions and guidelines relating to body fluids.
- Inform personnel about positioning needs of clients with specific limitations or therapeutic equipment, such as drains, casts, or traction.
- Clarify information that personnel are to report to the nurse about color, odor, amount, or incontinence of feces or urine.
- Verify that personnel are aware of proper hygiene.

IMPLEMENTATION FOR PROVIDING A BEDPAN AND URINAL

Steps	Rationale

1. See Standard Protocol (inside front cover).
2. **Providing a bedpan**
    a. Lower head of the bed so that it is nearly flat, and assist client with rolling toward you.
    b. Raise side rail, and have client grasp it if necessary to maintain the side-lying position.
    c. Go to opposite side of the bed, and place bedpan against buttocks as patient is on side; pan is not placed under hip. Lower end is just under the upper thighs.
    d. Press the bedpan firmly down into the mattress and against the buttocks. Keeping one hand against the bedpan, place the other on client's hip and assist client with rolling back onto the pan (see illustration).

Facilitates placement of the bedpan.

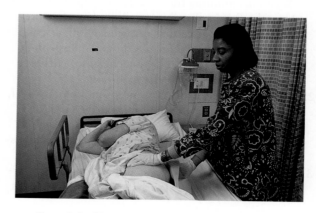

Step 2d   Placing client on regular bedpan.

Steps	**Rationale**

e. If client is able to lift buttocks, place the pan under the buttocks as they are lifted. Use of a fracture pan requires less lifting (see illustration). Check position of the pan by looking between client's legs. Front of the pan should be centered and visible.

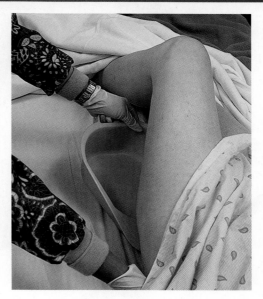

Step 2e   Placing client on fracture bedpan.

f. If not contraindicated, raise head of the bed at least 30 to 45 degrees. Have client bend knees to assume a squatting position (see illustration).

g. Raise the side rail, and place the call light and toilet paper within easy reach. Discard gloves. Provide privacy.

h. When client is finished, lower head of bed and side rail and assist client with rolling away from you onto one side as you hold the bedpan securely in place.

i. Assist client with wiping as needed; discard tissue in trash if on I&O. If necessary, clean perineum from front to back using a washcloth and warm soapy water.

j. Provide opportunity for client to wash hands.

k. Measure contents in graduated receptacle if on I&O. Then empty the contents into the toilet, and rinse thoroughly with spray faucet attached to the toilet.

This approximates the normal position for defecation as much as possible.

Privacy is essential for some clients to empty bowel and bladder successfully.

Prevents spilling contents on the bedding.

Cleaning front to back prevents transmission of microorganisms from anus to urethra, which may contribute to a urinary tract infection (UTI).

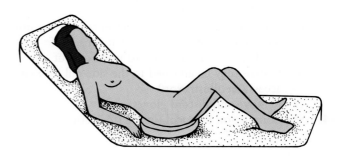

Step 2f   Proper positioning on a bed pan.

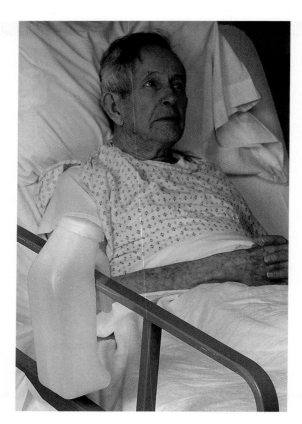

Step 3d   Urinal attached to side rail.

Steps	Rationale
l. Store bedpan and urinal in appropriate location, normally in the bathroom. Some clients need or want to have the bedpan within easy reach. If so, bedpan may be placed on a chair seat and covered with a disposable cover.	Promotes rapid accessibility when there is urgency or frequency of bowel or bladder elimination.
m. Discard gloves.	
3. Providing a urinal for a male client	
a. Position client on side, back, or sitting with head of the bed elevated, or assist to a standing position.	Men find it easier to void and empty the bladder while standing.
b. If lying in bed, client should hold urinal with base flat on the bed between the thighs, and if possible, client places penis into neck of the urinal. Assist as needed, and discard gloves.	Minimizes spilling.
c. Instruct client to notify caregiver so that the urinal can be emptied each time it is used. If needed, measure and record urine output.	Avoids overfilling; minimizes odors and growth of microorganisms. Provides accuracy in recording amount of each voiding.
d. Urinals may be attached to the side rail for easy access (see illustration).	
e. Remove and discard gloves.	
4. See Completion Protocol (inside front cover).	

• • • • • • • • • •

EVALUATION

1. Observe client's ability to assist with movement onto and off the bedpan and participate in self-cleaning.
2. Observe and record the appearance and characteristics of stool, including color, odor, consistency, frequency, amount, shape, and constituents.
3. Observe and record the appearance, odor, and amount of urine.
4. Observe skin integrity in the perineal and perianal area.

Unexpected Outcomes and Related Interventions

1. Client is unable to void using a bedpan or urinal.
   a. Provide sensory stimulation that promotes voiding, such as running water in the sink or warm water over perineum, stroking the inner thigh, placing hand in warm water, or providing a drink (if not contraindicated).
   b. Male clients may need to stand in order to void. Obtain adequate assistance if client is at risk of falling.
2. Client is unable to defecate using a bedpan.
   a. Assist to as normal a position as possible. Encourage client to massage upper abdomen from right to left to promote peristalsis.
   b. Provide reading materials, and allow ample time and privacy for the process.
   c. Consider use of a bedside commode rather than the bedpan if client is able to be up in a chair. Transfer client to commode as you would a chair. Client can sit on frame of commode in normal squatting position.
   d. Collaborate with physician to consider client's need to have a stool softener or laxative ordered.
3. Client is incontinent (see Skill 7.6, p. 177).
   a. Identify detailed information about episodes of incontinence, including how often, amount, and circumstances involved.
   b. Offer bedpan or urinal more frequently (e.g., every 2 hours).
   c. If client experiences the urge but cannot wait, place urinal within client's reach.
   d. Male clients may benefit from an external catheter (see Skill 9.3, p. 210).

Recording and Reporting

- Document client signs and symptoms.
- Describe feces and urine, including odor, consistency, amount, and any other pertinent characteristics.

Sample Documentation

0800 C/O abdominal cramping. Large, loose, light brown stool evacuated on bedpan.

SPECIAL CONSIDERATIONS

Pediatric Considerations

- Infants and young children who are not toilet trained will not be able to use a bedpan or urinal (Wong and others, 1991).
- Older children may be embarrassed or self-conscious when asked to use a bedpan or urinal (Wong and others, 1999).

Geriatric Considerations

- The aging process alters defecation and micturition (Lueckenotte, 2000). The older client may require the bedpan or urinal more frequently and more quickly or may not perceive the need to void or defecate.
- The older client may have a greater need for the "normal" position to empty the bowel or bladder because of long-ingrained cultural practices.
- The nurse may need to teach the older client the importance of diet and exercise in elimination.

Home Care Considerations

- Assess client and family for ability to carry out bowel and bladder care.
- Assess environment for accessibility of facilities and safety features such as elevated toilet seat.

Long-Term Care Considerations

- Provide personnel with a history of the client's elimination patterns to facilitate bowel and bladder care for the client when provided.
- Stress to personnel the importance of maintaining professional, respectful attitudes toward both cognitively impaired and alert clients requiring assistance with urine and bowel elimination.

Skill 9.3

Applying an External Catheter

The application of an external urinary drainage device is a convenient, safe method of draining urine in male clients. The external catheter is suitable for incontinent or comatose clients who have complete and spontaneous bladder emptying. The external catheter is a soft, pliable rubber sheath that slips over the penis. External catheters have elastic adhesive provided to secure them in place. The catheter may be attached to a leg drainage bag or a standard urinary drainage bag.

An external catheter should be assessed at least every 4 hours to detect potential problems such as skin irritation or inflammation of the urinary meatus and changed once every 24 hours for aseptic purposes. With each catheter change, the urethral meatus and penis are cleansed thoroughly and inspected for signs of skin irritation.

An external catheter has been developed that is held by a sheath attached to a brieflike man's undergarment. A clinical trial demonstrated ease of use by the client, increased dryness, decreased odor, and decreased skin irritation or breakdown (Peifer and Hanover, 1997).

ASSESSMENT

1. Assess urinary elimination patterns, ability to urinate voluntarily, and continence. *Rationale: External catheter is suitable for incontinent or comatose male clients with complete and spontaneous bladder emptying, who are at risk for skin breakdown.*
2. Assess mental status of client so appropriate teaching related to external catheter can be implemented. Teaching can include self-application. Assess client's knowledge of the purpose of an external catheter.
3. Assess condition of penis. *Rationale: Provides a baseline to compare changes in condition of skin after application of the external catheter.*

PLANNING

Expected outcomes focus on promoting dryness and preventing continual exposure of skin to urine.

Expected Outcomes

1. Client is continent with external catheter intact.
2. Client's penis remains free from skin irritation or breakdown.
3. Client's penis is without swelling or discoloration.

Equipment

- Urinary external catheter (appropriate size) with elastic or Velcro adhesive (if not using self-adhesive device)
- Urinary collection bag with drainage tubing or leg bag and straps
- Skin preparation (tincture of benzoin)
- Towels and washcloths
- Bath blanket
- Clean disposable gloves
- Scissors

Delegation Considerations

The skill of applying an external catheter can be delegated to assistive personnel (AP) in most settings, but assessment cannot. Consult agency policy. The method of applying the external catheter varies from manufacturer to manufacturer so it is critical that personnel understand how to apply and secure the catheter.

- Ensure that care provider follows standard precautions relating to body fluids.
- Stress the importance of showing respect for the client and sensitivity to the need for privacy.
- Instruct personnel to report to the professional nurse for further assessment before reapplying another external catheter if swelling, redness, or skin irritation or breakdown is noted.
- Stress the importance of securing the catheter to maintain adequate circulation.

IMPLEMENTATION FOR APPLYING AN EXTERNAL CATHETER

Steps	Rationale
1. See Standard Protocol (inside front cover).	
2. Assist client into supine position with a bath blanket over upper torso and lower extremities covered; only genitalia should be exposed.	Promotes comfort and prevents unnecessary exposure of body parts.

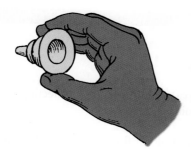

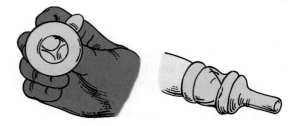

Step 7a   Positioning inner flap of self-adhesive external catheter.

Step 7b   Placing glans penis into opening of external catheter.

Steps	Rationale
3. Prepare urinary drainage collection bag and tubing. Clamp off drainage exit ports. Secure collection bag to bed frame; bring drainage tubing up between side rails and bed frame. Be sure tubing is not pulled when side rails are raised. Prepare leg bag for connection to external catheter, if necessary.	Provides easy access to drainage equipment. Positioning keeps drainage bag below level of client's bladder.
4. Using warm soapy water, remove all secretions from the penis and dry thoroughly.	Prevents skin breakdown from exposure to secretions. Rubber sheath rolls onto clean, dry skin more easily.
5. Clip hair at base of penis if necessary.	Hair adheres to adhesive and pulls during external catheter removal.
6. Apply skin preparation to length of penile shaft and allow to dry. In an uncircumcised male, be sure foreskin is in normal position. Do not apply preparation to glans of penis. The thin layer of plasticized skin spray protects skin from irritation.	Skin preparation has an alcohol base. Evaporation prevents irritation. Ensuring foreskin in normal position prevents foreskin from tightening around penile shaft, which impedes circulation to penis, and causes trauma to tissue.
7. Apply self-adhesive external catheter	
a. A plastic collar positions the inner flap for application (see illustration).	
b. Pinch catheter closed (see illustration). Place against glans as shown so tip, not entire glans, protrudes approximately 0.6 cm (¼ inch) into opening of catheter. Foreskin should remain in natural position so tip of glans and foreskin protrude 0.6 cm (¼ inch) into opening.	Allows free flow of urine into collecting tubing when client voids.
c. With nondominant hand, grasp penis along shaft. With the other hand, unroll catheter up the shaft of the penis with as little wrinkling as possible. Discard plastic collar.	Plastic collar is for application of external catheter. Wrinkling can cause skin irritation and impaired circulation.

NURSE ALERT   *Do not push collar onto the penis.*

---

d. Gently squeeze catheter to adhere sheath to skin. Once applied, do not attempt to reposition catheter. Pinch wrinkles to seal openings.	Catheter must be snug, but not tight enough to cause constriction of blood flow.

Steps	**Rationale**

8. **Apply external catheter without adhesive (see illustration)**
   a. Apply sheath to penis as in Step 7c.
   b. Allow 2.5 to 5 cm (1 to 2 inches) of space between tip of glans penis and end of external catheter.
   c. Encircle penile shaft with strip of elastic adhesive kept only in contact with sheath. Apply snugly, but not tightly.

Allows free passage of urine into collecting tubing when client voids.

Constriction of blood flow may occur if applied too tightly.

NURSE ALERT　*Do not apply standard adhesive tape or Velcro or elastic strips around the penis; this could interfere with circulation and cause necrosis of the skin and penis.*

---

9. Connect drainage tubing to the end of the external catheter. A urine drainage bag is used at night (see illustration *A*), and a leg bag attached above or below the knee may be used for ambulation (see illustration *B*).
10. Secure so that the tubing is not looped and the sheath is not twisted.
11. Remove sheath for 30 minutes every 24 hours to allow assessment and cleansing of skin. Remove and discard gloves, and wash hands.
12. See Completion Protocol (inside front cover).

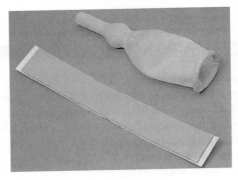

Step 8　External catheter without adhesive.

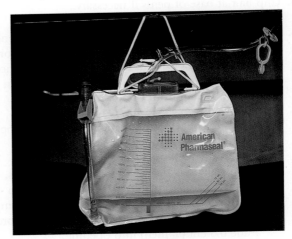

Step 9 (A)　Urine drainage bag attached to external catheter.

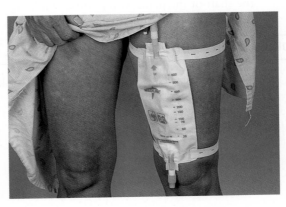

Step 9 (B)　Leg bag attached to external catheter.

EVALUATION

1. Observe amount and characteristics of urine in drainage container every 4 hours.
2. Remove sheath, and inspect skin on penile shaft for signs of breakdown or irritation at least daily during hygiene and when external catheter is reapplied.
3. Observe circulation of glans penis 1 hour after application and every 4 hours thereafter to determine that sheath has not been applied too tightly.

Unexpected Outcomes and Related Interventions

1. Urination is reduced or infrequent, indicating possible urinary retention.
   a. Check for urinary retention and bladder distention.
   b. Monitor urine output.
2. Skin irritation occurs. Client may have allergy to adhesive product or irritation from contact with urine.
   a. Increase frequency of skin cleansing, and remove external catheter for 30 minutes each shift to promote healing.
   b. Make sure urine drains readily rather than sitting in contact with penis.
   c. Investigate the availability of the new product with a sheath attached to undergarment instead of adhesive.
3. Urine accumulates in sheath, tubing becomes kinked.
   a. Unkink and straighten tubing.
4. Urine leaks from tubing.
   a. Remove catheter, and reapply more snugly.
5. Penile swelling occurs.
   a. Remove catheter, and allow swelling to decrease.
   b. Reapply more loosely.

Recording and Reporting

- Client response to condom application, including condition of the penis and scrotum
- Justification for use of the external catheter
- Description of product

Sample Documentation

0900 Urinary dribbling constant for 1 week. Perineal area reddened, even with frequent washing, drying, and application of barrier lubricant. Skin of penis intact without edema. Self-adhesive external catheter applied, connected to leg drainage bag.

1000 Voided 200 ml in leg bag without discomfort. Penis remains without swelling or discoloration. No changes in skin irritation on penis.

SPECIAL CONSIDERATIONS

Geriatric Considerations

- Clients with neuropathy must be carefully evaluated before application of an external catheter and at more frequent intervals, at least twice daily.
- The skin on the penis will be very delicate on the older person and prone to tearing; extreme caution is needed with the adhesives.
- External catheters are not recommended in clients with prostatic obstruction.

Home Care Considerations

- External catheters may contribute to UTIs; therefore teach the family signs and symptoms of infection, and emphasize medical asepsis.
- Encourage use of a leg bag during the day and a bedside drainage bag at night.
- Loose-fitting clothing may be needed to promote adequate drainage.
- Explain to the family that long-term use of external catheters may result in skin breakdown.

Long-Term Care Considerations

Teach personnel signs and symptoms of UTI and complications associated with external catheter use.

Skill 9.4

Administering an Enema

The primary reason for an enema is promotion of defecation. The volume and type of fluid instilled can lubricate or break up the fecal mass, stretch the rectal wall, and initiate the defecation reflex. Clients should not rely on enemas to maintain bowel regularity because they do not treat the cause of irregularity or constipation. Frequent enemas disrupt normal defecation reflexes, resulting in dependence on enemas for elimination. Fluid and electrolyte imbalances can occur with frequent enemas.

An enema is the instillation of a solution into the rectum and sigmoid colon. Cleansing enemas promote complete evacuation of feces from the colon by stimulating peristalsis through infusion of large volumes of solution. When "enemas until clear" is ordered in preparation for surgery or diagnostic testing, the water expelled should be colorless and contain no particles of feces.

An oil-retention enema lubricates the rectum and colon, softens the feces, and facilitates defecation. An oil-retention enema can be used alone or as adjunct therapy to manual removal of a fecal impaction. An impaction involves presence of a fecal mass too large or hard to be passed voluntarily. Either constipation or diarrhea can suggest the presence of an impaction.

Medicated enemas contain pharmacological therapeutic agents and are used to reduce dangerously high serum potassium levels, as with a sodium polystyrene sulfonate (Kayexalate) enema, or to reduce bacteria in the colon before bowel surgery, as with a neomycin enema.

A carminative enema, such as the Harris or return-flow enema, is used to relieve accumulated flatus. A small amount (100 to 200 ml) of enema solution is administered into the client's rectum and colon. The container is then lowered, and the solution flows back through the enema tubing to the container. Flatus will also return. The process can be repeated numerous times and results in reduced flatus and increased peristalsis (Potter and Perry, 2001).

Enema administration may be considered an evil practice in some cultures, thus introducing a conflict when the client is in need of an enema. A young child may be frightened by administration of an enema.

ASSESSMENT

1. Assess last bowel movement and presence or absence of bowel sounds. *Rationale: Reduced bowel motility may indicate need for enema.*
2. If client is expected to have decreased sphincter control, assess ability to control external sphincter by performing a rectal examination. Insert lubricated gloved finger gently into anus, and ask client to bear down around your finger. *Rationale: Client with paralysis and no sphincter control must be placed on bedpan because enema solution cannot be retained.*
3. Assess presence or absence of hemorrhoids, which may obscure the rectal opening and cause discomfort or bleeding with evacuation.
4. Assess for abdominal pain. *Rationale: Indicates an enema is contraindicated until further assessment rules out danger of bowel perforation.*
5. Determine client's level of understanding and previous experience with enemas in order to provide appropriate teaching measures.
6. Assess limitations of mobility.

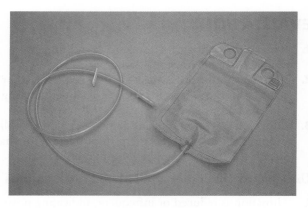

Figure 9-4   High-volume enema bag with tubing.

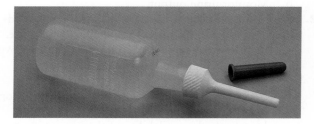

Figure 9-5   Prepackaged enema container with rectal tip(s).

PLANNING

Expected outcomes focus on establishing a normal pattern of bowel elimination and normal consistency of stools.

Expected Outcomes

1. Client verbalizes relief of abdominal discomfort.
2. Client empties rectum and lower colon of stool and fluid.

Equipment

- Enema bag (disposable or reusable) (Figure 9-4)
- Disposable gloves
- Waterproof absorbent underpads
- Adult: 750 to 1000 ml warm water or prepackaged disposable enema with prelubricated tip (Figure 9-5)
- Water-soluble lubricant
- Bath blanket
- Toilet tissue
- Bedpan, bedside commode, or access to toilet
- Wash basin, washcloths, towel, and soap
- IV pole

Delegation Considerations

The skill of administering an enema can be delegated to assistive personnel (AP).

- Stress importance of standard precautions for body fluids.
- Instruct care provider to use alternative positioning if there are mobility restrictions.
- Instruct personnel to stop and report inability to hold enema solution, severe cramping, bleeding, or severe abdominal pain.

IMPLEMENTATION FOR ADMINISTERING AN ENEMA

Steps	Rationale
1. See Standard Protocol (inside front cover).	
2. If using an enema bag, fill it with 750 to 1000 ml warm tap water as it flows from faucet. Check temperature of water by pouring small amount over inner wrist. Remove air from tubing by allowing solution to fill tubing. Clamp tubing.	Hot water can burn intestinal mucosa. Cold water can cause abdominal cramping and is difficult to retain.
3. Add castile soap if ordered.	Causes mild level of bowel irritation, facilitating mucus secretion.
4. Assist client into left side-lying (Sims') position with right knee flexed. Encourage client to remain in position until procedure is completed. Place client in as private and comfortable an environment as possible.	Allows enema solution to flow downward by gravity along natural curve of sigmoid colon and rectum, thus improving retention of solution (Potter and Perry, 2001).

NURSE ALERT *Clients with minimal sphincter control may not be able to retain all of enema solution and will require placement of a bedpan under the buttocks. Administering enema with client sitting on toilet is ineffective because solution will not effectively infuse against gravity into bowel.*

COMMUNICATION TIP

- *Adapt explanation of procedure to developmental level of client. If client is confused, use simple explanation and have AP assist with positioning.*
- *Ask a parent to assist if a child is to receive the enema.*

Steps	Rationale
5. Place waterproof pad absorbent side up under hips and buttocks to prevent soiling of linen.	
6. Cover client with bath blanket, exposing only rectal area, and clearly visualize anus.	Provides warmth, reduces exposure of body parts, allows client to feel more relaxed and comfortable. Presence of hemorrhoids obscures anal opening and increases discomfort with bowel elimination.

Steps	Rationale

7. If client will be expelling contents in toilet, ensure that toilet is available and place client's slippers and bathrobe in easily accessible location. If client is unable to get out of bed, place bedpan in easily accessible position.

8. Administer enema in prepackaged disposable container

   a. Remove plastic cap from rectal tip. Tip may be already lubricated. More lubricant can be applied if needed.

Lubrication provides for smooth insertion of rectal tube without rectal irritation or trauma.

   b. 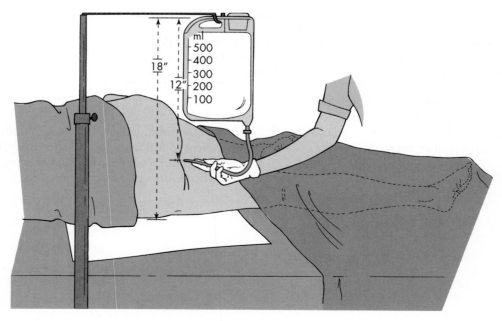 Gently separate buttocks and locate anus. Instruct client to relax by breathing out slowly through mouth.

Breathing out promotes relaxation of external rectal sphincter. Presence of hemorrhoids obscures location of anus. Probe gently with gloved finger to locate rectal opening if necessary.

   c. Insert lubricated tip of bottle gently into rectum approximately 7.5 to 10 cm (3 to 4 inches) for an adult.

Gentle insertion prevents trauma to rectal mucosa.

   d. Squeeze bottle continuously until all of solution has entered rectum and colon. (Most bottles contain approximately 250 ml solution.)

Hypertonic solutions require only small volumes to stimulate defecation. Intermittent squeezing results in return of solution to the bottle.

9. Administer enema in standard enema bag

   a. Lubricate 7.5 to 10 cm (3 to 4 inches) of tip of rectal tube with lubricating jelly.

Prevents trauma to rectal mucosa.

   b. Gently separate buttocks and locate anus. Instruct client to relax by breathing out slowly through mouth.

Breathing out promotes relaxation of external anal sphincter.

   c. Insert tip of rectal tube slowly by pointing tip in direction of client's umbilicus. *Adult:* 7.5 to 10 cm (3 to 4 inches) past the internal sphincter.

Careful insertion prevents trauma to rectal mucosa from accidental lodging of tube against rectal wall. Forceful insertion beyond 10 cm (4 inches) could cause bowel perforation.

   d. Hold tubing in rectum constantly until end of fluid instillation.

Bowel contraction can cause expulsion of rectal tube.

   e. With container at client's hip level, open regulating clamp and allow solution to enter slowly.

Rapid infusion can stimulate evacuation and cause cramping.

Step 9f Administering an enema. (From Sorrentino S: *Assisting with patient care,* St Louis, 1999, Mosby.)

Steps	Rationale
f. Raise height of enema container slowly to 30 to 45 cm (12 to 18 inches) above the anus. Infusion time varies with volume of solution administered (e.g., 1 L may take 7 to 10 minutes). Hang container on IV pole (see illustration).	Raising container too high causes rapid infusion and possible painful distention of colon.
g. Lower container or clamp tubing if client complains of cramping or if fluid escapes around rectal tube.	Temporary cessation of infusion minimizes cramping and promotes ability to retain all the solution.
h. Clamp tubing after all the solution is infused. Tell client that the procedure is completed and that you will be removing rectal tube. Then gently withdraw tube.	Clients may misinterpret the sensation of removing the tube as loss of control.
10. Explain to client that feeling of distention is normal. Ask client to retain solution as long as possible (5 to 10 minutes) while lying quietly in bed.	Solution distends bowel. Length of retention varies with type of enema and client's ability to contract rectal sphincter. Longer retention promotes more effective stimulation of peristalsis and defecation.
11. Discard enema container and tubing in proper receptacle, or rinse out thoroughly with warm soap and water if container is to be reused.	
12. Assist client to bathroom or commode if possible. If necessary to use the bedpan, assist to as near the normal position for evacuation as possible.	Normal squatting position promotes defecation.
13. Instruct clients with a history of cardiovascular disease to exhale while expelling enema to avoid the Valsalva maneuver (forced effort against a closed airway), especially if client is dehydrated.	The Valsalva maneuver in strenuously trying to move a constipated stool may result in cardiac arrest.
14. Instruct client to call for nurse to inspect results before flushing the toilet. Observe character of feces and solution.	When enemas are ordered "until clear," enemas are repeated until client passes fluid that is clear and contains no formed fecal matter. Usually three consecutive enemas are adequate.
15. Assist client as needed to wash anal area with warm soap and water.	Fecal contents can irritate skin. Hygiene promotes client's comfort.
16. Discard gloves.	
17. See Completion Protocol (inside front cover).	

• • • • • • • • • •

EVALUATION

1. Ask client if abdominal discomfort has been relieved.
2. Inspect color, consistency, and amount of stool and characteristics of fluid passed.

Unexpected Outcomes and Related Interventions

1. Client is unable to hold enema solution.
   a. If this occurs during instillation, slow rate of infusion.
   b. Position on bedpan while administering the solution.
2. Severe cramping, bleeding, or sudden severe abdominal pain occurs and is unrelieved by temporarily stopping or slowing flow of solution.
   a. Stop enema.
   b. Notify physician.
3. With an order for "enemas until clear," after three enemas the water is highly colored or contains solid fecal material.

   a. Notify the physician before continuing because excessive loss of electrolytes is a dangerous possibility.

Recording and Reporting

* Client signs and symptoms and response to enema
* Type of enema given
* Results, including color, amount, and appearance of stool

Sample Documentation

2000 Last BM 5 days ago. C/O abdominal fullness and rectal pressure. Abdomen distended, firm. Rectum free of fecal material on palpation. 900 ml tap water enema given with "mild" abdominal cramping during administration. Solution returned with large amount of dark brown, soft-formed stool.

   2100 States is comfortable with no fullness in abdomen. Abdomen soft, nondistended.

SPECIAL CONSIDERATIONS

Pediatric Considerations

- Infants and children do not usually receive hypertonic enemas or tap water enemas (McKinney and others, 2000).
- Infants and young children are unable to retain the enema solution so the buttocks must be held together after enema administration (Wong and others, 1999).
- The tip of the enema tubing is inserted a shorter distance in the rectum of infants and children to prevent rectal damage and perforation.
- The nurse may want to involve the parents of infants and children in the procedure.

Geriatric Considerations

- Older adults may become fatigued more quickly and are at greater risk for fluid and electrolyte imbalances; therefore caution is needed when administering enemas "until clear."
- Teach older adults and their caregivers dietary and activity measures to avoid constipation.

Home Care Considerations

- Assess client's and family's ability and motivation to administer enema in the home, and provide instruction as needed.
- Assess client's ability to manipulate equipment to self-administer enema.
- Assess client's environment to identify location where enema may be administered with privacy.
- Instruct client and family not to exceed number and volume of enemas.

Long-Term Care Considerations

Teach long-term care AP signs and symptoms (diaphoresis, pallor, shortness of breath, palpitations) that require stopping enema administration and to report immediately to the nurse.

Skill 9.5

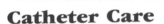

Catheter Care

Clients with altered urinary elimination may require an indwelling catheter (see Chapter 35). The catheter potentially provides a direct route for infection from the client's bladder to the outside, unless the catheter system remains intact and the catheter is cleansed. The urinary tract is the most common site of nosocomial (hospital-acquired) infections. To help reduce the risk of UTI, clients with indwelling catheters require regular catheter care that includes perineal care (see Chapter 7) and cleansing of the first 4 inches of the exposed catheter tubing at least every 8 hours. It is also recommended that catheter care be performed after each bowel movement (Evans, 1999).

ASSESSMENT

1. Assess the urethral meatus and surrounding tissues for inflammation, swelling, secretions, or encrustations at the catheter insertion site. *Rationale: Determines presence of infection and status of hygiene.*
2. Assess color, clarity, and odor of urine. *Rationale: Urine that is cloudy and has a strong odor may indicate UTI.*
3. Assess for any complaints of pain or discomfort in lower abdomen. *Rationale: May indicate inflammation of urinary tract mucosa caused by bacterial invasion (Lewis, Heitkemper, and Dirkson, 2000).*
4. Monitor client's temperature. *Rationale: Fever may indicate a UTI.*
5. Monitor client's fluid intake. *Rationale: Decreased fluid intake inhibits the natural flushing of urinary system and increases the possibility of bacterial growth.*
6. Assess client's understanding of the procedure. *Rationale: Identifies the need for client instruction.*

PLANNING

Expected outcomes focus on promoting perineal cleanliness and absence of UTI.

1. Urine is clear, and volume is adequate.
2. Urethral meatus is free of secretions and encrustations.
3. Client is afebrile.
4. Client verbalizes feeling of comfort after procedure is completed.

Equipment

- Soap
- Washcloths and towel
- Bath basin
- Warm water
- Disposable gloves
- Bath blanket
- Waterproof pad

Delegation Considerations

The skill can be delegated to assistive personnel (AP) and incorporated into routine perineal care. If the client has had trauma or surgical procedures that involve the perineal area, catheter care should not be delegated.

- Ensure that AP follows standard precautions related to body fluids.
- Instruct AP to report catheter drainage (color, odor, amount of urine), presence of secretions and encrustations at the catheter insertion site, and condition of perineum (presence of inflammation, contamination from fecal discharge).
- Stress the importance of sensitivity to client's privacy needs.
- Instruct the caregiver regarding any special positioning needs of client.

IMPLEMENTATION FOR CATHETER CARE

Steps	Rationale
1. See Standard Protocol (inside front cover)	

2. Position client comfortably, and cover with bath blanket, exposing only perineal area.
  a. Female in dorsal recumbent position
  b. Male in supine position
	Reduces client embarrassment. Ensures easy access to perineal area.

3. Place waterproof pad under client.	
4. Provide routine perineal care (see Skill 7.1, p. 150), being sure all perineal folds are cleansed thoroughly.	
5. Hold the catheter securely near the meatus with the gloved nondominant hand. Using a clean washcloth, soap, and water, take the dominant hand and wipe in a circular motion along the length of the catheter for about 10 cm (4 inches). Avoid placing tension on or pulling on the exposed catheter tubing.	Reduces presence of secretions, drainage, or fecal matter on exterior of catheter surface, decreasing risk of bacterial growth (Ebersole and Hess, 1998). Tension causes urethral trauma. Pulling on the catheter tubing may lead to accidental removal.
6. Replace as necessary the anchor device used to secure the catheter tubing to the client's leg or abdomen (see Skill 35.1, p. 840).	Anchoring of catheter reduces pressure on the urethra, reducing the possibility of tissue injury (Evans, 1999). Local irritation to the urethra predisposes tissues to bacterial invasion.

7. Check drainage tubing and bag to ensure that:
  a. Tubing is not looped or positioned above level of bladder
  b. Tubing is coiled and secured onto bed linen
  c. Tubing is not kinked or clamped
  d. Collection bag is positioned appropriately on bed frame (see Skill 35.1, p. 840)
	Ensures free flow of urine.
	
	Any interruption with the free flow of urine may cause UTI.

8. Empty collection bag as necessary or at least every 8 hours (see Skill 9.1, p. 200).	Urine in collection bag provides a medium for bacteria growth.
9. See Completion Protocol (inside front cover).	

• • • • • • • • • •

EVALUATION

1. Observe color and clarity of urine.
2. Inspect the catheter insertion site for secretions and encrustations.
3. Monitor the client's temperature.
4. Ask client about feelings of discomfort or burning.

Unexpected Outcomes and Related Interventions

1. Urethral or perineal irritation is present.
   a. Assess for leaking of catheter, and replace as needed.
   b. Ensure that the catheter is anchored correctly (see Skill 35.1, p. 840).
2. Notify physician if securing catheter does not improve urethral irritation.
3. Client develops a UTI (see Chapter 35) as evidenced by fever, cloudy and concentrated urine.
   a. Assess other signs of UTI.
   b. Increase fluid intake to at least 1500 ml/day.
   c. Monitor body temperature.
   d. Notify physician of findings.

Recording and Reporting

- Condition of the perineum, including any secretions or encrustations at catheter insertion site
- Characteristics of the urine

Sample Documentation

1000 Incontinent of large amount liquid brown stool after breakfast. Perineal area cleansed, and catheter care given. No inflammation of perineum. No secretions or encrustations at catheter insertion site. Urine in catheter tubing and bag light amber and clear.

⊛ SPECIAL CONSIDERATIONS ⊛

Pediatric Considerations
Describe the procedure to children at their level of understanding. The nurse may also need to explain the procedure to the parents of young children.

Geriatric Considerations
- The older adult client may exhibit atypical symptoms of a UTI such as change in mental status (Lueckenotte, 2000).
- Older adults have age-related changes in the immune system; therefore they are at high risk for nosocomial (hospital-acquired) infections (Lewis, Heitkemper, and Dirkson, 2000).

Home Care Considerations
- Teach client and family importance of catheter care.
- Teach client and family signs and symptoms to report to nurse or physician.

CRITICAL THINKING EXERCISES

1. Mrs. Meyers, 85, has colorectal cancer and is scheduled the next morning for a colon resection with a creation of a sigmoid colostomy. She has a history of cardiac disease and recent weight loss. The client states that although she has been eating, she has not been drinking many fluids lately. She is to be on clear liquids the evening prior to surgery. In addition, the physician ordered cleansing enemas until clear.
   a. Analyze the enema order. Is it appropriate? Give the rationale for your answer.
   b. Explain what assessments you should perform as an RN before enema administration for this client.
   c. What specific precautions should you communicate when you delegate to the AP before enema administration?
   d. You go into Mrs. Meyer's room and note that she is having abdominal cramping as the enema is being administered. Explain what you would assess. What instructions would you give the AP?
   e. After three enemas, Mrs. Meyers continues to pass semiformed stool. The AP is insisting that Mrs. Meyers needs more enemas. How would you respond? Include the rationale for your response and related intervention(s).

2. Mr. Jones, 90, is incontinent and has a stage I pressure ulcer on his sacrum. You as the RN decide to place an external catheter on the client.
   a. The AP asks why you do not obtain an order for catheterization. Explain your decision.
   b. Explain the assessments you would make before placing the external catheter by yourself or before delegating the task to AP.
   c. Mr. Jones tells you that he doesn't understand why the external catheter keeps getting "tighter." What could be the cause, and what interventions would be appropriate?

3. Mr. James Johnson, age 78, is hospitalized for gastroenteritis. He has been vomiting and had diarrhea for 3 days; he is unabe to tolerate oral food or fluids. On admission, IV fluids are started and run at 125 ml per hour. You notice that the output fot the first 8 hours of hospitalization includes 200 ml of concentrated urine; vomiting two times, 500 ml each time; and three diarrhea stools of 350 ml, 200 ml, and 500 ml.
   a. Based on this information what is his total intake and output?
   b. If he is dehydrated, what would you expect the hematocrit to be? Increased or decreased?
   c. What would be a significant weight loss after 24 hours if his admission weight was 200 pounds?

REFERENCES

Ebersole P, Hess P: *Human needs and nursing responses*, ed 5, St Louis, 1998, Mosby.

Evans E: Indwelling catheter care: dispelling the misconceptions, *Geriatr Nurs* 20(2):85, 1999.

Fox V: Postoperative education that works, *AORN J* 65(5): 1010, 1998.

Hockenberry MJ and others: *Wong's nursing care of infants and children*, ed 7, St Louis, 2003, Mosby.

Ignatavicius D, Workman M: *Medical-surgical nursing: critical thinking for collaborative care*, ed 4, St Louis, 2002, Saunders.

Lewis S, Heitkemper M, Dirkson S: *Medical surgical nursing: assessment and management of clinical problems*, ed 5, St Louis, 2000, Mosby.

Lueckenotte A: *Gerontological nursing*, ed 2, St Louis, 2000, Mosby.

McKinney E and others: *Maternal child nursing*, St Louis, 2000, Saunders.

Peifer D, Hanover R: Clinical evaluation of the Easy-Flow Catheter, *J Rehabil Res Dev* 34(20):215, 1997.

Potter P, Perry A: *Fundamentals of nursing: concepts, process, and practice*, ed 5, St Louis, 2001, Mosby.

Wong DL and others: *Whaley and Wong's nursing care of infants and children*, ed 6, St Louis, 1999, Mosby.

Promoting Comfort, Sleep, and Relaxation

Clients experience various forms of stress, undergo painful procedures, and experience painful illnesses. In addition, the experience of staying in a health care environment and the symptoms of various diseases can disrupt clients' sleep patterns. Assisting clients with acquiring rest and relaxation can be a challenge. Sleep research has shown that sleep is necessary for healing. One of the nurse's responsibilities in the basic care of all clients is to create a comfortable environment and apply principles of stress management to assist clients in gaining necessary sleep and rest.

The major problem in sleep disturbances is insufficient quantity and quality of sleep. Clients may experience difficulty falling asleep, frequent awakenings during sleep time, an inadequate duration of sleep, or a combination of all of these characteristics. The benefits of sleep often go unnoticed until a person develops problems resulting from sleep deprivation, which lead to changes in thought processes, memory, pain tolerance, and neurological function. Severity of symptoms such as agitation, disorientation, hyperactivity, and fatigue is highly variable and relates to the duration of the sleep deprivation. Research has shown that older adults tend to experience changes in sleep patterns, with a deterioration in the quality of sleep (Beck-Little and Weinrich, 1998). This can result in impaired judgment and concentration.

Pain and discomfort are subjective and highly individualized sensations. Acute pain protects an individual from a harmful stimulus, and it also can be a warning of tissue damage. Pain is greatly influenced by psychosocial and cultural factors. The gate-control theory suggests that pain impulses can be regulated or blocked by "closing gates" that transmit pain sensations to the spinal cord. A bombardment of sensory impulses, such as from a back rub, closes the gates to pain stimuli. This theory also suggests that gating mechanisms can be altered by thoughts, feelings, and memories. The nurse applies the gate-control theory in the use of noninvasive pain-control measures. The focus of this chapter is the nurse's role in providing basic comfort measures. (For additional information on pain management, refer to Chapter 11.)

Pain stimulates the autonomic nervous system as part of the stress response. Nurses must use and teach stress management techniques and comfort measures that can promote pain relief, relaxation, and falling and remaining asleep. Life-threatening illness, changes in family structure, job stress, depression, and grief increase the anxiety of clients and their families. Anxiety can increase a client's

level of pain and discomfort, interfere with learning, lower resistance to disease, and delay the recovery process. Stress-related conditions frequently bring clients into the health care system. Recent studies support the effectiveness of progressive relaxation and guided imagery in reducing self-reported pain and analgesic use (McCaffery and Pasero, 1999).

NURSING DIAGNOSES

Disturbed Sleep Pattern is a time-limited disruption of sleep amount and quality. Disturbed sleep can cause discomfort or interfere with a person's desired lifestyle. Related factors may include physical discomfort, emotional stress such as loneliness or grief, family stress, depression, medications, environmental or habit changes, and physical symptoms such as shortness of breath, nausea, or fever. The focus of care involves reducing factors that interfere with sleep. **Fatigue** is an overwhelming sustained sense of exhaustion and decreased capacity for physical and mental work. Related factors are psychological, environmental, situational, and physiological. The focus for clients with fatigue becomes conservation of energy and the provision of rest periods. **Anxiety** is a vague, uneasy feeling of discomfort or dread accompanied by an autonomic response: a feeling of apprehension caused by anticipation of danger or threat. Related factors include unmet needs, situational or maturational crises, and threat to self-concept. The nursing focus with anxiety is promoting relaxation and stress management. **Acute Pain** is an unpleasant sensory and emotional experience arising from actual or potential tissue damage with an anticipated or predictable end and a duration of less than 6 months. Related factors include biological, chemical, physical, and psychological injury agents. The nursing focus with pain is to promote comfort. **Chronic Pain** is constant or recurring without an anticipated or predictable end and a duration of greater than 6 months.

Powerlessness is a perception that one's own action will not significantly affect an outcome, or a perceived lack of control over a current situation or immediate happening. Related factors include the health care environment, interpersonal interaction, and illness-related regimen. The focus of care includes activities that empower the client by allowing the experiencing of an increased sense of control over life situations and personal activities.

Skill 10.1

Comfort Measures That Promote Sleep

Factors within a hospital environment are likely to influence clients' ability to fall and remain asleep. Acutely ill clients undergo frequent treatment and observation and are exposed to unavoidable environmental stimulation to the point of having difficulty attaining needed sleep. Disruptive sounds such as paging systems, alarms, monitors, telephones, flushing toilets, suctioning equipment, and nursing activities create an environment that is not conducive to sleep. This is especially problematic for clients in intensive care units (ICUs) where normal sleep-wake cycles are frequently disrupted.

In addition, any illness that causes pain, difficulty breathing or swallowing, itching, nausea, or nocturia (urination at night) results in discomfort. Discomfort, emotional stress, anxiety, and depression may interfere with falling asleep or may cause frequent awakening or early awakening. Symptom management, the elimination of factors that create stress or anxiety, and the management of the client's immediate environment become the focus for the nurse's efforts at promoting comfort and sleep.

ASSESSMENT

1. Ask client to describe character of any discomfort, including location, onset, severity, precipitating or aggravating factors, and quality. Use a pain rating scale to measure severity (see Chapter 11). *Rationale: Provides important baseline to determine efficacy of nursing measures.*

2. To identify client's normal sleep pattern, ask:
   a. What time do you usually go to sleep?
   b. How quickly do you fall asleep?
   c. What is the average number of hours you sleep?
   d. How many times do you awaken during that time?
   e. When do you typically awaken?
   f. Do you rise once you awaken, or do you stay in bed?
   Rationale: Enables nurse to adapt interventions specific to nature of client's sleep alteration.

3. When a sleep problem is identified, use open questions to help the client describe the problem more fully.
   a. What interferes with your sleep?
   b. What type of sleep problem do you experience?
   c. When did you notice the problem? How long has it lasted?
   d. How often do you have trouble sleeping?
   e. Compare your sleep now with your normal sleep.
   f. What do you do just before going to bed?

g. What do you think about as you fall asleep?
h. Have you had any recent changes at work or at home?
i. How has the loss of sleep affected you?
j. Have you or your partner noted any changes in behavior since the sleep problem started? Irritability, fatigue, trouble concentrating, others?

COMMUNICATION TIP *Before discussing specific sleep problems with the client, use this time to inform the client and family about factors, such as diet and exercise, that could positively or negatively affect sleep patterns.*

4. Identify medications that may influence sleep patterns (Table 10-1). *Rationale: Client may benefit from change in medication schedule or type of medication following further consultation with physician.*

5. Identify illnesses or conditions that can alter sleep (see Table 10-1, p. 225).

6. Identify indications of sleep apnea. *Rationale: Sleep apnea is the temporary cessation of airflow through the nose and mouth for 10 seconds or more during sleep (Barkauskas and others, 1998). The sleeping partner may be a better source of information than the client.*
   a. Snores loudly and irregularly?
   b. Stops breathing for a while and then starts up again?
   c. Has headaches after awakening?
   d. Awakens coughing or choking?
   e. Makes grunting or gurgling noises during sleep?

PLANNING

Expected outcomes focus on providing comfort and assisting the client in improving the quality of sleep.

Expected Outcomes

1. Client is relaxed and comfortable after intervention as evidenced by self-reported reduction in pain severity; slow, deep respirations; calm facial expression; calm tone of voice; relaxed muscles; and relaxed posture.
2. Client demonstrates and describes sleep-promoting measures.
3. Client reports receiving restful sleep.

Equipment

- Night-light
- Client's preferred reading material
- Compact disc (CD), audiotape, or radio to provide music

Table 10-1

Factors That Can Alter Sleep

MEDICATIONS

Drug Class	Effects on Sleep
Hypnotics	Interfere with reaching deeper sleep stages Provide only temporary (1 week) increase in quantity of sleep Eventually cause "hangover" feeling during day: excess drowsiness, confusion, decreased energy May worsen sleep apnea in adults
Beta-adrenergic blockers	Cause nightmares, insomnia, awakening from sleep
Benzodiazepines	Increase sleep time and daytime sleepiness.
Opiates (morphine, meperidine [Demerol])	Suppress REM sleep If discontinued quickly, can increase risk of cardiac dysrhythmias because of rebound Cause increased awakenings and drowsiness
Antidepressants and stimulants	Suppress REM sleep and decrease total sleep time
Alcohol	Speeds onset of sleep but disrupts REM sleep Awakens person during night and causes difficulty returning to sleep

ILLNESSES AND CONDITIONS

Type of Illness/Condition	Effects on Sleep
Respiratory disease	Rhythm of breathing may be altered; nasal congestion and sore throat impair breathing and ability to relax
Coronary heart disease with episodes of chest pain and irregular heart rate	Frequent awakenings and sleep stage changes
Hypertension	Early morning awakening and fatigue
Hypothyroidism	Decreases stage 4 sleep
Hyperthyroidism	Takes more time to fall asleep
Nocturia	Awakenings at night to urinate; difficulty returning to sleep
Gastric reflux	Burning pain in lower esophagus increases when lying flat in bed

Delegation Considerations

The nurse, in collaboration with the client, is responsible for the assessment, planning, implementation, and evaluation of needed comfort and sleep-enhancing measures. The following information is necessary when delegating skills to assistive personnel (AP) or family members:

- Have personnel report changes in client's condition.
- Identify and eliminate environmental conditions that might inhibit sleep.
- Plan comfort measures at a time during the day or night to provide maximum rest periods.
- Inform personnel of any restrictions related to client's condition that might affect positioning, use of hot or cold applications, and diet.

IMPLEMENTATION FOR COMFORT MEASURES THAT PROMOTE SLEEP

Steps	Rationale
1. See Standard Protocol (inside front cover).	
2. Promote usual bedtime routines (reading, listening to music, eating a snack, watching television). Encourage client to empty bladder. Provide opportunity to wash face and hands, brush teeth or dentures, and cleanse mouth.	Activities promote relaxation and remove any irritating physical stimuli.
3. Offer a bedtime snack such as a dairy product. Also encourage client to avoid caffeine at bedtime.	Dairy product that contains L-tryptophan may help promote sleep. Caffeine in coffee, tea, colas, and chocolate is a stimulant and can interfere with sleep. It also acts as a diuretic and may cause the need to void during the night.
4. Schedule diuretics early in the day. Decrease fluid intake 2 to 4 hours before bedtime.	Interventions decrease incidence of nocturia.
5. Teach client to eliminate/reduce physical activities 2 hours before bedtime.	Physical exertion can disrupt sleep. Completing rigorous exercise 2 hours before bedtime allows body to cool down and maintain a state of fatigue that promotes relaxation.
6. Encourage client to avoid ingestion of alcohol before bedtime.	Alcohol can interrupt sleep cycles and reduce the amount of deep sleep.
7. Make sure client's gown and linens are clean and dry. Change wet dressings. Tighten and smooth wrinkled bed linen. Provide adequate warmth, especially for feet and shoulders.	
8. Provide cutaneous stimulation such as a massage (see Skill 10.2, p. 228), a warm bath, or a warm or cold compress.	Massage promotes muscle relaxation. The gate-control theory suggests that cutaneous stimulation of certain nerve fibers closes gates to transmission of discomfort.
9. Assist client to a comfortable, anatomically correct position, providing support to body parts to minimize muscle tension. Place a pillow at the client's back to support in lateral position (see illustration). Position client off tubing and other equipment.	The lateral position is good for relaxation in general. Removal of painful stimuli reduces pain reception and perception.
10. Raise side rails if appropriate, and place call light within reach. Remind client to call for help if getting up for any reason is necessary. Assure client you will respond to calls as quickly as possible. If client is at risk for falls, use fall precaution guidelines (see Chapter 5).	Clients who have urinary urgency may attempt to go to the bathroom alone rather than experience soiling the bed. This is one of the most common factors associated with client falls.
11. Eliminate environmental noise as much as possible. Closing door to the hallway may minimize disturbing sounds. Some clients are accustomed to music or the sound of radio or television (Box 10-1).	
12. Provide an acceptable level of indirect light. Use of a night-light may be beneficial.	May reduce confusion if client awakens at night.
13. Schedule necessary nursing assessments, medications, and treatments to minimize the number of times client must be awakened, and assure client of this plan.	Increases the opportunity for quality sleep and rapid eye movement (REM)/non–rapid eye movement (NREM) sleep cycling.
14. See Completion Protocol (inside front cover).	

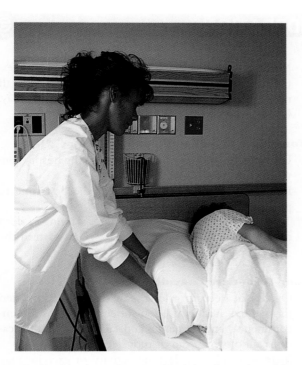

Step 9 Positioning client in side-lying lateral position for comfort.

Box 10-1

Control of Noise in the Hospital

Close doors to client's room.

Provide a sign on the door requesting avoidance of interruptions.

Reduce volume of nearby telephone and paging equipment.

Wear rubber-soled shoes.

Turn off equipment if possible (e.g., oxygen, suction).

Drain humidified oxygen tubing of water accumulation periodically.

Avoid flushing a toilet or moving beds if possible.

Keep talking at low levels, especially at night.

Conduct nursing reports and discussions in areas away from client rooms.

Turn off television or radio or provide soft music.

• • • • • • • • • •

EVALUATION

1. Ask client to rate discomfort level on a scale of 0 to 10 (10 is the worst).
2. Observe client for evidence of sleep 30 minutes after preparing for sleep and every hour thereafter.
3. Ask client to describe methods used to promote sleep, and discuss their effectiveness.
4. Assess client's perception of feeling rested on awakening.

Unexpected Outcome and Related Interventions

1. Client reports delay in falling asleep, frequent awakenings during the night, or not feeling rested on awakening.
   a. Have client keep a sleep-wake log. Each morning, record evening and bedtime rituals, the time attempting to begin sleep, number and length of awakenings, and time of morning awakening.
   b. Monitor for signs of sleep deprivation.
   c. Offer sedatives and hypnotics (if ordered) 30 to 40 minutes before usual bedtime. A low-dose, short-acting benzodiazepine for short-term use (no longer than 2 to 3 weeks) is recommended (Ancoli-Israel, 1997; Neubauer, 1999).
   d. Clients should avoid alcohol, smoking, and drinking caffeine while taking hypnotics. Alcohol can increase the sedation produced by these drugs and can dangerously depress brain function. Smoking and drinking caffeine interfere with effectiveness.

Recording and Reporting

• Report continued sleep pattern disturbance to charge nurse or physician.
• Record findings of ongoing assessment, interventions completed, and client's response to interventions.
• Report client's response to techniques to nurse in charge and to staff at change of shift.

Sample Documentation

0700 States awakened frequently when turning, when caregivers enter room, and with roommate movement. Lethargic with flat affect. Closes eyes repeatedly during interaction with nurse. Expresses desire for uninterrupted sleep. Discussed using soft music or a fan for distraction and obtaining pillow from home.

SPECIAL CONSIDERATIONS

Pediatric Considerations
- Place healthy infants on their back when being put to sleep (American Academy of Pediatrics, 1996). This position makes it more difficult for the infant to roll over in the prone position, a possible risk factor for sudden infant death syndrome (SIDS).
- Children vary in regard to comfortable room temperature but usually sleep best in cooler environments.
- Newborns and infants benefit from quiet activities such as holding them snugly in blankets, talking or singing softly, and gentle rocking. Reading stories, allowing children to sit in a parent's lap while listening to music or prayer, and coloring are routines that can be associated with preparing for bed.

Geriatric Considerations
- Older adults awaken more often during the night, and it may take more time for them to fall asleep. Their sleep efficiency is reduced, and the number of naps taken during the day is increased (Beck-Little and Weinrich, 1998).
- Use of benzodiazepines in the older adult population is potentially dangerous because of the drug's tendency to remain active in the body for a longer time. The drugs can potentially interact with other agents (Luekenotte, 2000). Short-acting benzodiazepines (e.g., oxazepam, lorazepam, or temazepam) at the lowest possible dose are recommended.

- Maintain a regular rising time. Eliminate naps unless they are a routine part of an older adult's schedule. If naps are used, limit to 20 minutes or less twice a day. Go to bed when sleepy.

Home Care Considerations
- Use same noise-control strategies as in the hospital environment (see Box 10-1, p. 227).
- Inform friends and relatives about the best time to phone or visit the client.
- Turn off ringer on phone when client is trying to sleep during the day. Be sure to instruct client to turn the phone ringer back on.

Long-Term Care Considerations
- Quality of sleep in a long-term care facility is often fragmented. Residents often suffer chronic disease, incontinence, and dementia and take multiple medications, all of which can disrupt sleep.
- Increase in client's daytime activity or exercise may improve self-reports of sleep (Stevenson and Topp, 1990).
- Limit time clients spend in bed. Serve meals in the resident dining area. Keep residents involved in social activities.
- Clients with dementia often have disrupted sleep-wake cycles. They often become easily fatigued and experience periods of insomnia (Luekenotte, 2000). In this situation, shorten activities and visits to allow client to maintain an adequate energy level.

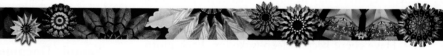

Skill 10.2

Relaxation Techniques

A number of nonpharmacologic therapies are used for pain relief, including massage, imagery, music therapy, biofeedback, hypnosis, exercise, and relaxation techniques (Freeman and Lawlis, 2001). Several of these therapies require special training or certification to perform, including biofeedback and hypnosis. Relaxation therapies, such as massage, imagery, and progressive relaxation, lessen the reception and perception of pain and can be used by nurses in a variety of health care settings. These therapies can and should be used in combination with pharmacological measures (see Chapter 11). The Agency for Health Care Research and Quality (AHRQ) guidelines for acute pain

management (1992) cite nonpharmacological interventions (1992) to be appropriate for clients who:

Find such interventions appealing

Express anxiety or fear

May benefit from avoiding or reducing drug therapy

Are likely to experience and need to cope with a prolonged interval of postoperative pain

Have incomplete pain relief from pharmacological therapies

As the nurse, you are responsible for evaluating the effects of nonpharmacological measures to ensure pain relief

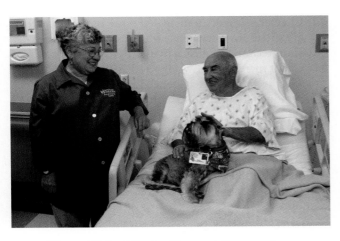

Figure 10-1   Client with a pet-therapy dog.

occurs so that clients are not excluded from use of pharmacological therapies.

DISTRACTION

With meaningful sensory stimuli, a client can ignore or become unaware of pain. Pleasurable sensory stimuli reduces pain perception by the release of endorphins. Distraction directs a client's attention to something else and thus can reduce the awareness of pain and even increase tolerance (Figure 10-1). Distraction may work best for short, intense pain lasting a few minutes such as during an invasive procedure or while waiting for an analgesic to work.

PROGRESSIVE RELAXATION

By teaching clients the use of progressive relaxation techniques, the nurse offers the client a sense of self-control when pain occurs. Progressive relaxation may be used independently or with other pain-relief measures. The technique is particularly effective for chronic pain, labor pain, and relief of procedure-related pain. Relaxation is less effective for episodes of acute or severe pain. Clients who use relaxation techniques successfully go through physiological and behavioral changes (e.g., decreased pulse and blood pressure, decreased muscle tension). Relaxation techniques may require a physician's order if the stability of a client's condition is in question. The nurse should be available to assist the client in performing relaxation techniques and in timing procedures (such as dressing changes) so that the technique can be most beneficial. The client's full participation and cooperation are necessary for progressive relaxation to be effective.

GUIDED IMAGERY

Guided imagery is a creative sensory experience that can effectively reduce pain perception and minimize reaction to pain. In guided imagery a client creates an image in the mind, concentrates on that image, and gradually becomes less aware of pain. The image created by the client results in a positive psychophysiological response. Pain relief associated with imagery may be related to the release of endorphins (Tiernan, 1994).

Assisting clients with guided imagery first involves creating a comfortable environment, controlling for factors such as noise, temperature extremes, or bright lighting. A nurse has clients choose an image that they find pleasant. For example, a scene of rolling waves at the seashore may be restful to one client but desolate or frightening to another. Imagery may be used with progressive relaxation or massage or as a distraction. To become competent in guided imagery, certification is available nationally through the Academy for Interactive Guided Imagery.

MASSAGE

Cutaneous stimulation is the stimulation of the skin to relieve pain. A gentle massage is a simple way to reduce pain perception. The mode of action for cutaneous stimulation is unclear, although the gate-control theory suggests that cutaneous stimulation activates large-diameter sensory nerve fibers in the skin, which decreases pain transmission through small-diameter pain fibers. Massage may also cause the release of endorphins. A proper massage not only blocks the perception of pain impulses but also helps relax muscle tension and spasm that otherwise might increase pain (Ferrell-Torry and Glick, 1993). The high state of relaxation often achieved with massage adds to the effects of other pain-relief measures (Ferrell-Torry and Glick, 1993; Meintz, 1995). A massage of the back, shoulders, and lower part of the neck is sometimes referred to as a back rub. A nurse should offer a back rub after a bath or before a client prepares for sleep to promote relaxation and comfort, relieve muscle tension, and stimulate circulation. An effective back rub takes several minutes and is an important intervention for decreasing pain and improving the sense of well-being.

ASSESSMENT

1. Assess character of client's discomfort, including severity of pain. *Rationale: Establishes baseline to evaluate efficacy of relaxation measures.*
2. Assess facial expressions and verbal indications of discomfort or distress. Clients may cry, moan, grimace, clench jaws, or tightly close or widely open mouth or eyes. *Rationale: Provide criteria to determine efficacy of relaxation measures.*
3. Observe body movement indicating physical or psychological distress. This may include restlessness, muscle tension, hand and finger movements, pacing, rhythmical or rubbing motions, or immobilization.
4. Observe social interactions that suggest physical or psychological distress. Clients may avoid conversa-

tion, have reduced attention span, avoid eye contact, or display irritability, anger, or withdrawal.

5. Assess for physiological signs of anxiety or stress, which may include tachycardia (increased heart rate), increased respirations or hyperventilation, elevated blood pressure, sweaty palms, trembling, and dry mouth.

6. Determine if client has a bleeding tendency or is receiving anticoagulants. *Rationale: May contraindicate use of massage as a relaxation technique.*

7. Assess the types of activities client normally uses to promote relaxation or provide distraction. *Rationale: Allows nurse to individualize relaxation technique to optimize results.*

8. Assess client's willingness to receive nonpharmacologic pain relief measures.

9. Assess for spiritual concerns or distress. *Rationale: May warrant spiritual intervention or referral to clergy.*

PLANNING

Expected outcomes focus on alleviating or reducing discomfort, increasing client's sense of control, and providing client empowerment through education.

Expected Outcomes

1. Client reports a reduction in pain severity (using pain scale).
2. Client demonstrates verbally and nonverbally a sense of well-being and relaxation.
3. Client verbalizes an increased sense of control over life situations as evidenced by integration of relaxation techniques into activities of daily living.
4. Client increases knowledge and skill of basic relaxation techniques as evidenced by ability to use and demonstrate techniques correctly.

Equipment

- Distraction: reading material, CD player or audiocassette, games
- Progressive muscle relaxation: cassette tape player, taped instructions for relaxation, nature sounds, or music
- Massage: lotion or oil, folded sheet, bath towel

 Delegation Considerations

The nurse, in collaboration with the client, is responsible for the assessment, planning, initial implementation, and evaluation of needed comfort measures. The following information is necessary when delegating skills to assistive personnel (AP) or family members:
- Instruct staff to alert nurse if signs of discomfort increase.
- Emphasize importance of controlling environment to ensure quiet and privacy.

IMPLEMENTATION FOR RELAXATION TECHNIQUES

Steps	Rationale
1. See Standard Protocol (inside front cover).	
2. Remove any noises or other irritating stimuli such as bright lights.	Promotes client's ability relax.
3. **Distraction**	
a. Ask client to close eyes or to focus on single object in room.	Directs attention inward and minimizes external distraction.
b. Apply activities determined in assessment that will direct client's attention away from pain, uncomfortable procedure, or uncomfortable thought (e.g., singing, listening to music, describing photos out loud, playing games).	Distraction reduces pain perception.
4. **Progressive muscle relaxation**	

NURSE ALERT *Teach relaxation technique only when the client is not in acute discomfort and is able to concentrate.*

Steps	Rationale

a. Assist client in assuming comfortable position in a chair in good alignment or lying in bed with entire body well supported. Encourage to settle in comfortably. Instruct client to notice areas of tension.

Adequate support enhances relaxation.

    (1) *Sitting:* Entire back rests against back of chair with head supported in line with spine, feet flat on floor, legs apart, and arms resting comfortably on arms of chair or lap (see illustration).

    (2) *Lying:* Keep head aligned with spine, with a thin small pillow under head, arms resting at sides without touching sides of body, legs separated, and toes slightly outward (see illustration).

b. Apply a light sheet or blanket to keep client warm and comfortable.

c. Tell client to close eyes, relax, and breathe slowly and deeply, allowing the abdomen to rise and fall with each breath.

Deep, regular breathing pattern creates a sensation of removing all discomfort and stress.

d. Instruct client to follow verbal cues for relaxation; use calm, soft voice.

Relaxation is guided verbally or by tape until individual is comfortable with sequence and no longer needs verbal guidance.

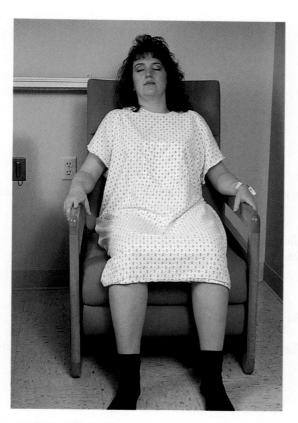

Step 4a(1)   Client sits in comfortable position before relaxation exercise.

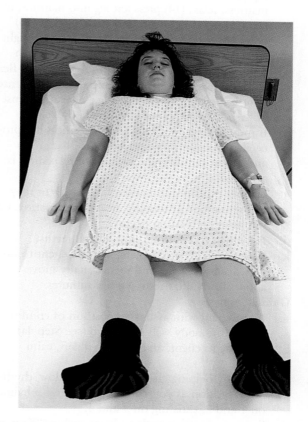

Step 4a(2)   The lying position provides support for the entire body and promotes relaxation.

Steps	Rationale
e. Begin series of alternating tightening and relaxing muscle groups: (1) clench right fist, relax; (2) clench left fist, relax; (3) clench both fists, relax; (4) tighten right biceps, relax; (5) tighten left biceps, relax. Continue with all muscle groups.	Alternating tension and relaxation in muscle groups allows client to feel difference.

NURSE ALERT *Tension of each muscle group is maintained for 5 to 7 seconds except for the feet. Allows time to focus on the muscle group; cramps can easily occur in the feet.*

Steps	Rationale
f. As each muscle group is completed, ask client to enjoy relaxed feeling and allow mind to drift and think how nice it is to be relaxed. Ask client to breathe deeply.	Distracts client from perceiving pain. Enhances the relaxation response. Breathing deeply prevents Valsalva response, which can increase intrathoracic pressure and compromise cardiac function.
g. Instruct client to repeat each step 2 times: (1) reach with right arm, relax; (2) reach with left arm, relax; (3) reach with both arms, relax; (4) wrinkle forehead, relax; (5) squint eyes, relax; (6) tighten jaw muscles, relax; (7) press head into pillow, relax; (8) bring right shoulder to earlobe, relax; (9) bring left shoulder to earlobe, relax; (10) bring both shoulders to earlobe, relax; (11) tighten abdominal muscles, relax; (12) tighten hips and buttocks, relax; (13) press right leg into mattress, relax; (14) press left leg into mattress, relax; (15) point right toes and stretch, relax; (16) point left toes and stretch, relax; (17) stretch right leg, relax; (18) stretch left leg, relax; (19) stretch both legs, relax; (20) flex right foot, relax; (21) flex left foot, relax; (22) flex both feet, relax; (23) tense right leg, relax; (24) tense left leg, relax; (25) tense both legs, relax; (26) tense entire body, relax.	Relaxation is integrated response associated with diminished sympathetic nervous system arousal; decreased muscle tension is desired outcome. Relaxation decreases pulse rate, respiration rate, and blood pressure and reduces anxiety.
h. If muscle group tightens after relaxation has proceeded to other muscles, return to that group and repeat tension-relaxation until relaxation is achieved.	
i. Calmly explain during exercise that client may feel sensations of tingling, heaviness, floating, or warmth as relaxation occurs.	Prevents anxiety should sensation occur without warning.
j. Ask client to continue slow, deep breaths.	Allows opportunity to enjoy feelings of relaxation.
k. When exercise is complete, instruct client to inhale deeply, exhale, and then initially move about slowly after resting a few minutes.	Returns client to more awake and alert state. When deeply relaxed, client may experience dizziness on arising too rapidly.

5. Guided imagery

Steps	Rationale
a. Assist client with assuming position of comfort with entire body well supported (see Step 4a).	The ability to relax physically promotes mental relaxation.
b. Sit close to client, and speak in a soft, calm voice.	The experience of discomfort can be altered by concentrating on a serene, tranquil voice.
c. Begin by helping client breathe in a slow, rhythmical fashion as you count, and suggest inhaling on 1 and 2, exhaling on 3 and 4.	
d. Suggest relaxation with a phrase such as "Your body is beginning to relax . . . think relax . . . continue to breathe slowly and relax."	Focusing on the sensation of relaxation enhances the ability to relax.

Steps	**Rationale**
e. Direct client through guided imagery exercise: the following is an example. Remember to use images meaningful and relaxing to client.	
(1) Instruct client to imagine that inhaled air is ball of healing energy.	Development of specific images assists in removal of pain perception.
(2) Imagine inhaled air travels to area of pain.	Client's ability to concentrate decreases pain perception.
f. Alternatively, nurse may direct imagery:	
(1) Suggest client think about going to pleasant place such as beach or mountains.	Directs imagery after selection of restful place by nurse and client.
(2) Direct client to experience all sensory aspects of restful place (e.g., for beach: warm breeze, warm sand between toes, warmth of sunshine, rhythmic sound of waves, smell of salt air, gulls gliding and swooping in air).	Helps client concentrate and relax. Promotes use of all senses.
(3) Describe the scene identified by client as pleasurable and relaxing; for example, "Imagine yourself lying on a cool bed of grass with the sounds of rushing water from a nearby stream. It's a sunny day, and there is a gentle cool breeze." Have client travel mentally to the scene.	Allows relaxation to progress.
(4) Ask questions to help client experience the scene: "How does this look? Sound? Smell? Feel? Taste?"	
g. Encourage client to practice the imagery. It may be helpful to tape record the imagined experience for repeated practice opportunities.	It takes repeated practice to master relaxation.
h. Continue deep, slow rhythmic breathing.	
i. End the experience: "Experience the comfort and relaxation. When you open your eyes, you will feel alert and renewed. Breathe deeply. Be aware of where you are now, stretch gently, and when you are ready, open your eyes."	
6. Massage	
a. Adjust bed to high, comfortable position, and lower side rail.	Ensures proper body mechanics and prevents strain on nurse's back muscles.
b. Place client in comfortable lying or sitting position.	Enhances relaxation and exposes area to be massaged.

NURSE ALERT *Clients with respiratory difficulties may lie on side with head of bed elevated.*

c. Turn on soft pleasing music of client's preference.	
d. Drape client as needed to expose only area to be massaged.	Maintains client's privacy and warmth.
e. Warm lotion in hands. (NOTE: If you choose to massage head and scalp, defer use of lotion until completed.)	Warm lotion is soothing, and warmth helps to produce local muscle relaxation (Meintz, 1995).
f. Select body part to be massaged. Massage each part at least 3 minutes.	Ensures fuller relaxation of part.

NURSE ALERT *Clients who are heavily medicated or unable to communicate verbally need very gentle massage because they cannot inform the nurse if massage becomes uncomfortable.*

Steps	Rationale
g. Select stroke technique based on desired effect: (1) Effleurage (see illustration)	Gliding stroke, used without manipulating deep muscles, smooths and extends muscles, increases nutrient absorption, and improves lymphatic and venous circulation (Meintz, 1995).
(2) Pétrissage (see illustration)	Use on tense muscle groups to "knead" muscles, promote relaxation, and stimulate local circulation.
(3) Friction	Strong circular strokes bring blood to surface of skin, thereby increasing local circulation and loosening tight muscle groups (Meintz, 1995).
h. Encourage client to breathe deeply and relax during massage.	
i. Make contact with the client's skin, first with one hand and then the other.	Avoids startling the client

j. Massage head and scalp. NOTE: Do not use lotion.
  (1) Standing behind client, stimulate scalp and temples.
  (2) Supporting client's head, rub muscles at base of head.
	Strong circular strokes (friction) stimulate local circulation and relaxation.

k. Massage hands and arms.	Releases tension in hands and arms. Studies indicate that anxious behaviors may be significantly reduced with hand massage (Snyder, Egan, and Burns, 1995).
(1) Using both hands, slowly open the palm, gliding your fingers over the palmar surface. While supporting the hand, use both thumbs to apply friction to the palm and use them in a circular motion to stretch the palm outward.	Encourages relaxation; enhances circulation and venous return.
(2) Massage each finger outward and then separately, using a corkscrewlike motion from base of finger to the tip.	
(3) With thumb and finger, knead each small muscle in the client's fingers. Glide hands smoothly from fingertips to wrists. Repeat for other hand.	

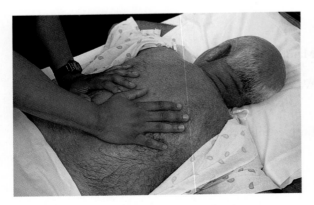

Step 6g(1)   Nurse massages back using effleurage.

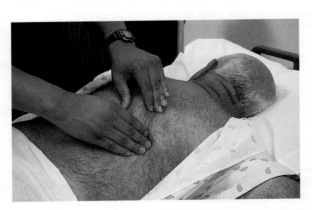

Step 6g(2)   The use of pétrissage involves kneading tight muscles.

Steps	Rationale
(4) Use a gliding stroke to massage from the client's wrist to forearm. With thumb and forefinger of both hands, knead muscles from forearm to shoulder. Continue kneading biceps, deltoid, and triceps muscles. Finish with gliding stroke from the wrist to the shoulder.	
l. Massage neck.	
(1) Support the neck at the hairline with one hand, and massage up it with a gliding stroke. Knead muscles on one side. Switch hands to support neck, and knead other side. Stretch the neck slightly, with one hand at the top and the other at the bottom.	Reduces tension that often localizes in neck muscles.
m. Massage back.	
(1) Place client in prone or side-lying position as tolerated.	Side-lying position is indicated for clients unable to lie prone.
(2) Do not allow hands to leave client's skin.	Continuous contact with skin's surface is soothing and stimulates circulation to tissues.
(3) Apply hands first to sacral area, and massage in circular motion (see illustration). Stroke upward from buttocks to shoulders. Massage over scapulae with smooth, firm stroke. Continue in one smooth stroke to upper arms and laterally along sides of back down to iliac crests. Use long, gliding strokes along muscles of spine. Knead any tense or tight muscles.	Gentle, firm pressure applied to all muscle groups promotes relaxation.

NURSE ALERT *Be certain to massage muscular region, not bones of the spine. Avoid bruised, swollen, or inflamed areas (Meintz, 1995).*

---

(4) Knead muscles of each shoulder toward front of client.	Area often tightens because of tension.
(5) Use palms in upward and outward circular motion from lower buttocks to neck.	

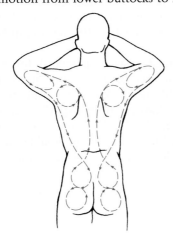

Step 6m(3)   Pattern to follow in massage of back.

Steps	Rationale
(6) Knead muscles of upper back and shoulder between thumb and forefinger.	These muscles are thick and can be vigorously massaged.
(7) End back massage with long stroking movements.	Most soothing of massage movements.
n. Massage feet, avoiding bunions or other sensitive areas.	
(1) Place client in supine position.	
(2) Hold foot firmly. Support ankle with one hand or support sides of foot with each hand while performing massage.	Prevents strain on ankle.
(3) Make circular motions with thumb and fingers around bones of ankle and top of foot.	
(4) Trace space between tendons with firm finger pressure, moving from toe to ankle.	
(5) Massage sides and top of each toe.	
(6) Use top of fist to make circular motions on bottom of foot.	
(7) Knead sides of foot between index finger and thumb.	
(8) Conclude with firm, sweeping motions over top and bottom of foot. Tell client you are ending massage.	Light strokes may tickle. Informs client.

7. When procedure is complete, instruct client to relax and breathe slowly. Wipe excess oil or lotion from client's back with towel.

8. See Completion Protocol (inside front cover).

• • • • • • • • • •

EVALUATION

1. Ask client to rate level of comfort using a scale of 0 to 10.
2. Inspect client's physiological (e.g., vital sign changes, posture) and behavioral (facial expressions, tone of voice, affect) responses to technique.
3. Observe when client performs relaxation technique.
4. Ask client to demonstrate relaxation technique at a time of low stress.

Unexpected Outcomes and Related Nursing Interventions

1. Client's level of comfort declines.
   a. Coach client with relaxation technique.
   b. Try different type of distraction or relaxation intervention.
   c. Consider analgesic.
2. Client is unable to perform relaxation technique.
   a. Reinstruct client and demonstrate procedure.
   b. Coach client through relaxation procedure.
   c. Try different relaxation intervention.

Recording and Reporting

• Record client's level of comfort before and after procedure, document relaxation technique used, client vital signs, and overall client response.
• Record type of guided image client uses.
• Report client's response to relaxation technique and any unusual responses to technique to charge nurse or physician.

Sample Documentation

2000 Client observed to be restless and reports a severe headache (7 on scale of 1 to 10). States cannot sleep. Tylenol #3, 2 tablets administered orally. Participated in 10-minute progressive relaxation exercise. States headache is relieved (3 on scale 1 to 10). Resting in bed with eyes closed.

2200 Guided imagery practiced for 5 minutes in preparation for sleep. States feeling "much more relaxed and comfortable now." Verbalizes plans to practice this regularly using "favorite fishing spot" as setting.

2330 Reports "dull ache in neck and shoulders" (8 on scale 1 to 10). Massage given to shoulder, neck, and back regions. Verbalizes pain decreasing (5 on 1 to 10 scale). Resting with eyes closed.

SPECIAL CONSIDERATIONS

Geriatric Considerations

- Massage communicates caring and can easily be taught to family members.
- Most forms of touch are pleasurable to older adults. Use with caution in clients with bone metastases or osteoporotic bones (Lueckenotte, 2000).
- Reminiscence is an effective form of distraction in older adults.

Home Care Considerations

- Teach family member how to perform distraction/relaxation/imagery techniques.
- Teach family how to reduce home environmental noises.

CRITICAL THINKING EXERCISES

1. Mrs. Jones is scheduled for an open laparotomy in the morning for a bowel obstruction. She verbalizes at 2100 that she feels quite anxious and cannot sleep. She describes her pain as 7 on a scale of 0 to 10. It is still 1 hour before her as-needed (prn) analgesic can be given. After assessing her source of anxiety, you learn that she has several unanswered questions about the procedure. Discuss the nursing interventions you will use to promote relaxation and sleep.

2. Mr. Jackson comes to the clinic and reports he is having trouble falling asleep at night and awakening during the night. In your assessment you find that he normally eats around 7 PM, and he enjoys coffee with his meal. He normally exercises in the mornings before going to work. He is currently on an antiinflammatory for arthritis and a diuretic for hypertension. What might you suggest to help Mr. Jackson to help improve the quality of his sleep?

3. Mr. Williams, a 70-year-old man, has chronic obstructive pulmonary disease (COPD). He states he feels "tense in my shoulders and neck" and would like a massage. He exhibits mild dyspnea. Discuss adaptations you would make in the massage technique to accommodate his respiratory problem?

4. Describe what you believe to be the most effective comfort measures for the following clients:
   a. Older adult with low back pain
   b. Young female in labor
   c. First day postoperative client

REFERENCES

American Academy of Pediatrics, Task Force on Infant Positioning: Positioning and sudden infant death syndrome (SIDS): update, *Pediatrics* 98(6):1218, 1996.

Ancoli-Israel S: Sleep problems in older adults: putting myths to bed, *Geriatrics* 52(1):20, 1997.

Barkauskas VH and others: *Health and physical assessment,* ed 5, St Louis, 1998, Mosby.

Beck-Little R, Weinrich S: Assessment and management of sleep disorders in the elderly, *J Gerontol Nurs* 24(4):21, 1998.

Ferrell-Torry A, Glick O: The use of therapeutic massage as a nursing intervention to modify anxiety and the perception of cancer pain, *Cancer Nurs* 16(2):93, 1993.

Freeman LW and Lawlis GF: *Mosby's complimentary and alternative medicine: a research based approach,* St Louis, 2001, Mosby.

Lueckenotte A: *Gerontologic nursing,* ed 2, St Louis, 2000, Mosby.

McCaffery M, Pasero C: *Pain: clinical manual,* ed 2, St Louis, 1999, Mosby.

Meintz S: Whatever became of the back rub? *RN* 58(4):49, 1995.

Neubauer D: Sleep problems in the elderly, *Am Fam Physician* 59(9):2551, 1999.

Snyder M, Egan EL, Burns KR: Efficacy of hard massage in decreasing agitation behavior associated with care activities in persons with dementia, *Geriatr Nurs* 16(2):60, 1995.

Tiernan P: Independent nursing interventions: relaxation and guided imagery in critical care, *Crit Care Nurse* 14(5):47, 1994.

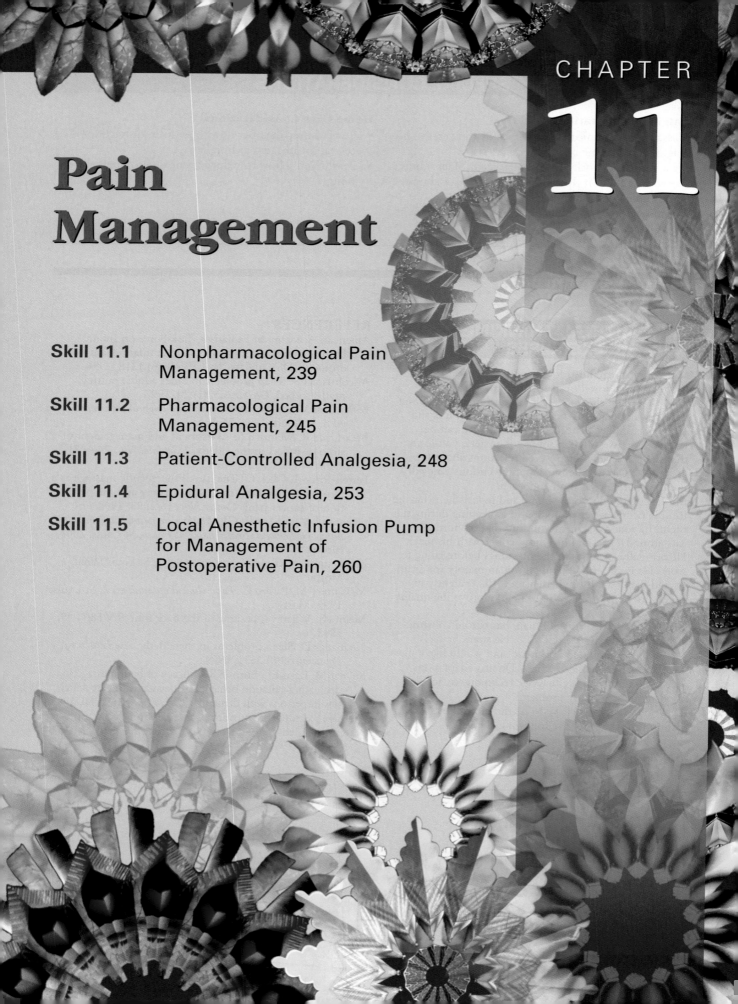

Pain Management

Pain can be described as "an unpleasant sensory and emotional experience associated with actual or potential tissue damage, or described in terms of such damage" (Merskey, 1986). It may be caused by disease, trauma, or certain therapeutic procedures or have no identifiable cause (Principles of Analgesic Use, 1999). Pain response is varied and is influenced by the individual's psychosocial, economic, and cultural experiences (Andrews and Boyle, 1999; Lasch, 2000).

Pain is classified as acute or chronic. Chronic pain may be noncancer or cancer pain. Acute and chronic pain are differentiated according to onset, duration, and cause. Acute pain is protective, has a sudden onset, an identifiable cause, and an anticipated duration. It may progress to chronic pain if not successfully treated. Chronic pain is a continuous or recurring pain that usually lasts longer than is typically expected or predicted. It may be associated with prolonged healing of an acute injury or disease; however, it may not have an identifiable pathologic cause. Chronic pain may be continuous or intermittent. Intermittent chronic pain is often associated with activity, other conditions, or it may have an unknown etiology. With all pain, but especially chronic pain, clients may become depressed, anxious, and/or frustrated. Unrelieved chronic pain affects every aspect of a client's life.

Adequate pain management has become a priority for health care agencies with the introduction of pain standards by the Joint Commission on Accreditation of Health Care Organizations (JCAHO). Written guidelines for pain management have been developed by several organizations, including the Agency for Healthcare Research and Quality, the American Pain Society, and the World Health Organization (WHO). Furthermore, the American Nurses Association's Code of Ethics (2001) states, "The nurse promotes, advocates for and strives to protect the health, safety and rights of the patient." This statement ethically obligates the nurse to provide clients with adequate pain management.

When managing a client's pain for palliative care, the nurse uses the same methodical approach and pain management guidelines used for clients with nonterminal acute and chronic pain. Many clients suffer needless pain months before dying and at the end of life. Appropriate use of nonopioids, nonsteroidal antiinflammatory drugs (NSAIDs), opioids, and adjuvants to manage pain should be maximized before resorting to highly technical, invasive procedures (Perron and Schonwetter, 2001).

NURSING DIAGNOSES

Impaired Physical Mobility related to pain applies to clients who have limited independent physical movement resulting from painful conditions. **Fatigue** related to pain applies to clients who experience a decreased capacity for physical and mental work. **Risk for Disuse Syndrome** is a state in which a client is at risk for deterioration of body systems and deconditioning resulting from inactivity associated with severe pain. Other nursing diagnoses may include **Anxiety, Ineffective Coping,** or **Powerlessness** when pain compromises a client's emotional resources. **Impaired Social Interaction** and **Spiritual Distress** apply to clients whose social awareness and spiritual health have been exhausted by chronic pain. Once the cause of the pain is identified, **Acute Pain** and **Chronic Pain** are nursing diagnoses in which the focus of care is on pain control rather than on the client's response to pain.

Skill 11.1

Nonpharmacological Pain Management

Controlling pain and promoting comfort are two of the most important goals of nursing practice. In 1965 Melzack and Wall proposed the gate control theory of pain. They suggested that pain transmission could be increased or decreased by opening or closing a gating mechanism in the central nervous system (CNS). In addition, it was the first theory to suggest that pain sensation has both physical and psychological components. Thus the nurse should use pharmacological and nonpharmacological interventions to manage both components of pain. Nonpharmacological strategies are varied (Table 11-1) and should be used in conjunction with and not instead of pharmacological interventions, and vice versa. If a pain management plan is to be successful, pain must continually be assessed, treated, and interventions evaluated to determine if a client is achieveing comfort.

ASSESSMENT

1. Identify possible factors for the discomfort/pain. Alterations in comfort may be acute (postoperative, associated with labor of childbirth, traumatic wounds, burns) or chronic (associated with cancer, migraine headaches, low back pain, joint pain). *Rationale: Causative factors influence the choice of interventions most likely to be successful.*

2. Assess factors that influence perception of pain (e.g., past pain history, depression, fatigue, loneliness, anxiety, helplessness, fear). *Rationale: These factors significantly reduce clients' ability to cope with pain.*

3. Assess clients' culturally determined beliefs about pain. *Rationale: Culture influences the meaning pain holds for a client and how a client reacts toward discomfort.*

Table 11-1

Nonpharmacological Interventions for Pain (Should Be Used With Analgesic Medication)

Interventions	Comments
Physical	
Progressive muscle relaxation	Reduces mild to moderate pain. Requires 3 to 5 minutes of staff time for instruction.
Massage	Effective for reduction of mild to moderate discomfort. May be firm, gentle, or light stroking of the body part involved or the opposite extremity. Requires 3 to 10 minutes of staff time.
Transcutaneous electrical nerve stimulation (TENS)	Effective in reducing mild to moderate pain by stimulating the skin with mild electrical current. Electrodes are placed over or near the site of pain. Requires special equipment (Figure 11-1). Requires physician order.
Heat/cold application	Selection of heat versus cold varies with the situation. Moist heat relieves stiffness of arthritis and relaxes muscles. Cold applications reduce acute pain associated with inflammation from arthritis or from acute injury. Requires physician order.
Psychological/Cognitive	
Music	Simple relaxation. Best taught preoperatively. Both client-preferred and "easy listening" music effective for mild to moderate pain.
Biofeedback	Effective in reducing mild to moderate pain and operative site muscle tension. Requires skilled personnel and special equipment.
Imagery	Effective for reduction of mild to moderate pain. Requires skilled personnel.
Education	Effective for reduction of all types of pain. Should include sensory and procedural information and instruction aimed at reducing activity-related pain. Requires 5 to 15 minutes of staff time.

4. Assess client's sensation of pain (PQRST assessment):
   a. **P:** *P*recipitating factors: position, movement, edema, constricting dressings, tubes or drains, invasive procedures, distended bladder. *Rationale: Assists in determining factors to avoid.*
   b. **Q:** *Q*uality: sharp, dull, burning, nagging, stabbing, aching, throbbing, shooting, or crushing. *Rationale: Helps determine type of pain (somatic, visceral, neuropathic) (Table 11-2).*
   c. **R:** *R*egion: localized, radiating, or generalized. Have client point to area of body affected. *Rationale: Assists in identifying cause of pain.*
   d. **S:** *S*everity: have client rate pain both at rest and with activity using an appropriate pain scale (Figure 11-2). For children ages 3 years and older use the Wong-Baker FACES Pain Rating Scale (Figure 11-3). Scales for neonates and infants include the CRIES Instrument and the FLACC Scale (Bildner, 1997). Different scales may be used with different clients; however, the same scale must be used consistently with each client. *Rationale: Provides a measurable means to determine if client's pain improves or worsens over time.*
   e. **T:** *T*iming/Duration: onset: sudden or gradual; constant or intermittent or both; procedural or nonprocedural. *Rationale: Assists in determining if pain is acute (a new pain or pain due to a complication) or chronic (same pain or escalating pain).*

5. Perform physical assessment of site of pain. *Rationale: This may reveal the nature of the pain and appropriate interventions.*
6. Assess physiological and psychological responses to pain. *Rationale: Physiological signs may assist in the etiology. However, due to physiological adaptation, overt and persistent physical responses (vital signs) to pain rarely occur, whereas lasting psychological distress is often evident.*
7. Assess behavioral responses to pain (Box 11-1). *Rationale: Nonverbal responses to pain may be especially useful in assessing pain in clients who are cognitively impaired or nonverbal. Before assuming that a change in behavior is due to pain, however, complete a physical assessment to rule out other possible causes for change in behavior such as pneumonia, urinary tract infection, constipation, or medication side effect. Once these are ruled out, a trial of short-acting pain medications should be initiated and the client's behavior observed (Wentz, 2001).*
8. In cognitively impaired clients, obtain a proxy pain intensity rating from the primary caregiver. (e.g., family member or friend). *Rationale: Proxy ratings may closely approximate the client's pain intensity.*

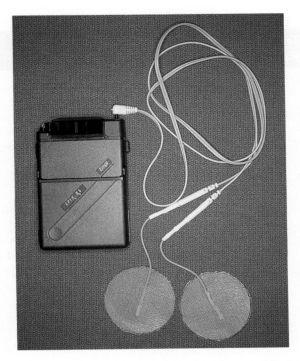

Figure 11-1   Transcutaneous Electrical Nerve Stimulator (TENS).

Numerical

0	1	2	3	4	5	6	7	8	9	10
No pain										Severe pain

Descriptive

No pain	Mild pain	Moderate pain	Severe pain	Unbearable pain

Visual analog

No pain	Unbearable pain

Client designates a point on the scale corresponding to his perception of the pain's severity at the time of assessment.

Figure 11-2   Sample pain intensity scales for use with cognitively intact adults.

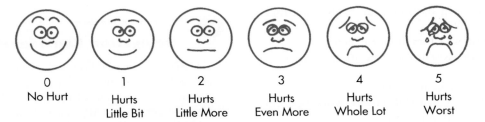

0	1	2	3	4	5
No Hurt	Hurts Little Bit	Hurts Little More	Hurts Even More	Hurts Whole Lot	Hurts Worst

Figure 11-3   Wong-Baker FACES Pain Rating Scale for use with children 3 years old and older. (From Wong DL, Hockenberry-Eaton M, Wilson D, Winkelstein ML, Schwartz P: *Wong's Essentials of pediatric nursing*, ed 6, St Louis, 2001, p. 1301.)

Table 11-2
Characteristics of Pain

Quality	Characteristics
Somatic (myofascial/joints)	Aching, deep, gnawing, throbbing, sharp, stabbing, constant, increases with movement, well localized
Visceral (organ-related, smooth muscle)	Cramping, squeezing, pressure-like, poorly localized, constant or intermittent, associated with symptoms of visceral discomfort
Neuropathic	Burning, searing, shooting, electric-like, numbing, radiating, stabbing, tingling, touch sensitive

Box 11-1
Behavioral Indicators of Pain

Facial expression: grimace, frowning, crying
Vocalizations: moaning, groaning
Posture: bent, leaning, guarding
Gait: favors one side, uneven
Activity level: increased, decreased, restless
Muscle: tense, guarded
Behavior: change in usual activities
Emotions: irritable, withdrawn
Change in ADLs: eating, sleeping, dressing, conversing

9. Assess environment for factors such as noise or bright lights that may aggravate the client's perception or tolerance of pain. *Rationale: Environmental factors may intensify perception of discomfort.*

10. Determine what does or may relieve the client's pain. Consider client's experience with over-the-counter drugs (including herbals and topicals) that have helped to reduce pain in the past.

11. Consider physician's orders regarding activity, oral intake, and prescribed medication.

PLANNING

Expected outcomes focus on attaining pain-intensity goal set by client and client's improved ability to participate in routine activities.

Expected Outcomes

1. Client understands and uses identified pain intensity scale appropriately (Box 11-2).
   a. Client and health care providers mutually agree on pain-intensity goal.
   b. Client rates pain at or below pain-intensity goal.

2. Clients who are unable to state a pain-intensity goal have a goal set at 4 or below (0 to 10 scale) because this level has been shown to minimally affect function (Feldt, 2000).

3. Client identifies factors that ease pain.

4. Client asks for assistance in repositioning when needed.

5. Client able to adequately function and perform activities of daily living (ADLs) (walk, work, perform hygiene, eat, sleep, interact).

Box 11-2

Teaching the Client/Family How to Use a Pain Rating Scale

- Show and briefly explain available pain rating scales, and ask which one the client prefers.
- Explain the purpose of the scale.
- Explain the parts of the scale: for example, 0 means no pain, whereas 10 means the worse pain you can imagine.
- Discuss pain as a broad concept that is not restricted to a severe or intolerable sensation. Discomfort, hurt, or ache are also considered pain sensations.
- Verify the client understands the concept of pain; ask client to give an example of pain experienced in the past.
- Ask the client to practice using the pain rating scale with present pain, or select one of client's examples. Also, ask to rate worse pain and average pain in past 24 hours.
- Set mutual goal for comfort and function/recovery.

Modified from McCaffery M, Pasero C: *Pain: clinical manual,* St Louis, 1999, Mosby.

 Delegation Considerations

The RN, in collaboration with the client, is responsible for the assessment, planning, initial implementation, and evaluation of needed comfort measures. Assistive personnel (AP) or family members may be delegated the following skills:

- Screening for pain and reporting to RN changes in client's behavior
- Identifying and eliminating environmental conditions that might enhance pain
- Providing maximum rest periods
- Turning or positioning of client

IMPLEMENTATION FOR NONPHARMACOLOGICAL PAIN MANAGEMENT

Steps	Rationale
1. See Standard Protocol (inside front cover).	
2. Teach client how to use pain intensity scale.	Accurate reporting by client improves pain assessment.
3. Set pain-intensity goal with client.	Pain is unique to each individual. When able, client should set goal for tolerable pain severity.
4. Remove or reduce painful stimuli.	
a. Reposition using pillows as needed for support and to prevent pressure areas.	Repositioning reduces stimulation of pain and pressure receptors.

Steps	**Rationale**
b. Reapply dressings if wet or constricting (see Skill 24.3, p. 588).	Clean, dry dressings minimize irritation to surrounding tissues.
c. Reapply or adjust equipment as needed: blood pressure (BP) cuff, intravenous (IV) arm board, Ace bandages, tubes, drains, or identification bands.	Constricting devices create discomfort.
5. Reduce or eliminate factors that increase the pain experience.	Fear or anxiety may cause muscle tension and vasoconstriction, which intensify the pain experience.
a. Relate acceptance of client, and acknowledge the client's report of pain.	

COMMUNICATION TIP   *This is a good time to use open-ended statements, such as "Tell me what your discomfort feels like" or "What makes your pain feel better (or worse)?"*

---

b. Explain the cause of pain (if known).	
6. Assist client in splinting painful area using firm pressure over a bath blanket or pillow during coughing, deep breathing, and turning (see Skill 19.2, p. 496).	Splinting reduces pain by minimizing muscle movement.
7. Massage painful area gently or firmly.	Cutaneous stimulation closes the "pain gate," thus reducing pain perception.

NURSE ALERT   *Do not massage in the presence of bleeding tendencies (low platelet count, low fibrinogen levels, receiving anticoagulants) or abnormal reactive hyperemia. Massage may cause tissue damage (see Chapter 24).*

---

8. Encourage relaxation using nonpharmacological strategies such as imagery, progressive relaxation, or deep rhythmical breathing (see Chapter 10).	Encourages active client participation in pain plan, enhances analgesic effect, reduces psychosocial aspect of pain.

9. Direct client's attention to something else that increases pain tolerance. Possible distractions include:
   a. Singing or music
   b. Praying
   c. Describing pictures
   d. Discussing pleasant memories
	The reticular activating system (RAS) in the brain, which is essential for concentration, inhibits painful stimuli if a person receives sufficient or excessive sensory input. With meaningful sensory input a person can ignore the pain. Pleasurable stimuli also increase endorphins, which relieve pain.

10. Following nonpharmacologic interventions, be sure client is positioned comfortably and room is left clean and pleasant.	Promotes client's ability to rest and fall asleep.
11. See Completion Protocol (inside front cover).	

• • • • • • • • • • •

EVALUATION

1. Ask client to rate pain intensity using appropriate pain scale both at rest and with activity.
2. Evaluate PQRST aspects of pain.
3. Observe client's facial expression, body language, position, mobility, relaxation, and ability to rest, sleep, eat, and participate in usual activities.

Unexpected Outcomes and Related Interventions

1. Client's pain intensity is greater than desired.
   a. Try an alternative nonpharmacologic intervention.
   b. Consult with physician if analgesic necessary.
2. Client continues to display nonverbal behaviors reflecting pain.

   a. Try an alternative nonpharmacologic intervention
   b. Consider if appropriate to administer an analgesic
   c. Discomfort that is unrelieved or is worse may indicate need for additional diagnostic, medical, or surgical intervention or a change in the pain management plan.

Recording and Reporting

- Pain documentation should be on a regular (every 4 to 12 hours) basis (agency dependent).
- Report significant changes in any of the PQRST parameters to physician. Box 11-3 lists suggestions for communicating with physician (Collins and others, 1999).

Box 11-3

Communicating With the Physician

- Identify the goals of care: function and comfort.
- Establish the client's pain-intensity goal.
- Know your agency's policies and standards (e.g., placebos not allowed).
- Use analgesic guidelines: WHO analgesic ladder, maximum doses.
- Consider equianalgesic dosing (conversion table available through American Pain Society).
- Complete the client's assessment.
- Formulate a plan: Consult with colleague; include nonpharmacological interventions; include client in plan; monitor for side effects.
- State to physician why you are calling.
- Give assessment.
- Suggest plan.
- Summarize concerns.

- Record findings of ongoing assessment, interventions completed (including notification of physician, if done), and client's response to interventions.

Sample Documentation

0700 Client rates pain along arch of left ankle at 6 (scale 0 to 10). Tylenol #3, 2 tablets administered. Foot elevated and gentle massage of ankle and knee for 5 minutes.

0730 Body more relaxed. Pain intensity now reported as 3.

SPECIAL CONSIDERATIONS

Pediatric Considerations

- Ask parents what nonpharmacological interventions their child might prefer.
- When possible, have parents help deliver the nonpharmacological intervention.

Geriatric Considerations

- Pain may be difficult to assess in older adults. Cognitive impairment or dementia may affect their ability to report pain; however, recent research studies have indicated that most cognitively impaired older adults can successfully use pain scales if given time and patience (Krulewitch, 2000).
- Pain is not a normal part of the aging process. Such a belief can lead to underreporting of pain by these clients and/or undertreatment of pain by health care providers.
- Pain assessment in older adults should include an evaluation of the effect of pain on the client's quality of life or ability to function (The Management of Chronic Pain, 1998).
- Many older clients have multiple sources of pain.

- Visual, hearing, cognitive, sensory, and motor impairments may make it difficult for older adults to effectively use procedures such as distraction, relaxation, or guided imagery (Agency for Health Care Policy and Research [AHCPR], 1992).
- Use terms other than *pain*, such as *hurt* or *pressure*, when assessing older adult clients because they may reserve the word *pain* for severe discomfort.

Home Care Considerations

- Family caregivers and nurses' aides require education with regard to screening for pain so that they can notify professional caregivers quickly of their suspicions of the presence of pain.
- A supportive bed and quiet environment will enhance sleep and promote the control of pain.

Long-Term Care Considerations

Nurses' aides should be taught how to deliver specific nonpharmacological therapies and how to recognize potential nonverbal pain behaviors that need to be reported.

Skill 11.2

Pharmacological Pain Management

Analgesics are the most common treatment for pain. Analgesics are classified as nonopioid (e.g., acetaminophen), nonsteroidal antiinflammatory drugs (NSAIDs), opioids (e.g., morphine sulfate, hydromorphone, oxycodone, and fentanyl), and adjuvant analgesics (e.g., anticonvulsants, antidepressants, muscle relaxants, and antiarrhythmics). There are misconceptions about the potential dangers of opioids. Concerns about addiction and misinformation about client behaviors in relation to pain have resulted in undertreatment of pain. According to the 2001 World Health Organization (WHO) pain guidelines, analgesics should be individualized, offered via various routes, given around-the-clock (ATC), and available for break-through pain.

Nonopioid analgesics provide relief for mild to moderate pain (minimally affects client function). They act primarily on peripheral receptors, diminishing transmission of pain stimuli by inhibiting the synthesis of prostaglandins at the site of injury. Inhibition of prostaglandins may also re-sult in reduced renal and gastric mucosa blood flow, which can lead to renal compromise and gastric bleeding. Be sure to monitor renal function and stools for occult blood. In addition, there is a limit on the amount of NSAIDs that can be administered per day (Table 11-3).

Opioid analgesics are usually used for moderate to severe pain, are available in short- and long-acting forms, and can be given via several routes, including oral, IV, intramuscular (IM), subcutaneous (SQ), rectal, transdermal, and intrathecal. Opioids act on higher centers of the CNS by blocking pain transmission and by modifying perception of pain. Opioids are appropriate for acute and chronic pain.

There is no maximum amount of opioid that may be titrated to relieve pain. Each client responds uniquely to opioids, and nurses must always be alert for possible respiratory depression. However, morphine and oxycodone, in high doses, do have nephrotoxic metabolites and thus should be used with caution in clients with renal compromise. In addition, once a client has been receiving ATC opioids for 1 to 2 weeks, when they are no longer needed the opioids must be reduced slowly over several days to prevent abstinence/withdrawal syndrome.

Opioids combined with drugs such as acetaminophen, aspirin, or ibuprofen are commonly ordered for mild to moderate pain. However, the nonopioid drug limits the number of opioid tablets that can be administered daily. Nonopioids also have significant side effects, including gastrointestinal (GI) bleeding, nephrotoxicity, and hepatotoxicity; thus they must be carefully monitored. In addition, clients may purchase OTC drugs containing acetaminophen, aspirin, or ibuprofen, thus escalating the risk for toxicity.

Opioids have several potential adverse effects (Box 11-4); however, with the exception of constipation, clients usually become tolerant to these side effects within a short time. Sedatives, antiemetics, antianxiety agents, and muscle relaxants may be prescribed to minimize responses to pain and other signs and symptoms associated with pain, such as depression and nausea. These drugs can cause drowsiness and impaired coordination, judgment, and mental alertness.

Adjuvants are medications originally prescribed for reasons other than pain relief but which also have analgesic properties. Examples are anticonvulsants and antidepressants, which are especially effective in treating neuropathic pain (Guay, 2001).

Table 11-3

Commonly Used Nonopioids and Their Maximum Doses per 24 Hours

Medication	Maximum Dose per 24 Hours
Acetaminophen (Tylenol,* Anacin-3,* Panadol,* Tempra*)	4000 mg
Aspirin (acetylsalicylic acid) (ASA,* Aspergum,* Bayer Aspirin,* Ecotrin,* Empirin,* Nuprin,* Excedrin*)	4000 mg
Ibuprofen (Motrin,* Advil,* and others)	3200 mg
Rofecoxib (Vioxx)	50 mg
Celecoxib (Celebrex)	400 mg

*May be purchased without a prescription.

Box 11-4

Adverse Effects of Opioids

Constipation	Sedation
Nausea and vomiting	Respiratory depression
Itching (pruritus)	Hallucinations/delirium
Urinary retention	Hypotension
Myoclonus	Dizziness

ASSESSMENT

1. Perform complete pain assessment as for Skill 11.1.
2. Check last time of administration of medication, including dose and degree of relief experienced. *Rationale: Determines if next dose can be administered.*
3. Determine if client has allergies to medications.
4. Determine an analgesic's prescribed route and frequency. Nonopioids can be alternated or given with opioids. Injectable medications generally act within 15 to 30 minutes. Immediate-release oral medications may take 1 hour to be effective, whereas some extended-release preparations may take up to 2 hours to be effective. *Rationale: Allows for planning pain relief measures with client activities; anticipating peak and duration of analgesic; and evaluating effectiveness of analgesic.*

PLANNING

Expected outcomes focus on elimination/reduction of pain and return to optimal functioning with minimal side effects.

Expected Outcomes

1. Client understands and uses identified pain intensity scale appropriately.
   a. Client and health care providers mutually agree on pain-intensity goal.
   b. Client rates pain at or below pain-intensity goal.

2. Clients who are unable to state a pain-intensity goal have a goal set at 4 or below (0 to 10 scale) because this level has been shown to minimally affect function (Feldt, 2000).
3. Client is able to adequately function and perform ADLs (walk, work, eat, sleep, interact).
4. Client does not experience intolerable or unmanageable adverse effects from the analgesic.

Equipment

- Prescribed medication
- Necessary administration device (see Chapter 18)
- Opioid/narcotic control sheet (for controlled substances only)

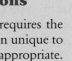

Delegation Considerations

The skill of administration of analgesics requires the critical thinking and knowledge application unique to a nurse. For this skill, delegation is inappropriate. However, assistive personnel (AP) should know behaviors suggestive of pain and notify the nurse when they occur.

IMPLEMENTATION FOR PHARMACOLOGICAL PAIN MANAGEMENT

Steps	Rationale
1. See Standard Protocol (inside front cover).	
2. Review six rights for administration of medications.	Ensures safe and appropriate medication administration.
3. Administer analgesics (see Chapters 16, 17, and 18). Consider NSAIDs, opioids, and adjuvants.	Nonopioids may be administered with opioids to improve opioid effectiveness. Adjuvants are more effective for neuropathic pain than opioids.

NURSE ALERT *If a client is unable to swallow or has a gastrostomy or jejunostomy tube in place, remember that the extended-release opioid formulations may not be crushed for administration.*

Steps	Rationale
a. As soon as pain occurs	Pain is easier to prevent than to treat.
b. Before pain increases in severity	Higher levels of pain may not respond to ordered analgesic.
c. Before pain-producing procedures or activities	Reduce or block pain transmission in the CNS.
d. Routinely, ATC	Maintains analgesic within therapeutic range, reducing pain intensity and minimizing side effects.
4. Include nonpharmacological pain control measures in addition to analgesics (see Skill 11.1, p. 239).	Increases effectiveness of pharmacological agents; treats nonphysiological aspects of pain.

Steps	Rationale
5. Identify expected time for peak effects and usual duration of action of analgesics.	Effects vary depending on the type of medication used; allows for anticipation of next dose; permits evaluation of effectiveness of analgesic.
6. Coordinate nursing care measures to maximize effectiveness (i.e., encourage to turn, cough, and deep breathe while medication effects are best).	Maximizes effectiveness of nursing measures to prevent complications.
7. Monitor for adverse effects.	

NURSE ALERT   *Clients receiving ATC opioids should also receive stimulant laxatives. Opioids decrease intestinal propulsion (peristalsis) but not intestinal motility (churning); thus stool softeners alone are ineffective. Recommend stimulant laxatives.*

---

8. Remove and dispose of gloves, if used.
9. See Completion Protocol (inside front cover).

• • • • • • • • • •

EVALUATION

1. Ask client to rate pain intensity using appropriate pain scale both at rest and with activity.
2. Evaluate PQRST aspects of pain (see Skill 11.1).
3. Observe client's position, mobility, relaxation, and ability to rest, sleep, eat, and participate in usual activities.

Unexpected Outcomes and Related Interventions

1. Client's pain intensity is greater than desired.
   a. Try an alternative nonpharmacologic intervention.
   b. Consult with physician if analgesic necessary.
2. Client continues to display nonverbal behaviors reflecting pain.
   a. Try an alternative nonpharmacologic intervention.
   b. Consider if appropriate to administer an analgesic.
   c. Discomfort that is unrelieved or is worse may indicate need for additional diagnostic, medical, or surgical intervention or a change in the pain management plan.

Recording and Reporting

- Record client's pain rating, response to analgesic, and additional comfort measures given. Incorporate pain-relief techniques in nursing care plan.
- Record alterations in client's condition and/or behavior.
- Report unsuccessful or untoward client response to analgesics to physician.

Sample Documentation

0800 Client reports severe aching pain in lower back, 9 (scale of 0 to 10). Unable to obtain relief in any position. Morphine 5 mg given IVP. Positioned on side with legs supported and back in alignment. Gentle massage provided to lower back.

0830 Is relaxed now. Pain described as 6 (scale 0 to 10).

SPECIAL CONSIDERATIONS

Pediatric Considerations

- Aspirin and aspirin-containing drugs should be avoided in children because of the increased risk for developing Reye's syndrome.
- Rectal formulations of analgesics should also be avoided if possible because this route is very uncomfortable.

Geriatric Considerations

- Cognitive impairment or dementia may affect an older adult's ability to report pain severity on a visual analog scale or numerical scale. Behavioral observations for pain (see Box 11-1, p. 241) may be confused with signs of dementia (AHCPR, 1992). Assess for potential causes of dementia, particularly if new symptom.
- Older adults may have liver or kidney impairment, resulting in faster onset and prolonged effect of analgesics because of reduced metabolism and excretion of these drugs. Dosage and frequency of analgesic administration should be titrated to the client's response to the specific analgesic agent (Buffum and Buffum, 2000; Chronic Pain Management, 1999). Rule of thumb: Start low, and go slow.
- IM analgesic administration should be avoided in older adults because IM injections hurt and because analgesic uptake from the muscle into the cardiovascular system is unpredictable, thus affecting therapeutic and side effect profile (The Management of Chronic Pain, 1998; Waitman, 2001; Perin, 2000).
- Specific analgesics are to be avoided in older adults because of cardiovascular, CNS, renal, and/or liver toxicity. These analgesics are propoxyphene hydrochloride (Darvon, Darvocet) and meperidine (Demerol) (The Management of Chronic Pain, 1998).

- Because of renal and liver decline associated with the aging process, maximum daily doses of NSAID and acetaminophen may need to be lower.
- If an older adult client is cognitively impaired and had a procedure that usually causes pain, the nurse should consult with the physician about ordering an appropriate analgesic ATC instead of as needed (prn).

Home Care Considerations

- Family members may need to understand the importance of ATC analgesic administration to maximize effect.
- Family members need to be encouraged to accept and acknowledge the client's report of pain.
- Family members who manage a client's pain while at home need to have access to health care providers on a 24-hour basis.

Long-Term Care Considerations

- Careful assessment of concurrent medical conditions that may affect pharmacological management of pain is essential.
- Because many older adults are also receiving several drugs for a variety of conditions, drug-drug interactions are a possibility.
- A variety of medical conditions require a variety of physicians. The nurse should facilitate information regarding prescribed medications among physicians.

Skill 11.3

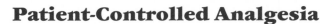

Patient-Controlled Analgesia

Patient-controlled analgesia (PCA) is based on the theory that clients are the best judges of their pain; it allows them to take active roles in controlling that pain (Pasero, 1998). PCA allows clients to self-administer small, frequent prescribed doses of IV opioids as they feel the need.

The equipment used includes a portable infusion pump with a timing device that can be set to limit the amount and frequency of medication. Most are battery operated, have locking mechanisms to prevent tampering and

overdosing, and have digital readouts that describe functions and store information about the amount of medication actually used (Pasero, 1999).

PCA enables a client to receive a prescribed continuous (bolus) dose or self-administered (demand) dose of analgesic intermittently. Both features may be used simultaneously. For demand dosing, clients must be able to understand the use of the PCA equipment and be physically able to press the button to deliver the dose. Instructions are best given when the client is not experiencing intense pain or sedated from anesthesia. If surgery is the reason for PCA analgesia, teaching should be done preoperatively if possible. The client should be aware that the analgesia may not eliminate all discomfort but will allow reasonable comfort to allow rest and movement with minimal pain (Wood, 2000; Reiff, 2001).

Not all clients are suitable candidates for PCA. Debilitated and cognitively impaired clients or clients with physical disabilities should be carefully assessed before initiating therapy. PCA should be used cautiously in clients with a history of opioid addiction or abuse (Compton, 1999; Newshan, 2000), neurological disease, hypovolemia, or impaired renal or pulmonary function. Several models of PCA devices are available; therefore the nurse must read the manufacturer's guidelines to obtain specific operating instructions.

ASSESSMENT

1. Check physician's orders for prescribed medication, dosage, and lockout settings. Verify that client is not allergic to prescribed medication. *Rationale: Ensures right drug is administered to client.*
2. Verify patency of the IV site and compatibility with the solution currently infusing. *Rationale: Other IV medication may not be compatible with PCA opioid. The PCA should never be attached to an IV with blood running or to IVs with cardiovascular drugs infusing. If necessary, start another IV site.*
3. Determine client's physical ability to manipulate PCA device and cognitive ability to understand directions. *Rationale: Determines if client can safely self-manage PCA.*
4. Assess baseline pain intensity, sedation level, and respiratory rate and quality. *Rationale: Provides a means to determine if client's condition improves or worsens following PCA use.*
5. Assess if client has history of sleep apnea. *Rationale: PCA may be contraindicated.*

PLANNING

Expected outcomes focus on proper use of the PCA device and adequate pain control without oversedation and with no or manageable adverse effects.

Expected Outcomes

1. Client demonstrates how to operate PCA device correctly.
2. Client rates pain at or below intensity goal.
3. Client remains cooperative and responsive to verbal instructions.
4. Client maintains respirations of greater than 12 breaths per minute.
5. Client's function improves.

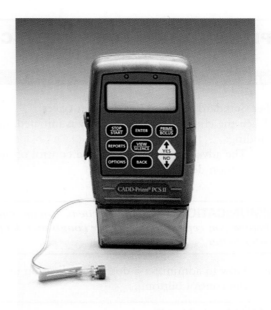

Figure 11-4 Patient-controlled analgesia (PCA) pump with cassette. (Courtesy Deltec, Inc, St Paul, Minnesota.)

Equipment

- PCA system and tubing (Figure 11-4)
- Prescribed medication in appropriate reservoir (varies with pump design.)

 Delegation Considerations

The skill of PCA administration requires the critical thinking and knowledge application unique to a nurse. For this skill, delegation is inappropriate. Assistive personnel (AP) should notify the RN if the client is confused about operating the PCA pump, if the PCA alarms, or if it is suspected that the PCA pump is not working properly. AP must not administer a PCA dose for the client under any circumstances.

IMPLEMENTATION FOR PATIENT-CONTROLLED ANALGESIA

Steps	Rationale
1. See Standard Protocol (inside front cover).	
2. Teach the client before the therapy is initiated, including:	Ensures client understands how to manipulate device and implications of therapy.
a. The advantages of self-initiated control of medication delivery.	Helps client to understand the value of controlling pain rather than waiting to receive an analgesic when pain severity is high.

COMMUNICATION TIP *Advise client, "Giving yourself a dose of pain medication before you reposition, walk, or cough and deep breathe will help you perform activities better."*

b. How to administer a dose of medication using the control button.	

COMMUNICATION TIP *Explain to client, "Press the PCA button to deliver a small dose of pain medication into your IV. Because you are administering your pain medication, you will not need to wait for a nurse to draw up and administer a pain shot; therefore your pain will decrease sooner. There is a lockout time between doses so you cannot give yourself an overdose."*

c. That the lockout feature prevents risk of overdose.	
d. Possible side effects, based on the medication prescribed.	
e. To notify the nurse for the following: if relief is not being obtained, severity or location of pain changes, alarms sound, or questions arise.	Ensures nurse's more timely response to developing problems.
3. Prepare medication for infusion.	
a. Attach prefilled medication reservoir to pump device.	
b. Prime the unit.	Air in the line will result in the analgesic not being delivered, the unit alarming, or a potential air embolus.
c. Adjust the PCA to reflect physician orders, and lock pump settings.	
4. Transport equipment to client's room, and plug into electrical outlet.	Battery backup is intended for transport only.
5. Verify client identity by checking identification band against medication administration record, and ask client to state name.	Following the five rights is essential for client safety.
6. Attach PCA tubing to client's maintenance IV tubing at Y-port closest to IV insertion site.	Because of small volume (0.5 to 1 ml) of analgesic delivered with each button push, PCA tubing must be close to IV insertion site.
a. Open all clamps.	
b. Start pump.	
c. Be sure maintenance IV rate is at least 50 ml/hr (Reiff and Niziolek, 2001).	If the IV maintenance fluid is infusing too slowly, the analgesic delivered into the tubing will not reach the client quickly, resulting in inadequate pain relief.
d. Place control device within easy reach of client.	
7. Reinforce previous teaching of proper use of PCA pump. Have client demonstrate ability to use PCA.	Repeating instructions and demonstration reinforces learning.

Steps	Rationale
8. Encourage client to self-administer medication without delay whenever discomfort is felt.	Prevents pain from escalating.
9. Instruct family to support and assist client, but not press button for client.	Effectiveness and appropriate dosage are able to be determined only with participation of client. Oversedation and respiratory depression can occur if another person administers PCA dose.
10. Involve client in planning care activities. Inform client of times when procedures are planned, and encourage use of PCA.	Ability to anticipate activities that may cause discomfort ensures more timely administration of PCA dose. Client likely to achieve good pain control during activities.

11. To discontinue PCA:
  a. Obtain necessary PCA information from pump for documentation.
  b. Turn pump off.
  c. Disconnect PCA tubing from IV maintenance line, but maintain IV access.
  d. Appropriately dispose of remaining opioid.	

NURSE ALERT *If pump is discontinued before container of opioid is completely empty, waste must be witnessed by another RN, with a notation on PCA medication record regarding date, time, and volume wasted (Figure 11-5, p. 252). Federal regulations specify guidelines for recording use and waste of controlled substances.*

12. See Completion Protocol (inside front cover).

· · · · · · · · · · ·

EVALUATION

1. Observe client manipulate control button.
2. Observe client's ability to cooperate and respond to verbal instructions.
3. Ask client to describe pain intensity using the selected pain scale.
4. Evaluate client's level of consciousness and respiratory rate and quality regularly.

Unexpected Outcomes and Related Interventions

1. Client's pain intensity is higher than goal.
   a. Make sure tubing of PCA device is not kinked.
   b. Reevaluate client's ability to use PCA.
   c. Physician may need to adjust the dosage parameters because blood levels of analgesics need to remain stable to be effective. A continuous rate of administration may be needed to provide coverage during hours of sleep, or the PCA dose may need to be increased. (See manufacturer's instructions to change PCA dose or start continuous administration.)

NURSE ALERT *Do not increase demand or basal dose and decrease the interval time (e.g., from 10 to 5 minutes) simultaneously because this will increase the risk for oversedation, respiratory depression, and other adverse effects.*

   d. Use nonpharmacological pain-relieving interventions.

   e. Suggest supplemental nonopioids, if not contraindicated.
2. Venipuncture site shows evidence of infiltration or inflammation.
   a. Start a new IV site.
3. Client is too sedated and unable to participate in activities (turning, coughing, deep breathing, ambulation).
   a. Determine how frequently the pump has been used and total dose administered.
   b. Dosage parameters may need to be reduced by the physician. (See manufacturer's instructions for changing parameters.)
4. Client is unable to manipulate device to maintain pain control.
   a. Reposition the PCA button.
   b. Use an alternative form of ATC analgesia.

Recording and Reporting

- Record drug, concentration, dose (basal and/or demand), time started, and lockout time. Many institutions have a separate flow sheet for PCA documentation.
- Dose calculation includes adding demand and continuous dose together. The following example is documented on a PCA flow sheet (see Figure 11-5, p. 252). A PCA pump of hydrocodone 0.5 mg/ml is initi~ at 1400 with the following parameters: PCA dose, 0.5 mg; continuous dose, 0.25 m lockout interval of 10 minutes. At 1800 amount of drug (1 mg from continuous/ of 0.25 mg/hr and 7 mg from PCA deman

Barnes-Jewish Hospital
BJC HealthCare℠

CONTROLLED DRUG RECORD

ADDRESSOGRAPH

PATIENT NAME	DIVISION	CONTROL NUMBER
SAM JACKSON	2 MAIN	183003

(IV/PCA)	EPIDURAL
☐ Morphine 1 mg/ml in NS, 100 ml in Casette	☐ Hydromorphone _____ mg/ml in NS 250 ml
☐ Meperidine 10 mg/ml in NS, 100 ml in Cassette	☐ Morphine 0.04 mg/ml in NS 250 ml
☒ Hydromorphone 0.5 mg/ml in NS, 100 ml in Cassette	☐ Fentanyl _____ mcg/ml/Bupivacaine _____ % in NS 250 ml
☐ Fentanyl 50 mcg/ml, 50 ml in Cassette	☐ Bupivacaine 0.8 mg/ml and Sufentanil 0.4 mcg/ml in 100 ml NS
☐ Lorazepam 1 mg/ml in D5W, 40 ml in Cassette	☐ Other: Drug/Diluent _____
☐ Other: Drug/Diluent _____	Concentration _____ mg/ml
Concentration _____ mg/ml	Total Volume _____ ml
Total Volume _____ ml	

ROUTE: ☐ Central Line ☐ Peripheral ☐ Epidural

METHOD: ☐ PCA ☐ Large Volume Infusion

DRUG DISPENSED BY: ☐ Pharmacy ☐ PYXIS

DISPENSING PHARMACIST SIGNATURE	DATE	TIME
M. Smith, Ph.D.	1-18-02	1330
DRUG STARTED BY: NURSE SIGNATURE Jill St. John	1-18-02	1400

STOP HERE, DETACH THIS SECTION AND ROUTE TO PHARMACY

DOCUMENT EVERY 8 HOURS

DATE/TIME	BASAL RATE	BOLUS RATE	VOLUME CC/ML INFUSED	CUMULATIVE VOLUME CC/ML INFUSED	AMOUNT MG/MCG INFUSED	CUMULATIVE MG/MCG INFUSED	ATTEMPTS/ DELIVERED	NURSE SIGNATURE
1-18 1800	0.25	0.50	16cc	16cc	8 mg	8 mg	20 14	J. Wills, RN
1-18 2200	0.25	0.50	8cc	24cc	4 mg	12 mg	10 6	J. Wills, RN
— PUMP DISCONTINUED								J. Wills, RN

☒ WASTAGE ☐ RETURNED	DATE 1-18-02	TIME 1800	VOLUME 76 cc
NURSE SIGNATURE: #1 J. Wills RN		NURSE SIGNATURE: #2 Susan Crow, RN	
PRINTED NURSE NAME #1 J. Wills, RN		PRINTED NURSE NAME #2 S. Crow, RN	

MUST BE COMPLETED BEFORE RETURNED TO PHARMACY

Figure 11-5 PCA Documentation form. (Courtesy Barnes-Jewish Hospital, St Louis, Mo.)

administered by the client) was 8 mg. In addition, the volume (ml/cc) of drug needs monitoring. The cumulative volume column alerts the nurse to the need for a new reservoir and to the possible diversion of opioids (volume administered and volume remaining in reservoir should total beginning volume).

Sample Documentation

1700 Client reports no pain when lying still and gnawing abdominal incisional pain intensity of 4 (goal is 4 on a scale of 0 to 10) when turning. Sleeping at intervals but arouses easily. Respiratory rate is 16. IV PCA infusing in left forearm without signs of infiltration.

SPECIAL CONSIDERATIONS

Pediatric Considerations

- Children 5 years of age and over can be taught how to use a PCA. Be sure to assess ability to operate pump.
- Use appropriate terminology when teaching children pump use.
- Include parents when teaching child.

Geriatric Considerations

- Older clients can use a PCA. Demand dose is preferred over continuous/basal dose; however, the dose should still be large enough to achieve pain relief (Loeb, 1999).
- Older adults should be assessed as to physical and cognitive ability to operate the PCA.

Home Care Considerations

- PCA should not be used in clients physically or cognitively unable to activate device.
- Professional support should be available to family members through regular telephone contact and scheduled nursing visits (Inyang and Kaplan, 1999).
- Provide instruction regarding appropriate dosage adjustment and potential errors teaching.
- Notify physician if after dosage adjustments pain intensity remains unacceptable.

Long-Term Care Considerations

- PCA pumps are generally not found in a long-term care facility, but when used should have the same precautions as for hospital use.
- Locking mechanisms are essential to prevent confused clients from changing pump settings.

Skill 11.4

Epidural Analgesia

The administration of analgesics into the epidural space has become an increasingly popular technique for managing acute postoperative pain, as well as chronic pain, especially for clients with cancer. Epidural opioids reduce the total amount of opioids required to control pain, thus producing fewer side effects.

The epidural space is located between the vertebral column and the dura mater, the outermost protective layer of the spinal cord (Figure 11-6). When an opioid is injected into the epidural space, it diffuses slowly into the cerebrospinal fluid (CSF) of the subarachnoid space, where it binds to opiate receptors located in the dorsal horn of the spinal cord. The binding of opioids on the dorsal horn results in a block of pain impulse transmission to the cerebral cortex.

The anesthesiologist or nurse anesthetist places a catheter into the epidural space, usually in the lower lumbar region, to administer analgesics. Opioids such as mor-

phine sulfate or fentanyl citrate (Sublimaze) are often used; however, adjuvants may also be given (Guay, 2001). When the epidural catheter is intended for short-term use, it does not need to be sutured in place and exits from the insertion site on the back (Figure 11-6). A catheter for long-term use, however, is tunneled under the subcutaneous tissue and exits on the side of the body or the abdomen (Figure 11-7). Tunneling reduces the risk of infection and dislodging of the catheter. In both cases the catheter is covered with a sterile occlusive dressing.

Although the use of epidural opioids for control of pain has many advantages for the client, it also requires astute nursing observation and care. Because of its anatomical location, the epidural catheter has potential for migration through the dura and disruption of spinal nerves and vessels. In many hospitals, anesthesiologists and nurse anesthetists are the only health care professionals who may initiate an epidural opioid infusion or administer a bolus.

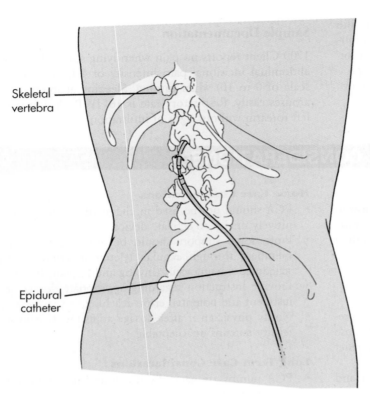

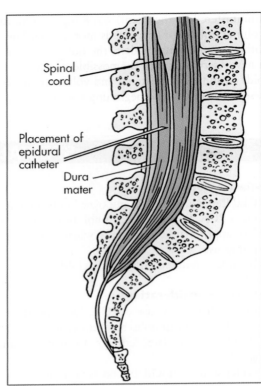

Spinal cord

Placement of epidural catheter

Dura mater

Skeletal vertebra

Epidural catheter

Figure 11-6   Tunneled epidural catheter.

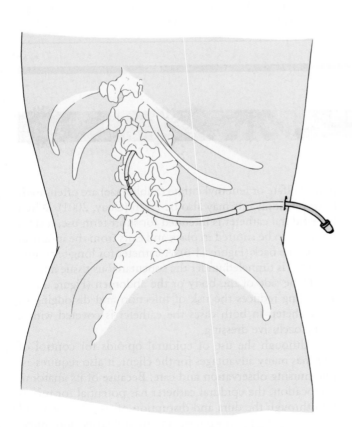

Figure 11-7   Epidural catheter taped in place.

Some hospitals have nurses who have successfully completed a certification program that enables them to begin the epidural opioid infusion or administer a bolus once the catheter has been placed (check agency policy).

ASSESSMENT

1. Assess client's pain (see Skill 11.1, p. 239). Certain conditions make epidural analgesia the method of choice for clients experiencing pain: postoperative states, trauma, and advanced cancer. *Rationale: Provides baseline for determining effectiveness of epidural analgesia.*

2. For cognitively impaired or non–English-speaking clients, assess nonverbal responses. *Rationale: Because client cannot verbalize pain intensity, nonverbal responses help the nurse to determine the presence of pain.*

3. Assess sedation level of client (see Chapter 15), including respiratory status and level of consciousness (LOC), to establish a baseline before first dose. *Rationale: The first sign of altered respiratory function from opioid use is a change in sedation level (Young-McCaughan and Misakowski, 2001).*

4. Check rate, depth, and pattern of respirations to establish a baseline (see Chapter 12). *Rationale: Slow, shallow, and irregular respirations are signs of respiratory depression, which may occur as late as 24 hours after epidural injection (Cox, 2001).*

5. Check blood pressure to establish a baseline. Small drop in blood pressure may be seen in the first hour after epidural injection. *Rationale: Hypotension after opioid use usually results from a decreased circulating catecholamine level that was elevated in response to pain (Cox, 2001).*

6. Assess mobility/motor and sensory function (see Chapter 13) before assisting client into or out of bed. Check for motor weakness and numbness and tingling of lower extremities (paresthesias). *Rationale: Prevents injury from falling that may occur from muscle weakness. In addition, rapid onset of motor weakness is an indication that the epidural catheter may have migrated from the dura into the subarachnoid space (Cox, 2001; Miller and Cosentino, 2000). If the catheter puts pressure on spinal nerves, paresthesias can result (Cosentino, 2000; Hall, 2000).*

7. Check to see if epidural catheter is secured to client's skin. *Rationale: Prevents dislodging or migration of catheter.*

8. Assess condition of client's skin, especially over those areas client is most often positioning self. *Rationale: The presence of an epidural catheter may limit client's mobility, increasing risk for pressure ulcer formation.*

9. Assess epidural catheter insertion site for redness, warmth, tenderness, swelling, and drainage. *Rationale: To identify early local inflammation or superficial skin infections at the insertion site (Cox, 2001). Purulent drainage is a sign of infection. Catheter will need to be removed.*

10. If continuous infusion, check infusion pump for proper calibration and operation. *Rationale ensures client obtains prescribed analgesic dose.*

11. If continuous infusion, check patency of IV tubing. *Rationale: IV tubing must be patent for medication to reach epidural space.*

12. Check client's history of drug allergies to avoid placing client at risk for allergic reaction.

PLANNING

Expected outcomes focus on the achievement of pain control or relief and the prevention of complications of epidural analgesia.

Expected Outcomes

1. Client verbalizes pain relief within 30 to 60 minutes of initiation of epidural infusion.
2. Client's epidural dressing remains dry and intact.
3. Client does not have headache while epidural catheter is in place or up to 72 hours after removal.
4. Client experiences no redness, warmth, exudate, tenderness, or swelling at catheter insertion site during time epidural catheter is in place. The client is afebrile.

5. Client's respirations are regular, unlabored, and equal to or greater than 12 breaths per minute.
6. Client is awake, alert, and oriented to person, place, and time.
7. Client voids without difficulty and in adequate amounts of 250 to 500 ml after administration of epidural opioid.
8. Client has no or manageable opioid adverse effects (see Box 11-4, p. 245).

Equipment

- Gloves

Bolus Medication

- 10- to 12-ml syringe
- Filter needle
- 20-gauge, 1-inch needle
- Povidone-iodine swabs
- Prediluted preservative-free opioid as prescribed by physician
- Label (for injection port)

Continuous Infusion

- Prediluted preservative-free opioid as prescribed by physician and prepared for use in IV infusion pump (usually prepared by pharmacy)
- Infusion pump
- Infusion pump–compatible IV tubing without Y-ports
- Tape
- Label (for tubing)

Delegation Considerations

Administration of epidural analgesia requires the critical thinking and knowledge application unique to an RN. Delegation to assistive personnel (AP) is inappropriate. However, staff must be instructed in how to reposition clients so as to prevent disruption of the catheter and to report to RN immediately any occurrence of headache, difficulty breathing, client report of itching, drainage on dressing, or symptoms of infection.

IMPLEMENTATION FOR EPIDURAL ANALGESIA

Steps	Rationale
1. See Standard Protocol (inside front cover).	
2. Check client's name on identification band with medication administration record. Ask client to state name.	Ensures right client receives right medication
3. Review six rights of administration of medications.	Ensures safe and appropriate medication administration.

4. Prepare and administer bolus injection.

a. Attach "epidural line" label close to injection cap on epidural catheter.

    Labeling helps to ensure opioid analgesic is administered into correct line and into epidural space.

b. Using a large syringe, draw up prediluted preservative-free opioid solution through a filter needle.

    A large volume of fluid permits opioid to contact the optimal number of receptors (Cox, 2001). Preservative may be toxic to neural tissue and could result in nerve damage (Miller and Cosentino, 2000). Filter needle removes any microscopic glass particles.

c. Change from filter needle to regular 20-gauge needle.

    Changing to regular needle prevents infusion of microscopic glass particles possibly lodged in lumen of filter needle and allows medication to be injected.

d. Clean injection cap with povidone-iodine. (Do not use alcohol.)

    Cleaning agent prevents introduction of microorganisms during needle insertion. Alcohol causes pain and is toxic to neural tissue.

e. Dry the injection cap with sterile gauze.

    Reduces possible injection of povidone-iodine.

f. Insert needle into injection cap. Or if using a needless system, attach syringe directly to injection cap. Aspirate.

    Aspiration of clear fluid of less than 1 ml is indicative of epidural catheter placement. More than 1 ml of clear fluid or bloody return means catheter may be in subarachnoid space or in a vessel; do not inject drug. Notify anesthesiologist/nurse anesthetist.

g. If less than 1 ml clear fluid returns, inject drug slowly (see Chapter 29). (Administer a bolus of an opioid via a pump at a rate of 1 ml/30 sec.)

    Slow injection helps prevent client discomfort by lowering the pressure exerted by fluid as it enters the subarachnoid space (Cox, 2001).

h. Remove needle or syringe from injection cap.

i. Dispose of uncapped needle and syringe in sharps container. Remove and discard gloves, and decontaminate hands.

NURSE ALERT *Keep an ampule of naloxone (Narcan), 0.4 mg/ml, a strong opioid antagonist, at the bedside to use in case of emergency to counteract respiratory depression (respiratory rate less than or equal to 8 breaths per minute). Dilute naloxone with 9 ml of preservative-free saline, and administer 0.5 ml over 2 minutes and assess respirations. Titrate to effect. When respiratory rate is 10 breaths per minute or above and depth is adequate, naloxone may be discontinued; however, continue to observe client because respiratory depression may reappear and thus more naloxone required (Pasero and McCaffery, 2000). If 0.8 mg of naloxone produces no effect, consider other causes. Naloxone will reverse the opioid's effect but will also reverse pain control. Client may require alternative medication for pain relief.*

---

5. Administer continuous infusion.

a. Attach "epidural line" label to IV tubing connected to epidural catheter. Use tubing without Y-ports.

    Prevents inadvertent administration of other drugs via epidural catheter.

Steps	Rationale
b. Attach container of diluted preservative-free opioid to infusion pump tubing and prime (see Chapter 29).	Tubing should be filled with solution and free of air bubbles to avoid air embolus.
c. Attach proximal end of tubing to infusion pump and distal end to epidural catheter. Tape all connections. Start infusion. (See Chapter 29 for use of infusion pump.)	Infusion pump propels fluid through tubing. Taping maintains a secure, closed system to help prevent infection and minimizes risk of separation of analgesic tubing from epidural catheter.
d. Check infusion pump for proper calibration and operation.	Maintains patency and ensures client is receiving proper dose.

6. Remove and dispose of gloves.
7. Explain that nurses will be monitoring client's response to epidural analgesic routinely. Also instruct client on signs or problems to report to nurse.

COMMUNICATION TIP *Explain to client, "Some potential side effects of epidural analgesia that we will be watching you for include excessive sleepiness or sedation, slowing of your respirations, inability to pass urine, and itching. Please let a nurse know if you experience any of these problems. Also let a nurse know if your pain level increases or if your epidural catheter feels wet or starts to peel off."*

---

8. See Completion Protocol (inside front cover).

• • • • • • • • • •

EVALUATION

1. Evaluate every hour for 24 hours then every 4 hours or more if needed, and report immediately changes in level of consciousness, increasing pain intensity, or changes in vital signs (BP less than 90 mm Hg, respiratory rate less than 10 breaths per minute). No additional opioids or sedatives should be administered unless approved by physician/Certified Registered Nurse Anesthetist (CRNA) initiating and/or monitoring therapy.
2. Ask client to rate pain intensity on selected pain scale.
3. Inspect epidural dressing for dryness and intactness.
4. Ask client if headache is present. Note nonverbal signs of headache.
5. Assess catheter insertion site for redness, warmth, exudate, tenderness, or swelling.
6. Assess rate, depth, and pattern of respirations. (When infusion started or if a bolus is given, check respiratory rate, depth, and pattern every 15 minutes for 2 hours, then every 30 minutes for 2 hours, then every 1 hour for 1 hour, then every 2 hours.)
7. Assess sedation level, LOC, and orientation.
8. Assess client's voiding pattern and amount. If voiding in amounts less than 150 ml at a time and is experiencing frequency, palpate for bladder distention.
9. Ask client if itching is present.

Unexpected Outcomes and Related Interventions

1. Client's respirations decrease to 6 breaths per minute and are shallow. Client is not easily aroused with verbal stimulation.
   a. Follow institution's policy, which may include:
      (1) Turn off pump to stop epidural infusion.
      (2) Administer 2 L of oxygen via nasal cannula.
      (3) Administer naloxone (Narcan) (see Nurse Alert on p. 256).
      (4) Notify anesthesiologist/nurse anesthetist.
      (5) Assess respiratory rate, rhythm, and depth until rate reaches 12 breaths per minute, then continue assessing every 15 minutes for 2 hours, every 30 minutes for 2 hours, every hour for 1 hour, then every 2 hours.
   b. Do not give other opioids or CNS depressants except as prescribed by the anesthesiologist/nurse anesthetist responsible for epidural analgesia.
2. Client states pain is not controlled.
   a. Check infusion pump for malfunction if receiving a continuous infusion.
   b. Check catheter insertion site for outward migration.
   c. Check tubing for kinks.

d. Teach client other pain management strategies that may enhance pharmacological intervention (e.g., imagery, distraction, relaxation).

e. Explain that pain relief begins within 30 to 60 minutes after epidural injection and may last between 6 and 24 hours.

3. Client experiences redness, warmth, tenderness, swelling, or exudate at catheter insertion site. Client is febrile.
   a. Notify anesthesiologist/nurse anesthetist for catheter to be discontinued.

4. Client reports a headache.
   a. Notify anesthesiologist/nurse anesthetist.

5. Clear drainage is present on epidural dressing, or more than 1 ml can be aspirated from catheter.
   a. Stop infusion or bolus injection.
   b. Notify anesthesiologist/nurse anesthetist

Recording and Reporting

- Record drug, dose, and time given (if injection) or time begun and ended (if infusion) on appropriate medication record. Specify concentration and diluent.
- Record medication on epidural opioid record.
- With continuous infusion, obtain and record pump readout hourly for first 24 hours after infusion is begun and then every 4 hours.
- Record regular periodic assessments of client's status in nurses' notes or on appropriate flow sheets (Figure 11-8).

Indicate:

    Vital signs
    Intake and output
    Sedation level
    Pain severity score
    Neurological status
    Assessment of epidural site
    Presence or absence of adverse reactions to medication
    Presence or absence of complications resulting from placement and maintenance of epidural catheter

- Report any adverse reactions or complications to physician.

Sample Documentation

0800 Fentanyl 2000 micrograms in 500 ml 0.9 normal saline infusing at 15 ml/hr into epidural catheter via infusion pump. Respiratory rate 10 with moderate depth and regular pattern. States abdominal surgical pain is a 5 (scale 0 to 10), compared with previous 7.

1000 Respiratory rate 6 with shallow depth and periods of apnea. Arouses with verbal stimulation. Epidural infusion stopped. Narcan 0.2 mg IV push given in titrated doses. Anesthesiologist notified.

1005 Respiratory rate 8, shallow depth, and regular pattern. Alert, awake, and oriented 3.

1020 Respiratory rate 12, moderate depth, regular pattern. Rates abdominal surgical incision pain a 4 on a 0 to 10 scale.

 SPECIAL CONSIDERATIONS

Pediatric Considerations

- Epidural analgesia may be used in all pediatric age groups.
- Dose of analgesic is by milligram or microgram per kilogram.
- Epidural analgesia in infants and children is generally used for acute pain conditions such as sickle cell crisis and heel cord tendon release in muscular dystrophy (Hockenberry, 2003).
- During epidural analgesia, infants and children require continuous cardiac, respiratory, and oxygen saturation monitoring,

Geriatric Considerations

Because older adult clients often receive medications for hypertension, evaluating for hypotension during epidural analgesia is essential.

Home Care Considerations

- Clients needing home therapy are discharged with a tunneled catheter (Figure 11-7). Before consideration of catheter placement in preparation for discharge and care in the home, several variables must be assessed, including fine motor skills, cognitive ability, stage of disease and prognosis, and degree of involvement of family or significant others. Inform the client and the caregiver how to contact clinician.

- Teach client and caregiver the proper dosage and technique for administration of medication. Evaluate client's or family member's technique for catheter care and administering medication, as well as reinforcing instructions.

- Teach client and caregiver aseptic technique for opioid administration and for all catheter care procedures. This includes dressing changes, signs and symptoms of infection to report, signs and symptoms of adverse reactions to opioid being used (see Box 11-4, p. 245), and actions to be taken.

- Provide client and family list of all supplies needed for procedures and where to purchase.

Long-Term Care

Epidural pain management is rarely used in long-term care settings.

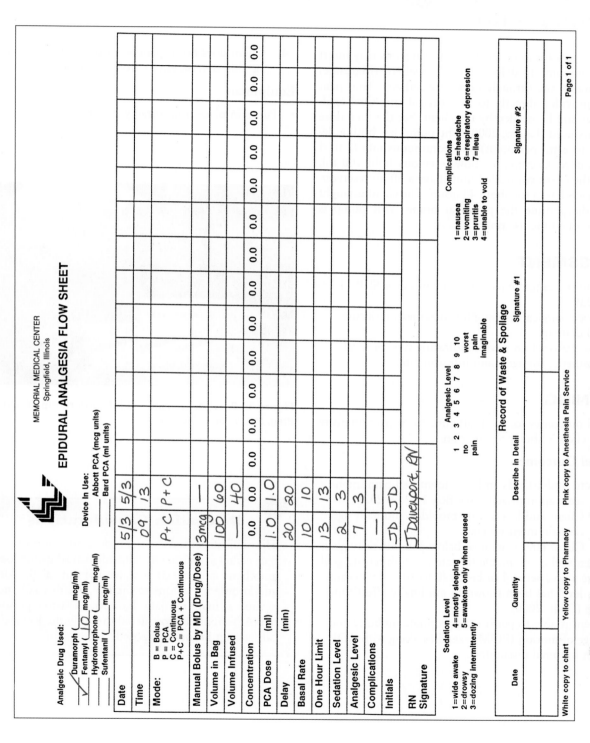

Figure 11-8   Epidural and analgesia documentation form. (Courtesy Memorial Medical Center, Springfield, Ill.)

Skill 11.5

Local Anesthetic Infusion Pump for Management of Postoperative Pain

During surgery for joint replacement, surgeons may insert an infusion pump to deliver a local anesthetic (Marcaine) to the surgical site through a one-way catheter. Thus pain relief is provided directly to the surgical site. Oral analgesics may still be needed by the client, but the total dose is often reduced (Pasero, 2000). The pump has both a demand (4 to 6 ml per bolus) and continuous rate (2 to 4 ml/hr) feature. Continuous flow reservoirs hold 100 ml, whereas the client-controlled units have a 50-ml reservoir. The device is left in for about 48 hours. The client is taught how to discontinue the pump at home. This pump is meant for one-time use only.

ASSESSMENT

1. Perform complete pain assessment as for Skill 11.1, p. 239.
2. Inspect surgical dressing for intactness, moisture, and drainage.
3. Observe label on device indicating type of local anesthetic, strength, and infusion rate.

PLANNING

Expected outcomes focus on attainment of pain-intensity goal and client's ability to function.

Expected Outcomes

1. Client understands and uses identified pain intensity scale appropriately (see Box 11-2, p. 242).
   a. Client and health care providers mutually agree on pain-intensity goal.
   b. Client rates pain at or below pain-intensity goal.
2. Clients who are unable to state a pain-intensity goal have a goal set at 4 or below (0 to 10 scale) because this level has been shown to minimally affect function (Feldt, 2000).
3. Client is able to perform appropriate mobility and range-of-motion (ROM) exercises along with ADL with minimal discomfort.

4. Client does not experience intolerable or unmanageable adverse effects from the analgesic.

Equipment

- Pump in place from surgery (Figure 11-9).

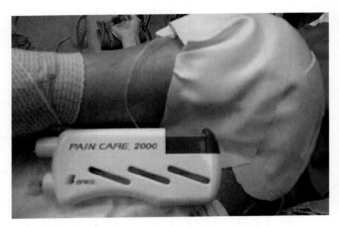

Figure 11-9 Local anesthetic infusion pump. (Courtesy Breg, Inc., Vista, California.)

 Delegation Considerations

The skill of pain assessment, determination of correct catheter placement, and identification of local anesthetic side effects requires the critical thinking and knowledge unique to the RN. For this skill, delegation is inappropriate. However, assistive personnel (AP) should be instructed to notify the RN if the catheter tip becomes exposed.

IMPLEMENTATION FOR LOCAL ANESTHETIC INFUSION PUMP FOR MANAGEMENT OF POSTOPERATIVE PAIN

Steps	Rationale
1. See Standard Protocol (inside front cover)	
2. Review surgeon's note.	Indicates reason for placement, anatomical area of catheter placement, and any initial bolus of local anesthetic given.
3. Assess surgical dressing and site of catheter insertion.	Dressing should be dry and intact. If not, stop infusion and notify physician. Catheter may not be properly placed.
a. Assess catheter connections.	Catheter connections should be firmly attached. If connections become detached, do NOT reattach because infection could result. Notify surgeon.
b. Assess for blood backing up tubing.	Stop infusion, and notify surgeon. Indicates possible displacement of catheter into blood vessel.
c. Read label on device.	Provides information regarding type of anesthetic, concentration, volume, flow rate, date and time prepared, and name of person who prepared it.
4. Determine extremity activity level from physician orders.	Excessive activity may cause catheter displacement.
5. Assess for signs of Marcaine toxicity: hypotension, dizziness, tremor, severe itching, swelling of the skin or throat, irregular heartbeat, palpitations, confusion, ringing in the ears, muscle twitching, numbness around the mouth, metallic taste, seizures.	Early identification of Marcaine toxicity prevents possible complications, including seizures.
6. For catheter removal order:	Clients may remove their own catheter at home with physician order. Provide verbal and written instructions to the client and/or family member.
a. Remove surgical dressing.	
b. Wash hands with soap and water for at least 2 minutes, and then **apply sterile gloves.**	Surgical apsepsis needed for catheter manipulation and removal.
c. Have client sit in relaxed position.	
d. Sit with leg up and supported if knee surgical site.	Relaxes joint.
e. Encourage client to take a few deep breaths and relax.	Provides distraction and relaxes joint muscles.
f. Grasp tube firmly, and pull outward from skin with a steady motion.	If there is resistance, stop pulling. Reposition extremity, and try again. If tubing continues to stretch and demonstrates resistance, stop pulling, cover area with sterile dressing, and notify surgeon.
g. Observe catheter tip for mark on end.	Indicates complete removal of entire catheter.
h. Place catheter in plastic bag using standard precautions.	Client is to bring catheter to physician's office on first visit.
i. Once catheter is removed, place a sterile dressing over the area and apply pressure for at least 2 minutes.	Prevents hematoma formation.
j. Observe site for excessive bleeding or fluid loss. If none, apply an adherent dressing (Band-Aid).	Protects insertion site and reduces chance of infection.
7. Document findings.	
8. Remind client of physician's follow-up appointment.	
9. See Completion Protocol (inside front cover).	

• • • • • • • • • •

EVALUATION

1. Ask client to rate pain intensity using appropriate pain scale both at rest and with activity.
2. Evaluate PQRST aspects of pain (see Skill 11.1, p. 239).
3. Observe client's position, mobility, relaxation, and ability to rest, sleep, eat, and participate in usual activities.
4. Inspect condition of surgical dressing.

Unexpected Outcomes and Related Interventions

1. Severe pain may indicate catheter displacement or pump malfunction.
   a. Have client notify surgeon.
2. Symptoms of Marcaine toxicity may occur.
   a. Stop pump, and call surgeon immediately.

Recording and Reporting

- Record client's pain rating, response to anesthetic, and additional comfort measures given.
- Record alterations in client's condition and/or behavior.
- Record condition of surgical dressing and catheter tubing.
- Report unsuccessful or untoward client response to analgesics to physician.

Sample Documentation

1000 Client returns from operating room following right total knee replacement. Dressing dry and intact. Anesthetic pump in place, catheter connections intact, receiving continuous morphine sulfate infusion at 4 ml/hr. Client currently rates knee pain at a 4 (scale 0 to 10).

SPECIAL CONSIDERATIONS

Geriatric Considerations
Clients with physical or mental disabilities are not candidates for this device.

Home Care Considerations
- Clients and their families should be taught to notify the surgeon if excessive bleeding or fluid on the dressing occurs.
- Instruct client and family not to reattach pump if catheter becomes disconnected, but to cover ending with sterile dressing and notify surgeon.
- Provide written instructions regarding side effects of Marcaine that should be reported to the surgeon immediately.
- Provide instructions regarding extremity movement.

Long-Term Care Considerations
Local anesthetic infusion pumps are rarely used in the long-term care setting.

CRITICAL THINKING EXERCISES

1. A 63-year-old woman underwent a colon resection and has just returned from the postanesthesia care unit (PACU) at 1300. Assessment reveals pain rated a 3 (on a scale of 0 to 10), which the client states is bearable for her at this time. Morphine sulfate is being administered via PCA, which was initiated by the PACU nursing staff.
   a. When is the best time to teach this client how to use PCA?
   b. The client uses the PCA appropriately for pain control and maintains a pain level of 4 or less until 2330, when she awakens with a pain intensity of 8 (0 to 10 scale). What interventions should the nurse implement to assist this client in gaining control over her pain?

2. A 72-year-old man has a continuous epidural analgesia infusion for pain management following a radical prostatectomy.
   a. What nursing interventions are associated with the use of epidural analgesia in the care of this client?
   b. If this client's respiratory rate decreases to 6 breaths per minute and he arouses easily with verbal stimulation, what should the nurse's response be?

3. An 80-year-old client who is confused and has global aphasia following a cerebrovascular accident (CVA) is admitted to your unit. He has a large sacral decubitus ulcer that the physician plans to surgically debride, at the bedside, in the next hour.
   a. How would you assess this client's pain?
   b. What pain management plan would be optimal for this client?

REFERENCES

Agency for Health Care Policy and Research, Acute Pain Management Guideline Panel: *Acute pain management in infants, children and adolescents: operative or medical procedures and trauma,* Clinical practice guideline, AHCPR Pub No. 92-0032, Rockville, Md, 1992, Agency for Health Care Policy and Research, Public Health Service, U.S. Department of Health and Human Services.

American Geriatric Society: *The management of chronic pain in older persons: clinical practice guidelines,* New York, 1998, The Society.

American Medical Directors Association: *Chronic pain management in the long-term care setting: clinical practice guidelines,* New York, 1999, The Association.

American Nurses Association: *Code for nurses with interpretative statements,* Kansas City, 2001, The Association.

Andrews A, Boyle J: *Transcultural concepts in nursing care,* ed 3, Philadelphia, 1999, Lippincott.

Bildner J: CRIES Instrument, 1997, City of Hope Pain Resource Center, Los Angeles, California.

Buffum M, Buffum J: Nonsteroidal anti-inflammatory drugs in elderly, *Pain Manag Nurs* 1(2):40, 2000.

Collins P and others: Talking with physicians about pain, *Am J Nurs* 99(10):20, 1999.

Compton P: Managing a drug abuser's pain, *Nursing* 29(5):26, 1999.

Cosentino B: Epidural pain management, *Nurs Spect* 12A(4):NJ1, 2000.

Cox F: Clinical care of patients with epidural infusions, *Prof Nurse* 16(10):1429, 2001.

Feldt K: The checklist of nonverbal pain indicators (CNPI), *Pain Manag Nurs* 1(1):35, 2000.

Guay D: Adjunctive agents in the management of chronic pain, *Pharmacotherapy* 21(9):1070, 2001.

Hall J: Epidural analgesia management, *Nurs Times* 96(28):38, 2000.

Hockenberry, MJ and others: *Wong's nursing care of infants and children,* ed 7, St Louis, 2003, Mosby.

Inyang A, Kaplan R: Patient-controlled analgesia in the home care setting, *Home Health Care Consultant* 6(10):19, 1999.

Krulewitch H and others.: Assessment of pain in cognitively impaired older adults: a comparison of pain assessment tools and their use by nonprofessional caregivers, *J Am Geriatr Soc* 48(12):1607, 2000.

Lasch K: Culture, pain, and culturally sensitive pain care, *Pain Manag Nurs* 1(3):S16, 2000.

Loeb J: Pain management in long-term care, *Am J Nurs* 99(2):48, 1999.

Melzack R, Wall P: Pain mechanisms: a new theory, *Science* 150:971, 1965.

Merskey H: Classification of chronic pain: description of chronic pain syndromes and definitions of pain terms, *Pain* 1986(Suppl 3):S217.

Miller M, Cosentino B: Epidural pain management, *Nurs Spect* 9(17):12, 2000.

Newshan G: Pain management in the addicted patient: practical considerations, *Nurs Outlook* 48(2):81, 2000.

Pasero C: Teaching patients how to use PCA, *Am J Nurs* 98(9):14, 1998.

Pasero C: Using continuous infusion with PCA, *Am J Nurs* 99(2):22, 1999.

Pasero C: Continuous local anesthetics, *Am J Nurs* 100(8):22, 2000.

Pasero C, McCaffery M: Reversing respiratory depression with naloxone, *Am J Nurs* 100(2):26, 2000.

Perin, M: Problems with propoxyphene, *Am J Nurs* 100(6):22, 2000.

Perron V, Schonwetter R: Assessment and management of pain in palliative care patients, *JMCC* 8(1):15, 2001.

Principles of analgesic use in the treatment of acute pain and cancer pain, ed 4, Glenview, Ill., 1999, American Pain Society.

Reiff P, Niziolek M: Troubleshooting tips for PCA, *RN* 64(4):33, 2001.

Waitman J: Meperidine—a liability, *Am J Nurs* 101(1):57, 2001.

Wentz J: Assessing pain in the cognitively impaired adult, *Nursing* 31(7):26, 2001.

Wood M: Advanced skills update: patient-controlled analgesia, *Prof Nurs* 15(6):404, 2000.

Wong D and others: *Whaley and Wong's essentials of pediatric nursing,* ed 6, St Louis, 1999, Mosby.

Wong DL, Hockenberry-Eaton M, Wilson D, Winkelstein ML, Schwartz P: *Wong's essentials of pediatric nursing,* ed 6, St Louis, 2001, Mosby.

Young-McCauthan S, Miaskowski C: Definition of and mechanism for opioid-induced sedation, *Pain Manag Nurs* 2(3):84, 2001.

Vital Signs

Temperature, pulse, respirations, and blood pressure (BP) are the vital signs, which indicate the body's ability to regulate body temperature, maintain blood flow, and oxygenate body tissues. Oxygen saturation is an additional vital sign obtained through pulse oximetry that reflects the ability of the cardiac and respiratory system to maintain adequate oxygenation. Measurement of temperature, pulse, respirations, BP, and oxygen saturation are obtained by the nurse. Recently the Joint Commission on Accreditation of Healthcare Organizations and pain management experts have advocated for making pain the fifth vital sign to ensure routine screening for pain (Lynch, 2001). Pain is the symptom most likely to lead clients to seek health care. A client's pain status is critical to understanding a client's state and progress. Chapter 11 summarizes pain assessment and interventions.

Vital signs indicate clients' responses to physical, environmental, and psychological stressors. Vital signs may reveal sudden changes in a client's condition. A change in one vital sign (e.g., pulse) can reflect changes in the other vital signs (temperature, respirations, BP, and oxygen saturation). The nurse's findings aid in determining whether it is necessary to assess specific body systems more thoroughly. The nurse must be able to measure vital signs correctly, to understand and interpret the values, to begin interventions as needed, and to report findings appropriately. Keeping clients informed of their vital signs promotes understanding of their health status.

Part of the nurse's clinical judgment involves deciding which vital signs to measure, when measurements should be made (Box 12-1), and when measurements can be safely delegated to assistive personnel (AP). For example, after assessing an abnormal respiratory rate, the nurse also auscultates lung sounds. In certain situations, vital sign assessment may be limited to measurement of a single vital sign for the purpose of monitoring a specific aspect of a client's condition. For example, after administering an antihypertensive medication, the nurse measures the client's BP to evaluate the drug's effect.

 ## TEMPERATURE

Body tissues and cell processes function best within a relatively narrow temperature range between 36° and 38° C (96.8° and 100.4° F). The temperature range of a normal adult depends on age, physical activity, status of hydration, and state of health, including the presence of infection (Table 12-1). Temperature fluctuates in a 24-hour cycle, being lowest between 1 and 4 AM, rising steadily throughout the day, and peaking at about 6 PM. Body temperature is physiologically regulated by vasodilatation, vasoconstriction, shivering, and sweating. A client's behavior can adjust body temperature by avoiding temperature extremes, adding or removing external clothing or coverings, and ingesting fluids and drugs. Average body temperature varies depending on the measurement site

---

Box 12-1

When to Take Vital Signs

1. On client's admission to a health care facility
2. In a hospital or care facility on a routine schedule according to a physician's order or institution's standards of practice
3. When assessing client during home health visits
4. Before and after a surgical or invasive diagnostic procedure
5. Before and after the administration of medications or application of therapies that affect cardiovascular, respiratory, and temperature-control functions
6. When the client's general physical condition changes (e.g., loss of consciousness or increased severity of pain)
7. Before and after nursing interventions influencing a vital sign (e.g., before and after a client previously on bed rest ambulates or before and after client performs range-of-motion exercises)
8. When the client reports specific symptoms of physical distress (e.g., feeling "funny" or "different")

Table 12-1

Vital Signs: Normal Ranges	
Vital Sign	**Normal Range**
Temperature	Range 36°-38° C; 98.6°-100.4° F
Oral/Tympanic	37.0° C; 98.6° F
Rectal	37.5° C; 99.5° F
Axillary	36.5° C; 97.7° F
Pulse	60-100 beats per minute, strong and regular
Respirations	Adult: 12-16 breaths per minute, deep and regular
Blood Pressure*	Systolic: less than 130 mm Hg Diastolic: less than 85 mm Hg Average BP 120/80 mm Hg
Pulse Pressure	30-50 mm Hg

*In some clients, BP is consecutively measured lying, sitting, and standing or in both arms. In normal individuals the change from lying to standing causes a decrease in systolic BP of less than 15 mm Hg (Barkauskas and others, 2002). Record the position and extremity, and compare the measurements for significant differences.

Table 12-2

Considerations for Frequently Selected Temperature Measurement Sites

Site Advantages	Site Limitations
Oral Site	
Easily accessible—requires no position change	Affected by ingestion of fluids or foods, smoke, and oxygen delivery
Comfortable for client	
Provides accurate surface temperature reading	Should not be used with clients who have had oral surgery, trauma, history of epilepsy, or shaking chills
Reflects rapid change in core temperature	
Shown to be reliable route to measure temperature in intubated clients.	Should not be used with infants, small children, or confused, unconscious, or uncooperative clients
	Risk of body fluid exposure
Tympanic Membrane Sensor	
Easily accessible site	Hearing aids must be removed before measurement
Minimal client repositioning required	Only one size sensor cover available
Provides accurate core reading because eardrum close to hypothalamus; sensitive to core temperature changes	Should not be used with clients who have had surgery of the ear or tympanic membrane
Can be obtained without disturbing, repositioning, or waking client	Does not accurately measure core temperature changes during and after exercise
Unaffected by oral intake of food, fluids, or smoking	Otitis media and cerumen impaction can distort readings
Can be used for clients with tachypnea without affecting breathing	
Can be used in newborns to reduce infant handling and heat loss (Bailey and Rose, 2001)	
Rectal Site	
Contended to be more reliable when oral temperature cannot be obtained	May lag behind core temperature during rapid temperature changes
	Should not be used with clients who have had rectal surgery, bleeding tendencies, or diarrhea
	Requires positioning and may be a source of client embarrassment and anxiety
	Risk of body fluid exposure
Axillary Site	
Safe and noninvasive	Not recommended to detect fever in infants and young children
Can be used with unconscious clients	Long measurement time (3 minutes)
	Requires continuous positioning by nurse
	Measurement lag behind core temperature during rapid temperature changes
	Requires exposure of thorax, which can result in temperature loss, especially in newborns
Skin	
Inexpensive	Lags behind other sites during temperature changes, especially during hyperthermia
Provides continuous reading	Can be affected by environmental temperature
Safe and noninvasive	Diaphoresis or sweat can impair adhesion

used. Each site and type of thermometer has unique techniques, contraindications, or limitations and norms (Table 12-2). The measurement of body temperature is aimed at obtaining a representative average of the core body tissues. Sites reflecting core temperatures include rectal, tympanic, esophageal, pulmonary artery, and urinary bladder. These sites tend to be more reliable indictors of body temperature than sites reflecting surface temperatures which are the skin, oral, and axillary sites. Several types of thermometers are commonly available to measure body temperature (Box 12-2). Temperature can be measured on a Celsius or Fahrenheit scale (Figure 12-1). Although some

Box 12-2

Types of Thermometers

ELECTRONIC THERMOMETERS

- A rechargeable battery-powered display unit with a thin wire cord and a temperature-processing probe covered by a disposable cover.
- Within 1 minute after placement, the thermometer displays a digital temperature reading.
- Separate probes are used for oral temperature measurement (blue tip) and rectal temperature measurement (red tip) (see illustration A).

TYMPANIC ELECTRONIC THERMOMETER

- The tympanic membrane reflects core body temperature because it shares its blood supply with the hypothalamus, the body's temperature-control center in the brain.
- The probe consists of an otoscope-like speculum with an infrared sensor tip that detects heat radiated from the tympanic membrane of the ear (see illustration B).
- Within 2 to 5 seconds after placement in the ear canal and depressing the scan button, a digital reading appears on the display unit. A sound signals when the peak temperature has been measured.

CHEMICAL DOT SINGLE-USE OR REUSABLE THERMOMETERS

- Thin strips of plastic with a temperature sensor at one end and chemically impregnated dots formulated to change color at different temperatures (see illustration C).
- Chemical dots on the thermometer change color to reflect temperature reading, usually within 60 seconds.
- Useful for screening temperatures, especially in infants and during invasive procedures.
- Not appropriate for measuring temperature in acutely ill clients or monitoring temperature therapies.
- Chemical dot thermometers may underestimate oral temperature by 0.4° C or more in 50% of adults (Erickson and others, 1996).

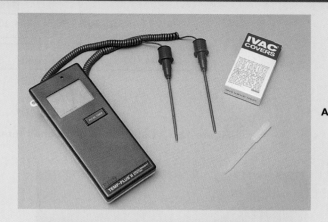

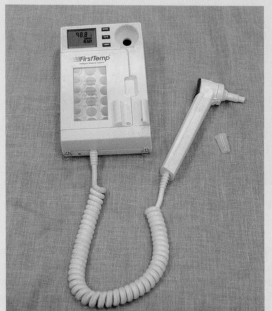

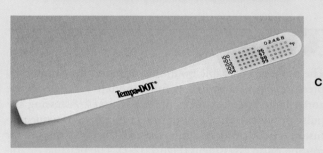

A, Electronic thermometer. Blue probe for oral or axillary use. Red probe for rectal use. B, Electronic tympanic thermometer. C, Chemical dot disposable single-use thermometer.

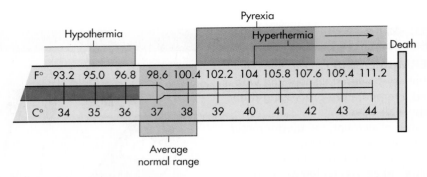

Figure 12-1 Celsius and Fahrenheit temperatures related to temperature ranges.

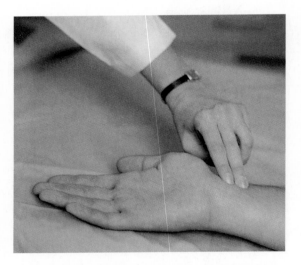

Figure 12-2 Palpating the right radial pulse.

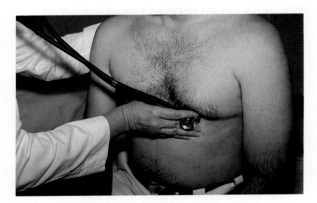

Figure 12-3 Assessing apical pulse.

electronic thermometers can display both Celsius and Fahrenheit readings, conversion charts are also available to convert from one system to the other. To ensure accuracy and client safety, each type of thermometer must be used correctly and appropriately.

PULSE

The pulse is a palpable bounding of blood flow caused by pressure wave transmission from the left ventricle to the aorta, large arteries, and peripheral arteries. Assessing the pulse provides indications of heart function and tissue perfusion (circulation). In adults the radial pulse is the site for routine pulse assessment (Figure 12-2). The brachial or apical pulse is the site for routine pulse assessment in infants.

The pulse should be easily palpable, regular in rhythm, and range between 60 and 100 beats per minute in adults. When palpated, a normal pulse does not fade in and out and is not easily obliterated by pressure. Pulse abnormalities include bradycardia (pulse less than 60 beats per minute), tachycardia (pulse greater than 100 beats per minute), and dysrhythmia (irregular pulse). *Weak, feeble,* and *thready* are de-

scriptive words for a pulse of low volume that is difficult to palpate. *Bounding* is the term used to describe a pulse that is easy to palpate. Strength (amplitude) of pulses may be rated by the following scale: 4+, bounding; 3+, full; 2+, normal; 1+, weak; 0, absent. Changes in the pulse can reflect the client's metabolic rate and physiological responses to stress, exercise, blood loss, and pain. If abnormalities are identified, such as an irregular rhythm or an inability to palpate the radial pulse, an apical pulse must be obtained (Figure 12-3). The apical pulse, the most accurate measure of heart rate and rhythm, is obtained using a stethoscope (see Chapter 13). Familiarity and practice using a stethoscope improve assessment skills (Box 12-3). The stethoscope magnifies the sounds as they are transmitted from the chest wall, through the tubing, to the listener. The apical pulse is auscultated (heard with a stethoscope) by placing the diaphragm over the point of maximum impulse at the fifth intercostal space on the left midclavicular line (Figure 12-4).

RESPIRATIONS

Movement of air between the environment and the lungs involves three interrelated processes: ventilation, which is mechanical movement of air in and out of the lungs; diffusion, which involves movement of respiratory gases (oxygen and carbon dioxide) between the alveoli and red

Box 12-3

Learning to Use a Stethoscope

1. Place earpieces in both ears with tips of earpieces turned toward the face. Lightly blow against the diaphragm (flat side of chestpiece). Now place the earpieces in both ears with the tips turned toward the back of the head, and again blow against the diaphragm. Compare comfort in the ears and amplification of sounds with earpieces in both directions. Most people find pointing earpieces toward the face more comfortable and effective.

2. If the stethoscope has both a diaphragm (flat side) and a bell (bowl shaped with a rubber ring) (see illustration below), put earpieces in ears and lightly blow against the diaphragm. The chestpiece can be turned to allow sound to be carried through either side (bell or diaphragm) of the chestpiece. If sound is faint, lightly blow into the bell. Then turn the chestpiece, and blow again against both the diaphragm and the bell. NOTE: The diaphragm is used for higher-pitched heart sounds, bowel sounds, and lung sounds. The bell is used for lower-pitched heart sounds and vascular sounds (see illustration below).

3. With earpieces in place and using the diaphragm, move the diaphragm lightly over the hair on your arm. The bristling sound mimics a sound heard in the lungs. When listening for significant sounds, hold the diaphragm firmly and still, eliminating extraneous sounds.

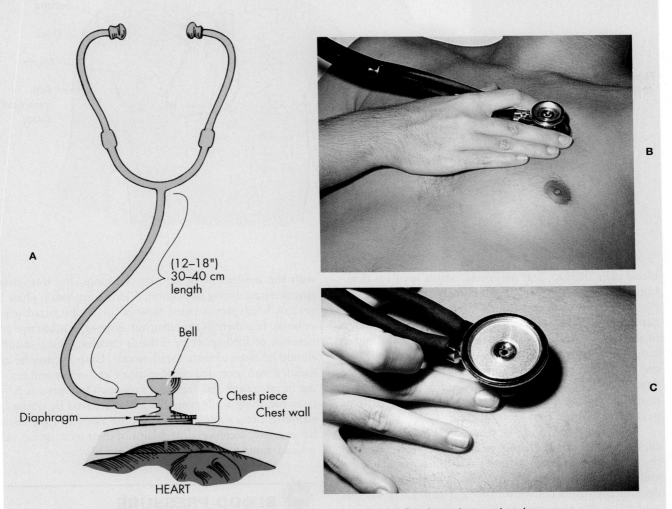

A, Parts of a stethoscope. B, The diaphragm is placed firmly and secretly when auscultating high-pitched lung and bowel sounds. C, The bell must be placed lightly on the skin to hear low-pitched vascular and heart sounds.

Continued

Learning to Use a Stethoscope—cont'd

4. Place the diaphragm over the front of your chest, and listen to your own breathing, comparing the bell and the diaphragm. Repeat the process while listening to your heartbeat. Ask someone to speak in a conversational tone, and note how the speech detracts from hearing clearly. When using a stethoscope, both the client and the examiner should remain quiet.

5. With the earpieces in your ears, gently tap tubing. Note that this also generates extraneous sounds. When listening to a client, maintain a position that allows tubing to extend straight and hang free. Movement may allow tubing to rub or bump objects, creating extraneous sounds. Kinked tubing muffles sounds.

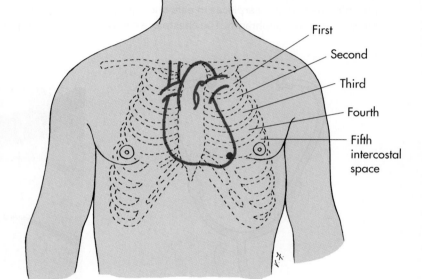

First
Second
Third
Fourth
Fifth intercostal space

Figure 12-4 Point of maximum impulse is at fifth intercostal space.

blood cells (RBCs); and perfusion, which involves distribution of blood through the pulmonary capillaries.

These processes are evaluated by observing the rate, depth, and rhythm of respiratory movements. Rate refers to the number of times the person breathes in and out in 1 minute. Depth of respirations is estimated by observing the movement of the chest during inspiration and can be described as deep or shallow. Rhythm of respirations is normally regular; however, irregular respiration patterns may occur (Table 12-3).

Breathing patterns can be determined by observing the chest or the abdomen. Diaphragmatic breathing results from the contraction and relaxation of the diaphragm and is most visible in the abdomen. Healthy men and children usually demonstrate diaphragmatic breathing (Figure 12-5), whereas women breathe more with the thorax, most apparent in the upper chest. Labored respirations usually involve the accessory muscles of respiration in the neck. The breathing cycle consists of a period of inspiration followed by a period of expiration. When something such as a foreign body interferes

with the movement of air into the lungs, the intercostal spaces retract during inspiration. A longer expiration phase is evident when the outward flow of air is obstructed (e.g., asthma). If a client is experiencing dyspnea, a subjective experience of inadequate or difficult breathing, lung sounds should be assessed with a stethoscope. Dyspnea may be associated with increased effort to inhale and exhale and active use of intercostal and accessory muscles. Orthopnea is difficulty breathing while lying flat and is relieved by sitting or standing. Lung sounds should also be assessed if the client has excessive secretions, complains of chest pain, or has sustained trauma to the chest (see Chapter 13).

 BLOOD PRESSURE

BP is the force exerted by the blood against the vessel walls. The systolic BP is the peak pressure occurring during the heart's contraction as blood is forced under high pressure into the aorta. The diastolic BP is the pressure present

Table 12-3

Alterations in Breathing Pattern

Alteration	Description	Alteration	Description
Bradypnea	Rate of breathing is regular but abnormally slow (less than 12 breaths per minute).	Cheyne-Stokes respiration	Respiratory rate and depth are irregular, characterized by alternating periods of apnea and hyperventilation. Respiratory cycle begins with slow, shallow breaths that gradually increase to abnormal rate and depth. The pattern reverses, and breathing slows and becomes shallow, climaxing in apnea before respiration resumes.
Tachypnea	Rate of breathing is regular but abnormally rapid (greater than 20 breaths per minute).	Kussmaul's respiration	Respirations are abnormally deep but regular.
Hyperpnea	Respirations are increased in depth. Hyperpnea occurs normally during exercise.	Biot's respiration	Respirations are abnormally shallow for two to three breaths followed by irregular period of apnea.
Apnea	Respirations cease for several seconds. Persistent cessation results in respiratory arrest.		
Hyperventilation	Rate and depth of respirations increase. Hypocarbia may occur.		
Hypoventilation	Respiratory rate is abnormally low, and depth of ventilation may be depressed. Hypercarbia may occur.		

when the ventricles are relaxed and the minimal pressure exerted against the arterial wall. The pulse pressure is the difference between the systolic and diastolic pressure. For a BP of 120/80, the pulse pressure is 40.

BP reflects many factors within the circulatory system, including cardiac output, peripheral resistance, blood volume, blood viscosity, and vessel wall elasticity. For example, a decreased cardiac output related to congestive heart failure or a low blood volume related to dehydration can result in a low BP. An increase in peripheral resistance related to stress or arteriosclerosis (loss of elasticity of the vessel walls) can result in a high BP. Drug therapy can decrease or increase BP by acting on any one or all of the factors regulating the circulatory system.

A diagnosis of hypertension in nonpregnant adults is made when an average of two or more diastolic readings on at least two subsequent visits is 90 mm Hg or higher or when the average of multiple systolic BP on two or more

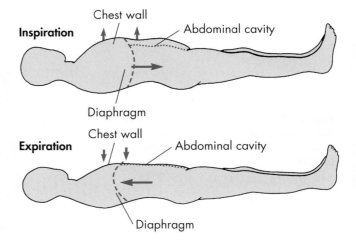

Figure 12-5   Illustration of a diaphragmatic and chest wall movement during inspiration and expiration.

subsequent visits is consistently higher than 140 mm Hg (National High Blood Pressure Education Program, 1997). One BP recording does not qualify as a diagnosis of hypertension. Over 50 million Americans have high BP, and hypertension is a major contributing factor for death, heart attack, and cerebrovascular accident (CVA, stroke) in the United States and Canada (Futterman and Lemberg, 2002). Factors that increase the risk of hypertension include obesity, increased sodium intake, smoking, and lack of exercise.

Two methods are available to determine BP: auscultatory and oscillometric. The ausculatatory method detects the sounds of the rush of blood (Korotkoff phases) as blood resumes its flow through the artery. The auscultatory method can be performed manually with the use of a sphygmomanometer and a stethoscope or electronically with an auscultatory BP machine. The electronic auscultatory BP machine uses a microphone to detect the Korotkoff phases.

A sphygmomanometer includes a pressure manometer, an occlusive cloth or vinyl cuff that encloses an inflatable rubber bladder, and a pressure bulb with a release valve that inflates the bladder. It can be portable or wall mounted (Figure 12-6). The manometer has a glass-enclosed circular gauge containing a needle that registers millimeter calibrations. The needle of the aneroid gauge should point to zero when not in use and move freely when the cuff pressure is released. The metal parts of an aneroid gauge are subject to temperature expansion and contraction; routine maintenance for calibration is required.

The cloth or disposable vinyl compression cuff of the sphygmomanometer contains an inflatable bladder. The cuff is placed around the arm or thigh. Cuffs come in several different sizes, and the BP measurement will not be accurate unless the correct size BP cuff is used (Figure 12-7). The cuff is quickly inflated until blood flow ceases. The cuff is slowly deflated while the aneroid needle begins to fall. Korotkoff phases are auscultated by placing the stethoscope over the artery distal to the BP cuff. In some clients, the sounds are clear and distinct, whereas in others, only the beginning and ending sounds are heard (Figure 12-8). The BP is recorded with the systolic and diastolic numbers written as a fraction. The systolic pressure is the first heart sound. Before the sounds cease, they may become distinctly muffled (second sound). The diastolic pressure is the last sound heard. In adults the systolic and diastolic BP readings are identified and recorded by the pressures corresponding to the first of two consecutive sounds heard and the disappearance of sounds (not muffling), respectively. Confirm the last sounds by continuing to listen for 10 to 20 mm Hg below the last sound heard. The nurse promotes

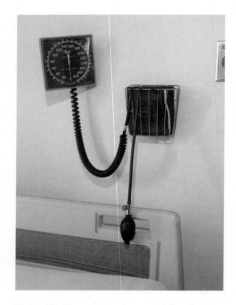

Figure 12-6   Wall-mounted aneroid sphygmomanometer.

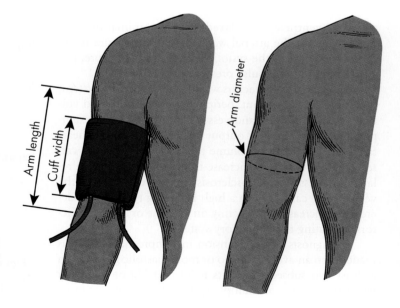

Figure 12-7   Proper cuff size: Width of cuff is 20% more than upper arm diameter, or 40% of arm circumference and two thirds of arm length.

accuracy in measurement by being aware of the various factors that influence accurate BP values when a stethoscope and sphygmomanometer are used (Table 12-4).

The oscillometric method of obtaining BP relies on an electronic sensor to detect the vibrations caused by the rush of blood through the artery. When the cuff is deflated, some oscillometric BP machines determine the initial burst of oscillations and translate the information into a systolic pressure reading. The diastolic measurement is made when the oscillations are lowest, just before they stop (Bridges and Middleton, 1997). Other oscillometric BP machines record the mean BP and compute systolic and diastolic BP from a programmed formula (Yucha, 2001).

Many different styles of auscultatory and oscillometric electronic BP machines are available to determine BP automatically (Figure 12-9). These devices are used when frequent BP assessment is required, such as in critically ill or potentially unstable clients, during or after invasive procedures, or when therapies require frequent monitoring (e.g., trials of new drugs). Electronic BP machines can be found in public areas such as shopping malls or in clients' homes. Although electronic BP machines are fast and free the nurse for other activities, they do have disadvantages. Auscultatory electronic BP machines are sensitive to external noise and are less

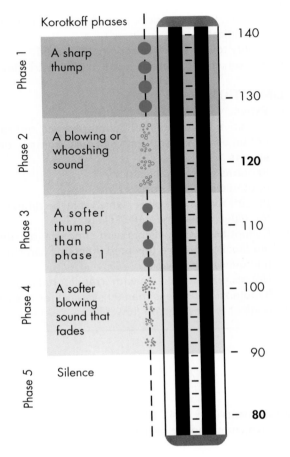

Korotkoff phases

Phase 1	A sharp thump	— 140
Phase 2	A blowing or whooshing sound	— 130 / **120**
Phase 3	A softer thump than phase 1	— 110
Phase 4	A softer blowing sound that fades	— 100 / — 90
Phase 5	Silence	**80**

Figure 12-8   Sounds auscultated during blood pressure measurement can be differentiated into five Korotkoff phases. In this example the blood pressure is 140/90.

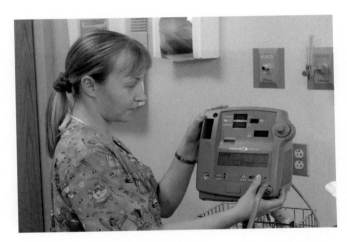

Figure 12-9   Electronic BP machines vary in appearance.

Table 12-4

Common Mistakes in Blood Pressure Assessment

Error	Effect
Bladder cuff too narrow	False-high reading
Cuff wrapped too loosely or unevenly	False-high reading
Deflating cuff too slowly	False-high diastolic reading
Arm below heart level	False-high reading
Arm not supported	False-high reading
Bladder cuff too wide	False-low reading
Deflating cuff too quickly	False-low systolic, false-high diastolic
Arm above heart level	False-low reading
Muffled sounds as a result of stethoscope that fits poorly or impairment of examiner's hearing	False-low systolic and false-high diastolic readings
Stethoscope applied too firmly against antecubital fossa	False-low diastolic reading
Repeating assessments too quickly	False-high systolic reading

Procedural Guideline 12-1

Obtaining Blood Pressure From Lower Extremity by Auscultation

Equipment: Stethoscope, sphygmomanometer, large-leg BP cuff, wide and long enough to allow for larger girth of thigh.

1. Assist client to prone position that provides the best access to the popliteal artery. If client is unable to assume prone position, assist client to supine position with knee slightly flexed.
2. Move aside bed linen and any constrictive clothing to ensure proper cuff application.
3. Locate and palpate the popliteal artery just below the thigh in the back of the knee in the popliteal space.
4. Apply BP cuff 2.5 cm (1 inch) above popliteal artery around middle thigh, centering arrows marked on BP cuff over the artery (see illustration). If there are no center arrows on the BP cuff, estimate the center of the cuff bladder and place this center over the artery.

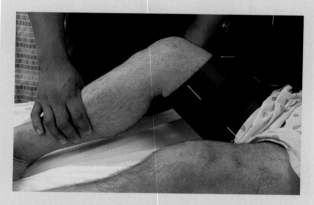

Lower extremity BP cuff positioned above popliteal artery at midthigh.

5. Obtain BP using auscultatory method. Systolic pressure in the legs is usually 10 to 40 mm Hg higher than the brachial artery, but the diastolic pressure is the same.

---

measurements (Box 12-4). The importance of accuracy in BP measurement cannot be overemphasized.

NURSING DIAGNOSES

Hyperthermia is the nursing diagnosis when a client's body temperature is above the upper range of normal (over 38° C or 100.4° F). Conversely, **Hypothermia** is the nursing diagnosis for a body temperature below the lower value of 36° C (96.8° F). **Risk for Imbalanced Body Temperature** is an appropriate nursing diagnosis for a client who demonstrates risk factors for hypothermia because the client is unable to maintain a body temperature within a normal range. Clients at risk include those at the extremes of age (older adults and the young) and the extremes in weight (obese and malnourished) and those with exposure to environmental extremes. Altered health status, including dehydration, infection, surgery, compromised neurological status, medication use, and alcohol consumption can affect body temperature. **Ineffective Thermoregulation** is an appropriate nursing diagnosis when an individual's body temperature fluctuates between hyperthermia and hypothermia. This may be related to ineffective temperature-regulating mechanisms.

---

precise on clients with obese upper extremities. (Anwar and White, 2001). Oscillometric electronic BP machines are less affected by external noise but cannot be used in clients who are shivering, have tremors, or have seizures. The oscillometric method may be less accurate in clients with high and low BP (Anwar and White, 2001). Any abnormal BP obtained by an electronic BP machine should be verified by obtaining a BP with the sphygmomanometer and stethoscope. The nurse must know the appropriate applications, advantages, and limitations of these devices to ensure accurate

Decreased Cardiac Output is manifested by decreased BP, decreased or irregular peripheral pulses, and/or difficulty breathing. Decreased cardiac output to meet body demands increases the **Risk for Activity Intolerance. Activity Intolerance** should be considered when an individual has insufficient energy to endure or complete required or desired daily activities.

Ineffective Airway Clearance is appropriate for clients who are unable to clear secretions or obstructions and maintain airway patency. **Ineffective Breathing Pattern** is appropriate when the client's rate, depth, and rhythm of respirations or chest and abdominal movements are not adequate for gas exchange to occur. Decreased energy, pain, musculoskeletal disease, or neurological dysfunction can contribute to ineffective breathing patterns.

Impaired Gas Exchange refers to altered oxygen or carbon dioxide exchange in the lungs or at the cellular level. The lowered oxygen level can be assessed by noting circumoral, nail bed, or mucous membrane cyanosis; tachycardia; dizziness; and mental confusion.

Ineffective Tissue Perfusion (cardiopulmonary, peripheral) should be considered when a client exhibits decreased pulses, cold extremities, and BP changes. A decreased BP, increased pulse rate, and increased body temperature can characterize a state of **Deficient Fluid Volume.** In this condition, clients have decreased body fluids from hemorrhage or failure of body regulatory mechanisms (e.g., diabetes insipidus). **Excess Fluid Volume** is noted by altered respirations, BP changes, and abnormal breath sounds (see Chapter 13).

Skill 12.1

Assessing Temperature, Pulse, Respirations, and Blood Pressure

The nurse routinely obtains a baseline measurement of vital signs at initial contact with a client to provide a means for comparison with subsequent vital sign values. This skill routinely includes temperature measurement with an electronic thermometer using the oral, rectal, or axillary sites; palpating the radial pulse; and auscultating an upper extremity BP.

ASSESSMENT

1. Consider normal daily fluctuations in vital signs. *Rationale: BP and body temperature tend to be lowest in early morning, peak in late afternoon, and gradually decline during the night. When temperatures are taken between 5 PM and 7 PM, fever is more accurately assessed.*

2. Identify medications or treatments that may influence vital signs. *Rationale: Antiarrhythmics, cardiotonics, antihypertensives, vasodilators, and vasoconstrictors affect BP and pulse rate. Antiinflammatory drugs, steroids, warming or cooling blankets, and fans affect temperature. Oxygen and bronchodilators affect respiratory assessment.*

3. Identify factors that influence vital signs. *Rationale: Exercise increases metabolism and heat production, resulting in increased temperature, pulse, respirations, and BP. Vital signs also tend to increase through hormonal and neural stimulation related to anxiety and pain.*

4. Identify factors likely to interfere with accuracy of vital signs. *Rationale: Oral temperature can be altered by intake of hot or cold food and fluid and by smoking. BP and pulse can be altered by caffeine and nicotine. Coffee increases BP within 15 minutes and can last up to 3 hours*

(Pickering, 2001). BP and pulse rate are immediately increased by smoking, which lasts up to 15 minutes (Pickering, 2001).

5. Identify conditions that influence BP. *Rationale: High BP is associated with pain, rapid intravenous (IV) infusion of fluids or blood products, increased intracranial pressure, cardiovascular disease, and renal disease. Low BP is associated with rapid vasodilation, shock, hemorrhage, and dehydration.*

6. Assess pertinent laboratory values, including complete blood count (CBC) and arterial blood gases (ABGs). *Rationale: Low values for hemoglobin, hematocrit, and RBC count are associated with decreased oxygen transport to tissues and hypoxia. ABG levels reflect adequacy of oxygenation and ventilation. Low hemoglobin levels, decreased oxygenation, and decreased ventilation can increase pulse rate, BP readings, and respiratory rate. A WBC count greater than 12,000/mm³ in a nonpregnant adult suggests the presence of infection, which can lead to hyperthermia; a WBC count less than 5000/mm³ suggests that the body's ability to fight infection is compromised, which can lead to ineffective thermoregulation.*

7. Determine previous baseline vital signs from client's record. *Rationale: This allows the nurse to assess for change in condition by comparing future vital sign measurements.*

8. Determine appropriate temperature site for client, considering advantages and disadvantages of each site (see Table 12-2, p. 266).

9. Determine BP device most appropriate for client. *Rationale: Electronic BP device can be used when frequent measurements are required.*

PLANNING

Expected outcomes focus on identifying abnormalities and restoring homeostasis.

Expected Outcomes

1. Client's vital signs are within normal range for client's age group.
2. Client identifies factors that influence vital signs.
3. A baseline must be established for clients with chronic diseases that alter vital signs such as arteriosclerosis.
4. Client states strategies to reduce personal risk factors for hypertension.

Equipment

- Thermometer (select based on site used, see Table 12-2, p. 266)
- Disposable probe covers
- Water-soluble lubricant (for rectal measurements only)
- Stethoscope
- Sphygmomanometer
- BP cuff of appropriate size
- Alcohol swab
- Watch that displays seconds
- Vital signs flow sheet

Delegation Considerations

The skill of vital sign measurements for stable clients can be delegated to assistive personnel (AP) with instructions including:

- Appropriate route and device for assigned client to measure temperature.
- Restrictions for limb to be used for BP measurement.
- Appropriate-size BP cuff for designated extremity.
- Frequency of specific vital sign measurements.
- To report any significant changes or abnormalities to the nurse.

IMPLEMENTATION FOR ASSESSING TEMPERATURE, PULSE, RESPIRATIONS, AND BLOOD PRESSURE

Steps	Rationale
1. See Standard Protocol (inside front cover).	
2. Assist client to comfortable position either lying or sitting. When obtaining BP, avoid injured arm or one with IV infusion, previous breast or axilla surgery, cast, or arteriovenous shunt for renal dialysis.	Good circulation facilitates accuracy in BP measurement. BP measurement temporarily disrupts circulation.
3. **Oral temperature**	
a. Remove thermometer pack from charging unit; attach oral (blue tip) probe to thermometer unit. Grasp top of probe stem, being careful not to apply pressure on the ejection button. Slide disposable plastic probe cover over thermometer probe stem until cover locks in place (see illustration).	Ejection button releases plastic cover from probe.
b. Ask client to open mouth; then gently place thermometer probe under tongue in posterior sublingual pocket lateral to center of lower jaw (see illustration). Ask client to hold thermometer with lips closed.	Heat from superficial blood vessels in sublingual pocket produces temperature reading. With electronic thermometer, temperatures in right and left posterior sublingual pockets are significantly higher than in area under front of tongue.
c. Leave thermometer probe in place until audible signal indicates completion and client's temperature appears on digital display; remove thermometer probe from under client's tongue. Inform client of temperature reading, and record measurement.	Ensures accurate reading.
d. Inform client of temperature reading. Push ejection button on thermometer probe stem to discard plastic cover into an appropriate receptacle. Return thermometer stem to storage position of thermometer unit. Return thermometer to charger.	Returning thermometer stem automatically causes digital reading to disappear. Charger maintains battery charge of unit.

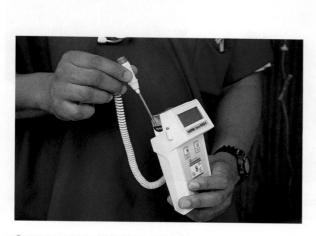

Step 3a Inserting thermometer stem in to plastic probe cover.

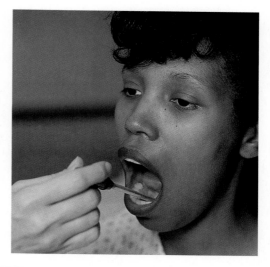

Step 3b Probe under tongue in posterior sublingual pocket.

Steps	**Rationale**

NURSE ALERT *If temperature is abnormal, repeat measurement. If indicated, select an alternative site or instrument.*

4. **Tympanic temperature**
   a. Assist client in assuming a comfortable position with head turned toward side, away from nurse.

   b. Remove thermometer handheld unit from charging base, being careful not to apply pressure to the ejection button. Slide disposable speculum cover over otoscope-like tip until it locks in place. Be careful not to touch lens cover.

   c. If holding handheld unit with right hand, obtain temperature from client's right ear; left-handed persons should obtain temperature from client's left ear.

   d. For an adult, pull ear pinna back, up, and out to straighten the external auditory canal. Note an obvious presence of earwax in the client's ear canal; if present, switch to other ear or choose alternate site.

   e. Pointing toward the nose, insert speculum into ear canal snugly to seal the ear canal from ambient air temperature. Some manufacturers recommend moving the speculum in a rocking or figure-eight pattern to scan the tympanic membrane. Refer to manufacturer's instructions for each instrument.

   f. As soon as the probe is in place, depress scan button on handheld unit. Leave thermometer probe in place until audible signal occurs and client's temperature appears on digital display (see illustration).

   g. Carefully remove speculum from auditory meatus. Push ejection button on thermometer stem to discard speculum cover into appropriate receptacle.

Rationale:

- Facilitates visualization of the ear canal.

- Dust, fingerprints, or earwax on lens can impede optical pathway.

- Facilitates correct angle of approach for a better probe position and seal.

- Allows maximum exposure of the tympanic membrane.

- Signal indicates infrared energy has been detected.

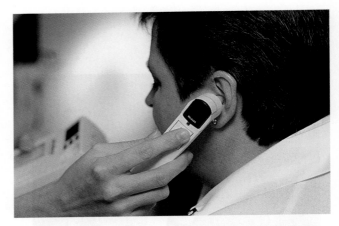

Step 4f   Tympanic membrane thermometer with probe cover positioned in client's ear.

Steps	Rationale

h. If temperature is abnormal, repeat measurement in other ear, or wait 2 to 3 minutes to repeat in same ear. Consider an alternate site or instrument.

i. Inform client of temperature reading. Return handheld unit to charging base, which will cause digital reading to disappear and protect sensor tip from damage.

5. Rectal temperature

a. Draw curtain around bed and/or close room door. Assist client to Sims' position with upper leg flexed. Move aside bed linen to expose only anal area. Keep client's upper body and lower extremities covered with sheet or blanket.

    Maintains client's privacy, minimizes embarrassment, and promotes comfort.

b. Remove thermometer pack from charging unit, and attach rectal (red tip) probe to thermometer unit. Grasp top of probe stem, being careful not to apply pressure on the ejection button. Slide disposable plastic probe cover over thermometer probe stem until cover locks in place.

    Ejection button releases plastic cover from probe.

c. Squeeze liberal portion of lubricant on tissue. Dip thermometer probe end into lubricant, covering 2.5 to 3.5 cm (1 to 1½ inches) for adult.

    Lubrication minimizes trauma to rectal mucosa during insertion. Tissue avoids contamination of remaining lubricant in container.

d. With nondominant hand, separate client's buttocks to expose anus. Ask client to breathe slowly and relax.

    Relaxes anal sphincter for easier thermometer insertion.

e. Gently insert thermometer into anus in direction of umbilicus 3.5 cm (1½ inches) for adult. Do not force thermometer. If resistance is felt during insertion, withdraw thermometer immediately.

f. Hold thermometer probe in place until audible signal occurs and client's temperature appears on digital display; remove thermometer probe from anus.

    Probe must stay in place until signal occurs to ensure accurate reading.

g. Push ejection button on thermometer probe stem to discard plastic cover into appropriate receptacle. Return thermometer stem to storage position of thermometer unit.

    Returning thermometer stem automatically causes digital reading to disappear.

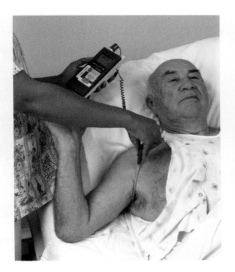
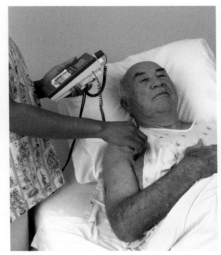

Step 6c   Thermometer tip in axilla.

Steps	Rationale

h. Wipe client's anal area with soft tissue to remove lubricant or feces. Discard tissue and remove gloves.

i. Inform client of temperature reading, and record measurement. Return thermometer to charger.

Maintains battery charge.

6. Axillary temperature

a. Draw curtain around bed and/or close room door. Assist client to supine or sitting position, and move clothing or gown away from shoulder and arm.

Maintains client's privacy, minimizes embarrassment, and promotes comfort. Exposes axilla for correct thermometer probe placement.

b. Remove thermometer pack from charging unit; attach oral (blue tip) probe to thermometer unit. Grasp top of thermometer probe stem, being careful not to apply pressure on the ejection button. Slide disposable plastic probe cover over thermometer stem until cover locks in place.

Ejection button releases plastic cover from probe.

c. Raise client's arm away from torso; dry axilla if excess perspiration is present; insert thermometer probe into center of axilla, lower arm over thermometer, and place arm across client's chest (see illustrations).

Maintains proper placement of thermometer against blood vessels in axilla.

NURSE ALERT *In an infant or young child it may be necessary to hold the arm against the child's side when using the axillary method. If infant is in a side-lying position, the lower axilla will record the higher temperature.*

---

d. Hold thermometer in place until audible signal occurs and client's temperature appears on digital display; remove thermometer probe from axilla. Inform client of temperature reading, and record measurement.

Probe must stay in place until signal occurs to ensure accurate reading.

e. Push ejection button on thermometer probe stem to discard plastic cover into appropriate receptacle. Return thermometer probe stem to storage position of thermometer unit. Return thermometer to charger.

Returning thermometer stem automatically causes digital reading to disappear. Maintains battery charge.

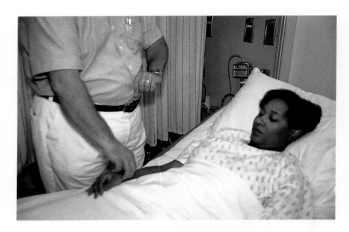

Step 7a   Client position during pulse assessment.

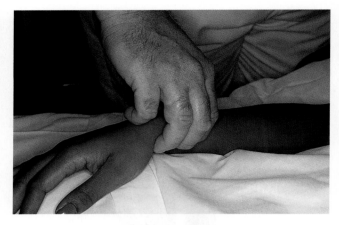

Step 7b   Fingers of hand over radial groove.

Steps	Rationale
7. Pulse	
a. If client is supine, place client's forearm straight alongside or across lower chest or upper abdomen with wrist extended straight (see illustration). If sitting, bend client's elbow 90 degrees and support lower arm on chair or on nurse's arm. Slightly extend or flex the client's wrist with palm down until strongest pulse is felt.	Relaxed position of lower arm and extension of wrist permits full exposure of artery to palpation.
b. Place tips of first two or middle three fingers of hand over groove along the radial or thumb side of the client's inner wrist (see illustration).	Fingertips are most sensitive parts of hand to palpate arterial pulsation. Nurse's thumb has pulsation that may interfere with accuracy.
c. Lightly compress against radius, obliterate pulse initially, and then relax pressure so pulse becomes easily palpable.	
d. Determine strength of pulse. Note whether thrust of vessel against fingertips is bounding, strong, weak, or thready.	
e. After pulse can be felt regularly, look at watch's second hand and begin to count rate; when sweep hand hits number on dial, start counting with zero, then one, two, and so on.	Rate is determined accurately only after nurse is assured pulse can be palpated. Timing begins with zero. Count of one is first beat palpated after timing.
If pulse is regular, count rate for 30 seconds and multiply total by 2.	It requires 30 seconds to discern if the pulse is regular in rhythm.
If pulse is irregular, count rate for 60 seconds. Assess frequency and pattern of irregularity.	Inefficient contraction of heart fails to transmit pulse wave, interfering with cardiac output, resulting in irregular pulse. Longer time period ensures more accurate count.

NURSE ALERT   *If pulse is irregular, assess for a pulse deficit. Count apical pulse (see Chapter 13) while colleague counts radial pulse. Begin apical pulse, initiating counting by a signal to simultaneously assess pulses for a full minute. If pulse count differs by more than 2 beats per minute, a pulse deficit exists, which may indicate alteration in cardiac output.*

---

8. Respirations	
a. Without changing the position of your hand on the pulse, observe one complete respiratory cycle (one inspiration and one expiration) (see illustration).	Maintaining the same position keeps client from being aware that you are counting respirations. Inconspicuous assessment prevents client from consciously or unintentionally altering rate and depth of breathing. Viewing an entire respiratory cycle promotes accurate measurement.

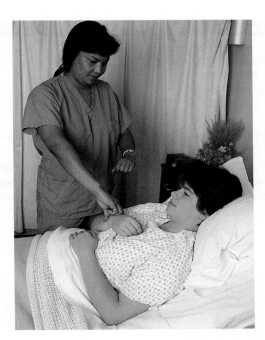

Step 8a Assessing respirations after pulse count.

Steps	Rationale
b. After cycle is observed, look at watch's second hand and begin to count rate; when sweep hand hits number on dial, begin time frame, counting one with first full respiratory cycle.	Timing begins with count of one. Respirations occur more slowly than pulse; thus timing does not begin with zero.
c. If rhythm is regular, count number of respirations in 30 seconds and multiply by 2. If rhythm is irregular, less than 12 respirations per minute, or greater than 20 respirations per minute, count for 1 full minute.	Respiratory rate is equivalent to number of respirations per minute. Suspected irregularities require assessment for at least 1 minute (see Table 12-3, p. 271).
d. Note depth of respirations, subjectively assessed by observing degree of chest wall movement while counting rate. Nurse can also objectively assess depth by palpating chest wall or auscultating the posterior chest during respiratory excursion (see Chapter 13) after rate has been counted. Depth is shallow, normal, or deep.	Characteristics of ventilation may reveal specific disease state, restricting volume of air from moving into and out of the lungs.

NURSE ALERT *Position of discomfort may cause client to breathe more rapidly. Respiratory rate less than 12 breaths per minute or greater than 20 breaths per minute and shallow and slow respirations (hypoventilation) may require immediate intervention.*

---

e. Note rhythm of ventilation. Normal breathing is regular and uninterrupted. Sighing should not be confused with abnormal rhythm. Periodically people unconsciously take single deep breaths or sighs to expand small airways prone to collapse.	
f. Observe for evidence of dyspnea (increased effort to inhale and exhale). Ask client to describe subjective experience of shortness of breath compared with usual breathing pattern.	Clients with chronic lung disease may experience difficulty breathing all the time and can best describe their own discomfort from shortness of breath.

Steps	Rationale

NURSE ALERT *Occasional periods of apnea are a symptom of underlying disease in the adult and must be reported to the physician or nurse in charge. Irregular respirations and short episodes of apnea are normal in a newborn.*

---

9. **Manual auscultation of upper extremity BP**

    a. Determine the best site for BP assessment. Avoid applying cuff to extremity when IV fluids are being infused; when an arteriovenous shunt or fistula is present; when breast or axillary surgery has been performed on that side; or when extremity has been traumatized, diseased, or requires a cast or bulky bandage. The lower extremities may be used when the brachial arteries are inaccessible (see Procedural Guideline 12-1).

    Inappropriate site selection may result in poor amplification of sounds, causing inaccurate readings. Application of pressure from inflated bladder temporarily impairs blood flow and can further compromise circulation in extremity that already has impaired blood flow.

    b. Select appropriate cuff size (see Figure 12-7, p. 272).

    Improper cuff size results in inaccurate readings (see Table 12-4, p. 273). If cuff is too small, it results in false-high readings and tends to come loose as it is inflated. If the cuff is too large, false-low readings may be recorded.

    c. Expose upper arm by removing restrictive clothing.

    Ensures proper cuff application. Tight clothing causes congestion of blood and can falsely elevate BP readings.

    d. With client sitting or lying, position client's forearm, supported, with palm turned up at level of the heart (see illustration).

    If arm is unsupported, client performs isometric exercise that can increase diastolic pressure 10%. Placement of arm above the level of the heart causes false-low reading. Placement of arm lower than the level of the heart causes false-high readings.

NURSE ALERT *Client should be seated or lying in a quiet environment, free from temperature extremes, for at least 5 minutes before BP is obtained. Eliminate extraneous noise, such as television and conversation. Noise interferes with accuracy. Falsely elevated readings will be obtained if client moves, talks, or coughs during BP measurement (Pickering, 2001).*

---

    e. Palpate brachial artery (see illustrations).

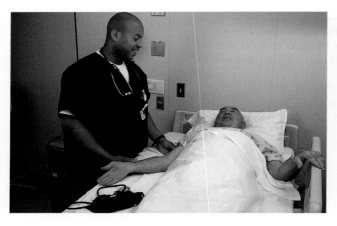

Step 9d Client's forearm supported in bed.

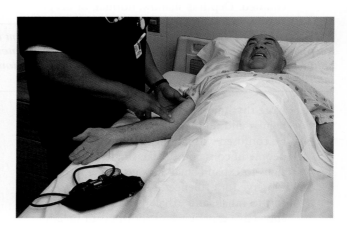

Step 9e Palpating the brachial artery.

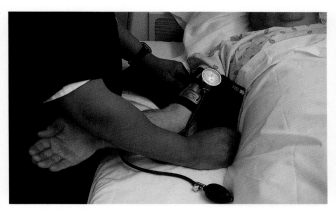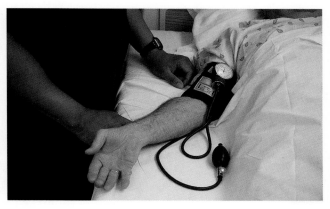

Step 9f   A, Center bladder of cuff above artery. **B,** Blood pressure cuff wrapped around upper arm.

Steps	Rationale
f. Position cuff 2.5 cm (1 inch) above site of brachial pulsation (antecubital space). Apply bladder of cuff above artery by centering arrows marked on cuff over artery. If there are not any center arrows on cuff, estimate the center of the bladder and place this point over artery (see illustration). With cuff fully deflated, wrap cuff evenly and snugly around upper arm (see illustration).	Inflating bladder directly over brachial artery ensures proper pressure is applied during inflation. Loose-fitting cuff causes false-high readings.
g. Position manometer gauge vertically at eye level. Observer should be no farther than 1 m (approximately 1 yard) away.	Ensures accurate reading.
h. If you do not know client's baseline BP, estimate systolic pressure. Palpate the brachial or radial artery with fingertips of one hand while inflating cuff rapidly to pressure 30 mm Hg above point at which pulse disappears. Slowly deflate cuff, and note point when pulse reappears.	Estimating prevents false-low readings, which may result from the presence of an auscultatory gap (inaudible sounds below the actual systolic pressure). This phenomenon occurs in about 5% of adults and is prevalent in individuals with hypertension.
i. Deflate cuff fully, and wait 30 seconds.	Deflating cuff prevents venous congestion and false-high readings.
j. Place stethoscope earpieces in ears.	
k. Relocate brachial artery, and place bell or diaphragm chestpiece of stethoscope lightly over it. Do not allow chestpiece to touch cuff or clothing (see illustration).	Excess pressure results in falsely low diastolic BP readings.
l. Close valve of pressure bulb clockwise until tight.	
m. Rapidly inflate cuff to 30 mm Hg above palpated systolic pressure.	Rapid inflation ensures accurate reading.
n. Slowly release pressure bulb valve, and allow needle to fall at rate of 2 to 3 mm Hg/sec. Make sure there are no extraneous sounds at this point (see illustration).	Too rapid or slow a decline in pressure can cause inaccurate readings. Noise interferes with precise hearing of Korotkoff phases.

NURSE ALERT *If you hear sounds immediately, release the pressure, wait 60 seconds, and estimate systolic pressure at higher reading. Reinflate the cuff to 30 mm Hg above the sound first heard. Reinflation of a partially deflated cuff is uncomfortable for client and may render an inaccurate reading.*

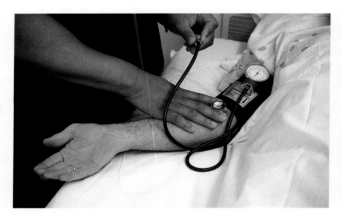

Step 9k Stethoscope over brachial artery to measure BP.

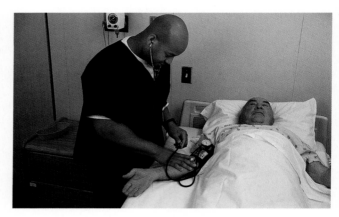

Step 9n Auscultating blood pressure.

Steps	Rationale
o. Note point on manometer when first clear sound is heard. The sounds will slowly increase in intensity.	First Korotkoff phase reflects systolic BP.
p. Continue to deflate cuff gradually, noting point at which sound disappears in adults. Note pressure to nearest 2 mm Hg. Listen for 10 to 20 mm Hg after the last sound, and then allow remaining air to escape quickly.	Beginning of the fifth Korotkoff phase is an indication of diastolic pressure in adults. The fourth Korotkoff phase involves distinct muffling of sounds, and in children it is recorded as the diastolic pressure.
q. If this is first assessment of client, repeat procedure on other arm.	Comparison of BP in both arms detects circulatory problems. (Normal difference of 5 to 10 mm Hg exists between arms.)
r. Remove cuff from client's arm unless measurement must be repeated.	Continuous cuff inflation causes arterial occlusion, resulting in numbness and tingling of client's arm.
s. Record readings from both arms. Use arm with highest BP measurement for all subsequent BP recordings.	
t. Inform client of the BP. If possible, discuss risk factors for high BP. If BP is elevated, inquire as to any factors that may have affected BP, including general health, life stress, or diet changes. If client takes BP medication, determine if anything has interfered with prescribed regimen.	

COMMUNICATION TIP *This is a good time to discuss with client the benefits of exercise and weight control in reducing the risks for hypertension and coronary artery disease or lowering an existing BP elevation.*

---

10. See Completion Protocol (inside front cover).

• • • • • • • • • •

EVALUATION

1. Compare vital signs with client's baseline and normal expected ranges.
2. Ask client to identify factors that influence vital signs.
3. Identify a baseline for clients with chronic diseases that alter vital signs.
4. Ask client to describe changes in vital signs related to therapies (e.g., ambulation, medications).

Unexpected Outcomes and Related Interventions

1. Client has a temperature 1° C or more above normal range.
   a. Assess for additional related data suggesting systemic infection, including loss of appetite; headache; hot, dry skin; flushed face; thirst; general malaise; or chills.
   b. Further assess for possible site of localized infection, including pain or tenderness, purulent drainage, redness, or area of unusual warmth.

c. Increase fluid intake to at least 3 L daily (unless contraindicated by client's condition).

d. Control environmental temperature at 21° to 27° C (70° to 80° F).

e. Reduce external covering on client's body to promote heat loss. Do not induce shivering.

f. Keep clothing and bed linen dry.

g. Limit physical activity and sources of emotional stress.

h. Initiate measures to stimulate appetite and provide nutrients to meet increased energy needs (see Chapter 8).

i. Encourage oral hygiene because oral mucous membranes dry easily from dehydration (see Chapter 7).

j. Implement measures to determine etiology of fever; for example, obtain necessary culture specimens for laboratory analysis (e.g., urine, blood, sputum, and wound sites) (see Chapter 14).

k. Implement measures to prevent or control spread of infection; for example, pulmonary hygiene and postural drainage (see Chapter 31), wound care (see Chapter 22), and adequate urinary elimination (see Chapter 9).

l. If fever persists or reaches unacceptable level as defined by physician, administer antipyretics and antibiotics as ordered and apply hypothermia blanket.

2. Client has a temperature 1° C or more below normal range.

a. Cover client with warm blankets.

b. Close room doors or windows to eliminate drafts.

c. Encourage warm liquids.

d. Hyperthermia blankets may be ordered by the physician.

e. Remove wet clothes, and replace with dry garments.

f. Monitor apical pulse rate and rhythm (see Chapter 13), because hypothermia may cause bradycardia, cardiac dysrhythmias, and electrolyte imbalances.

3. Client has a weak or difficult-to-palpate radial pulse.

a. Assess both radial pulses, and compare findings. Local obstruction to peripheral blood flow (e.g., clot or edema of hand and wrist) may cause pulse to be difficult to palpate.

b. Have another nurse assess pulse.

c. Perform complete assessment of all peripheral pulses (see Chapter 13).

d. Observe for symptoms associated with altered peripheral tissue perfusion, including pallor or cyanosis of tissue distal to pulse and cold extremities.

e. Auscultate the apical pulse to determine a pulse deficit (see Chapter 13).

f. Observe for factors associated with a decrease in cardiac output that result in diminished peripheral pulses, such as hemorrhage, hypothermia, or heart muscle damage.

4. Client has pulse greater than 100 beats per minute (tachycardia).

a. Identify related data, including pain, fear or anxiety, recent exercise, low BP, blood loss, elevated temperature, or inadequate oxygenation.

b. Observe for symptoms associated with abnormal cardiac function, including dyspnea, fatigue, chest pain, orthopnea, syncope, palpitations (unpleasant awareness of pulse), jugular vein distention, edema of dependent body parts, cyanosis, or pallor of skin (see Chapter 13).

5. Client has pulse less than 60 beats per minute (bradycardia).

a. Auscultate the apical pulse (see Chapter 13).

b. Observe for factors that may alter heart rate and regularity, including medications such as digoxin and antiarrhythmics; it may be necessary to withhold prescribed medications until the physician can evaluate the need to alter the dosage.

6. Client has irregular rhythm.

a. Auscultate the apical pulse (see Chapter 13), and identify the pattern of irregularity. Assess for the presence of a pulse deficit.

b. Clients with an irregular rhythm may require an electrocardiogram (ECG) or 24-hour heart monitor per physician's order to detect heart abnormalities.

7. Client has abnormal respiratory rate, depth, or pattern of dyspnea with complaints of feeling short of breath.

a. Observe for related factors, including obstructed airway; noisy respirations; cyanosis of nail beds, lips, mucous membranes, and skin; restlessness; irritability; confusion; dyspnea (labored breathing); shortness of breath; productive cough; and abnormal breath sounds (see Chapter 13).

b. Consider possible effects of anesthesia or medications such as narcotic analgesics (pain relievers).

c. Assist client to a supported sitting position (semi-Fowler's or high-Fowler's unless contraindicated), which improves ability to take a deep breath.

d. Provide oxygen as ordered by physician (see Skill 31.1, p. 748) if client exhibits signs or symptoms of respiratory distress.

8. Client has elevated BP, as evidenced by pressure greater than 140 mm Hg systolic or 90 mm Hg diastolic. NOTE: A diagnosis of hypertension involves two or more elevated readings on separate occasions.

a. Assess BP in other arm and compare findings. Recheck or have another nurse recheck readings.

b. Observe for related symptoms. Often symptoms are not apparent unless BP is extremely high. Client may have a headache (usually occipital), flushing of face, or nosebleed; older adult client may notice fatigue.

c. Be certain size of cuff is appropriate. A cuff that is too small gives false-high readings. Recheck or have another nurse recheck readings.

d. Administer antihypertensive medication as ordered. If none is ordered, report BP to initiate appropriate evaluation and treatment.

9. Client is hypotensive when BP is not sufficient for adequate perfusion and oxygenation of tissues.

a. Compare to baseline. A systolic reading of 90 may be normal for some persons and cause no ill effects.

b. Observe for symptoms associated with hypotension related to decreased cardiac output, which include tachycardia; weak, thready pulse; weakness, dizziness, or confusion; pale, dusky, or cyanotic skin; or cool, mottled skin over extremities.

c. Position client in supine position to enhance circulation, and restrict activity that may drop BP further.

d. Increase rate of IV infusion, or administer vaso-constricting drugs if ordered.

e. Observe for factors that would contribute to a low BP such as hemorrhage, dilation of blood vessels resulting from hyperthermia or anesthesia, and medication side effects.

10. Client BP is inaudible or difficult to obtain.

a. Determine that no immediate crisis is present by obtaining respiratory rate and pulse rate.

b. Implement palpation method to obtain systolic BP (see Procedural Guideline 12-2).

c. Use an ultrasonic Doppler instrument to obtain BP.

d. Auscultate BP in lower extremity (see Procedural Guideline 12-1, p. 274).

Recording and Reporting

- Record vital signs promptly on vital sign flow sheet (see Appendix A), computer database, or nurses' notes. Record associated findings and related factors in narrative from nurses' notes.
- Record position of client, pulse, and method and site of BP and temperature measurements.
- Report abnormal findings to nurse in charge or physician.

Sample Documentation

2300 BP 104/56 right arm, supine, dropping from baseline of 124/72. Tachycardia noted with radial pulse 112, weak and thready. Respirations 24 and regular. Temperature 36.8° C tympanic. Reports dizziness. Skin pale. Client denies dyspnea, nausea, or pain. Physician notified. Orders received.

SPECIAL CONSIDERATIONS

Pediatric Considerations

- Axillary temperature cannot be relied on to detect fevers in infants and young children.
- Temperature is best taken as the last vital sign with children who cry or become restless.
- Children often have a sinus dysrhythmia, which is an irregular heart beat that speeds up with inspiration and slows down with expiration. Breath holding in a child affects pulse rate.
- Acceptable average respiratory rate for newborns is 35 to 40 breaths per minute; infant (6 months) is 30 to 50 breaths per minute; toddler (2 years) is 25 to 32 breaths per minute; and child is 20 to 30 breaths per minute.
- Infant's respirations are primarily diaphragmatic and best observed by abdominal movement.
- Infants tend to breathe less regularly.
- BP is not a routine part of assessment in children under 3 years.
- Average width of BP cuff bladder for infant is 2.4 to 3.2 inches; for child, cuff bladder is 4.8 to 5.4 inches.

Geriatric Considerations

- Temperatures considered within normal range may reflect a fever in an older adult.
- Older adults are very sensitive to slight changes in temperature.
- Adults who wear dentures and who do not have them in place or older adults with muscle weakness may be unable to close their mouth tightly enough to obtain accurate oral temperature readings.
- A decrease in sweat gland reactivity in the older adult results in higher threshold for sweating at high temperatures, which can lead to hyperthermia (Maas and others, 2001).
- Older adults are at high risk for hypothermia because of diminished sensation to cold, abnormal vasoconstrictor responses, and impaired shivering.
- With aging, a loss of subcutaneous fat reduces the insulating capacity of the skin.
- With aging, cerumen is drier and cilia become coarse and stiff, contributing to the buildup of cerumen. It is estimated that one third or more of older adults may have occlusive amounts of cerumen in one or both ear canals that affects tympanic temperature.

Geriatric Considerations—cont'd

- Once elevated, the pulse rate of an older adult takes longer to return to normal resting rate (Lueckenotte, 2000).
- Depth of respirations tends to decrease with aging.
- A change in lung function with aging results in respiratory rates that are generally higher in older adults with a normal of 16 to 25 breaths per minute (Lueckenotte, 2000).
- Older adults, especially the frail elderly, who have lost upper arm mass, require special attention to selection of smaller BP cuff.
- Skin of older adults is more fragile and susceptible to cuff pressure when BP measurements are frequent. More frequent assessment of skin under cuff or rotation of BP sites is recommended.
- Older adults have an increase in systolic pressure related to decreased vessel elasticity (Lueckenotte, 2000).
- Older adults often experience a fall in BP after eating.
- Older adults are instructed to change position slowly and wait after each change to avoid postural hypotension and to prevent injuries.

- It is often difficult to palpate the pulse of an older adult or obese client. A Doppler device provides a more accurate reading.
- The arteries of an older adult may feel stiff and knotty because of atherosclerosis and decreased elasticity.

Home Care Considerations

- Assess temperature and ventilation of environment to determine existence of any conditions that may influence client's temperature.
- Assess home noise level to determine the room that will provide the quietest environment for assessing BP.
- Assess family's financial ability to afford a sphygmomanometer for performing BP evaluations on a regular basis.
- Consider an electronic BP cuff with large digital display for home if client or caregiver has hearing or vision difficulties.
- Clients taking certain prescribed cardiotonic or antidysrhythmic medications should learn to assess their own pulse rates to detect side effects of medications.
- Assess for environmental factors in the home that may influence client's respiratory rate such as secondhand smoke, inadequate ventilation, or gas fumes.

Procedural Guideline 12-2

Electronic Blood Pressure Measurement

Equipment: Electronic BP machine, BP cuff of appropriate size as recommended by manufacturer

1. See Standard Protocol (inside front cover).
2. Clients requiring continuous electronic BP measurement frequently have unstable vital signs, or their vital signs need to be closely monitored for evaluating response to medications (e.g., antihypertensive medications). For these reasons this skill usually requires problem-solving and critical-thinking skills unique to the professional nurse and should not be delegated to AP.
3. Determine appropriateness of using electronic BP measurement. Clients with irregular heart rates, peripheral vascular obstructions, seizures, tremors, and shivering are not candidates for this device.
4. Determine best site for cuff placement (see Skill 12-1, step 9a, p. 282).

5. Assist client to comfortable position, either lying or sitting. Place electronic BP machine near client because length of connector hose between cuff and machine is limited; plug machine in to source of electricity.
6. Locate on/off switch and turn machine on, which allows machine to self-test computer systems.
7. Select appropriate cuff size for client extremity (Table 12-5) and appropriate cuff for machine. Electronic BP cuff and machine must be matched by the manufacturer. Do not interchange BP cuffs from machines of different manufacturers. If an ideal cuff size is not available, a larger cuff will result in the smallest measurement error (Bridges and Middleton, 1997).
8. Expose extremity by removing restrictive clothing that can cause congestion of blood and distention of vessel walls.

Continued

Electronic Blood Pressure Measurement—cont'd

Table 12-5
Proper Cuff Size for Electronic Monitor*

Cuff Type	Limb Circumference (cm)
Small adult	17-25
Adult	23-33
Large adult	31-40
Thigh	38-50

*It is mandatory for the 12- to 24-foot cord to be used for adult monitoring.

9. Prepare BP cuff by manually squeezing all the air out of the cuff and connecting cuff to connector hose.
10. Wrap cuff snugly around extremity, verifying that only one finger can fit between cuff and client's skin. Make sure the "artery" arrow marked on the outside of the cuff is correctly placed (see illustration).
11. Verify that connector hose between cuff and machine is not kinked.
12. Following manufacturer's directions, set the frequency control for automatic or manual, then press the start button. The first BP measurement sequence will pump the cuff to a peak pressure of about 180 mm Hg. After this pressure is reached, the machine begins a deflation sequence that determines the BP. The first reading determines the peak pressure inflation for additional measurements.
13. Determine the frequency of measurement and client-specific alarm limits by physician order or nursing clinical judgment. Follow manufacturer's directions to set frequency of BP measurements and upper and lower alarm limits for systolic, diastolic, and mean BP readings. Additional readings can be determined at any time by pressing the start button. Pressing the cancel button immediately deflates the cuff. Intervals between BP measurements may be set from 1 to 90 minutes. The monitor displays the most recent reading and flashes the time in minutes that has elapsed since that measurement occurred (see illustration).
14. When BP determinations are frequent, the cuff may be left in place. Remove cuff at least every 2 hours to assess underlying skin integrity, and if possible, alternate sites.

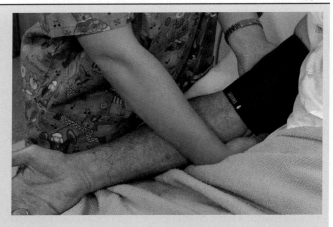

Step 10 Aligning BP cuff arrow with brachial artery.

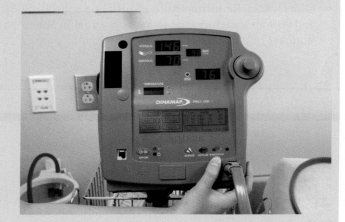

Step 13 Monitor displays reading. Verify electronic alarm settings.

15. Compare electronic BP readings with auscultatory BP as ordered, usually every 1 to 2 hours.
16. When electronic BP measurements are difficult to obtain or appear inaccurate, use the auscultatory method and immediately report your findings.
17. See Completion Protocol (inside front cover).

Skill 12.2

Measuring Oxygen Saturation With Pulse Oximetry

Pulse oximetry is a noninvasive measurement of arterial oxygen saturation (SaO_2) that assesses the level of oxygen in the blood available to the body tissues. SaO_2 reflects the percentage of hemoglobin that is bound with oxygen in the arteries and is expressed as a percentage; for example, an SaO_2 of 96% indicates that 96% of the hemoglobin molecules are carrying oxygen molecules. The more the hemoglobin is saturated with oxygen, the higher the SaO_2. Normally the SaO_2 is over 90%. The pulse oximeter is a device that measures pulse saturation (SpO_2), a reliable estimate of SaO_2. For an SaO_2 over 70% the SpO_2 is accurate to 2% (Tittle and Flynn, 1997). The measurement of SpO_2 is simple, is painless, and has fewer risks than obtaining an arterial blood gas (ABG) level, an invasive procedure. Pulse oximetry is indicated in clients who have an unstable oxygen status or in those who are at risk for alterations in oxygenation. Conditions that can require SpO_2 monitoring are listed in Box 12-5.

A pulse oximeter includes a probe with a light-emitting diode (LED) connected by cable to an oximeter (Figure 12-10). Light waves emitted by the LED are absorbed and then reflected back by oxygenated and deoxygenated hemoglobin molecules. The reflected light is processed by the oximeter, which calculates SpO_2. In adults the oximeter sensor is applied to the finger, toe, earlobe, or bridge of the nose. In addition, sensors for infants and children can be applied to the palm or the sole of the foot. New oximeters are being developed with sensors applied to the forehead. The nurse selects the appropriate sensor site for the client's condition (Box 12-7). SpO_2 can be assessed continuously, intermittently, or with spot checks, depending on the client's condition.

ASSESSMENT

1. Identify clients at risk for unstable oxygen status (e.g., clients recovering from conscious sedation,

clients requiring oxygen therapy, clients with chronic respiratory conditions, clients with chest wall injury or chest pain).

2. Identify medications or treatments that may influence oxygen saturation. *Rationale: Oxygen therapy, respiratory therapy such as postural drainage and percussion, and bronchodilators will affect client's ability to ventilate and perfuse lung tissue.*

3. Identify factors that influence oxygen saturation. *Rationale: Any abnormalities in the type or amount of hemoglobin affect the ability of oxygen to be carried to the tissues (see Box 12-6).*

4. Identify factors likely to interfere with accuracy of pulse oximeter. *Rationale: Skin pigmentation affects the ability of SpO_2 to predict SaO_2. Darker pigments can result in false-high readings (Tittle and Flynn, 1997).*

5. Assess pertinent laboratory values, including hemoglobin and ABGs if available. *Rationale: Anemia affects the ability of oxygen to attach to the hemoglobin molecule. ABG levels measure SaO_2, which serves as a standard and provides a basis for comparison to assist in the assessment of respiratory status.*

6. Determine client-specific site appropriate to place pulse oximeter sensor by measuring capillary refill (see Chapter 13). If less than 3 seconds, select alternative site; note presence of moisture or nail polish. *Rationale: Site must have adequate local circulation for sensor to detect hemoglobin molecules that absorb emitted light. Changes in SpO_2 are reflected in the circulation of finger capillary bed within 30 seconds and earlobe capillary bed within 5 to 10 seconds. Moisture, dark nail polish, and acrylic nails impede sensor detection of emitted light and produce falsely elevated SpO_2 levels (Tittle and Flynn, 1997).*

Box 12-5
Conditions That Can Require SpO_2 Monitoring

Acute respiratory disease (e.g., pneumonia or asthma)
Chronic respiratory disease (e.g., emphysema)
Ventilator dependence
Chest pain
Activity intolerance
Recovery from general anesthesia after surgery
Recovery from conscious sedation after procedures
    such as endoscopy, bronchoscopy, or cardiac
    catheterization
Traumatic injury to chest wall
Changes in supplemental oxygen therapy

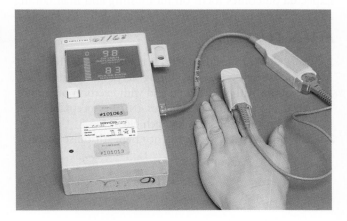

Figure 12-10   LED connected to pulse oximeter.

Box 12-6

Factors Affecting Determination of Pulse Oxygen Saturation

INTERFERENCE WITH LIGHT TRANSMISSION
- Outside light sources can interfere with the oximeter's ability to process reflected light.
- Carbon monoxide (caused by smoke inhalation or poisoning) artificially elevates SpO_2 by absorbing light similar to oxygen.
- Client motion can interfere with the oximeter's ability to process reflected light.
- Jaundice may interfere with the oximeter's ability to process reflected light.
- Intravascular dyes (methylene blue) absorb light similar to deoxyhemoglobin and artificially lower saturation.

REDUCTION OF ARTERIAL PULSATIONS
- Peripheral vascular disease (Raynaud's disease, atherosclerosis) can reduce pulse volume.
- Hypothermia at assessment site decreases peripheral blood flow.
- Pharmacological vasoconstrictors (epinephrine, phenylephrine, dopamine) will decrease peripheral pulse volume.
- Low cardiac output and hypotension decrease blood flow to peripheral arteries.
- Peripheral edema can obscure arterial pulsation.

Box 12-7

Characteristics of Pulse Oximeter Sensors and Sites

REUSABLE SENSORS
Digit Sensors
- Easy to apply, conform to various sizes
- Yield strong correlation with SaO_2

Earlobe Sensors
- Clip-on is smaller and lighter, although more positional than digit sensor
- Research suggests greater accuracy at lower saturations (Tittle and Flynn, 1997)
- Yield strong correlation with SaO_2
- Good when uncontrollable movements are a problem, such as hand tremors seen with Parkinson's disease
- Site least affected by decreased blood flow (Carroll, 1997)

DISPOSABLE SENSORS
- Can be applied to variety of sites: earlobe of adult or nose bridge, palm, or sole of infant
- Less restrictive for continuous SpO_2 monitoring
- Expensive
- Contain latex
- Skin under adhesive may become moist and harbor pathogens
- Available in variety of sizes, pad can be matched with infant weight

7. Determine previous baseline SpO_2 from client's record. *Rationale: Baseline information provides basis for comparison and assists in assessment of current status and evaluation of interventions.*

PLANNING

Expected outcomes focus on monitoring and maintaining adequate oxygenation when client is at risk for hypoxemia.

Expected Outcomes

1. SaO_2 level greater than 90% is maintained, with or without oxygen therapy, during sleep, after removal of secretions with suctioning, and with exertion of ambulating in the hall for 5 minutes. (NOTE: Acceptable level must be individualized for each client.)
2. Client maintains skin integrity beneath pulse oximeter sensor.

Equipment

- Oximeter
- Oximeter sensor appropriate for client and recommended by the manufacturer (see Box 12-7)
- Acetone or nail polish remover

Delegation Considerations

The skill of measuring oxygen saturation with a pulse oximeter can be delegated to assistive personnel (AP). Be sure to inform AP of:
- Appropriate sensor and measurement site for client
- Client-specific factors that can falsely lower SpO_2
- Frequency of SpO_2 measurement
- Need to report any measurement lower than 90% to nurse

IMPLEMENTATION FOR MEASURING OXYGEN SATURATION WITH PULSE OXIMETRY

Steps	Rationale
1. See Standard Protocol (inside front cover).	
2. Select site, which may include ear, nail bed, or bridge of nose. If finger is selected, remove fingernail polish and acrylic nail (if worn) with acetone or polish remover.	Opaque coatings decrease light transmission, and nail polish containing blue pigments can absorb light emissions and falsely alter saturation.

NURSE ALERT *Mixing probes from different manufacturers can result in burn injury to the client. If client has a latex allergy or latex sensitivity, avoid adhesive sensor, which contains latex.*

Steps	Rationale
3. Determine capillary refill at site. If less than 3 seconds, select alternative site.	Cold temperature with vasoconstriction or vascular disease may decrease circulation, impair refill, and prevent sensor from measuring SpO_2.
4. Position client comfortably. If finger is chosen as monitoring site, support lower arm. Instruct client to keep sensor probe site still.	Movement interferes with SpO_2 determination. Pressure of sensor probe's spring tension on finger or earlobe may be uncomfortable.
5. Attach sensor to selected site (see illustration), making sure photodetectors of light sensors are aligned opposite each other.	Pulse waveform/intensity display enables detection of valid pulse or presence of interfering signal. Pitch of audible beep is proportional to SpO_2 value. Double-check pulse rate to ensure oximeter accuracy.
6. Turn on oximeter by activating power. Observe pulse waveform/intensity display and audible beep. Compare oximeter pulse rate with client's radial pulse.	Ensures oximeter accuracy.

COMMUNICATION TIP *Inform client that oximeter alarm will sound if the sensor falls off or if he or she moves the sensor.*

NURSE ALERT *Do not attach probe to finger, ear, or bridge of nose if area is edematous or skin integrity is compromised. Do not place sensor on same extremity as electronic BP cuff. Blood flow to finger will be temporarily interrupted when cuff inflates and cause inaccurate reading and trigger alarms.*

NURSE ALERT *If oximeter pulse rate, client's radial pulse rate, and apical pulse rate are different, reevaluate oximeter sensor placement and reassess pulse rates.*

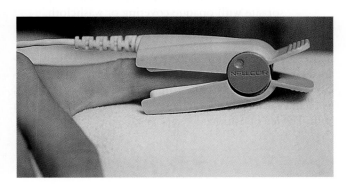

Step 5 Digit sensor to measure oxygen saturation.

Steps	Rationale
7. Leave sensor in place until oximeter reaches constant value and pulse display reaches full strength during each cardiac cycle. Read SpO_2 on digital display.	Reading may take 10 to 30 seconds, depending on site selected.
8. If continuous SpO_2 monitoring is planned, verify SpO_2 alarm limits, which are preset by the manufacturer at a low of 85% and a high of 100%. Limits for SpO_2 and pulse rate should be determined as indicated by client's condition. Verify that alarms are on. Assess skin integrity under sensor every 2 hours. Relocate sensor at least every 4 hours, and more frequently if skin integrity is altered.	Spring tension of sensor or sensitivity to disposable sensor adhesive can cause skin irritation and lead to disruption of skin integrity.
9. If intermittent or spot-checking SpO_2 measurements are planned, remove and turn oximeter power off. Store probe in appropriate location.	Sensor probes are expensive and vulnerable to damage.
10. See Completion Protocol (inside front cover).	

• • • • • • • • • • •

EVALUATION

1. Compare SpO_2 levels whenever oxygen therapy is initiated or discontinued, before and during sleep, before and after removal of secretions with suctioning, and during activity.
2. Assess skin integrity under sensor every 2 hours.

Unexpected Outcomes and Related Interventions

1. Client's SpO_2 is less than 90%.
   a. Observe for indications of hypoxemia, which include the presence of cyanosis, restlessness, altered respiratory patterns, and tachycardia. Skin beneath oximeter sensor is intact without irritation.
   b. Compare SpO_2 with SaO_2 on ABG. An SpO_2 of 85% to 89% may be acceptable for certain chronic disease conditions and reflects the client's baseline oxygen saturation. An SpO_2 less than 85% is abnormal and is often accompanied by changes in respiratory rate, depth, and rhythm. Immediate medical intervention is required.
   c. Observe for and minimize factors that decrease SpO_2, such as lung secretions, increased activity, altered neurological status, and hyperthermia.
   d. Assist client to a position that maximizes ventilation effort, for example, placing an obese client in a high-Fowler's position.
   e. Verify appropriate oxygen delivery system and liter flow; administer oxygen according to physician's orders.

   f. Implement measures to reduce client's energy consumption by avoiding unnecessary activity, anxiety, or emotional stress.
2. Pulse rate indicated on oximeter is less than radial or apical pulse rate.
   a. Change sensor site. Clients who have cold hands or peripheral vascular disease may have decreased blood flow to extremity.
   b. Check sensor for excessive spring pressure, which can constrict blood flow.
   c. Assess apical and radial pulse along with other signs and symptoms that would indicate compromised cardiac status or decreased peripheral blood flow.
3. Pulse rate intensity display indicated on oximeter is dampened or irregular.
   a. Request that client not move extremity or area with sensor because movement interferes with measurements. Motion artifact is most common cause of inaccurate readings.
   b. Reposition sensor for better contact with underlying skin.
   c. Protect sensor from room light by covering sensor site with opaque covering or washcloth.

Sample Documentation

1715 Continuous pulse ox on right index finger. Sensor relocated to left index finger. Capillary refill R = L, 2 seconds. Skin intact, no redness noted. SpO_2 93% with 3 L O_2 via nasal cannula. RR 24, client denies dyspnea, remains in semi-Fowler's position.

SPECIAL CONSIDERATIONS

Pediatric Considerations

Infant and toddler sensors attached to adhesive sensor pads are available and conform to fingers, palm of hand, and sole of foot.

Geriatric Considerations

• Identifying an acceptable sensor site may be difficult on older adults because of the likelihood of peripheral vascular disease, cold-induced vasoconstriction, and anemia.

• Older adults require more frequent assessment of sensor site because of tissue fragility and decreased elasticity caused by aging.

Home Care Considerations

Pulse oximetry is used in home care to noninvasively monitor oxygen therapy or changes in oxygen therapy.

CRITICAL THINKING EXERCISES

1. Mr. Charles is a 45-year-old computer programmer who is admitted to your home health agency for follow-up care and teaching of newly diagnosed type 2 diabetes. The client lives alone and was discharged from an acute care facility with a healing foot ulcer. His vital signs upon discharge were BP, 160/90 mm Hg right arm; pulse, 88 beats per minute; respirations, 24 breaths per minute; and tympanic temperature, 97.8° F. Mr. Charles is 64 inches tall and weighs 340 pounds. During your initial assessment Mr. Charles reports that he has been feeling tired and short of breath.
    a. What would be your priorities for assessing this client?
    b. You obtain a BP of 142/86 mm Hg in the client's left arm. What might explain the difference between this BP and the BP upon discharge?
    c. How would you assess the client's respiratory system?

2. As the team leader in the ambulatory surgical unit, you have just received Mrs. Roberts, a 35-year-old client from the postanesthesia care unit (PACU) who has recovered from a diagnostic laparoscopy. She is asking for some pain medication and something to drink. In addition, Mr. Woody, a 75-year-old client, has just arrived from the endoscopy suite. Mr. Woody had a colonoscopy with conscious sedation and is very sleepy.
    a. What vital sign activities and in what priority do you delegate to the AP?
    b. Mr. Woody's vital signs are BP, 170/92 mm Hg; heart rate, 64 beats per minute; respiratory rate, 14 breaths per minute; SpO_2, 90%; and oral temperature, 96.8° F. What actions would you take? What factors may have affected each of these vital signs?
    c. An hour later the AP reports that before home discharge Mrs. Roberts's oral temperature was 96.0° F. What is your response to the AP, and what actions would you take?

REFERENCES

Anwar YA, White WB: Ambulatory monitoring of the blood pressure: devices, analysis and clinical utility. In White WB, ed: *Blood pressure monitoring in cardiovascular medicine and therapeutics,* Totowa, NJ, 2001, Humana Press.

Bailey J, Rose P: Axillary and tympanic membrane temperature recording in the pre-term neonate: a comparative study, *J Adv Nurs* 34(4):465, 2001.

Barkauskas VH and others: Health and physical assessment, ed 3, St Louis, 2002, Mosby.

Bridges EJ, Middleton R: Direct arterial oscillometric monitoring of blood pressure: stop comparing and pick one, *Crit Care Nurse* 17(3):58, 1997.

Carroll P: Using pulse oximetry in the home, *Home Healthc Nurse* 15(2):89, 1997.

Erickson RS and others: Accuracy of chemical dot thermometers in critically ill adults and young children, *IMAGE J Nurs Scholarship* 28:23, 1996.

Futterrman LG, Lemberg L: Hypertension in the aged population, *Am J Crit Care* 11(1):80, 2002.

Lueckenotte AG: *Gerontologic nursing,* ed 3, St Louis, 2000, Mosby.

Lynch M: Pain as the fifth vital sign, *J Intraven Nurs* 24(2):85, 2001.

Maas ML and others: *Nursing care of older adults,* St Louis, 2001, Mosby.

National High Blood Pressure Education Program: *Sixth report of the Joint National Committee on the Prevention, Detection, Evaluation and Treatment of High Blood Pressure,* NIH Publication No. 98-4080, Bethesda, Maryland Public Health Service National Insitute of Health, 1997.

Pickering TG: Self-monitoring of blood pressure. In White WB, ed: *Blood pressure monitoring in cardiovascular medicine and therapeutics,* Totowa, NJ, 2001, Humana Press.

Tittle M, Flynn MB: Correlation of pulse oximetry and co-oximetry, *Dimens Crit Care Nurs* 16(2):88, 1997.

Yucha CB: Ambulatory blood pressure monitoring: measurement implications for research, *J Nurs Meas* 9(1):49, 2001.

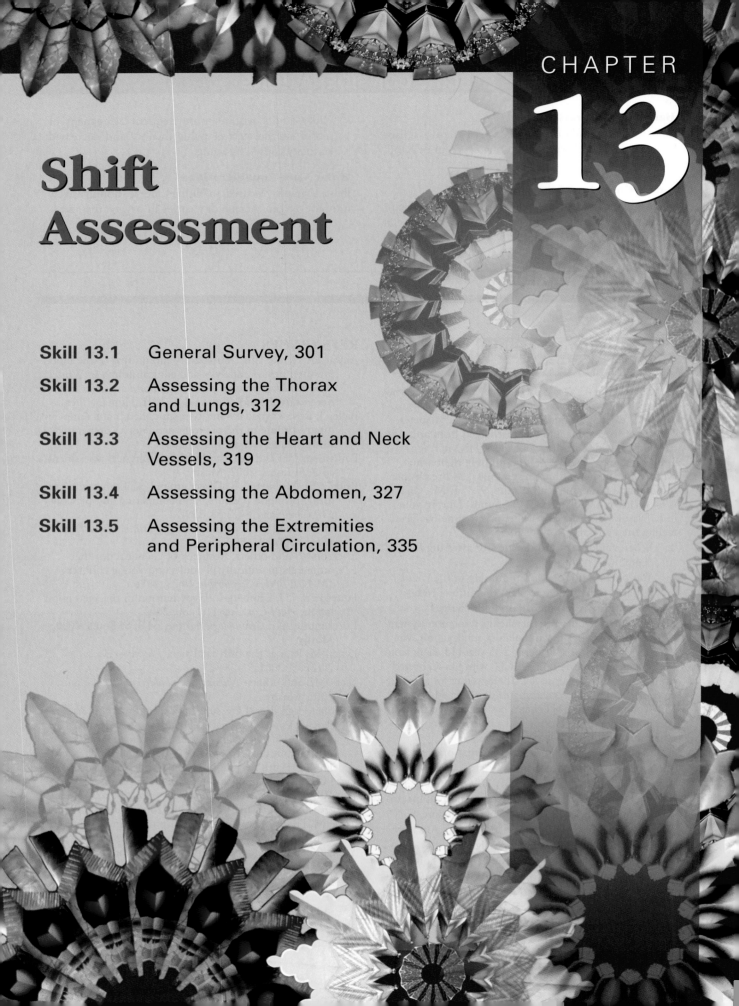

Shift
Assessment

Periodic systematic assessments are done on a regular basis in nearly every health care setting (e.g., hospitals, home health, nursing homes). In acute care settings a brief assessment is done at the beginning of each shift to identify changes in the client's status compared with the previous assessment. This routine assessment takes 10 to 15 minutes and reveals information that supplements the database for the client (Box 13-1). In nursing homes and home health, similar assessments are done weekly or monthly and more frequently when a change in health status occurs.

A more comprehensive assessment is done on admission to a health care agency. This assessment involves a detailed review of a client's condition, with the nurse collecting a nursing history and performing a behavioral and physical examination. The health history involves an interview with a client to gather subjective data about any presenting conditions. A physical assessment is a head-to-toe review of each body system that of-fers objective information about the client. The client's condition and response affect the extent of the examination. Once data are gathered, the nurse groups significant findings into patterns of data that reveal actual or potential nursing diagnoses (see Chapter 1). Each abnormal finding directs the nurse to gather additional data. Information gathered during an initial assessment and examination provides the baseline for a client's clinical status abilities and serves as a comparison for future assessment findings. In addition, the information helps the nurse select the best nursing measures to manage the client's health problems.

Nurses are often the first to detect changes in clients' conditions, regardless of the setting. For this reason the ability to think critically and interpret client behaviors and physiological changes is essential. The skills of physical assessment are powerful tools with which to detect subtle, as well as obvious, changes in a client's health.

Box 13-1

Checklist for Routine Shift Assessment

1. **MENTAL STATUS/NEUROLOGICAL STATUS**
   a. Level of consciousness/responsiveness
   b. Alertness/orientation
   c. PERRLA ("pupils equal, round, reactive to light, accomodative")
   d. Mood
   e. Behavior

2. **VITAL SIGNS**
   a. Blood pressure
   b. Pulse
   c. Respiration
   d. Temperature
   e. Pain and comfort level

3. **MOTOR SENSORY FUNCTION**
   a. Range of motion
   b. Paralysis
   c. Weakness
   d. Numbness or tingling

4. **INTEGUMENTARY (SKIN/MUCOUS MEMBRANES)**
   a. Color
   b. Temperature
   c. Turgor
   d. Moisture
   e. Edema
   f. Integrity

5. **CARDIOPULMONARY**
   a. Heart sounds
   b. Apical rate and rhythm
   c. Lung sounds
   d. Breathing pattern
   e. Peripheral pulses
   f. Capillary refill

6. **GASTROINTESTINAL**
   a. Bowel sounds
   b. Abdominal palpation
   c. Degree of abdominal distension
   d. Bowel elimination problems (i.e., diarrhea/constipation/flatulence)
   e. Nausea

7. **WOUND**
   a. Cleanliness
   b. Swelling/redness/infection
   c. Drainage
   d. Bandage dressing

8. **INVASIVE TUBES (E.G., INTRAVENOUS LINES, NASOGASTRIC TUBES, WOUND DRAINS, CATHETERS)**
   a. Device and location
   b. Intravenous line: Correct medicine infusing
   c. Patency and position
   d. Redness, swelling, or tenderness at site
   e. Drainage rate or infusion rate
   f. Date of last tubing change

ASSESSMENT TECHNIQUES

Inspection, palpation, percussion, auscultation, and olfaction are assessment techniques that enable the nurse to collect a broad range of physical data about clients. Experience is needed to recognize normal variations among clients, as well as ranges of normal in an individual. Cultural diversity needs to be recognized as one of the factors that influences both normal variations and potential alterations. It is extremely important to methodically take the time necessary to carefully assess each body part. If the nurse becomes hurried, significant signs may be overlooked and incorrect conclusions may be made about a client's condition.

Inspection is the process of visual examination of body parts/areas. An experienced nurse learns to make many observations, almost simultaneously, while becoming very perceptive of abnormalities. The secret is to always pay attention to the client. Watch all movements, and look carefully at any body part being inspected. It is important to recognize normal physical characteristics of clients of all ages before trying to distinguish abnormal findings.

Inspection requires good lighting and full exposure of body parts. Each area is inspected for size, shape, color, symmetry, position, and the presence of abnormalities. If possible, each area inspected is compared with the same area on the opposite side of the body. When necessary, use additional light, such as a penlight, to inspect body cavities such as the mouth and throat. *Do not hurry. Pay attention to detail.* Verify and clarify all abnormalities with subjective client data. In other words, ask the client for further information about each abnormality or change.

Palpation involves use of the sense of touch. Through palpation the hands can make delicate and sensitive measurements of specific physical signs, including resistance, resilience, roughness, texture, temperature, and mobility. Palpation is often used with or after visual inspection. The nurse uses different parts of the hand to detect specific characteristics. For example, the dorsum (back) of the hand is sensitive to temperature variations. The pads of the fingertips detect subtle changes in texture, shape, size, consistency, and pulsation of body parts. The palm of the hand is especially sensitive to vibration. The nurse measures position, consistency, and turgor by lightly grasping the body part with the fingertips.

Assist the client in being relaxed and positioned comfortably because muscle tension during palpation impairs the nurse's ability to palpate correctly. Asking the client to take slow, deep breaths enhances muscle relaxation. Tender areas are palpated last. The nurse asks the client to point out areas that are more sensitive and notes any nonverbal signs of discomfort. Clients appreciate clean, warm hands; short fingernails; and a gentle approach. Palpation may be either light or deep and is controlled by the amount of pressure applied with the fingers or hand. Light palpation precedes deep palpation. The nurse must consider the client's condition, the area being palpated, and the reason for using palpation. For example, when a client is admitted to the emergency department following an automobile accident, the nurse should consider the factors surrounding the client's injury and inspect the chest wall carefully before performing any palpation around the area of the ribs.

To palpate, the nurse applies pressure slowly, gently, and deliberately, depressing about 1 cm (½ inch). Tender areas are examined further using light intermittent pressure. After light palpation, deeper palpation may be used to examine the condition of organs (Figure 13-1). The nurse depresses the area being examined approximately 2 cm (1 inch). Caution is the rule. Bimanual palpation involves one hand placed over the other while pressure is applied. The upper hand exerts downward pressure as the other hand feels the subtle characteristics of underlying organs and masses. A student nurse seeks the assistance of a qualified instructor before attempting deep palpation.

Percussion involves tapping the body with the fingertips to evaluate the size, borders, and consistency of body organs and to discover fluid in body cavities (Figure 13-2). It requires practice and skill. Percussion helps identify the location, size, and density of underlying structures. The nurse strikes the body's surface with a finger to create a vibration, and sound waves are heard as percussion tones arising from vibrations in body tissues (Seidel and others, 1999). The character of sound depends on the density of

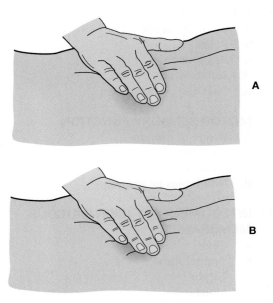

Figure 13-1 A, During light palpation, gentle pressure against underlying skin and tissues can be used to detect areas of irregularity and tenderness. **B,** During deep palpation, depress tissue to assess condition of underlying organs.

underlying tissues. For example, the normal lung transmits sounds with high intensity and low pitch, whereas the solid liver transmits a high-pitched sound of soft intensity.

There are two methods of percussion: direct and indirect. The direct method involves striking the body surface directly with one or two fingers. The indirect technique is performed by placing the middle finger of the examiner's nondominant hand firmly against the body surface. With palm and fingers remaining off the skin, the tip of the middle finger of the dominant hand strikes the base of the distal joint of the finger. The examiner uses a quick, sharp stroke, keeping the forearm stationary. The wrist remains relaxed to deliver the proper blow. Once the finger has struck, the wrist snaps back. If the blow is not sharp, if the hand is held loosely, or if the palm rests on the body surface, the sound is softened and the nurse cannot detect the presence of underlying structures. A light, quick blow produces the clearest sounds. Table 13-1 describes the five different percussion sounds.

Auscultation is listening with a stethoscope to sounds produced by the body. To auscultate correctly, listen in a quiet environment for both the presence of sound and its characteristics. The nurse is more successful in auscultation after knowing normal sounds from each body structure, including the passage of blood through an artery, heart sounds, and movement of air through the lungs. These sounds vary according to the location in which they can most easily be heard. Likewise, the nurse becomes familiar with areas that normally do not emit sounds. It is important for a student to listen to many normal sounds in order to recognize abnormal sounds when they arise.

To auscultate, the nurse needs good hearing acuity, a good stethoscope, and knowledge of how to use the stethoscope properly (see Chapter 12). Nurses with hearing disorders may purchase stethoscopes with greater sound amplification and may need to ask colleagues to verify some findings through auscultation. It is more effective to place the stethoscope directly on a client's naked skin because clothing obscures and changes sound.

Through auscultation the nurse notes the following characteristics of sound:

Pitch—Number of sound wave cycles generated per second by a vibrating object. The higher the frequency, the higher the pitch of a sound and vice versa.

Loudness—Amplitude of a sound wave. Auscultated sounds are described as loud or soft.

Quality—Sounds of similar frequency and loudness from different sources. Terms such as *blowing* or *gurgling* describe quality of sound.

Duration—Length of time that sound vibrations last. Duration of sound is short, medium, or long. Layers of soft tissue dampen the duration of sounds from deep internal organs.

A nurse cannot be successful at auscultation without knowing how to use a stethoscope properly. Chapter 12 describes the parts of the acoustic stethoscope and use of the bell and diaphragm.

Olfaction is using the sense of smell to detect abnormalities that go unrecognized by any other means. Some alterations in body function and certain bacteria create characteristic odors (Table 13-2).

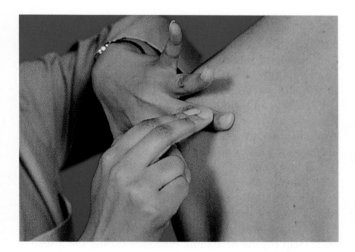

Figure 13-2 Indirect percussion. (From Barkauskas VH and others: *Health and physical assessment*, ed 3, St Louis, 2002, Mosby.)

Table 13-1

Sounds Produced by Percussion

Sound	Intensity	Pitch	Duration	Quality	Common Location
Tympany	Loud	High	Moderate	Drumlike	Enclosed, air-containing space; gastric air bubble, puffed-out cheek
Resonance	Moderate to loud	Low	Long	Hollow	Normal lung
Hyperresonance	Very loud	Very low	Longer than resonance	Booming	Emphysematous lung
Dullness	Soft to moderate	High	Moderate	Thudlike	Liver, spleen, gallbladder
Flatness	Soft	High	Short	Flat	Muscle

Table 13-2

Assessment of Characteristic Odors

Odor	Site or Source	Potential Causes
Alcohol	Oral cavity	Ingestion of alcohol
Ammonia	Urine	Urinary tract infection
Body odor	Skin, particularly in areas where body parts rub together (e.g., underarms, beneath breasts)	Poor hygiene, excess perspiration (hyperhidrosis), foul-smelling perspiration (bromhidrosis)
Feces	Wound site	Wound abscess
	Vomitus	Bowel obstruction
	Rectal area	Fecal incontinence
Foul-smelling stools in infant	Stool	Malabsorption syndrome
Halitosis	Oral cavity	Poor dental and oral hygiene, gum disease
Sweet, fruity ketones	Oral cavity	Diabetes acidosis
Stale urine	Skin	Uremic acidosis
Sweet, heavy, thick odor	Draining wound	*Pseudomonas* (bacterial) infection
Musty odor	Casted body part	Infection inside cast
Fetid, sweet odor	Tracheostomy or mucous secretions	Infection of bronchial tree (*Pseudomonas* bacteria)

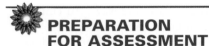 **PREPARATION FOR ASSESSMENT**

The process of assessment begins the moment the nurse sees the client and continues with each encounter. It is important to have as much awareness as possible of the client's health history and the reason the client sought care. Also be alert for any changes or problems that may have developed since the last assessment.

Preparation of the environment, equipment, and client facilitates a smooth assessment. To promote client comfort and efficiency it is essential to provide privacy for the client. In a health care facility the nurse closes the room door or pulls privacy curtains. In the home an examination is conducted in the bedroom. A comfortable environment includes: a warm, comfortable temperature; a loose-fitting gown or pajamas for the client; adequate direct lighting; control of outside noises; precautions to prevent interruptions by visitors or health care personnel; and placing the bed at the nurse's waist level if possible.

Preparing the Client

To facilitate an accurate assessment, prepare the client both physically and psychologically. A tense, anxious client may have difficulty understanding or following directions or cooperating with the nurse's instructions. To prepare the client the nurse needs to do the following:

1. Provide for client's physical comfort by allowing the opportunity to empty the bowel or bladder (a good time to collect needed specimens).

2. Provide privacy. This may involve asking friends or family to step out of the room.

3. Minimize client's anxiety and fear by conveying an open, receptive, and professional approach. The nurse, using simple terms, thoroughly explains what will be done, what the client should expect to feel, and how the client can cooperate. Even if the client appears unresponsive, it is still important that the nurse's actions be explained.

4. Provide access to body parts while draping areas that need not be exposed.

5. Eliminate drafts, control room temperature, and provide warm blankets.

6. Help the client assume positions during the assessment so that body parts are accessible and the client stays comfortable. A client's ability to assume positions will depend on physical strength and limitations. Some positions are uncomfortable or embarrassing; keep a client in position no longer than is necessary.

7. Pace assessment according to the client's physical and emotional tolerance.

8. Use a relaxed voice tone and facial expressions to put the client at ease.

9. Encourage the client to ask questions and report discomfort felt during the examination.

10. Have a family member or a third person of the client's gender in the room during assessment of genitalia. This prevents the client from accusing the nurse of behaving in an unethical manner.

11. At the conclusion of the assessment, ask the client if he or she has any concerns or questions.

PHYSICAL ASSESSMENT OF VARIOUS AGE-GROUPS

Children and Adolescents

1. Routine assessment of children has a focus on health promotion and illness prevention, particularly for care of well children with competent parenting and no serious health problems (Wong and others, 1999). The focus is on growth and development, sensory screening, dental examination, and behavioral assessment.
2. Children who are chronically ill, disabled, in foster care, or foreign-born adopted may require additional assessments.
3. When obtaining histories of infants and children, gather all or part of information from parents or guardians.
4. Parents may think they are being tested or judged by the examiner. Offer support during examination, and do not pass judgment.
5. Call children by their preferred name, and address parents as "Mr. and Mrs. Brown" rather than by first names.
6. Open-ended questions often allow parents to share more information and to describe more of the child's problems.
7. Older children and adolescents tend to respond best when treated as adults and individuals and often can provide details about their health history and severity of symptoms.
8. The adolescent has a right to confidentiality. After talking with parents about historical information, the nurse arranges to be alone with the adolescent to speak further privately and to perform the examination.

Older Adults

1. Do not assume that aging is always accompanied by illness or disability. Most older adults are able to adapt to change and maintain functional independence (Lueckenotte, 2000).
2. Allow extra time, and be calm, relaxed, and unhurried with older adults.
3. Provide adequate space for an examination, particularly if the client uses a mobility aid.
4. Plan the history and examination, taking into account the older adult's energy level, physical limitations, pace, and adaptability. More than one session may be needed to complete the assessment (Lueckenotte, 2000).
5. Measure performance under the most favorable of conditions. Take advantage of natural opportunities for assessment (e.g., during bathing, grooming, and mealtime) (Lueckenotte, 2000).

6. Sequence an examination to keep position changes to a minimum. Be efficient throughout the examination to limit client movement.
7. Be sure an examination of an older adult includes review of mental status.

GUIDELINES

1. Set priorities for assessment based on a client's presenting signs and symptoms or health care needs. For example, a client who develops sudden shortness of breath should first undergo an assessment of the lungs and thorax. If a client is acutely ill, the nurse may choose to assess only the involved body systems. The nurse's judgment is needed to ensure that an examination is relevant and inclusive.
2. Organize the examination. Compare both sides of the body for symmetry. If a client becomes fatigued, offer rest periods. Perform painful procedures near the end of the examination.
3. Use a head-to-toe approach following the sequence of inspection, palpation, percussion, and auscultation (except for abdominal assessment). This sequence facilitates an effective assessment.
4. Encourage the client to be an active participant. Clients are usually knowledgeable about their physical condition. Often the client can let the nurse know when certain findings are normal or when actual changes have occurred.
5. Respect the client's race, gender, age, and cultural beliefs. These important variables often influence assessment findings and approaches to use. A client's health beliefs, use of alternative therapies, nutritional habits, relationships with family, and comfort with close physical contact during an assessment must be considered (Box 13-2).
6. Follow standard precautions for infection control. Assessments may require the nurse to have contact with body fluids and discharge. When there are breaks in the skin, lesions, or wounds, gloves must be worn. In some circumstances the nurse must wear a gown.
7. Consider the possibility of latex allergy. The incidence of serious allergic reaction to latex has recently increased dramatically (Seidel and others, 1999).
8. Record quick notes to facilitate accurate documentation.
9. Continue to use assessment skills during each contact, including activities such as bathing, administration of medications, or other therapies, or while conversing with a client.
10. Integrate health promotion and education into physical assessment activities. There are "teachable moments" when the nurse can share findings and educate clients about health promotion.

Box 13-2

Cultural Awareness of Touch During Physical Examination

Physical contact with a client can convey a variety of meanings, depending on the client's cultural background. Consider these guidelines, but remember that each client is an individual and may respond differently.

HISPANICS
Highly tactile
Very modest (men and women)
May ask for health care provider of same gender
Women may refuse to be examined by male health care provider

ASIANS/PACIFIC ISLANDERS
Avoid touching (patting head is strictly taboo)
Touching during an argument equals loss of control (shame)
Public display of affection toward members of same gender is permissible (but not toward members of opposite gender)

AFRICAN-AMERICANS
May not like to be touched without permission
May exercise level of distrust or caution initially in care provider

NATIVE AMERICANS
Shake hands lightly
May not like to be touched without permission
Nonverbal communication is important

Data from Lueckenotte A: *Gerontologic nursing*, ed 2, St Louis, 2000, Mosby; Seidel HM and others: *Mosby's guide to physical examination*, ed 5, St Louis, 2003, Mosby.

11. Record a summary of the assessment using appropriate medical terminology and in the sequence that findings are gathered. Use commonly accepted medical abbreviations to keep notes concise.

NURSING DIAGNOSES

Shift assessment involves gathering data about the client's status and changes in comparison to the previous shift. It is important to be aware of nursing diagnoses previously established. The client may present many nursing diagnoses. However, the following are easily screened for during shift assessment.

Impaired Skin Integrity or **Risk for Impaired Skin Integrity** is appropriate when the client is at risk for or has experienced skin breakdown. Influencing factors may include immobility, moisture from incontinence, or circulatory alterations, or the client is unconscious or has impaired voluntary movement.

Ineffective Airway Clearance is appropriate when the client is unable to clear secretions or obstructions from the respiratory tract. **Ineffective Breathing Pattern** involves altered inhalation or exhalation and may include either hypoventilation or hyperventilation. Influencing factors may include decreased muscle strength or energy, pain, and anxiety.

Activity Intolerance applies when physiological energy is inadequate for the completion of desired activities because of altered cardiac function. Activity intolerance may also be related to prolonged immobility, weakness, and muscle atrophy. **Decreased Cardiac Output** is appropriate when there is a need to reduce cardiac workload or improve cardiac performance.

Acute or **Chronic Pain** related to unknown etiology may be appropriate when the focus of nursing care involves identifying factors that contribute to pain. An example would be when the client has signs and symptoms of discomfort and/or suffers a condition that may cause pain. Abdominal pain is one of the most common symptoms clients have.

Constipation or **Diarrhea** may be associated with abdominal pain or cramping and altered peristalsis resulting in either infrequent hard stools or frequent unformed stools and fluid loss.

Ineffective Peripheral Tissue Perfusion involves a chronic deficit in blood supply to the extremities and is appropriate when findings reveal alteration in arterial or venous circulation.

Disturbed Thought Processes is appropriate when the client lacks orientation to time, place, person, and/or event or demonstrates an abnormality in any of the six components of the mental health examination. **Acute Confusion** is appropriate when the client has an abrupt onset of global, transient changes and disturbances in attention, cognition, sleep-wake cycle, and psychomotor activity (Kim, McFarland, and McLane, 1997). **Impaired Memory** is appropriate when the client experiences the inability to remember or recall information or behavioral skills (Kim, McFarland, and McLane, 1997).

Risk for Injury is appropriate when the client has muscle weakness or altered level of consciousness. **Impaired Physical Mobility** may apply when clients have indications of cerebellar disease, Parkinson's paresis, and any form of plegia (e.g., paraplegia or hemiplegia). **Unilateral Neglect** applies when a client who has suffered a stroke is perceptually unaware of and inattentive to one side of the body.

Skill 13.1

General Survey

The general survey begins a review of the client's primary health problems, and it includes assessment of the client's vital signs, height and weight, general behavior, and appearance. The survey provides information about characteristics of an illness, a client's hygiene, skin and body image, emotional state, recent changes in weight, and developmental status. The survey can reveal important information about the client's behavior that can influence how the nurse communicates instructions to the client and continues the assessment.

ASSESSMENT

1. Note if client has had any acute distress: difficulty breathing, pain, or anxiety. If such signs are present, defer general survey until later. *Rationale: Signs establish priorities regarding what part of the examination to conduct first.*

NURSE ALERT *Findings may change the direction of the examination. Any client in acute distress will require an immediate assessment of the body system(s) affected.*

---

2. Review graphic sheet for temperature, pulse, respirations, and blood pressure, and consider factors or conditions that may alter reading of vital signs (see Chapter 12).
3. Determine client's primary language. If need for an interpreter is identified, determine availability of family members. It is best to have an interpreter of the same gender who is older and more mature. Have the interpreter translate verbatim if possible.
4. Reconfirm (after reviewing history) primary reason client has sought health care. *Rationale: Keeps assessment focused on client to ensure that client's expectations are addressed.*
5. Identify client's normal height and weight. If a sudden gain or loss in weight has occurred, determine amount of weight change and period of time in which it occurred. Assess if client has recently been dieting or following exercise program. *Rationale: Generally, weight of 15% to 20% above standard indicates excess body fat; however, fluid retention is one factor that must be ruled out. A person's weight can fluctuate daily because of fluid loss or retention (1 L of water weighs 1 kg or 2.2 pounds).*
6. Review client's past fluid intake and output (I&O) records. *Rationale: Fluid and electrolyte balance maintains health and function in all body systems. Intake includes all liquids taken orally, by feeding tube, and parenterally. Liquid output includes urine, diarrhea stool, fistulas, vomitus, drainage from gastric suction, and drainage from postsurgical tubes, such as chest tubes or Jackson-Pratt drains.*
7. Identify client's general perceptions about personal health. *Rationale: Assessment of client's general appearance coupled with client's own perceptions may reveal specific problem areas.*
8. Assess for evidence of latex allergy, which may include contact dermatitis or systemic reactions. *Rationale: Gloves will be worn during certain aspects of the assessment. Repeated exposure may result in more serious reactions, including asthma, itching, and anaphylaxis (Seidel and others, 1999).*

PLANNING

Expected outcomes focus on accuracy in collection of assessment data.

Expected Outcomes

1. Client demonstrates alert, cooperative behaviors without evidence of physical or emotional distress during assessment.
2. Client provides appropriate subjective data related to physical condition.

Equipment

- Stethoscope
- Sphygmomanometer and cuff
- Thermometer
- Digital watch or wristwatch with second hand
- Tape measure
- Clean gloves (use nonlatex if necessary)
- Tongue blade

Delegation Considerations

The general survey requires the critical thinking skills and knowledge application unique to an RN. It should not be delegated to assistive personnel (AP). However, the following activities may be delegated: measuring height and weight, oral intake, urinary output, and vital signs and reporting a client's subjective signs and symptoms. All monitoring data must be reported to an RN.

IMPLEMENTATION FOR GENERAL SURVEY

Steps	Rationale
1. See Standard Protocol (inside front cover).	
2. *Prepare client:* Tell the client you will be doing a routine process to check for areas of concern. Ask if any area you examine hurts when touched, and explain that pain is an important finding during your assessment.	Gains client's cooperation.
3. Throughout the assessment note the client's verbal and nonverbal behaviors. Determine the level of consciousness and orientation by observing and talking to the client (Box 13-3).	Behaviors may reflect specific physical abnormalities. Dementia and level of consciousness influence ability to cooperate. Timing of recent medications, especially pain medication and sedatives, may alter assessment data.
4. Obtain temperature, pulse, respirations, and blood pressure unless routinely taken within last 3 hours or a serious potential change is noted (e.g., change in level of consciousness or difficulty breathing [see Chapter 12]). Inform client of vital signs.	Vital signs provide important information regarding physiological changes in relation to oxygenation and circulation.
5. Observe the following aspects of appearance: gender, race, and age. Note the client's physical features.	Gender influences type of examination performed and manner in which assessments are made. Different physical characteristics and predisposition to illnesses are related to gender and race.
6. If uncertain whether client understands a question, rephrase or ask a similar question.	Inappropriate response from a client may be caused by language or deterioration of mental status, preoccupation with illness, or decreased hearing acuity.
7. If a client's responses are inappropriate, ask short, to-the-point questions regarding information the client should know, for example: "Tell me your name." "What is the name of this place?" "Tell me where you live." "What day is this?" "What month is this?" or "What season of the year is this?"	Measures client's orientation to person, place, and time. This may be noted in documentation as "Oriented × 3." If disoriented in any way, include subjective and/or objective data rather than just documenting disoriented.

Box 13-3
Symptoms That May Indicate Dementia

LEARNING AND RETAINING NEW INFORMATION
Trouble remembering recent conversations, events, and appointments
Frequently misplaces objects

HANDLING COMPLEX TASKS
Difficulty following a complex train of thought
Difficulty performing tasks that require many steps

REASONING ABILITY
Unable to develop plan to address problems at work or home
Displays uncharacteristic disregard for rules of social conduct

SPATIAL ABILITY AND ORIENTATION
Difficulty driving
Difficulty in organizing objects around the house
Difficulty finding way around familiar places

LANGUAGE
Increasing difficulty with expressing self
Difficulty following conversations

BEHAVIOR
Appears more passive and less responsive
More irritable and suspicious than usual
Misinterprets visual and auditory stimuli

Steps	Rationale
8. If client is unable to respond to questions of orientation, offer simple commands, for example, "Squeeze my fingers" or "Move your toes."	Levels of consciousness exist along a continuum that include full responsiveness, inability to consciously initiate meaningful behaviors, and unresponsiveness to stimuli.

NURSE ALERT   *When client responds inappropriately to questions or requests or family members comment on client's change in memory or confusion, you may want to consider a more specialized assessment for cognitive function such as the Mini-Mental State Examination (MMSE) (Box 13-4). When a client exhibits a marked change in mental status, notify the physician immediately.*

Steps	Rationale
9. Assess affect and mood. Note if verbal expressions match nonverbal behavior and if appropriate to situation.	Reflects client's mental status, consciousness, feelings, and emotional status.
10. Observe client interaction with spouse or partner, older adult child, or caregiver. Be alert for indications of fear, hesitancy to report health status, or willingness to let caregiver control assessment interview. Does partner or caregiver have a history of violence, alcoholism, or drug abuse? Is the person unemployed, ill, or frustrated with caring for client? Note if client has any obvious physical injuries.	Abuse is often first suspected in clients who have suffered obvious physical injury or neglect, show signs of malnutrition, or have bruises on the extremities or trunk. Evidence of abuse is often identified first by health care providers, because clients often are unable to tell family or friends. Partners or caregivers often have history of abusive or addictive behaviors.

NURSE ALERT   *Be discreet in how interview is handled. It may be necessary to delay assessment to a later time, when the partner or caregiver is not present. Asking a partner or caregiver to leave during an assessment may create an awkward situation.*

Box 13-4

MMSE Sample Items

Orientation to Time
  "What is the date?"
Registration
  "Listen carefully, I am going to say three words. You say them back after I stop. Ready? Here they are . . .
  HOUSE (pause), CAR (pause), LAKE (pause). Now repeat those words back to me." [Repeat up to 5 times, but score only the first trial.]
Naming
  "What is this?" [Point to a pencil or pen.]
Reading
  "Please read this and do what it says." [Show examinee the words on the stimulus form: CLOSE YOUR EYES.]

Reproduced by special permission of the Publisher, Psychological Assessment Resources, Inc., 16204 North Florida Avenue, Lutz, FL 33549, from the Mini-Mental State Examination, by Marshal Folstein and Susan Folstein, Copyright 1975, 1998, 2001 by Mini-Mental LLC, Inc. Published 2001 by Psychological Assessment Resources, Inc. Further reproduction is prohibited without permission of PAR, Inc. The MMSE can be purchased from PAR, Inc. by calling (800) 331-8378 or (813) 968-3003.

Steps	**Rationale**
11. Assess posture, noting alignment of shoulders and hips. Observe whether the client has a slumped, erect, or bent posture (see illustration).	May reflect neuromuscular disease or emotional status if deviation from erect posture and correct alignment.
a. Body movements: Are they purposeful? Are there tremors of the extremities? Are any body parts immobile?	May indicate neurological or muscular problem or emotional stress.
b. Note if movements are coordinated or uncoordinated.	May indicate neurological, muscular , or emotional problem.
12. Assess speech. Is it understandable and moderately paced? Is there an association with the person's thoughts?	May reflect neurological impairment, injury or impairment of mouth, improperly fitting dentures. In addition, differences in dialect and language may also affect client's speech patterns.
13. Observe hygiene and grooming for presence or absence of makeup, type of clothes (hospital or personal), and cleanliness.	Grooming may reflect activity level before examination, resources available to purchase grooming supplies, client's mood, and self-care practices. May also reflect culture, lifestyle, economic status, and personal preferences.
a. Observe the color, distribution, quantity, thickness, texture, and lubrication of hair.	Changes in hair distribution may reflect hormonal changes, changes from aging, poor nutrition, or use of certain hair care products.
b. Inspect the condition of nails.	Changes may indicate inadequate nutrition or grooming practices, nervous habits, or systemic diseases.
c. Assess the presence or absence of body odor.	Body odor may result from physical exercise, deficient hygiene, or physical or mental abnormalities. Inadequate oral hygiene or unhealthy teeth may cause bad breath.
14. Assess the eyes.	
a. Inspect position of eyes, color of conjunctivae and sclera, and movement.	Asymmetrical positioning may reflect trauma or tumor growths. Differences in color may be congenital; changes in color of conjunctivae may be due to local infection or symptomatic of another abnormality (e.g., pale conjunctivae is associated with anemia).
b. Note client's near vision (ability to read newspaper or magazines) and far vision (follow movement, ability to read the clock, television, or signs at a distance).	If client has visual acuity or visual field loss, make adjustments to support self-care measures (e.g., feeding, bathing and hygiene, dressing) and teaching.
c. Inspect pupils for size, shape, and equality (see illustration).	Normal pupils are round, clear, and equal in size and shape.
d. Test pupillary reflexes. To test reaction to light, dim room lights. If light cannot be dimmed, cup hand over eye to temporarily shield the light. As client looks straight ahead, move penlight from side of client's face, and direct light on pupil. Observe pupillary response of both eyes, noting briskness and equality of reflex (see illustration).	Darkened room normally ensures brisk response of pupils to light. Pupil that is illuminated constricts. Pupil in other eye should constrict equally (consensual light reflex).

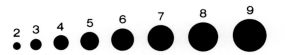

Step 14c   Pupil size in millimeters.

Steps	Rationale

15. Assess hearing. Note the client's response to questions and the presence/use of a hearing aid. If hearing loss is suspected, ask client to repeat random numbers with two equally accented syllables (e.g., nine, four). Repeat, gradually increasing voice intensity until client correctly repeats the numbers.

Seidel and others (1999) report that clients normally hear numbers clearly when whispered, responding correctly at least 50% of the time. For client with obvious hearing impairment, speak clearly and concisely, stand so that client can see face, and speak toward client's good ear, using a low pitch, and without yelling.

NURSE ALERT *If hearing deficit is present, inspect client's ears because impaired hearing may be due to impacted cerumen, external otitis, or swelling in ear canal due to allergic reactions to materials in hearing aids.*

---

16. In clients with a nasogastric, nasointestinal, or nasotracheal tube, inspect nares for excoriation or inflammation. Stabilize tube as needed.

Swallowing or coughing reflex causes movement of tubes against nares, and pressure against tissues and mucosa can result in tissue erosion.

17. Assess the mouth. Inspect oral mucosa. Retract mouth to inspect the tongue, teeth, and gums for hydration and obvious lesions (see illustration). Determine if client wears dentures or retainers and if they are comfortable. Dentures may be removed to visualize and palpate gums.

Ill-fitting dentures and retainers chronically irritate mucosa and gums and may pose risk for mouth cancer.

18. Ask if client has noted any changes in the skin, including:
   a. Pruritus, oozing, bleeding.
   b. Change in the appearance of a bump or nodule.
   c. Change in sensation (itchiness, tenderness, pain).

Incidence of melanoma, an aggressive form of skin cancer, has increased significantly. It is more than 10 times higher among whites than blacks (American Cancer Society, 2001). The cancer can spread to other parts of the body quickly. Early detection and prompt treatment are critical (Box 13-5).

   d. Petechiae (pinpoint-size, red or purple spots on the skin caused by small hemorrhages in the skin layers).

Petechiae may indicate serious blood clotting disorder, drug reaction, or liver disease.

19. Inspect skin surfaces. Compare color of symmetrical body parts, including areas unexposed to sun. Look for any patches or areas of skin color variation.

Changes in color can be indicative of pathological alterations (Table 13-3). Bluish discoloration of mucosa at base of tongue (central cyanosis) indicates low oxygen saturation, seen in lung disease and congenital heart defects of children. Peripheral cyanosis (bluish discoloration of lips and nail beds) results from low cardiac output or local vasoconstriction.

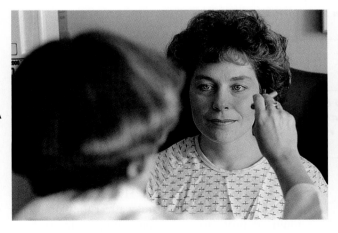
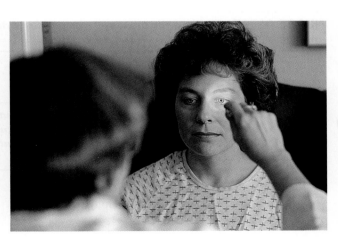

Step 14d **A,** To check pupil reflexes, first hold penlight to side of client's face. **B,** Illumination causes pupillary constriction.

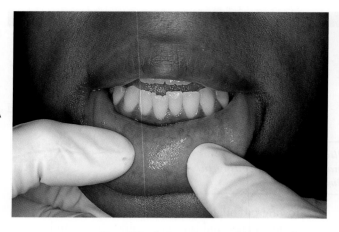
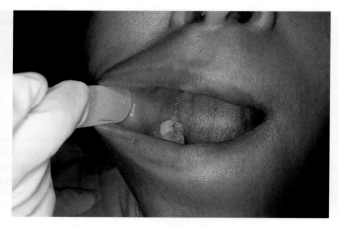

A   B

Step 17   **A,** Inspection of inner oral mucosa of lower lip. **B,** Retraction with tongue blade allows for clear view of buccal mucosa.

Box 13-5

Malignant Melanoma

MNEMONICS
The ABCD Rule of Melanoma
Here is a simple way to remember the characteristics that should alert you to the possibility of malignant melanoma.

A *A*symmetry of lesion
B *B*orders; irregular
C *C*olor blue/black or variegated
D *D*iameter >6 mm

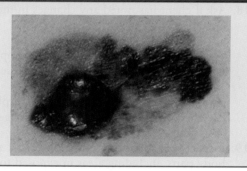

Illustration from Zitelli B, Davis H: *Atlas of pediatric physical diagnosis,* ed 3, St Louis, 1997, Mosby.

Steps	Rationale

NURSE ALERT   *Be alert for basal cell carcinomas, often seen in sun-exposed areas, which frequently occur in sun-damaged skin.*

20. Carefully inspect color of face, oral mucosa, lips, conjunctivae, sclerae, palms of hands, and nail beds.	Nurse can more readily identify abnormalities in areas of body where melanin production is lowest.

NURSE ALERT   *When assessing the skin of a client with bandages, cast, restraints, or other restrictive devices, note areas of pallor and decreased temperature, which may indicate impaired circulation. Immediate release of pressure from the restrictive device may be necessary.*

21. Use fingertips to palpate skin surfaces to feel texture and moisture of intact skin (nurse may remove a glove temporarily if worn).	Changes in texture may be the first indication of skin rashes in dark-skinned clients. Hydration, body temperature, and environment may affect the skin. Older adults are prone to serosis, presenting as dry, scaly skin (Lueckenotte, 2000).

Table 13-3

Pathological Color Changes

Color Changes	Light Skin	Dark Skin
Cyanosis: related to hypoxia (late sign of decreased oxygen), heart or lung disease, cold environment	Blue tinge, especially in conjunctivae, nail beds, earlobes, oral membrane, soles, and palms	Ashen-gray lips and tongue
Pallor: related to decreased perfusion (blood flow, anemia, shock)	Loss of rosy glow in skin, especially face	Ashen-gray appearance in black skin
Erythema: related to increased blood flow (fever, irritation)	Redness easily seen anywhere on body	Difficult to assess; palpate for warmth or edema
Jaundice: related to deposits of biluribin in tissue, liver disease	Yellow staining in sclerae of eyes, skin, fingernails, soles, palms, and oral mucosa	Most reliably assessed in sclerae, hard palate, palms, and soles
Ecchymoses: related to bleeding into skin, often due to trauma	Purple to yellowish green areas resulting from bleeding into skin, usually related to trauma	Difficult to see except in mouth or conjunctivae
Petechiae: minute hemorrhages into skin	Purple pinpoints most easily seen on buttocks, abdomen, and inner surfaces of arms or legs	Usually invisible except in oral mucosa, conjunctivae, or eyelids and covering eyeballs

Steps	Rationale
a. Using dorsum (back) of hand, palpate for temperature of skin surfaces. Compare symmetrical body parts. Compare upper and lower body parts. Note distinct temperature differences. Note localized areas of warmth.	Skin on dorsum of hand is thin, which allows detection of subtle temperature changes. Cool skin temperature often indicates decreased blood flow. A stage I pressure ulcer may cause warmth and erythema (redness) of an area. Environmental temperature and anxiety may also affect skin temperature.
b. Assess skin turgor by grasping fold of skin on the sternum, forearm, or abdomen with the fingertips. Release skinfold, and note ease and speed with which skin returns to place (see illustration).	With reduced turgor, skin remains suspended or "tented" for a few seconds before slowly returning to place, indicating decreased elasticity and possible dehydration. With altered turgor it is essential to provide measures for prevention of pressure ulcers.

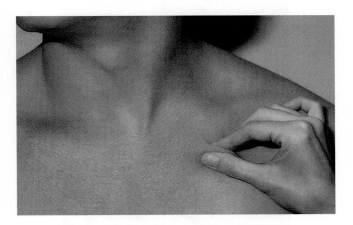

Step 21b   Assessment of skin turgor. (From Seidel HM and others: *Mosby's guide to physical examination,* ed 4, St Louis, 1999, Mosby.)

Steps	**Rationale**

22. 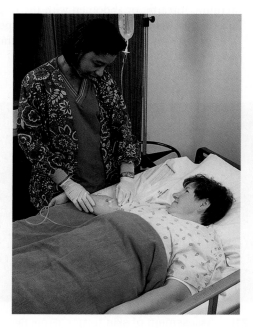 Inspect character of any secretions; note color, odor, amount, and consistency (e.g., thin and watery or thick and oily).

Description of secretions helps to indicate whether infection is present or the wound is healing.

23. Assess condition of skin for pressure areas, paying particular attention to regions of pressure (e.g., sacrum, greater trochanter, heels, occipital area, clavicles). If areas of redness are noted, place fingertip over area and apply gentle pressure, then release.

Normal reactive hyperemia (redness) is a visible effect of localized vasodilation, the body's normal response to lack of blood flow to underlying tissue. Affected area of skin will blanch with fingertip pressure. If pressure is not relieved, tissue damage can occur in as little as 90 minutes because of tissue hypoxia.

NURSE ALERT *Evidence of normal reactive hyperemia must result in repositioning the client and development of turning schedule if client is dependent (see Chapter 23).*

24. When a lesion is detected, with adequate lighting inspect color, location, texture, size, shape, and type (Box 13-6). Note also grouping (e.g., clustered or linear) and distribution (localized or generalized).

Observation of the lesion allows for accurate description and identification.

   a.   Gently palpate any lesion to determine mobility, contour (flat, raised, or depressed), and consistency (soft or hard). If lesion is moist or draining, apply disposable gloves before palpation.

   b.   Note if client reports tenderness during palpation.

Tenderness may be indicative of inflammation or pressure on body part.

   c.   Measure size of lesion (height, width, depth) with centimeter ruler.

Provides for baseline to assess changes in lesion over time.

25. Using clean gloves, palpate intravenous (IV) site (see illustration) for evidence of inflammation (redness, heat, swelling, drainage, tenderness) or infiltration (puffiness, pallor, coolness). Note when site is due to be changed.

Agency policy will indicate how often tubing is to be changed to prevent infections. Intravenous (IV) site changes are usually performed every 72 hours.

Step 25 Palpate IV site for tenderness.

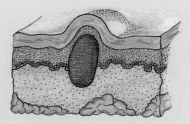

Box 13-6

Types of Skin Lesions

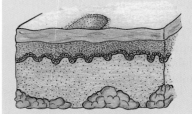

Macule: flat, nonpalpable, change in skin color, smaller than 1 cm (e.g., freckle or petechia)

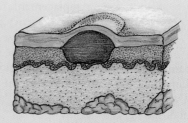

Papule: palpable, circumscribed, solid elevation in skin, smaller than 0.5 cm (e.g., elevated nevus)

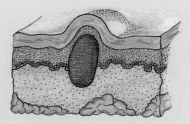

Nodule: elevated solid mass, deeper and firmer than papule, 0.5 to 2.0 cm (e.g., wart)

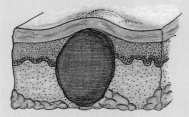

Tumor: solid mass that may extend deep through subcutaneous tissue, larger than 1 to 2 cm (e.g., epithelioma)

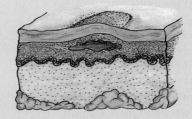

Wheal: irregularly shaped, elevated area or superficial localized edema, varies in size (e.g., hive or mosquito bite)

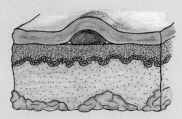

Vesicle: circumscribed elevation of skin filled with serous fluid, smaller than 0.5 cm (e.g., herpes simplex or chickenpox)

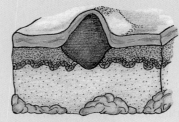

Pustule: circumscribed elevation of skin similar to vesicle but filled with pus, varies in size (e.g., acne or staphylococcal infection)

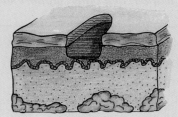

Ulcer: deep loss of skin surface that may extend to dermis and frequently bleeds and scars, varies in size (e.g., venous stasis ulcer)

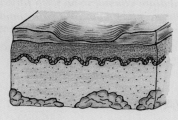

Atrophy: thinning of skin with loss of normal skin furrow with skin appearing shiny and translucent, varies in size (e.g., arterial insufficiency)

Steps	Rationale
26. Check the IV fluid and any added medications (apply six rights of medication administration). Note the rate of infusion.	Infusion rate that is too rapid may result in fluid volume excess; a rate too slow can result in inadequate fluid replacement. Changing the fluids and tubing according to agency policy helps prevent IV-related infections (Pugliese, 1997).
27. Observe for signs of abuse. a. For a child: Blood on underclothing, pain in genital area, or difficulty sitting or walking may be indicative of child sexual abuse. b. For a female client: Injury or trauma inconsistent with reported cause or obvious injuries to face or neck (black eyes, broken nose, lip lacerations, broken teeth, strangulation marks or burns) may indicate domestic abuse. c. For an older adult: Injury or trauma inconsistent with reported cause, injuries in unusual locations (such as neck or genitalia), pattern injuries (left when an object with which a person is struck leaves an imprint), parallel injuries (such as bilateral bruises on the upper arms suggesting the person was held and shaken) and burns (shaped like a cigarette, iron, rope, or immersion with a clear line of demarcation), and prolonged interval between injury and time medical care was sought are signs indicative of older adult abuse or neglect (Lynch, 1997).	Assessment of the individual client, whether child, woman, or older adult, is specifically directed and is based upon common findings of abuse in those populations.

NURSE ALERT *A pattern of findings indicating abuse usually mandates a report to a social service center (refer to state guidelines). Nurse should obtain immediate consultation with physician, social worker, and other support staff to facilitate placement in a safer environment.*

---

28. See Completion Protocol (inside front cover).

. . . .

EVALUATION

1. Observe throughout the assessment for evidence of physical or emotional distress.
2. Compare assessment findings with previous observations.
3. Ask the client if there is information about physical condition that has not been discussed.

Unexpected Outcomes and Related Interventions

1. Client demonstrates acute distress such as shortness of breath, acute pain, or severe anxiety.
   a. Respond immediately to identified need (repositioning, oxygen, or medication as appropriate).
   b. Notify charge nurse or physician if orders are needed for relief of acute symptoms.
2. Client has abnormal skin condition (dry texture, reduced turgor, lesions, or erythema).
   a. Identify contributing factors, and prevent continued irritation or damage as appropriate (see Chapter 22).
3. Client is unwilling or unable to provide adequate information relating to identified concerns.
   a. Seek information from family members if present, and review client's record for baseline data.

Recording and Reporting

- Record client's vital signs on vital sign flow sheet. Compare to previous data for significant changes (see Chapter 12).
- Document significant changes in level of consciousness, mood, speech, and body movements on neurological flow sheet.
- Describe abnormal skin conditions, noting size, location, color, whether raised or indented, and presence or absence of drainage.

- Describe abnormal sensations such as pruritus, pain, burning, or numbness, including specific location and bilateral comparison as subjective data using quotes. Determine if sensation changes are related to inappropriately applied therapy (e.g., cast or dressings).
- Report any skin breakdown and draining lesions to physician and/or clinical specialist.
- Record condition of IV site on IV flow sheet including presence/absence of redness, tenderness, swelling, or leakage.

Sample Documentation

Documentation routinely involves use of an assessment flow sheet (see Appendix A). Changes in condition need a description in nurses' notes.

08:30 Client reports a "painful bottom." A 2-cm flat, round, erythematic area is noted on the sacrum. Skin integrity is intact. Client is repositioned to left side and will be rotated every 2 hours.

SPECIAL CONSIDERATIONS

Pediatric Considerations

- Measurement of physical growth is a key element in evaluation of a child's health status. An effort sponsored by the World Health Organization has resulted in the revision of growth charts for young children from birth to 5 years of age. This was constructed from an international longitudinal study including breast-fed infants (Garza and De Onis, 1999).
- Infants are weighed nude. Children may be weighed in light underclothes or gown.
- A child's interactions with parents provide valuable information regarding the child's behavior.

Geriatric Considerations

- An older adult's presenting signs and symptoms can be deceiving. An older adult has a diminished physiological reserve that may mask the usual, or "classic," signs and symptoms of a disease. In older adults signs and symptoms are often blunted or atypical (Lueckenotte, 2000).
- Postural hypotension is common in older clients. Vital signs should be checked in lying, sitting, and standing positions, especially when positional dizziness and light-headedness is reported.
- Nutritional problems are frequently noted in older adults. Skipping meals is a common practice. The amount of food eaten diminishes, and the adequacy of nutrition becomes questionable. The following factors pose risks for malnutrition in older adults: limited income, loneliness, abuse of alcohol and other central nervous system depressants, forgetfulness, inability to feed self, reduced strength and mobility, and decreased vision (Ebersole and Hess, 1998).
- Common skin changes with aging include dryness, wrinkling, reduced elasticity, and "liver spots" in areas exposed to sun. Common lesions include seborrheic keratosis (pigmented macular-papular lesion that can be warty, scaly, or greasy); cherry angioma (bright, ruby-red or purplish papular lesion); skin tags (soft pinkish-tan to light-brown pedunculated lesions); and senile lentigines (gray-brown irregular macular lesions on sun-exposed areas) (Lueckenotte, 2000).
- Inspection of the feet is critically important in the presence of impaired circulation, impaired vision, and diabetes. Common podiatric conditions include ulceration, fungal infection, calluses, bunions, and plantar warts (Sitzman, 1999).

Home Care Considerations

- In the home the focus may be on the client's ability to perform basic self-care tasks. The nurse should ensure that the home assessment builds on all health concerns identified in other settings.
- Transport of small portable scale may be required to monitor weight changes.
- Measurement of visual acuity helps determine level of assistance client requires with daily living activities and ability of client to safely ambulate and function independently within home. Client and family may need help to adjust room arrangement at home and to obtain self-help aids.
- Older adults may report problems with sense of smell during examination. Stress the importance of installing smoke detectors throughout home and checking/dating food labels for possible spoilage.
- Consult referring physician as to the assessment findings and proposed plan of care.

Long-Term Care Considerations

The Minimum Data Set (MDS) is a tool that includes a comprehensive assessment of residents in the long-term care setting. It is meant to provide a total picture of a resident and to provide an ongoing comprehensive assessment of each resident, emphasizing functional ability and both a physical and a psychosocial profile. Only an RN can function as the assessment coordinator. Contributions are made by licensed vocational or practical nurses, the dietary supervisor, social worker, recreational therapist, physical therapist, and occupational therapist (Lueckenotte, 2000).

Skill 13.2

Assessing the Thorax and Lungs

Assessment of respiratory function is one of the most critical assessment skills because alterations can be life threatening. Routine shift assessment is essential because changes in respirations and or breath sounds can occur quickly as a result of a variety of factors, including immobility, infection, and fluid overload. Shift assessment includes auscultation, which assesses the movement of air through the tracheobronchial tree. Normally air flows through the airways unobstructed. Recognizing the sounds created by normal airflow allows the nurse to detect sounds caused by obstruction of the airways. Auscultation of the lungs requires familiarity with landmarks of the chest (Figure 13-3). During the assessment, the nurse should keep a mental image of the location of the lung lobes. To locate the position of each rib, the nurse locates the angle of Louis by palpating the "speed bump" on the

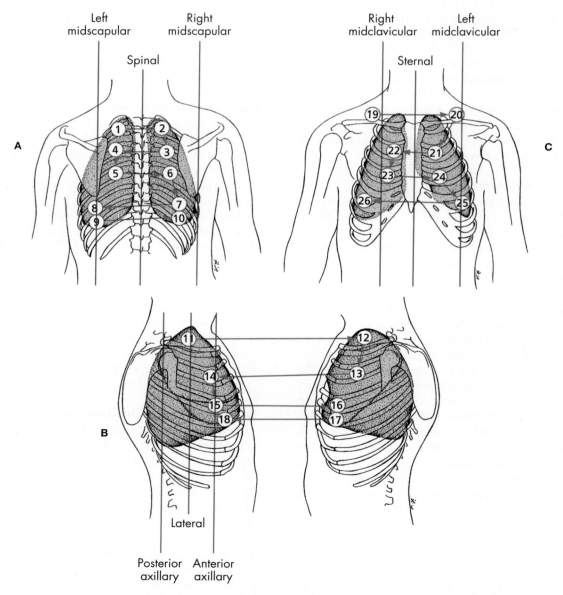

Figure 13-3 Anatomical landmarks and order of progression for examination of the thorax. **A,** Posterior thorax. **B,** Lateral thorax. **C,** Anterior thorax.

sternum where the second rib articulates with the sternum. The ribs and intercostal spaces are counted from this point. Auscultation involves listening to breath sounds using a stethoscope; the sounds are best heard when the person breathes deeply through the mouth.

Adventitious sounds are abnormal sounds resulting from air passing through moisture, mucus, or narrowed airways; alveoli suddenly reinflating; or an inflammation between the pleural linings. The four types of adventitious sounds include crackles (also referred to as rales), gurgles (also referred to as rhonchi), wheezes, and pleural friction rub (Table 13-4). The location and characteristics of the sounds should be noted, as well as diminished breath sounds or the absence of breath sounds (found with collapsed or surgically removed lobes).

ASSESSMENT

1. Assess history of tobacco or marijuana use, including type of tobacco, duration, and amount in pack years. Pack years equal number of years smoking times the number of packs per day (e.g., ½ pack per day times 4 years equals 2 pack years). If client has quit, determine the length of time since smoking stopped. *Rationale: Smoking is a risk factor linked with the incidence of lung cancer, heart disease, and chronic lung disease (emphysema and chronic bronchitis). Cigarette smoking is responsible for 87% of all lung cancers in the United States (American Cancer Society, 2001).*

2. Ask if client experiences any of the following: persistent cough (productive or nonproductive), sputum

Table 13-4

Adventitious Sounds

Sound	Site Auscultated	Cause	Character
Crackles (also called rales)	Are most commonly heard in dependent lobes: right and left lung bases	Random, sudden reinflation of groups of alveoli*	Are fine, short, interrupted crackling sounds heard during inspiration, expiration, or both; vary in pitch: high or low; may or may not change with coughing*; sound like crushing cellophane
Ronchi	Are primarily heard over trachea and bronchi; if loud enough, can be heard over most lung fields	Fluid or mucus in larger airways, causing turbulence	Are low-pitched, continuous sounds heard more during expiration; may be cleared by coughing; sounds like blowing air through milk with a straw
Wheezes	Can be heard over all lung fields	Severely narrowed bronchus	Are high-pitched, musical sounds heard during inspiration or expiration; do not clear with coughing†
Pleural friction rub	Is heard best over anterior lateral lung field (if client is sitting upright)	Inflamed pleura, parietal pleura rubbing against visceral pleura	Has grating quality heard best during inspiration; does not clear with coughing

*Data from Forgacs P: The functional basis of pulmonary sounds, *Chest* 73:399, 1978.

production, chest pain, shortness of breath, orthopnea, dyspnea during exertion, activity intolerance, and recurrent attacks of pneumonia or bronchitis. *Rationale: Warning signs of lung cancer include persistent cough, bloody sputum, and recurrent lung infections.*

3. Check for history of allergies to pollens, dust, or other airborne irritants, as well as to any foods, drugs, or chemical substances. Determine if client works in environment containing pollutants such as asbestos, coal dust, or chemical irritants. Does client have exposure to secondhand cigarette smoke? *Rationale: Clients with chronic respiratory disease, particularly asthma, have symptoms aggravated by change in temperature and humidity, irritating fumes or smoke, emotional stress, and physical exertion. Allergies are associated with wheezes on auscultation, dyspnea, cyanosis, and diaphoresis.*

4. Review history for known or suspected human immunodeficiency virus (HIV) infection, substance abuse, low income, and residence in nursing home. *Rationale: Known risk factors for exposure to and/or development of tuberculosis.*

5. Ask if client has history of cough, hemoptysis, weight loss, fatigue, night sweats, and/or fever. *Rationale: Signs and symptoms for both tuberculosis and HIV infection.*

6. Review family history for cancer, tuberculosis, allergies, or chronic obstructive pulmonary disease (COPD). *Rationale: The most common symptom of pulmonary tuberculosis is a cough. Initially cough is nonproductive. If untreated, it becomes productive with mucoid or mucopurulent sputum. Other symptoms include night sweats and weight loss. The condition may be diagnosed by chest x-ray examination, sputum for acid-fast bacillus, and sputum for culture and sensitivity.*

PLANNING

Expected outcomes focus on identifying alterations in respiratory function.

Expected Outcomes

1. Respirations are passive, diaphragmatic or costal, and regular (12 to 20 breaths per minute in adult) with symmetrical expansion.
2. Breath sounds are clear to auscultation in all lung fields.

Equipment

- Stethoscope
- Disposable gloves

Delegation Considerations

Assessment skills of the lung and thorax require the critical thinking and knowledge application unique to an RN. For these skills, delegation is inappropriate. For clients with abnormal lung sounds, assistive personnel (AP) must be instructed to observe client's respirations and report any changes in rate and depth and to keep head of bed elevated for client to breathe.

IMPLEMENTATION FOR ASSESSING THE THORAX AND LUNGS

Steps	Rationale
1. See Standard Protocol (inside front cover).	
2. Position client sitting upright. For bedridden client, elevate head of bed 45 to 90 degrees.	Promotes full lung expansion during examination.
a. If unable to tolerate sitting, supine position and side-lying positions are used.	Clients with chronic respiratory disease will likely need to sit up throughout the examination because of shortness of breath. Assistance of another caregiver may be required to position unresponsive clients.
b. Remove gown or drape first from posterior chest, keeping legs covered. As examination progresses, remove gown from area being examined.	Avoids unnecessary exposure and provides full visibility of thorax. Allows direct placement of diaphragm or bell of stethoscope on the client's skin, which enhances clarity of sounds.
c. Explain all steps of procedure, encouraging client to relax and breathe normally through the mouth.	Anxiety may alter respiratory function. Breathing through the mouth decreases extraneous sounds from air passing through the nose.

Steps	Rationale
3. *Posterior thorax:* If possible, stand behind client to inspect thorax for shape, deformities, position of the spine, slope of the ribs, retraction of intercostal spaces during inspiration, and bulging of intercostal spaces during expiration.	Allows for identification of any factors that may impair chest expansion and any symptoms of respiratory distress. In a child, shape of chest is almost circular, with anteroposterior diameter in 1:1 ratio. In adult, chest is twice as wide as deep, with 1:2 anteroposterior diameter. Chronic lung disease results in 1:1 ratio. This is referred to as a "barrel chest." Clients with breathing problems assume postures that improve ventilation.

NURSE ALERT *Localized chest pain may be evidenced by the client holding the chest wall during breathing. Assess the nature of pain, including onset, precipitating factors, quality, region, and radiation.*

---

4. Determine the rate and rhythm of respiration (see Chapter 12).	This is a good time to count respirations, with client relaxed and unaware of inspection. Awareness could alter respirations.
5. Systematically palpate posterior chest wall, costal spaces, and intercostal spaces, noting any masses, pulsations, unusual movement, or areas of localized tenderness (see illustration). If suspicious mass or swollen area is detected, palpate for size, shape, and typical qualities of lesion (see Skill 13-1, p. 301). Do not palpate painful areas deeply.	Palpation assesses further characteristics and confirms or supplements findings from assessment. Localized swelling or tenderness may indicate trauma to ribs or underlying cartilage. A fractured rib fragment could be displaced.
6. Standing behind client, place thumbs along the spinal processes at the tenth rib, with the palms lightly contacting the posterolateral surfaces (see illustration *A*). The nurse's thumbs should be about 2 inches (5 cm) apart, with the thumbs pointing toward the spine and the fingers pointing laterally. Press hands toward client's spine to form small skinfold between thumbs. After exhalation, client takes deep breath. Note movement of thumbs (see illustration *B*), and note symmetry of chest wall movement. Normally thumbs separate 3 to 5 cm (1½ to 2 inches) during chest excursion.	Palpation of chest excursion assesses depth of client's breathing. This technique is good measure to evaluate client's ability to perform deep breathing exercises (see Chapter 21). Limited movement on one side may indicate that client is voluntarily splinting during ventilation because of pain. Avoid allowing the hands to slide over the skin, which gives a false measure of excursion.

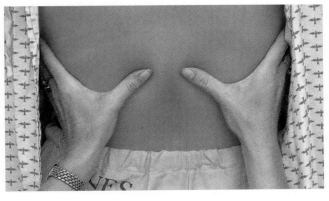
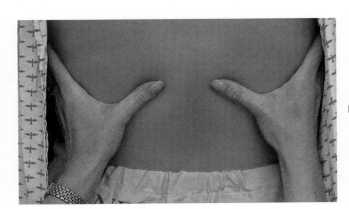

A

B

Step 6 **A,** Position of hands for palpation of posterior thorax excursion. **B,** As client inhales, movement of chest excursion separates nurse's thumbs.

Steps	Rationale
7. Percuss the chest wall moving from side to side and top to bottom following the same pattern as with palpation (see Step 5). Using indirect percussion, percuss intercostal spaces over symmetrical area of the lungs. Compare percussion notes for all lung lobes.	Determines density of underlying lung tissue. Ask client to fold arms forward across chest. This position separates scapulae to expose more lung tissue to assessment.
8. Auscultate breath sounds. Have client take slow deep breaths with the mouth slightly open. For adult, place diaphragm of stethoscope firmly on chest wall over intercostal spaces (see illustration). Listen to entire inspiration and expiration at each stethoscope position. Systematically compare breath sounds over right and left sides. If sounds are faint, ask client to breathe a little deeper temporarily.	Assesses movement of air through tracheobronchial tree (Table 13-5). Recognition of normal airflow sounds allows detection of sounds caused by mucus or airway obstruction. Sounds are characterized by length of inspiratory and expiratory phases. Gurgles caused by fluid or mucus in larger airways can be diminished or eliminated by effective coughing. Crackles may or may not change with coughing.

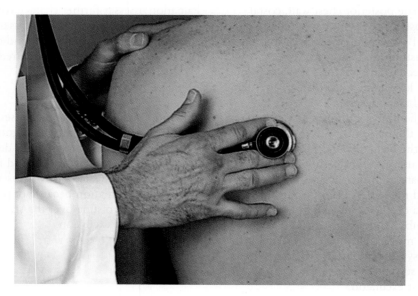

Step 8   Use of diaphragm of stethoscope to auscultate breath sounds. (From Seidel HM, and others: *Mosby's guide to physical examination,* ed 5, St Louis, 2003, Mosby.)

Table 13-5

Normal Breath Sounds

Description	Location	Origin
Vesicular Vesicular sounds are soft, breezy, and low pitched. Inspiratory phase is 3 times longer than expiratory phase.	Best heard over lung's periphery (except over scapula)	Created by air moving through smaller airways
Bronchovesicular Bronchovesicular sounds are medium-pitched and blowing sounds of medium intensity. Inspiratory phase is equal to expiratory phase.	Best heard posteriorly between scapulae and anteriorly over bronchioles lateral to sternum at first and second intercostal spaces	Created by air moving through large airways
Bronchial Bronchial sounds are loud and high pitched with hollow quality. Expiration lasts longer than inspiration (3:2 ratio).	Best heard over trachea	Created by air moving through trachea close to chest wall

Steps	Rationale
9. If adventitious sounds are auscultated, have client cough. Listen again with stethoscope to determine if sound has cleared with coughing (see Table 13-4, p. 313).	Improves access to lateral thoracic structures.
10. *Lateral thorax:* Instruct client to raise arms, and inspect chest wall for same characteristics as reviewed for posterior chest.	Allows for location of abnormalities in lateral lung fields.
11. Extend palpation, percussion, and auscultation of posterior thorax to lateral sides of chest, except for excursion measurement (Figure 13-3, *B*, p. 312).	Extent to which accessory muscles are used reveals degree of effort to breathe. Generally these muscles are not used for breathing.
12. *Anterior thorax:* Inspect accessory muscles of breathing: sternocleidomastoid, trapezius, and abdominal muscles, noting effort to breathe.	Indicates congenital, acquired, or traumatic alterations that may influence client's chest expansion.
13. Inspect width or spread of angle made by costal margins and tip of sternum. Angle is usually larger than 90 degrees between margins.	Assesses client's effort to breathe; symmetrical, passive movement indicates no respiratory distress.
14. Observe the client's breathing pattern, observing symmetry and degree of chest wall and abdominal movement. Respiratory rate and rhythm are more often assessed on the anterior chest wall.	Localized swelling or tenderness may indicate trauma to underlying ribs or cartilage.
15. Palpate anterior thoracic muscles and ribs for lumps, masses, tenderness, or unusual movement.	Assesses depth of client's breathing and ability to perform deep breathing exercises. Certain abnormalities are evident if expansion is not symmetrical.

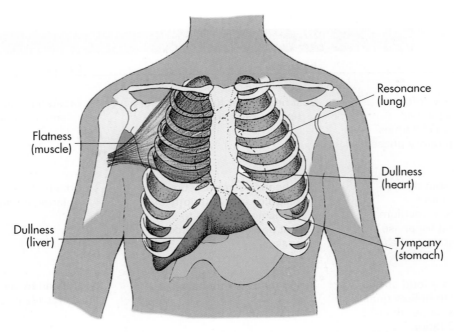

Step 17   Variations in percussion notes in normal thorax and upper abdomen.

Steps	Rationale
16. Palpate anterior chest excursion. Place hands over each lateral rib cage, with thumbs approximately 5 cm (2 inches) apart and angled along each costal margin. Thumbs are pushed toward client's midline to create skinfold between thumbs. As client inhales deeply, thumbs should normally separate approximately 3 to 5 cm (1½ to 2 inches), with each side expanding equally.	Can determine presence of underlying fluid, air, or mass.
17. Percuss anterior thorax between intercostal spaces with the client lying or sitting (procedure is easier when client is lying down). Begin above the clavicles; move across and then down as during palpation (see illustration).	Sitting allows the client to be more comfortable.
18. With client sitting, auscultate anterior thorax. Begin above the clavicles, and move across and then down (see Figure 13-3, p. 312).	
19. See Completion Protocol (inside front cover).	

• • • • • • • • • •

EVALUATION

1. Compare respirations (depth, regularity, and breath sounds) with findings of previous shift.

Unexpected Outcomes and Related Interventions

1. Client demonstrates PaO_2 <80 or $PaCO_2$ >35, hypoventilation, cyanosis, and/or altered LOC.
  a. Stay with the client and call for help.
  b. Position client in semi-Fowler's or other comfortable position to maximize lung expansion.
  c. Initiate oxygen therapy.
  d. Monitor vital signs.
  e. Notify physician; ABGs may need to be drawn for blood gas analysis.

2. Client has copious mucous production, audible wheezing, congested cough with thick, tenacious mucous.
   a. Assist client to cough by splinting chest, teach to inhale slowly through nose, exhale and cough; encourage expectoration of sputum.
   b. Auscultate breath sounds before and after cough to evaluate the effectiveness of cough in eliminating secretions.
   c. Encourage increased fluid intake (if permitted).
   d. If unable to clear airway by coughing, suctioning is indicated (see Chapter 31).
   e. Monitor vital signs.
   f. Notify physician.
3. Client demonstrated weakness, fatigue, dyspnea, altered vital signs, and dizziness with exertion.
   a. Provide bed rest and limited activity to conserve oxygen.
   b. Assess response to activity.
   c. Plan interventions alternately with periods of rest.
   d. Monitor for restlessness, anxiety, confusion, and respiratory status.

Recording and Reporting

- Record adventitious breath sounds, including type; location; presence on inspiration, expiration, or both; and changes noted after coughing.
- If client has a productive cough and mucus is purulent, obtaining a specimen is appropriate (see Chapter 14). Record amount, color, consistency, and odor of mucus.

- Report increased dyspnea and acute respiratory distress immediately.

Sample Documentation

730 Wheezing noted over anterior upper lobes bilaterally. Respiratory rate 26. C/O shortness of breath even at rest. Head of bed raised to 90 degrees. M.D. notified.

SPECIAL CONSIDERATIONS

Pediatric Considerations
Children younger than 6 years of age exhibit noticeable abdominal or diaphragmatic movement. Older children and adults exhibit more costal or thoracic movement. Use bell to auscultate breath sounds in children. Breath sounds are louder in children because of their thin chest walls.

Geriatric Considerations
Older adults have a costal angle (anteriorly) of slightly less than 90 degrees. The anteroposterior diameter may be increased from kyphosis. In older adults, chest expansion is reduced because of calcification of rib cartilage and partial contraction of inspiratory muscles. Older adults should be vaccinated against the flu in the early fall (Lueckenotte, 2000).

Skill 13.3

Assessing the Heart and Neck Vessels

A client who presents with signs or symptoms of heart (cardiac) problems, such as chest pain, may be suffering a life-threatening condition requiring immediate attention. In this situation the nurse acts quickly and decides on the portions of the examination that are absolutely necessary. When a client's condition is stable, a more thorough assessment can reveal baseline heart function and any risks for heart disease. Clients tend to seek information about heart disease because it remains a leading cause of death in the United States. The heart and neck vessels can be assessed together because the two systems work in unison and are in close proximity.

The nurse may begin assessment of the heart after examining the lungs because the client is already in a suitable position with the chest exposed. Assessment then proceeds to the neck vessels. The nurse uses inspection, palpation, auscultation, and percussion during the examination.

ASSESSMENT

1. Assess client for history of smoking, alcohol intake, caffeine intake (coffee, tea, soft drinks, chocolate), use of "recreational" drugs, exercise habits, and dietary patterns and intake. *Rationale: These can contribute to risk factors for cardiovascular disease.*
2. Determine if client is taking medications for cardiovascular function (e.g., antiarrhythmics, antihypertensives, antianginals) and if client knows their purpose, dosage, and side effects. *Rationale: Allows nurse to assess client's compliance with and understanding of drug therapies. Medications for cardiovascular function cannot be taken intermittently.*
3. Ask if client has experienced dyspnea, chest pain or discomfort, palpitations, excess fatigue, cough, leg pain or cramps, edema of the feet, cyanosis, fainting,

and orthopnea. Ask if symptoms occur at rest or during exercise. *Rationale: These are the cardinal symptoms of heart disease. Cardiovascular function may be adequate during rest but not during exercise.*

4. If client reports chest pain, determine onset (sudden or gradual), precipitating factors, quality, region, severity, and if it radiates. Angina pain is usually a deep pressure or ache that is substernal and diffuse, radiating to one or both arms, neck, or jaw. *Rationale: Symptoms may reveal myocardial infarction or coronary artery disease.*

5. Assess family history for heart disease, diabetes, high cholesterol levels, hypertension, stroke, or rheumatic heart disease. *Rationale: Family history of heart problems increases risk for heart and vascular disease, as do these other factors.*

6. Ask client about a history of heart trouble (e.g., heart failure, congenital heart disease, coronary artery disease, dysrhythmias, murmurs), heart surgery, or vascular disease (hypertension, phlebitis, varicose veins). *Rationale: Knowledge reveals client's level of understanding of condition. A preexisting condition influences examination techniques used by nurse and expected findings.*

PLANNING

Expected outcomes focus on identifying alterations in cardiovascular function.

Expected Outcomes

1. Heart is in normal sinus rhythm (NSR) with rate from 60 to 100 beats per minute (adolescent through adult), and S_1 and S_2 are heard clearly, without extra sounds or murmurs.

2. Point of maximal impulse (PMI) is palpable at fifth intercostal space at left midclavicular line in adult. PMI is at third or fourth intercostal space at left midclavicular line in infant or child (Figures 13-4 and 13-5).

3. Client describes changes in own behavior that may improve cardiovascular function.

4. Client describes schedule, dosage, purpose, and benefits of medications being taken for cardiovascular function. Information related to health benefits may improve compliance with therapy.

5. Blood pressure is within normal limits for client (see Chapter 12).

6. Carotid pulse is localized, strong, elastic, and equal bilaterally. No change occurs during inspiration or expiration without carotid bruit present. This indicates a patent vessel.

7. Jugular veins distend when client lies supine and flatten when client is in sitting position. Venous pressure is normal.

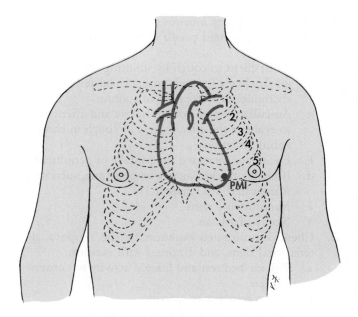

Figure 13-4 Location of PMI in adult.

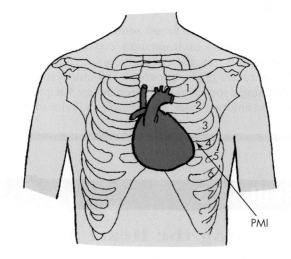

Figure 13-5 Location of PMI in child under 7 years old. (From Wong DL and others: *Whaley and Wong's nursing care of infants and children,* ed 6, St Louis, 1999, Mosby.)

Equipment

- Stethoscope
- Doppler stethoscope (optional)
- Conducting gel (if a Doppler stethoscope is used)

IMPLEMENTATION FOR ASSESSING THE HEART AND NECK VESSELS

Steps	Rationale

1. See Standard Protocol (inside front cover).
2. Assist client to be as relaxed and comfortable as possible.

An anxious or uncomfortable client can have mild tachycardia that may lead the nurse to confounding findings.

3. Have client assume semi-Fowler's or supine position.

Provides adequate visibility and access to left thorax and mediastinum. Client with heart disease often experiences shortness of breath while lying flat.

4. Explain procedure. Avoid facial gestures reflecting concern.

Client with previously normal cardiac history may become anxious if nurse shows concern.

5. Be sure that room is quiet.

Subtle, low-pitched heart sounds are difficult to hear.

6. Form a mental image of the exact location of the heart (see illustration). The base of the heart is the upper portion, and the apex is the bottom tip. The surface of the right ventricle composes most of the heart's anterior surface.

Visualization improves ability to assess findings accurately and determine possible source of abnormalities.

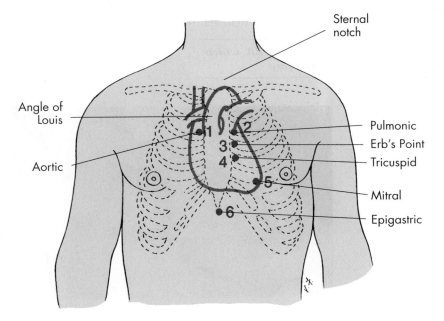

Step 6   Anatomical sites for assessment of cardiac function.

Steps	Rationale
7. Find the angle of Louis, felt as a ridge in the sternum approximately 5 cm (2 inches) below the sternal notch (between the sternal body and manubrium). Slip fingers down each side of angle to feel adjacent ribs. The intercostal spaces are just below each rib.	Provides examiner with landmarks for cardiac assessment.

8. Find the following anatomical landmarks (see illustration for Step 6):
  a. The aortic area is at the second intercostal space on the client's right *(1)*;
  b. The pulmonic area is at the second intercostal space on left *(2)*.
  c. The second pulmonic area is found by moving down left side of sternum to the third intercostal space *(3)*, also referred to as Erb's point.
  d. The tricuspid area *(4)* is located at the fourth left intercostal space along the sternum.
  e. The mitral area is found by moving fingers laterally to client's left to locate fifth intercostal space at left midclavicular line *(5)*.
  f. The epigastric area *(6)* is at the inferior tip of the sternum.
	Familiarity with landmarks allows nurse to describe findings more clearly and ultimately may improve assessment.

9. Stand to the client's right, and look first at the precordium with the client supine. Note any visible pulsations and more exaggerated lifts. Inspect closely at the area of the apex.	May reveal size and symmetry of the heart. The apical impulse is normally visible at the midclavicular line in the fifth intercostal space. The apical impulse (PMI) may become visible only when the client sits up, bringing the heart closer to the anterior wall. It is easily obscured by obesity.

NURSE ALERT   *Presence of a thrill is not normal and may indicate a disruption of blood flow caused by a defect in closure of a heart valve or atrial septal defect.*

10. Locate the PMI by palpating with fingertips along fifth intercostal space in midclavicular line (see illustration). Note a light, brief pulsation in an area 1 to 2 cm (½ to 1 inch) in diameter at the apex.	In the presence of serious heart disease, the PMI will be located to the left of the midclavicular line related to enlarged left ventricle. In chronic lung disease the PMI may be to the right of the midclavicular line as a result of right ventricular enlargement.

NURSE ALERT   *A stronger than expected impulse may be a heave or lift, which may indicate increased cardiac output or left ventricular hypertrophy.*

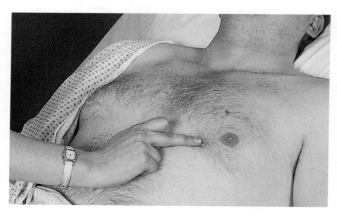

Step 10   Palpation of PMI.

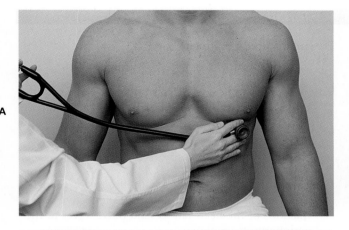

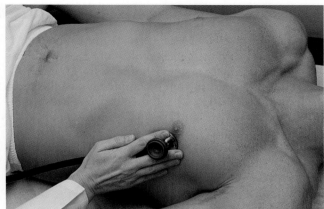

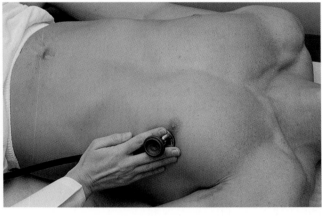

Step 13 Sequences of client positions for heart auscultation. **A,** Sitting. **B,** Supine. **C,** Left lateral. (From Seidel HM and others: *Mosby's guide to physical examination,* ed 4, St Louis, 1999, Mosby.)

Steps	Rationale
11. If palpating PMI is difficult, turn client onto left side.	Maneuver moves the heart closer to the chest wall.
12. Inspect the epigastric area, and palpate the abdominal aorta. Note a localized strong beat.	Rules out reduced blood flow or diffuse pulse, which may indicate a number of abnormalities.
13. Auscultate heart sounds. Begin by having client sit up and lean slightly forward; then have client lie supine; and end the examination with client in a left lateral recumbent position (see illustration). In a female client it may be necessary to lift the left breast to hear heart sounds more effectively.	Different positions help to clarify type of sounds heard. Sitting position is best to hear high-pitched murmurs (if present). Supine is common position to hear all sounds. Left lateral recumbent is best position to hear low-pitched sounds.
14. While auscultating sounds, ask client not to speak but to breathe comfortably. Begin with the diaphragm of the stethoscope; then alternate with the bell. Use very light pressure for the bell. Inch the stethoscope along; avoid jumping from one area to another. Do not try to hear all heart sounds at once.	Auscultation requires the examiner to isolate each heart sound at all auscultation sites.
a. Begin at the apex or PMI; then move systematically to the tricuspid area, second pulmonic area, and pulmonic and aortic areas. (NOTE: Some examiners use reverse sequence.) S_1 is best heard at the apex and is simultaneous with the carotid pulse.	At normal slow rates S_1 is high pitched and dull in quality and sounds like a "lub." This sound precedes the systolic phase of heart contraction.
b. Listen for S_2 at each site. It precedes the diastolic phase and sounds like "dub." This sound is best heard at the aortic area. Heart sounds will vary by pitch, loudness, and duration, depending on the auscultatory site.	Normal sounds S_1 and S_2 are high pitched and best heard with diaphragm.

Steps	Rationale
c. After both sounds are heard clearly as "lub-dub," count each combination of S_1 and S_2 as one heartbeat. Count the number of beats for 1 minute.	Determines apical pulse rate.
d. Assess heart rhythm by noting the time between S_1 and S_2 (systole) and then the time between S_2 and the next S_1 (diastole). Listen to the full cycle at each auscultation area. Note regular intervals between each sequence of beats. There should be a distinct pause between S_1 and S_2.	Failure of heart to beat at regular intervals is a dysrhythmia, which interferes with heart's ability to pump effectively.
e. When heart rate is irregular, compare apical and radial pulses (Table 13-6). Auscultate the apical pulse, and then immediately palpate the radial pulse. A colleague can assess the radial pulse while the nurse assesses the apical.	Determines if a pulse deficit (radial pulse is slower than apical) exists. Deficit indicates that ineffective contractions of the heart fail to send pulse waves to the periphery.
15. Continue to auscultate for extra heart sounds at each site. If any abnormal sounds are heard, note pitch, loudness, duration, and timing (when in relation to the cardiac cycle). Note location on the chest wall.	Abnormal sounds include murmurs. Characteristics of murmurs help to identify contributing factors.
a. Use the bell of the stethoscope, and listen for low-pitched extra heart sounds such as S_3 and S_4 gallops, clicks, and rubs. S_3, or a ventricular gallop, occurs just after S_2 at the end of ventricular diastole. It may sound like "lub-dub-ee" or "Kentuc-ky." S_4, or an atrial gallop, occurs just before S_1 or ventricular systole. It sounds like "dee-lub-dub" or "Ten-nes-see."	Gallops may be caused by premature rushes of blood into a ventricle that is stiff or dilated or an atrial contraction pushing against a ventricle that is not accepting blood.
b. Listen for clicks as short high-pitched extra sounds.	Clicks are caused by abnormalities such as mitral valve prolapse or prosthetic valves.
c. With client leaning forward or lying on the left side, listen for friction rubs as squeaky or rubbing sounds. Instruct client to hold breath as you continue to listen.	Rubs may result from lungs or inflamed visceral and parietal layers of the pericardium of the heart rubbing against one another. If the sound is present only while the client is breathing, the origin of the rub is pulmonary rather than cardiac.

Table 13-6

Common Types of Dysrhythmias

Definition	Cause
Sinus dysrhythmia: Pulse rate changes during respiration, increasing at peak of inspiration and declining during expiration.	Blood is momentarily trapped in lungs during inspiration, causing fall in heart's stroke volume.
Sinus tachycardia: Pulse rhythm is regular, but rate is accelerated to more than 100 beats per minute.	Exercise, emotional stress, and caffeine or alcohol ingestion are common factors that cause increased firing of sinoatrial nodes.
Sinus bradycardia: Pulse rhythm is regular, but rate is slower than normal at 40 to 60 beats per minute.	Sinoatrial node fires less frequently. This is common in well-conditioned athletes and with use of antidysrhythmic medications.
Premature ventricular contraction: Premature beat occurs before regularly expected heart contraction.	Ventricle contracts prematurely because of electrical, impulse bypassing normal conduction pathway. It may occur so early that it is difficult to detect as second beat. It may be followed by a pause.
Atrial fibrillation: Rapid, random contractions of atria cause irregular ventricular beats at 130 to 150 beats per minute.	Atria discharge very rapidly, with some impulses not reaching ventricles. This condition occurs in rheumatic heart disease and mitral stenosis. It causes reduced cardiac output.

Steps	Rationale
16. Auscultate for heart murmurs over each of the auscultation sites.	Murmurs are sustained swishing or blowing sounds heard at the beginning, middle, or end of systole or diastole. They are caused by increased blood flow through a normal valve, forward flow through a stenotic valve or into a dilated vessel or chamber, or backward flow through a valve that fails to close.
17. When a murmur is detected, listen carefully to note where the murmur can be heard best. Note the intensity of the murmur.	Intensity is related to rate of blood flow through the heart or the amount of blood regurgitated. A thrill is a continuous palpable sensation like the purring of a cat. A thrust is the upward lift felt when palpating the chest wall.
18. Note if the murmur is low, medium, or high in pitch using the bell for low-pitched sounds.	Pitch depends on velocity of blood flow through the valves.
19. Assess carotid arteries: Have client remain in sitting position.	Allows easier mobility of neck to expose artery for inspection and palpation.
20. Inspect neck on both sides for obvious pulsations of artery. Ask client to turn head slightly away from artery being examined. Sometimes pulse wave can be seen.	Carotids are the only sites to assess quality of pulse wave. Experience is required to evaluate wave in relation to events of cardiac cycle.
21. Palpate each carotid artery separately with index and middle fingers around medial edge of sternocleidomastoid muscle. Ask client to raise chin slightly, keeping the head straight (see illustration). Note rate and rhythm, strength, and elasticity of artery. Also note if pulse changes as client inspires and expires.	If both arteries were occluded simultaneously, client could lose consciousness from reduced circulation to brain. Turning head improves access to artery. Change may indicate a sinus dysrhythmia.

NURSE ALERT *Do not vigorously palpate or massage the artery. Stimulation of carotid sinus may cause a reflex drop in heart rate and blood pressure.*

Steps	Rationale
22. Place bell of stethoscope over each carotid artery, auscultating for blowing sound (bruit) (see illustration).	Narrowing of carotid artery's lumen by athrosclerotic plaques causes disturbance in blood flow. Blood passing through narrowed section creates turbulence and emits blowing or swishing sound.

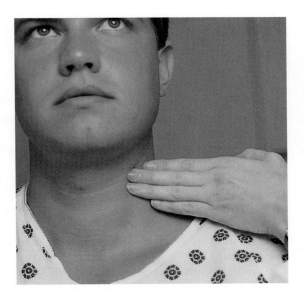

Step 21 Palpation of internal carotid artery.

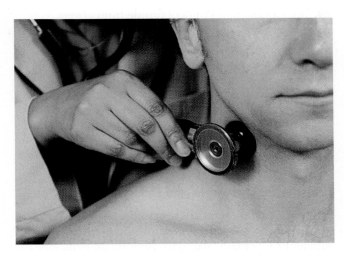

Step 22 Auscultation for carotid bruit. (From Barkauskas VH and others: *Health and physical assessment*, ed 2, St Louis, 1998, Mosby.)

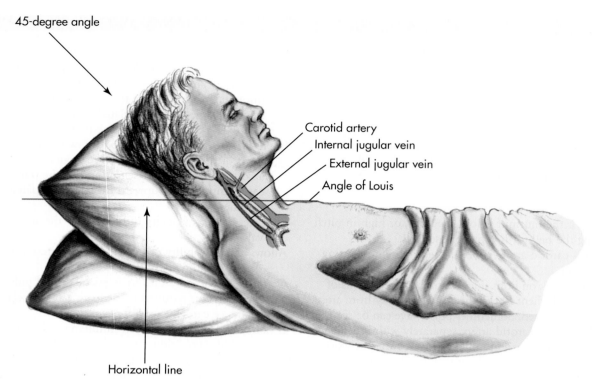

45-degree angle

Carotid artery
Internal jugular vein
External jugular vein
Angle of Louis

Horizontal line

Step 23   (Modified from Thompson JM and others: *Mosby's manual of clinical nursing,* ed 5, St Louis, 2001, Mosby.)

Steps	Rationale
23. With client's head and neck elevated 45 to 90 degrees in Fowler's position, observe for level of venous filling and visible jugular pulsation (see illustration). Observe for cyanosis (bluish discoloration of lips, mouth, conjunctivae, nail beds).	The level above a line drawn along the angle of Louis at which the jugular venous pulse is visible indicates right atrial pressure.

NURSE ALERT   *Visible jugular pulsation suggests need for immediate treatment.*

24. See Completion Protocol (inside front cover).

• • • • • • • • • •

EVALUATION

1. Compare findings with normal assessment characteristics of heart and vascular system.
2. If heart sounds are not audible or pulses are not palpable, ask another nurse to confirm assessment.
3. Ask client to describe behaviors that increase risk for heart and vascular disease.

Unexpected Outcomes and Related Interventions

Abnormal findings that are new to the client's assessment data require physician notification. Be prepared to assist with an EKG; obtain vital signs. Abnormalities include the following:

a. Pulsations, vibrations, or both are palpable. These are result of valvular problem, murmur, or both.

b. PMI is found to left of midclavicular line, which is the result of cardiomegaly.
2. Pulse is irregular and/or the rate less than 60 beats per minute or more than 100 beats per minute.
   a. Check blood pressure. If low, dysrhythmia is contributing to inadequate cardiac output.
   b. Observe for sensations or reports of dizziness or feeling "faint."
3. Pulse deficit is noted. There is risk for inadequate cardiac output.
4. Extra heart sounds S_3 or S_4 are auscultated. Extra sounds indicate atrial or ventricular gallop.
5. Murmur is auscultated. Impaired blood flow through heart may indicate need for immediate medical attention. Some murmurs are benign.

Recording And Reporting

- Document quality (clear or muffled), intensity (weak or pounding), rate, and rhythm (regular, regularly irregular, or irregularly irregular).
- Document activity level and subjective data related to fatigue, shortness of breath, and chest pain.
- Document preferred position, medications and/or treatments used, and client's response.
- Report immediately to physician any irregularities in heart function and indications of impaired arterial blood flow.

Sample Documentation

0730 Pulse rate 104 and irregularly irregular. Blood pressure 120/70. Client denies discomfort. Resting quietly in bed without complaints of distress. (See Routine Nursing Assessment: Cardiovascular, Appendix A.)

⊛ SPECIAL CONSIDERATIONS ⊛

Pediatric Considerations

Perform cardiac assessment on infant or toddler while quiet, before more uncomfortable procedures. The PMI is at third or fourth intercostal space at left midclavicular line in infants or children. It is not uncommon for children to have third heart sounds (S_3). Sinus dysrhythmia occurs normally in many children (Wong and others, 1999). Children have louder, higher-pitched heart sounds because of their thin chest walls.

Geriatric Considerations

PMI may be difficult to find in an older adult because anteroposterior diameter of the chest deepens. Accidental massage of the carotid sinus during palpation of the carotid artery can be a particular problem for older adults, causing a sudden drop in heart rate from vagal nerve stimulation (Lueckenotte, 2000). Older adults with hypertension may benefit from regular monitoring of blood pressure (daily, weekly, or monthly). Home monitoring kits are available. Teach client how to use them.

Skill 13.4

Assessing the Abdomen

Abdominal assessment is complex because of the multiple organs located within and near the abdominal cavity. This area of the body is associated with many health complaints, and many people are embarrassed by bowel or bladder dysfunction, reproductive problems, or urinary elimination problems. Abdominal pain is one of the most common symptoms clients report when seeking medical care. Abdominal pain could be caused by alterations in organs such as the stomach, gallbladder, or intestines, or the pain may be the result of spinal or muscular injury. An accurate assessment requires matching the client's history with a careful assessment of the location of physical symptoms (Table 13-7).

To perform an effective abdominal assessment the nurse needs a detailed knowledge of the underlying structures involved, including the lower pelvis, kidneys, rectum, genitalia, liver, gallbladder, stomach, spleen, intestines, and reproductive organs (Figure 13-6). An abdominal assessment is routine after abdominal surgery and for any client who has undergone invasive diagnostic tests of the gastrointestinal tract (see Chapter 14).

The order of an abdominal assessment differs from that of other assessments. The nurse begins with inspection and follows with auscultation. It is important to auscultate before palpation and percussion because these maneuvers may alter the frequency and character of bowel sounds.

ASSESSMENT

1. If client has abdominal or low back pain, assess the character of pain in detail (location, onset, frequency, precipitating factors, aggravating factors, type of pain, severity, course). *Rationale: Knowing pattern of characteristics of pain helps determine its source.*
2. Carefully observe client's movement and position, such as:
   a. Lying still with knees drawn up
   b. Moving restlessly to find a comfortable position
   c. Lying on one side or sitting with knees drawn up to chest
   Rationale: Positions assumed by the client may reveal nature and source of pain (e.g., peritonitis, renal stone, pancreatitis).
3. Assess client's normal bowel habits: frequency of stools; character of stools; recent changes in character of stools; measures used to promote elimination,

Table 13-7

Common Causes for Abdominal Pain

Conduction	Physical Alteration	Physical Signs and Symptoms
Appendicitis	Obstruction of the appendix associated with inflammation, perforation, and peritonitis.	Sharp pain directly over the irritated peritoneum 2-12 hours after onset. Often pain localizes at McBurney's point in the right lower quadrant between the anterior iliac crest and the umbilicus. Associated with rebound tenderness.
Cholecystitis	Obstruction of the cystic duct causing inflammation or distention of the gallbladder.	Murphy's sign: Apply gentle pressure below the right subcostal arch and below the liver margin. Sharp pain and inspiratory arrest occur when the client takes a deep breath (Wright, 1997).
Constipation	Disruption in normal bowel pattern, which may occur with narcotic use or inadequate fiber and fluid intake.	Generalized discomfort accompanied by distention and palpation of a hard mass in the left lower quadrant. Nausea and vomiting may begin after several days.
Crohn's disease	A chronic inflammatory lesion of the ileum. Cause is unknown.	Steady colicky pain in the right lower quadrant, with cramping, tenderness, flatulence, nausea, fever, and diarrhea. Often associated with bloody stools, weight loss, weakness, and fatigue.
Gastroenteritis	Inflammation of the stomach and intestinal tract.	Generalized abdominal discomfort accompanied by nausea, vomiting, diarrhea.
Intestinal obstruction	Blockage of the lumen of the intestine.	Colicky pain, nausea, vomiting, constipation, and abdominal distention. Bowel sounds are hyperactive with a rushng sound or absence of bowel sounds.
Pancreatitis	Inflammation of the pancreas associated with alcoholism and gallbladder disease.	Steady epigastric pain close to the umbilicus radiates to the back. Associated with abdominal rigidity and vomiting. Pain is unrelieved by vomiting.
Paralytic ileus	Obstruction of the small bowel that occurs after abdominal surgery or use of anticholinergic medications.	Generalized severe abdominal distention, nausea, and vomiting.
Peptic ulcers	Damage of gastrointestinal (GI) mucosa at any area of the GI tract. May be caused by bacterial infection or nonsteroidal antiinflammatory drugs. Believed to be unrelated to stress. Aggravated by smoking and excessive alcohol use.	Localized midepigastric pain with heartburn that develops 2 hours or more after meals, when the stomach is empty. Eating may relieve the pain. Acidic liquid, such as orange juice or coffee, may aggravate the pain (Daly, 1997).

such as laxatives, enemas, dietary intake; and eating and drinking habits. *Rationale: These data, compared with information from physical assessment, may help to identify cause and nature of elimination problems.*

4. Determine if client has had abdominal surgery, trauma, or diagnostic tests of the gastrointestinal tract. *Rationale: Surgery or trauma to abdomen may result in altered position of underlying organs.*

5. Assess if client has had any nausea, vomiting, or cramping, especially in last 24 hours. *Rationale:*

Changes may indicate alterations in upper gastrointestinal tract (e.g., stomach, gallbladder) or lower colon.

6. Assess for difficulty in swallowing, belching, flatulence, bloody emesis (hematemesis), black or tarry stools (melena), heartburn, diarrhea, or constipation. *Rationale: Indicative of gastrointestinal alterations.*

7. Determine if client takes antiinflammatory medications (e.g., aspirin, steroids, nonsteroidal antiinflammatory drugs), or antibiotics. *Rationale: These pharmacological agents may cause gastrointestinal upset or bleeding.*

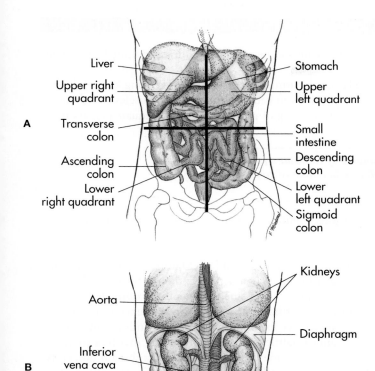

A

Liver

Upper right quadrant

Transverse colon

Ascending colon

Lower right quadrant

Stomach

Upper left quadrant

Small intestine

Descending colon

Lower left quadrant

Sigmoid colon

B

Aorta

Inferior vena cava

Descending colon

Ureters

Kidneys

Diaphragm

Ascending colon

Bladder

Figure 13-6   A, Anterior view of abdomen divided by quadrants. **B,** Posterior view of abdominal sections.

8. Inquire about family history of cancer, kidney disease, alcoholism, hypertension, or heart disease. *Rationale: Data may reveal risk for significant abdominal alterations. Chronic alcohol ingestion can cause gastrointestinal and liver problems.*

9. Determine if female client is pregnant. *Rationale: Pregnancy may cause nausea and vomiting, as well as changes in abdominal shape and contour.*

10. Review client's history for health care occupation, hemodialysis, IV drug use, household or sexual contact with hepatitis B virus (HBV) carrier, sexually active (heterosexual person with more than one sex partner in previous 6 months), sexually active homosexual or bisexual man, or international traveler in area of high HBV prevalence. *Rationale: These are risk factors for HBV exposure.*

PLANNING

Expected outcomes focus on identifying alterations in the abdomen.

Expected Outcomes

1. Abdomen is soft and symmetrical with smooth and even contour. No mass, distention, or tenderness is palpable. No forceful visible pulsations are noted.
2. Bowel sounds are active and audible in all four quadrants.
3. No costovertebral angle tenderness is present.
4. Client denies discomfort or worsening of existing discomfort following examination.

Equipment

- Stethoscope
- Tape measure
- Examination light
- Marking pen

 Delegation Considerations

This skill requires the critical thinking and knowledge application unique to an RN. For this skill, delegation is inappropriate. However, assistive personnel (AP) need to report to the RN the development of abdominal pain and changes in the client's bowel habits or dietary intake.

IMPLEMENTATION FOR ASSESSING THE ABDOMEN

Steps	Rationale
1. See Standard Protocol (inside front cover).	
2. Prepare client:	
a. Ask if client needs to empty bladder or defecate.	Palpation of full bladder can cause discomfort and feeling of urgency and make it difficult for client to relax.
b. Keep upper chest and legs draped.	Expose only areas to be examined.
c. Be sure that room is warm.	Provides for client comfort.

Steps	**Rationale**
d. Expose area from just above the xiphoid process down to the symphysis pubis.	Exposes areas to be examined during abdominal assessment.
e. Have client lie supine or in a dorsal recumbent position with arms down at sides and knees slightly bent. A small pillow may be placed under client's knees.	Placing the arms under the head or keeping knees fully extended can cause the abdominal muscles to tighten. Tightening of muscles prevents adequate palpation.

NURSE ALERT   *Observe respirations as position is changed. If abdomen is distended, lying flat may result in increased respiratory difficulty because of pressure on the diaphragm (Daly, 1997).*

f. Maintain conversation during assessment except during auscultation. Explain steps calmly and slowly.	Informs client of assessment technique to be used.
g. Ask client to point to tender areas.	Painful areas are assessed last. Manipulation of body part can increase client's pain and anxiety and make remainder of assessment difficult to complete.
3. Identify landmarks that divide abdominal region into quadrants; from the tip of xiphoid process to symphysis pubis crosses line intersecting umbilicus, dividing abdomen into four equal sections (see Figure 13-6, p. 329).	Location of findings by common reference point helps successive examiners to confirm findings and locate abnormalities. Normal ventilation involves rhythmic movement of abdomen as diaphragm descends and rises and a slight pulsation of aorta with each beat of systole.
4. Inspect skin of abdomen's surface for color, scars, venous patterns, rashes, lesions, silvery white striae (stretch marks), and artificial openings. Observe lesions for characteristics described in Skill 13-1, p. 308.	Scars reveal evidence that client has had past trauma or surgery. Striae indicate stretching of tissue from growth, obesity, pregnancy, ascites, or edema. Venous patterns may reflect liver disease (portal hypertension). Artificial openings indicate bowel or urinary diversion.
5. If bruising is noted, ask if client self-administers injections (e.g., heparin or insulin).	Frequent injections can cause bruising and hardening of underlying tissues.

NURSE ALERT   *Bruising may also indicate physical abuse, accidental injury, or bleeding disorders.*

6. Inspect the contour, symmetry, and surface motion of the abdomen. Note any masses, bulging, or distention. (Flat abdomen forms a horizontal plane from xiphoid process to symphysis pubis. Round abdomen protrudes in convex sphere from horizontal plane. Concave abdomen sinks into muscular wall. All are normal.)	Changes in symmetry or contour may reveal underlying masses, fluid collection, or gaseous distention. An everted (pouch extends outward) umbilicus may indicate distention. A hernia can also cause the umbilicus to protrude upward.
7. If abdomen appears distended, note if distention is generalized. Look at the flanks on each side.	Distention may be caused by one or more of the six *F*s (fat, flatus, feces, fluids, fibroid, and fetus). If gas causes distention, flanks do not bulge. If fluid causes distention, flanks bulge. A tumor may cause a unilateral bulging or distention. Pregnancy causes symmetrical bulge in lower abdomen.
8. If distention is suspected, measure size of abdominal girth by placing tape measure around abdomen at level of umbilicus (see illustration). Use the marking pen to indicate where tape measure was applied.	Consecutive measurements will show any increase or decrease in abdominal distention. All subsequent measurements are taken at same level of umbilicus to provide objective means to evaluate changes. A water-based pen can be used to make a mark on abdomen for subsequent measurements.
9. If nasogastric or intestinal tube is connected to suction, turn off momentarily.	Sound obscures bowel sounds.

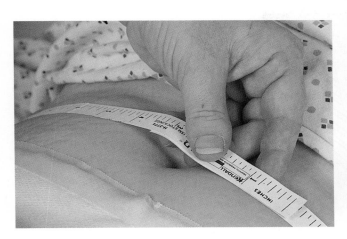

Step 8   Measuring abdominal girth at the level of the umbilicus.

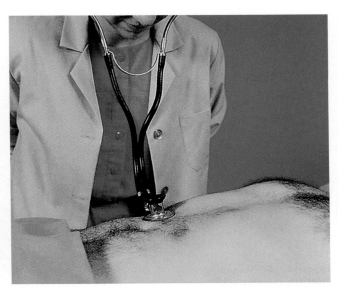

Step 10   Auscultation of bowel sounds. (From Barkauskas VH and others: *Health and physical assessment,* ed 3, St Louis, 2002, Mosby.)

Steps	Rationale
10. To auscultate bowel sounds, place the diaphragm of the stethoscope lightly over each of the four abdominal quadrants. Ask client not to talk. Listen until repeated gurgling or bubbling sounds are heard in each quadrant (minimum of once in 5 to 20 seconds). Describe sounds as normal, hyperactive, hypoactive, or absent. Listen 5 minutes over each quadrant before deciding that bowel sounds are absent (see illustration).	Normal bowel sounds occur irregularly every 5 to 15 seconds. Absence of sounds indicate cessation of gastric motility. Hyperactive bowel sounds not related to hunger or a recent meal may indicate diarrhea or early intestinal obstruction. Hypoactive or absent bowel sounds may indicate paralytic ileus or peritonitis (Daly, 1997). It is common for bowel sounds to be hypoactive postoperatively for 24 hours or more, especially following abdominal surgery.

NURSE ALERT   *Severe paralytic ileus may be accompanied by nausea and vomiting, increasing distention, and inability to pass flatus.*

11. Place the bell of the stethoscope over the epigastric region of the abdomen and each quadrant. Auscultate for vascular sounds.	Determines presence of turbulent blood flow (bruit) through thoracic or abdominal aorta.

NURSE ALERT   *If aortic bruit is auscultated, suggesting presence of an aneurysm, stop assessment and notify physician immediately. Percussion or palpation over abdominal bruit can cause rupture of an already weakened vessel wall in the presence of an abdominal aneurysm.*

12. With client supine, gently percuss each of four abdominal quadrants systematically. Note areas of tympany and dullness.	Reveals presence of air or fluid in stomach and intestines. Normal percussion is tympanic because of swallowed air in gastrointestinal tract. Presence of fluid or underlying masses is revealed by dull percussion.
13. Ask client if abdomen feels unusually tight, and determine if this is a recent development.	Continued sensation of fullness helps to detect distention. A feeling of fullness after a heavy meal causes only temporary distention. Tightness is not felt with obesity.

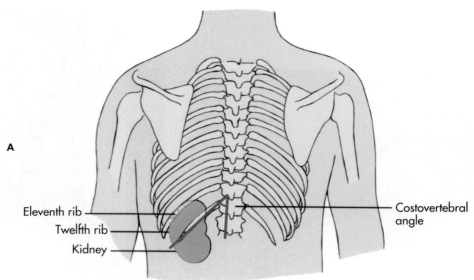

A

Eleventh rib ⎯⎯
Twelfth rib ⎯⎯
Kidney ⎯⎯

⎯⎯ Costovertebral angle

Step 14 A, Assessing for CVA tenderness. **B,** Percussion of the kidney. (From Seidel HM: *Mosby's guide to physical examination,* ed 4, St Louis, 1999, Mosby.)

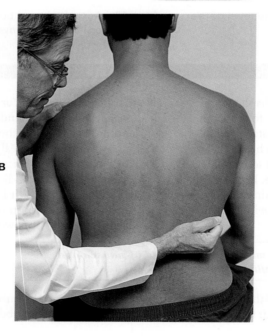

B

Steps	Rationale
14. With client sitting, gently but firmly percuss over each costovertebral angle along scapular lines (see illustration *A*). Use ulnar surface of fist to percuss directly against client's skin, or percuss indirectly by placing nondominant hand flat against costovertebral angle and percussing hand with dominant hand (see illustration *B*). Note if client experiences pain.	In the presence of kidney infection the client usually experiences pain on palpation.
15. Lightly palpate over each abdominal quadrant, laying the palm of the hand with fingers extended and approximated lightly on the abdomen. Keep the palm and forearm horizontal. The pads of the fingertips depress the skin approximately 1 cm (½ inch) in a gentle dipping motion (see illustration).	Detects areas of localized tenderness, degree of tenderness, and presence and character of underlying masses. Palpation of sensitive area causes guarding (voluntary tightening of underlying abdominal muscles).

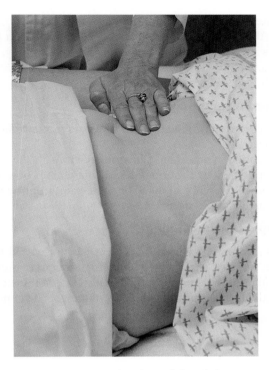

Step 15   Light palpation of the abdomen.

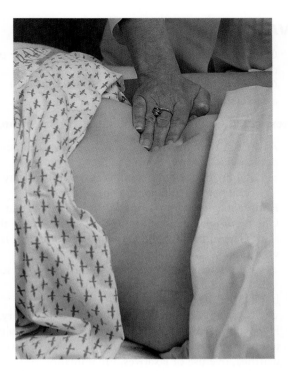

Step 19   Deep palpation of the abdomen.

Steps	Rationale

NURSE ALERT   *Palpate painful areas last. Avoid quick jabs. To avoid tickling, place the client's hand on the abdomen with the nurse's hand on the client's.*

a. Note muscular resistance, distention, tenderness, and superficial masses or organs while observing client's face for signs of discomfort.

b. Note if abdomen is firm or soft to touch.

16. Just below umbilicus and above symphysis pubis, palpate for a smooth, rounded mass. While applying light pressure, ask if client has sensation of need to void.

Client's verbal and nonverbal cues may indicate discomfort from tenderness. Firm abdomen may indicate active obstruction with fluid or gas building up.

Soft abdomen is normal or reveals that obstruction is resolving.

Detects presence of dome of distended bladder.

NURSE ALERT   *Routinely check for distended bladder if client has been unable to void, client has been incontinent, or an indwelling Foley catheter is not draining well.*

17. If masses are palpated, note size, location, shape, consistency, tenderness, mobility, and texture.

18. When tenderness is present, test for rebound tenderness by pressing slowly and deeply into the involved area and then let go quickly. Note if pain is aggravated.

19. Perform deep palpation, being sure the client is relaxed. Depress the palm and fingers approximately 2.5 to 7.5 cm (1 to 3 inches) into the abdomen (see illustration).

20. See Completion Protocol (inside front cover).

Descriptive characteristics help to reveal type of mass.

Results are positive if pain increases. May indicate appendicitis.

Detects less obvious masses and delineates abdominal organs.

• • • • • • • • • •

EVALUATION

1. Observe throughout the assessment for evidence of discomfort.
2. Compare assessment findings with previous shift assessment.

Unexpected Outcomes and Related Interventions

1. Abdomen is asymmetrical, with palpable mass, and dull to percussion.
   a. Report to the physician because findings may indicate enlarged liver, spleen, or tumor.
2. Abdomen protrudes symmetrically, with skin taut. Client complains of tightness. Bowel sounds are absent. Gastrointestinal motility has ceased. Client is vomiting.
   a. Keep client on "nothing by mouth" (NPO) status, and encourage ambulation.
   b. Notify physician.
   c. Gastric decompression may become necessary.
3. Hyperactive bowel sounds are evident with gastrointestinal motility. Commonly they result from anxiety, diarrhea, overuse of laxatives, inflammation of the bowel, or reaction of the intestines to certain foods.
   a. Client may need to be NPO.
   b. Contact physician if client may need antidiarrheal medications.
4. Rebound abdominal tenderness is found. Results from peritoneal irritation (e.g., appendicitis, pancreatitis) (Wright, 1997).
   a. Avoid palpating area.
   b. Notify physician if this is a new finding.
   c. Keep client on NPO status until physician can evaluate.
5. Bladder is palpable over symphysis pubis. Bladder is distended.
   a. Facilitate voiding.
   b. If unable to void, urinary catheterization may be necessary.
6. Internal organs (liver, spleen) are enlarged or tender. Do not continue to palpate area.
   a. Tenderness is indicative of hepatitis.
   b. Enlargement may be due to cancerous involvement or cirrhosis.
   c. Notify physician.
7. Keep client NPO until physician evaluates.
8. Abdominal girth is increased, accompanied by a fluid wave. Fluid has built up within peritoneal cavity.
   a. Notify physician.
   b. Place client on NPO status.

Recording and Reporting

- Record results of assessment in nurses' notes or flow sheet.
- Record content of any client instruction.
- Report serious abnormalities, such as absent bowel sounds, presence of mass, or acute pain, to nurse in charge and physician.

Sample Documentation

0800 Abdomen is distended. Client has not passed flatus since surgery, and bowel sounds are not present. Encouraged to sip on warm fluids and ambulate frequently. Denies nausea, vomiting, or pain at this time.

SPECIAL CONSIDERATIONS

Pediatric Considerations

Most common palpable mass in child is feces, usually felt in right lower quadrant (Wong and others, 1999). Have a child stand erect and then lie supine during inspection of abdominal surface. Normal abdomen of infants and young children is cylindrical in erect position and flat in supine position. In infants and children skin is usually taut and without wrinkles or creases.

Geriatric Considerations

Older adults often lack abdominal tone; underlying organs are more easily palpable. A weakened intestinal musculature and decreased peristalsis affect the large intestine. Constipation, nausea, flatulence, and heartburn are common. Stress to older adults the importance of adequate fluid intake, regular exercise, and a diet with at least four servings daily of fresh fruit and vegetables and high-fiber foods to promote normal defecation.

Skill 13.5

Assessing the Extremities and Peripheral Circulation

The nurse's assessment of the extremities and peripheral circulation uses inspection and palpation to examine the musculoskeletal, circulatory, and neurologic systems. Initial assessment involves a general inspection of gait, posture, and body position. A more thorough assessment of major bone, joint, and muscle groups is indicated in the presence of abnormalities. Much of the assessment can be performed while the nurse examines other body systems; for example, while assessing neck structures, the nurse can also assess neck range of motion (ROM). It is effective for the nurse to integrate assessment into routine activities of care, for example, while bathing or positioning the client. Assessment is especially important when the client reports pain or loss of joint or muscle function. Neurological assessment is often conducted simultaneously because muscles may be weakened as result of nerve involvement.

Inadequate tissue perfusion results in an inadequate delivery of oxygen and nutrients to cells, a condition called ischemia. This can be caused by constriction of the vessels or by occlusion (blockage) from clot formation. The effects of the ischemia depend on the duration of the problem and the metabolic needs of the tissues. Ischemia results in pain. If lack of oxygen to tissues is unrelieved, tissue necrosis (death) occurs. An embolus is a blood clot that breaks loose and travels through the circulation. If the clot obstructs circulation to the lungs or the brain, it can be life threatening. The nurse's assessment is designed to determine the integrity of the circulatory system.

ASSESSMENT

1. Review client history (particularly with female clients) for risk of osteoporosis, including heavy alcohol use, cigarette smoking, constant dieting, calcium intake less than 1000 mg daily, thin and light body frame, females who have never been pregnant, occurrence of menopause before age 45, being postmenopausal, bilateral oophorectomy (ovary removal), family history of osteoporosis, or European American, Asian, or Native American descent. *Rationale: These factors increase the risk for osteoporosis.*

2. Ask client to describe history of alteration in bone, muscle, or joint function (e.g., recent fall, trauma, lifting heavy objects, bone or joint disease with sudden or gradual onset) and location of alteration. *Rationale: Assists in assessing nature of musculoskeletal problem.*

3. Assess nature and extent of client's pain: location, duration, severity, predisposing and aggravating factors, relieving factors, and type of pain. If pain or cramping is reported in the lower extremities, ask if it is relieved or aggravated by walking. Assess the distance walked and characteristics of pain before, during, and after activity. *Rationale: Alterations in bone, joints, or muscle are frequently accompanied by pain. Pain has implications not only for comfort but also ability to perform activities of daily living. Pain caused by certain vascular conditions tends to increase with activity.*

4. Determine how client's alteration influences ability to perform activities of daily living (e.g., bathing, feeding, dressing, toileting, ambulating) and social functions (e.g., household chores, work, recreation, sexual activities). *Rationale: Level of nursing care is determined by extent to which client can perform self-care. Type and degree of restriction in continuing social activities influence topics for client education.*

5. Assess height decrease of woman older than 50 by subtracting current height from recall of height at age 30. *Rationale: A loss of height more than 2 inches from the height at age 30 strongly suggests the presence of osteoporosis (American Medical Directors Association, 1998).*

6. Ask if client experiences dyspnea, chest pain or discomfort, palpations, excessive fatigue, fainting, cyanosis, orthopnea, or edema of the feet. *Rationale: These are the cardinal symptoms of activity intolerance associated with heart disease. Cardiovascular function may be adequate during rest but not during exercise.*

7. Ask if client has noted signs of reduced sensation or weakness in extremities. *Rationale: Signs indicative of neurologic changes.*

8. Ask if client experiences leg cramps, numbness or tingling in extremities, or sensation of cold appendages. Also determine if client has noted any swelling of feet, ankles, or hands. *Rationale: These are common signs and symptoms of peripheral vascular disease.*

PLANNING

Expected outcomes focus on identifying deficits in neuromuscular, neurologic, and circulatory function.

Expected Outcomes

1. Client demonstrates erect posture, strong grasp, and steady gait, with arms swinging freely at side.

2. There is bilateral symmetry of extremities in length, circumference, alignment, position, and skinfolds.

3. Full active ROM is present in all joints with good muscle tone and absence of contractures, spasticity, or muscular weakness.

4. Peripheral pulses are equal and strong (3+), extremities are warm and pink, with capillary refill less than 3 seconds. There is no dependent edema. Peripheral hair growth is normal, and the skin is free of lesions.

Equipment

- Tape measure
- Doppler
- Reflex hammer

Delegation Considerations

Physical examination of musculoskeletal function is a skill that requires the critical thinking and knowledge application unique to an RN. For this skill, delegation is inappropriate. Assistive personnel (AP) may assist clients with ambulation, transfer, and positioning. In addition, AP can recognize problems with gait and ROM. The RN informs AP to report any problems noted in ROM or muscle strength. AP need to be aware of the importance of gentleness during ROM to avoid forcing a joint beyond the client's current ROM. The RN also informs AP of clients at risk for falls and provides instructions for clients with muscular weakness who require special assistance with transfer and ambulation.

IMPLEMENTATION FOR ASSESSING THE EXTREMITIES AND PERIPHERAL CIRCULATION

Steps	Rationale
1. See Standard Protocol (inside front cover).	
2. Prepare client:	
a. Integrate musculoskeletal and neurologic assessment during other portions of physical assessment or during nursing care. As in assessment of integument, nurse can conduct assessment as client moves in bed, rises from chair, walks, or goes through movements required during complete physical examination.	Assessment integrated with nursing care conserves client's energy and allows observation of the client performing activities more naturally.
b. Plan time for short rest periods during assessment.	Movement of body parts and various maneuvers may fatigue client. It is particularly important to consider rest periods with older adults and very ill clients.
3. Observe ability to use arms and hands for grasping objects.	Assesses coordination and muscle strength.
4. Assess muscle strength of upper extremities by applying gradual increase in pressure to muscle group.	Upper and lower extremity on client's dominant side is normally stronger than that on nondominant side. Pain, rather than weakness, may cause reduced muscle strength; however, long-term pain can lead to muscle weakening.
5. To assess hand grasp strength, have the client grasp the fingers of both of your hands and squeeze them as hard as possible. To avoid discomfort, the nurse may cross hands.	It is common for the client's dominant hand to be slightly stronger than the nondominant hand. By crossing hands, client's right hand grasps your right hand.
6. Have client resist pressure applied by attempting to move against resistance (e.g., flex elbow). Have client maintain resistance until told to stop. Compare symmetrical muscle groups. Note weakness, and compare right with left.	Evaluates strength of symmetrical muscle groups. Rate muscle strength on scale of 0 to 5: Grade as follows: 0 = No voluntary contraction 1 = Slight contractility, no movement 2 = Full range of motion, passive 3 = Full range of motion, active 4 = Full range of motion against gravity, some resistance 5 = Full range of motion against gravity, full resistance

Steps	Rationale
7. If muscle weakness is identified, measure muscle size with tape measure placed around body of muscle. Compare with same muscle on opposite side of body.	Indicates degree of atrophy.
8. Observe position for sitting, supine, prone, or standing. Muscles and joints should be exposed and free to move to allow for accurate measurement.	Each joint or muscle group may require different position for measurement.
9. Inspect gait as client walks and stands. Observe for foot dragging, shuffling or limping, balance, and presence of obvious deformity in lower extremities, and position of the trunk in relation to the legs.	Gait is more natural if client is unaware of nurse's observation.
10. Stand behind client, and observe postural alignment (position of hips relative to shoulders). Look sideways at cervical, thoracic, and lumbar curves (see illustration, p. 338).	Abnormal curves of posture include lordosis (swayback, increased lumbar curvature), kyphosis (hunchback, exaggerated posterior curvature of thoracic spine), and scoliosis (lateral spinal curvature) (see illustration). Postural changes may indicate muscular, bone, or joint deformity; pain; or muscular fatigue. Head should be held erect.
11. Make a general observation of the extremities. Look at overall size, gross deformity, bony enlargement, alignment, and symmetry.	General review helps to pinpoint areas requiring in-depth assessment.

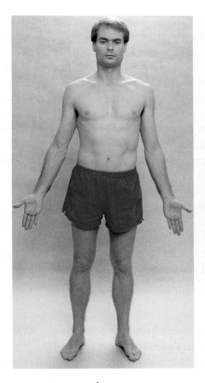
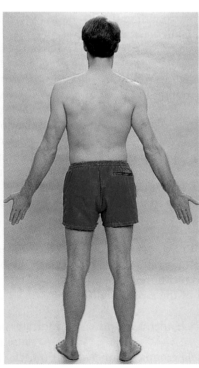
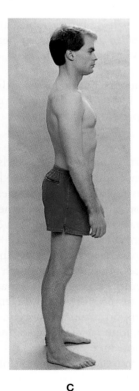

A	B	C

Step 10 Inspection of overall body posture. **A,** Anterior view. **B,** Posterior view. **C,** Lateral view. (From Seidel HM, and others: *Mosby's guide to physical examination,* ed 5, St Louis, 2003, Mosby).

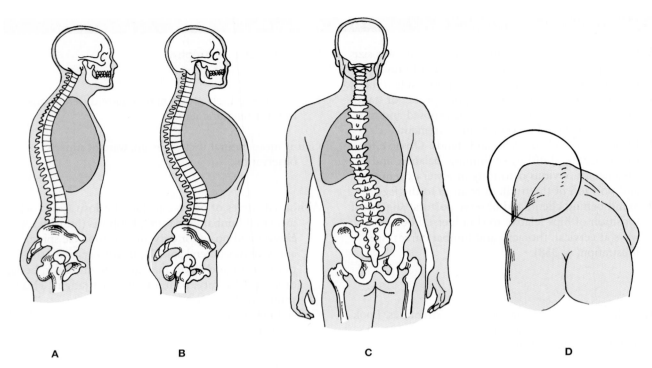

Step 10   Spinal deformities. **A,** Kyphosis. **B,** Lordosis. **C,** Scoliosis. **D,** Scoliosis with client bending forward.

Steps	Rationale

12. Gently palpate bones, joints, and surrounding tissue in involved areas. Note any heat, tenderness, edema, or resistance to pressure.

May reveal changes resulting from trauma or chronic disease. Do not attempt to move joint when fracture is suspected or when joint is apparently "frozen" by lack of movement over a long period of time.

13. Ask client to put major joint through its full ROM (Table 13-8). Observe equality of motion in same body parts:

Assessment of client's normal ROM provides baseline for assessing later changes after surgery or inactivity. Clients with deformities, reduced mobility, joint fixation or weakness may require passive motion assessment.
Identifies muscle strength, as well as detecting altered strength or limited ROM.

    a. *Active motion.* (Client needs no support or assistance and is able to move joint independently.) Instruct client in moving each joint through its normal range. It may be necessary to demonstrate movements and ask client to mimic your movements.

    b. *Passive motion.* (Joint has full ROM, but client does not have the strength to move it independently.) Have client relax and move the same joints passively until the end of the range is felt. Support extremity at joint.

Determines ability to perform joint motion in the presence of muscle weakness.

14. Palpate joint for swelling, stiffness, tenderness, and heat; note any redness.

Indicates acute or chronic inflammation. ROM may cause pain or injury.

15. Assess muscle tone in major muscle groups. Normal tone causes mild, even resistance to movement through entire ROM.

If muscle has increased tone (hypertonicity), any sudden movement of joint is met with considerable resistance. Hypotonic muscle moves without resistance. Muscle feels flabby.

16. Inspect lower extremities for changes in color and condition of the skin (Table 13-9). Note skin and nail texture, hair distribution, venous patterns, edema, and scars or ulcers. Compare skin color lying and standing.

Changes may reflect impaired peripheral circulation.

Table 13-8

Assessing Range of Motion (ROM)*

Body Part	Assessment Procedure	ROM
Upper Extremities		
Shoulders	Raise both arms to a vertical position at the sides of the head.	Flexion.
	Place both hands behind the neck, with elbows out to the sides.	External rotation and abduction.
	Place both hands behind the small of the back (internal rotation).	Internal rotation.
	Have client make small circles with hands with arms extended at shoulder level.	Circumduction.
Elbows	Bend and straighten the elbows.	Flexion and extension.
	Place hands at waist with elbows flexed.	
Wrist	Flex and extend wrist.	Flexion and extension.
	Bend wrist to radial then ulnar side—radial and ulnar deviation.	
	Turn palm upward, then downward.	Supination and pronation.
Hand	Make a fist with both hands; open hand.	Flexion and extension.
	Extend and spread fingers and thumb outward; bring back together.	Adduction and abduction.
Lower Extremities		Flexion: Expect 90 degrees.
Hips (with client supine)	With knees extended, raise one leg upward.	
	Repeat with knee flexed.	Abduction: Expect 45 degrees.
	Swing legs laterally.	Adduction: Expect 30 degrees.
		Internal and external rotation: Expect 40-45 degrees.
	With knee flexed hold the ankle and rotate the leg inward and outward.	Extension: Expect full extension and up to 15 degrees hyperextension.
Knees (with client sitting)	Raise the foot, keeping the knee in place.	Plantar flexion: Expect 45 degrees.
Ankle	With foot held off the floor, point toes, then bring toes back toward the knee.	Dorsiflexion: Expect 20 degrees.
	Turn foot inward and then outward.	Inversion ad eversion: Expect to reach 5 degrees.
		Expect to reach 40 degrees.
Toes	Bend toes down and back.	

*This may be done actively by the client (AROM) or passively by the nurse (PROM).

Table 13-9

Signs of Venous and Arterial Insufficiency

Assessment Criterion	Venous	Arterial
Color	Normal or cyanotic	Pale; worsened by elevation of extremity; dusky red when extremity lowered
Temperature	Normal	Cool (blood flow blocked to extremity)
Pulse	Normal	Decreased or absent
Edema	Often marked	Absent or mild
Skin changes	Brown pigmentation around ankles	Thin, shiny skin; decreased hair growth; thickened nails

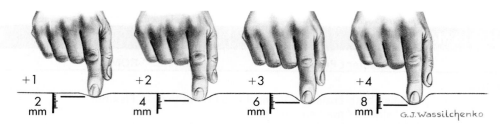

Step 18 Assessing for pitting edema. (From Cannobio MM: *Cardiovascular disorders*, St Louis, 1990, Mosby.)

Steps	Rationale
17. Palpate edematous areas, noting mobility, consistency, and tenderness.	Assists in determining extent of edema. Edema results from fluid in tissues. Inadequate venous return causes edema in the sacrum if client is confined to bed or in the feet and ankles if sitting.
18. Assess for pitting edema by pressing area firmly for 5 seconds, then releasing. Depth of indentation determines severity (see illustration): 2 mm: 1+ edema 4 mm: 2+ edema 6 mm: 3+ edema 8 mm: 4+ edema	In some settings a tape measure may be used to observe the extent of edema by measuring the circumference of the extremity daily.
19. Check capillary refill by grasping client's fingernail or toenail and noting color of nail bed. Next, apply gentle firm pressure to the nail bed. Release quickly, watching for color change. Circulation is restored and normally returns to pink color in less than 3 seconds.	Cold environmental temperature with vasoconstriction and vascular disease can delay refill. Local pressure from a cast or bandage may also deter refill.
20. Ask if the client experiences tenderness, and then palpate for heat, firmness, or localized swelling of the calf muscle, which are signs of deep venous thrombosis (DVT).	Clients who have been immobilized for several days and those who have bone or joint disease, surgical correction of joint or bone, or pain are at risk for altered tissue perfusion (Breen, 2000). Some clients have DVTs and only complain of calf pain (Urbano, 2001).

NURSE ALERT   *The Homan's sign is no longer a reliable indicator for the presence or absence of DVT (Breen, 2000; Urbano, 2001; Delis and others; 2001) and should not be considered a reliable parameter. Trauma to the vein or muscle, reduced mobility, and increased blood clotting are reliable risk factors. If the calf is swollen, red, or tender, notify client's physician for further assessment and evaluation.*

21. Starting at the most distal part of each extremity, palpate each peripheral artery for equality, comparing side to side; elasticity of vessel wall: depress and release artery, noting ease with check if it springs back to shape; and strength of pulse (force of blood against arterial wall) using the following rating scale (Seidel and others, 1999): No pulse palpable 1+ Pulse difficult to palpate, weak and thready, and easy to obliterate 2+ Stronger than 1+, located with light pressure 3+ Easy to palpate and not easily obliterated 4+ Strong, bounds against fingertips, and cannot be obliterated	Comparison of both arteries allows nurse to determine any localized obstruction or disturbance in blood flow. Pulses should be symmetrical side to side. If asymmetry is noted, look for other factors related to impaired circulation.

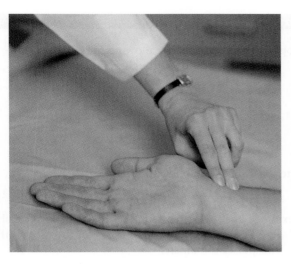

Step 22 Palpation of radial pulse.

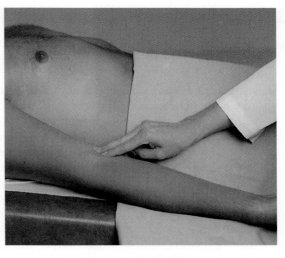

Step 24 Palpation of brachial pulse.

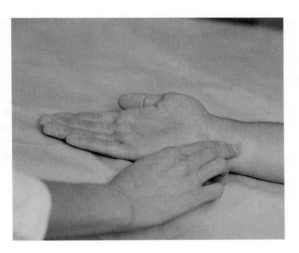

Step 23 Palpation of ulnar pulse.

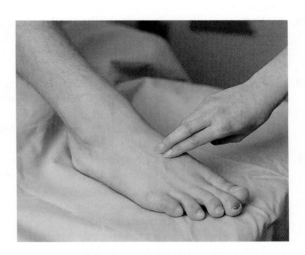

Step 25 Palpation of pedal pulse.

Steps	Rationale
22. Palpate radial pulse by lightly placing tips of first and second fingers in groove formed along radial side of forearm, lateral to flexor tendon of wrist (see illustration).	Pulse is relatively superficial and should not require deep palpation.
23. Palpate ulnar pulse by placing fingertips along ulnar side of forearm (see illustration).	Palpated when arterial insufficiency to hand is expected or when nurse assesses effects that radial occlusion (e.g., during arterial blood gas sampling) might have on circulation to hand (see Chapter 14).
24. Palpate brachial pulse by locating groove between biceps and triceps muscles above elbow at antecubital fossa (see illustration). Place tips of first two fingers in muscle groove.	Artery runs along medial side of extended arm, requiring moderate palpation.
25. Have client lie supine with feet relaxed, and palpate dorsalis pedis pulse. Gently place fingertips between great and first toe; slowly move fingers along groove between extensor tendons of great and first toe until pulse is palpable (see illustration).	Artery lies superficially and does not require deep palpation. Pulse may be congenitally absent.

Steps	Rationale

26. If the pedal pulse is difficult to palpate or it is not palpable at all, use a Doppler instrument over the pulse site:
 	
  a. Apply conducting gel to the client's skin over the pulse site or onto transducer tip of probe.
 	
  b. Turn Doppler on. Gently apply ultrasound probe to the skin, changing Doppler angle until pulsation is audible. Adjust volume as needed.
	Doppler amplifies sounds, allowing nurse to hear low-velocity blood flow through peripheral arteries.

27. Palpate posterior tibial pulse by having client relax and slightly extend feet. Place fingertips behind and below medial malleolus (ankle bone) (see illustration).	Artery is easily palpable with foot relaxed.
28. Palpate popliteal pulse by having client slightly flex knee with foot resting on table or bed. Instruct client to keep leg muscles relaxed. Palpate deeply into popliteal fossa with fingers of both hands placed just lateral to midline. Client may also lie prone to achieve exposure of artery (see illustration).	Flexion of knee and muscle relaxation improve accessibility of artery. Popliteal pulse is one of the more difficult pulses to palpate.
29. With client supine, palpate femoral pulse by placing first two fingers over inguinal area below inguinal ligament, midway between pubic symphysis and anterosuperior iliac spine (see illustration).	Supine position prevents flexion in groin area, which interferes with artery access.
30. In clients with back pain or surgery, a cerebrovascular accident, or spinal cord compression, it is appropriate to monitor deep tendon reflexes (DTR) (McHugh and McHugh, 1990). In most settings this is not part of the routine shift assessment.	Muscle spasticity and hyperactive reflexes may result from disorders such as stroke and paralysis. Diminished DTRs and muscle weakness may suggest lower motor neuron disorders such as amyotrophic lateral sclerosis (ALS) or Guillain-Barré syndrome.
31. If indicated, test DTR: For each reflex tested, compare sides and assign a grade on the following scale: No response 1+ Sluggish or diminished response 2+ Normal, active or expected response 3+ More brisk than expected; slightly hyperactive 4+ Very brisk; hyperactive, with clonus a. *Knee reflex:* Palpate the patellar tendon just below the patella. Tap the pointed end of the reflex hammer briskly on the tendon. The normal response is knee extension (see illustration).	Clonus is described as repeated spasms of muscular contraction and relaxation. Knee reflex is the most common DTR assessment performed.

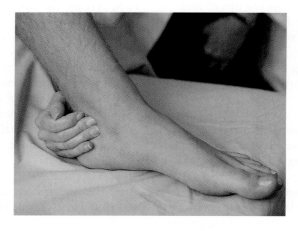

Step 27   Palpation of posterior tibial pulse.

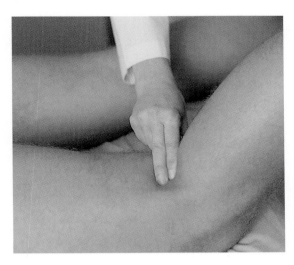

Step 28   Palpation of popliteal pulse with client prone.

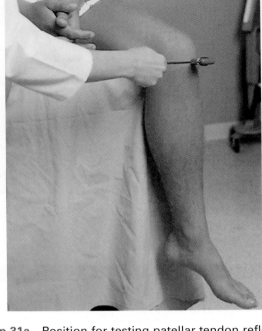

Step 31a   Position for testing patellar tendon reflexes. Lower leg will normally extend.

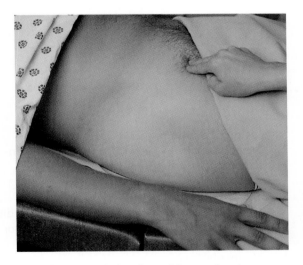

Step 29   Palpation of femoral pulse.

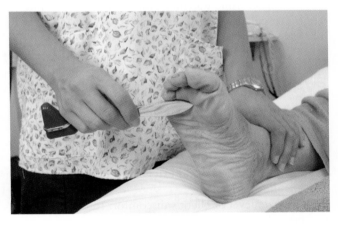

Step 31b   Toes should flex inward and downward.

Steps	Rationale
b. *Plantar response (Babinski's reflex):* Using the handle end of the reflex hammer, stroke the lateral aspect of the sole, from the heel to the ball of the foot. The toes should flex inward and downward (see illustration).	This is usually considered abnormal in adults.
c. If Babinski's reflex is present, which is normal in a newborn, the great toe will dorsiflex, accompanied by fanning of the other toes.	Positive Babinski is considered abnormal in the adult. It indicates central nervous system dysfunction.

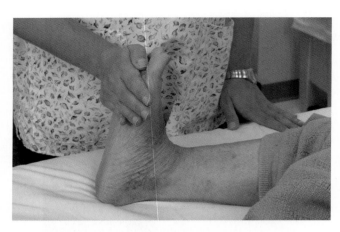

Step 31d   Maintain position while watching and feeling for rhythmic oscillations.

Steps	Rationale
d. *Ankle clonus:* If reflexes seem hyperactive, testing ankle clonus is indicated. Support the knee in a slightly flexed position, and move the forefoot in a circular motion several times, ending with a sharp dorsiflexion of the foot. Maintain that position while watching and feeling for rhythmic oscillations (see illustration).	Sustained clonus with continued repeated movement indicates pathological condition.

32. See Completion Protocol (inside front cover).

• • • • • • • • • •

EVALUATION

1. Compare muscle strength and range of motion with previous shift assessment.
2. Compare pulses and capillary refill bilaterally with previous shift assessment.
3. Compare presence and extent of edema with previous shift assessment.
4. Evaluate level of client's discomfort following procedure.

Unexpected Outcomes and Related Interventions

1. Previously palpable pedal pulses are diminished or absent indicating circulatory compromise.
   a. Notify physician.
   b. Elevate extremity.
2. Client's lower extremities have pale, cool, thin, and shiny skin, with reduced hair growth and thickened nails, indicating chronic arterial insufficiency.
   a. Instruct client in proper foot care.
   b. Refer to podiatrist for nail trimming.
   c. Inspect feet for signs of impaired skin integrity.
3. Joints are prominent, swollen, and tender with nodules or overgrowth of bone in distal joints, indicating signs of arthritis.

   a. Instruct client in proper ROM.
   b. Determine client's knowledge regarding antiinflammatory medications.
4. Reduced ROM in one or more major joints—shoulder, elbow, wrist, fingers, knee, hip.
   a. Assess for pain during movement, with joint unstable, stiff, painful, or swollen or with obvious deformity.
   b. Notify physician.
   c. Reduce mobility in extremity until cause of abnormal joint motion is determined.
5. Client demonstrates weakness in one or more major muscle groups, or gait demonstrates unsteady balance with shuffling or stumbling of feet.
   a. Assess client's musculoskeletal and neurological functioning.
   b. Provide for client safety when ambulating.
6. Postural abnormalities such as lordosis, kyphosis, or scoliosis are noted. Reduced ROM in spine is observed. Alteration may be caused by congenital or traumatic conditions.

Recording And Reporting

- Record all findings in nurses' notes or appropriate assessment flow sheet.
- Report acute pain or sudden muscle weakness to nurse in charge or physician; it may be indicative of condition requiring immediate treatment.
- Report changes in peripheral circulation evidenced by edema, diminished or absent pulses or capillary refill, which may indicate circulatory compromise that can result in permanent nerve damage or tissue death if untreated.

Sample Documentation

1530 Right lower leg red, warm, and tender to touch. Circumference of right leg 16 inches and left leg 14 inches. Client instructed to remain in bed. Findings reported to Dr. H.

SPECIAL CONSIDERATIONS

Pediatric Considerations

- Infants must be carefully examined for musculoskeletal anomalies resulting from genetic or fetal insults. An examination includes review of posture, generalized movement, symmetry and skin creases of the extremities, muscle strength, and hip alignment.
- Normally the back of a newborn is rounded or C-shaped from the thoracic and pelvic curves.
- Scoliosis, lateral curvature of the spine, is an important childhood problem, especially in females apparent at puberty. (For closer examination, have child stand erect, wearing only underclothes. Observe from behind, looking for asymmetry of shoulders and hips. Then observing from the back as the child bends forward.) Uneven dress hems or pant leg hems or uneven fit of clothing at the waist may be noted.
- The shape of bones may vary in children. Most conditions are benign, for example, valgus of the lower legs (lateral bowing of tibia), which is common in toddlers until they have well-developed lower back and leg muscles; varus of the knee (opposite of valgus) is normal in children from age 2 to 7 years (Wong and others, 1999). If either of these conditions is excessive, further evaluation is needed.

- Watching a child during play can reveal information about musculoskeletal function.

Geriatric Considerations

- Older adult's gait normally has smaller steps and a wider base of support.
- Older adults tend to assume a stooped, forward-bent posture, with hips and knees somewhat flexed and arms bent at the elbows and the level of the arms raised (Ebersole and Hess, 1998).
- In older adults, joints often become swollen and stiff, with reduced ROM resulting from cartilage erosion and fibrosis of synovial membranes.
- Older adults may develop kyphosis because of osteoporosis.
- Functional assessment is a measure of older person's ability to perform basic self-care tasks (Lueckenotte, 2000). When client is unable to perform self-care easily, determine the need for assistive devices (e.g., zippers on clothing instead of buttons, elevation of chairs to minimize bending of knees and hips). Creativity by the nurse is often needed (Kee, 2000).

CRITICAL THINKING EXERCISES

1. Sara Williams, 36 years of age, was admitted yesterday with right lower quadrant abdominal pain. Describe the most important points to include relating to her pain in her morning shift assessment. List the assessment techniques to be used in the order of priority.
2. A postoperative client is becoming more distended and refuses breakfast. It is the second postoperative day following a cholecystectomy. What additional assessment data should be gathered during your initial shift assessment?
3. As you begin your shift assessment of Jane Jacobs, a 45-year-old woman recovering from a hysterectomy, she reports discomfort at her IV site. How would you proceed with your assessment?
4. Jim Lewis, a 76-year-old man with arthritis who lives alone at home, reports difficulty walking. What physical assessments could you perform while he is in bed in relation to this concern?

REFERENCES

American Cancer Society: *Cancer facts and figures 2001,* Atlanta, 2001, The Society.

American Medical Directors Association: *Osteoporosis: clinical practice guidelines,* 1998, http://www.amda.com.

Barkauskas VH and others: *Health and physical assessment,* ed 2, St Louis, 1998, Mosby.

Breen P: DVT: what every nurse should know, *RN* 63(4):58, 2000.

Daly S: *Expert 10 minute physical examinations,* St Louis, 1997, Mosby.

Delis KT and others: Incidence, natural history and risk factors of deep vein thrombosis in elective knee arthroscopy, *Thromb Haemost* 86(3):817, 2001.

Ebersole P, Hess P: *Toward healthy aging: human needs and nursing response,* ed 5, St Louis, 1998, Mosby.

Folstein MF, Folstein S, McHugh PR: Mini-mental state: a practical method for grading the cognitive state of patients for the clinician, *J Psychiatr Res* 12:189, 1975.

Forgacs P: The functional basis of pulmonary sounds, *Chest* 73(3):399, 1978.

Garza C, De Onis M: A new international growth reference for young children, *Am J Clin Nutr* 70(1):169S, 1999.

Kee C: Osteoarthritis: manageable scourge of aging, *Nurs Clin North Am* 35(1):199, 2000.

Kim MJ, McFarland GK, McLane AM: Pocket guide to nursing diagnosis, ed 7, St Louis, 1997, Mosby.

Lueckenotte A: *Gerontologic nursing,* ed 2, St Louis, 2000, Mosby.

Lynch SH: Elder abuse: what to look for, how to intervene, *Am J Nurs* 97(1):26, 1997.

McHugh J, McHugh W: How to assess deep tendon reflexes, *Nursing* 20(8):62, 1990.

Mosby's expert ten minute physical examinations, ed 4, St Louis, 1999, Mosby.

Pugliese G: Reducing risks of infection during vascular access, *J Intraven Nurs* 20(6 suppl):511, 1997.

Seidel HM and others: *Mosby's guide to physical examination,* ed 4, St Louis, 1999, Mosby.

Sitzman K: Feet first, *Home Healthc Nurse* 17(5):328, 1999.

Urbano FL: Homan's sign in the diagnosis of deep venous thrombosis, *Hosp Physician* 37(3):22, 2001.

Wong DL and others: *Whaley & Wong's nursing care of infants and children,* ed 6, St Louis, 1999, Mosby.

Wright JA: Seven abdominal assessment signs every emergency nurse should know, *J Emerg Nurs* 23(5):446, 1997.

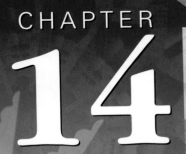

CHAPTER 14

Laboratory Tests

Skill and judgment in obtaining specimens and assisting with diagnostic procedures affect client safety and comfort and ensure the quality of diagnostic information. Nurses are accountable for monitoring, recognizing, and reporting significant alterations. Laboratory tests are often expensive. Current health care economics insist that laboratory and diagnostic procedures be performed accurately and within an appropriate time frame.

Laboratory test results aid in the diagnosis of health care problems, provide information about the stage and activity of a disease process, and measure the response to therapy. Nurses are often responsible for collecting specimens of body secretions and excretions such as urine, stool, blood, or sputum. When there are questions about laboratory tests, the nurse should consult the institution's procedure manual or call the laboratory.

Before collecting any specimen, the nurse needs to know the purpose of the specimen, how much of the specimen is needed, what collection container is appropriate, and how it is to be transported to the laboratory (Parini, 2000). Clients may experience embarrassment or discomfort when giving a sample of body excretions or secretions. It is important to handle excretions discreetly and to provide the client with as much comfort and privacy as possible. The nurse needs to be aware that sociocultural variations may affect the client's response and willingness to participate in various diagnostic procedures. Anxiety is also provoked by the invasive nature of some collection procedures or by fear of unknown test results. Clients who are given a clear explanation about the purpose of a specimen and how it is to be obtained will be more cooperative in its collection. With clear instructions many clients are able to obtain their own specimens of urine, stool, and sputum, thus avoiding embarrassment.

A laboratory requisition is needed for each specimen to be certain that the appropriate tests are performed on each specimen and to facilitate accurate reporting of the results. Each requisition must include the following information: the date and time the specimen is obtained, the name of the test, and the source of specimen/culture for each container. After the specimen is collected, the container itself (not the lid) must also be labeled with the client's name, hospital identification number, specimen source, collection date and time, series number (if more than one specimen), and anatomical site if appropriate (e.g., wound culture from knee versus abdominal incision). Often a label is stamped with a client's Addressograph and applied to the container.

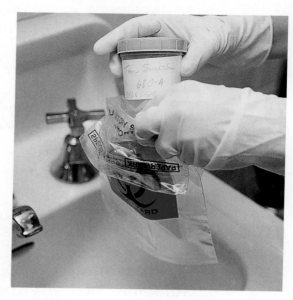

Figure 14-1 Enclose all specimens in a biohazard plastic bag.

Nurses and assistive personnel (AP) are at risk for exposure to body fluids regardless of what specimen is being collected. Therefore special attention is needed regarding the use of clean gloves. Agencies require the use of a small plastic bag for delivery of all specimens to the laboratory (Figure 14-1). Specimens need to be delivered promptly to the laboratory. If the specimen is left at room temperature too long, the results of the test may be skewed by additional bacterial growth. Normal values for laboratory tests can be found in reference books, but the nurse should know that each laboratory establishes its own values for each test. These values are usually printed on the laboratory slips of the agency. The nurse must know what magnitude of deviation is significant in order to know how quickly physician notification is required.

NURSING DIAGNOSES

Anxiety may be related to anticipating embarrassment, discomfort, or pain as a specimen is obtained. **Fear** may be related to anticipation of unfavorable or unknown test results. **Risk for Infection** exists when skin or tissue integrity is altered. **Ineffective Airway Clearance** is appropriate for a client who cannot expectorate a sputum specimen.

Skill 14.1

Urine Specimen Collection—Midstream, Sterile Urinary Catheter

Laboratory examination of urine provides valuable information about body system functions. A urinalysis provides information about kidney or metabolic function, nutrition, and systemic diseases. Urine may be collected using a variety of methods depending upon the purpose of the urinalysis and the presence or absence of a urinary catheter. Regardless of the method of collection, guidelines for assessment, planning, and evaluation are similar. Routine urinalysis includes the following measurements:

1. pH value (4.6 to 8): Indicates acid-base balance.
2. Protein level (not normally present in urine): Presence suggests renal disease or damage.
3. Glucose level (not normally present): Elevated in diabetes.
4. Ketones (not normally present): Present with dehydration, starvation, and poorly controlled diabetes mellitus.
5. Blood (<2 RBC): Elevated with kidney disease or damage, trauma, and surgery.
6. Specific gravity (1.010 to 1.025): Reflects urine concentration. Increased with dehydration, decreased with overhydration, altered with kidney damage and abnormal antidiuretic hormone (ADH) secretion.
7. White blood cell (WBC) count (0 to 4 per low-power field): Elevated with urinary tract infection.
8. Bacteria (not normally present): Presence indicates urinary tract infection.
9. Casts (not normally present): Presence indicates kidney abnormality.

A random urine specimen is a method for collecting urine that involves using a specimen "hat" (Figure 14-2) that is placed under a toilet seat to collect voided urine. Approximately 120 ml of urine is then placed in a specimen container, labeled, and sent to the laboratory.

A culture and sensitivity (C&S) of urine is a test performed to identify urinary tract infection and to determine the most effective antibiotic for treatment. As a result, it is necessary to collect a sterile urine specimen to ensure that any microorganisms present originate in the urine and not from the client's skin. Specimens for C&S may be collected either as a clean-voided midstream specimen or under sterile conditions from a urinary catheter. Urine collected by these sterile methods may also be analyzed for the same components as the routine urinalysis.

Timed urine specimens for quantitative analysis require urine to be collected over 2 to 72 hours. The 24-hour timed collection is most common and allows for measurement of the exact amount of elements such as amino acids, creatinine, hormones, glucose, and adrenocorticosteroid

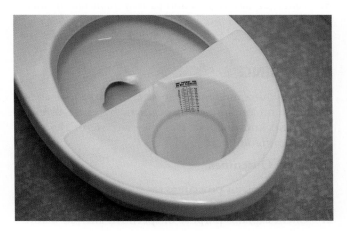

Figure 14-2   Specimen "hat."

excreted. Procedural Guideline 14-1 on p. 355 describes the steps for collecting urine for a 24-hour timed test for quantitative analysis.

Testing chemical properties of urine can also be done by immersing a specially prepared strip of paper (Chemstrip) into a clean urine specimen to detect the presence of glucose, ketones, protein, or blood, not normally present in the urine. When the screening test for the presence of substances in the urine is positive, additional laboratory tests are used to determine the client's diagnosis or to measure the effectiveness of treatment. This type of quick screening may be done as described in Procedural Guideline 14-2 on p. 355 when laboratory testing is not readily available, for example, in a physician's office or clinic and in the outpatient, long-term care, or home setting. It may also be done for pregnant women on admission to the hospital in labor.

ASSESSMENT

1. Assess client's ability to assist with urine specimen collection: able to position self and hold container. *Rationale: This determines client's ability to cooperate and level of assistance required.*
2. Assess client's understanding of need for the specimen. *Rationale: This determines the need for health teaching. Client's understanding of purpose promotes cooperation.*
3. Determine if fluid, dietary requirements, or medications need to be administered in conjunction with test. *Rationale: Certain substances affect excretion and levels of urinary constituents. Specific amounts of fluid may be required for concentration/dilution tests. Drugs such as cor-*

tisone preparations, diuretics, and anesthetics increase glucose levels. Anticoagulants increase risk of blood in the urine.

4. Assess for signs and symptoms of urinary tract infection (frequency, urgency, dysuria, hematuria, flank pain, cloudy urine with sediment, foul odor, fever). *Rationale: Indicators of urinary tract infection (UTI).*

5. Assess urinary elimination pattern. *Rationale: Indicators of urinary tract infection (UTI). Knowledge of frequency of urination facilitates effective planning of specimen collection.*

PLANNING

Expected outcomes focus on the collection of an appropriate uncontaminated specimen by nurse or client with client knowledgeable of the purpose of the specimen examination.

Expected Outcomes

1. Client explains procedure for specimen collection before collection is attempted.
2. Client explains purpose of specimen analysis before collection is attempted.
3. Client's specimen is appropriate and free of contaminants, such as toilet tissue or stool.

Equipment

- Disposable gloves

Collecting Clean-voided Urine Specimen

- Commercial kit for clean-voided urine (Figure 14-3) containing:

  Antiseptic towelettes
  Sterile specimen container

- Soap, water, washcloth, and towel
- Bedpan (for nonambulatory client), specimen "hat" (for ambulatory client)
- Sterile water and cotton balls (optional)

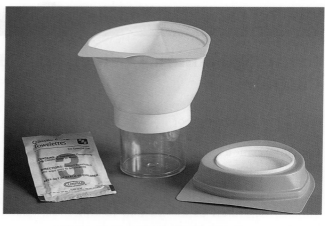

Figure 14-3   Clean voided urine kit.

Sterile Urine Specimen From a Urinary Catheter

- 3-ml syringe with 1-inch needle (21 to 25 gauge) for culture
- 20-ml syringe with 1-inch needle (21 to 25 gauge) for routine urinalysis
- Metal clamp or rubber band
- Alcohol, povidone-iodine, or other disinfectant swab
- Specimen container (nonsterile for routine urinalysis, sterile for culture)

 Delegation Considerations

The collection of urine specimens may be performed by assistive personnel (AP) familiar with aseptic and sterile technique. Inform AP of when to collect specimen and proper transport of specimen. Direct AP to notify nurse immediately if appearance of urine specimen is abnormal (e.g., presence of blood, cloudiness, or excess sediment).

IMPLEMENTATION FOR COLLECTING URINE SPECIMEN COLLECTION— MID-STREAM, STERILE URINARY CATHETER

Steps	Rationale
1. See Standard Protocol (inside front cover)	
2. Explain to client and/or family member reason specimen is needed, how client can assist (when applicable), and how to obtain specimen free of tissue and stool.	Promotes cooperation and client participation. In some cases clean-voided specimen can be collected independently by client.
3. **Collect clean-voided urine specimen**	
a. Give client or family member towel, washcloth, and soap to cleanse perineum, or assist client (following application of disposable gloves) with cleansing perineum. If client is bedridden, this may be done with the client positioned on the bedpan to facilitate access to the perineum.	Clients usually prefer to wash their own perineal area when possible.

Steps	Rationale
b. Using sterile technique, open commercial specimen kit, maintaining sterility of inside of specimen container.	Maintains sterility of inside of specimen container.
c. Open specimen container, and place cap with sterile inside surface up. Do not touch inside of container.	Contaminated specimen is the most frequent reason for inaccurate reporting of urine cultures and sensitivities.
d. Have client cleanse perineum and collect specimen independently if possible. If necessary, provide assistance:	Cleansing with an antiseptic solution prevents contamination of urine after it passes from the urethra.

COMMUNICATION TIP *Inform client that antiseptic solution will feel cold. Tell female to wipe from front to back. Tell male client to retract foreskin for effective cleansing of urinary meatus.*

Steps	Rationale
(1) *Male:* Hold penis with one hand; using circular motion and antiseptic towelette, cleanse meatus, moving from center to outside (see illustration). In uncircumcised males, foreskin must be retracted for effective cleansing of meatus and during voiding.	
(2) *Female:* Spread labia minora with fingers of nondominant hand. Use dominant hand to cleanse area with antiseptic towelette, moving from front (above urethral orifice) to back (toward anus) (see illustration on p. 352).	
e. If agency procedure indicates, rinse area with sterile water and dry with cotton.	Prevents contamination of specimen with antiseptic solution.
f. While retracting foreskin of penis or continuing to hold labia apart (see illustration on p. 352), client initiates urine stream while holding specimen container.	Initial urine flushes out microorganisms that normally accumulate at the urinary meatus and provides uncontaminated urine from the bladder itself.

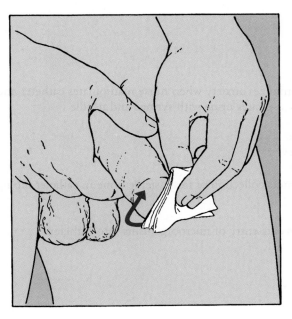

Step 3d(1)   Cleanse penis with circular motion. (Modified from Grimes D: *Infectious diseases,* Mosby's clinical nursing series, St Louis, 1991, Mosby.)

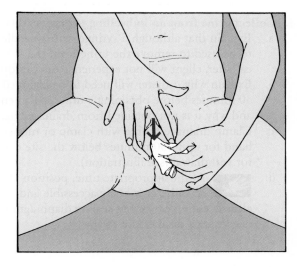

Step 3d(2)   Cleanse from front to back, holding labia apart. (Modified from Grimes D: *Infectious diseases,* Mosby's clinical nursing series, St Louis, 1991, Mosby.)

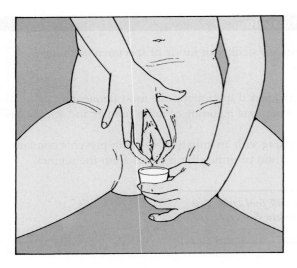

Step 3f Continue to hold labia apart while collecting specimen. (Modified from Grimes D: *Infectious diseaes,* Mosby's clinical nursing series, St Louis, 1991, Mosby.)

Steps	Rationale
g. After stream is achieved, pass specimen container into stream and collect 30 to 60 ml of urine without touching the inside or rim of the container.	Collects sterile specimen.
h. Remove specimen container before flow of urine stops and before releasing labia or penis. Client finishes voiding into bedpan or toilet.	Prevents contamination of specimen with skin flora.
i. Replace cap securely on specimen container, touching only outside.	Avoids contamination and prevents spilling.
j. Cleanse urine from exterior surface of container.	

NURSE ALERT *Indicate on the laboratory slip if client is menstruating.*

4. Collect urine from an indwelling urinary catheter	
a. Explain that although a syringe with a needle is to be used to remove the urine from the catheter, client will not experience discomfort.	Minimizes anxiety when nurse manipulates catheter and aspirates urine with syringe and needle.
b. Explain why catheter will need to be clamped for 30 minutes before obtaining a urine specimen and why it is not obtained from drainage bag.	
c. Clamp drainage tubing with clamp or rubber band for up to 30 minutes below the site chosen for withdrawal (see illustration).	Permits collection of fresh, sterile urine in catheter tubing.
d. At the appropriate time, position client so catheter is easily accessible and cleanse entry port or self-sealing diaphragm for needle with disinfectant swab.	Prevents entry of microorganisms into catheter.

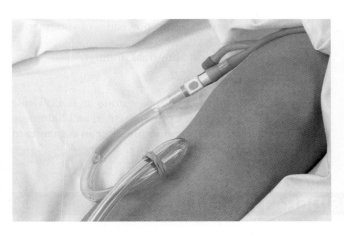

Step 4c   Clamp catheter drainage tubing.

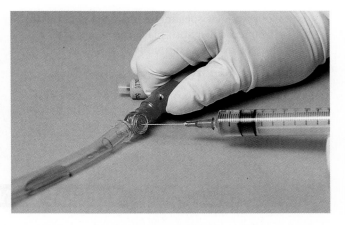

Step 4e   Accessing catheter port to withdraw urine.

Steps	Rationale
e. Insert needle of syringe at 90-degree angle through entry port (see illustration) or 30-degree angle for self-sealing diaphragm, and withdraw necessary volume of urine (3 ml for culture, 20 ml for routine urinalysis).	Angle of insertion ensures tip of needle enters catheter lumen for withdrawal of urine.

NURSE ALERT *Do not insert a needle into the catheter where a port or diaphragm is not present. This will cause urine to leak from catheter.*

Steps	Rationale
f. Transfer urine from syringe into nonsterile urine container for routine urinalysis, or transfer urine from syringe into sterile urine container for culture.	
g. Do not recap needle. Dispose of needle and syringe in proper receptacle.	Reduces risk of needle-stick injury.
h. Place lid tightly on container.	
i. Unclamp catheter, and allow urine to flow into drainage bag. Ensure urine flows freely.	Prevents backup of urine, which can potentially cause renal damage.

5. Securely attach properly completed identification label to the side of specimen container (not the lid).
6. Send specimen and requisition to laboratory as soon as possible and within no more than 2 hours (Parini, 2000).
7. See Completion Protocol (inside front cover).

• • • • • • • • • •

EVALUATION

1. Ask client to identify steps in specimen collection procedure.
2. Ask client to state purposes of specimen collection.
3. Inspect clean voided specimen for contamination with toilet tissue or stool.

Unexpected Outcomes and Related Interventions

1. Client is unable to void, or urine does not collect in drainage tube.
    a. Offer fluids (if permitted) to enhance urine production.
2. Client's urine specimen is contaminated with stool and tissue.
    a. Reinforce importance of obtaining specimen free of contaminants.

b. Collect a new specimen, and assist client with specimen collection: place specimen "hat" as close to front of commode as possible.

Recording and Reporting

- Record method used to obtain specimen, date and time collected, type of test ordered, and laboratory receiving specimen.
- Describe characteristics of specimen.

- Describe client's tolerance to procedure of specimen collection.
- When available, report abnormal findings.

Sample Documentation

1214 Voided 140 ml of dark amber urine at 1145. Urine discarded. 24-hour urine for protein started at 1200 noon. Client instructed to save all urine and place in container in bathroom. Verbalized understanding.

 SPECIAL CONSIDERATIONS

Pediatric Considerations

It is not possible to obtain a midstream urine collection on a non–toilet-trained child; consequently, urine for culture should be obtained by use of a sterile plastic urine-collecting bag that adheres to the perineum (Figure 14-4). The same cleansing procedure of the perineum as described in Skill 14.1, Steps 3d and 3e, is followed.

Geriatric Considerations

- Older adults may need assistance in positioning to obtain specimen. In confused clients, AP may be necessary to hold client's hands while sample is being obtained.

- The older client may need a written reminder placed on the bathroom mirror to collect all urine.

Home Care Considerations

When a specimen for culture is collected at home, the specimen is kept on ice until it reaches the laboratory to minimize bacterial growth before applying it to a culture medium in a laboratory setting.

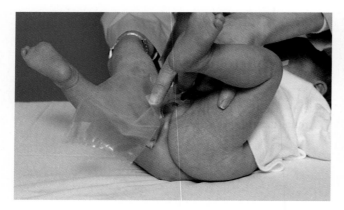 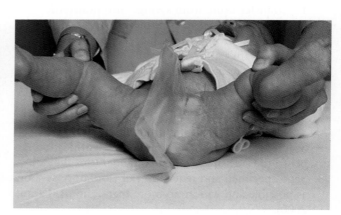

Figure 14-4 Application of pediatric urine collection bag. (From Wong DL and others: *Whaley and Wong's nursing care of infants and children,* ed 6, St Louis, 1999, Mosby.)

Procedural Guideline 14-1

Collecting 24-Hour Timed Urine Specimens

Equipment: Large collection bottle with cap that usually contains a chemical preservative for urine, bedpan, urinal, specimen "hat," graduated measuring cup, if intake and output (I&O) are to be recorded, basin large enough to hold collection bottle surrounded by ice if immediate refrigeration is required, signs that remind client and staff of timed urine collection, clean disposable gloves.

1. See Standard Protocol (inside front cover).
2. Explain the reason for specimen collection, how client can assist, and that urine must be free of feces and toilet tissue.
3. Have client drink two to four glasses of water about 30 minutes before timed collection to facilitate ability to void at the appropriate time for the test to begin.
4. Discard this first specimen as test begins. Print time that test began on laboratory requisition. For accurate results the client must begin the test with an empty bladder.
5. Place signs indicating timed urine specimen collection on client's door and toileting area.
6. Measure volume of each voiding if intake and output is being recorded.
7. Place all voided urine in labeled specimen bottle with appropriate additive.

NURSE ALERT *It is essential for all urine to be collected for accurate test results. Restart timed period if urine is accidentally lost, discarded, or contaminated.*

8. Unless instructed otherwise, keep specimen bottle in specimen refrigerator or in container of ice in bathroom to prevent decomposition of urine.
9. To facilitate voiding at the time the test ends, encourage client to drink two glasses of water 1 hour before timed urine collection ends.
10. Encourage client to empty bladder during last 15 minutes of urine collection period.
11. Intermittently during the 24-hour collection period, observe/ask if all urine has been saved.
12. Remove signs, and inform client that specimen collection period is completed.
13. Securely attach properly completed identification label to the side of specimen container (not the lid). Send specimen and requisition to laboratory as soon as possible.
14. See Completion Protocol (inside front cover).

Procedural Guideline 14-2

Urine Screening for Glucose, Ketones, Protein, Blood, and pH

Equipment: Disposable gloves; reagent test strip; test strip color chart; specimen "hat," bedpan, urinal, or commode; watch with second hand or digital counter; clean disposable gloves (if person other than client tests urine).

1. See Standard Protocol (inside front cover).
2. Ask client to collect a fresh random urine specimen (see Skill 14.1, p. 349). If client is catheterized, a 5-ml specimen from catheter is adequate.
3. 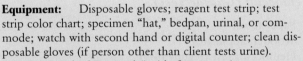 Immerse end of chemically impregnated test strip into urine. Remove the strip immediately, and tap it gently against container's side to remove excess urine.
4. Hold strip in horizontal position to prevent mixing of chemical reagents.
5. Precisely time the number of seconds specified on container, then compare color of strip with color chart on container (see illustration).
6. Remove and discard gloves.

7. Discuss test results with client.
8. See Completion Protocol (inside front cover).

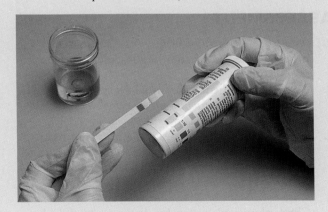

Step 5 Compare multistix with color chart.

Skill 14.2

Testing for Gastrointestinal Alterations (Stool Specimen, Hemoccult test, Gastroccult test)

Analysis of stool or gastric secretions from the gastrointestinal (GI) tract can provide useful information about pathological conditions such as the presence of tumors, infection, and malabsorption problems. Clients can often assist in providing stool specimens. The collection of gastric secretions generally involves obtaining a specimen via a nasogastric (NG) or nasointestinal tube. When a client has emesis, the nurse tests the material for the presence of blood.

As with 24-hour timed urine collection, a 24-hour stool collection can be performed. Although infrequent, the test is used to measure the constituents of stool to determine the status of GI absorption.

The term *occult blood* refers to blood that is not visible but is present in microscopic amounts. Tests are done to detect the presence of occult blood in stool (guaiac test) or emesis and gastric secretions (Gastroccult test), revealing bleeding in the esophagus, stomach, small intestine, or large intestine. The tests verify the presence of blood when the nurse notices red or black coloration of stool or gastric contents, or coffee-grounds appearance of gastric contents in emesis or with NG suction (see Chapter 32).

Hemoccult testing is a useful diagnostic tool for detecting the presence of occult blood in the stool for conditions such as colon cancer, bleeding GI ulcers, and localized gastric or intestinal irritation. The stool may appear bloody in the presence of certain foods. Hemoccult testing differentiates between blood and other questionable substances in stool. When blood is present, further testing is indicated to determine the source of the bleeding.

ASSESSMENT

1. Assess client's medical history for GI disorders (e.g., history of bleeding, hemorrhoids, colitis, malabsorption disorders).
2. Assess female client's menstrual cycle. *Rationale: A woman who is menstruating may accidentally provide a stool specimen contaminated with blood.*
3. Review medications for drugs that can contribute to GI bleeding. *Rationale: Anticoagulants, steroids, nonsteroidal antiinflammatory drugs (NSAIDs), and acetylsalicylic acid (ASA) commonly cause increased bleeding tendency or irritation of GI mucosa.*
4. Check physician's orders for dietary restrictions before testing. *Rationale: Diets rich in red meats, green leafy vegetables, poultry, and fish may produce false-positive guaiac results (Chernecky and Berger, 1997).*

PLANNING

Expected outcomes focus on the collection of an appropriate specimen, with client knowledgeable of the purpose of the specimen test. Arrange for dietary and/or medication restrictions as indicated.

Expected Outcomes

1. Client will discuss the purpose of test before specimen collection is attempted.
2. Client will maintain dietary/medication restrictions for specified period.
3. Client's specimen is appropriate for testing analysis.

Equipment

- Disposable gloves
- Soap, water, washcloth, and towel

Stool Specimens

- Plastic container with lid
- Two tongue blades
- Paper towel
- Bedpan, specimen "hat," or bedside commode
- "Save stool" signs (24-hour timed specimen)
- Sterile test tube and swab (for culture)
- Completed specimen identification label
- Completed laboratory requisition form

Hemoccult (Guaiac Test)

- Paper towel
- Wooden applicator
- Hemoccult test (Figure 14-5)

  Cardboard Hemoccult slide
  Hemoccult developing solution

Gastroccult Test

- Facial tissues
- Emesis basin
- Wooden applicator or 3-ml syringe
- 60-ml bulb or catheter tip syringe
- Gastroccult test (Figure 14-6)

  Cardboard Gastroccult slide
  Gastroccult developing solution

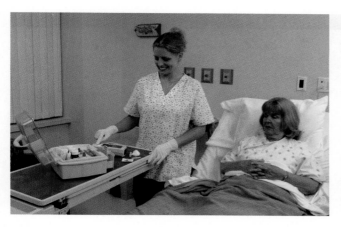

Figure 14-5 Cardboard Hemoccult slide, wooden applicator, and developing solution.

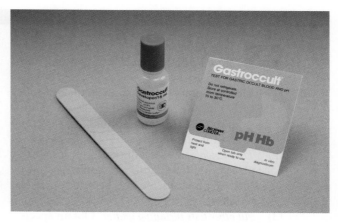

Figure 14-6 Cardboard Gastroccult slide and developing solution.

Delegation Considerations

The collection of stool and emesis for testing may be performed by assistive personnel (AP). The skills of assessing the significance of test results require the critical thinking and knowledge application unique to a nurse. Delegation of the analysis of test results is inappropriate. Inform AP to notify nurse immediately if results are positive, so the nurse may repeat the testing.

The skills of obtaining and testing gastric secretions from an NG or nasoenteral tube require the critical thinking and knowledge application unique to a nurse. Delegation of these skills is inappropriate.

IMPLEMENTATION FOR TESTING FOR GASTROINTESTINAL ALTERATIONS (STOOL SPECIMEN, HEMOCCULT TEST, GASTROCCULT TEST)

Steps	Rationale
1. See Standard Protocol (inside front cover).	
2. Discuss reason specimen is needed, how client can assist in collecting an uncontaminated specimen (if stool specimen), and how the gastric specimen will be obtained.	Promotes client cooperation.
3. **Obtaining stool specimens**	
a. Assist client as needed into bathroom or onto commode or bedpan. Instruct client to void into toilet before defecating (discard urine before collecting specimen in bedpan). Provide client clean, dry bedpan or specimen "hat" in which to defecate.	Feces should not be mixed with urine or toilet tissue. Urine inhibits fecal bacterial growth. Toilet tissue contains bismuth, which interferes with test results. Feces should not be mixed with urine or water.
b. If needed, assist client in washing after toileting, and leave in safe, comfortable position after defecation.	Promotes comfort and safety.

Steps	**Rationale**

c. Take covered bedpan or container with stool to bathroom or utility room, and gather specimen:

(1) *Culture.* Remove swab from sterile test tube, gather bean-sized piece of stool, and return swab to tube. If stool is liquid, soak cotton swab in it and return to tube.

Stool is touched only by sterile swab to prevent introduction of bacteria.

(2) *Timed stool specimen.* All of each stool is placed in waxed cardboard containers for specific time ordered and kept in specimen refrigerator.

Tests for dietary products and digestive enzymes such as fat content or bile require analysis of all feces over select time period.

(3) *All other tests including guaiac.* Obtain specimen by using tongue blades to transfer portion of stool to container (2.5 cm [1 inch] of formed stool or 15 ml of liquid stool).

d. For timed test, place signs that read "Save all stool (with appropriate date or time)" over client's bed, on bathroom door, and above toilet.

Helps prevent any accidental disposal of stool.

e. Once specimen going to the laboratory is obtained, immediately place lid on container tightly.

Prevents spread of microorganisms by air or contact with other articles.

4. Perform hemoccult test.

a. Use tip of wooden applicator to obtain small portion of feces.

Small specimen is sufficient for measuring blood content.

b. Open flap of Hemoccult slide, and apply thin smear of stool on paper in first box.

Guaiac paper inside box is sensitive to fecal blood content.

c. Using the other end of the wooden applicator, obtain a second fecal specimen from different portion of stool and apply thinly to slide's second box (see illustration).

Occult blood from upper GI tract is not always equally dispersed through stool. Findings of occult blood are more conclusive when entire specimen is found to contain blood.

d. Close slide cover, and turn slide over to reverse side. Open cardboard flap, and apply 2 drops of Hemoccult developing solution on each box of guaiac paper (see illustration).

Developing solution penetrates underlying fecal specimen. Blood is indicated by change in color of guaiac paper.

e. Read results of test after 30 to 60 seconds. Note color changes.

Bluish discoloration indicates occult blood (guaiac positive). No change in color of guaiac paper indicates negative results.

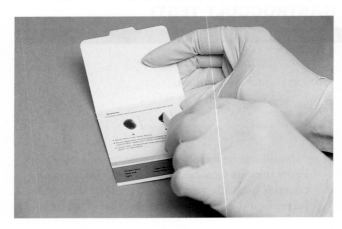

Step 4c Apply stool to both spots on cardboard slide.

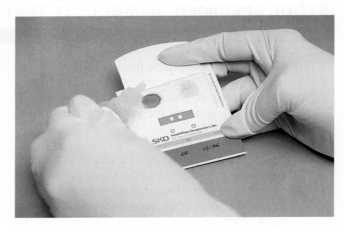

Step 4d Apply developing solution to Hemoccult slide.

Steps	Rationale

5. Perform gastroccult test.

a. To obtain specimen of gastric contents using NG or nasoenteral tube, position client in high Fowler's position in bed or chair.

Minimizes chance of aspiration of gastric contents. Position relieves pressure on abdominal organs. If client is nauseated, flat position in bed or one in which client cannot sit straight may cause abdominal discomfort.

b. Verify NG tube placement (see Chapter 32).

Ensures aspiration of gastric contents.

c. 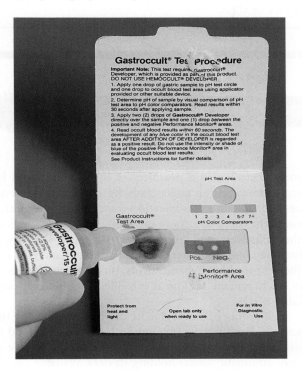 Collect gastric contents via NG or nasoenteral tube (see Chapter 32). Disconnect tube from suction or gravity drainage. Attach bulb- or cone-tipped syringe. Aspirate 5 to 10 ml. To obtain sample of emesis, use a 3-ml syringe or wooden applicator.

Only small amount of specimen is needed for pH and occult blood testing.

d. Using applicator or syringe, apply 1 drop of gastric sample to Gastroccult blood test slide.

Sample must cover test paper for test reaction to occur.

e. Apply 2 drops of commercial developer solution over sample and 1 drop between positive and negative performance monitors (see illustration).

f. After 60 seconds compare color of gastric sample with that of performance monitors.

Positive performance monitor turns blue in 30 seconds, and negative monitor remains white or beige. If sample turns blue, test is positive for occult blood. If sample turns green, test is negative.

g. Verify that performance monitor turns blue in 30 seconds, which indicates slide is working properly.

6. Explain test results to client.

7. Dispose of test slides, wooden applicator, and 1-ml syringe in proper receptacle.

Reduces spread of infection.

Step 5e Apply developing solution to Gastroccult test area.

Steps	Rationale
8. Reconnect NG tube to drainage system, suction, or clamp as ordered.	NG tube serves to decompress abdomen by promoting drainage. Clamping may be ordered to determine tolerance to stomach filling.
9. Remove and discard gloves.	
10. See Completion Protocol (inside front cover).	

• • • • • • • • • • •

EVALUATION

1. Observe quantity, character, and color of stool, emesis, or gastric secretions.
2. Compare test findings with normal expected results.
3. Ask client to explain the purpose of the test.

Unexpected Outcomes

1. Occult blood test results are positive.
   a. Monitor vital signs.
   b. Determine if client has pain, and evaluate the onset, characteristics, and severity of pain if present.
   c. Assess client for presence of hemorrhoids that can cause bleeding and false-positive Hemoccult test. (Bleeding could be misinterpreted as upper GI bleeding.)
   d. Repeat Hemoccult at least 3 times while client is on a meat-free, high-residue diet. (Red meats cause false-positive results.)

Recording and Reporting

• Record results of test in appropriate records (check agency policy).

• Record characteristics of stool/gastric contents in nurses' notes.
• Report positive results to physician.

Sample Documentation

1600 Large, liquid, dark brown stool tested positive for occult blood. Physician notified. Client informed that test is to be repeated × 2.

⚙ SPECIAL CONSIDERATIONS ⚙

Home Care Considerations
Clients are instructed to collect Hemoccult specimens at home and return them to clinic or physician's office. To collect stool specimen a piece of plastic wrap can be draped over the toilet. If possible the specimen should not be contaminated with urine. The client prepares slide with feces, closes cardboard slide, and returns it to office or clinic.

Skill 14.3

Blood Glucose Monitoring

Obtaining capillary blood by skin puncture is less painful than venipuncture, and the ease of the skin puncture method to obtain blood samples makes it possible for clients to perform this procedure. The capillary blood glucose test is used to measure blood glucose levels for monitoring the control of diabetes mellitus. Test results are used to direct diet, amount and type of medication, and exercise prescription. Along with the development of reagent strips and home glucose monitors, the skin puncture method has revolutionized home care of clients with diabetes. Self-monitoring of blood glucose is now recognized as an essential component of managing diabetes and is associated with improved glycemic control (Cunningham, 2001). By providing immediate feedback on glucose status, glucose monitoring helps clients prevent diabetic emergencies by prompt detection and treatment of hypoglycemia and hyperglycemia. Setting target goals for blood glucose levels needs to take into consideration the capacity and motivation of the client to achieve the goals, the age of the client, other illnesses, and the potential danger that hypoglycemia causes for the individual (Cunningham, 2001). In otherwise healthy diabetic clients, blood glucose levels often are to remain as close as possible to the normal range (Table 14-1).

Self-testing of blood glucose can be performed by two methods. Both require obtaining a large drop of blood by skin puncture. A hand-held single-use lancet or one of many automatic lancet-holding devices available on the market may be used. The blood is applied to a specially prepared chemical reagent strip.

Table 14-1

Goals for Glucose Control			
Biochemical Index	**Normal**	**Goal**	**Intervention Required**
Fasting glucose (mg/dl)	<115	<120	<80 or >140
Postprandial (mg/dl)	<140	<180	>180
Bedtime glucose (mg/dl)	<120	100-140	<100 or >160
Glycosylated hemoglobin (%)	<6%	<7%	>8%

From Cunningham MA: Glucose monitoring in type 2 diabetes, *Nurs Clin North Am* 36(2):361, 2001.

Table 14-2

Glucose Meters Currently Available				
Meter	**Glucose Range (mg/100 ml)**	**Test Strip Used**	**Test Time**	**Memory**
Accu-Chek Advantage	10-600	Advantage	40 seconds	100 readings
Accu-Chek Easy	20-500	Easy Test Strips	14-60 seconds	350 readings
Glucometer Elite	20-500	Glucometer Elite	30 seconds	Last reading recall
One Touch Basic	0-600	Genuine One Touch	45 seconds	Last reading recall

Data from American Diabetes Association: 1998 Buyer's guide to diabetes products, *Diabetes Forecast* 50(10):68, 1997. Copyright © 1997 American Diabetes Association. From *Diabetes Forecast*, October, 1997. Reprints with permission from *The American Diabetes Association*.

The first method involves visually reading the reagent strip by comparing it to the color chart on the container. Examples of such strips include Chemstrip bG, Gluostix, and Trendstrips. If the color on the strip falls between two reference blocks on the chart, the results may need to be estimated. Thus accurate results of blood glucose measurement may not always be obtained. The second type of blood glucose monitoring is done by the use of reflectance meters. A variety of meters are on the market (Table 14-2). Glucose monitors vary in size, shape, weight, ease of use, size of the display readout, size of blood sample required, and other features. A number of glucose monitors now have memory and data management capabilities. Glucose monitors and supplies are readily available and competitively priced. Accuracy of glucose monitors depends on several factors. A monitor is considered accurate when the results are comparable to laboratory test results. Accuracy of the client's technique and the monitoring system is assessed during hospital admissions and at least yearly. This skill describes the techniques used to measure blood glucose with a meter using the dry-wipe method. Specific steps in using meters will vary, depending on brand of equipment used. Follow manufacturer's instructions.

ASSESSMENT

1. Assess client's understanding of procedure and purpose and importance of glucose monitoring. *Rationale: Diabetes is a chronic disease. This assessment provides nurse with a database on which to provide necessary teaching.*

2. Assess client for types of medications received. *Rationale: Drugs such as cortisone preparations, diuretics, and anesthetics increase blood glucose levels.*

3. Determine if client has a low platelet count, is receiving anticoagulants, or has a bleeding disorder. *Rationale: Determines if client at risk for local ecchymosis and bleeding from skin puncture.*

4. Determine if specific conditions need to be met before or after sample collection (e.g., with fasting, after meals, or before insulin doses). *Rationale: Dietary intake of carbohydrates and concentrated glucose preparations alter blood glucose levels.*

5. Assess area of skin to be used as puncture site. Inspect fingers, toes, and heel. Avoid areas of bruising and open lesions. *Rationale: Sides of fingers, toes, and heels are commonly selected because of fewer nerve endings and vascularity. Puncture site should not be edematous, inflamed, or recently punctured because these factors cause increased interstitial fluid and blood to mix and also increase the risk of infection (Malarkey and McMorrow, 2000).*

6. Review physician's order for time of frequency of measurement. *Rationale: Physician determines test schedule on basis of client's physiological status and risk for glucose imbalance.*

7. For clients who test themselves at home, assess ability to handle skin-puncturing lancet, manipulate monitor, and read results. *Rationale: Client's physical health (e.g., vision, fatigue, neuropathy) may prevent client from performing test.*

8. Assess client for related signs and symptoms of glucose alterations (Table 14-3), which help reveal nature of the problem.

Table 14-3

Signs and Symptoms of Blood Glucose Alterations	
Blood Glucose Alteration	**Assessment Findings**
Hyperglycemia (elevated blood glucose)	Thirst, polyuria, polyphagia, weakness, fatigue, headache, blurred vision, nausea, vomiting, abdominal cramps
Hypoglycemia (low blood glucose)	Sweating, tachycardia, palpitations, nervousness, tremors, weakness, headache, mental confusion, fatigue

9. Check the calibration of the equipment for accuracy. This may be required daily or weekly according to agency policy.

PLANNING

Expected outcomes focus on minimizing tissue damage with finger stick, achieving accurate results, and maintaining glucose levels within goal range.

Expected Outcomes

1. Puncture site shows no evidence of bleeding or tissue damage.
2. Blood glucose measurement results are accurate and within established goal range for client.
3. Client demonstrates procedure and explains test results.

Equipment

- Blood glucose meter (Figure 14-7)
- Disposable gloves
- Antiseptic swab
- Cotton ball or 2 × 2 gauze
- Sterile lancet or bloodletting device
- Paper towel
- Sharps box
- Blood glucose reagent strips (brand determined by meter used)

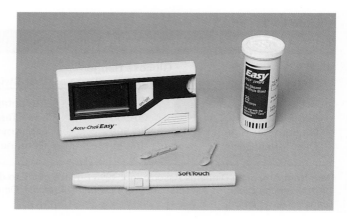

Figure 14-7 Blood glucose monitor, container of test strips, and bloodletting device.

 Delegation Considerations

The skill of obtaining and testing blood glucose level after skin puncture may be delegated to assistive personnel (AP) who have been certified in performing the skill. The client must be assessed to determine that his or her need for glucose monitoring is appropriate for delegation. If the client's condition changes frequently, this skill should not be delegated to AP.

IMPLEMENTATION FOR BLOOD GLUCOSE MONITORING

Steps	Rationale
1. See Standard Protocol (inside front cover).	
2. Instruct client to wash hands with soap and warm water.	Reduces presence of microorganisms. Promotes vasodilation at selected puncture site. Establishes practice for client when test is performed at home.
3. Position client comfortably in chair with hand lower than the heart for a short time.	Promotes vasodilation at selected puncture site.
4. Remove reagent strip from container, and tightly seal cap. Observe expiration date.	Reagent strips deteriorate with exposure to air over time.
5. Turn on glucose meter.	

Steps	Rationale

6. Insert strip into glucose meter, and make necessary adjustments as indicated.

7. Remove unused reagent strip from meter, and place on paper towel or clean, dry surface with test pad facing up. Avoid touching exposed reagent materials.

Moisture on strip can change its color, altering reading of final test results. These factors influence the accuracy of test results.

8. 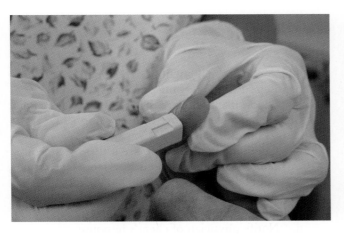 Choose a vascular area as a puncture site. In adult, select lateral side of finger; be sure to avoid central tip of finger, which has a dense nerve supply (Pagana and Pagana, 1998).

Side of finger is less sensitive to pain.

9. Hold finger to be punctured in dependent position while gently massaging finger toward puncture site (Malarkey and McMorrow, 2000).

Increases blood flow to area before puncture.

10. Cleanse site with warm water or alcohol wipe and *allow to dry completely.* Use alcohol sparingly.

Alcohol can cause blood to hemolyze.

11. Remove cover of bloodletting device. Some agencies use lancet devices with an automatic blade retraction system to reduce needle sticks.

12. Place bloodletting device firmly against side of finger and push release button, causing needle to pierce skin (see illustration). Hold lancet perpendicular to puncture site, and pierce finger quickly in one continuous motion (do not force lancet).

Pierces skin to appropriate depth, ensuring adequate blood flow. Shallow penetration minimizes tissue damage (Bloom, 1999).

13. Wipe away first droplet of blood with cotton ball. (See manufacturer's directions for meter used.)

First droplet of blood generally contains tissue fluids (Malarkey and McMorrow, 2000), which can dilute specimen and cause false results.

14. Lightly squeeze (but do not touch) puncture site until large droplet of blood has formed.

Large drop of blood ensures proper coverage of test pad on reagent strip.

15. Hold reagent strip test pad close to drop of blood, and lightly transfer droplet to test pad without smearing it (see illustration).

Smearing may alter chemical action and cause inaccurate test results.

NURSE ALERT   *Repuncturing may be necessary if large enough droplet does not form to ensure accurate test results. Diabetics frequently have peripheral vascular disease, making it difficult to produce a large droplet of blood.*

Step 12   Pierce skin with bloodletting device.

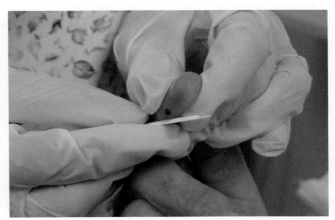

Step 15   Transfer droplet to test pad.

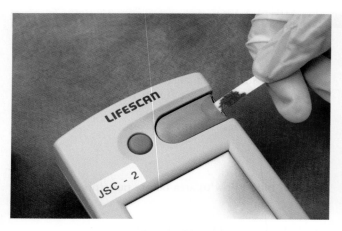

Step 19 Place strip into meter.

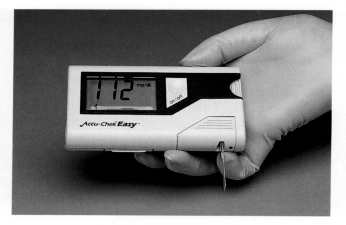

Step 20 Read results.

Steps	**Rationale**
16. Immediately press timer on glucose meter, and place reagent strip on paper towel or on side of timer. (See manufacturer's directions for meter used.) Strip must lie flat so blood does not pool on only one part of pad.	Accurate timing is necessary for accurate results. Some meters (e.g., One Touch) require blood sample to be applied to test strip already in meter.
17. Apply pressure to skin puncture site for at least 10 seconds and only to the area directly over the puncture. Check for continued bleeding. If present, continue to apply pressure until no blood leaks onto the tissue.	Promotes hemostasis and prevents development of painful bruises at the site (Bloom, 1999).
18. When timer displays 60 seconds (for Accu-Chek III model) or sounds, use moderate pressure to wipe blood from test pad with dry cotton ball.	For meter to read glucose levels, some strips must be dry. Refer to product directions for timing used with each type of meter.
19. While timer continues to count, place reagent strip into meter (see illustration).	
20. Read results on meter display (see illustration).	
21. Turn meter off.	Conserves the battery.
22. Dispose of test strip, cotton balls, and bloodletting device in proper receptacles.	Proper disposal reduces risk of needle-stick injury and the spread of microorganisms.
23. Remove and discard gloves.	
24. Share test results with client, and encourage questions. Plan next testing as client demonstration.	Promote client participation and adherence to glucose monitoring.
25. See Completion Protocol (inside front cover).	

• • • • • • • • • •

EVALUATION

1. Observe puncture site for evidence of bleeding or bruising.
2. Compare glucose meter reading with normal blood glucose levels.
3. Ask client to discuss procedure and test results.
4. Observe client performing self-testing.

Unexpected Outcomes and Related Interventions

1. Puncture site continues to bleed or is bruised.
   a. Apply pressure to site for at least 1 minute.
   b. Apply pressure to site for at least 5 minutes if client is taking anticoagulants or acetylsalicylic acid.

2. Glucose meter malfunctions.
   a. Repeat test, following directions.
   b. Follow manufacturer's directions for malfunctions.
3. Blood glucose level above or below normal range.
   a. Continue to monitor client.
   b. Check medical record to see if there are medication orders for deviations in glucose level; if not, notify physician.
   c. Administer insulin or carbohydrate source as ordered (depending on glucose level).
   d. Notify physician of client's response.

4. Client expresses misunderstanding of procedure and results.
  a. Reevaluate client knowledge base, and explain steps again if needed.
  b. Provide printed information if necessary.

Recording and Reporting

- Record glucose results on appropriate flow sheet or in nurses' notes.
- Describe response, including presence or absence of pain or excessive oozing of blood at puncture site.
- Report abnormal blood glucose levels, and take appropriate action for hypoglycemia or hyperglycemia (see Table 14-3).

Sample Documentation

0730 Blood glucose 110. No sliding-scale insulin administered.

  1200 Blood glucose 240. Regular insulin (4 U) administered subcutaneously as ordered per sliding scale.

SPECIAL CONSIDERATIONS

Geriatric Considerations

- Older adults may have difficulty seeing color charts. Clients with visual impairments can still perform glucose testing independently because there are several audio blood glucose meters on the market that give verbal instructions to guide the client through the procedure.
- Older adults with musculoskeletal alterations may not have fine motor coordination necessary to obtain samples on reagent strips.
- Warming fingertips may facilitate obtaining blood specimen.

Home Care Considerations

- Blood glucose levels are usually assessed before meals, before taking medication, and at bedtime to monitor effectiveness of treatment plan.
- In the home the client washes hands with soap and warm water before the finger stick, rather than using an antiseptic swab. Ongoing use of antiseptic swabs can aggravate callus formation.
- Verify that the client is able to complete the blood glucose monitoring independently or if a family member needs to perform the testing.
- It is generally recommended that one or more family members be able to monitor blood glucose levels in the event that the client is unable to do so independently.

Skill 14.4

Collecting Blood Specimens—Venipuncture With Vacutainer, Blood Cultures

Blood tests, one of the most commonly used diagnostic procedures, can yield valuable information about a client's nutritional, hematological, metabolic, immune, and biochemical status. Tests allow physicians and other health care providers to screen clients for early signs of physical illness, monitor changes in acute or chronic diseases, and monitor responses to therapies.

The nurse may be responsible for collecting blood specimens, although some institutions have specially trained technicians whose sole responsibility is to draw blood. Nurses must be familiar with their institution's policies and procedures and their state's Nurse Practice Act regarding guidelines for drawing blood samples. The nurse must be competent in performing phlebotomy to prevent client injury. Veins are major sources of blood for laboratory testing and routes for intravenous (IV) fluid or blood replacement; therefore maintaining their integrity is essential. When a client is at risk for loss of the integrity of the veins and it is anticipated that multiple access sites will be required, it is important to use the most distal sites first, and retain one or more appropriate sites for IV access. Blood is not drawn from a site proximal to an IV insertion. If the attempt to draw blood has failed after two attempts, ask for assistance.

The primary method for obtaining blood specimens is venipuncture. Venipuncture involves inserting a hollow-bore needle into the lumen of a large vein to obtain a specimen. The nurse may use a needle and syringe (see Procedural Guideline 14-3, p. 374) or a special Vacutainer tube that allows the drawing of multiple blood samples. Once a specimen is obtained, it is placed directly into the appropriate blood tube. A color-coding system for the tops of the collection tubes is used to indicate the type of specimen that can be collected within that tube. Special blood tubes are available, containing anticoagulants, because some tests cannot be performed on clotted or hemolyzed specimens.

The blood-borne pathogens standard of the Occupational Safety and Health Administration (OSHA) requires that "Each employer having an employee(s) with occupational exposure . . . shall establish a written Exposure Control Plan designed to eliminate or minimize employee exposure" (OSHA, 2001). As a result, phlebotomy equipment includes needle safety devices. Using standard precautions and appropriate personal protective equipment provides a barrier to protect skin and mucous membranes from contact with blood; however, most barriers are easily penetrated by needles. New safety devices are designed to protect health care workers as follows:

- Provide a barrier between the hands and the needle after use
- Allow or require the worker's hands to remain behind the needle at all times
- Are an integral part of the device and not an accessory
- Are simple to operate and require little training to use effectively

Regardless of the type of safety device in use, never recap needles and always carefully discard them in puncture-resistant containers close to the client. A major significant exposure occurs when a deep puncture is caused by a needle that has been used to collect blood. Report all needle-stick injures. All needle-stick injuries are not preventable; however, the use of needles with safety features has substantially decreased the risk of exposure to blood-borne pathogens for health care workers (Centers for Disease Control and Prevention, 1997).

Blood culture, a specific blood test used to detect the presence of bacteria in the blood (bacteremia), requires a special phlebotomy technique. Because bacteremia may be accompanied by fever and chills, blood cultures should be drawn when symptoms are present. It is important that at least two culture specimens be drawn from two different sites. Bacteremia exists when both cultures grow an infecting agent. If only one culture produces bacteria, the assumption is that the bacteria were skin contaminants rather than the infecting agent. Because culture specimens obtained through an IV catheter are frequently contaminated, tests using them should not be performed unless catheter sepsis is suspected. Blood cultures are always drawn before antibiotic therapy is started, because the antibiotic may interrupt the organism's growth in the laboratory.

ASSESSMENT

1. For a blood specimen, assess if special conditions need to be met for specimen collection (e.g., client allowed nothing by mouth [NPO], a specific time for collection in relation to time medication is given, need to ice specimen). *Rationale: Conditions may be required for accurate measurement of blood elements (e.g., fasting blood sugar, drug peak and trough, ammonia levels).*

2. Assess client for possible risks of venipuncture, which include anticoagulant therapy, low platelet count, or bleeding disorder. *Rationale: Abnormal clotting caused by low platelet count, hemophilia, or medications increases risk for bleeding and hematoma formation.*

3. Assess client for contraindicated sites for venipuncture: presence of IV infusion, hematoma at potential site, arm on side of mastectomy or axillary surgery, or hemodialysis shunt. *Rationale: Drawing specimens from such sites can result in false test results or may injure client.*

4. Review physician's order for type of blood tests. *Rationale: Multiple samples may be needed; physician's order is required.*

5. Determine client's understanding of purpose of test and ability to cooperate with procedure. *Rationale: Some clients may need assistance of another member of the health care team. Procedure can appear threatening to client.*

6. When drawing blood cultures, assess for systemic evidence of bacteremia, including fever and chills. *Rationale: Blood should be drawn when client is experiencing these clinical signs.*

PLANNING

Expected outcomes focus on the collection of an uncontaminated, appropriate blood specimen by the nurse or trained technician.

Expected Outcomes

1. Client explains purpose of blood collections before collection is attempted.
2. Client's venipuncture site shows no evidence of continued bleeding or hematoma.
3. Client reports minimal anxiety or discomfort.
4. Test results are within normal limits (see agency report or appropriate laboratory manual). Culture results are negative for bacteremia, or test identifies pathogen needing to be treated.

Equipment

All Procedures

- Alcohol or antiseptic swab (check agency policy for specific antiseptic solution)
- Disposable gloves
- Small pillow or folded towel
- Sterile gauze pads (2 × 2 inch)
- Tourniquet
- Adhesive bandage or adhesive tape
- Completed identification labels

- Completed laboratory requisition
- Plastic bag for specimen delivery to laboratory (or container as specified by agency)

Venipuncture—Vacutainer

- Vacutainer and safety access device
- Sterile double-ended needles: 20 to 21 gauge for adults; 23 to 25 gauge for children
- Appropriate blood tubes (depends upon tests being done)

Blood Cultures

- Povidone-iodine (Betadine) (check agency policy for antiseptic to use)
- 70% alcohol (check agency policy)
- Two 20-ml syringes
- Sterile needles: 20 to 21 gauge for adults; 23 to 25 gauge for children.
- Anaerobic and aerobic culture bottles (Figure 14-8)

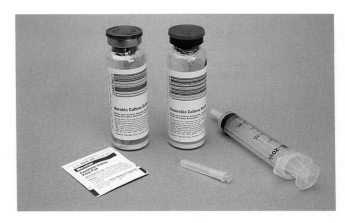

Figure 14-8 Blood culture bottles and syringe for venipuncture.

Delegation Considerations

Phlebotomy staff and RNs may obtain venipuncture samples. RNs who draw blood samples are usually certified by the agency that employs them. However, check agency policy to determine who may perform blood drawing.

IMPLEMENTATION FOR COLLECTING BLOOD SPECIMENS—VENIPUNCTURE WITH VACUTAINER, BLOOD CULTURES

Steps	Rationale
1. See Standard Protocol (inside front cover).	
2. Assist client with sitting or lying supine or in semi-Fowler's position with arm supported and elbow extended. Place small pillow or towel under upper arm.	Helps to stabilize extremity. Supported position in bed reduces chance of injury to client if fainting occurs.
3. Explain procedure to client. Explain how sensation of tourniquet, alcohol swab, and needle stick will feel.	

COMMUNICATION TIP *"As I begin, you are going to feel a tightness around your arm when I place this rubber tourniquet. The alcohol will feel cool and wet. I will tell you just as I insert the needle; it will feel like an insect sting."*

4. Quickly inspect extremity for best venipuncture site, looking for straight, prominent vein without swelling or hematoma. Of the three veins located in the antecubital area, the median cubital vein is preferred (see illustration on p. 358).	This vein is large, well anchored (does not easily move), is closer to the surface of the skin, and less painful to puncture. Straight and intact veins are easiest to puncture. The veins of the lower arm and hand are preferred for administering IV fluids.
5. Apply tourniquet so that it can be removed by pulling end with single motion	Tourniquet blocks venous return to heart from extremity, causing veins to dilate for easier visibility.
a. Position the tourniquet 5 to 10 cm (3 to 4 inches) above venipuncture site selected.	
b. Cross the tourniquet over the client's arm, holding the tourniquet between your fingers close to the arm (see illustration on p. 358).	

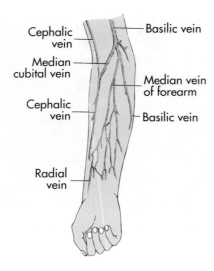

Step 4 Location of antecubital veins.

Cephalic vein
Basilic vein
Median cubital vein
Median vein of forearm
Cephalic vein
Basilic vein
Radial vein

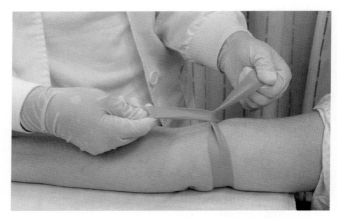

Step 5b Cross tourniquet over the arm.

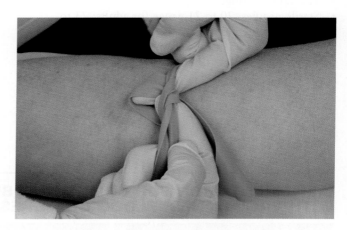

Step 5c Tuck a loop between the client's arm and tourniquet.

Steps	Rationale
c. Tuck a loop between the client's arm and the tourniquet so that the free end can be easily grasped (see illustration). d. Free end can be pulled to release tourniquet following venipuncture.	
6. Palpate distal pulse (e.g., radial) below tourniquet. If pulse is not palpable, reapply tourniquet more loosely.	If tourniquet is too tight, pressure will impede arterial blood flow.

NURSE ALERT *To prevent injury to skin and vein, it is recommended to not apply tourniquet on older adult with poor skin turgor and fragile veins.*

7. Keep tourniquet in place no longer than 1 minute. If this happens, remove and wait 60 seconds before reapplying or assess other extremity.	Minimizes effects of hemoconcentration and hemolysis. Prolonged time may alter test results and cause pain and venous stasis (e.g., falsely elevated serum potassium level) (Malarkey and McMorrow, 2000).
8. Apply warm, wet compress over extremity for 10 minutes if unable to visualize or palpate vein.	Heat causes local dilation.
9. Ask the client to gently open and close fist several times, finally leaving fist clenched.	Facilitates distention of veins by forcing blood up from distal veins. If done too vigorously, this may alter test results.

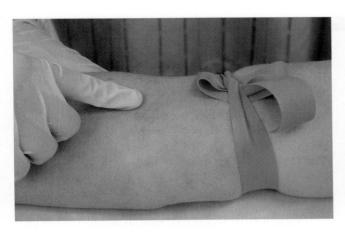

Step 10   Palpate vein.

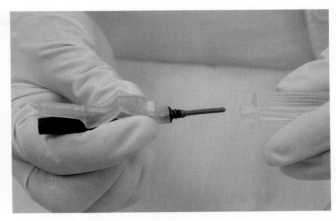

Step 11a(1)   Attach double-ended needle.

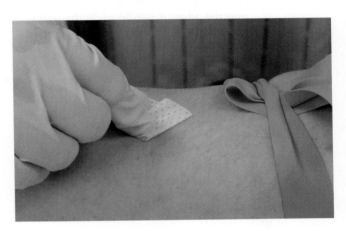

Step 11a(3)   Cleanse venipuncture site with alcohol.

Steps	Rationale
10. Palpate selected vein with finger (see illustration). Note if vein is firm and rebounds when palpated or if vein feels rigid and cordlike and rolls when palpated.	A healthy vein is elastic and rebounds on palpation. Thrombosed vein is rigid, rolls easily, and is difficult to puncture.

NURSE ALERT *Do not vigorously tap or slap veins because this can cause vasospasm.*

---

11. Obtain blood specimen:

   a. Vacutainer specimen

     (1) Attach double-ended needle to Vacutainer tube (see illustration).

     (2) Select proper blood specimen tubes, and place the first tube inside vacuum tube, but do not puncture rubber stopper.

     Tubes are usually color coded to indicate intended use based on size of tube and presence or absence of a chemical additive. Puncture of stopper results in loss of vacuum.

     (3) Cleanse venipuncture site with alcohol swab (70% isopropyl alcohol) using a circular motion out from site for approximately 5 cm (2 inches) (see illustration). Allow to dry.

     Antimicrobial agent cleans skin surface of resident bacteria so organisms do not enter puncture site. Allowing alcohol to dry reduces "sting" of venipuncture. Alcohol left on skin can cause hemolysis of sample.

     (4) Remove needle cover, and inform client that "stick" lasting only a few seconds will be felt.

     Client has better control over anxiety when prepared about what to expect.

Steps	**Rationale**
(5) Place thumb or forefinger of nondominant hand 2.5 cm (1 inch) *below* site, and pull skin taut. Stretch skin down until vein is stabilized.	Position of finger below site prevents accidental needle stick. Stretching helps to stabilize vein and prevent rolling during needle insertion.
(6) With dominant hand, hold Vacutainer needle at 15- to 30-degree angle from arm with bevel of needle up (see illustration).	Reduces chance of penetrating both sides of vein during insertion and is less trauma to vein.
(7) Slowly insert needle into vein until there is a decrease in resistance that indicates the vein has been entered.	Prevents puncture on opposite side.
(8) With the dominant hand braced against the client's arm to hold it still, use the thumb of the nondominant hand that anchored the vein to push the vacuum tube into the adaptor needle while the index and middle fingers grasp the flared ends of the adapter (see illustration).	Pushing needle through stopper breaks vacuum and causes flow of blood into tube. If needle in vein advances, vein may become punctured on other side.
(9) Note flow of blood into tube, which should be fairly rapid (see illustration).	Failure of blood to appear indicates that vacuum in tube is lost or needle is not in vein.

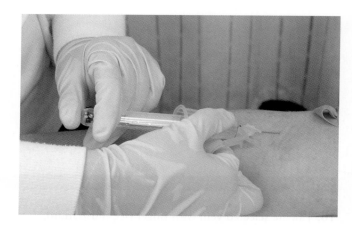

Step 11a(8) Use thumb of nondominant hand to push vacuum tube into needle.

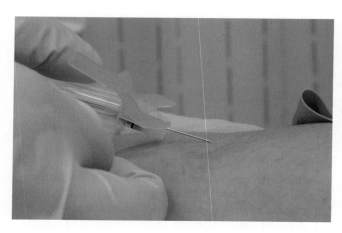

Step 11a(6) Hold Vacutainer needle at 15- to 30-degree angle.

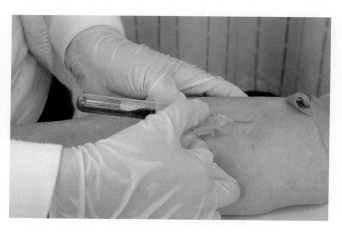

Step 11a(9) Note rapid flow of blood into tube.

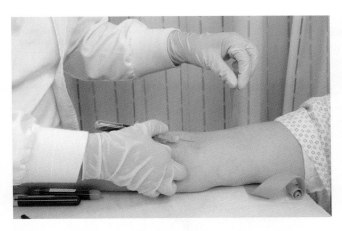

Step 11a(11)   Release tourniquet before removing needle.

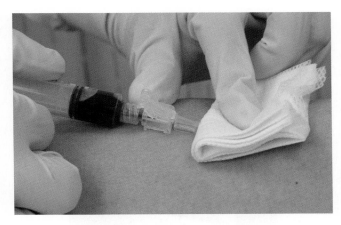

Step 12   Apply gauze over puncture site.

Steps	Rationale
(10) After specimen tube is filled, grasp vacuum tube firmly and remove specimen tube. Insert additional specimen tubes as needed.	Prevents needle from advancing or dislodging. Tubes with additives should be inverted as soon as possible.
NURSE ALERT *When filling tubes with an anticoagulant additive, let tube fill until the vacuum is exhausted. Ratio of blood to additive is important. Gently rotate the tube back and forth 8 to 10 times.*	Prevents clotting as additives are mixed with blood. Shaking can cause hemolysis of red blood cells, producing inaccurate test results.
(11) After last tube is filled, release tourniquet (see illustration).	Reduces bleeding at site when needle is withdrawn.
b. **Blood culture**	
(1) Cleanse venipuncture site with povidone-iodine or appropriate antiseptic. Allow to dry.	Antimicrobial agent cleans skin surface so organisms do not enter puncture site or contaminate culture.
(2) Clean bottle tops of vacuum tubes or culture bottles with appropriate antiseptic (check agency policy).	Ensures specimen is sterile.
(3) Collect 10 to 15 ml of venous blood by venipuncture (see Procedural Guideline 14-3, p. 374) from each venipuncture site.	Cultures must be obtained from two sites.
(4) Discard needle on syringe; replace with new sterile needle before injecting blood sample into culture bottles.	Maintains sterile technique and prevents contamination of specimen.
(5) If both aerobic and anaerobic cultures are needed, inoculate anaerobic first (Pagana and Pagana, 1998).	Anaerobic organisms may take longer to grow.
(6) Mix medium gently after inoculation.	Mixes medium and blood.
12. After venipuncture, apply 2 × 2 inch gauze pad over puncture site without applying pressure, and quickly but carefully withdraw needle from vein (see illustration).	Pressure over needle can cause discomfort. Careful removal of needle minimizes discomfort and vein trauma.

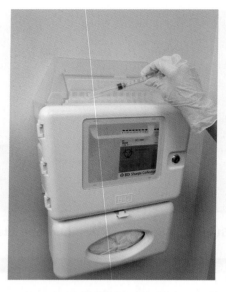

Step 16   Needle with safety cover.

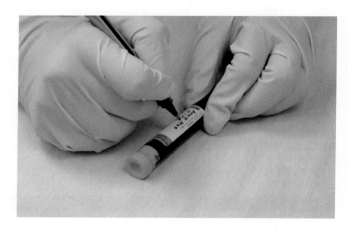

Step 18   Affix requisition to labeled blood tube.

Steps	Rationale
13. Immediately apply pressure over venipuncture site with gauze or antiseptic pad for 2 to 3 minutes or until bleeding stops. Inspect site for bleeding, and then tape gauze dressing securely over site.	Minimizes bleeding and prevents hematoma.
14. Take blood tubes containing additives; gently rotate back and forth 8 to 10 times	Additives should be mixed with blood to prevent clotting. Shaking can cause hemolysis of blood, cells producing inaccurate results (Pagana and Pagana, 1998).
15. If tubes have any sign of external presence of blood, decontaminate with 70% alcohol.	
16. Carefully discard uncapped sharps into appropriate container. If needle has built-in safety device, activate (see illustration) and then discard.	One-handed technique helps to avoid needle-stick injury (OSHA, 2001).
17. Remove and discard gloves.	
18. Label the specimen with the client's name, date, and time. Affix proper requisition (see illustration). For a culture specimen, include tentative diagnosis and antibiotics client may be receiving. Place in appropriate bag for transfer.	Ensures diagnostic information reported on correct client. Antibiotics may affect test results.
19. Transport cultures immediately to laboratory (or at least within 30 minutes) (Pagana and Pagana, 1998).	
20. See Completion Protocol (inside front cover).	

• • • • • • • • • •

EVALUATION

1. Ask client to explain purposes of tests.
2. Inspect venipuncture site for hemostasis.
3. Determine if client is anxious or fearful.
4. Check laboratory report for test results.

Unexpected Outcomes and Related Interventions

1. Client continues to have bleeding or develops hematoma at venipuncture site.
   a. Apply pressure to site, and document size and color.
   b. Apply pressure dressing.
   c. Reinspect site within 15 minutes.
2. Laboratory tests reveal significantly abnormal blood results (see laboratory report or laboratory manual for norms).
   a. Report to physician.
   b. Institute medical regimen as ordered.
3. Signs and symptoms of infection at venipuncture site occur.
   a. Notify physician.
   b. Apply heat to site.

Recording and Reporting

- Record method used to obtain blood specimen, date and time collected, type of test ordered, and laboratory receiving specimen.
- Describe venipuncture site after specimen collection.
- Describe client's tolerance to procedure of specimen collection.
- Report any stat results to physician or charge nurse.
- Report any abnormal results to physician or charge nurse.

Sample Documentation

1000 Serum chemistry and complete blood count specimens drawn from L antecubital fossa. 2-cm hematoma noted. Pressure applied using 2 × 2 gauze. Encouraged client to elevate arm and continue pressure and to notify nurse if bleeding occurs or hematoma enlarges.

SPECIAL CONSIDERATIONS

Pediatric Considerations

- If possible take child to a procedure room to perform venipuncture. Maintain hospital room as a "safe place." Allow parents to remain present if desired to provide emotional support.
- When performing venipuncture on children, the nurse needs to explore a variety of sources for vein access: scalp, antecubital fossa, saphenous veins, hand veins.
- Application of local anesthetic cream 30 minutes before procedure may be ordered to reduce pain in infants and young children.
- Since venipuncture can be difficult with small veins in infants and small children, collection of blood using a capillary heel stick are frequently used.
- Heel warming can be used to facilitate obtaining blood specimen from the heel of a neonate.

Geriatric Considerations

Older adults have fragile veins that are easily traumatized during venipuncture. Sometimes application of warm compresses may help in obtaining samples. Using a small-bore catheter also may be beneficial.

Home Care Considerations

- In the home care setting a blood pressure cuff, rather than a tourniquet, can be used for venipuncture.
- Instruct client to notify nurse or physician if persistent or recurrent bleeding or expanding hematoma occurs at venipuncture site.

Procedural Guideline 14-3
Venipuncture With Syringe

Equipment: Alcohol or antiseptic swab, disposable gloves, sterile needles (20- to 21-gauge for adults, 23- to 25-gauge for children), sterile syringe of appropriate size, small pillow or folded towel, sterile gauze pads (2 × 2 inch), rubber tourniquet, adhesive bandage or tape, appropriate blood tubes, completed laboratory identification labels and laboratory requisition, plastic bag for delivery of specimen.

1. See Standard Protocol (see inside front cover)
2. Prepare for venipuncture following Steps 2 to 10, Skill 14.4, pp. 367-369.
3. Have syringe with appropriate needle securely attached.
4. Cleanse venipuncture site with alcohol swab, moving in circular motion from site for approximately 5 cm (2 inches). Allow to dry.
5. Remove needle cover, and inform client that "stick" will last only a few seconds.
6. Place thumb or forefinger of nondominant hand 2.5 cm (1 inch) below site, and gently pull skin taut. Stretch skin down to stabilize vein.
7. Hold syringe and needle at 15- to 30-degree angle from client's arm with bevel up.
8. Slowly insert needle into vein (see illustration). With experience, nurse will feel "pop" as needle enters vein.
9. Hold syringe securely, and pull back gently on plunger while watching for a blood return (see illustration). If plunger is pulled back too quickly, ressure may cause vein to collapse.
10. Obtain appropriate amount of blood, keeping needle stabilized.
11. Release tourniquet, remove needle, and apply pressure with 2 × 2 gauze (see illustration, Step 12, Skill 14.4, p. 371).
12. Continue with Steps 13 to 19, Skill 14.4, pp. 371-372.
13. See Completion Protocol (inside front cover).

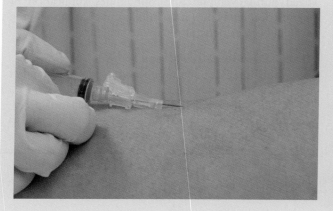

Step 8 Perform venipuncture.

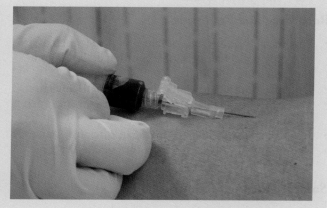

Step 9 Pull back on plunger.

Skill 14.5

Collecting Specimens From the Nose and Throat

When clients have signs and symptoms of upper respiratory or sinus infection, a nose or throat culture is a simple diagnostic tool for determining the nature of the client's problem. The laboratory staff places the specimen on a culture medium to determine if pathogenic microorganisms will grow. Regardless of what body fluids are cultured, certain principles apply. Cultures should be drawn before antibiotic therapy is started, because the antibiotic may in-

terrupt the organism's growth in the laboratory. If the client is receiving antibiotics, the laboratory needs to be notified and told what specific antibiotics the client is receiving (Pagana and Pagana, 2001).

Collection of a nose and throat specimen can cause the client discomfort because of sensitive mucosal membranes. Likewise, collection of a throat culture may cause gagging. For that reason it is important to collect a throat culture before mealtime or at least 1 hour after eating to lessen the chance of inducing vomiting. Clients should clearly understand how each specimen is to be collected to minimize anxiety or discomfort.

ASSESSMENT

1. Assess condition of and drainage from nasal mucosa and sinuses. *Rationale: Reveals physical signs that may indicate infection or allergic irritation.*
2. Determine if client has experienced postnasal drip, sinus headache or tenderness, nasal congestion, or sore throat. *Rationale: Further clarifies nature of problem.*
3. Assess condition of posterior pharynx (see Chapter 13).
4. Assess for systemic indications of infection, including fever, chills, and malaise.

PLANNING

Expected outcomes focus on obtaining an uncontaminated specimen in the appropriate amount for diagnosis and appropriate treatment.

Expected Outcomes

1. Client verbalizes understanding of purpose of specimen and how specimen is obtained.
2. Culture specimen is obtained without contamination from adjacent skin or tissues.

3. Client does not experience bleeding of nasal mucosa.
4. Client will maintain comfort level and experience minimal anxiety.

Equipment

- Disposable gloves
- Two sterile swabs in sterile culture tubes (flexible wire swab with cotton tip may be used for nose cultures)
- Nasal speculum (optional)
- Tongue blades
- Penlight
- Emesis basin or clean container (optional)
- Facial tissues
- 2 × 2 gauze
- Completed identification labels and laboratory requisition

Delegation Considerations

The skills of obtaining throat, nasal, and nasal pharyngeal cultures require the critical thinking and knowledge application unique to a nurse. Delegation of these skills is inappropriate.

IMPLEMENTATION FOR COLLECTING SPECIMENS FROM THE NOSE AND THROAT

Steps	Rationale
1. See Standard Protocol (inside front cover).	
COMMUNICATION TIP *Explain that client may have tickling sensation or gag during swabbing of throat. Nasal swab may create urge to sneeze. State that procedure takes only a few seconds.*	
2. Ask client to sit erect in bed or chair facing you. Acutely ill client may lie supported at a 45-degree angle in semi-Fowler's position.	Provides easy access to oral structures.
3. Have swab in tube ready for use. You may want to loosen top so swab can easily be removed.	Most commercially prepared tubes have a top that fits securely over end of swab, which allows nurse to touch outer top without contaminating swab stick.
4. Collect specimen.	
a. **Throat culture**	
(1) Instruct client to tilt head backward. For clients in bed, place pillow behind shoulders.	
(2) Ask client to open mouth and say "ah."	Permits exposure of pharynx, relaxes throat muscles, and minimizes gag reflex.

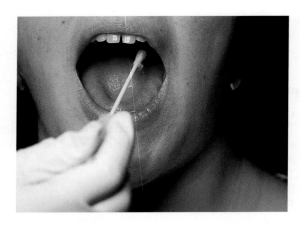

Step 4a(4)   Collecting a throat culture.

Steps	Rationale
(3) Depress tongue with tongue blade if unable to expose pharynx, and note inflamed areas of pharynx or tonsils. Depress anterior third of tongue only, and illuminate with penlight as needed.	Area to be swabbed should be clearly visualized.
(4) Insert swab without touching lips, teeth, tongue, or cheeks (see illustration).	
(5) Gently but quickly, swab tonsillar area side to side, making contact with inflamed or purulent sites and withdraw without touching mouth, teeth, or tongue.	Collects microorganisms from the throat tissues without contamination from mouth or tongue.
b. **Nose culture**	
(1) Ask client to blow nose, and then check nostrils for patency with penlight. Select nostril with greatest patency.	Clears nasal passage of mucus that contains resident bacteria.
(2) Ask client to tilt head back. Clients in bed should have pillow behind shoulders.	
(3) Gently insert nasal speculum in one nostril *(optional)*. Carefully pass swab into nostril until it reaches that portion of mucosa that is inflamed or containing exudate. Rotate swab quickly. NOTE: If nasopharyngeal culture is to be obtained, use a special swab on a flexible wire that can be flexed downward to reach nasopharynx	Swab should remain sterile until it reaches area to be cultured. Rotating swab covers all surfaces where exudate is present.
(4) With dominant hand remove swab without touching sides of speculum or nasal canal.	Prevents contamination by resident bacteria.
(5) With nondominant hand carefully remove nasal speculum (if used), and place in basin. Offer client facial tissue.	
5. Immediately place swab in culture tube.	
6. Take 2 × 2 gauze and cover end of tube, then crush ampule at bottom of tube to release culture medium. Push tip of swab into liquid medium.	Placing tip within culture medium maintains life of bacteria for testing.
7. Place top on tube securely.	
8. Discard supplies into trash.	

Steps	Rationale
9. Securely attach properly completed identification label and laboratory requisition to side of specimen container (not lid).	Incorrect identification of specimen could result in diagnostic or therapeutic errors.
10. Enclose specimen in a plastic bag.	
11. Send specimen immediately to laboratory, or refrigerate.	
12. Remove and discard gloves.	
13. See Completion Protocol (inside front cover).	Reduces transmission of microorganisms.

• • • • • • • • • •

EVALUATION

1. Ask client to describe purpose of culture.
2. Monitor technique of culture collection process for potential contamination.
3. Inspect specimen for traces of blood, and reinspect mucosa if bleeding apparent.
4. Ask client to describe comfort level and level of anxiety.

Unexpected Outcomes and Related Interventions

1. Cultures reveal heavy bacterial growth.
   a. Notify physician of results.
   b. Administer antibiotics as ordered.
2. Culture was contaminated by bacteria from adjacent skin or tissues.
   a. Notify physician.
   b. Repeat collection of cultures.
3. Client experiences minor nasal bleeding.
   a. Apply mild pressure and ice pack over bridge of nose.
   b. Notify physician of client's condition.
4. Client experiences increased pain and anxiety.
   a. Provide nonpharmacological comfort measures such as active listening, reassurance, and support.
   b. Provide analgesia as ordered.

Recording and Reporting

• Record types of specimen obtained, source, and time and date sent to laboratory.
• Describe appearance of site, presence or absence of signs of local or systemic infection noted.
• Record client's response to procedure and level of discomfort and anxiety noted.

Sample Documentation

0930 Client experiencing sore throat, oral temp 100° F. Pharynx inflamed with green-colored exudate noted on inspection. Obtained throat culture per order. Client tolerated without gagging or discomfort. Specimen sent to lab.

SPECIAL CONSIDERATIONS

Pediatric Considerations

• Ask parents if they wish to help hold child or if they prefer nurse to do so.
• Immobilization of child's head and arms is important when obtaining nose or throat culture and should be done in firm, gentle, kind manner. Ask another nurse to assist, if necessary. Ask parents to act as coach with their child.
• Showing tongue blade and penlight to child and demonstrating how to say "ah" helps to decrease anxiety.
• School-age child will be more cooperative if given opportunity to ask questions about procedure and results.
• Throat cultures should not be attempted if acute epiglottitis is suspected, because trauma from swab might cause increase in edema and resulting occlusion of airway (Wong and others, 1999).
• Children of school age and older are often very curious and may ask many questions about specimen collection. Questions should be answered honestly and at the child's level of understanding. Allow child to watch, if desired, while test is performed.

Skill 14.6

Collecting a Sputum Specimen by Suction

Sputum is produced by cells that line the respiratory tract. Although production is minimal in the healthy state, disease can increase the amount and change the appearance of sputum. Examination of sputum can aid in the diagnosis and treatment of conditions including bronchitis, tuberculosis (TB), and lung cancer.

Sputum specimens may be collected for three purposes. Cytology specimens are used to identify cancer cells. Sputum for C&S can be used to identify specific pathogens and to determine the antibiotics to which they are most sensitive. Sputum for acid-fast bacilli (AFB) is examined to support the diagnosis of TB.

Nasotracheal suctioning is required to collect a sputum specimen when a client cannot expectorate sputum. Suctioning can provoke violent coughing, which can induce vomiting and constriction of pharyngeal, laryngeal, and bronchial muscles. Suctioning can also cause direct stimulation of vagal nerve fibers, resulting in cardiac arrhythmias and increased intracranial pressure (Beare and Myers, 1998). Procedural Guideline 14-4 on p. 381 describes the steps for collecting an expectorated sputum.

ASSESSMENT

1. Check physician's orders for number and type of specimens needed, time and method of collection.
2. Assess client's understanding of procedure and its purpose.
3. Assess client's ability to cough and expectorate sputum. *Rationale: Suction is avoided when an expectorated specimen can be obtained.*
4. Determine when client last ate a meal. *Rationale: It is best to obtain the specimen 1 to 2 hours after a meal or 1 hour before to minimize gagging, which can cause vomiting and aspiration.*
5. Assess client's respiratory status, including respiratory rate, depth, pattern, lung sounds, and color. *Rationale: Changes in respiration may indicate the presence of secretions in tracheobronchial tree and potential need for supplementary oxygenation.*
6. Assess client's anxiety level. *Rationale: Obtain a premedication order (i.e., sedative) if client is extremely anxious. This procedure may be contraindicated in clients who cannot cooperate or remain still during the procedure (Pagana and Pagana, 2001).*

PLANNING

Expected outcomes focus on collecting an uncontaminated specimen while maintaining a patent airway, adequate oxygenation, and client comfort.

Expected Outcomes

1. Client's respirations are same rate and character as before procedure.
2. Client verbalizes understanding of the purpose and process of specimen collection.
3. Client maintains comfort level and experiences minimal anxiety.
4. Sputum is not contaminated by saliva or oropharyngeal flora.

Equipment

- Suction device (wall or portable)
- Sterile suction catheter (size 14, 16, or 18 Fr [not large enough to cause trauma to nasal mucosa])
- Sterile gloves
- Sterile saline in container
- In-line specimen container (sputum trap)
- Oxygen therapy equipment if indicated
- Protective eyewear (if required)

Delegation Considerations

Collection of expectorated sputum specimens may be delegated to assistive personnel (AP). Collection of a sputum specimen using sterile suction requires the critical thinking and knowledge application unique to a nurse and should not be delegated.

IMPLEMENTATION FOR COLLECTING A SPUTUM SPECIMEN BY SUCTION

Steps	Rationale
1. See Standard Protocol (inside front cover).	
2. Position client in high- or semi-Fowler's position for suctioning.	Promotes full lung expansion and facilitates ability to cough.
3. Explain steps of procedure and purpose. Encourage client to breathe normally to prevent hyperventilation.	
4. ✋ Prepare suction machine or device, and make sure it is functioning properly	Adequate amount of suction is necessary to aspirate sputum.
5. Connect suction tube to adapter on sputum trap.	
6. Apply sterile glove to dominant hand.	Allows handling of suction catheter without introducing microorganisms into the tracheobronchial tree, which is a sterile body cavity.
7. Preoxygenate for 1 minute with 100% oxygen (if available).	Use caution if client has chronic obstructive pulmonary disease (COPD), because 100% oxygen can depress respiratory effort.
8. Using gloved hand, connect sterile suction catheter to rubber tubing on sputum trap.	Aspirated sputum will go directly to trap instead of to suction tubing.
9. Gently insert tip of suction catheter prelubricated with sterile water through nasopharynx, endotracheal tube, or tracheostomy without applying suction (see Chapter 30) (see illustration).	Minimizes trauma to airway as catheter is inserted. Lubrication allows for easier insertion.
10. Gently and quickly advance catheter into trachea.	Triggers cough reflex.

COMMUNICATION TIP *Warn client to expect to cough. Entrance of catheter into larynx and trachea triggers cough reflex.*

---

11. As client coughs, apply suction for 5 to 10 seconds, collecting 2 to 10 ml of sputum.	Suctioning longer than 10 seconds can cause hypoxia and mucosal damage.
12. Release suction and remove catheter, then turn off suction.	Releasing suction avoids unnecessary trauma to mucosa as the catheter is withdrawn.
13. Detach catheter from specimen trap, and dispose of catheter into appropriate receptacle.	
14. Connect rubber tubing on sputum trap to plastic adapter (see illustration).	

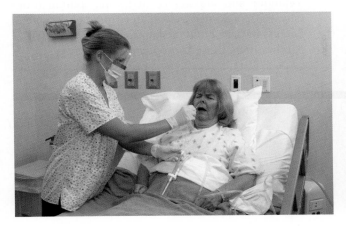

Step 9   Insert catheter through nasopharynx.

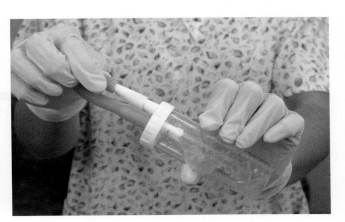

Step 14   Closing sputum trap.

Steps	Rationale
15. If any sputum is present on outside of container, wash it off with disinfectant.	Prevents spread of infection to persons handling specimen.
16. Offer client tissues after suctioning. Dispose of tissues in emesis basin or trash container. Remove and dispose of gloves.	
17. Securely attach properly completed identification label and laboratory requisition to side of specimen container (not lid).	Incorrect client identification could lead to diagnostic or therapeutic error.
18. Enclose specimen in a plastic bag.	
19. Send specimen immediately to laboratory.	Bacteria multiply quickly. Specimen should be analyzed promptly for accurate results.
20. Offer client mouth care if desired.	
21. See Completion Protocol (inside front cover).	

• • • • • • • • • •

EVALUATION

1. Observe respiratory and oxygenation status throughout procedure.
2. Ask client to describe the purpose and process of specimen collection.
3. Ask client to report level of comfort and anxiety.
4. Evaluate technique of collection process for sterility.

Unexpected Outcomes and Related Interventions

1. Client becomes hypoxic with increased respiratory rate and shortness of breath.
   a. Discontinue suctioning immediately.
   b. Administer oxygen.
   c. Monitor vital signs and oxygen saturation
   d. Notify physician if distress is unrelieved.
2. Inadequate amount of sputum is collected, or specimen contains saliva.
   a. Repeat collection procedure after client has rested.
   b. Encourage client to deep breathe and cough.
3. Client remains anxious or complains of discomfort from suction catheter.
   a. Discontinue procedure until client is stable.
   b. Provide oxygen as needed (if ordered).
   c. Notify physician of client's condition.
   d. Continue to monitor client's vital signs. Consider measuring oxygen saturation.

Recording and Reporting

- Record method used to obtain specimen, date and time collected, type of test ordered, and how specimen was transported to the laboratory.
- Describe characteristics of sputum specimen.
- Describe client's oxygenation and respiratory status.

Sample Documentation

0730 Expectorated 14 ml thick green sputum before breakfast. Specimen collected in sterile container and immediately transported to lab for C&S. Reports slightly short of breath. Respirations 26. Rales noted bilaterally in all lung fields.

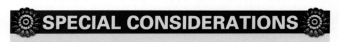

Home Care Considerations

- If client is to produce sputum specimen at home, instruct client and/or family member regarding proper technique and importance of having sputum (not saliva) specimen sent to laboratory in timely manner.
- Discuss ways to avoid contaminating specimen (e.g., handwashing, using appropriate equipment).

Procedural Guideline 14-4
Collecting a Sputum Specimen by Expectoration

Equipment: Sterile specimen container with cover, clean disposable gloves, facial tissues

1. See Standard Protocol (inside front cover).
2. Explain importance that client coughs and expectorates sputum. Client cannot simply clear throat and expectorate saliva.
3. Provide opportunity to cleanse or rinse mouth with water.
4. Provide sputum cup, and instruct client not to touch the inside of the container.
5. Have client take three to four deep breaths. Instruct client to emphasize slow, full exhalation. Then after a full inhalation ask client to cough forcefully, expectorating sputum directly into specimen container (see illustration).
6. Repeat until 5 to 10 ml (1 to 2 teaspoons) of sputum (not saliva) has been collected.
7. Secure top on specimen container tightly. If any sputum is present on outside of container, wash it off with disinfectant.
8. Offer client tissues after expectorating, dispose of tissues, and offer mouth care.
9. Remove and dispose of gloves.
10. Securely attach properly completed identification label and laboratory requisition to side of specimen container (not lid).
11. Enclose specimen in a plastic bag.
12. Send specimen immediately to laboratory.
13. See Completion Protocol (inside front cover).

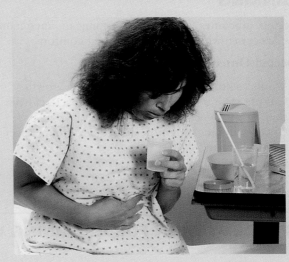

Step 5   Expectorating sputum. (From Grimes D: *Infectious diseases,* Mosby's Clinical Nursing Series, St Louis, 1991, Mosby.)

Skill 14.7

Obtaining Wound Cultures

When caring for a client with a wound, the nurse assesses the wound's condition and observes for the development of infection. Localized inflammation, tenderness, warmth at the wound site, and purulent drainage are signs and symptoms of wound infection. Infection cannot be confirmed or treated accurately without confirmation from a wound culture.

The nurse should never collect a wound culture sample from old drainage. Resident colonies of bacteria on the skin grow in wound exudate and may not be the true causative organisms causing infection. Separate techniques are used to collect specimens for measuring aerobic versus anaerobic microorganism growth. Aerobic organisms grow in superficial wounds exposed to the air. Anaerobic organisms grow deep within body cavities, where oxygen is not normally present.

ASSESSMENT

1. Assess client for fever, chills, malaise, elevated white blood cell count (WBC). *Rationale: Signs and symptoms indicate systemic infection.*
2. Assess severity of pain at wound site (scale of 0 to 10). *Rationale: If client requires analgesic before dressing change, ideally medication is given 30 minutes before dressing change to reach peak effect.*
3. Review physician's order for aerobic or anaerobic culture.
4. Determine when dressing change is scheduled. *Rationale: This step may be performed as part of the specimen collection procedure.*
5. Assess client's understanding of need for wound culture and ability to cooperate with procedure.

6. While wearing disposable gloves, remove any soiled dressing. Apply sterile gloves, and inspect for swelling, opening of wound edges, inflammation, and drainage. Palpate along wound edges and note tenderness.

PLANNING

Expected outcomes focus on obtaining an uncontaminated specimen while maintaining client comfort.

Expected Outcomes

1. Wound culture does not reveal bacterial growth.
2. Culture swab is not contaminated by bacteria from skin.
3. Client will discuss purpose and procedure for specimen collection.
4. Client experiences minimal discomfort (e.g., pain severity 4 or less on scale of 0 to 10).

Equipment

- Culture tube with swab and transport medium for aerobic culture
- Anaerobic culture tube with swab (tubes contain carbon dioxide or nitrogen gas)
- 5- to 10-ml syringe and 21-gauge needle
- Sterile gloves, protective eyewear, antiseptic swab, sterile dressing materials (determined by type of dressing)
- Paper or plastic disposable bag

 Delegation Considerations

Obtaining a wound culture requires the critical thinking and knowledge application unique to a nurse. Delegation of these skills is inappropriate.

IMPLEMENTATION FOR OBTAINING WOUND CULTURES

Steps	Rationale
1. See Standard Protocol (inside front cover).	
2.  Remove old dressing. Observe drainage. Fold soiled sides of dressing together, and then dispose of in bag.	
3. Cleanse area around wound edges with antiseptic swab, removing old exudate.	Ensures that culture will consist of fresh wound secretions.
4. Discard swab, and dispose of soiled gloves in bag.	
5. Open package containing sterile culture tube and dressing supplies.	Provides sterile field from which nurse can handle supplies.
6. Apply sterile gloves.	
7. Obtain culture:	
a. **Aerobic culture**	
(1) Take swab from culture tube, insert tip into wound in area of drainage, and rotate swab gently.	
(2) Remove swab, and return to culture tube. Using a gauze pad between gloved fingers and the ampule, crush the ampule of medium and immediately push swab into fluid. Place top on culture tube securely.	Prevents accidental injury should glass inside ampule break through tube
b. **Anaerobic culture**	
(1) Take swab from special anaerobic culture tube, swab deeply into body cavity where oxygen is not present, and rotate gently. Remove swab, and immediately return to culture tube to minimize exposure to oxygen. Place top on culture tube securely.	

or

Steps	Rationale

    (2)   Insert tip of syringe (without needle) into wound, and aspirate 5 to 10 ml of exudate. Attach 21-gauge needle, expel all air, and inject drainage into special culture tube where carbon dioxide or nitrogen gas keeps organisms alive. Place top on culture tube securely.

8. Clean wound as ordered, and apply new sterile dressing.

9. Ask another nurse or AP to securely attach properly completed identification label and laboratory requisition to side of specimen container (not lid).

                  Allows primary nurse to complete dressing change while specimen is promptly sent to the laboratory.

10. Enclose culture tube in a plastic bag.

11. Send specimen to laboratory within 15 minutes (Parini, 2000).

12. Remove and discard gloves and supplies.

13. See Completion Protocol (inside front cover).

• • • • • • • • • •

EVALUATION

1. Ask client to rate severity of pain during and after procedure (scale of 0 to 10).

2. Observe character of wound drainage, and note edges of wound.

3. During procedure ask patient to describe purpose of culture.

4. Obtain laboratory report for results of cultures.

Unexpected Outcomes and Related Interventions

1. Wound cultures reveal heavy bacterial growth.
    a. Monitor client for fever, chills, increased WBC.
    b. Inform physician of findings.

2. Laboratory report indicates wound culture is contaminated with superficial skin cells.
    a. Monitor client for fever and pain.
    b. Inform physician.
    c. Repeat collection of specimen as ordered.

Recording and Reporting

- Record type of specimen obtained, source, and time and date specimen sent to laboratory.
- Describe appearance of wound and characteristics of drainage.
- Record client's tolerance to procedure and response to analgesia.
- Report any evidence of infection to nurse in charge and physician.

Sample Documentation

1420 Client complains of pain from surgical site. 4-cm wound is separated at top with yellow purulent drainage. Lower half of dressing remains approximated. Incisional area tender to touch. Aerobic culture obtained from site of drainage, sent to lab.

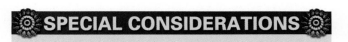

SPECIAL CONSIDERATIONS

Pediatric Considerations

If procedure is to be performed on a child and it is anticipated to be painful, some agencies perform procedure in area other than child's room, keeping child's room a same place (Wong and others, 1999).

Home Care Considerations

- Teach client or family caregiver proper aseptic technique for performing dressing changes.
- Educate client and family regarding signs and symptoms of wound infection and when to notify physician.

Long-Term Care Considerations

Carefully monitor wound drainage to prevent spread of infection to other residents.

CRITICAL THINKING EXERCISES

1. The assistive personnel reports to you that Mr. X had a positive Hemoccult test on a stool sample. What assessment do you as the RN make on this client?

2. You are to collect a clean-voided specimen from your client, who is an obese 76-year-old woman with osteoarthritis, which creates constant aching pain in the hip joints. The pain is rated 4 to 6 (scale 0 to 10) and is worsened with movement. She is also very weak after undergoing recent chemotherapy. How would you collect this specimen?

3. At 1030 you have admitted a client with a diagnosis of diabetes out of control who has a wound infection. Orders include BGM (blood glucose monitoring) before meals and at bedtime with sliding-scale insulin orders; culture wound for C&S; complete blood count stat; and IV antibiotics stat and q6h. The patient reports nausea, weakness, and fatigue and not having eaten breakfast. The routine morning insulin dose was taken as usual at home. What is your first priority and why? Which of the above orders must be completed before giving the antibiotic and why?

REFERENCES

American Diabetes Association: 1998 Buyer's guide to diabetes products, *Diabetes Forecast* 50(10):68, 1997.

Beare PG, Myers JL: *Adult health nursing,* ed 3, St Louis, 1998, Mosby.

Bloom AH: 5 Tips for your fingertips, *Nursing,* 29(5):59, May, 1999.

Centers for Disease Control and Prevention: Evaluation of safety devices for preventing percutaneous injuries among health care workers during phlebotomy procedures, Minneapolis, St Paul, New York City, and San Francisco, 1993-1995, *MMWR Morb Mortal Wkly Rep* 46(2):21, Jan 21, 1997.

Chernecky C, Berger B: *Laboratory tests and diagnostic procedures,* ed 2, Philadelphia, 1997, WB Saunders.

Cunningham MA: Glucose monitoring in type 2 diabetes, *Nurs Clin North Am* 36(2):361, 2001.

Malarkey L, McMorrow C: *Nurse's manual of laboratory tests and diagnostic procedures,* ed 2, Philadelphia, 2000, WB Saunders.

Occupational Safety and Health Administration (OSHA): Occupational exposure to bloodborne pathogens: final rule, *Federal Register* 66(12):5318, Jan 18, 2001.

Pagana KD, Pagana TJ: *Mosby's manual of diagnostic and laboratory tests,* St Louis, 1998, Mosby.

Pagana KD, Pagana TJ: *Mosby's diagnostic and laboratory test reference,* St Louis, 2001, Mosby.

Parini S: Combating infection: how to collect specimens, *Nursing* 30(5):66, 2000.

Wong DL and others: *Whaley and Wong's nursing care of infants and children,* ed 6, St Louis, 1999, Mosby.

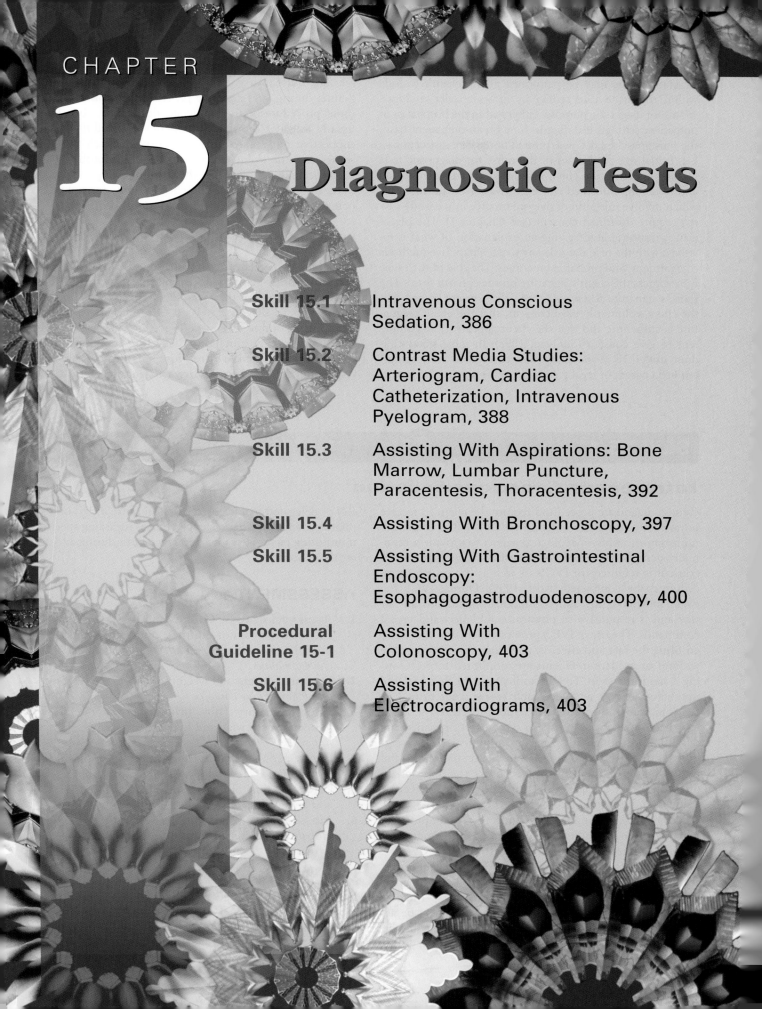

Diagnostic Tests

Diagnostic tests may be performed at the client's bedside within the acute care setting or in specifically equipped rooms for diagnostic purposes either within the hospital or in outpatient settings. If testing is done on an outpatient basis, the nurse provides detailed, printed home care instructions.

Initial responsibilities of the nurse for diagnostic tests include assessing the client's knowledge of the procedure and obtaining informed consent. Invasive diagnostic tests, which involve injection of dye or entrance into a body cavity, require informed consent (see Chapter 1). The physician is responsible for giving an explanation of what is involved with the test, the risks involved, alternative methods of treatment, and probable outcomes. The role of the nurse is to witness the client's signature on the consent form. The nurse's signature when witnessing the consent means that the client voluntarily gave consent, that the client's signature is authentic, and that the client appears to be competent to give consent (Sullivan, 1998). In most states children under 18 years of age are considered minors and require a parent or legal guardian to give informed consent.

The nurse also assesses and records the client's status before, during, and after the procedure. Because most of these procedures cause moderate discomfort, the client usually tolerates the procedure better if a well-informed, supportive nurse stays close and explains each step. In some cases the client receives nothing by mouth (NPO) for a specified period before the test. Following the procedure, the nurse monitors the client's status for potential complications.

NURSING DIAGNOSES

Anxiety may be related to anticipating discomfort or pain as a procedure is performed. **Fear** may be related to the unknown test results or the invasive nature of several procedures. Nursing diagnoses related to promoting optimum oxygenation during diagnostic procedures that affect pulmonary function include **Risk for Impaired Gas Exchange, Ineffective Breathing Pattern, Risk for Aspiration,** and **Ineffective Airway Clearance.**

Skill 15.1

Intravenous Conscious Sedation

Certain diagnostic procedures require the client to receive intravenous conscious sedation (IVCS). IVCS is the administration of pharmacological agents to provide a minimally depressed level of consciousness (LOC). Informed consent is required for IVCS, as well as the invasive procedure to be completed (Kost, 1999). During IVCS the client independently and continuously maintains an airway and is responsive to physical stimulation and verbal commands. The use of IVCS provides client comfort while ensuring the safe and effective performance of a procedure without oversedation. Clients are monitored for LOC using a scoring system. For the tool shown in Box 15-1 the optimal score is 4, and acceptable scores range from 3 to 5. More than 5 suggests oversedation, whereas a score of less than 3 may indicate risk for discomfort or inadequate relaxation. Although IVCS may be administered by a registered nurse (RN) with a physician in attendance, it is the responsibility of the physician to order the appropriate drugs and their dosages. Check agency policy for recommended and maximum doses of medications.

Client risks during IVCS include airway compromise, hemodynamic instability, and/or altered LOC. Emergency equipment must be immediately accessible where IVCS is administered (see Chapter 37). After IVCS, clients need continuous monitoring of vital signs, electrocardiogram (ECG), and oxygen saturation by pulse oximetry. In addition, the client's level of sedation and LOC must be assessed and documented according to agency policy by the RN or delegated to a licensed practical nurse (LPN) or respiratory therapist. Check agency policies regarding specific monitoring parameters and frequency both during and after the procedure.

ASSESSMENT

1. Assess vital signs, ECG, LOC and skin color, presence of chest pain or shortness of breath. *Rationale: Establishes baseline assessment. Physician must be notified of abnormalities.*
2. Determine height and weight. *Rationale: Needed for calculation of drug dosages.*
3. Assess respiratory status, including airway and ability to open mouth wide and hyperextend neck. *Rationale: Factors that influence intubation if needed.*
4. Palpate peripheral pulses, and check for peripheral edema. *Rationale: Signs of compromised circulation.*
5. Determine time of last oral intake. *Rationale: Clients need to be NPO for at least 4 hours before the procedure.*
6. Assess level of anxiety. *Rationale: The lower the anxiety level, the less sedation likely to be needed.*

PLANNING

Expected outcomes focus on client's knowledge of the procedure, client's level of anxiety, and prevention of complications.

Box 15-1

Assessment of Level of Consciousness for Conscious Sedation

Assign the number that best describes the client's response to each category. An optimal score is 4, with acceptable scores ranging from 3 to 5.

EMOTIONAL AFFECT

0 anxious/uneasy
1 calm/tolerant
2 unresponsive/flat affect

LEVEL OF CONSCIOUSNESS

0 awake or awakening
1 follows commands/intermittent arousal
2 unresponsive

VITAL SIGNS

0 increased/requires intervention
1 within acceptable limits
2 decreased/requires intervention

PHYSICAL REACTION TO PROCEDURE

0 resistive or intense response
1 tempered or intermittent response
2 no response

Modified from Kost M: Conscious sedation: guarding your patient against complications, *Nursing,* 29(4):34, April 1999.

Expected Outcomes

1. Client explains the purpose and basic steps of the procedure before it begins..
2. Client remains relaxed and comfortable (pain less than 2 on a scale of 0 to 10) *and* is responsive to physical and verbal stimuli with protective airway reflexes intact.
3. Client does not experience complications, such as respiratory depression, decreased cardiovascular function, confusion, and diminished reflexes, which are side effects of drugs used for IV sedation.

Equipment

- Equipment for IV start (see Chapter 29)
- Sedatives for IV sedation (e.g., diazepam [Valium], midazolam [Versed], and fentanyl [Sublimaze] are commonly used; however, others may be ordered)
- Equipment for resuscitation: oxygen, pulse oximeter, cardiac monitor, and appropriate reversal drugs.

Delegation Considerations

Assistive personnel (AP) may transport stable clients to the testing department. Monitoring vital signs following the procedures may be delegated to AP, but assessment cannot. Monitoring during IVCS requires the critical thinking and knowledge application unique to a nurse. Delegation is inappropriate.

IMPLEMENTATION FOR INTRAVENOUS CONSCIOUS SEDATION

Steps	Rationale
1. See Standard Protocol (inside front cover).	
2. Establish IV access (see Skill 29.1, p. 676).	Medications are given intravenously for rapid onset of action.
3. Monitor and record vital signs every 5 to 15 minutes.	Changes in vital signs signal level of sedation.
4. Observe for verbal or nonverbal evidence of pain, facial grimacing, and eye opening.	Physical responses signal level of sedation.
5. Monitor LOC (see Box 15-1), and notify physician of unacceptable scores.	Careful monitoring for excessive medication response is essential during conscious sedation.
6. Monitor ECG, oxygen saturation, and skin color.	
7. See Completion Protocol (inside front cover).	Reflects possible respiratory compromise due to client's response to sedation medications.

• • • • • • • • • •

EVALUATION

1. Ask client to explain purpose and basic steps of procedure before it begins.
2. Ask client to rate level of pain severity (scale of 0 to 10).
3. Assess client for low oxygen saturation, rate and/or depth of respirations, cyanosis or mottled skin, hypotension, changes in heart rate and/or rhythm (usually bradycardia), and decreased or nonpalpable peripheral pulses, reflexes, and LOC complications related to conscious sedation.

Unexpected Outcomes

1. Client develops respiratory distress evidenced by decreased oxygen saturation, cyanosis, and slow, shallow respirations with periods of apnea.
   a. Monitor vital signs and O_2 saturation.
   b. Notify physician immediately.
2. Client develops cardiac instability as evidenced by irregular heart rate, change in pulse rate, change in BP.
   a. Monitor BP, heart rate, peripheral pulses, and O_2 saturation.
   b. ECG as ordered.
   c. Notify physician immediately.

Recording and Reporting

- Record condition upon return to the unit including vital signs, O_2 saturation, depth of respirations, LOC, color, and level of comfort.
- Report to physician immediately any respiratory distress, cardiac compromise, or altered mental status.

Sample Documentation

1500 returned to unit post esophagogastroduodenoscopy (EGD) with conscious sedation, alert and awake. BP 120/60, P92, R26, O_2 sat 98%. Resp. deep and reg. Color pale. Rates pain as 6 (0-10) in Ⓡ rib cage, worse at 8 with deep breaths. Demerol 50 mg given IV.

  1530 Resting. Rates pain at 1 (0-10). Vital signs unchanged. O_2 sat 97%-99%.

SPECIAL CONSIDERATIONS

Geriatric Considerations

Older adult clients may have reduced drug clearance from decreased renal function or decreased hepatic function. Therefore the nurse must monitor the effects of narcotics and hypnotics that may interfere with breathing (Phipps, 1999).

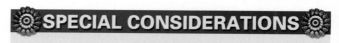

Skill 15.2

Contrast Media Studies: Arteriogram, Cardiac Catheterization, Intravenous Pyelogram

Contrast media studies involve visualization of blood vessels of a system of the body by the intravascular injection of a contrast medium. An arteriogram (angiogram), permits visualization of the blood vessels of the arterial system (Figure 15-1). This provides diagnosis of occlusions, stenosis, emboli, thromboses, aneurysms, tumors, congenital malformations, or trauma of the arteries of the brain, heart, lung, kidneys, or lower extremities.

Cardiac catheterization is a specialized form of angiography in which a catheter is inserted into either the left or right side of the heart via a peripheral major blood vessel (subclavian or femoral vein). The test studies pressures within the heart, cardiac volumes, valve function, and patency of coronary arteries.

An intravenous pyelogram (IVP) is done to visualize the kidneys or renal pelvis, ureters, and bladder. The client is given a cathartic on the evening before the test and is usually NPO after midnight. Clients with preexisting renal insufficiency are at risk.

The diagnostic procedures addressed in this skill are performed in radiology or a special procedures department by a variety of specially trained technicians and physicians (Figure 15-2). Roles of the nurse include assisting with the preparation of the client before the procedure, providing support during the procedure if indicated, and monitoring for complications after the procedure.

ASSESSMENT

1. Assess client's knowledge of the procedure. *Rationale: Determines level of understanding and what teaching may be necessary.*
2. Observe verbal and nonverbal behaviors to determine level of client's anxiety.
3. Assess for allergy to iodine dye or shellfish; if so, notify cardiologist or radiologist. *Rationale: A hypoallergenic contrast medium can sometimes be used.*
4. Assess vital signs to provide baseline data for comparison with findings during and after procedure.

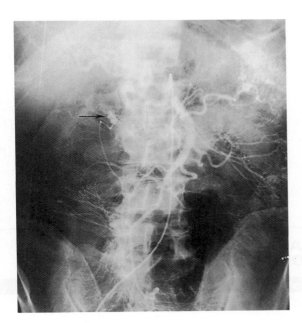

Figure 15-1 Arteriogram. (From Dougherty DB, Jackson DB: *Gastrointestinal disorders,* Mosby's clinical nursing series, St Louis, 1993, Mosby.)

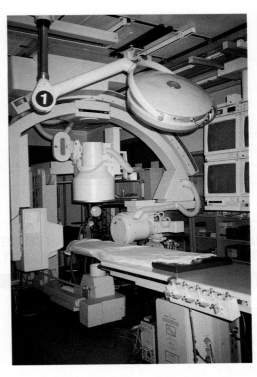

Figure 15-2 Cardiac catheterization laboratory. (From Wong and others: *Whaley and Wong's nursing care of infants and children,* ed 6, St Louis, 1999, Mosby.)

5. Assess peripheral pulses (for clients undergoing angiography) to provide baseline data for comparison with findings during and after procedure.

6. Assess hydration status of client. *Rationale: Severe dehydration can cause renal shutdown and failure (Pagana and Pagana, 2001).*

7. Assess client's coagulation status (e.g., use of anticoagulants, platelet count, prothrombin time) to determine factors that can increase risk of bleeding. *Rationale: Use of anticoagulants and abnormal clotting factors may contraindicate the procedure at that time.*

8. Auscultate heart and lung sounds (for clients undergoing angiography) to provide baseline data for comparison with findings during and after procedure.

9. Verify that client has signed consent form (check agency policy).

10. Assess time of last ingested fluid or food. *Rationale: Excessive hydration causes dilution of contrast medium, making structure more difficult to visualize. Iodine dye may cause nausea.*

11. Assess client's ability to remain still and cooperate throughout the procedure.

PLANNING

Expected outcomes focus on improving the client's knowledge of the procedure, reducing client's level of anxiety, prevention of complications, and control of discomfort during and after the procedure.

Expected Outcomes

1. Client explains the purpose and basic steps of the procedure before it begins.

2. Client assumes the correct position and remains still throughout the entire procedure.

3. Client has pain less than 2 (on a scale of 0 to 10).

4. Client does not experience postprocedural discomfort or complications, such as the following:
   a. Flushing, itching, and urticaria, which signify possible allergic reaction to dye
   b. Diminished or absent peripheral pulses, which may signify thrombosis or embolism
   c. Hypotension and tachycardia, which may signify hemorrhage or allergic reaction to dye
   d. Decreased or absent urine output related to renal failure

Equipment

- Sterile packs containing various sizes and types of catheters/equipment for performing the procedures
- Equipment for IV start (see Chapter 29)
- Diazepam, midazolam, or other sedative for IV sedation if indicated
- Equipment for resuscitation: oxygen, pulse oximeter, cardiac monitor
- Sterile gown, sterile gloves, mask, and goggles

Delegation Considerations

Assistive personnel (AP) may transport stable clients to the testing department. Monitoring vital signs following the procedures may be delegated to AP, but assessment cannot. Diagnostic studies requiring the use of contrast medium are subject to potentially life-threatening complications. Inform AP to report to the nurse any complications (e.g., allergic reactions and bleeding). If IVCS is used, delegation is inappropriate.

IMPLEMENTATION FOR CONTRAST MEDIA STUDIES: ARTERIOGRAM, CARDIAC CATHETERIZATION, INTRAVENOUS PYELOGRAM

Steps	Rationale
1. See Standard Protocol (inside front cover).	
2. Assist client with emptying bladder before procedure.	Ensures that client will not need to void during procedure.
3. Client may be monitored continuously during the procedure including ECG, oxygen saturation, and blood pressure. Assist with equipment application and setup.	
4. Provide IV access using large-bore cannula (see Chapter 29).	Provides access for delivery of IV fluids and/or drugs.
5. Assist client in assuming comfortable position on x-ray table.	Position may need to be maintained for 1 to 3 hours.
6. Physician cleanses site for catheter insertion (femoral, carotid, or brachial) with antiseptic.	
7. All members of the team apply sterile gown and gloves, and the client is draped with sterile drapes, leaving puncture site exposed.	
8. The skin at the puncture site is anesthetized with a local anesthetic.	
9. Physician inserts needle and guide wire. Catheter is advanced to area to be visualized, and contrast medium is injected.	

COMMUNICATION TIP *Tell client that the dye injection often causes a transitory flushing of the face, a feeling of warmth, a salty taste in the mouth, or even transient nausea (Pagana and Pagana, 2001).*

Steps	Rationale
10. If iodinated dye is administered, the nurse observes client for signs of anaphylaxis, including respiratory distress, palpitations, itching, and diaphoresis.	Allergic reactions can be life threatening.
11. During the dye injection, specialized equipment provides visualization of the dye moving through blood vessels and takes rapid sequence of x-ray films.	Provides radiographic visualization of structures and abnormalities.
12. For cardiac catheterization, the nurse assists with measuring cardiac volumes and pressures.	Provides data related to cardiac output, central venous pressure (CVP), ventricular pressures, and pulmonary artery pressure.
13. The physician withdraws catheter and applies pressure to puncture site for at least 5 minutes.	Pressure on puncture site promotes clotting and prevents bleeding.

Steps	Rationale
14. Remove and discard gloves.	
15. After the procedure, keep client in a position so that the insertion site extremity is kept straight. Clients often remain in bed for 4 to 6 hours (Ignatavicius and Workman, 2002).	Prevents bleeding.
16. Apply a pressure dressing or bandage over the insertion site (Ignatavicius and Workman, 2002). A 5- or 10-pound sandbag or a C-clamp may be applied over the insertion site.	Ensures hemostasis at insertion site.
17. See Completion Protocol (inside front cover).	

• • • • • • • • • •

EVALUATION

1. Ask client to explain purpose and basic steps of the procedure before it begins.
2. Assess client's body position and comfort during procedure.
3. Ask if client has questions or concerns about the procedure before it begins and later about test results. Assess nonverbal behaviors of anxiety before, during, and after procedure.
4. Evaluate client's level of comfort on a scale of 0 to 10.
5. Monitor for complications.
   a. Vital signs every 15 minutes for 1 hour, then every 30 minutes for 2 hours or until vital signs are stable, then every 4 hours (see agency policy) (Ignatavicius and Workman, 2002).
   b. Monitor insertion site for bloody drainage or hematoma formation.
   c. Assess peripheral pulses in the affected extremity, as well as skin temperature and color. Monitor each time vital signs are checked. Changes can indicate altered circulation.
   d. Auscultate heart and lungs, and compare findings with preprocedure findings. Monitor ECG recording.
   e. Monitor the client for allergic reactions.
      (1) Assess client for flushing, itching, and urticaria.
      (2) Assess client's respiratory status for sudden, severe shortness of breath.
      (3) Assess for decreased output, which may be an indication of renal failure.
   f. Monitor client's LOC and neurological status.

Unexpected Outcomes and Related Interventions

1. Client's dorsalis pedis pulses are nonpalpable bilaterally 2 hours after an angiogram.
   a. Assess dorsalis pedis pulses with a Doppler scope.
   b. Notify physician immediately.
2. Hematoma or hemorrhage is present at catheter insertion site.
   a. Maintain direct pressure over insertion site.

   b. Contact physician immediately.
   c. Monitor catheter site every 30 minutes for 2 to 3 hours, then as ordered.
3. Client experiences chest pain or dysrhythmias.
   a. Contact physician immediately.
4. Client experiences allergic reaction to dye.
   a. Assess vital signs.
   b. Administer antihistamine if ordered.
   c. Notify physician.
5. Client develops neurological changes such as visual disturbances, slurred speech, or swallowing difficulties, indicating possible cerebral vascular accident.
   a. Contact physician immediately.

Recording and Reporting

- Record client's condition on return to nursing unit: vital signs, status of pulses for equality, and temperature of extremities. Record type and appearance of dressing, type and amount of drainage, and client's level of comfort.
- Report to physician or charge nurse immediately: changes in vital signs and/or oxygen saturation, urine output, and level of client responsiveness.
- Also report excessive bleeding or development of hematoma, decreased or absent peripheral pulses.

Sample Documentation

0800 Client returned from angiogram via stretcher. Dorsalis pedis and posterior tibial pulses are 2 bilaterally. No bleeding, swelling, or discoloration noted at catheter insertion site in left groin. Sandbag in place over left groin. Left leg extended. Complains of mild discomfort at left groin, but denies need for analgesics.

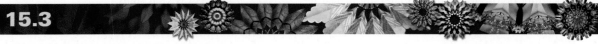

SPECIAL CONSIDERATIONS

Geriatric Considerations

- In the older adult, slight alterations in vital signs or behavior may be precursors to impending problems; therefore skilled observations are critical (Phipps, 1999).
- Be aware that NPO status in the older adult client may result in dehydration.

Home Care Considerations

- Upon discharge, client will be instructed to contact the physician (or affiliated emergency department) if the following occurs after cardiac catheterization:
  - Bleeding from the catheterization puncture site; apply gentle pressure with a clean gauze or cloth.

- Formation of a knot or lump under the skin that increases in size.
- Worsening of a bruise or its movement down the extremity rather than disappearing.
- Pain at puncture site or in the extremity used for the catheterization.
- Extremity where arterial puncture is made becomes pale and cool to touch.
- Appearance of redness, swelling, or warmth of the affected extremity.
- Bathing or showering may be allowed the day after the catheterization.

Skill 15.3

Assisting With Aspirations: Bone Marrow, Lumbar Puncture, Paracentesis, Thoracentesis

Aspirations involve removal of body fluids or tissue for diagnostic purposes. They are usually performed by a physician at the client's bedside or in a treatment room by a physician assisted by a nurse or other health care personnel. Informed consent is legally required for these invasive procedures. Most of these procedures cause moderate discomfort, and the client may tolerate the procedure better if a well-informed nurse stays at the bedside and explains each step. Table 15-1 includes information about preparation, site of entry and body position, and special considerations for each of these procedures.

A bone marrow aspiration involves the removal of a small amount of marrow, the liquid material from the bone. The site of aspiration is usually the sternum or the superior iliac crest. In children the proximal tibia may be used. A bone marrow aspiration may be done to diagnose leukemias, certain malignancies, anemias, and thrombocytopenia. The marrow is examined in a laboratory to reveal the number, size, shape, and development of red blood cells (RBCs) and platelet precursors. This test takes about 20 minutes.

A lumbar puncture, also called a spinal puncture or spinal tap, involves the introduction of a needle into the subarachnoid space of the spinal column. The purpose is to measure the pressure in the subarachnoid space, to obtain cerebrospinal fluid for visual and laboratory examination and to inject anesthetic, diagnostic, or therapeutic agents. Lumbar puncture is used for the diagnosis of

meningitis, encephalitis, brain or spinal cord tumors, and cerebral hemorrhage.

Abdominal paracentesis involves removal of peritoneal fluid from the abdomen for diagnostic analysis. The fluid may be analyzed for the presence of bacteria, blood, fungi, glucose, and protein and may be cytologically analyzed to detect tumors. This procedure may also be done to reduce intraabdominal pressure for palliative reasons. There may be increased intraabdominal pressure from the buildup of fluid (ascites) secondary to liver disease or bleeding resulting from blunt trauma. This increased pressure may cause respiratory distress from pressure against the diaphragm. The procedure takes 30 minutes or less.

Thoracentesis involves the removal of pleural fluid for gross appearance and consistency; measurement of protein, glucose, amylase, lactic dehydrogenase (LDH) levels; and cytological examination for malignancy. It also may be cultured for pathogens. Therapeutic thoracentesis is used to relieve pain, dyspnea; and signs of pleural pressure. Diagnostic thoracentesis is used in the presence of pleural effusion of unknown etiology and generally takes 30 minutes or less.

ASSESSMENT

1. Assess client's knowledge of procedure to determine level of teaching required.
2. Observe verbal and nonverbal behaviors to determine client's anxiety.

Table 15-1

Summary of Aspiration Procedures

Aspiration Procedure	Preparation/Assessment Specific to Test	Position and Site	Special Considerations
Bone marrow aspiration	Assess complete blood count for abnormalities.		Clients with arthritis or orthopnea may have difficulty assuming this position. Pressure is applied to the site following procedure.
Lumbar puncture	Assess neurological status, including movement, sensation, and muscle strength of legs to provide a baseline for comparison. Assess bladder for distention, and determine last voiding. Weigh client, assess abdomen, and measure abdominal girth at largest point. Mark location.		**Risk of spinal headache:** Instruct client to remain flat and log roll according to physician orders. Observe for excessive drainage at the site. Fluid loss at the site can predispose client to headache and infection.

(From Ignatavicius D, Workman L: *Medical-surgical nursing: critical thinking for collaborative care*, ed 4, St Louis, 2002, Mosby.)

Continued

Table 15-1

Summary of Aspiration Procedures—cont'd

Aspiration Procedure	Preparation/Assessment Specific to Test	Position and Site	Special Considerations
Paracentesis	Assess bladder for distention, and determine last voiding. Weigh client, assess abdomen, and measure abdominal girth at largest point. Mark location.		After removing fluid, pressure on diaphragm is released and breathing becomes much easier. **Risk of trauma:** Have client empty urinary bladder before procedure.
Thoracentesis	Assess respiratory rate and depth, symmetry of chest on inspiration and expiration, cough and sputum. Assist client with remaining still during the procedure to prevent trauma to the visceral pleura. Client will need to hold breath and avoid coughing during the procedure.	Area for needle insertion	Monitor blood pressure for hypotension if large quantity of fluid is removed. **Risk of pneumothorax:** Observe for sudden shortness of breath, tracheal deviation, anxiety, and altered vital signs and decreased oxygen saturation.

(From Beare P, Myers J: *Adult health nursing,* ed 3, St Louis, 1998, Mosby.)

Ribs, Parietal pleura, Visceral pleura, Lung tissue (parenchyma), Pleural effusion, Diaphragm

3. Assess client's ability to understand and follow directions. *Rationale: Procedures require client to follow directions closely and assume proper position. The procedures may be contraindicated in clients who cannot cooperate or remain still during the procedure (Pagana and Pagana, 2001).*

4. Assess client's ability to physically assume position required for procedure and ability to remain still. *Rationale: Client must maintain position, without moving, to avoid complications during needle or trochar insertion.*

5. Determine whether client is allergic to antiseptic or anesthetic solutions. *Rationale: Common allergic reactions to local anesthetic agents include central nervous system depression, respiratory difficulties, and hypotension. Allergic reactions to antiseptic solutions are usually skin irritations.*

6. Assess whether client has signed consent form (check agency policy).

7. Assess vital signs to provide baseline data for comparison with postprocedural vital signs.

8. Assess client's coagulation status (use of anticoagulants, platelet count, prothrombin time) to determine factors that can increase risk of bleeding.

9. Assess according to aspiration or diagnostic procedure being performed (see Table 15-1).

10. Assess need for preprocedural pain medication. *Rationale: Procedure may be painful, and pain control helps client remain still throughout procedure.*

PLANNING

Expected outcomes focus on improving client's knowledge of the procedure, including the need to remain still to prevent complications; reducing client's anxiety regarding procedure and results; and control of discomfort during and after the procedure.

Expected Outcomes

1. Client explains purpose and basic steps of the procedure before it begins.

2. Client verbalizes decreased anxiety about the procedure before it begins.

3. Client assumes the correct position and remains still throughout the entire procedure.

4. Client verbalizes pain at less than 2 on a scale of 0 to 10 after the procedure.

5. Client maintains respirations, heart rate, and blood pressure within normal limits during and after aspiration procedure.

6. Puncture site dressing remains clean, dry, and intact.

7. Client does not experience postprocedural complications

8. Client is able to explain position and activity restrictions after aspirations.

Equipment

Aspiration trays: Most institutions purchase trays with contents appropriate for the specific aspiration, or the trays are assembled by the institution's central supply department. Contents of trays may differ from one institution to another.

Equipment needed but not found in aspiration trays includes:
- Two pair of sterile gloves of appropriate size for physician
- Laboratory requisitions and labels
- Mask, goggles, and gowns for physician and nurse

Standard aspiration trays may contain:
- Antiseptic solution (e.g., povidone-iodine)
- Gauze sponges (4 × 4)
- Sterile towels
- Anesthetic agent (e.g., lidocaine 1%)
- Two 3-ml sterile syringes with 23- to 25-gauge needles
- 2-inch adhesive tape
- Adhesive bandages

Delegation Considerations

Diagnostic studies are invasive and can result in potentially life-threatening complications. Monitoring of vital signs after the procedures may be delegated to assistive personnel (AP), but assessment cannot. Inform AP to report immediately to the nurse indications of allergic reactions, respiratory distress, or bleeding.

IMPLEMENTATION FOR ASSISTING WITH ASPIRATIONS: BONE MARROW, LUMBAR PUNCTURE, PARACENTESIS, THORACENTESIS

Steps	Rationale
1. See Standard Protocol (inside front cover).	
2. Explain steps of skin preparation, anesthetic injection, needle insertion, and position required.	Anticipation of expected sensation reduces anxiety.
3. Set up sterile tray or open supplies to make accessible for physician.	Reduces risk of contamination of sterile field and promotes prompt completion of procedure.

Steps	Rationale
4. Obtain a premedication order (i.e., sedative) if client is extremely anxious.	
5. Assist client in maintaining correct position. Reassure client while explaining procedure.	Decreases chance of complications during procedure. Explanations increase client comfort and relaxation.
6. Physician cleanses site with antiseptic solution and drapes site with sterile drape.	
7. Physician injects local anesthetic and waits for area to become numb.	Discomfort and pressure may still occur when deep tissues are disrupted.
8. Explain each step that may cause discomfort.	Client should know exactly what is occurring so that discomfort can be anticipated and surprises eliminated.
9. Physician inserts trochar or needle into body cavity involved (see Table 15-1).	
10. To aspirate tissue or body fluid for specimens, a syringe is attached to the trochar or needle and aspirate is placed into appropriate specimen container.	
11. If excess fluid is being drained, as for thoracentesis or paracentesis, physician attaches drainage tubing and container and fluid drains by gravity flow.	
12. Properly label specimens with client information and name of test desired.	Nurse is responsible for labeling tubes with client's name and tests desired. Test tubes are numbered in sequence of collection (e.g., 1 through 4).
13. Physician removes needle or trochar and immediately applies pressure over insertion site until drainage ceases. Pressure dressing may be applied. Nurse may be asked to continue to apply pressure for a specific time period.	
14. Place antiseptic ointment with 2 × 2 gauze over site.	Minimizes risk of infection.
15. Note characteristics of fluid/tissue aspirate (e.g., amount, color).	Characteristics are used for observation, reporting, and recording.
16. Remove and discard gloves.	
17. See Completion Protocol (inside front cover).	

• • • • • • • • • • •

EVALUATION

1. Ask client to state purpose and explain steps of the procedure before it is started.
2. Ask if client has questions or concerns about the procedure before it begins and later about test results. Assess nonverbal behaviors of anxiety before, during, and after procedure.
3. Observe client body position throughout procedure, and assist with maintaining position as necessary.
4. Ask client to describe level of comfort using a scale of 0 to 10 during and after procedure.
5. Monitor client's respiratory status: rate, rhythm, and depth of respirations; symmetry of chest movement. Compare client's heart rate and blood pressure during and after procedure to preprocedure baseline. (Check agency policy; this may be as often as every 15 minutes for 2 hours.)
6. Inspect dressing over puncture site for drainage every hour after the procedure as ordered.
7. Observe client for postprocedural complications:
   a. Decrease in blood pressure and tachycardia (could signify hemorrhage or allergic reaction to dye)
   b. Flushing, itching, and urticaria (could signify allergic reaction to dye)
   c. Abdominal pain, fever, and bleeding (could signify perforation of abdominal structures)
8. Ask client to describe postprocedural positioning and activity restrictions.

Unexpected Outcomes and Related Interventions

1. Client develops a suboccipital headache after lumbar puncture.
   a. Instruct client to lie flat in bed.
   b. Encourage fluid intake of at least one glass per hour if not contraindicated.
   c. Administer analgesics as prescribed.
   d. Apply ice pack to area of discomfort.
2. Client is unable to assume correct position or moves during procedure.
   a. Reassure client, and reinforce the importance of maintaining position and not moving.
   b. Further assess client to determine if sedation might be necessary.

3. Client experiences tenderness and erythema at aspiration site, decreased blood pressure, and increased pulse.
   a. Continue to monitor vital signs and aspiration site.
   b. Notify physician of findings, and obtain further orders.
4. Client develops shortness of breath, anxiety, and tachypnea following thoracentesis or paracentesis.
   a. Elevate head of bed, and administer oxygen (if ordered).
   b. Monitor vital signs.
   c. Notify physician of findings, and obtain further orders.
5. Client complains of light-headedness while sitting at side of bed after aspiration.
   a. Assist client to supine position.
   b. Check blood pressure and pulse.
   c. Inspect abdominal dressing for bleeding or peritoneal fluid.

Recording and Reporting

* Record preprocedure client preparation.
* Record name of procedure, location of puncture site (if applicable), amount and color of fluid drained or specimen obtained, client's tolerance to procedure (e.g., vital signs, comfort), laboratory tests ordered, type of dressing, and drainage.
* Report to physician or charge nurse immediately:

   Significant changes in vital signs or oxygen saturation status
   Unexpected drainage

Sample Documentation

0930 Client voided 300 ml. Abdominal girth measures 42 inches at umbilicus. Assisted with sitting on side of bed.

Dr. X completed abdominal paracentesis with 1100 ml cloudy liquid aspirated. Respirations 18 with moderate depth, pulse 98, and blood pressure 138/86. Rates pain at 6 on scale of 0 to 10. 22-inch gauze dressing applied to puncture site; remains dry and intact.

0940 Morphine sulfate 10 mg given in right dorsal gluteal for abdominal pain

1010 States pain has decreased to 2, which is tolerable. Abdominal girth measures 34 inches at umbilicus. Weight decreased to 158 pounds.

◉ SPECIAL CONSIDERATIONS ◉

Pediatric Considerations
* Very young children may receive conscious sedation or general anesthetic for aspiration procedures.
* Allow child to practice procedure beforehand, using doll as a model.

Geriatric Considerations
Older adults with arthritis may have difficulty sustaining the position required for the procedure.

Home Care Considerations
* Instruct client that some clients experience tenderness at the puncture site for several days, and mild analgesia may be ordered by the physician.
* If paracentesis is done on an outpatient basis, inform client to notify physician of fever or any swelling, pain, or drainage at puncture site. In males, scrotal edema should be reported to the physician.

Skill 15.4

Assisting With Bronchoscopy

Bronchoscopy is the examination of the tracheobronchial tree through a lighted tube containing mirrors (Figure 15-3). The bronchoscope most commonly used is a flexible fiberoptic bronchoscope with lumens for visualization of lesions, to determine the source of bloody sputum, and for obtaining sputum, foreign bodies, and biopsy specimens.

Bronchoscopy may be an emergency or scheduled procedure and is performed for both diagnostic and therapeutic reasons. The procedure is usually performed by a physician, pulmonary specialist, or surgeon, and takes about 30 to 45 minutes. It may be done in a specially equipped room. This is an invasive procedure, and informed consent is required.

ASSESSMENT

1. Assess client's knowledge of procedure to determine level of teaching required.
2. Assess level of anxiety, observing verbal and nonverbal cues.

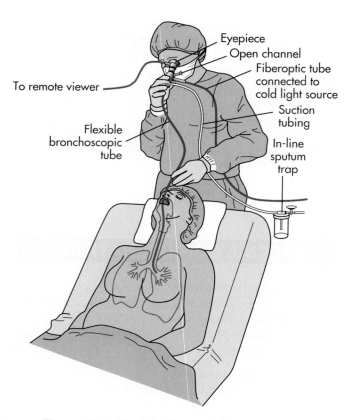

To remote viewer — Eyepiece
— Open channel
— Fiberoptic tube connected to cold light source
— Suction tubing
Flexible bronchoscopic tube
— In-line sputum trap

Figure 15-3 Flexible fiberoptic bronchoscopy.

3. Assess time of last ingested fluid or food. Clients should be NPO 8 hours before bronchoscopy. *Rationale: Excessive hydration causes dilution of contrast medium, making structures more difficult to visualize. NPO decreases chance of aspiration of stomach contents.*
4. Assess vital signs to provide baseline data for comparison with findings during and after procedure.
5. Assess client's allergies. Determine if client previously received topical anesthetic.
6. Assess respiratory status—lung sounds, type of cough, and sputum produced to provide baseline data for comparison with respiratory status during and after procedure.

PLANNING

Expected outcomes focus on improving client's knowledge of the procedure, including position; reducing client's anxiety regarding procedure and results; and early detection of potential complications.

Expected Outcomes

1. Client explains what to expect during the procedure before it is begun.
2. Client verbalizes willingness to talk about anxiety and fears.
3. Client has stable respiratory status without distress.
4. Client has vital signs within normal limits.
5. Client does not experience complications, including severe shortness of breath resulting from laryngospasm or bronchospasm in response to irritation from bronchoscope or topical anesthetic.

Equipment

- Bronchoscopy tray, if available from central supply, may include:

  Flexible fiberoptic bronchoscope
  Gauze sponges
  Local anesthetic spray (lidocaine)
  Sterile tracheal suction catheters
  Sterile gloves
  Sterile water-soluble lubricating jelly

- Mask, goggles, and gown
- Emesis basin
- Tracheal suction equipment
- Oxygen equipment

Delegation Considerations

Monitoring vital signs may be delegated to assistive personnel (AP), but assessment cannot. Inform assistive personnel to report indications of allergic reactions, respiratory distress, or coughing up blood to the nurse immediately.

IMPLEMENTATION FOR ASSISTING WITH BRONCHOSCOPY

Steps	Rationale
1. See Standard Protocol (inside front cover).	
2. Remove and safely store client's dentures and eyeglasses (if applicable).	
3. Establish IV access using large-bore cannula (see Chapter 29).	Provides access for delivery of IV fluids and/or drugs.
4. Assist client in maintaining position desired by physician, usually semi-Fowler's.	Provides maximal visualization of lower airways and adequate lung expansion.

Steps	Rationale
5. Physician sprays nasopharynx and oropharynx with topical anesthetic. Lidocaine is commonly used for throat spraying, which is done 10 to 15 minutes before the procedure.	
6. Instruct client not to swallow local anesthetic; provide emesis basin.	Swallowed anesthetic may be absorbed systemically and cause central nervous system and cardiovascular reactions.
7. Physician applies goggles, mask, and sterile gloves and then introduces bronchoscope into mouth to pharynx. The scope is passed through the glottis and then into trachea and bronchi.	
8. The nurse assists the client through procedure by explanations, verbal reassurance, and support.	Although premedicated and drowsy, clients need to be reminded not to change position and to cooperate.
9. Monitor ECG, pulse, and blood pressure for changes every 5 minutes during procedure.	See Skill 15.1 on p. 386 for monitoring clients with IVCS.
10. Monitor client's respiratory status every 5 minutes during procedure: observe degree of restlessness and respiratory rate; observe capillary refill and color of nail beds; monitor pulse oximetry (oxygen saturation).	Bronchoscope may cause feelings of suffocation; also, because airway is partially occluded, client may become hypoxic during observations.
11. Note characteristics of suctioned material.	Information used to record and report and to make further client observations.
12. Wipe client's nose to remove lubricant after bronchoscope is removed.	Promotes hygiene and comfort.
13. Monitor LOC, gag reflex, pulse oximetry, respiratory rate, blood pressure, pulse, heart rate, and capillary refill after the procedure.	Indications of postprocedural complications.
14. Use tongue depressor to touch pharynx to test for presence of gag reflex.	Prevents aspiration of food or fluid, which could cause pneumonia.

NURSE ALERT   *Do not allow client to eat or drink until the tracheobronchial anesthesia has worn off and gag reflex returns.*

15. Remove and discard gloves.
16. See Completion Protocol (inside front cover).

• • • • • • • • • •

EVALUATION

1. Monitor vital signs.
2. Observe character and amount of sputum. Physician may order serial sputum collection for 24 hours for cytological examination.
3. Observe respiratory status closely.
4. Assess level of sedation and LOC.
5. Monitor for return of gag reflex, which usually returns within 2 hours.

Unexpected Outcomes and Related Interventions

1. Client experiences laryngospasm and bronchospasm indicated by sudden, severe shortness of breath.
   a. Call physician immediately.
   b. Emergency resuscitation equipment must be readily available.
2. Client experiences hypoxemia, indicated by shortness of breath, and altered LOC.
   a. Maintain airway.
   b. Monitor oxygen saturation
   c. Notify physician immediately.
3. Client hemorrhages.
   a. Call physician immediately.
   b. Emergency resuscitation equipment must be readily available.

Recording and Reporting

• Record the name of procedure, duration of procedure, vital signs, oxygen saturation, respiratory status including ease of respirations, color, lung sounds, presence or absence of cough and sputum (color, amount, and consistency). Note time gag reflex returns. Include client's response to procedure and level of anxiety.

Sample Documentation

0900 To bronchoscopy via stretcher.

1030 Returned from bronchoscopy. Alert and oriented. Vital signs stable. Oxygen saturation 88%. Resting in semi-Fowler's position. Denies dyspnea. Color pale. Respirations 28; rhonchi noted bilaterally at bases, clears some with cough. Occasional cough noted productive of small amount bright red sputum. No gag reflex present.

1130 Vital signs stable and recorded q15min × 4 (see graphic). No change in assessment.

1230 Vital signs stable. Gag reflex present. Taking sips of clear liquids.

SPECIAL CONSIDERATIONS

Pediatric Considerations
- In children the procedure is most frequently performed to remove foreign bodies from larynx or trachea and may be done under general anesthesia.
- Because of the smaller airways, children are at higher risk of hypoxemia than adults. The bronchoscope further decreases the available breathing space (Pagana and Pagana, 2001).

Geriatric Considerations

Postprocedure restlessness in the older adult client could indicate either hypoxemia or pain. Thoroughly assess oxygenation status before administration of a narcotic analgesic, which could further deplete the body's oxygen supply.

Home Care Considerations
- Outpatients should be instructed to notify the physician if the following symptoms develop: fever, chest pain, dyspnea, wheezing, or hemoptysis.
- Throat discomfort is normal following this procedure. Warm saline gargles or throat lozenges may be helpful (Phipps, 1999).

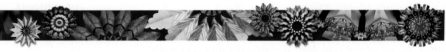

Skill 15.5

Assisting With Gastrointestinal Endoscopy: Esophagogastroduodenoscopy (EGD)

Gastrointestinal (GI) endoscopy involves introduction of an instrument through the mouth (upper GI viewing, or UGI) to allow the physician to inspect the integrity of mucosa, blood vessels, and organ parts. Informed consent is required for these invasive procedures. IVCS is often used. Endoscopies are performed by a physician, usually in a specially equipped endoscopy room (Figure 15-4).

UGI endoscopy or gastroscopy allows visualization of the esophagus, stomach, and duodenum (Figure 15-5). The physician inspects for tumors, vascular changes, mucosal inflammation, ulcers, hernias, and obstructions. A gastroscope enables the physician to perform a biopsy of tissue, remove abnormal tissue growth such as polyps, and coagulate sources of bleeding.

To examine the lower GI tract a colonoscopy is usually the test of choice and employs the use of a fiber optic endoscope with a lens viewer, a long flexible tube, and a light source at the end. It allows viewing of structures at the tip of the tube and insertion of special instruments for biopsy throughout the colon. In some cases the physician may choose to do a more limited approach, to view only the rectum using a proctoscope or the sigmoid colon using a sigmoidoscope. This visualization uses rigid, tube-shaped instruments with attached light sources that allow visualization of only the distal portion of the lower GI tract. See Procedural Guideline 15-1 on p. 403 for the basic steps for assisting with a colonoscopy. The assessment, planning, and evaluation are similar to those outlined for EGD.

ASSESSMENT

1. Assess client's knowledge of the procedure. *Rationale: Determines level of teaching required.*
2. Observe anxiety level, including verbal and nonverbal behaviors.
3. Observe character of emesis, stool, and nasogastric tube drainage for frank blood or black material that looks like coffee grounds. *Rationale: Determines if GI bleeding is present.*
4. Establish baseline vital signs.

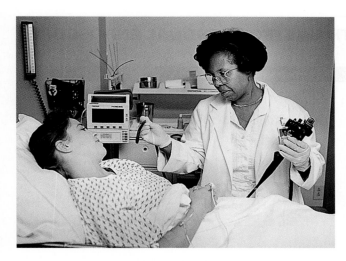

Figure 15-4   Physician preparing for endoscopy.

5. Verify that client has been NPO for at least 8 hours for UGI. *Rationale: Promotes adequate visualization and helps prevent vomiting.*
6. Assess client's ability to understand and follow directions. *Rationale: Procedures require client to follow directions closely and assume proper position.*

PLANNING

Expected outcomes focus on improving client's knowledge of the procedure, minimizing anxiety about the procedure and the results, and preventing procedural complications.

Expected Outcomes

1. Client explains purpose and basic steps of the procedure before it begins.
2. Client verbalizes decreased fear of procedure after the nurse reviews the procedure.
3. Client assumes the correct position and remains cooperative throughout the procedure.
4. Client has little discomfort (pain less than 2 on a scale of 0 to 10) and does not aspirate.
5. Gag reflex is effectively suppressed with local anesthetic during the procedure.
6. Client has stable vital signs with no postprocedure bleeding.

Equipment

- Endoscopy tray with fiberoptic endoscope
- Solutions for biopsy specimens

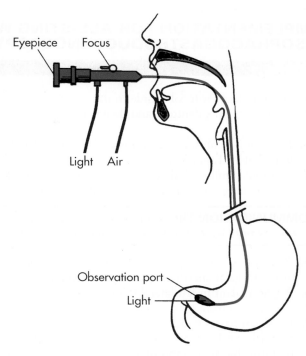

Figure 15-5   Flexible endoscope to visualize stomach.

- Local anesthetic spray
- Tracheal suction equipment
- Blood pressure equipment
- Sterile gloves for physician
- Emesis basin
- IV fluid and equipment for IV access
- Equipment and medications for IVCS
- Oxygen, resuscitative equipment, pulse oximeter, cardiac monitor
- Mask, gown, gloves, goggles

Delegation Considerations

Assistive personnel (AP) may transport stable clients to the testing department and may monitor vital signs and assist with positioning during the procedure. Vital signs following the procedures may be delegated to AP, but assessment cannot. If the client requires IVCS, has active GI bleeding, or is unstable, assisting with endoscopy requires the critical thinking and knowledge application unique to a nurse and delegation is inappropriate.

IMPLEMENTATION FOR ASSISTING WITH GASTROINTESTINAL ENDOSCOPY: ESOPHAGOGASTRODUODENOSCOPY

Steps	Rationale
1. See Standard Protocol (inside front cover).	
2. Remove client's dentures and dental appliances.	Prevents dislodgment of dental structures during intubation phase.
3. Monitor IV fluids, and administer IVCS as ordered (see Skill 15-1, p. 386).	
4. Promote comfort, and keep client informed of what is happening, using a calm and reassuring voice.	Helps to minimize client's anxiety.

COMMUNICATION TIP *Inform the client that while the tube is in place the client will be unable to speak.*

Steps	Rationale
5. Assist physician to spray nasopharynx and oropharynx with local anesthetic (usually xylocaine).	
6. Position client in left lateral (Sims') position.	Maintains open airway if client gags and vomits gastric contents.
7. Physician passes endoscope into mouth, esophagus, stomach, or duodenum; examines structures; and performs biopsy if appropriate.	
8. Place tissue specimens in proper laboratory containers, and label for microscopic examination.	
9. Suction airway if client begins to vomit or accumulate saliva.	Prevents aspiration of gastric contents or oral secretions.
10. Inform client that it is unsafe to attempt to eat or drink until after gag reflex returns.	Absence of gag reflex increases risk of aspiration.
11. See Completion Protocol (inside front cover).	

• • • • • • • • • •

EVALUATION

1. Ask client to describe purpose and basic steps of the procedure before it begins.
2. Observe for verbal and nonverbal signs of fear and anxiety.
3. Observe positioning and ability to cooperate throughout the procedure.
4. Ask client to describe discomfort and breathe without difficulty.
5. If local anesthetic was used to numb the throat, observe for return of gag reflex, usually within 2 to 4 hours.
6. Monitor vital signs for signs of bleeding.

Unexpected Outcomes and Related Interventions

1. Client develops dyspnea or respiratory distress.
   a. Notify physician immediately. This can be life threatening.
2. Client develops hypotension, tachycardia, or tachypnea, associated with or without visible signs of hemorrhage.
   a. Notify physician immediately. This can be life threatening.
3. Client develops sharp intense pain in chest, stomach, or abdomen and cool, pale skin.
   a. Notify physician immediately. These can be signs of GI perforation.

Reporting and Recording

- Record preparation, time of transport, procedure done, duration, collection and disposition of specimen.
- Report onset of bleeding, abdominal pain, dyspnea, and significant vital sign changes to physician.

Sample Documentation

0800 NPO since midnight. Transported to endoscopy department via wheelchair for EGD. Vital signs within normal limits (WNL). Consent signed. Client reports that MD explained procedure, and he has no questions at present.

1000 Returned from endoscopy. Reports no discomfort. Vital signs WNL. No apparent bleeding.

SPECIAL CONSIDERATIONS

Pediatric Considerations

Because of the small airway, the risk of respiratory distress is intensified following insertion of the endoscope through the throat.

Geriatric Considerations

*   Older adults have increases in the incidence of irritation and ulceration of gastric mucosa because of age-related changes (Phipps, 1999).
*   Older adults who undergo bowel evacuation with electrolyte laxative solution are at risk of dehydration and exhaustion from test preparation.

Home Care Considerations

*   Following insertion of the endoscope through the throat the client may be hoarse or have a sore throat. Ice chips or anesthetic lozenges can be used after the gag reflex returns.
*   After colonoscopy a warm tub bath may be soothing to minimize rectal discomfort.

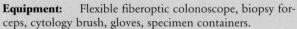

Procedural Guideline 15-1
Assisting With Colonoscopy

Equipment: Flexible fiberoptic colonoscope, biopsy forceps, cytology brush, gloves, specimen containers.

1. See Standard Protocol (inside front cover).
2. *Preparation:* Lower GI tract is cleansed by maintaining a liquid diet for 2 days before procedure. On the day before the test the client takes a chilled electrolyte laxative solution, usually 8 ounces every 15 minutes until 1 gallon is taken. Client may experience nausea and may be at risk of fluid/electrolyte imbalance.
3. Premedicate client with narcotic as ordered. IVCS is often used.
4. In the endoscopy department client is positioned on left side with legs and hips flexed (Sims' position).

5.   Physician inserts scope through the rectum and through the sigmoid, descending, transverse, and ascending colon.
6. Air is instilled to distend the colon as scope is advanced.
7. Biopsy forceps and cytology brush may be used to obtain specimens for study. Complete laboratory slips, and send specimens to the laboratory.
8. Scope is removed, and rectal area cleaned and dried.
9. See Completion Protocol (inside front cover).

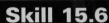

Skill 15.6

Assisting With Electrocardiograms

An ECG is a graphic representation of the heart's electrical activities, or conduction system. The conduction system originates with the sinoatrial (SA) node, the "pacemaker" of the heart. The SA node is in the right atrium. The rate of impulses initiated at the SA node for an adult at rest is about 75 beats per minute. The electrical impulses are then transmitted through the atria to the atrioventricular (AV) node. The AV node assists with atrial emptying by delaying the impulse before transmitting it through the bundle of His and the ventricular Purkinje network.

The electrical activity of the conduction system is recorded on an ECG. An ECG monitors the regularity and path of the electrical impulse through the conduction system; however, it does not reflect muscular work of the heart. The normal sequence on the ECG is called normal sinus rhythm (NSR) (Figure 15-6, p. 405). Disturbances in conduction may result when impulses cannot travel through the normal pathways. These rhythm disturbances are called dysrhythmias, meaning a deviation from the normal sinus heart rhythm (Table 15-2). Dysrhythmias may occur as a response to ischemia, valvular abnormality, anxiety, drug toxicity, or acid-base or electrolyte imbalance. Some common dysrhythmias include tachycardia (greater than 100 beats per minute), bradycardia (less than

Table 15-2

Common Basic Cardiac Dysrhythmias

Rhythm Characteristics	Appearance	Clinical Significance
A. Sinus tachycardia: Regular rhythm, rate 100-180 beats per minute, normal PQRS complex		Normal response to exercise, emotion, or pain, fever, hyperthyroidism, and certain drugs.
B. Sinus bradycardia: Regular rhythm, rate less than 60 beats per minute, normal P, PR interval, and QRS complex		May be associated with decreased cardiac output, dizziness, syncope, chest pain.
C. Premature ventricular contractions (PVCs): Irregular rhythm followed by compensatory pause		Caused by irritable focus. If more than 6 per minute or in pairs, indicates increased ventricular irritability.
D. Ventricular tachycardia: Rhythm slightly irregular, rate 100-200 beats per minute, P wave absent, PR interval absent, QRS complex wide and bizarre		Often a forerunner of ventricular fibrillation; may cause decreased cardiac output because of decreased ventricular filling time.

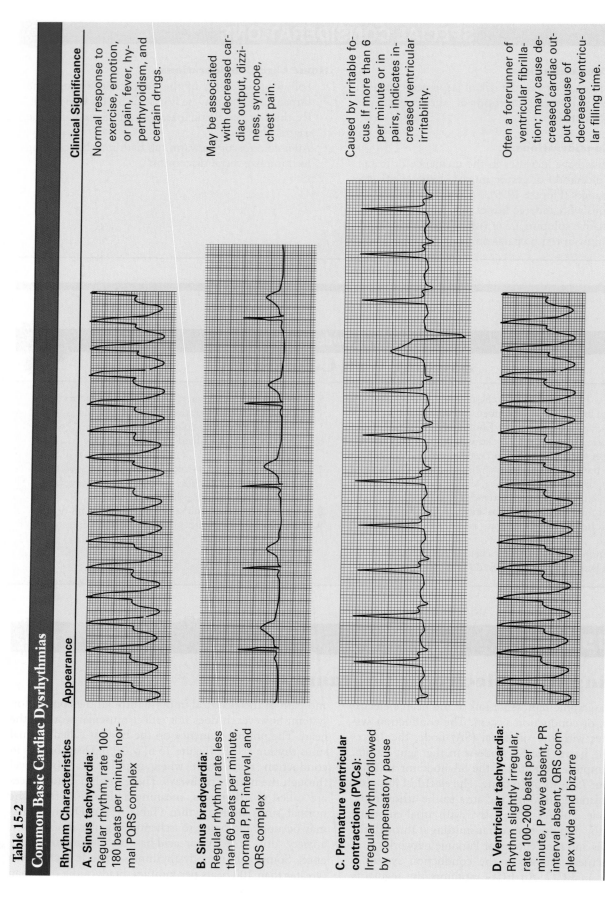

Modified from Potter PA, Perry AG: *Basic nursing: a critical thinking approach*, ed 4, St Louis, 1999, Mosby.

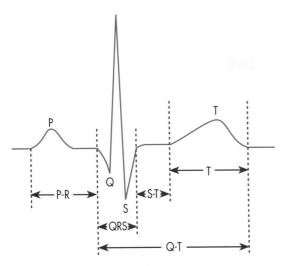

Figure 15-6 Normal sinus rhythm. (From Canobbio MM: *Cardiovascular disorders,* St Louis, 1990, Mosby.)

60 beats per minute), premature ventricular contractions (early beat), or heart block (delayed or absent beat).

A Holter monitor is a small, portable device that records electrical activity of the heart for up to 24 hours. This makes it possible for ambulatory clients to monitor cardiac rhythm during activity, rest, and sleep. Clients keep a diary of activity, noting when they experience rapid heartbeats or periods of dizziness. Correlation between activities and abnormal electrical activity can then be determined.

ASSESSMENT

1. Assess client's knowledge of the procedure. *Rationale: Determines level of teaching required.*
2. Observe anxiety level, including verbal and nonverbal behaviors.

3. Assess client's ability to follow directions closely and remain still in a supine position. *Rationale: Provides clear accurate recording without artifacts.*

PLANNING

Expected outcomes focus on improving client's knowledge of the procedure and minimizing anxiety about the procedure and the results.

Expected Outcomes

1. Client explains purpose and basic steps of the procedure before it begins.
2. Client verbalizes decreased fear of procedure after the nurse reviews the procedure.
3. Client lays supine and remains still throughout the procedure.

Equipment

- ECG machine
- Electrode paste (gel)
- ECG leads or electrodes
- Alcohol wipes
- Razor

Delegation Considerations

ECGs are often done by technicians specifically trained for this test. Nurses with advanced training may monitor ECG patterns continuously in intensive care settings, in the emergency department, or on units where telemetry is utilized. Stable clients may have vital signs monitored by assistive personnel (AP). AP need to report chest pain or altered vital signs immediately to the nurse.

IMPLEMENTATION FOR ASSISTING WITH ELECTROCARDIOGRAMS

Steps	Rationale
1. See Standard Protocol (inside front cover).	
2. Expose client's chest and arms, and cleanse and prepare skin using alcohol wipes.	Alcohol defats the skin and minimizes artifact due to inadequate contact with the skin (Chernecky and Berger, 1997).
3. If large amounts of hair are present, it may be necessary to clip hair at the placement sites.	Promotes adherence of leads (electrodes) to chest or extremity.

4. Apply self-sticking electrodes, or apply electrode paste and attach leads. For 12-lead ECG (see illustration):
(a) Chest (precordial leads)
     V_1—Fourth intercostal space (ICS) at right sternal border
     V_2—Fourth ICS at left sternal border
	Position of leads promotes proper display of ECG on paper.

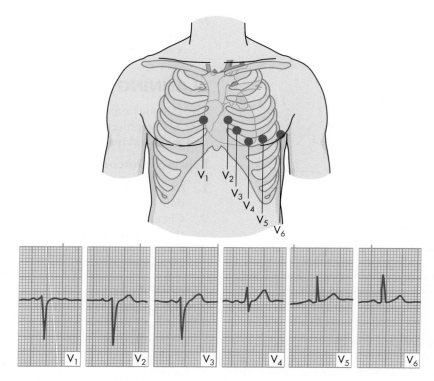

Step 4 Placement of ECG leads. (From Phipps W, Wands J, Mardk J: *Medical-Surgical nursing*, ed 7, St Louis, 2003, Mosby.)

Steps	Rationale

V_3—Midway between V_2 and V_4
V_4—Fifth ICS at midclavicular line
V_5—Left anterior axillary line at level of V_4
    horizontally
V_6—Left midaxillary line at level of V_4
    horizontally

(b)   Extremities: one on lower portion of each
    extremity
    aV_R—Right wrist
    aV_L—Left wrist
    aV_F—Left ankle

5. Turn on machine, and obtain tracing; 12-lead ECG may be obtained without removing precordial leads.

Transfers electrocardiac conduction on ECG tracing paper for subsequent analysis by cardiologist.

COMMUNICATION TIP   *Tell client to lie quietly until a reading is obtained.*

6. Disconnect leads, wipe excess electrode paste from chest, and wash hands.

Promotes comfort and hygiene.

7. Deliver ECG tracing to appropriate laboratory or nursing unit.

Provides for review of ECG by cardiologist.

8. See Completion Protocol (inside front cover).

• • • • • • • • • •

EVALUATION

1. Ask client to explain the procedure.
2. Discuss anxiety and fears related to test process and results.
3. Observe client's ability to understand and follow directions.
4. Observe client's ability to maintain position required for procedure and ability to remain still.

Unexpected Outcomes and Related Interventions

1. Client experiences chest pain (not result of test, but client's condition).
   a. Continue to monitor
   b. Follow specific orders related to findings.
   c. Notify physician
2. Client experiences severe anxiety
   a. Stay with the client.
   b. Utilize active listening to try to understand reasons for distress.
   c. Encourage stress management and relaxation techniques (see Chapter 10)

Recording and Reporting

- Record ECG completed, date and time, rationale for obtaining (e.g., chest pain, discomfort, preoperative, postoperative), and vital signs.
- Include a rhythm strip in the client's chart according to agency policy.

Sample Documentation

1030 c/o chest pain 4 (0-10) for 30 minutes with "heaviness" and "aching" in epigastric region. Pain radiates to $\widehat{L}$ shoulder blade. Very restless. Reports some short episodes of more severe pain 7-8 (0-10) lasting 30-60 sec. and relieved some by position changes. BP 160/90. P110. R20. O_2 sat 98%. HOB↑. ECG done, c̄ sinus tachcardia noted. (See rhythm strip.) Physician notified.

SPECIAL CONSIDERATIONS

Geriatric Considerations

- Many factors can contribute to dysrhythmias, including medications such as digitalis and quinidine, hypertrophy of cardiac muscle, alcohol, thyroid dysfunction, coffee, tea, tobacco, electrolyte imbalances, edema, acid-base imbalances, and myocardial ischemia.
- Clients with dysrhythmias are at risk for cardiac arrest. The nurse needs to be familiar with crash cart location and well prepared with knowledge of emergency equipment, medications, and cardiopulmonary resuscitation (CPR) skills.

CRITICAL THINKING EXERCISES

1. One hour after gastroscopy, the client attempts to drink water furnished by a family friend. What action should you take?
2. In the recovery room after an endoscopy, the client is sleepy but responds to verbal stimulation. Respirations are shallow at a rate of 10 breaths per minute, oxygen saturation is 85%, and the ECG reading shows NSR. What are the priorities for nursing intervention?
3. An 86-year-old woman has an IVP because of repeated urinary tract infections. As you prepare her for the test and inform her of what to expect, what assessments are indicated? What sensations should she expect when the dye is injected?
4. The role of the nurse during a thoracentesis involves what primary responsibilities?

REFERENCES

Cannobio MM: *Cardiovascular disorders,* St Louis, 1990, Mosby.

Chernecky CC, Berger BJ: *Laboratory tests and diagnostic procedures,* ed 4, Philadelphia, 2001, WB Saunders.

Doughty DB, Jackson DB: *Gastrointestinal disorders,* St Louis, 1993, Mosby.

Ignatavicius DD, Workman ML: *Medical-surgical nursing: critical thinking for collaborative care,* ed 4, Philadelphia, 2002, Saunders.

Kost M: Conscious sedation: guarding your patient against complications, *Nursing,* 29(4):34, April 1999.

Pagana K, Pagana T: *Mosby's diagnostic and laboratory test reference,* ed 5, St Louis, 2001, Mosby.

Perry AG, Potter PA: *Clinical nursing skills and techniques,* ed 5, St Louis, 2002, Mosby.

Phipps W: *Medical-surgical nursing: concepts and clinical practice,* ed 5, St Louis, 1999, Mosby.

Potter PA, Perry AG: *Basic nursing: a critical thinking approach,* ed 4, St Louis, 1999, Mosby.

Sullivan G: Getting informed consent: role of nurses in obtaining informed consent from patients, *RN* 61(4):59, 1998.

Van Riper S, Van Riper J: *Cardiac diagnostic tests: a guide for nurses,* Philadelphia, 1997, WB Saunders.

Wong DL, Hockenberry-Eaton M, Wilson D, Winkelstein ML, Ahmann E, and DiVito-Thomas AA: *Whaley and Wong's nursing care of infants and children,* ed 6, St Louis, 1999, Mosby.

Preparation for Medication Administration

Safe and accurate administration of medications is one of the nurse's most important responsibilities. The nurse is responsible for understanding the action of the medication, dosage, desired effects, possible adverse reactions, drug interactions, contraindications, and precautions. The nurse uses the nursing process as a framework for nursing care related to medication administration. This includes assessment and planning to identify the need for and effectiveness of medications. Nursing diagnoses help communicate concerns related to drug therapy and direct interventions for appropriate nursing care. Implementation includes administering drugs correctly, monitoring the client's response, and in many cases, teaching the client how to self-administer drugs safely with an appropriate knowledge base. Evaluation involves continued monitoring of drug effectiveness. This chapter includes basic information needed when preparing to administer medications. Subsequent chapters address administration of nonparenteral medications and injections.

 DRUG EFFECTS

When administering medications, the nurse needs to know the mechanism of action, the therapeutic effects of the drugs, the purpose for the specific client, and the desired effect. The therapeutic effects of drugs include health maintenance, disease prevention and treatment, diagnosis, and cure. It is also important for the nurse to know possible side effects, adverse reactions, contraindications, and toxic effects.

Mechanism of Action

When a drug is administered to a client, a predictable chemical reaction is expected that changes the physiological activity of the body. This most commonly occurs as the medication bonds chemically at a specific site called a receptor site. The reactions are possible only when the receptor site and the chemical fit together like a key in a lock. When the chemical fits well, the chemical response is good. We call these drugs agonists (Skidmore-Roth, 2002). Some drugs attach at the receptor site but do not produce a new chemical reaction. These drugs are called antagonists. Other drugs attach and produce only a small response or prevent other reactions from occurring. These drugs are called partial agonists (Box 16-1).

 DRUG ACTIONS

Pharmacokinetics is the study of how drugs enter the body, reach the site of action, and are metabolized and excreted from the body. Absorption describes how a drug enters the body and passes into body fluids and tissues and influences route of drug administration. Distribution addresses the ways the drugs move to the sites of action in the body. Metabolism refers to the chemical reactions by which medication is broken down until it becomes chemically inactive. Excretion is the process of drug elimination from the body via the gastrointestinal tract, kidneys, or other body secretions (Skidmore-Roth, 2002).

A drug dose response includes onset of drug action, peak (its highest effective concentration), and duration of action (length of time the drug is present in a concentration great enough to produce a response). This information is useful in planning drug administration schedules. Most agencies have standard administration schedules (see Abbreviations and Equivalents, Appendix B) and allow for administration of the drug one half hour before or after the scheduled time without concern for altering the effectiveness of the medication. Some medications are ordered for administration as needed (prn) within certain parameters prescribed by the physician.

Therapeutic Effects

A single medication may have many therapeutic effects. For example, aspirin creates analgesia, reduces inflammation, reduces fever, and affects blood clotting. Other drugs have more specific therapeutic effects. For example, an antihypertensive medication controls high blood pressure, and antibiotics treat a bacterial infection.

Side Effects

Predictably, a drug causes unintended secondary effects. Side effects may be harmless or injurious. In the example of codeine phosphate, a client may experience constipation. If the side effects are serious enough to outweigh the beneficial effects of a drug's therapeutic action, the prescriber may discontinue the drug. Clients may stop taking medications because of side effects; for example, some cardiac and antihypertensive medications may initially worsen the client's fatigue, and the client feels worse on the drug and stops taking it.

Box 16-1

Mechanisms of Action

Agonist: Chemical fits receptor site well; chemical response is good.

Antagonist: Drug attaches at a reeptor site and then is chemically inctive; no drug response.

Partial Agonist: Drug attaches at a receptor site, and a slight chemical action is produced.

Data from Skidmore-Roth L, McKenry: *Mosby's drug guide for nurses,* ed 4, St Louis, 2002, Mosby.

Toxic Effects

After prolonged intake of high doses of medication, ingestion of drugs intended for external application, or when a drug accumulates in the blood because of impaired metabolism or excretion, a toxic effect may develop. Toxic effects may be lethal, depending on the drug's action. For example, morphine, a narcotic analgesic, relieves pain by depressing the central nervous system. However, toxic levels of morphine cause severe respiratory depression and death.

Idiosyncratic Reactions

Medications may cause unpredictable effects, such as an idiosyncratic reaction in which a client overreacts or underreacts to a drug or has a reaction different from normal. Predicting which clients will have an idiosyncratic response is impossible. For example, lorazepam, an antianxiety medication, when given to the older adult may worsen anxiety and cause agitation and delirium.

Allergic Reactions

Allergic reaction is another unpredictable response to a drug. Exposure to an initial dose of a medication may cause an immunological response. The drug acts as an antigen, which causes antibodies to be produced. With repeated administration the client develops an allergic response to the drug, its chemical preservatives, or a metabolite of it.

An allergic reaction may be mild or severe. Allergic symptoms vary, depending on the client and the drug. Among the different classes of drugs, antibiotics cause a high incidence of allergic reactions. Common, mild allergy symptoms are summarized in Table 16-1. Severe, or anaphylactic, reactions are characterized by sudden constriction of bronchiolar muscles, edema of the pharynx and larynx, and severe wheezing and shortness of breath. The client may become severely hypotensive, necessitating emergency resuscitation measures (Box 16-2).

It is common practice for clients who are hospitalized and have a known drug allergy to have this information recorded in a clearly identifiable place. This allows everyone involved in the client's care to be aware of the known allergy. In many institutions this information is recorded on the front of the client's medical record on an eye-catching sticker. Clients also wear a type of wristband that indicates that the client has an allergy. Client allergies should always be recorded on the client's medication administration record (MAR). Clients cared for in other settings (e.g., home) and who have a known history of an allergy to a medication should be encouraged to wear an identification bracelet or medal, which alerts all health care providers to the allergies in case the client is unconscious when receiving medical care.

Drug Tolerance and Dependence

Drug tolerance occurs when clients receive the same drug for long periods of time and require higher doses to produce the same desired effect. Clients who are taking various pain medications may develop tolerance over time.

Generally, clients hospitalized for acute episodes of illness do not develop tolerance to pain medications. It may take a month or even longer for this phenomenon to occur (McCaffery and Ferrell, 1999). Drug tolerance is not the same as drug dependence. Two types of drug dependence exist: psychological (or addiction) and physical. In psychological dependence the client desires the medication for some benefit other than the intended effect. Physical dependence implies that a client will suffer some

Table 16-1	
Mild Allergic Reactions	
Symptom	**Description**
Urticaria (hives)	Raised, irregularly shaped skin eruptions with varying sizes and shapes; eruptions have reddened margins and pale centers.
Eczema (rash)	Small, raised vesicles that are usually reddened; often distributed over the entire body.
Pruritus	Itching of the skin; accompanies most rashes.
Rhinitis	Inflammation of mucous membranes lining the nose, causing swelling and a clear watery discharge.
Wheezing	Constriction of smooth muscles surrounding bronchioles that decreases diameter of airways; occurs primarily on inspiration because of severely narrowed airways; development of edema in pharynx and larynx further obstructs airflow.

Box 16-2
Severe Allergic Reactions With Anaphylactic Shock
Constriction of bronchioles with wheezing
Edema of pharynx and larynx
Shortness of breath
Severe hypotension
In severe cases, may result in death

ill effect if the medication is not given. When clients receive medications for a short term (such as for postoperative pain), dependence is rare (McCaffery and Ferrell, 1999).

Drug Interactions

When one drug modifies the action of another drug, a drug interaction occurs. Drug interactions are common in individuals taking many medications. A drug may potentiate or diminish the action of other drugs and may alter the way in which another drug is absorbed, metabolized, or eliminated from the body.

When two drugs are given simultaneously, they can have a synergistic or additive effect. With a synergistic reaction the physiological action of the two drugs in combination is greater than the effect of the drugs when given separately. Alcohol is a central nervous system depressant that has a synergistic effect with antihistamines, antidepressants, and narcotic analgesics.

A drug interaction may be desirable. Often a physician orders combination drug therapy to create a drug interaction for therapeutic benefit. For example, a client with moderate hypertension may receive several drugs, such as diuretics and vasodilators, which act together to keep blood pressure at a desirable level.

Drug Dose Responses

After the nurse administers a drug, it undergoes absorption, distribution, metabolism, and excretion. These processes determine how much of the administered dose reaches the site of action. These processes are influenced by factors such as body surface area, body water content, body fat content, and body protein stores.

When certain medications such as antibiotics are prescribed, the goal is to achieve a constant drug blood level within a safe therapeutic range. The client and nurse must follow regular dosage schedules and administer prescribed doses at correct intervals. Knowledge of the following time intervals of drug action also helps to anticipate a drug's effect:

1. Onset of drug action—Time it takes after a drug is administered for it to produce a response
2. Peak action—Time it takes for a drug to reach its highest effective concentration
3. Duration of action—Length of time during which the drug is present in a concentration great enough to produce a response
4. Plateau—Blood serum concentration reached and maintained after repeated, fixed doses

The therapeutic levels of certain drugs, such as antibiotics, can be monitored by laboratory tests. A blood sample is drawn to identify the peak serum level of a drug, which varies according to the specific drug involved. The lowest serum level is known as the trough level. Blood samples for trough levels are usually drawn just before the next scheduled dose of medication. Precise coordination with the laboratory is essential for obtaining meaningful information. These data allow physicians to modify drug dosages.

Routes of Administration

The route chosen for administering a drug depends on its properties and desired effect and on the client's physical and mental condition. The nurse is often the best person to judge the route most desirable for a client. Table 16-2 summarizes the routes of drug administration.

 RECEIVING MEDICATION ORDERS

A physician's order is required for all medications to be administered by the nurse (except in states where Nurse Practice Acts allow advanced practice nurses and nurse practitioners to prescribe in specific situations).

A physician's order sheet is a form on which the physician writes the date, time, and drug order, including:

1. The name of the drug, which may be either the trade name (e.g., Percocet) or the generic name (e.g., oxycodone).
2. The dose (e.g., 5 mg).
3. The form (e.g., tabs).
4. The route (e.g., PO [by mouth]).
5. The frequency (e.g., q4h [every 4 hours]).
6. Orders for drugs to be given prn also include the reason they are to be given (e.g., for pain).
7. The signature of the prescriber.

Verbal orders and telephone orders are orders received by the nurse and written on the physician's order sheet

Table 16-2

Routes of Drug Administration	
NonParenteral	
Oral	By mouth
Sublingual	Under the tongue
Topical	On the skin (as a cream or patch), and eye/ear drops
Parenteral	
Intramuscular	Into the muscle
Subcutaneous	Into the subcutaneous tissue
Intradermal	Into the dermis
Intravenous	Into the vein

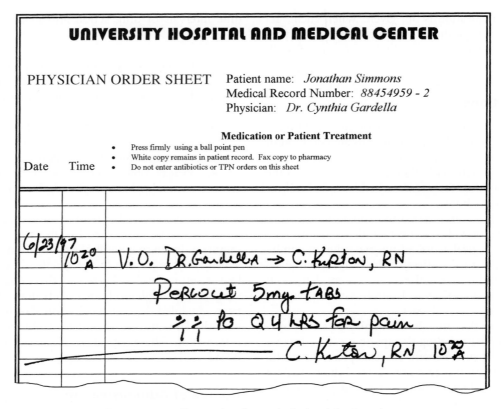

Figure 16-1 Example of a verbal physician's order.

(Figure 16-1). The name of the prescriber and the signature of the nurse are included. Most institutions require the prescriber to sign verbal and telephone orders within 24 hours after giving the order. In many settings there are "routine physician's orders," which are preprinted and individualized according to the client's history and circumstances. In the long-term care setting there also are "standing orders" that can be implemented when appropriate, for example, if a client needs a laxative.

COMMUNICATION AND TRANSCRIPTION OF ORDERS

After new medication orders are written, the drugs must be obtained from the pharmacy. Usually the copy of the physician's order sheet is sent to the pharmacy. The pharmacist is responsible for providing the correct medications and delivering them to the nursing unit.

Unit-Dose System

In acute care settings each client on the nursing unit has a medication bin or drawer that contains all the medications for a 24-hour period. Many times this is in a medication cart that can be pushed from room to room to facilitate administration of medications at routine times. The cart is kept locked when not attended. In some settings the medications are kept in a locked cabinet in the client's room.

Newer medication dispensing systems, such as computer-assisted or electronic devices, are variations of unit-dose and floor stock systems. For example, the Pyxis Corporation designs the MedStation. This system can carry a variety of medications, housed in individual compartments that are accessed by the nurse after requesting the medication from a computerized screen. Access can be restricted to only those medications specifically ordered for a client. All medications retrieved from the MedStation are recorded in the system's computer and can be automatically charged to the client. Baxter Healthcare Corporation manufactures the Sure-Med Unit-Dose Center, which provides single doses of floor stock medications. Some drugs may be distributed as floor stock, although this is no longer a common practice. Floor stock medications are distributed to the nursing unit in bulk (either individually wrapped or in bottles). Generally, medications that are appropriate for floor stock are those that are routinely prescribed or prescribed on a prn basis. Examples of these medications are stool softeners, antacids, and antipyretics.

Medication Administration Record

An MAR is a form used to verify that the right medications are being administered at the correct times. Examples of different forms are given in Figures 16-2 and 16-3. Every 24 hours an MAR is distributed for each client

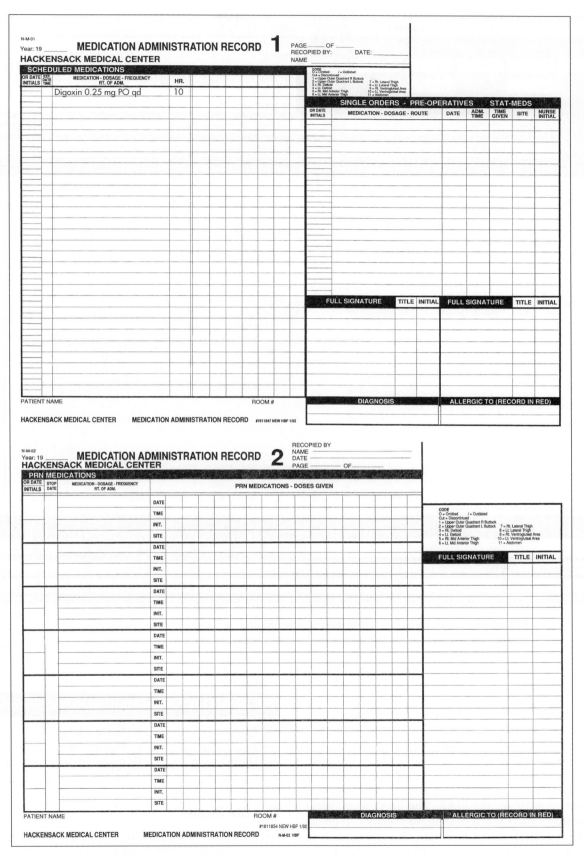

Figure 16-2 Medication administration record. (Courtesy Hackensack University Medical Center, Hackensack, NJ.)

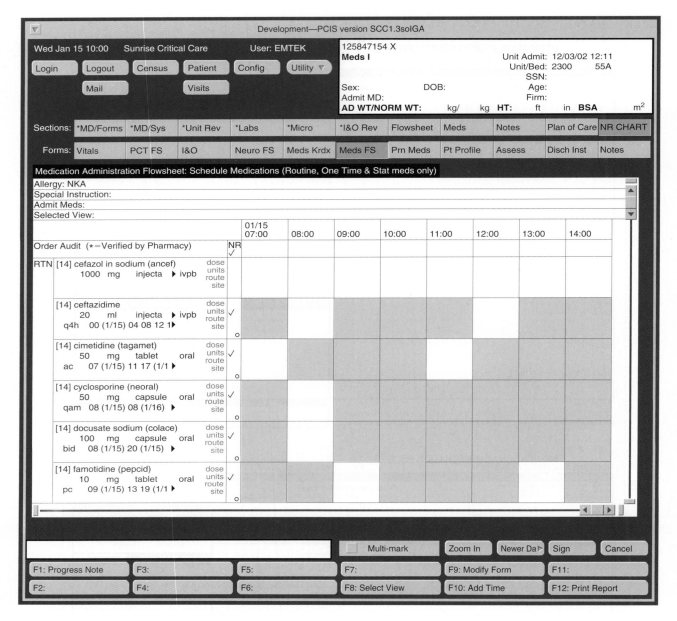

Figure 16-3 Computer list of ordered medications. (Courtesy Barnes-Jewish Hospital, St Louis, Mo.)

for that day. The nurse is responsible for verifying that the MAR is accurate and up-to-date by comparing each medication to the original order, including drug name, dose, route of administration, and times to be given. If a medication is to be given before the computer printout is available, the nurse or a designated unit secretary writes the complete order on the MAR. The nurse who checks all transcribed orders is responsible for accuracy. If an order seems incorrect or inappropriate, the nurse needs to consult the prescriber. The nurse who gives the wrong medication or an incorrect dosage is legally responsible for the error.

Box 16-3

Six Rights for Administration of Medication

- Right drug
- Right dose
- Right client
- Right route
- Right time
- Right documentation

The Six Rights

Preparing and administering medications requires accuracy and the full attention of the nurse. The six rights is a traditional checklist to promote accuracy in drug administration (Box 16-3).

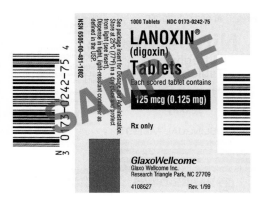

Figure 16-4   Sample drug label. (Reproduced with permission of Glaxo Welcome, Inc., Research Triangle Park, NC.)

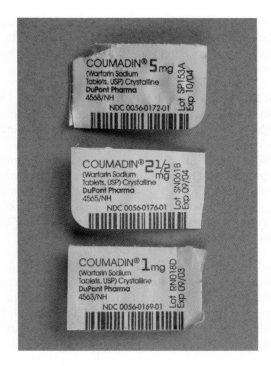

Figure 16-5   Coumadin in three strengths.

Right Drug. The nurse is responsible for verifying that the order was accurately transcribed. Many institutions have a policy that requires that registered nurses (RNs) on a specific shift verify the accuracy of MAR forms printed for each client each day. Whenever new orders are handwritten on the MAR, the RN adding the orders must verify that they are accurately added to the MAR. When verification is done, the MAR is initialed and signed by the RN.

The nurse compares the label of the drug with the MAR at least 3 times: (1) Before removing the drug from the storage bin; (2) before placing the drug in the medicine cup for distribution; and again (3) before giving the drug to the client. If the drug is ordered by trade name and dispensed from the pharmacy by generic name, the nurse must verify that there is no discrepancy (Figure 16-4).

If a client questions the medication, stop and recheck to be certain there is no mistake. In most cases the drug order has been changed or is manufactured by a different company than the client has been using at home. Sometimes, however, attention to a client's question is how errors are identified and prevented.

Right Dose. When a medication must be prepared from a dose other than what is ordered, the chance of errors increases. After calculating the dose, having a second nurse check the calculations is recommended, especially if it is an unusual calculation or involves a potentially toxic drug, such as Coumadin (an anticoagulant preparation that can be life threatening if an incorrect dose is given). Coumadin is available in a variety of strengths (Figure 16-5).

After calculating dosages, the nurse preparing the medication needs to use appropriate measuring devices. Liquid preparations may be measured using a medicine cup marked in ml (cc) or a syringe for oral use. Some pediatric medications come with a scaled dropper (Figure 16-6).

Right Client. To identify clients correctly, the nurse checks the MAR against the client's identification (ID) bracelet and asks the client to state his or her full name.

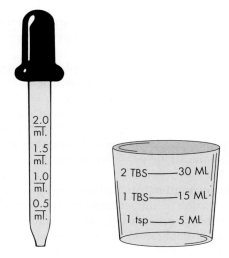

Figure 16-6   Scaled dropper for pediatric use and cup to measure oral liquids. (From Clayton BD, Stock YN: *Basic pharmacology for nurses*, ed 12, St Louis, 2000, Mosby.)

In some agencies the nurse also compares the medical record number on the MAR with the ID bracelet. When nursing students are caring for one client, this process may seem awkward; however, when a nurse is giving medications to many clients, this practice is invaluable. This is essential even after caring for the same client for several days. By forming this identification routine systematically every single time, it will become a good habit that can prevent serious medication errors. If the client questions the practice, the nurse should explain that this is the routine practice for making sure the client is getting the correct medication.

Right Route. The prescriber's order must designate a route of administration. If the route of administration is missing or if the specified route is not the recommended route, the nurse must consult the prescriber immediately.

When injections are administered, the nurse must use only preparations intended for parenteral use. Injection of a liquid intended for oral use can produce local complications, such as sterile abscess, or fatal systemic effects. Medication companies label parenteral medication "for injectable use only."

Right Time. Each agency has routine time schedules for medications ordered at standard intervals. For example, medications to be given tid (3 times a day) may be routinely scheduled for 0800, 1400, and 2000, or 0900, 1300, and 1900, depending on the agency policy. A drug may also be ordered q8h (every 8 hours), which is also 3 times a day; however, the medication ordered q8h needs to be given around-the-clock to maintain adequate therapeutic levels and would, for example, be given at 0800, 1600, and 2400. All routinely ordered medications should be given within 30 minutes before or after the scheduled time; however, nursing judgment may allow some variance, depending on the medication involved.

The medication may also be ordered for special circumstances. A preoperative medication may be ordered "stat" (to be given immediately); "now," which means as soon as available, usually within an hour; or "on call," which means the operating room will notify the nurse when it is the appropriate time. A drug may be ordered "ac" (before meals) or "pc" (after meals).

Right Documentation. After administering a medication, the nurse records it immediately on the administration form. Recording immediately after administration prevents errors of duplication (see postadministration activities [p. 420] and medical administration record [p. 415]). When a prn analgesic is ordered q3-4h the nurse needs to assess the characteristics and severity of the pain to determine whether it is given every 3 hours or less frequently. It is important to teach clients to ask for the medication when they are beginning to feel discomfort. If the client waits until the pain is severe, the medication may not be effective. A prn medication at hs (bedtime) should be given when the client is prepared for sleep.

PREPARING FOR MEDICATION ADMINISTRATION

It is legally advisable to administer only medications personally prepared. Administering a drug prepared by another

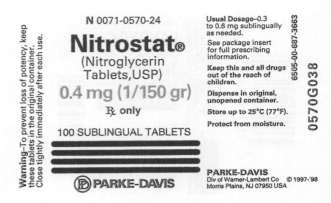

Figure 16-7 Interpreting a drug label. (Reproduced with permission of Warner-Lambert Company.)

nurse greatly increases the opportunity for error. The nurse who gives the wrong medication or an incorrect dose is legally responsible for the error. Physicians may order a drug using the trade name, and the pharmacist may dispense it using the generic name. Many drugs have both names on the label. The importance of checking similar names and verifying for the correct drug cannot be overemphasized.

Some medications are also available as either tablets or capsules and in liquid form. Liquid forms are appropriate when the client has difficulty swallowing or must be given medications via a nasogastric (NG) tube or gastric (G) tube (see Skill 33.2, p. 805). Liquid medications include elixirs, suspensions, syrups, and tinctures. Liquids are more quickly absorbed than solids.

Interpreting Drug Labels

Drug labels include several basic pieces of information: the trade name of the drug in large letters, the generic name in smaller letters, the form of the drug, the dosage, the expiration date, the lot number, and the name of the manufacturer. The trade name given by the manufacturer often suggests the action of the drug, and the generic name is the chemical name (Figure 16-7).

Conversions

Drugs are not always dispensed in the unit of measure in which they are ordered. Drug companies package and bottle certain standard equivalents. The nurse often must convert available units of volume and weight to desired dosages or vice versa. The nurse must know approximate equivalents in all of the measurement systems or make use of conversion tables. An example follows:

The nurse receives an order: vancomycin 1 g IV.
The pharmacy supplies: vancomycin in 500-mg vials.
Because the drug dose on the drug label is in milligrams, conversion should be from grams to milligrams.

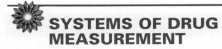
SYSTEMS OF DRUG MEASUREMENT

The proper administration of medication depends on the nurse's ability to compute drug dosages accurately and measure medications correctly. A careless mistake in placing a decimal point or adding a zero to a dosage can lead to a fatal error. The prescriber and client depend on the nurse to check the dosage before administering a drug. The most common system used in the measurement of medications is the metric system. The apothecary and household systems can also be used.

Metric System

As a decimal system, the metric system is the most logically organized of the measurement systems. Each basic unit of measure is organized into units of 10. Multiplying or dividing by 10 forms secondary units. In multiplication, the decimal point moves to the right; in division, the decimal moves to the left.

The basic units of measure in the metric system are the meter (length), the liter (volume), and the gram (weight). For drug calculations the nurse uses primarily volume and weight units. In the metric system small or large letters are used to designate the basic units:

Gram: g or Gm
Liter: l or L
Small letters are abbreviations for subdivisions of major units:
Milligram: mg
Milliliter: ml

Apothecary System

The apothecary system is one of the oldest systems of measurement. It is seldom used; however, some drug companies still include the apothecary measure in addition to the metric. The basic units of measure in the apothecary system include weight (grains) and volume (minims, drams, and ounces). The measures used in this system are approximate, and a 10% variance has become acceptable in preparation and administration of most medications. The apothecary system often uses roman numerals and fractions. The symbol "ss" is used for the fraction ½. Unlike the metric system, in the apothecary system the abbreviation or symbol for a unit of measure is written before the amount or quantity.

Household Measurements

Household measures are familiar to most people and are used when more accurate systems of measure are unnecessary. Included in household measures are drops, tea-

spoons, tablespoons, cups, and glasses for volume; and ounces and pounds for weight.

Before the actual administration of medication, the nurse may need to carry out several steps, namely, conversion of units within a system or between systems and calculation of drug dosages (Box 16-4).

NURSE ALERT   *Drugs ordered in units and milliequivalents are not convertible to metric, apothecary, or household measurements.*

Dosage Calculations

Dosage calculations are necessary when the dose on the drug label differs from the dosage ordered. There are several methods used for calculating dosages. The most common methods are ratio-proportion or use of a formula (Box 16-5). Dimensional analysis is becoming a popular method for dosage calculation because it involves simple multiplication and division and does not require algebra (Box 16-6).

Box 16-4
Approximate Equivalents

$$1 \text{ g}^* = 60 \text{ mcg}$$
$$1 \text{ g} = 1000 \text{ mg}$$
$$1000 \text{ mcg } (\mu g) = 1 \text{ mg}$$
$$1 \text{ kg} = 2.2 \text{ lb}$$
$$1 \text{ mL or ml (1 cc)} = 15\text{-}16 \text{ minims}^*$$
$$5 \text{ mL} = 1 \text{ tsp}^\dagger$$
$$3 \text{ tsp}^\dagger = 1 \text{ tbs}^\dagger$$
$$30 \text{ mL} = 1 \text{ oz}^\dagger$$
$$1000 \text{ mL} = 1 \text{ L}$$

*Apothecary measure.
†Household measure.

Box 16-5
Formula Method

$$\frac{D}{H} \times V = \text{amount to give}$$

D is the desired dose or the dose ordered by the physician for the client.
H is the drug dose on hand or available for use. The dose is on the drug label.
V is the volume (liquid) or vehicle (tablets, capsules) that delivers the available dose.

NOTE: the desired dose **(D)** and the on-hand **(H)** dose must be in the same unit of measurement. If they are in different units, then conversions must be done before completing the formula.

Box 16-6

Dimensional Analysis

Step 1: Identify the starting factor (amount ordered), which is the first item of the equation, and the answer label (tablets, capsules, or ml), which is the last item.

Step 2: Identify appropriate equivalents with a 1:1 ratio (e.g., 1 g = 1000 mg). Set up the equation so that labels can be canceled; for example, if mg is in the numerator, mg must be in the denominator to cancel.

Step 3: Solve the equation.
   a. Cancel labels first, the answer label should not cancel.
   b. Reduce numbers to lowest terms.
   c. Multiply/divide to solve equation.
   d. Reduce answer to lowest terms, convert to decimal, and round to a measurable quantity.

$$\text{Starting factor} \times \frac{\text{Equivalent}}{\text{Equivalent}} = \text{Answer label}$$

Example 1
When the dose ordered has the same label as the dose available:

Step 1. The starting factor is 0.5 g.
The answer label is tablets; that is, How many tablets should be given?

Step 2. Formulate the conversion equation:
The equivalent needed is 1 tablet = 0.25 g.

$$\frac{0.5 \text{ g}}{1} \times \frac{1 \text{ tab}}{0.25 \text{ g}} = \text{tabs}$$

Cancel labels (g).
NOTE: If properly written, all labels except the answer label will cancel.

Step 3. Solve the equation:
Reduce the numerical values, and multiply the numerators and the denominators.

$$\frac{\overset{2}{\cancel{0.5 \text{ g}}}}{1} \times \frac{1 \text{ tab}}{\cancel{0.25 \text{ g}}} = 2 \text{ tabs}$$

Example 2
When the dose ordered has a different label than the dose available:

Dose ordered: 0.5 g
Tablets available: 250 mg per tablet

Step 1. The starting factor is 0.5 g.
The answer label is tablets; that is, How many tablets should be given?

Step 2. Formulate the conversion equation:
The equivalents needed are 1 g = 1000 mg and 1 tab = 250 mg.

$$\frac{0.5 \text{ g}}{1} \times \frac{1000 \text{ mg}}{1 \text{ g}} \times \frac{1 \text{ tab}}{250 \text{ mg}} = \text{tabs}$$

Cancel labels (g, mg).

Step 3. Solve the equation:
Reduce the values, and multiply the numerators and the denominators.

$$\cancel{0.5 \text{ g}} \times \frac{\overset{4}{\cancel{1000 \text{ mg}}}}{\underset{2}{\cancel{1 \text{ g}}}} \times \frac{1 \text{ tab}}{\cancel{250 \text{ mg}}} = \frac{4}{2} = 2 \text{ tabs}$$

Example 3
When the dose ordered is available in a liquid form:

Dose ordered: Keflex 250 mg PO
Available: 125 mg per 5 ml

Step 1. The starting factor is 250 mg.
The answer label is ml.

Step 2. Formulate the conversion equation:

$$\frac{250 \text{ mg}}{1} \times \frac{5 \text{ ml}}{125 \text{ mg}} = \text{ml}$$

Cancel labels (mg).

Step 3. Solve the equation:
Reduce and multiply.

$$\frac{\overset{2}{\cancel{250 \text{ mg}}}}{1} \times \frac{5 \text{ ml}}{\cancel{125 \text{ mg}}} = 10 \text{ ml}$$

Example 4
When dosage is ordered based on body surface area (commonly done for pediatric dosages): The body surface area is estimated on the basis of weight, using standard charts or nomogram. The formula is a ratio of the child's body surface area compared with the body surface area of an average adult (1.7 square meters, or 1.7 m^2).

$$\text{Child's dose} = \frac{\text{Surface area of child}}{1.7 \text{ m}^2} \times \text{Normal adult dose}$$

Physician orders ampicillin for a child weighing 12 kg, and the nomogram chart shows that the body surface area for this child is 0.54 m². The normal single adult dose is 250 mg.

1) Child's dose $= \dfrac{0.54 \text{ m}^2}{1.7 \text{ m}^2} \times 250 \text{ mg}$

2) The m² units cancel out and can be ignored.

3) Child's dose $= \dfrac{0.54}{1.7} \times 250 \text{ mg}$

$$0.3 \times 250 \text{ mg} = 75 \text{ mg}$$

Child's dose = 75 mg

NURSING PROCESS AND MEDICATIONS

The nurse's role extends beyond simply giving drugs to a client. The nurse is responsible for monitoring clients' responses to medications, providing education to the client and family about the medication regimen, and informing the physician when medications are effective, ineffective, or no longer necessary. The nurse uses the nursing process to integrate drug therapy into client care.

ASSESSMENT

Nursing assessment relating to drug therapy includes a history of allergies to medication. In acute care settings clients wear ID bands listing medication allergies, and allergies are conspicuously noted on the front of the chart, as well as on the MAR. It is important to differentiate between allergies, such as anaphylactic shock, which can be life threatening, and drug intolerances, such as nausea and vomiting, which are uncomfortable side effects.

Nursing assessment also involves identifying drugs the client takes every day at home, including over-the-counter (OTC) preparations and herbal supplements. The client should know the name, purpose, dosage, route, and side effects of medications and supplements that are being taken. Often clients take many drugs and carry a list that includes this information. Clients have different levels of understanding. One client may describe a diuretic as a "water pill," whereas another describes it as a drug to minimize swelling and lower blood pressure. Still another may describe it as "the little white pill I take in the morning." By assessing the client's level of knowledge, the nurse determines the need for teaching. If a client is unable to understand or remember pertinent information, it may be necessary to involve a family member.

NURSING DIAGNOSES

Nursing diagnoses may be identified based on therapeutic effects or side effects of specific prescribed medications or factors affecting the client's ability to self-administer drugs.

Ineffective Therapeutic Regimen Management may be related to a knowledge deficit of the purpose of prescribed medications, the complexity of a drug schedule, or unpleasant side effects. **Health-Seeking Behaviors (medications)** is a useful nursing diagnosis when clients have a knowledge deficit and want to learn how to provide self-medication. **Noncompliance** involves a person's informed decision not to adhere to a therapeutic regimen of medication administration, which may be related to economic, cultural, or spiritual beliefs. Certain medications, such as chemotherapeutic agents, steroids, and anticoagulants, may contribute to **Ineffective Protection,** in which therapy alters the client's ability to respond normally to infection or bleeding. **Disturbed Sensory Perception (visual or auditory)** may be appropriate in clients receiving eye or ear medications.

PLANNING

When a nurse assumes responsibility for administering medications, the following general goals should be met:

1. Achievement of the therapeutic effect of the prescribed medication
2. Absence of complications related to the prescribed medication
3. Client and/or family understanding of drug therapy

IMPLEMENTATION

Nursing interventions focus on safe and effective drug administration. This includes careful drug preparation, accurate and timely administration, and client education.

Preadministration Activities

1. Identify the drug action and purpose, side effects, and nursing implications for administering and monitoring. Ensure that the medication order has not expired.
2. Complete appropriate assessments, which may include and are not limited to vital signs, laboratory

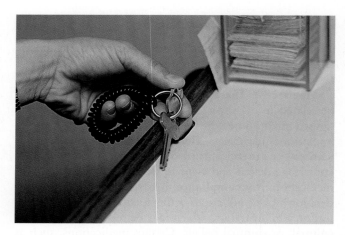

Figure 16-8 Medication carts must be kept locked when unattended and the key kept by an authorized person.

data, or nature and severity of symptoms. If data contraindicates medication administration, the drug should be withheld and the prescriber notified.

3. Calculate drug doses accurately, and use appropriate measuring devices. Verify that the dose prescribed is appropriate for the client situation.

4. Give medications within 30 minutes before or after the scheduled time to maintain a therapeutic level. NOTE: Medications ordered stat should be given immediately. Preoperative medications may be ordered "on call" and are given when the operating room personnel notify the nurse of the appropriate time. Certain drugs, such as insulin, should be given at a precise interval before a meal, whereas others should be given with meals or on an empty stomach.

5. Use good hand-hygiene technique for nonparenteral medications. Avoid touching tablets and capsules. Use sterile technique for parenteral medications. Gloves are worn during the administration of parenteral medications.

6. Administer only those medications you personally prepare. Do not ask another person to administer drugs you prepare. Keep drugs secure (Figure 16-8).

7. When preparing medications be sure the label is clear and legible, the drug is properly mixed, has not changed in color, clarity, or consistency, and has not expired.

8. Tablets and capsules should be kept in their wrappers and opened at the client's bedside. This allows the nurse to review each drug with the client. If a client refuses medication, there is no question about which one should be withheld.

Drug Administration

1. Follow the six rights for medication administration (see Box 16-3, p. 414).

2. Inform the client of each drug's name, purpose, action, and common side effects. Evaluate the client's knowledge of the drug, and provide appropriate teaching.

3. Remain with the client until the medication is taken. Provide assistance as necessary. Do not leave medication at the bedside without a prescriber's order to do so. For example, some clients may take their own vitamins or birth control pills while in the hospital.

4. Respect the client's right to refuse medication. If the medication wrapper is intact, the medication may be returned to the client's storage bin. When medication is refused, determine the reason for this, and take action accordingly. If, for example, the client has unpleasant side effects, it may be possible to eliminate them by giving the pills with food or using a different time schedule. Refusal of medications must be documented, and the physician is notified within 24 hours or according to institutional policy.

Postadministration Activities

1. Record medications immediately according to agency policy, including drug name, dose, route, time, and signature of person administering the drug.

2. Document data pertinent to the client's response. This is particularly important when giving drugs ordered prn.

3. If a drug is refused, document that it was not given, the reason for the refusal, and when the physician was notified.

EVALUATION

1. Monitor for evidence of therapeutic effects, side effects, and adverse reactions. This may involve monitoring physical response (e.g., heart rhythm, blood pressure, urine output, relief of symptoms) or laboratory results.

2. Observe injection sites for bruises, inflammation, localized pain, numbness, or bleeding.

3. Evaluate client's understanding of drug therapy and ability to self-administer medication.

 ## CLIENT AND FAMILY TEACHING

A properly informed client is more likely to take medications correctly. The nurse provides information about the purpose of medications, their actions, desired effects, side effects, dosage schedules, and actions to take in case side or toxic effects develop. Special instructional booklets or leaflets are often available as teaching aids. When teaching clients about their medications it is best to include persons identified as being significant to the client's recovery. This may include family members, partners, or home care providers. There are specific nursing interventions that are appropriate in the home setting (Box 16-7).

Box 16-7

Home Care

1. During each home visit, assess both the prescription and nonprescription medications being taken by the client.
2. Document and notify the primary health care provider of the client's medication regimen and of multiple physician sources for medications.
3. Teach the complications and interactions of all over-the-counter medications to clients and their caregivers.
4. Collaborate with social workers to identify community resources for financial assistance with pharmceutic needs.
5. Use laboratory parameters to monitor overuse and underuse of medications, as well as interactive states of medications.
6. Monitor urinary output status of clients, because changes in renal excretion may require a decrease or increase in drug dosage.
7. Teach the homebound older client to set up a daily or weekly schedule of medications using a method or tool that fosters safe, independent administration.
8. Reduce the chance of medication error by labeling or color coding medication bottles.
9. Keep an accurate record of the homebound client's weight, especially the older adult, because many medication dosages are calculated by body weight.
10. Teach drug safety in the home environment by instructing clients to do the following:

    - Keep drug in original, labeled container.
    - Dispose of outdated medications in a sink or toilet only; never dispose of them in the trash within reach of children.
    - Never "share" drugs with friends or family members.
    - Always finish a prescribed medication; do not save it for a future illness.
    - Read labels carefully and follow all instructions.

11. Instruct clients with muscle weakness and older adults who have difficulty opening childproof containers to request health care providers ask for nonchildproof containers when writing prescription.

Data from Lueckenotte A: *Gerontological nursing*, ed 2, St Louis, 2000, Mosby.

Teaching Clients About Side Effects

All medications have side effects. The nurse teaches the client and family members about side effects associated with each medication prescribed. Because medications can have many side effects, teaching the client about all of them can overwhelm the client and impede learning; remember, client learning is a continual process. When beginning to teach a client about a new medication, evaluate each of the side effects and teach the client about the ones that are the most likely to occur and occur early after administration. For example, some antibiotics cause hypersensitivity reactions, hepatotoxicity, nephrotoxicity, and platelet dysfunction. Hypersensitivity reactions are likely to occur shortly after taking a few doses of an antibiotic. The other side effects tend to occur after long-term antibiotic administration. Teach clients about side effects in terms of things that they can see, feel, touch, or hear. For example, thrombocytopenia, a reduction in the number of platelets in the blood, can be a side effect of a drug. The client cannot see, feel, touch, or hear thrombocytopenia. However, thrombocytopenia can cause bleeding. The nurse teaches the client how to look for evidence of bleeding. Be sure to teach the client what to do about side effects when they are discovered.

Medications and the Client's Activities of Daily Living

The nurse evaluates the client's activities of daily living and the effect they will have on the client's ability to comply with medication schedules. When medications are initiated in the acute care setting, they are often administered around-the-clock. In the community it may not be reasonable to think clients can administer medications according to this schedule. In collaboration with the prescriber or the pharmacist, the nurse teaches the client and family members how to adjust medication schedules that are consistent with the client's lifestyle, including what to do if doses are missed.

Evaluating the effectiveness of teaching ensures that the client can administer drugs in a safe manner. One method of evaluating client understanding is to create medication cards with the name of the drug on the front of the card and all pertinent drug information on the back of the card. The nurse flashes the card in front of the client and asks the client to read the name of the medication (this also ensures that the client can read the names of the medication). If the client correctly identifies the name of the medication, ask the client the following questions:

- Why are you taking this medication?
- How often do you take this medication?

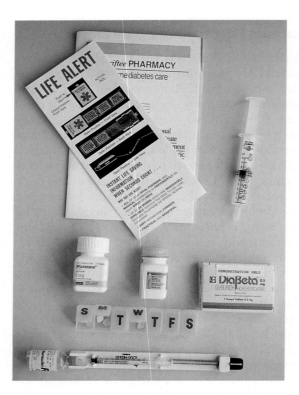

Figure 16-9 Self-help devices for managing medications at home. *Clockwise from top:* Life Alert, syringe for liquid medication, various oral medications with weekly pill sorter, insulin syringe with electronic dispenser.

Box 16-8

Storage and Accountability for Controlled Substances

- All narcotics are stored in a locked cabinet or container (Figure 16-8, p. 420).
- Authorized nurses carry a set of keys or computer entry code for the narcotics cabinet.
- An inventory record is kept to record all narcotics used, including client's name, date, name of drug, and time of drug administration.
- Before removing any drug from the cabinet, the number actually available is compared with the number indicated on the narcotic record. If incorrect, the discrepancy must be rectified before proceding.
- If any part of a dose of a controlled substance is discarded, a second nurse witnesses disposal of the unused portion, and the record is signed by both nurses.
- At change of shift one nurse going off duty counts all narcotics with a nurse coming on duty. Both nurses sign the narcotic record to indicate the count is correct. (Computerized storage has eliminated this process.)
- Discrepancies in narcotic counts are reported immediately.

- What side effects can occur with this medication?
- If this side effect occurs, what are you going to do about it?

It may be helpful to have actual labeled medication bottles with the drug name. Drug bottles often have fine print and may not be easily read by the client with impaired visual acuity.

Be sure to evaluate the client's sensory, motor, and cognitive functions which, when impaired, may affect the client's ability to safely self-administer medications. When impairments are assessed, family members, friends, or home health aides may be available to assist with medication administration. Many self-help devices are also available for purchase (e.g., pill boxes with times displayed and electronic dispensers) (Figure 16-9).

SPECIAL HANDLING OF CONTROLLED II SUBSTANCES

The nurse is responsible for following legal regulations when administering controlled II substances (drugs with potential for abuse). Violations of the Controlled Substances Act may result in fines, imprisonment, and loss

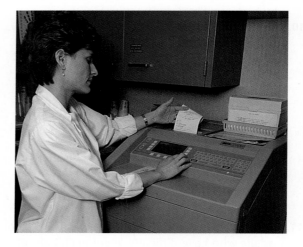

Figure 16-10 Computerized system for medication distribution.

of license. Health care institutions have policies for the proper storage and distribution of controlled substances, including narcotics (Box 16-8). Many agencies use computerized systems for medication access and distribution (Fig 16-10).

MEDICATION ERRORS

A medication error is any preventable medication-related event that occurs as a result of actions by a health care professional that could cause client harm (Pape, 2001). Medication errors can be made by anyone involved in the prescribing, transcribing, preparation, dispensing, and administration of medications (Smetzer, 2001). Hospital medication delivery systems are designed so that there is a system of checks that help prevent medication errors. Conscientious adherence to the six rights of medication administration helps prevent errors.

When an error occurs, it should be acknowledged immediately, and the client should be assessed. The nurse has an ethical and professional obligation to report the error to the client's physician, the nurse manager, and any other persons as indicated by the institution's policy regarding errors. Appropriate follow-up may include administering an antidote, withholding a subsequent dose, and monitoring the effects of the drug. The client's record should include a notation including what was given, who was notified, the observed effects of the drug, and follow-up measures taken.

The nurse is also responsible for completing a report describing the incident. Most institutions have a policy or protocol for reporting adverse events. This report provides an objective analysis of what went wrong and provides information for the risk management team to identify factors contributing to errors and ways to avoid similar errors in the future (Benner, 2001).

Table 16-3

Drug Effects in Older Adults

Drug Effect	Related Interventions
Difficulty swallowing large tablets or capsules; tissue damage related to uncoated medications such as aspirin and potassium chloride	Position client sitting upright. Give full glass of liquid (if unrestricted). Crush tablets and mix with food, or give liquid form if available.
Slowing of drug excretion; overuse and abuse of laxatives by client	Instruct client to increase fluid intake, eat high-fiber foods, and avoid daily use of laxatives.
Longer biotransformation of drugs by the liver with greater risk for drug sensitivity and toxicity	Monitor for signs of liver dysfunction (laboratory tests, jaundice, dark urine). Monitor for contraindications in clients with known liver disease.
Risk of drug accumulation and toxicity related to altered kidney function or renal blood flow	Monitor for renal impairment (decreased urine output) and contraindications dosage in clients with known renal disease.

SPECIAL CONSIDERATIONS FOR SPECIFIC AGE-GROUPS

Pediatric Considerations

Children vary in age, weight, and the ability to absorb, metabolize, and excrete medications. Children's dosages are lower than those of adults, and caution is needed in preparing medications. Drugs may or may not be prepared and packaged in doses appropriate for children. Preparing appropriate doses often requires calculation based on body weight (Wong, 1999). A child's parents may be helpful in determining the best way to give a child medication. Sometimes it is more effective to have the parent give the drug as the nurse stands by.

Geriatric Considerations

Individual over the age of 65 years are the largest users of drugs (Lueckenotte, 2000). Because of physiological changes associated with the aging process, special nursing interventions are needed to promote safe and effective medication administration (Table 16-3). Be aware of the following patterns related to drug use:

1. *Polypharmacy.* The client takes many medications in an attempt to treat several disorders. This increases the risk of drug interactions with other drugs or with foods.
2. *Self-prescribing.* Older adults often attempt to seek relief from a variety of problems with OTC preparations, folk medicines, and herbs.
3. *Misuse of drugs.* Misuse by older adults includes overuse, underuse, erratic use, and contraindicated use.
4. *Noncompliance.* Defined as a deliberate misuse of medication. Older adults alter dose because of ineffectiveness or unpleasant side effects.

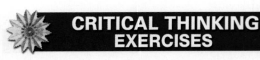

CRITICAL THINKING EXERCISES

1. Janet Janes, RN, is orienting a newly hired nurse to the division. This is the third day that the nurse has passed medications on this division. After preparing medications at the medicine cart, the nurse enters a two-bed room to administer the medications to the client in bed A. The nurse then begins to prepare the medications for the client in bed B. Janet Janes reminds the new nurse that bed B is the one on the right when entering the room. The nurse suddenly says, " I just gave the last medications to the wrong client!" Prioritize and discuss the activities that are indicated.

2. A clinic client is diagnosed with a bacterial upper respiratory infection and is given a prescription for an antibiotic. Two weeks later the client is seen in clinic again complaining of the same symptoms. The client states, "I was getting better, and now I'm sick again." When assessing the client, the nurse learns that the client took the medication for only 5 of the 10 days that it was prescribed because he was feeling better. What is an appropriate nursing diagnosis for this client?

3. You are caring for an 89-year-old woman. She has a history of hypertension and was switched to a single beta blocker to control her blood pressure. During a home visit you are asked to see all medications the patient is taking each day. She shows you 3 medicines, the prescribed beta blocker, a diuretic, and an ACE inhibitor. Your client states that her previous doctor ordered the diuretic and ACE inhibitor and she was going to continue taking these until "all the pills are gone because they cost money." What are your actions?

REFERENCES

Benner P: Creating a culture of safely and improvement: a key to reducing medical error, *Am J Crit Care* 10(4):281, 2001.

Clayton B, Stock Y: *Basic pharmacology for nurses,* St Louis, 2000, Mosby.

McCaffery M, Ferrell B: Opioids and pain management: what do nurses know? *Nursing* 29(3):48, 1999.

Lueckenotte A: *Gerontologic nursing,* ed 2, St Louis, 2000, Mosby.

Pape T: Searching for the final answer: factors contributing to medication administration errors, *J Contin Educ Nurs* 32(4):152, 2001.

Skidmore-Roth L: *Mosby's drug guide for nurses,* ed 2, St Louis, 2002, Mosby.

Smetzer J: Take 10 giant steps to medication safety, *Nursing* 31(11):49, 2001.

Wong D: *Essentials of pediatric nursing,* St Louis, 1999, Mosby.

Administration of Nonparenteral Medications

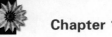

Nonparenteral medications are given by several routes that do not invade the skin, including oral, topical, inhalation, or instilled into the eye, ear, rectum, or vagina. The route chosen depends on the properties and desired effects of the medication, as well as the physical and mental condition of the client. Each route has advantages and disadvantages (Table 17-1). There are many reasons a nurse may find it necessary to change from one route to another. When this occurs, the nurse is responsible for consulting with the physician and pharmacist to safely meet the client's needs.

The easiest and most desirable way to administer medications is orally (by mouth). Clients usually are able to ingest or self-administer oral drugs with a minimum of problems. Situations, however, may arise that contraindicate clients' receiving medications by mouth, the presence of gastrointestinal (GI) alterations, the inability of a client to swallow food or fluids, and the use of gastric suction. An

Table 17-1

Nonparenteral Routes of Administration

Route	Advantages	Disadvantages
Oral (swallowed)	Easy, comfortable, economical; may produce local or systemic effects.	Some drugs are destroyed by gastric secretions. Cannot be given if client is NPO, unable to swallow, has gastric suction, or is unconscious or confused and unwilling to cooperate. May irritate lining of GI tract, discolor teeth, or have unpleasant taste.
Skin: topical application or transdermal patches	Provides primarily local effect; painless; limited side effects. Transdermal application provides systemic effects, and bypasses the liver and its first-pass effects.	Extensive topical applications may be bulky or cause difficulty in maneuvering. May leave oily or pasty substance on skin; may soil clothing. Systemic absorption can be unreliable. Allergies to the adhesive in transdermal patches may develop.
Mucous membranes: eyes, ears, nose; vaginal, rectal, buccal, sublingual	Local application to involved site; limited side effects. Buccal and sublingual rapidly absorbed. Rectal route an alternative when oral route not available.	Insertion of vaginal or rectal products may cause embarrassment. Rectal suppositories are contraindicated with rectal surgery or active rectal bleeding.
Inhalation	Provides direct effects on lung tissues and rapid relief of respiratory distress.	Difficult for some clients to administer correctly. Clients must be taught how to use equipment.

Modified from Lilley LL, Aucker RS: *Pharmacology and the nursing process,* ed 3, St Louis, 2002, Mosby.

Box 17-1

Dysphagia

Dysphagia, or difficulty in swallowing, may lead to aspiration of food or fluid into the lungs. A variety of signs and symptoms may be associated with dysphagia:

- Choking while eating or drinking
- Facial droop
- Drooling or leakage of food from the mouth
- Coughing during or after meals
- Holding pockets of food in the cheeks
- Absent or diminished gag reflex
- Gurgly voice quality
- Increased congestion or secretions after eating or drinking

The client's swallow, cough, and gag reflexes must be carefully assessed. Swallowing can be assessed at the bedside by placing the thumb and index finger on both sides of the client's Adam's apple and feeling for elevation of the larynx when the client tries to swallow. The elevation should be the same on both sides.

If swallowing difficulties are suspected or detected, a referral to a speech pathologist is needed for definitive diagnosis. Dysphagia that is not recognized or managed may lead to dangerous complications such as aspiration pneumonia.

Modified from Kayser-Jones J, Pengilly K: Dysphagia among nursing home residents, *Geriatr Nurs* 20(2):77, 1999; Mahan LK, Escott-Stump S: *Krause's food, nutrition, and diet therapy,* ed 10, Philadelphia, 2000, WB Saunders.

important precaution to take when administering any oral preparation is to protect clients from aspiration. Aspiration occurs when food, fluid, or medication intended for GI administration inadvertently is administered into the respiratory tract. The nurse can protect the client from aspiration by evaluating the client's ability to safely swallow (Box 17-1). Properly positioning the client is also essential in preventing aspiration. Unless contraindicated, the nurse positions the client in a seated position when administering oral medications. The lateral position can also be used when the client's swallow, gag, and cough are intact. A client who has difficulty swallowing should be evaluated by appropriate personnel (e.g., speech therapist) before receiving oral preparations.

Topical administration of medications involves applying drugs locally to skin, mucous membranes, or tissue membranes. The nurse applies medications to the skin by painting, spraying, or spreading medication over an area, applying moist dressings, soaking body parts in solution, or giving medicated baths. Adhesive-backed medicated disks (or transdermal patches) can also be applied to the skin to provide a continuous release of medication over several hours or days. Systemic effects from topical agents can occur if the skin is thin, if the drug concentration is high, or if contact with the skin is prolonged. Topical administration avoids puncturing the skin and lessens tissue injury and risk of infection that may occur with injections. The risk of serious side effects is generally low, but they can occur.

Drugs applied to membranes such as the cornea of the eye or rectal mucosa are absorbed quickly because of the membrane's vascularity. When drug concentrations are high, systemic effects can occur. For example, bradycardia may occur following atropine instillation to the eye. Mucous and other tissue membranes differ in their sensitivity to medications. The cornea of the eye, for example, is extremely sensitive to chemicals. Clients commonly experience burning sensations during administration of eye and nose drops. Medications are generally less irritating to vaginal or rectal mucosa.

Medications for topical use can be administered in the following ways:

1. Direct application of a liquid—eye drops, gargling, swabbing the throat
2. Insertion of a drug into body cavity—suppository into rectum or vagina; creams and foams into the vagina
3. Instillation of fluid into body cavity (fluid is retained)—ear drops, nose drops, bladder and rectal instillation
4. Irrigation of body cavity (fluid is not retained)—flushing eye, ear, vagina, bladder, or rectum with medicated fluid
5. Spray—instillation into nose or throat, or sublingually
6. Inhalation of medicated aerosol spray—distributes medication throughout the nasal passages and tracheobronchial airway
7. Direct application to skin or mucosa—lotion, ointments, creams, patches, and disk

NURSING DIAGNOSES

Nursing diagnoses may be identified based on factors affecting the client's ability to self-administer drugs. For example, **Ineffective Therapeutic Regimen Management** may be related to a knowledge deficit of the purpose of prescribed medications, the complexity of a drug schedule, or unpleasant side effects. **Health-Seeking Behaviors** is useful when clients want to learn how to provide self-medication. Nursing diagnoses may also be identified based on therapeutic effects or side effects of specific prescribed medications. For example, **Impaired Skin Integrity** may be used when topical medications are used to treat rashes and skin injury, and **Impaired Gas Exchange** may be appropriate when medications are administered by inhalation. Certain medications such as chemotherapeutic agents, steroids, and anticoagulants may contribute to **Ineffective Protection,** in which the client's ability to respond normally to infection or bleeding is decreased.

Skill 17.1

Administering Oral Medications

The majority of medications the nurse administers in many health care settings are given by mouth. The nurse usually prepares the oral medications for the client to self-administer in an area designed for medication preparation or at the unit-dose cart. Some agencies have a locked cabinet for medications in each client's room.

The ability of an oral medication to be absorbed after it is ingested depends largely on its form or preparation. Solutions and suspensions that are already in a liquid state (Figure 17-1) are absorbed more readily than tablets or capsules. Oral medications are absorbed more easily when administered between meals, when the

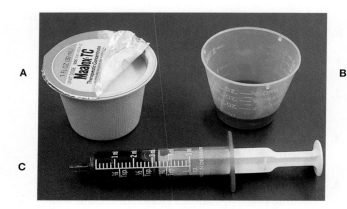

Figure 17-1 A, Liquid medication in single-dose package. **B,** Liquid measured in medicine cup. **C,** Oral liquid medicine in syringe.

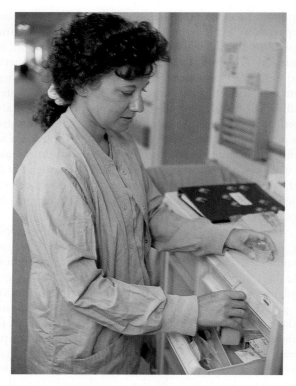

Figure 17-2 The nurse removes medications from a drawer in a medication cart, which is kept locked when not in use.

stomach is not filled with food which would slow the absorption process. When effective absorption in the stomach is required for certain drugs, they should be given at least 1 hour before or 2 hours after meals or antacids. Acidic drugs are absorbed quickly in the stomach.

Some drugs are not absorbed until reaching the small intestine. Enteric coatings on some tablets resist dissolution in gastric juices and prevent digestion in the upper GI tract. The coating protects the stomach lining from irritation by the medication. Eventually the drug is absorbed in the intestine. Enteric-coated medication should not be crushed or dissolved before administration.

ASSESSMENT

1. Identify the drug(s) ordered: action, purpose, normal dosage and route, common side effects, time of onset and peak action, and nursing implications. *Rationale: This allows nurse to anticipate effects of drug and to observe client's response.*
2. Assess for any contraindications to oral medication, including inability to swallow, nausea/vomiting, bowel inflammation, reduced peristalsis, GI surgery, and gastric suction. *Rationale: Alterations in gastrointestinal function can interfere with drug absorption, distribution, and excretion. Giving oral medication to clients with impaired swallowing increases their risk of aspiration.*
3. Check for a history of allergies and related response (rash or anaphylactic shock.).
4. Assess for identification bracelet or photograph. Replace any missing, outdated, or faded identification tools. *Rationale: Identification bracelets or photographs provide positive client identification.*
5. Assess client's knowledge regarding each medication. *Rationale: Determines need for drug education and assists in identifying client's compliance with drug therapy at home.*
6. Assess client's preferences for fluids. Maintain fluid restrictions as prescribed. *Rationale: Offering fluids during drug administration is an excellent way to increase*

client's fluid intake. Fluids ease swallowing and facilitate absorption from the GI tract. However, fluid restrictions must be maintained.

PLANNING

Expected outcomes focus on safe, accurate, and effective drug therapy.

Expected Outcomes

1. Client takes medications as prescribed, with evidence of improvement in condition (e.g., relief of pain, regular heart rate, stable blood pressure).
2. Client explains purpose of medication and drug dose schedule.

Equipment

- Medication administration record (MAR) or computer printout
- Medication cart (Figure 17-2) or locked cabinet in client's room
- Disposable medication cups
- Glass of water, juice, or preferred liquid and drinking straw
- Device for crushing or splitting tablets (optional)

Delegation Considerations

In acute care settings, administration of oral medication requires the critical thinking and knowledge application unique to a nurse, therefore delegation to assistive personnel (AP) is not appropriate. The nurse needs to inform providers about potential adverse effects of medications and to inform them of the need to report their occurrence. In some long-term care settings AP are trained and certified to administer nonnarcotic, nonparenteral medications to stable residents; however, knowledge of desired effects and adverse reactions is very limited; therefore assessment and evaluation of medication effects remains primarily the responsibility of the nurse.

IMPLEMENTATION FOR ADMINISTERING ORAL MEDICATIONS

Steps	Rationale
1. See Standard Protocol (inside front cover). 2. **Preparing medications** a. Compare MAR with scheduled medication list or physician's orders. If discrepancies exist, check against original physician orders (Ignatavicius, 2000).	Physician's order is most reliable source and only legal record of drugs client is to receive. Orders should be checked at least every 24 hours and when client questions a drug order. Often this is done during the night shift.

NURSE ALERT *Incomplete or unclear orders should be clarified with the prescriber before implementation.*

Steps	Rationale
b. Arrange medication tray and cups in medication preparation area, or move medication cart to position outside client's room.	Organization of equipment saves time and reduces error.
c. Unlock medicine drawer or cart (see illustration).	Unauthorized access to medications is safeguarded when locked in cabinet or cart.
d. Prepare medications for one client at a time. Follow the six rights of medication administration. Keep all pages of MARs or computer printouts for one client together.	Prevents preparation errors.

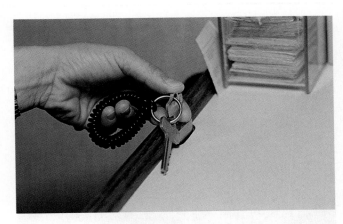

Step 2c The nurse unlocks the medication cart.

Steps	Rationale
e. Select correct drug from stock supply or unit-dose drawer. Compare label of medication with MAR or computer printout (see illustration).	Reading label and comparing it against transcribed order reduces errors. **This is the first check for accuracy.**
f. Check drug dose. If dose printed on the package differs from ordered dose, calculate correct amount to give.	Double-checking pharmacy calculations reduces risk of error. Some agencies require nurses to check calculations of certain medications with another nurse.
g. To prepare unit-dose tablets or capsules, place prepackaged tablet or capsule directly into medicine cup without removing wrapper (see illustration). Give medications only from containers with labels that are clearly marked and legible.	Wrapper identifies drug name and dosage, which can facilitate teaching.
h. To prepare tablets or capsules from a floor stock bottle, pour required number into bottle cap and transfer medication to medication cup. Do not touch medication with fingers. Extra tablets or capsules may be returned to bottle.	Floor stock bottles are often used in long-term care settings for common over-the-counter (OTC) drugs such as laxatives and nonnarcotic analgesics.
i. Check the expiration date of each drug. Return all outdated drugs to pharmacy.	Outdated drugs cannot be safely administered.
j. Place all tablets or capsules requiring preadministration assessments (e.g., pulse rate, blood pressure) in a separate cup.	Serves as a reminder to complete appropriate assessment and facilitates withholding drugs (if necessary.)
k. Medications that must be broken to administer half the dose can be broken using a gloved hand or cut with a cutting device. Tablets that are broken in half should be scored, as identified by a manufactured line across the center of the tablet. Unused portions of divided tablets or capsules may be discarded or returned to the original container, depending on agency policy.	Discarding prevents mislabeling by placement in the incorrect container. Returning unused portion is more cost-effective.
l. If client has difficulty swallowing, use a mortar and pestle to grind pills or a pill-crushing device (see illustrations). Mix ground tablet in small amount of soft food (custard or applesauce).	Ground tablet mixed with palatable soft food is usually easier to swallow.

NURSE ALERT *Not all drugs can be crushed (e.g., capsules, enteric-coated, and long-acting/slow-release drugs). The coating of these drugs is designed to protect the stomach from irritation or protect the drug from destruction from stomach acids. Consult with the pharmacist when in doubt or to determine if the medication is available in a liquid, injection, or suppository form that would be more appropriate (Miller and Miller, 2000).*

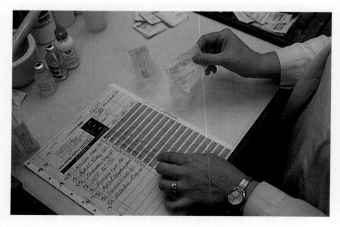

Step 2e The nurse compares the MAR to the medication label.

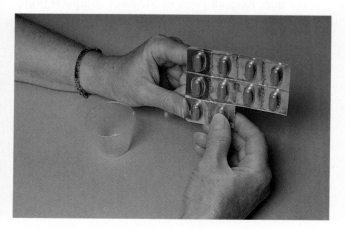

Step 2h Place tablet into medicine cup without removing wrapper.

Steps	Rationale
m. When using a blister pack, "pop" medications through foil or paper backing into a medication cup.	Many long-term care agencies use blister packs, which provide about 1 month's supply of prescription drugs for an individual client. Each "blister" usually contains a single dose. Blister packs are prepared by a pharmacist.
n. When preparing liquids, thoroughly mix before administering. Check and discard medications that are cloudy or have changed color.	Liquid medications packaged in single-dose cups need not be poured into medicine cups.
(1) Remove bottle cap from container, and place cap upside down.	
(2) Hold bottle with label against palm of hand while pouring.	Spilled liquid will not soil or obscure label.
(3) Place medication cup at eye level on countertop, or when necessary, in hand, and fill to desired level (see illustration).	Ensures accurate measurement.
(4) Wipe lip of bottle with paper towel.	Prevents contamination of bottle's contents and prevents bottle cap from sticking.
(5) If giving less than 5 ml of liquids, prepare medication in a sterile syringe without a needle (see Figure 17-1, p. 418).	Allows more accurate measurement of small amounts.
o. When administering narcotic preparation, check narcotic record for previous drug count and compare with supply available. Narcotics may be stored in a computerized locked cart (see Chapter 16).	Controlled substance laws require careful monitoring of dispensed narcotics. In most agencies, cosignature by an RN is required when students administer narcotics.
p. Check expiration date on all medications.	Medications used past expiration date may be inactive or harmful to client.

A

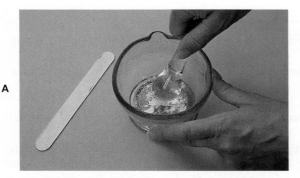

B

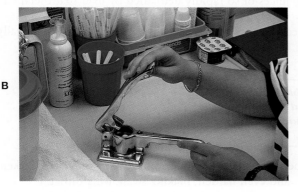

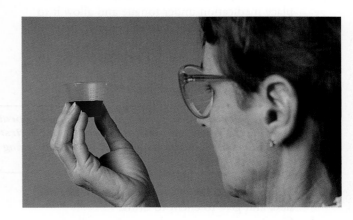

Step 2l **A,** Using a mortar and pestle to grind pills. **B,** Using a pill-crushing device.

Step 2n(3) Measuring liquid medication. Look at meniscus at eye level.

Steps	Rationale

3. Administer medications

a. Take medications to client within 30 minutes be-fore or after scheduled time. Stat and single-order medications are given at the exact time ordered.

Promotes intended therapeutic effect.

NURSE ALERT   *Apply the six rights of medication administration (see Chapter 16, p. 408).*

---

b. Identify client.
(1) Compare name on MAR or computer printout with name on client's identification bracelet.

Identification bracelets are made at the time of the client's admission and are the most reliable source of identification. In many long-term care settings pictures maybe used along with arm bands. **This is the second check for accuracy.**

(2) Ask client to state name.

This is the third check for accuracy.

COMMUNICATION TIP   *Asking client to state name may elicit a surprised reaction, especially when you have previously established a relationship; however, it is a routine practice that has prevented identification errors. Simply state: "I just want to verify that I am giving you the correct medications."*

---

c. Perform necessary preadministration assessment for specific medications (e.g., blood pressure or pulse).

Assessment data determine whether specific medications should be withheld at that time.

d. Discuss the purpose of each medication and its action with client. Allow client to ask any questions about drugs.

Client has the right to be informed, and client's understanding of purpose of each medication improves compliance with drug therapy.

e. Assist client to sitting or side-lying position.

Sitting position prevents aspiration during swallowing.

NURSE ALERT   *If in doubt about client's ability to swallow, check cough and gag reflexes (see Box 17-1, p. 426). If client is unable to swallow pills without choking, consider administering the drug in another form (crushed, oral liquid, suppository, or by injection).*

---

f. Client may wish to hold solid medications in hand or cup before placing in mouth.

Client can become familiar with medications by seeing each drug.

g. If client is unable to hold medications, place medication cup to the lips and gently introduce each drug into the mouth, one at a time. Do not rush.

Administering single tablet or capsule eases swallowing and decreases risk of aspiration.

h. Offer water or juice to help client swallow medications.

Choice of fluid promotes client's comfort and can improve fluid intake.

i. For sublingual-administered drugs, have client place medication under tongue and allow it to dissolve completely. Caution client against swallowing tablet.

Drug is absorbed through blood vessels of undersurface of tongue. If swallowed, drug is destroyed by gastric juices or so rapidly detoxified by liver that therapeutic blood levels are not attained.

j. For buccal-administered drugs, have client place medication in mouth against mucous membranes of the cheek until it dissolves.

Buccal medications act locally on mucosa or systemically as they are swallowed in saliva.

NURSE ALERT   *If client is to receive a combination of oral tablets, capsules, and sublingual or buccal drugs, administer tablets/capsules first and have client take sublingual and buccal medications last. Avoid administering liquids until buccal medication has dissolved.*

---

k. Mix powdered medications with liquids at bed-side, and give to client to drink.

When prepared in advance, powdered drugs may thicken and even harden, making swallowing difficult.

l. Caution client against chewing or swallowing lozenges.

Drug acts through slow absorption through oral mucosa, not gastric mucosa.

Steps	Rationale
m. Give effervescent powders and tablets immediately after dissolving.	Effervescence improves unpleasant taste of drug and often relieves GI problems.
n. Stay until client has completely swallowed each medication. If concerned about ability or willingness to swallow, ask client to open mouth and inspect for presence of medication.	Nurse is responsible for ensuring that client receives ordered dosage. If left unattended, client may forget to take it, drop it, or intentionally not take dose without nurse's awareness.
o. For certain medications that should not be given on an empty stomach (e.g., aspirin), offer client nonfat snack (e.g., crackers) if not contraindicated by client's condition.	Reduces gastric irritation. The fat content of foods may delay absorption of the medication.
4. Replenish stock such as cups and straws, return cart to medicine room, and clean work area.	Well-stocked, clean working space assists other staff in completing duties efficiently.
5. See Completion Protocol (inside front cover).	

• • • • • • • • • •

EVALUATION

1. Return within appropriate time to determine client's response to medications, including therapeutic effects, side effects or allergy, and adverse reactions. Sublingual/buccal medications take effect in 15 minutes; most oral medications take effect in 30 to 60 minutes.
2. Ask client or family member to identify drug name and explain purpose, action, dosage schedule, and potential side effects of drug.

Unexpected Outcomes and Related Interventions

1. Client exhibits toxic effects as a result of prolonged high doses or altered excretion.
   a. Withhold further doses.
   b. Notify physician and provide supportive therapy as prescribed.
2. Tablet or capsule falls to the floor.
   a. Discard it.
   b. Repeat preparation.
   c. Replacement may need to be obtained from pharmacy with unit-dose systems.
3. Client exhibits side effects common to medication.
   a. Identify comfort measures that relieve symptoms.
   b. Report severe or intolerable side effects to physician. Dosage or form of medication may be changed.
4. Client experiences allergic response that could be related to medication. Symptoms such as urticaria, pruritus, rhinitis, and wheezing may indicate allergic reaction.
   a. Withhold further doses.
   b. Notify the physician. If symptoms are severe, drugs may be prescribed to counteract adverse effects.
5. Client is unable to explain drug information and is unable or unwilling to remember information about purpose, schedule, or adverse effects.
   a. Identify family member willing to assume responsibility.
   b. Refer to home health agency for follow-up after discharge if needed.
   c. Utilize appropriate aids to facilitate accurate self-administration which may include: homemade calendars for each week that contain plastic bags containing medications to take at specific times, egg cartons divided into color-coded sections with medications for day, clock faces for clients who cannot read or see clearly, color coding for drug types (e.g., blue for sedative, red for pain pill).
6. Administration error is made (wrong drug, dose, client, route, or time).
   a. Acknowledge it immediately. Nurses have an ethical and professional responsibility to report the error to the client's physician.
   b. Institute measures to counteract the effects of the error if necessary.
   c. Monitor client for untoward effects according to the drug action and side effects.
   d. Complete medication error form as required by the agency. These reports can assist in preventing additional similar errors.

Recording and Reporting

• Record actual time each drug was administered on the MAR or computer printout. Do not chart medication administration until *after* it is given to the client. Include initials or signature (see Figure 16-3, p. 415).
• If drug is withheld, record reason in nurses' notes. Circle time the drug normally would have been given on the MAR or computer printout.
• Report adverse effects/client response and/or withheld drugs to nurse in charge or physician.

Sample Documentation

0900 Apical pulse 50. Client c/o nausea. Digoxin held and Dr. Jay notified.

SPECIAL CONSIDERATIONS

Pediatric Considerations

- Oral liquids available in colorful and palatable forms are preferred for administration of medications to children. Small pills may be aspirated.
- Pediatric doses are usually calculated based on body weight. Professional nurses are responsible for verifying that the prescribed dose is safe.
- Bitter or distasteful oral preparations will be rejected by the child. Mix the drug with a small amount (about 1 teaspoon) of a sweet-tasting substance, such as jam, applesauce, honey, or fruit puree. Do not use honey in infants because of the risk of botulism. The nurse can also offer the child juice or an ice pop after medication administration. Do not place medication in a favorite food; the child may refuse the food at a later time.
- Measure small amount of liquid medications using a plastic calibrated syringe. Amounts less than a teaspoon are impossible to measure accurately with a molded medicine cup. (Wong and others, 1999).

Geriatric Considerations

Physiological changes of aging may influence how oral medications are absorbed, distributed, and excreted. Common changes include loss of elasticity in oral mu-

cosa; reduction in parotid gland secretion, causing dry mouth; delayed esophageal clearance, impairing swallowing; reduction in gastric acidity and stomach peristalsis, increasing susceptibility to highly acidic drugs; and reduced colon motility, slowing drug excretion.

- Administer with a full glass of water (unless restricted) to aid passage of the drug. Give client time to swallow.
- Older adults may have several health problems or chronic conditions that require the use of multiple drugs, often prescribed by different health care providers. Polypharmacy creates a high risk for drug interactions and adverse reactions.
- The most common adverse reactions that may occur in older adults are lethargy, sedation, falls, and confusion.
- When instructing clients about their medication regimen, include the client's spouse or caregiver.
- If possible, provide a written medication schedule for client to follow at home (Ebersole and Hess, 1998).

Home Care Considerations

Instruct client in specific information pertaining to drug regimen (purpose, action, dose, dosage intervals, side effects, food to avoid or take with drugs).

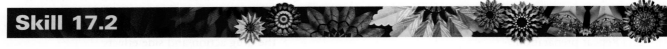

Skill 17.2

Applying Topical Medications

Topical administration of medications involves applying drugs locally to skin, mucous membranes, or tissue membranes. The client is unlikely to experience GI disturbances, and the risk of serious side effects is generally low, although serious systemic effects can occur.

Many topically applied drugs such as lotions, patches, pastes, and ointments can create systemic and local effects if absorbed through the skin. Adhesive-backed medicated patches applied to the skin provide sustained, continuous release of medication over several hours or days. Systemic effects from topical agents can occur if the skin is thin, if drug concentration is high, or if contact with the skin is prolonged.

The skin should be cleansed gently and thoroughly with soap and water before applying topical medications. When applied over skin encrustations, the dead tissues harbor microorganisms and block contact of medications with the tissues to be treated. Simply applying new medications without cleansing does not offer maximum therapeutic benefit.

ASSESSMENT

1. Review physician's order for client's name, name of drug, strength, time of administration, and site of application.
2. Review information pertinent to medication: action, purpose, side effects, and nursing implications.
3. Assess condition of client's skin. Cleanse skin if necessary to visualize adequately. Note if client has symptoms of skin irritation, such as pruritus or burning. *Rationale: Assessment provides baseline to determine change in condition of skin after therapy. Application of certain topical agents can lesson or aggravate these symptoms.*
4. Further inspect the condition of the skin or membranes. Do not administer topical medications to skin whose integrity is altered unless indicated. *Rationale: Break in skin integrity can affect drug absorption. In addition, medication preparation can further irritate or damage non-intact skin.*

5. Determine whether client has a known allergy to latex or topical agent. Ask if client has had reaction to a cream or lotion applied to the skin. *Rationale: Allergic contact dermatitis is relatively common and can intensify existing dermatological condition.*

6. Determine amount of topical agent required for application by assessing skin site, reviewing physician's order, and reading application directions carefully (a thin, even layer is usually adequate). *Rationale: An excessive amount of topical agent can cause chemical irritation of skin, negate drug's effectiveness, and/or cause adverse systemic effects, such as decreased white blood cell counts.*

7. Determine if client is physically able to apply medication by assessing grasp, hand strength, reach, and coordination. *Rationale: This is necessary if client is to self-administer drug in the home.*

PLANNING

Expected outcomes focus on safe, accurate, and effective drug therapy.

Expected Outcomes

1. Client has evidence of improvement in condition (e.g., relief of pain, inflammation, and itching).

2. Client self-administers topical medication or patch correctly.

3. Client explains purpose of medication, dosage schedule, and possible side effects.

Equipment

- Clean gloves (for intact skin) or sterile gloves (for nonintact skin)
- Cotton-tipped applicators or tongue blades
- Ordered agent (powder, cream, ointment, spray, patch)
- Basin of warm water, washcloth, towel, nondrying soap
- Sterile dressing, tape (if needed)
- MAR or computer printout

Delegation Considerations

Periodic evaluation of affected areas is the responsibility of the nurse, and delegation is inappropriate. Application of *some* lotions and ointments to irritated skin or for the protection of the perineum may be delegated to assistive personnel (AP) (check agency policy).

IMPLEMENTATION FOR APPLYING TOPICAL MEDICATIONS

Steps	Rationale
1. See Standard Protocol (inside front cover).	

NURSE ALERT: *Apply six rights of drug administration (see Chapter 16, p. 408).*

Steps	Rationale
2. **Apply topical creams, ointments, and oil-based lotions.**	
a. Expose affected area while keeping unaffected areas covered.	Adequate visualization is necessary for evaluation of the effectiveness of treatment.
b. Wash affected area, removing all debris, encrustations, and previous medication.	Removal of debris enhances penetration of topical drug through skin. Cleansing removes microorganisms resident in remaining debris.
c. In some cases, soaking is needed to remove crusted tissues using plain warm water and rinsing without soap.	Minimizes inflammation and irritation of underlying tissue.
d. Pat skin dry, or allow area to air dry.	Excess moisture can interfere with even application of topical agent.
e. If skin is excessively dry and flaking, apply topical agent while skin is still damp.	Retains moisture within skin layers.
f. Remove gloves, and apply new clean or sterile gloves.	Sterile gloves are used when applying agents to open, noninfectious skin lesions. Disposable gloves prevent cross-contamination of infected or contagious lesions and protect nurse from drug effects.

COMMUNICATION TIP *Tell client what to expect (e.g., "Your skin will feel soothed after the topical application.").*

Steps	Rationale
g. Place approximately 1 to 2 teaspoons of medication in palm of gloved hand and soften by rubbing briskly between hands.	Softening of topical agent makes it easier to apply to skin.
h. Once medication is thin and smooth, smear it evenly over skin surface, using long, even strokes that follow direction of hair growth. Discard gloves, and wash hands.	Ensures even distribution of medication. Technique prevents irritation of hair follicles.
i. Explain to client that skin may feel greasy after application.	Application often contains oil.

3. Apply antianginal (nitroglycerin) ointment.

Steps	Rationale
a. Remove previous dosage paper, and wipe off residual medication with a tissue.	Prevents overdose that can occur with multiple dosage papers or excess medication left in place.
b. Apply desired number of inches of ointment over paper measuring guide (see illustration).	Application of gloves prevents absorption of antianginal ointment on the nurse's skin. Ensures correct dose of medication.
c. Antianginal (nitroglycerin) ointments are usually ordered in inches and can be measured on small sheets of paper marked off in $\frac{1}{2}$-inch markings.	

NURSE ALERT *Unit-dose packages are available. (Warning: One package equals 1 inch; smaller amount should not be measured from this package.)*

Steps	Rationale
d. Antianginal medication may be applied to the chest area, back, upper arm, or legs. Do not apply on hairy surfaces or over scar tissue. If client complains of headaches, apply ointment away from head.	Application on hairy surfaces or scar tissue may interfere with absorption.
e. Be sure to rotate application sites.	Minimizes skin irritation.
f. Apply ointment to skin surface by holding edge or back of the paper wrapper and placing ointment and wrapper directly on the skin (see illustration).	Minimizes chance of ointment covering gloves and later touching nurse's hands.
g. Do not rub or massage ointment into skin.	Medication is designed to absorb slowly over several hours; massaging may increase absorption.
h. Write date, time, and nurse's initials on application paper.	Promotes accuracy.
i. Cover ointment and paper with plastic wrap and tape securely, or follow manufacturer's directions. Discard gloves, and wash hands.	Prevents staining of clothes or accidental removal of the medication (Lilley and Aucker, 2001).

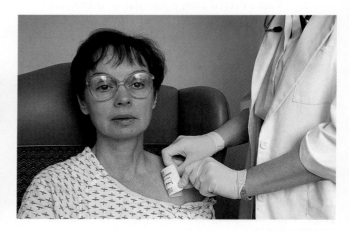

Step 3b Ointment is spread in inches over the measuring guide paper.

Step 3f Nurse applies dosage paper with medication to client's skin.

Steps	Rationale

4. **Apply transdermal patches (e.g., analgesic, nitro-glycerin, nicotine, estrogen)** (see Step 4).

   a. Choose a clean, dry area of the body that is free of hair. Do not attempt to apply the patch on skin that is oily, burned, cut, or irritated in any way.

   b. Carefully remove the patch from its protective covering. Hold the patch by the edge without touching the adhesive edges.

      Rationale: Touching only the edges ensures that the patch will adhere and that the medication dosage has not been changed.

   c. Immediately apply the patch, pressing firmly with the palm of one hand for 10 seconds. Make sure it sticks well, especially around the edges. Date and initial patch, and note time.

      Rationale: Adequate adhesion prevents loss of the patch, which results in decreased dosage and effectiveness. Visual reminders of dose applications prevent missing doses.

NURSE ALERT *Estrogen patches should never be applied to the breast tissue.*

---

   d. Advise clients not to use heating pads anywhere near the site.

      Rationale: Heat increases circulation and the rate of absorption.

   e. After appropriate time, remove the patch and fold it so the medicated side is on the inside. Discard safely according to agency policy. Discard gloves, and wash hands.

      Rationale: Residual medication can be a hazard to children and pets (Willens, 1998).

NURSE ALERT *It is recommended that nitroglycerin transdermal patches be removed after 10 to 12 hours to allow for a nitrate-free interval and reduce the chance of tolerance to the medication. Check with the client's prescriber (Lilley and Aucker, 2001).*

---

   f. Avoid previously used sites for at least 1 week.

      Rationale: Minimizes skin irritation.

   g. Clients should be cautioned not to use alternative forms of medications or drugs when using patches. For example, clients should not smoke while using a nicotine patch. Clients should not apply nitroglycerin ointment in addition to the patch unless specifically ordered to do so by their physician.

      Rationale: Use of patch with an additional/alternative preparation of drug can result in toxicity and other side effects.

5. **Administer aerosol sprays (e.g., local anesthetic sprays).**

   a. Shake container vigorously.

      Rationale: Mixes contents and propellant to ensure distribution of a fine, even spray.

   b. Read container's label for distance recommended to hold spray away from area, usually 6 to 12 inches (15 to 30 cm).

      Rationale: Proper distance ensures fine spray hits skin surface. Holding container too close results in thin, watery distribution.

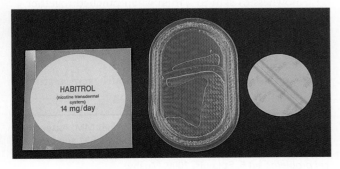

Step 4 A variety of medications are available as transdermal (skin) patches.

Steps	Rationale
c. If neck or upper chest is to be sprayed, ask client to turn face away from spray or briefly cover face with towel.	Prevents inhalation of spray.
d. Spray medication evenly over affected site (in some cases, spray is timed for period of seconds).	Entire affected area of skin should be covered with thin spray.
6. Apply suspension-based lotion.	
a. Shake container vigorously.	Mixes powder throughout liquid to form well-mixed suspension.
b. Apply small amount of lotion to small gauze dressing or pad, and apply to skin by stroking evenly in direction of hair growth.	Method of application leaves protective film of powder on skin after water base of suspension dries. Technique prevents irritation of hair follicles.
c. Explain to client that area will feel cool and dry.	Water evaporates to leave thin layer of powder.
7. Apply medicated powder.	
a. Be sure skin surface is thoroughly dry.	Minimizes caking and crusting of powder.
b. Fully spread apart any skin folds such as between toes or under axilla.	Fully exposes skin surface for application.
c. Dust skin site lightly using dispenser so that area is covered with fine, thin layer of powder.	Thin layer of powder is more absorbent and reduces friction by increasing area of moisture evaporation.
d. Cover skin area with dressing if ordered by physician.	May help prevent agent from being rubbed off skin. Protects clothing from being stained.
8. Instruct client to dispose of applicators, patches, and similar materials into cardboard or plastic disposable containers. Remove and dispose of gloves when appropriate.	Careful disposal is necessary to ensure the safety of client, others, pets, and children.
9. See Completion Protocol (inside front cover).	

• • • • • • • • • •

EVALUATION

1. Inspect condition of skin between applications to determine if skin condition improves.
2. Observe client applying topical medication or patch.
3. Ask the client or significant other to name the medication and its purpose, dosage, schedule, and side effects.

Unexpected Outcomes and Related Interventions

1. Skin site may appear inflamed and edematous with blistering and oozing of fluid from lesions, indicating subacute inflammation or eczema that can develop from worsening of skin lesions. Notify prescriber.
2. Client continues to complain of pruritus and tenderness.
   a. Indicates slow or impaired healing.
   b. Notify prescriber; alternative therapies may be needed.
3. Client is unable to explain information about topical application or does not administer as prescribed.
   a. Identify possible reasons for noncompliance.
   b. Explore alternative approaches or options.

Recording and Reporting

• Describe objective data (appearance of abnormal skin, including size, shape, and characteristics of lesions).
• Include subjective data such as pain and itching.

• Report and record changes in appearance and condition of skin lesions.

Sample Documentation

0930 Skin on the back of both hands and wrists is dry, red, and flaky. Client complains of itching. Hydrocortisone cream 1% applied sparingly to affected areas as prescribed. 1000 Client reported itching is relieved.

❖ SPECIAL CONSIDERATIONS ❖

Geriatric Considerations

Handle older persons gently, and observe for changes that may occur in the skin of the older client including:
• Increased wrinkling
• Slowness of skin to flatten when pinched together (tenting)
• Dry, flaking skin with possible signs of excoriation caused by pruritus
• Increased tendency to bruise
• Diminished awareness of pain, touch, temperature
• Diminished rate of wound healing

Modified from Lewis SM, Collier IC, Heitkemper MM: Assessment and management of clinical problems. In Lewis SM and others: *Medical-surgical nursing: assessment and management of clinical problems,* ed 5, St Louis, 2000, Mosby.

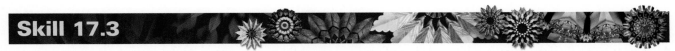

Skill 17.3

Instilling Eye and Ear Medications

Eye (ophthalmic) medications commonly used by clients include both drops and ointments. Recently intraocular disks have been developed as a third type of medication delivery option. Medications delivered this way resemble a contact lens. The disk is placed into the conjunctival sac, where it remains in place for up to 1 week.

Many clients receive prescribed ophthalmic drugs after cataract extraction and for eye conditions such as glaucoma. Eye medications come in a variety of concentrations. Instilling the wrong concentration may cause local irritation to eyes, as well as systemic effects. Certain eye medications that dilate or constrict the pupil, such as mydriatics and cycloplegics, temporarily blur a client's vision. Use of the wrong drug concentration can prolong these undesirable effects.

Orders will indicate administration to one or both eyes, and abbreviations are often used to indicate the site. The abbreviation for right eye is O.D.; left eye, O.S.; and both eyes, O.U.

The eye is extremely sensitive because the cornea is richly supplied with sensitive nerve fibers to protect the eye. The conjunctival sac is much less sensitive and thus a more appropriate site for medication instillation. Care must be taken to prevent instilling medication directly onto the sensitive cornea.

Clients receiving topical eye medication should learn correct self-administration of the medication. Clients with glaucoma, for example, usually require lifelong eye drops for control of their disease. At times it may become necessary for family members to learn how to administer eye drops or ointment, particularly immediately after eye surgery, when clients' vision is so impaired that it is difficult for them to assemble needed supplies and handle applicators correctly.

Medications used in the ear are usually in a solution and instilled by drops. Internal ear structures are very sensitive to temperature extremes, and therefore solutions are administered at room temperature. When drops are instilled cold from a refrigerator, the client may experience vertigo (severe dizziness) or nausea.

Although structures of the outer ear are not sterile, it is wise to use sterile drops and solutions because the eardrum could be ruptured without the awareness of the client or nurse. Introduction of nonsterile solutions into the middle ear can cause serious infection.

Avoid forcing solution into the ear or occluding the ear canal with a medicine dropper, because medication administered under pressure within the canal can injure the eardrum.

ASSESSMENT

1. Review physician's medication order, including client's name, drug name, concentration, number of drops (if a liquid), time, and eye/ear that is to receive the medication.

2. Review information pertinent to medication, including action, purpose, side effects, and nursing implications. Tell clients receiving mydriatics or cycloplegics that vision will be temporarily blurred, and that photophobia (sensitivity to light) may occur. They should temporarily not drive or attempt to perform any activity that requires acute vision, or sensitivity to light. *Rationale: Injury or accidents may result from temporarily reduced vision.*

3. Assess condition of external eye or ear structures (see Chapter 13). *Rationale: This may also be done just before drug instillation to provide a baseline to determine later if local response to medications occurs. This also indicates the need to clean the area before drug application.*

4. Determine whether client has symptoms of discomfort or hearing or visual impairment. *Rationale: Certain eye medications can act to either lessen or increase symptoms. Occlusion of external ear canal by swelling, drainage, or cerumen can impair hearing acuity and is painful. Nurse must be able to recognize changes in client's condition.*

5. Determine whether client has any known allergies to medications. Also, ask if client has allergies to latex, if using latex gloves.

6. Assess client's level of consciousness and ability to follow instructions. *Rationale: Client must lie still during drug administration. Sudden movements can cause injury from eye or ear dropper.*

7. Assess client's knowledge regarding drug therapy and desire to self-administer medication. Assess client's ability to manipulate and hold dropper. *Rationale: Client's level of understanding may indicate need for health teaching. Motivation influences teaching approach. Reflects client's ability to learn to self-administer medication.*

PLANNING

Expected outcomes focus on relief of symptoms without unpleasant adverse reactions.

Expected Outcomes

1. Symptoms (e.g., irritation, intraocular pressure) are relieved.
2. Client denies unpleasant side effects or adverse reactions.

3. Client describes medication effects and technique of application.
4. Client correctly demonstrates self-installation of eye drops, ear drops.

Equipment

- Appropriate medication (eye drops with sterile dropper, ointment tube, medicated intraocular disk, or ear drops)
- Cotton-tipped applicator, cotton balls or tissue
- Warm water and washcloth
- Disposable clean gloves
- Eye patch and tape (optional)

Delegation Considerations

Administration of eye and ear drops requires the critical thinking and knowledge application unique to a nurse and should not be delegated to assistive personnel (AP). AP should be instructed about potential side effects of medications and to report their occurrence. In addition, the care providers should be notified if vision impairment is possible after administration of eye medications.

IMPLEMENTATION FOR INSTILLING EYE AND EAR MEDICATIONS

Steps	Rationale
1. See Standard Protocol (inside front cover).	
2. Compare MAR with label of eye/ear medication.	Verifies correct concentration of drug.

NURSE ALERT *Review six rights of drug administration (see Chapter 16, p. 408).*

Ensures correct client receives medication.

Steps	Rationale
3. Explain procedure to client. Clients experienced in self-instillation may be allowed to give drops under nurse's supervision (check agency policy).	Clients often become anxious about medication being instilled into eye because of potential discomfort.
4. For eye medications, ask client to lie supine or sit back in chair with neck slightly hyperextended.	Position provides easy access to eye/ear for medication instillation. Correct positioning minimizes drainage of eye medication into tear duct.
5. If crusting or drainage is present along eyelid margins or inner canthus, gently wash away from inner to outer canthus. If indicated, soak any crusting with a damp washcloth for several minutes.	Cleansing eye from inner to outer canthus avoids introducing microorganisms into lacrimal ducts. Soaking allows easy removal of crusts that harbor microorganisms.

NURSE ALERT *Do not hyperextend the neck of a client with a cervical neck injury.*

Steps	Rationale
6. Instill eye drops.	
a. Hold clean tissue in nondominant hand on client's cheekbone just below lower eyelid.	Tissue absorbs medication that escapes eye. Avoid cotton balls, which may leave fibers that may get into the eyes.
b. With tissue resting below lower lid, gently press downward with thumb or forefinger against bony orbit, exposing conjunctival sac (see illustration).	Prevents pressure and trauma to eyeball and prevents fingers from touching eye.
c. Ask client to look at ceiling.	Moves the sensitive cornea up and away from conjunctival sac and reduces stimulation of blink reflex.
d. Rest dominant hand gently on client's forehead, and hold filled medication eyedropper approximately 1 to 2 cm (½ to ¾ inch) above conjunctival sac.	Resting hand helps prevent accidental contact of eyedropper with eye and reduces risk of injury and transfer of microorganisms to dropper. Contact of eyedropper with eye contaminates the container (ophthalmic medications are sterile).

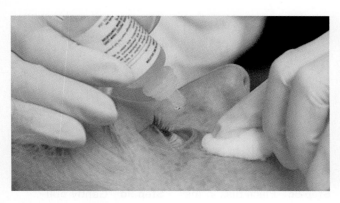

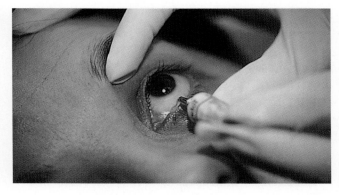

Step 6b   Instilling eye drops into the conjunctival sac.

Step 7b   Applying eye ointment along the inside edge of the lower eyelid on the conjunctiva from the inner to outer canthus.

Steps	Rationale
e. Drop prescribed number of medication drops into conjunctival sac.	Conjunctival sac normally holds 1 or 2 drops. Applying drops to sac provides even distribution of medication across eye.
f. If client blinks or closes eye or if drops land on outer lid margins, repeat procedure.	Therapeutic effect of drug is obtained only when drops enter conjunctival sac.
g. When administering drugs that may cause systemic effects, apply gentle pressure to client's nasolacrimal duct with a cotton ball or tissue for 30 to 60 seconds. Avoid pressure directly against client's eyeball.	Prevents overflow of medication into nasal and pharyngeal passages. Minimizes absorption into systemic circulation.
h. After instilling drops, ask client to close eyes gently. Discard gloves, and wash hands.	Helps to distribute medication. Squinting or squeezing of eyelids forces medication from conjunctival sac. Distributes medication evenly across eye and lid margin.

7. Instill eye ointment.

a.   Ask client to look up.

Moves the sensitive cornea up and away from the conjunctival sac and reduces stimulation of the blink reflex during ointment application.

b. Apply thin stream of ointment along upper lid margin on inner conjunctiva (see illustration).

Distributes medication evenly across eye and lid margin.

c. Have client close eye, and rub lid lightly in circular motion with cotton ball, if rubbing is not contraindicated.

Further distributes medication without traumatizing eye. Avoid pressure directly against client's eyeball.

d. If excess medication is on eyelid, gently wipe it from inner to outer canthus.

Promotes comfort and prevents trauma to eye.

8. If client needs an eye patch, apply clean one by placing it over affected eye so entire eye is covered. Tape securely without applying pressure to eye (see illustration).

Clean eye patch reduces chance of infection.

9. Intraocular disk application

a. Open package containing the disk. Gently press your fingertip against the disk so that it adheres to your finger. Position the convex side of the disk on your fingertip. It may be necessary to moisten gloved finger with sterile saline.

Allows nurse to inspect disk for damage or deformity.

b. With your other hand, gently pull the client's lower eyelid away from his eye. Ask client to look up.

Prepares conjunctival sac for receiving medicated disk and moves sensitive cornea away.

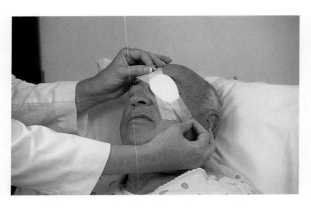

Step 8 Application of eye patch.

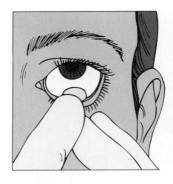

Step 9c Place disk in the conjunctival sac between the iris and lower eyelid.

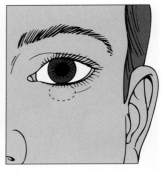

Step 9d Gently pull lower eyelid over the disk.

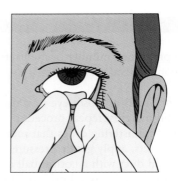

Step 10b Carefully pinch the disk to remove it from client's eye.

Steps	Rationale
c. Place the disk in the conjunctival sac, so that it floats on the sclera between the iris and lower eyelid (see illustration).	Ensures delivery of medication.
d. Pull the client's lower eyelid out and over the disk. You should not be able to see the disk at this time. Repeat if you can see the disk (see illustration).	Ensures accurate medication delivery.
10. Remove intraocular disk.	
a. Gently pull downward on the lower eyelid.	Exposes the disk.
b. Using your forefinger and thumb of your opposite hand, pinch the disk and lift it out of the client's eye (see illustration).	
c. If excess medication is on eyelid, gently wipe it from inner to outer canthus.	Promotes comfort and prevents trauma to eye.
d. If client had eye patch, apply clean one by placing it over affected eye so entire eye is covered. Tape securely without applying pressure to eye.	Clean eye patch reduces chance of infection.
11. Instill ear drops.	

NURSE ALERT: *Apply the six rights of medication administration (see Chapter 16, p. 408).*

---

a. Apply gloves if drainage is present.

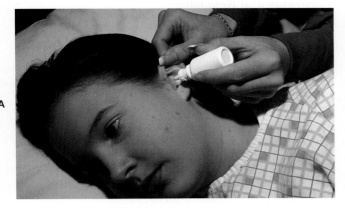
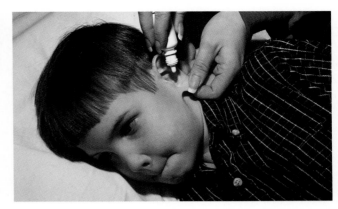

Step 11d A, Pull the pinna up and back for adults and children over age 3 years. **B,** Pull the pinna down and back for children age 3 years or less. (From Lilley LL, Aucker RS: *Pharmacology and the nursing process,* ed 3, St Louis, 2001, Mosby.)

Steps	Rationale
b. Warm ear drops to body temperature. Hold bottle in hands or place in warm water.	Ear structures are very sensitive to temperature extremes.
c. Position client on side or sitting in a chair with affected ear facing up.	
d. Straighten ear canal by pulling auricle upward and outward (adult or child over age 3 years) or down and back (child) (see illustrations).	Straightening of ear canal provides direct access to deeper external ear structures.
e. If cerumen or drainage occludes outermost portion of ear canal, wipe out gently with cotton-tipped applicator, taking care not to force wax inward.	Cerumen and drainage harbor microorganisms and can block distribution of medication into canal. Occlusion blocks sound transmission.
f. Instill prescribed drops holding dropper 1 cm (½ inch) above ear canal.	Avoiding contact avoids contamination of the dropper, which could contaminate the medication in the container.
g. Ask client to remain in side-lying position 5 to 10 minutes, and apply gentle massage or pressure to tragus of ear with finger.	Allows complete distribution of medication. Pressure and massage move medication inward.
h. If ordered, gently insert a portion of cotton ball into outermost part of canal.	Prevents escape of medication when client sits or stands.
i. Remove cotton after 15 minutes.	Allows adequate time for drug distribution and absorption.

12. See Completion Protocol (inside front cover).

• • • • • • • • • •

EVALUATION

1. Observe effects of medication by assessing desired changes.
2. Note client's response to instillation and observe for side effects, and ask if any discomfort was felt.
3. Ask client to discuss drug's purpose, action, side effects, and technique of administration.
4. Observe client demonstrate self-administration of next dose.

Unexpected Outcomes and Related Interventions

1. Client complains of burning or pain after administration of eye drops.

   a. Use greater caution during next instillation to instill drops into conjunctival sac and not onto the cornea.

2. Client experiences local side effects, for example, headache, bloodshot eyes, and local eye irritation.

   a. Drug concentration and client's sensitivity both influence chances of side effects developing.

3. Client experiences systemic effects from eye drops, for example, increased heart rate and blood pressure from epinephrine or decreased heart rate and blood pressure from timolol.

   a. Systemic absorption through tear duct can cause potentially dangerous effects. Local anesthetics and antibiotics may cause anaphylaxis.

4. Client experienced increased ear pain. Rupture of eardrum may have occurred.
   a. Notify prescriber immediately.
5. Ear canal remains occluded with cerumen.
   a. Irrigation may be required.
6. Client lacks confidence or ability to instill medication without supervision.
   a. If client is unable to manipulate the dropper or is unable to see, instruct a family member in the technique.

Recording and Reporting

- Include objective data related to condition of tissues involved (redness, drainage, irritation) and subjective data (discomfort, itching, altered vision or hearing).
- Include evaluation related to desired effects of medications instilled and evidence of any side effects experienced.

Sample Documentation

1300 Cyclopentolate ophthalmic 1% solution, 2 drops instilled in each eye. No side effects of tachycardia, drowsiness, or confusion noted.

SPECIAL CONSIDERATIONS

Pediatric Considerations

- When instilling drops in an infant or young child, have parent gently restrain child's head with child in parent's lap. Be sure that the child's hands do not interfere with instillation.
- Infants often clench the eyes tightly to avoid eye drops. To administer drops in an uncooperative infant, with the head gently restrained, place the drops at the nasal corner where the lids meet. When the infant opens the eye, the medication will flow into the eye.
- Cotton pledgets may be used to prevent medication from flowing out of external canal. They should be inserted loosely enough to allow any discharge to exit from ear. To prevent cotton from absorbing medication in ear, premoisten cotton with a few drops of medication (Wong and others, 1999).

Geriatric Considerations

Many older adults experience excessive accumulation of cerumen in the ear. This should be removed before administration of medication.

Home Care Considerations

- Clients with chronic health problems should consult with their health care provider before using OTC eye medications.
- When using prescribed or OTC eye drops, clients should not share medications with other family members. Risk of infection transmission is high.

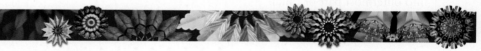

Skill 17.4

Using Metered-Dose Inhalers

Metered-dose inhalers (MDIs) are handheld inhalers that dispense a measured dose of aerosol spray, mist, or fine powder to penetrate lung airways. The deeper passages of the respiratory tract provide a large surface area for drug absorption. The alveolar-capillary network absorbs medication rapidly.

Inhaled medications are designed to produce local effects; for example, bronchodilators open narrowed bronchioles, and mucolytic agents liquefy thick mucous secretions. However, because these medications are absorbed rapidly through the pulmonary circulation, most create systemic side effects. For example, isoproterenol (Isuprel) dilates bronchioles and can also cause cardiac dysrhythmias.

Clients who receive drugs by inhalation frequently have chronic respiratory disease, and because clients depend on medications for airway management, they need to know how to administer them safely. It is NOT appropriate to try to teach a client how to use an inhaler during an episode of shortness of breath, because the client's ability to learn is greatly diminished.

Drugs can be delivered by MDIs, which deliver a measured dose of drug with each push of a canister. Because use of an MDI requires coordination during the breathing cycle, clients may spray only the back of their throats and not receive a full dose. The inhaler must be depressed to expel medication just as the client inhales. This ensures the medication reaches the lower airways. Difficulty with coordination can be resolved by the use of spacer devices or the use of a breath-activated MDI (Weilitz and Van Sciver, 2000).

ASSESSMENT

1. Assess respiratory pattern and auscultate breath sounds. *Rationale: Establishes baseline of airway status for comparison during and after treatment.*
2. Assess client's ability to hold, manipulate, and depress canister and inhaler. *Rationale: Impairment of grasp or presence of tremors of hands interferes with client's ability to depress canister within inhaler.*
3. Assess client's readiness to learn: client asks questions about medication, disease, or complications; client requests education in use of inhaler; is mentally alert; client participates in own care.
4. Assess client's ability to learn: client should not be fatigued, in pain, or in respiratory distress; assess level of understanding of terms.
5. Assess client's knowledge and understanding of disease and purpose and action of prescribed medications. *Rationale: May assist in assessing client's potential for compliance with self-administration.*
6. Assess physician's order for drug schedule and number of inhalations prescribed for each dose.

PLANNING

Expected outcomes focus on relief of symptoms and promoting knowledge for self-administration of inhalers.

Expected Outcomes

1. Client manipulates mouthpiece, canister, and inhaler correctly and cleans inhaler after use.
2. Client describes proper time during respiratory cycle to inhale spray and number of inhalations for each administration.

3. Client experiences effects of medication within 10 to 15 minutes, which validates proper administration technique.
4. Client lists side effects of medications and criteria for calling health care professional if dyspnea develops.

Equipment (Figure 17-3)

- MDI with medication canister
- Spacer device, such as AeroChamber or InspirEase (optional)
- Facial tissues (optional)
- MAR or computer printout
- Stethoscope

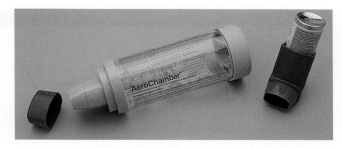

Figure 17-3   Example of an MDI spacer device *(left)* and MDI *(right).*

 Delegation Considerations

Administration of metered-dose inhalers requires the critical thinking and knowledge application unique to the nurse and should not be delegated to assistive personnel (AP). AP should be instructed about potential side effects of medications and to report their occurrence.

IMPLEMENTATION FOR USING METERED-DOSE INHALERS

Steps	Rationale
1. See Standard Protocol (inside front cover).	
NURSE ALERT *Review six rights of drug administration (see Chapter 16, p. 408).*	
2. Allow client opportunity to manipulate inhaler, canister, and spacer device. Explain and demonstrate how canister fits into inhaler.	Client must be familiar with how to assemble and use equipment.
3. Explain what metered dose is, and warn client about overuse of inhaler, including drug side effects.	Client needs to know the dangers of excessive inhalations because of risk of serious side effects. If drug is given in recommended doses, side effects are minimal.
4. Remove mouthpiece cover from inhaler.	
5. Shake inhaler well for 2 to 5 seconds.	Ensures mixing of medication in canister.

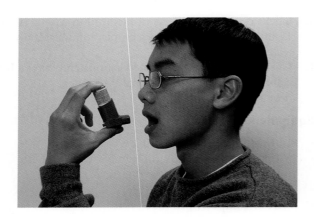

Step 6　Using an MDI.

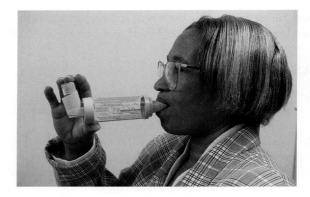

Step 7　Use of an MDI with a spacer device.

Steps	Rationale
6. *Without spacer device:* Have client take a deep breath and exhale completely. Open lips and place inhaler 1 to 2 cm ($\frac{1}{2}$ to 1 inch) from mouth with opening toward back of throat. Lips should not touch inhaler (see illustration).	Avoids rapid influx of inhaled medication and subsequent airway irritation. Positioning the mouthpiece 1 to 2 cm from the mouth is considered the best way to deliver the medication without a spacer.
7. *With spacer device:* Exhale fully, then grasp spacer mouthpiece with teeth and lips while holding inhaler with thumb at the bottom of spacer and fingers at the top of inhaler (see illustration).	Spacers are recommended because the device allows particles of medication to "ride" the breath into the airways rather than hit the back of the throat (Owen, 1999).
8. Instruct client to tilt head back slightly, inhale slowly and deeply through mouth, and depress medication canister fully.	Medication is distributed to airways during inhalation.
9. Breathe in slowly for 2 to 3 seconds. Hold breath for approximately 10 seconds.	As client inhales, particles of medication are delivered to airway. Holding breath allows tiny drops of aerosol spray to reach deeper branches of airways.
10. Exhale slowly through pursed lips.	Pursed-lip breathing keeps small airways open during exhalation.
11. Instruct client to wait 2 to 5 minutes between puffs. More than one puff is usually prescribed.	First inhalation opens airways and reduces inflammation. Second or third inhalations penetrate deeper airways.
12. If more than one type of inhaled medications is prescribed, wait 5 to 10 minutes between inhalations or as ordered by physician.	Drugs are prescribed at intervals during day to promote bronchodilation and minimize side effects.

COMMUNICATION TIP　*Explain that there should not be a gagging sensation in the throat. These sensations occur when inhalant is used incorrectly.*

13. If steroid medications are administered via MDI, instruct client to rinse mouth.	Removing medication residue from oral cavity area reduces risk of oral yeast infection (oral candidiasis).
14. Instruct client to remove medication canister, and clean inhaler in warm water after each use.	Accumulation of spray around the mouthpiece can interfere with proper distribution during use.
15. Instruct client against repeating inhalations before next scheduled dose.	Drugs are prescribed at intervals during the day to provide constant drug levels and minimize side effects.
16. Teach client to measure the amount of medication remaining in the canister by immersing it in a large bowl or pan of water. The position the canister takes in the water determines the amount remaining (see illustration).	
17. See Completion Protocol (inside front cover).	

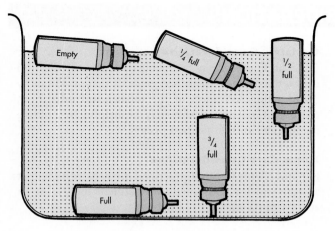

Step 16 Measuring the amount of medication remaining in the inhaler canister by immersion in water.

• • • • • • • • • •

EVALUATION

1. Have client explain and demonstrate steps in use of inhaler.
2. Ask client to explain drug schedule and dose of medication.
3. After medication instillation, assess client's respirations and auscultate lungs.
4. Ask client to list side effects and criteria for calling physician.

Unexpected Outcomes and Related Interventions

1. Client's breathing pattern is ineffective; respirations are rapid and shallow. Client's need for a bronchodilator more than every 4 hours can signal respiratory problems.
   a. Reassess type of medication or delivery method. Make sure client shakes canister before administration.
   b. Determine fullness of canister, using displacement in water.
   c. Wait adequate time between puffs to allow deeper penetration into the lungs.
   d. Observe whether the canister is releasing a spray. If not, the valve may need to be cleaned.
2. Client experiences gags or paroxysms of coughing from inability to inhale.
   a. Reinstruct on proper way to inhale.
3. Client is experiencing cardiac dysrhythmias. Signs and symptoms of overuse of xanthines and sympathomimetic drugs include tachycardia, palpitations, headache, restlessness, and insomnia.
   a. Notify physician; monitor heart rate and rhythm.

4. Client is unable to depress medication canister because of weakened grasp or presses the canister before or after taking a breath. Both should be done simultaneously for maximum effectiveness.
   a. Client may need practice with assistance for several different steps of procedure before being able to perform each skill independently.
   b. Alternative delivery routes or methods may need to be explored.

Recording and Reporting

- Include objective data related to the desired effects of the MDI (e.g., respiratory rate and pattern and breath sounds).
- Include evidence of side effects (e.g., heart rate, client's description of feelings experienced [anxiety and others]).
- Include ability to demonstrate correct use of the MDI.

Sample Documentation

0900 Coughing violently and reports difficulty breathing. Wheezing noted throughout all lung fields. Respirations 32/min, pulse 98. Self-administered MDI (2 puffs) correctly with no verbal coaching. Reported relief from shortness of breath within 1 minute. Respirations 24/min, pulse 96.

SPECIAL CONSIDERATIONS

Pediatric Considerations

- Because of difficulty with coordination of activating inhaler and inhaling, the use of a spacer device is recommended for young children (Wong and others, 1999).
- Educate child and parent about the need to use inhaler during school hours. Help family find resources within the school or day care facility. Keep in mind that many school systems do not permit self-administration of MDIs. Follow the school's policy regarding having the MDI available for use during school hours. A physician's order may be necessary.

Geriatric Considerations

Older adult client may be unable to depress medication canister because of weakened grasp. If there is difficulty coordinating activation of the inhaler and inhalation, the use of a spacer device may be helpful by holding medication until inhalation occurs.

Home Care Considerations

Remind clients to carry prescribed inhalers with them at all times to use as immediate treatment in case of an acute asthma attack.

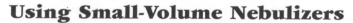

Skill 17.5

Using Small-Volume Nebulizers

Nebulization is a process of adding medications or moisture to inspired air by mixing particles of various sizes with air. Adding moisture to the respiratory system through nebulization may improve clearance of pulmonary secretions. Medications such as bronchodilators, mucolytics, and corticosteroids are often administered by nebulization. Small-volume nebulizers provide medications in an aerosolized form that can be inhaled by the client into the tracheobronchial tree and possibly into the bloodstream through the alveoli. As a result, systemic effects from the medications may occur.

Clients who receive drugs by nebulization frequently suffer from chronic lung disease characterized by airway hyperreactivity or constriction. Because clients depend on these medications for adequate oxygenation, they must learn how they work and how to administer them safely.

ASSESSMENT

1. Assess client's medical history, history of allergies, and medication history. *Rationale: These factors can influence how certain drugs act. Information also reflects client's need for medications.*
2. Assess client's ability to assemble, hold, and manipulate the nebulizer equipment. *Rationale: Impaired grasp or presence of hand tremors interferes with client's ability to use the equipment.*
3. Assess drug ordered, including amount, type, and amount of diluent (if unit dose is not available), and frequency. *Rationale: Unit-dose medications do not require dilution; however, a diluent may be used along with*

a unit-dose medication if a different percentage of drug is desired.

4. Assess pulse, respirations, and breath sounds before beginning treatment. *Rationale: Establishes a baseline for comparison during and after treatment.*

PLANNING

Expected outcomes focus on relief of symptoms and promoting knowledge for self-administration of small-volume nebulizers.

Expected Outcomes

1. Client's vital signs trend toward normal baseline.
2. Client describes techniques for use of small-volume nebulizers.
3. Client correctly self-administers medication using small-volume nebulizer.
4. Client correctly describes care of and cleaning of small-volume nebulizer and equipment.
5. Client lists side effects of medications and criteria for calling health care professional if dyspnea develops.

Equipment

- Medication ordered
- Diluent (if needed)
- Nebulizer bottle and tubing assembly
- Small-volume nebulizer machine (often called hand-held nebulizer or, simply, nebulizer)
- Stethoscope

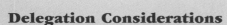

Delegation Considerations

The skill of administering medications by nebulizer requires the critical thinking and knowledge application unique to a nurse. In many institutions the respiratory therapist, as well as the nurse, perform administration of nebulizer medications. Because of the purpose of the prescribed medication and potential need for instructions to promote correct use of the small-volume nebulizer, this skill requires the critical thinking and knowledge application of a nurse and should not be delegated to assistive personnel (AP). Instruct AP on the side effects to report, should they develop.

IMPLEMENTATION FOR USING SMALL-VOLUME NEBULIZERS

Steps	Rationale
1. See Standard Protocol (inside front cover).	

NURSE ALERT *Review the six rights of drug administration (see Chapter 16, p. 408).*

Steps	Rationale
2. Explain the use of the nebulizer, and describe possible drug side effects (see illustration on p. 450).	Helps to make the client more knowledgeable about the treatment and the medication.

NURSE ALERT *Some respiratory medications can cause systemic effects such as restlessness, nervousness, and palpitations. Administer these medications with caution to clients with cardiac disease because of the possibility of hypertension, dysrhythmias, or coronary insufficiency. If severe bronchospasm occurs during treatment, discontinue drug immediately, and notify physician.*

COMMUNICATION TIP *Do not try to teach client how to use a nebulizer during an episode of shortness of breath.*

Steps	Rationale
3. Assemble the nebulizer equipment per manufacturer's directions.	Assembly may vary slightly with different manufacturers. Proper assembly ensures safe delivery of medication.
4. Add the prescribed medication and diluent (if needed) to the nebulizer.	Ensures proper dosage and delivery of ordered medication.
5. Have client hold the mouthpiece between the lips with gentle pressure (see illustration).	
a. A face mask is used for a child, an infant, or an adult who is fatigued, who cannot follow instructions, or who is unable to follow instructions.	Use of a face mask does not require the client to remember to hold mouthpiece correctly. Correct delivery ensures sufficient deposition of medication.
b. Use special adaptors for clients with a tracheostomy.	
6. Have client take a deep breath, slowly, to a volume slightly greater than normal. After inspiration have the client pause briefly, then have the client exhale passively.	Promotes greater deposition of medication in the airways.
a. If client is dyspneic, encourage client to hold every fourth or fifth breath for 5 to 10 seconds.	Improves effectiveness of medication.

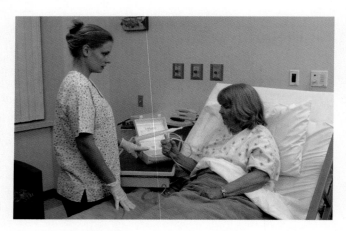

Step 2 Small-volume nebulizer machine, tubing, reservoir, and mouthpiece.

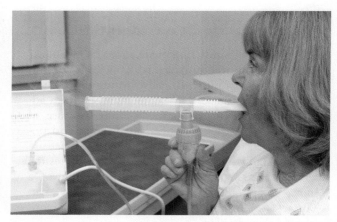

Step 5 Nebulizer mouthpiece placed between client's lips during treatment.

Steps	Rationale
7. Turn on the small-volume nebulizer machine, and ensure that a sufficient mist is formed.	Verifies that the equipment is working properly during delivery of medication.
a. Tap the nebulizer cup occasionally during treatment and toward the end of the treatment.	Releases droplets that may be clinging to the side of the cup, thus allowing for renebulization of the solution.
b. Remind client to repeat the breathing pattern described in Step 7 until the drug is completely nebulized. Some practitioners prefer to set a time limit as the length of the treatment (e.g., 20 minutes) rather than waiting for the medication to completely nebulize.	Maximizes effectiveness of medication.
c. Monitor client's pulse for tachycardia during procedure, especially if beta-adrenergics are used.	To observe for potential side effects of medications.
8. When medication is completely nebulized and liquid is gone, turn off machine and store tubing assembly per agency policy.	Proper storage reduces transfer of microorganisms.
a. Shake the nebulizer bottle, attempting to remove all remaining solution.	Tap water may contain microorganisms.
b. Teach client not to store medication in nebulizer for later use (Ashwill and Droske, 1997).	Stored medication may contain microorganisms, and medication may lose effectiveness.
9. If steroids are nebulized, encourage client to rinse mouth and gargle with warm water after nebulizer treatment.	Removes medication residue from oral cavity and helps to prevent thrush, a possible side effect of therapy with these drugs.
10. See Completion Protocol (inside front cover).	

• • • • • • • • • •

EVALUATION

1. Assess client's pulse, respiratory rate, and breath sounds after procedure.
2. Have client describe techniques for use of small-volume nebulizers.
3. Observe while client self-administers medication using small-volume nebulizer.
4. Ask client to explain and demonstrate care of and cleaning of small-volume nebulizer and equipment.
5. Ask client to describe side effects of medications and criteria for calling physician.

Unexpected Outcomes and Related Interventions

1. Client's breathing pattern is ineffective; respirations are rapid and shallow.
   a. Reassess type of medication or delivery method.
2. Client experiences paroxysms of coughing.
   Aerosolized particles irritate posterior pharynx.
   a. Notify prescriber; may need to reassess type of medication or delivery method.
3. Client experiences cardiac dysrhythmias. Client may experience side effects from medication.
   a. Notify prescriber; monitor heart rate and rhythm.

4. Client is unable to self-administer medication properly.
   a. Alternative delivery routes or methods may need to be explored.
5. Client is unable to explain technique and risks of drug therapy.
   a. Further teaching may be required.
   b. Include family in any instruction; they can serve as coaches.

Recording and Reporting

- Record the drug used, the dosage and concentration, and the time and date of administration on the MAR or computer printout immediately after administration.
- Record the client's baseline pulse, respirations, and breath sounds.
- Record the client's response to the medication, including pulse, respirations, and breath sounds assessed.
- Document skills taught and client's ability to perform them.

Sample Documentation

0900 Client reports that he "cannot catch his breath" after getting up to the bathroom. Dyspnea noted, with respiration rate 32, pulse 95, and scattered wheezes throughout lung fields. Albuterol 2.5 mg given by nebulizer over 20 minutes. Postnebulizer respiration rate 26, pulse 102, wheezes decreased. Client states he is "breathing easier now."

 SPECIAL CONSIDERATIONS

Pediatric Considerations
- A mask may be used for the nebulizer treatment if the child is too young to hold the mouthpiece correctly for the duration of the treatment.
- Instruct the child to breathe normally with the mouth open to provide a direct route to the airways for the medication (Wong and others, 1999).
- Use a peak flowmeter before and after the treatment to monitor the child's airway status (Schultz, 2000).
- Educate child and parent about the need to use nebulizer during school or day care hours. Help family find resources within the school or day care facility. Follow the school's policy regarding having the nebulizer and medication available for use during school hours. A physician's order may be necessary

Home Care Considerations
- When used at home, the nebulizer parts should be rinsed after each use with clear water and air dried. In addition, the parts should be cleaned daily with warm, soapy water, rinsed, and allowed to dry.

- Once a week the nebulizer parts should be soaked in a solution of vinegar and water (one part white vinegar to four parts water) for 30 minutes, rinsed thoroughly with clean water, and air dried. Nebulizer parts should never be stored until totally dried. Wet equipment encourages the growth of bacteria and mold (Ashwill and Droske, 1997).
- Follow manufacturer's recommendations for maintenance of small-volume nebulizer machine, including changing the filters when they become discolored (grayish).
- Advise clients taking long-acting beta-agonists, which are used for long-term control of symptoms, about possible adverse effects: nervousness, restlessness, tremor, headache, nausea, rapid or pounding heart rate, and dizziness. Emphasize that the drug should only be taken as ordered so that a tolerance to the drug is not developed (Owen, 1999).

Skill 17.6

Inserting Rectal and Vaginal Medications

Drugs administered rectally may exert either a local effect on GI mucosa, such as promoting defecation, or systemic effects, such as relieving nausea or providing analgesia. The rectal route is not as reliable as oral or parenteral routes in terms of drug absorption and distribution. However, the medications are relatively safe and rarely cause local irritation or side effects. Rectal medications are contraindicated in clients who have had rectal surgery or have active rectal bleeding.

Female clients may develop vaginal infections requiring topical application of antiinfective agents. Vaginal medications are available in foam, jelly, cream, or suppository form. Medicated irrigations or douches can also be given. However, their excessive use can lead to vaginal irritation.

Suppositories come individually packaged in foil wrappers and are usually stored in a refrigerator to prevent melting. *Caution:* Rectal and vaginal suppositories may be stored together in a refrigerator. Rectal suppositories are thinner than vaginal suppositories and bullet shaped. The rounded end prevents anal trauma during insertion. During administration, the nurse places the suppository past the internal sphincter and against the rectal mucosa.

After a suppository is inserted into either the rectum or vagina, body temperature melts the suppository so it can be distributed. Clients may prefer self-administering suppositories. If possible, allow privacy when the client is capable of self-administering without difficulty. Proper placement is important to promote retention of the medication until it dissolves and is absorbed into the mucosa. Avoid placing a rectal suppository into a mass of fecal material. If necessary, obtain a physician's order to administer a small cleansing enema to evacuate the lower bowel before the suppository is inserted.

ASSESSMENT

1. Review physician's order, including client's name, drug name, form (cream or suppository), route, dosage, and time of administration.
2. Review pertinent information related to medication, including action, purpose, side effects, and nursing implications.
3. Inspect condition of external genitalia and vaginal canal or rectum (may be done just before insertion). *Rationale: Provides a baseline to determine later if local response to medication occurs.*
4. Ask if client is experiencing any symptoms of pruritus, burning, rectal bleeding, or discomfort. *Rationale: May indicate adverse effects.*
5. Review client's knowledge of purpose of drug therapy, as well as ability and willingness to self-administer medication.
6. Review medical record for history of rectal surgery or bleeding. *Rationale: May alter tissue integrity and level of discomfort.*

PLANNING

Expected outcomes focus on relief of symptoms without unpleasant side effects.

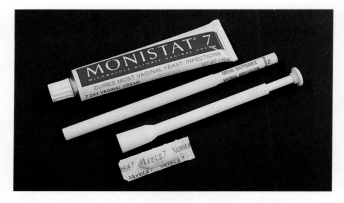

Figure 17-4 *From top:* Vaginal cream and applicator, applicator and vaginal suppository.

Expected Outcomes

1. Client reports relief of symptoms (e.g., discomfort, itching, constipation).
2. Client is able to self-administer suppository correctly.
3. Client explains purpose of medication, side effects, and steps to use for proper suppository insertion.

Equipment

- Disposable clean gloves
- Suppository
- Lubricant (water soluble)
- Suppository inserter (vaginal only)
- Vaginal creams or foam instillation (Figure 17-4)
- Vaginal cream or foam in plastic tube or can
- Perineal pad (optional)
- MAR or computer printout

Delegation Considerations

This skill requires assessment that uses the critical thinking and knowledge application unique to a nurse and should not be delegated to assistive personnel (AP). Judgment must be used regarding allowing the client to self-administer rectal or vaginal medications.

IMPLEMENTATION FOR INSERTING RECTAL AND VAGINAL MEDICATIONS

Steps	Rationale

1. See Standard Protocol (inside front cover).

NURSE ALERT *Review the six rights of medication administration (see Chapter 16, p. 408).*

2. Administer rectal suppository.

a. Assist client in assuming a left side-lying Sims' position with upper leg flexed upward.

Position exposes anus and helps client to relax external anal sphincter. Left side lessens the likelihood of the suppository or feces being expelled.

b. Keep client covered with only anal area exposed.

Maintains privacy and facilitates relaxation.

c. 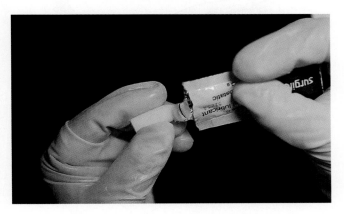 Examine condition of anus externally, and palpate rectal walls as needed (see Chapter 13).

Determines presence of active rectal bleeding. Palpation determines whether rectum is filled with feces, which may interfere with suppository placement.

NURSE ALERT *Do not palpate a client's rectum after rectal surgery. For clients with hemorrhoids use a liberal amount of lubricant and gently manipulate the tissues to visualize the anus. Generally, rectal suppositories are contraindicated in the presence of active rectal bleeding and diarrhea (McHenry and Salerno, 2001).*

d. Discard soiled gloves, and apply clean disposable gloves.

Minimizes contact with fecal material to reduce transmission of infection.

e. Remove suppository from foil wrapper, and lubricate rounded end (see illustration).

Lubrication reduces friction as suppository enters rectal canal.

f. Retract client's upper buttock with nondominant hand. Ask client to take slow, deep breaths through mouth and to relax anal sphincter.

Forcing suppository through constricted sphincter causes discomfort.

g. With gloved index finger of dominant hand, insert suppository, rounded end first gently through anus, past internal sphincter, and against rectal wall, 10 cm (4 inches) in adults.

Inserting the suppository against the rectal wall will enhance the effectiveness of the medication; inserting the suppository into a mass of fecal material will reduce the medication's effectiveness.

h. Wipe client's anal area, and discard gloves by turning them inside out and disposing of them in appropriate receptacle.

Inverting the gloves contains the microorganisms and prevents contamination of other articles.

i. Ask client to remain on side for 5 to 10 minutes or until urge to eliminate is strong.

Prevents expulsion of suppository. Provides sufficient time for the effects of the suppository to reach maximum effectiveness.

Step 2e Lubricate tip of suppository with water-soluble lubricant.

Steps	**Rationale**

j. If suppository contains laxative or fecal softener, place call light within reach so client can obtain assistance to reach bedpan or toilet.

Ability to call for assistance provides client with sense of control over elimination.

3. **Administer vaginal suppository.**

a. 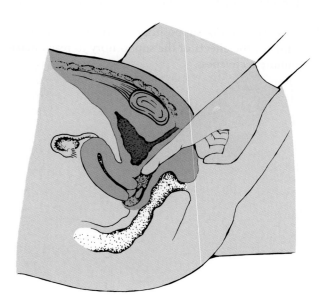 Assist client with lying in dorsal recumbent position with abdomen and lower extremities covered.

Provides easy access to vaginal canal and allows suppository to dissolve in vagina without leaking out.

b. Be sure vaginal orifice is well illuminated.

Proper insertion requires visualization of external genitalia if not self-administered.

c. Remove suppository from foil wrapper, and apply liberal amount of water-soluble lubricant. Lubricate gloved index finger of dominant hand.

Lubrication reduces friction against mucosal surfaces during insertion. Use of petroleum jelly may leave a residue that harbors bacteria and fungi.

d. With nondominant gloved hand, gently retract labial folds to expose vaginal orifice.

e. Insert rounded end of suppository along posterior wall of vaginal canal entire length of finger (7.5 to 10 cm, or 3 to 4 inches) (see illustration).

Proper placement of suppository ensures equal distribution of medication along walls of vaginal cavity.

f. Wipe away remaining lubricant from around orifice and labia. Remove and discard gloves.

g. Tell client there may be a small amount of discharge that is the color of medication exiting from vaginal canal. Client may wish to use disposable panty liners.

As the medication liquefies at body temperature, it is absorbed; however, small amounts may ooze from the vaginal canal.

4. **Administer vaginal cream or foam.**

a. Fill cream or foam applicator following package directions.

Dose is instilled based on volume in applicator.

b. With nondominant gloved hand, gently retract labial folds to expose vaginal orifice.

c. With dominant gloved hand, insert applicator approximately 5 to 7.5 cm (2 to 3 inches). Push applicator plunger to deposit medication into vagina (see illustration).

Step 3e Vaginal suppository insertion.

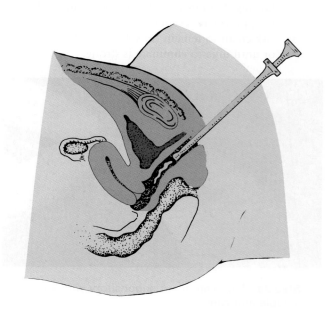

Step 4c Applicator inserted into vaginal canal.

Steps	Rationale
d. Withdraw applicator, and place on paper towel. Wipe off residual cream from labia or vaginal orifice, and remove and discard gloves.	Residual cream on applicator may contain microorganisms.
e. Instruct client to remain supine for at least 10 minutes.	Medication will be distributed and absorbed more evenly.
f. Offer disposable panty liners for use during ambulation.	Small amounts of medication may ooze from the vaginal orifice.
5. See Completion Protocol (inside front cover).	

• • • • • • • • • •

EVALUATION

1. Ask client about relief of symptoms for which medication was prescribed.
2. Inspect condition of vagina or rectum and external genitalia between applications. Ask about the presence of itching, burning, or discomfort.
3. Ask client to discuss purpose, side effects, and method of administration of medication.

Unexpected Outcomes and Related Interventions

1. Vaginal yeast infections may develop following extensive systemic antibiotic therapy. These are characterized by thick, white, patchy, curdlike discharge that clings to vaginal walls. Vaginal walls appear bright pink or inflamed.
   a. Report findings to physician; vaginal infections often are treated with topical application of antiinfective agents.
2. Client reports localized pruritus and burning, which may indicate infection or inflammation.
   a. Report symptoms to physician. Antiinfective agent may be ordered.
3. Client reports rectal pain during insertion of a rectal suppository.
   a. Use more lubrication before inserting suppository.
   b. The rectal route may be contraindicated; consult with physician.

Recording and Reporting

- Record appearance of rectum or vaginal canal and genitalia in nurses' notes, and report any unusual findings.
- Record drug name, dosage, time administered, and route on MAR.
- Record and report client's response to medication.

Sample Documentation

0800 Client complains of constipation. Has not had bowel movement for 3 days. Dulcolax suppository given per rectum as ordered. Expelled large, hard, dark-brown stool. States feeling much relieved. Encouraged to drink more fluids, to choose high-fiber foods from menu, and to ambulate as much as possible to prevent further problems. Verbalized understanding and willingness to comply.

SPECIAL CONSIDERATIONS

Pediatric Considerations
With children it may be necessary to gently hold the buttocks together for 5 to 10 minutes to relieve pressure on the anal sphincter until the urge to expel the suppository is gone (Wong and others, 1999).

Geriatric Considerations
Older adult clients with loss of sphincter control may have difficulty retaining suppository.

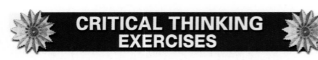

CRITICAL THINKING EXERCISES

1. Mrs. Jones is a 76-year-old widow who has been taking eye drops 3 times a day for several months. When you observe her self-administration, you realize she often does not get the drops into the conjunctival sac. What interventions might be appropriate?

2. A client has orders for eye drops, a cough syrup, a topical cream to the perineum for itching and skin breakdown, and 4 tablets (to swallow). What is the correct sequence for administration of these medications?

3. Your client has the following medications ordered: digoxin, 0.125 mg 4 times a day; Slow-K, 1 tablet twice a day; furosemide, 40 mg 4 times a day; Nitro-Bid, 1 capsule every 8 hours. His family caregiver calls you to tell you that she has had to crush all of his medications and give them with applesauce or pudding because the pills are too big. What would you tell her, and what suggestions do you have for his medication administration? (Check a pharmacology text to help you answer this question.)

4. When you go in the room to give the morning doses of medications, you note that Mr. C., your client, has not eaten his breakfast and is very short of breath. He is asking for his "treatment." You check his medication list and find that the medications due are as follows: metformin, 1 tablet with breakfast; erythromycin, 1 tablet q 6h, which he prefers to take with meals due to GI upset; and Lanoxin, 0.125 mg, 1 tablet daily. He also received albuterol via his nebulizer every 4 to 6 hours, and his last treatment was around midnight the night before. How would you prioritize his medication schedule this morning?

REFERENCES

Ashwill JW, Droske SC: *Nursing care of children,* Philadelphia, 1997, WB Saunders.

Ebersole P, Hess P: *Toward healthy aging,* ed 5, St Louis, 1998, Mosby.

Ignatavicius DD: Asking the right questions about medication safety, *Nursing* 30(9):51, 2000.

Kayser-Jones J, Pengilly K: Dysphagia among nursing home residents, *Geriatr Nurs* 20(2):77, 1998.

Lewis SM, Collier IC, Heitkemper MM: Assessment and management of clinical problems. In Lewis SM and others: *Medical-surgical nursing: assessment and management of clinical problems,* ed 5, St Louis, 2000, Mosby.

Lilley LL, Aucker RS: *Pharmacology and the nursing process,* ed 3, St Louis, 2001, Mosby.

Mahan LK, Escott-Stump S: *Krause's food, nutrition, and diet therapy,* ed 10, Philadelphia, 2000, WB Saunders.

McKenry LM, Salerno E: *Pharmacology in nursing,* ed 21, St Louis, 2001, Mosby.

Miller D, Miller H: To crush or not to crush, *Nursing* 30(2):51, 2000.

Owen CL. New directions in asthma management, *Am J Nurs* 99(3):6, 1999.

Schultz TR: Airing differences in pediatric nebulizer therapy, *Nursing* 30(9):55, 2000.

Weilitz PB, Van Sciver T: Obstructive pulmonary disease. In Lewis SM and others: *Medical-surgical nursing: assessment and management of clinical problems,* ed 5, St Louis, 2000, Mosby.

Willens JS: Giving fentanyl for pain outside the OR, *Am J Nurs* 98(2):24, 1998.

Wong D and others: *Whaley and Wong's nursing care of infants and children,* ed 6, St Louis, 1999, Mosby.

Administration of Injections

Box 18-1

Types of Injections

- *Subcutaneous (SQ, SC):* injection into tissues just below the dermis of the skin
- *Intramuscular (IM):* injection into the body of a muscle
- *Intradermal:* injection into the dermis just under the epidermis

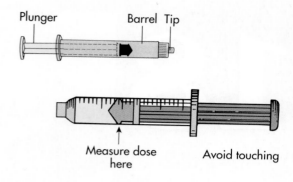

Figure 18-1 Parts of a syringe.

Injections instill medications into body tissues for systemic absorption (Box 18-1). Injected drugs act more quickly than oral medications, and these routes may be used when clients are vomiting, cannot swallow, and/or are restricted from taking oral fluids.

Injections are invasive, and strict aseptic technique is required during preparation and administration to minimize the risk of infection. Injections involve some discomfort. Because risk of tissue or nerve damage exists, site selection is an important nursing concern. The nurse must monitor the client's response closely and be aware of potential side effects or allergic reactions.

SYRINGES

Disposable syringes are packaged separately, with or without a sterile needle. The parts of a syringe are shown in Figure 18-1. Syringes come in various sizes, ranging in capacity from 0.3 to 60 ml. In selecting a syringe, it is important to choose the smallest syringe size possible to improve accuracy of medication preparation. In addition, the nurse must avoid injecting a large volume of fluid into tissues. It is unusual to use a syringe larger than 5 ml for intramuscular (IM) injections. A larger volume creates discomfort. Syringes are marked in two scales along the barrel; one side is divided by minims and the other by tenths of a milliliter (Figure 18-2, *A*). Tuberculin (TB) syringes, which are marked in hundredths, are used to measure very small dosages (Figure 18-2, *B*).

Syringes are classified as being Luer-Lok or non–Luer-Lok. Luer-Lok syringes (Figure 18-2, *A*) require special needles, which are twisted onto the tip and lock themselves in place. This prevents accidental removal of the needle. Non–Luer-Lok syringes (Figure 18-2, *B*) require needles that slip onto the tip.

Insulin syringes (Figure 18-2, *C* and *D*) hold 0.3 to 1 ml and are calibrated in units. Insulin syringes that hold 0.3 and 0.5 ml are known as low-dose syringes. These syringes are designed for more accurate dosages. Most insulin syringes are designed for use with U-100 strength insulin. Each milliliter of solution contains 100 units of insulin. Only insulin syringes are to be used for insulin administration.

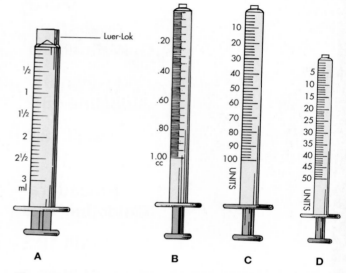

Figure 18-2 Types of syringes. **A,** 3-ml Luer-Lok syringe marked in 0.1 (tenths). **B,** Tuberculin syringe marked in 0.01 (hundredths) for doses of less than 1 ml. **C,** Insulin syringe marked in units (100 U). **D,** Insulin syringe marked in units (50) low dose.

Needles

Needles come packaged in individual sheaths to allow flexibility in choosing the right needle for a client. A needle has three parts: the hub, which fits onto the tip of the syringe; the shaft, which connects to the hub; and the bevel, or slanted tip (see Figure 18-1). The bevel creates a narrow slit when injected into tissue and quickly closes when the needle is removed, to prevent leakage of medication, blood, or serum. The nurse may handle the needle hub to ensure a tight fit on the syringe; however, the shaft and bevel must remain sterile.

Needles vary in length from ¼ to 3 inches (Figure 18-3). Often they are color coded for ease of selection. Longer needles (1 to 1½ inches) are used for IM injections and shorter needles (⅜ to ⅝ inch) for subcutaneous (SQ)

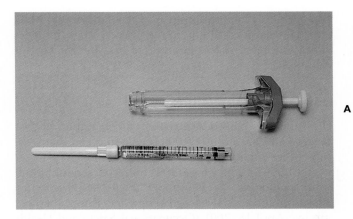

A

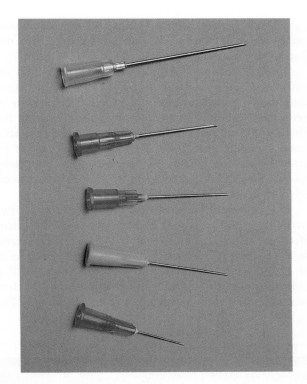

Figure 18-3 Needles *(top to bottom):* 19-gauge, 1¹/₂, inch length; 20-gauge, 1-inch length; 21-gauge, 1-inch length; 23-gauge, 1-inch length; and 25-gauge, ⁵/₈-inch length.

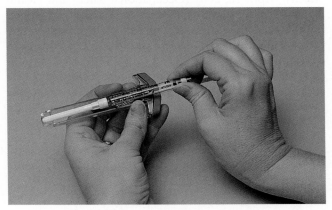

B

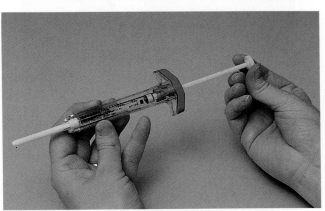

C

Figure 18-4 **A,** Carpuject syringe and prefilled sterile cartridge with needle. **B,** Assembling the Carpuject. **C,** Cartridge locks at needle end; plunger screws into opposite end.

injections. The nurse chooses the needle length according to the client's size and weight and the type of tissue into which the drug is to be injected. Children and very small, thin adults generally require a shorter needle.

The smaller the needle gauge is, the larger the needle diameter. The selection of a gauge depends on the viscosity of fluid to be injected. For example, a typical 22-gauge 1¹/₂-inch needle used for IM injections is larger than a 25-gauge ⁵/₈-inch needle used for SQ injections.

Filter needles are recommended for drawing medications from vials or ampules to prevent the withdrawing of glass and rubber particles into the syringe (Rodger and King, 2000). When a filter needle is used, the nurse must change the filter needle before administering the medication to prevent any unwanted particles from being injected into the client.

Disposable Injection Units

Single-dose, prefilled, disposable syringes are available for some medications. The nurse must carefully check the medication and concentration, because prefilled syringes appear very similar. When using a prefilled syringe, the nurse may need to expel some of the medication to deliver the correct dose. Some nurses prefer to transfer medication in prefilled syringes into regular syringes, especially when

it is necessary to mix the medication in the prefilled syringe with another medication.

The Tubex and Carpuject injection systems include a reusable plastic mechanism that holds prefilled, disposable, sterile cartridge-needle units (Figure 18-4). The nurse slips the cartridge into the holder, secures it (following product directions), and checks for air bubbles in the cartridge. The nurse advances the plunger to expel air and excess medication as in a regular syringe. Most cartridges have a little more medication than the label indicates; therefore it is essential to measure the correct volume.

Needle-Stick Prevention

The American Nurses Association (1999) estimated that between 600,000 and 1,000,000 needle-stick and sharps injuries occur among health care workers annually. Of these, at least 1,000 health care workers contracted serious blood-borne pathogens. In November 2000 the Needlestick Injury Prevention Act was signed into law. This act became effective April 18, 2001 (Occupational Safety and Health Administration [OSHA], 2001). As a result, employers must update their exposure control plans and seek employees' input when evaluating and selecting safer medical devices (OSHA, 2001).

Needleless injection systems prevent accidental needle sticks and should be used whenever possible. For example, a safety syringe is equipped with a plastic guard or sheath. The guard or sheath slips over the needle after an injection

is given to a client (Figure 18-5). Box 18-2 lists recommendations for health care workers to use to reduce their risk of sustaining a needle-stick injury.

Special puncture-proof and leak-proof containers are available in health care agencies for the disposal of sharps. Containers are made so that only one hand needs to be used when disposing of uncapped needles. Keeping the other hand well away from the container prevents accidental injury (Figure 18-6). A needle should never be forced by anyone into a full needle-disposal receptacle. Used needles and syringes should be disposed of immediately and in the appropriate container.

In administering injections with syringes that do not have safety sheaths, it may become necessary, for client safety reasons, to recap a contaminated needle. For example, the nurse may be assisting with emergency measures at the bedside and cannot reach a disposal container. If a commercially made recapping device is not available, then the nurse may use a one-handed recapping technique. The

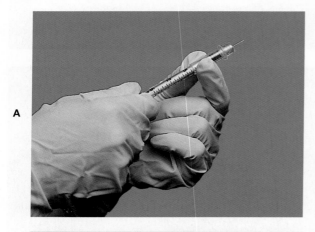

A

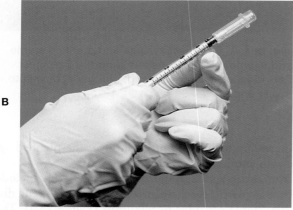

B

Figure 18-5 Needle with plastic guard to prevent needle sticks. **A,** Position of guard before injection. **B,** After injection the guard locks in place, covering the needle.

Box 18-2

Recommendations for the Prevention of Needle-Stick Injuries

1. Avoid using needles when effective needleless systems or Sharps with Engineered Sharps Injury Protection (SESIP) safety devices are available.
2. Do not recap needles.
3. Plan safe handling and disposal of needles before beginning a procedure that requires the use of a needle.
4. Immediately dispose of used needles, needleless systems, and SESIP into puncture-proof and leak-proof sharps disposal containers.
5. Maintain a Sharps Injury Log that includes:
   a. Type and brand of device involved in the incident
   b. Location of the incident (e.g., department or work area)
   c. Description of the incident
   d. Methods to maintain privacy of employees who have experienced sharps injuries
6. Participate in educational offerings regarding blood-borne pathogens, and follow recommendations for infection prevention, including receiving the hepatitis C vaccine.
7. Support legislation that promotes the safe use of needles and sharps.

Data from Occupational Safety and Health Administration (OSHA): Occupational exposure to bloodborne pathogens; needlestick and other sharps injuries; final rule, *Federal Register,* CFR 29, part 1910 (*Federal Register* 66:5317, Jan 18, 2001), and National Institute for Occupational Safety and Health (NIOSH): *NIOSH alert: preventing needlestick injuries in health care settings,* NIOSH Publications Dissemination DHHS (NIOSH) Pub No. 2000-108, Nov 1999.

needle cap is placed on a firm surface, and using one hand only, the nurse slips the tip of the needle into the cap (Figure 18-7). The nurse then presses the syringe, needle, and cover against a flat, vertical surface (e.g., cabinet door) to get the cap firmly in place.

If a nurse is accidentally stuck with a sterile needle while preparing medication, there is no risk of infection. The contaminated needle must be replaced before proceeding with the injection. If, however, a nurse is injured with a contaminated needle, the client is tested for hepatitis and acquired immunodeficiency syndrome (AIDS), and appropriate follow-up for the nurse is required (check agency policy). Regardless of whether the nurse is stuck with a sterile needle or a contaminated needle, an injury or occurrence report is filed according to institutional policy.

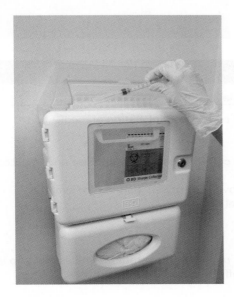

Figure 18-6 Sharps disposal using only one hand.

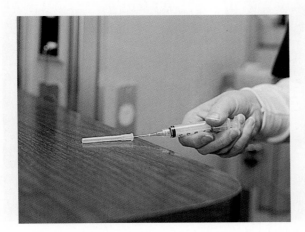

Figure 18-7 The scoop technique to prevent needle-stick injuries.

 ## PREPARATION OF INJECTABLE MEDICATIONS

Ampules contain single doses of injectable medication in a liquid form (Figure 18-8). They are available in several sizes, from 1 ml to 10 ml or more. An ampule is made of glass with a constricted neck that must be snapped off to allow access to the medication. The fluid enters the syringe easily with aspiration because no vacuum exists within the ampule.

A vial is a single-dose or multidose container with a rubber seal at the top (Figure 18-9). A cap protects the seal until it is used and cannot be replaced. Vials may contain liquid or dry forms of medications; drugs that are unstable in solution are packaged in dry form. The vial label specifies the liquid to use to dissolve the dry drug and the amount needed to prepare a desired drug concentration. Air must be injected into the vial to permit easy withdrawal of the solution.

Tables 18-1 and 18-2 describe the steps and rationale for drawing up medications from ampules and vials. Procedural Guideline 18-1 on p. 466 describes the steps for reconstituting medication from a powder.

Text continued on p. 466

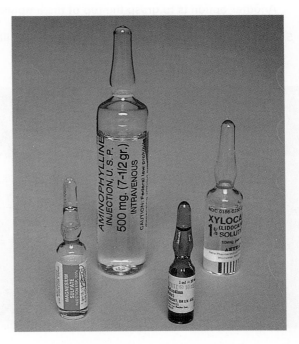

Figure 18-8 Medication in ampules.

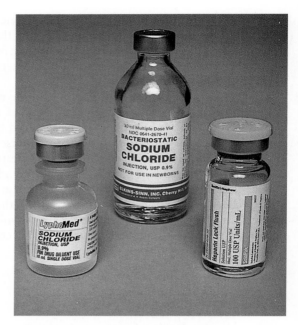

Figure 18-9 Medication in vials. Rubber top must be cleansed with alcohol when vial is reused.

Table 18-1

Drawing up Medication From an Ampule

Steps	Rationale
1. Check client's name, drug name, dosage, route of administration, and time of administration.	Ensures correct administration of medication.
2. Wash hands, and prepare supplies.	
3. Check medication order or MAR against label on medication.	Ensures correct medication and dose are prepared.
4. Remove fluid from neck of ampule by tapping top of ampule lightly and quickly with finger, quickly moving down in vertical direction (see illustration). Another option is to grasp the top of the ampule and shake it downward like a thermometer.	Fluid moves into lower chamber for eventual aspiration.
5. Small gauze pad placed to protect fingers (see illustration).	Protects nurse's fingers from trauma as glass tip is broken off.

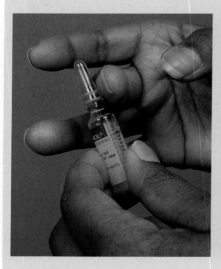

Step 4 Tapping ampule moves fluid down neck.

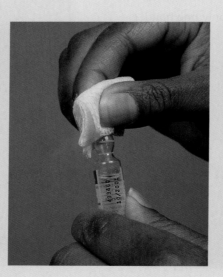

Step 5 Gauze pad placed to protect fingers.

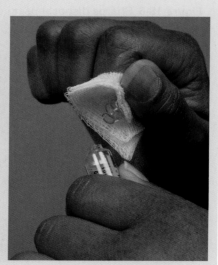

Step 6 Snapping neck away from hands.

Table 18-1

Drawing up Medication From an Ampule—cont'd

Steps	Rationale
6. Break neck of ampule quickly and firmly away from hands and body (see illustration).	Prevents shattering glass toward or in nurse's fingers or face.
7. Place ampule on countertop (see illustration). Using a filter needle, draw up medication, keeping the needle tip below the surface of liquid. Tip ampule to bring fluid within reach of needle.	Filter needle prevents withdrawal of glass or rubber particulate (Rodger and King, 2000).
8. Option for holding ampule and syringe: Insert filter needle into center of ampule opening and invert ampule (see illustration).	Solution dribbles out if shaft touches rim of ampule.
9. Aspirate medication from ampule into syringe by gently pulling back on plunger. Do not draw up the last drop in the ampule.	Do not allow needle shaft to touch rim of ampule. Leaving last drops reduces chance of withdrawing foreign particles (Beyea and Nicoll, 1995).
10. If air bubbles are aspirated, remove needle from ampule and hold syringe with needle pointing directly up. Tap side of syringe so that air bubbles rise toward needle (see illustration, p. 464). Draw back slightly on plunger, and then push the plunger upward to eject air until 1 drop of fluid is visible on the tip of the needle.	Pulling back on plunger allows fluid within needle to enter barrel so fluid is not expelled. Air at top of barrel and within needle is then expelled.

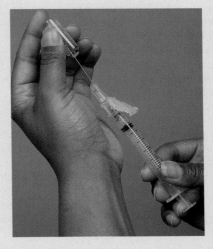

Step 8 Medication aspirated with ampule inverted.

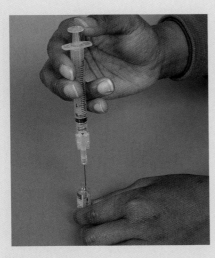

Step 7 Medication aspirated with ampule on flat surface.

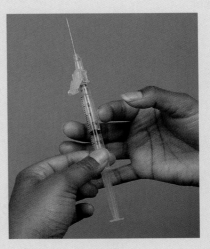

Step 10 Hold syringe upright; tap barrel to dislodge air bubbles from syringe.

Continued

Table 18-1

Drawing up Medication From an Ampule—cont'd

Steps	Rationale
11. If syringe contains excess fluid, hold syringe vertically with needle tip up and slanted slightly toward sink or receptacle, and eject excess fluid into sink. Recheck fluid level in syringe by holding it vertically at eye level at a 90-degree angle to measure accurate dose.	Position of needle allows medication to be expelled without it flowing down needle shaft. If necessary, flick syringe and needle sharply to eliminate fluid from outside of needle.
12. Remove filter needle, and dispose of in proper receptacle. Apply a new needle to syringe.	Prevents injection of glass or rubber particulate into client (Rodger and King, 2000).
13. Dispose of used supplies, and take medication to client's bedside for administration.	

Table 18-2

Drawing up Medication From a Vial

1. Check client's name, drug name, dosage, route of administration, and time of administration.	Ensures correct administration of medication.
2. Wash hands, and prepare supplies. Check date and time of any opened vials.	Drugs cannot be used after expiration dates (check agency policy).
3. Remove cap covering top of unused vial. Firmly wipe off surface of rubber seal with alcohol swab using friction. Allow alcohol to dry.	Vial comes packaged with cap that cannot be replaced after removal. Not all drug manufacturers guarantee that seals of unused vials are sterile (Posey and Long, 1996). Therefore seals must be swabbed before drawing up medication.
4. Pick up syringe with needle or needleless adapter (see illustration) and remove cap. Pull back on plunger to draw amount of air into syringe equivalent to volume of medication to be aspirated from vial.	Air must be injected into the vial to prevent buildup of negative pressure in vial when aspirating medication.
5. With vial on a flat surface, insert tip of needle through center of rubber seal (see illustration).	Center of seal is thinner and easier to penetrate.
6. Inject air into vial, holding on to plunger.	Plunger may be forced backward by air pressure within vial.
7. Invert vial while keeping firm hold on syringe and plunger.	Allows fluid to settle in lower half of container.

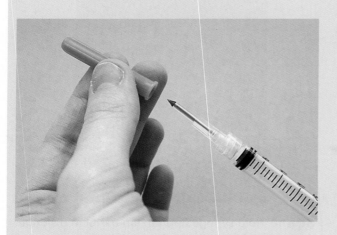

Step 4 Syringe with needleless adapter.

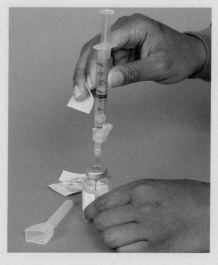

Step 5 Insert tip of needle through center of vial diaphragm (with vial flat on table).

Table 18-2

Drawing up Medication From a Vial—cont'd

8. Keep tip of needle below fluid level (see illustration).	Prevents aspiration of air.
9. Allow air pressure to fill syringe gradually with medication, or pull back slightly on plunger to obtain correct amount of solution (see illustration).	Positive pressure within vial forces fluid into syringe.
10. When desired volume has been obtained, position tip of needle into vial's air space. Tap side of syringe barrel carefully to dislodge any air bubbles. Eject any air remaining at top of syringe into vial.	Accumulation of air displaces medication and may cause dosage errors. Draw up the exact volume of medication.
11. Remove needle from vial by pulling on barrel of syringe. Hold syringe at eye level at a 90-degree-angle to ensure correct volume.	Pulling plunger rather than barrel causes separation from barrel and loss of medication.
12. If medication is to be injected into a client's tissue, change adapter or needle with a new needle of appropriate gauge and length according to route of medication.	Adapters must be changed with needles for injection into client's tissue. Needles become dull as they enter rubber stoppers. Changing needles also prevents tracking of medication through client's tissues, minimizing pain.
13. Label multidose vial with date, time, and initials.	Check agency policy for expiration regulations.

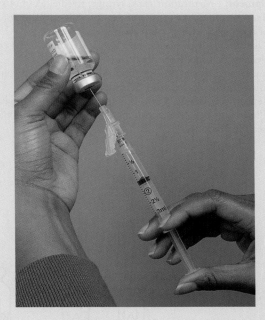

Steps 8 and 9 Withdraw fluid with vial inverted.

Procedural Guideline 18-1
Reconstituting Medications From a Powder

Equipment: Vial with medication, vial with diluent solution, syringe, needle, alcohol swab

1. Remove cap covering vial containing powdered medication and vial containing diluent. Label may specify use of sterile water, normal saline, or special diluent provided with the medication.
2. Firmly swab both rubber seals with alcohol swab and allow alcohol to dry.
3. Draw up diluent into syringe with needle (see Table 18-2, Steps 4 to 11).
4. Insert tip of needle through center of rubber seal of vial of powdered medication and inject diluent into vial.
5. Remove needle.
6. Mix medication by gently rolling vial between hands until completely dissolved.
7. Reconstituted medication in vial is ready to be drawn into syringe. Read label carefully to determine concentration after reconstitution.
8. Draw up medication into syringe (see Table 18-2, Steps 4 to 11).

Procedural Guideline 18-2
Mixing Medications From a Vial

Equipment: Medication vials, syringe, needle, alcohol swabs

1. Remove protective caps from top of vials, and cleanse seals of both vials with alcohol swab.
2. Take syringe with needle, and aspirate volume of air equivalent to first medication's dosage (vial A).
3. Inject air into vial A, making sure needle does not touch solution (see illustration). Withdraw needle.
4. Repeat with vial B. Without removing needle from vial B, fill syringe with proper volume of medication from vial B (see illustration).
5. Calculate total volume of medication by adding volume of both prescribed medications.
6. Insert needle of syringe into vial A, being careful not to push plunger and expel medication into vial. Invert vial, and carefully withdraw the exact amount of medication required into syringe (see illustration).

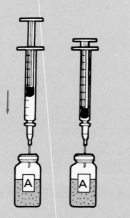
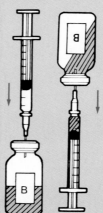
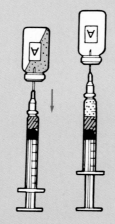

Step 3 Injecting air into vial A.

Step 4 Injecting air into vial B and withdrawing dose.

Step 6 Withdrawing medication from vial A; medications are now mixed.

Mixing Medications in One Syringe

To avoid giving two injections at one time, some medications can be mixed in the same syringe. It is essential that any medications mixed be compatible. Compatibility charts are available in most pharmacology books or the pharmacy. When mixing medications, observe for changes in the appearance of the solution, which suggests incompatibility. Whenever two medications are mixed in one syringe, it is essential to avoid injecting the contents from one vial or ampule into the other vial or ampule. When mixing medications from a vial and an ampule, the medication from the vial should be prepared first. Then medication from the ampule is withdrawn.

To mix medications in a syringe when one of the two is in a prefilled cartridge, draw back on the plunger of the syringe. Remove the needle from the syringe. Fill the syringe with the correct volume of medication from the prefilled cartridge by inserting the cartridge needle into the syringe tip. Procedural Guideline 18-2 describes the steps for mixing medications in the same syringe.

NURSING DIAGNOSES

Nursing diagnoses may be identified based on therapeutic effects or side effects of specific prescribed medications and effect of injection into tissues. **Acute Pain** is a diagnosis that may apply when clients are receiving medications to help control pain. **Anxiety** is a common diagnosis for clients who are uncomfortable with having injections. **Deficient Knowledge** regarding self-administration of medications is appropriate for clients who need to learn or review injection techniques. **Ineffective Therapeutic Regimen Management** is appropriate when the client is having difficulties complying with prescribed medication schedules. **Risk for Injury** applies because it is important to select injection sites carefully and to administer all injections correctly.

Skill 18.1

Subcutaneous Injections (Includes Insulin)

A SQ injection involves depositing medication into the loose connective tissue underlying the dermis (Figure 18-10). SQ tissue is not as richly supplied with blood vessels as muscle; thus drugs are usually absorbed more slowly than those given IM. Drugs commonly given SQ include insulin, heparin, and allergy medications.

The rate of absorption is influenced by factors that affect blood flow to tissues, such as physical exercise or the local application of hot or cold compresses. Conditions such as circulatory shock or occlusive vascular disease impair client's blood flow and may prevent or delay absorption, thus contraindicating SQ injections in these situations.

Only small doses of medications (up to 1 ml) should be given SQ. The SQ tissue is sensitive to irritating solutions and large volumes of medications. Medications collecting within the tissues can cause sterile abscesses, which appear as hardened, painful lumps.

The best sites for SQ injections include vascular areas around the outer aspect of the upper arms, the abdomen from below the costal margins to the iliac crests, and the anterior aspect of the thighs (Figure 18-11). These areas are easily accessible, especially for clients who must self-administer medications. When using the abdominal site, it is important to avoid the 2-inch diameter around the umbilicus because of the vascularity of this area. Other sites include the scapular areas of the upper back and the upper ventral or dorsal gluteal areas.

Injection sites should be free of infection, skin lesions, scars, bony prominences, and large underlying muscles or nerves. Rotation prevents the formation of lipohypertrophy or lipoatrophy in the skin. Body weight influences the depth of the SQ layer and is the criterion for selecting needle length and angle of insertion. Generally a 25-gauge $\frac{1}{2}$- to $\frac{5}{8}$-inch needle, with a medium bevel, inserted at a 90-degree an-

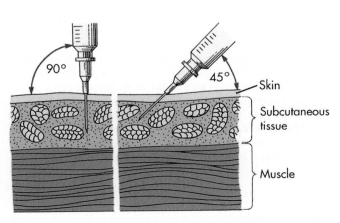

Figure 18-10 Subcutaneous injection. Angle and needle length depend on the thickness of skinfold.

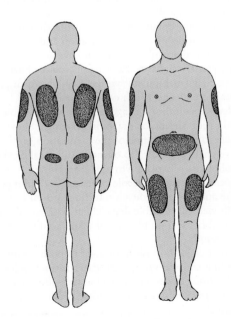

Figure 18-11 Sites recommended for subcutaneous injections.

gle (see Figure 18-10), deposits medication into the SQ tissue of a normal-size client. If a client is obese, the nurse pinches the tissue and uses a needle long enough to insert through the fatty tissue at the base of the skinfold. The nurse may need to pinch the skin and inject the SQ medication at a 45-degree angle when giving SQ injections to thin or cachectic clients and children. The preferred needle length is one half the width of the skinfold. A ⅞-inch needle is the longest needle for SQ use. To ensure medication reaches SQ tissue, this rule is followed: If 2 inches of tissue can be grasped, the needle is inserted at a 90-degree angle; if 1 inch of tissue can be grasped, the needle is inserted at a 45-degree angle.

Aspiration of any medication, including heparin and insulin, after injecting an SQ medication is not necessary. Piercing a blood vessel in a SQ injection is very rare and may cause hematoma formation (American Diabetes Association [ADA], 2001; McConnell, 2000; Peragallo-Dittko, 1997).

Some clients must take SQ medications at home. Common SQ medications include insulin and enoxaparin, an anticoagulant. In these cases the nurse must teach the client how to prepare and administer self-injections. Procedural Guideline 18-3 summarizes the steps necessary to teach this important skill to clients.

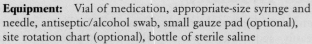

Procedural Guideline 18-3
Teaching Self-Injections

Equipment: Vial of medication, appropriate-size syringe and needle, antiseptic/alcohol swab, small gauze pad (optional), site rotation chart (optional), bottle of sterile saline

1. Determine if client is ready and able to learn this skill.
2. Determine client's ability to read and see medication label and syringe markings clearly. Provide assistive devices such as a syringe magnifier or enlist the help of the client's significant other if difficulties with vision are discovered.
3. Assess client's ability to hold and manipulate a syringe and medication vial. If client cannot manipulate syringe, an alternative plan must be developed (e.g., have significant other prepare medication).
4. Include significant other in teaching if possible.
5. Assemble teaching materials and equipment needed. Provide a comfortable, quiet, well-lit setting, free of distractions. Have client sit at table where all equipment is displayed; make sure equipment is within easy reach and organized logically.
6. Describe appropriate storage of medication and supplies. Help client decide where medication and syringes will be secured so that children will not have access to them.
7. Have client wash hands. Explain importance of handwashing.
8. Have client manipulate syringe. Explain which parts must remain sterile and which can be touched.
9. Discuss medication dosage, and show client how much medication should be drawn into syringe. Show client where to find the name of the medication on the vial.
10. Have client wipe off top of medication vial or vials with alcohol swab. Explain why this is important.
11. Have client remove needle cover and pull plunger out to same amount of medication to be removed from vial.
12. With vial still on table, have client push needle slowly into rubber seal on top of vial while holding syringe barrel carefully.
13. Instruct client to push in plunger to push air into bottle.
14. Holding vial and syringe together; instruct client to turn both upside down. Hold vial between thumb and forefinger, supporting syringe with other hand.

15. Teach client to slowly pull back on plunger until the correct amount of medication is transferred into the syringe. Be sure client keeps the needle under fluid in vial.
16. Have client check for and remove air bubbles inside syringe. To clear bubbles the client should tap the syringe lightly and expel them back into the vial. Before withdrawing the syringe, have client verify one more time that the amount of medication in the syringe is the accurate dose.
17. If client must mix two medications into one syringe, teach client to put the desired amount of air into one vial and remove the needle. Then instruct the client to put the desired amount of air into the second vial and pull up the desired amount of medication. Once all air bubbles are eliminated, the syringe should be pulled out and reinserted into the first vial. The client then should draw out the appropriate amount of medication from the vial into the syringe. Discuss with the client how much medication should be in the syringe at the end.
18. Instruct client to put cap or sheath back over needle without touching it.
19. Show client appropriate and accessible sites for injection. Discuss systematic rotation of sites, using all the sites in one area before changing to another. Help client choose an appropriate site and wipe it with alcohol. Explain that if a limb will be exercised shortly after the injection, that site should not be used because the medication will absorb more quickly than desired.
20. Once alcohol is dry, have client remove cap and explain that client should hold the syringe like a pencil or a dart.
21. If a SQ injection is given, have client grasp or pinch injection site between thumb and forefingers of free hand. To give SQ injections on the posterior upper arm, have client press back of arm against wall or back of chair and have client "roll" arm down to push up the skin. If IM injection is being taught, have client hold skin taut.

Procedural Guideline 18-3

Teaching Self-Injections—cont'd

22. Teach client to insert needle with a quick jab into prepared site all the way to the hub. Most injections should be given at 90-degree angle. A 45-degree angle may be used for children or thin adults receiving SQ injections.
23. Once needle is in, instruct client to let go of skin and transfer free hand to barrel of syringe.
24. If client is administering an IM injection, explain importance of aspirating before injecting the medication. Show client how to aspirate syringe and how to discontinue injection if blood is aspirated. If client is giving SQ injections, there is no need to aspirate.
25. Have client push plunger all the way in at a slow and steady rate to administer the medication.
26. Once medication has been administered, teach client to pull needle out quickly at same angle it was inserted. A small gauze pad may be held over the site if desired after the needle is removed.

27. Teach client appropriate disposal of used syringe. Syringe and uncapped needle or needle enclosed in safety shield should be placed in a puncture-proof box or a plastic receptacle, such as a hard plastic fabric softener bottle or soda bottle.
28. Explain safe reuse of needles. If client has adequate immune system and does not contaminate the needle during the injection process, the needle may be recapped and used for the next injection. Syringes and needles should be disposed of whenever the needle gets dull or if the syringe or needle becomes contaminated.
29. Have client indicate on record chart where injection was given.
30. Encourage client to ask questions about procedure, and provide client with written and visual guidelines.
31. Give client a bottle of sterile saline to practice preparing medication and avoid wasting of medication.

SPECIAL CONSIDERATIONS FOR ADMINISTRATION OF INSULIN

Insulin is the hormone used to treat diabetes mellitus. Clients with diabetes often receive a combination of different types of insulin to control their blood glucose levels. Regular, short-acting, unmodified insulin comes in a clear solution. The other intermediate-acting insulins (e.g., Lente, NPH) are cloudy solutions because of the addition of a protein, which slows absorption.

Rotation of insulin injections from major site to major site with each injection, once a common practice, is no longer necessary when clients use human insulin. Human insulins carry a much lower risk for hypertrophy and are most frequently prescribed for clients. Therefore clients can choose one region (e.g., the abdomen) and systematically rotate sites within that region, thus maintaining consistency in absorption from day to day. Once all potential sites within that area are used, the client may choose either to move to another anatomical site (e.g., the thigh) or to start the rotation pattern over in the same anatomical area (ADA, 2001).

An important nursing consideration with insulin administration is the timing of injections. When planning insulin injection times, the nurse must verify the client's current blood glucose level. Also, the peak action and duration of the client's insulin must be determined when developing an effective diabetes management plan. Table 18-3 compares the onsets, peaks, and durations of various insulin preparations. General guidelines related to insulin administration are listed in Box 18-3.

SPECIAL CONSIDERATIONS FOR ADMINISTRATION OF HEPARIN

Heparin therapy is used to provide therapeutic anticoagulation to reduce the risk of thrombus formation. It is administered subcutaneously or intravenously. Heparin suppresses clot formation. Therefore it creates a risk for bleeding. Nurses should be alert for signs of bleeding (e.g., bleeding gums, hematemesis, hematuria, melena) in clients receiving long-term anticoagulation therapy. A blood test measuring activated partial thromboplastin time (APTT) is used in monitoring the desired therapeutic range for intravenous (IV) heparin therapy.

Before administering heparin, the nurse assesses for preexisting conditions that may contraindicate the use of heparin, including threatened abortion, cerebral or aortic aneurysm, cerebrovascular hemorrhage, severe hypertension, blood dyscrasias, and recent ophthalmic surgery or neurosurgery. In addition, the nurse assesses for conditions in which increased risk of hemorrhage is present: recent childbirth, severe diabetes, severe renal disease, liver disease, severe trauma, vasculitis, and active ulcers or lesions of the gastrointestinal (GI), gastrourinary (GU), or respiratory tract. The client's current medication regimen must be assessed for possible drug interactions with heparin. Drugs that interact with heparin include aspirin, nonsteroidal antiinflammatory drugs (NSAIDs), cephalosporins, antithyroid agents, probenecid, and thrombolytics (McKenry and Salerno, 2001).

Table 18-3

Pharmacokinetics of Insulin Preparations

Insulins*	Onset (Hours)	Peak Effect (Hours)	Duration of Action (Hours)
Rapid Acting			
Insulin lispro (Humalog)	¼	1	4
Insulin injection (regular insulin)†	½-1	2-4	5-7
Prompt insulin zinc suspension (Semilente)	1-3	2-8	12-16
Intermediate Acting			
Insulin zinc suspension (Lente insulin)	1-3	8-12	18-28
Isophane insulin suspension (NPH insulin)	3-4	6-12	18-28
Combination Insulins			
Isophane insulin suspension (70%) plus insulin injection (30%) (Humulin 70/30, Novolin 70/30)	½	4-8	24
Isophane human insulin (50%) and human insulin (50%) (Humulin 50/50)	½	3	22-24
Long Acting			
Extended insulin zinc suspension (Ultralente)	4-6	18-24	36
Protamine zinc insulin suspension (PZI)	4-6	14-24	36
Insulin glargine (Lantus)	1	None	24

From McKenry LM, Salerno E: *Pharmacology in nursing,* ed 21, St Louis, 2001, Mosby.
*All above insulins are available in 100-unit strengths. Beef, pork, beef-pork, and human insulins are available in rapid-acting insulins and the two insulins listed under intermediate acting.
†This is the only insulin for IV use. Intravenously the onset of action is within 10 to 30 minutes, peak effect within 15 to 30 minutes, and duration of action within 30 minutes to 1 hour.

Box 18-3

General Guidelines for Insulin Administration

- Vials of insulin not in use should be refrigerated. Insulin may be kept at room temperature for 30 days from the date opened. Always time and date a vial when it is first opened.
- Inspect a vial of insulin before each use for changes (e.g., clumping, frosting, precipitation, change in clarify or color) that may signify a loss in potency.
- Be certain the correct form of insulin is prepared. Do not interchange insulin species or types without the approval of the prescriber.
- Raid-acting insulin should be injected within 15 minutes before a meal. The most commonly recommended interval between injection of short-acting insulin and a meal is 30 minutes.
- If client is allowed nothing by mouth (NPO) for diagnostic tests, insulin may be withheld depending on the time of the test and the client's blood glucose level. Check with prescriber about insulin administration before surgery or diagnostic tests.
- Before administering insulin, review available laboratory data (e.g., serum glucose level, blood glucose monitoring—normal range is 80 to 120. for nonpregnant adults). Abnormal results may indicate need for dosage adjustment.
- When a dose of insulin is being adjusted, watch for signs of hypoglycemia or hyperglycemia and encourage the client to report symptoms (e.g., weakness, shakiness, sweating, headache, visual disturbances).
- All individuals requiring insulin should carry at least 15 g carbohydrate to be eaten or taken in liquid form in the event of a hypoglycemic reaction (e.g., 4 ounces juice, 8 ounces milk).
- Administer mixed insulin (e.g., regular and NPH) within 5 minutes of preparation. Regular insulin binds with NPH, which reduces the action of the regular insulin.
- When mixing insulin, be sure to inject sufficient air into both vials before drawing up the dose. When mixing rapid- or short-acting insulin with intermediate- or long-acting insulin, the clear rapid or short-acting insulin should be drawn into the syringe first (see Procedural Guideline 18-2).

ASSESSMENT

1. Review physician's medication order for client's name, drug name, dose, and time and route of administration. *Rationale: Ensures safe and accurate drug administration.*
2. Review information pertinent to drug(s) ordered: action, purpose, appropriate route, time of onset and peak action, normal dosage, common side effects, and nursing implications.
3. Check expiration date of medication.
4. Assess for factors that may contraindicate SQ injections, such as circulatory shock or reduced local tissue perfusion.
5. Assess indications for SQ injections: unconscious or confused client, client who is unable to swallow or has GI disturbances, presence of gastric suction.
6. Assess client's medical history, history of allergies, and medication history.
7. Assess adequacy of adipose tissue; note presence of hardening or reduction in amount of tissue. *Rationale: Physiological changes of aging or repeated injections may create changes in SQ tissue affecting absorption.*
8. Assess client's knowledge regarding medication to dosage schedule. *Rationale: Information may pose implications for client education.*
9. Observe client's verbal and nonverbal response toward injection. *Rationale: Injections can cause anxiety, which may increase pain.*
10. Ask if client prefers to administer own injection if accustomed to doing so. If learning to do own injections, reinforce learning process.

PLANNING

Expected outcomes focus on safe, effective administration of injections with minimal anxiety and discomfort.

Expected Outcomes

1. Client demonstrates improved clinical condition after medication administration without evidence of adverse effects.
2. Client experiences no pain or mild burning at injection site.
3. Client's tissues remain soft and supple at injection site.
4. Client explains purpose, dosage, and effects of medication.

For Insulin

5. Client maintains serum glucose levels between 80 and 120 mg/100 ml or in an individualized targeted range.
6. Client describes symptoms and treatment of hypoglycemia and hyperglycemia and states blood glucose values and symptoms that should be reported to health care provider.

For Heparin

7. Client shows no signs of new thrombus formation or evidence of abnormal bleeding.
8. Client describes symptoms of bleeding to report to health care provider.

Equipment

*   Syringe (1 to 3ml)

    For insulin: 0.3- to 1-ml insulin syringe (needles are usually permanently attached to syringe)
    For heparin: tuberculin or 1- to 3-ml syringe

*   Needle (31 to 25 gauge, $\frac{3}{8}$ to $\frac{5}{8}$ inch)
*   Small gauze pad (optional)
*   Alcohol swab
*   Medication ampule or vial
*   Disposable gloves
*   Medication administration record (MAR) or computer printout

Delegation Considerations

The skill of administering SQ injections requires the critical thinking and knowledge application unique to a nurse. Delegation is inappropriate. Be sure assistive personnel (AP) know the unexpected changes in a client's condition to report to a nurse as soon as possible.

IMPLEMENTATION FOR SUBCUTANEOUS INJECTIONS (INCLUDES INSULIN)

Steps	Rationale
1. See Standard Protocol (inside front cover).	

NURSE ALERT *Review six rights for administration of medications.*

Steps	Rationale
2. Prepare medication in syringe (see Tables 18-1 and 18-2 and Procedural Guideline 18-1 and 18-2).	Ensures right client receives right medication.
3. Identify client by checking identification arm band and asking client's name, compare with MAR.	Ensures right client receives right medication.
4. Close room door or curtain. Explain steps of procedure and tell client injections will cause a slight burn or sting.	
5. Select appropriate injection site. Inspect surface of skin over sites for bruises, inflammation, or edema. Palpate site for masses, edema, or tenderness.	
6. Be sure needle size is correct by grasping skinfold at site with thumb and forefinger. Measure skinfold from top to bottom, and be sure needle is approximately half this length.	SQ injections can be inadvertently given in the muscle, especially in the abdomen and thigh sites (Peragallo-Dittko, 1997). Appropriate needle size ensures that needle will be injected into SQ tissue.
7. Assist client to comfortable position, and ask client to relax arm, leg, or abdomen depending on site chosen for injection.	Relaxation of area minimizes discomfort during injection. Promoting client's comfort through positioning and distraction helps reduce anxiety.
8. Talk with client about subject of interest. Keep syringe out of line of vision.	Minimizes anxiety.
9. Relocate site using anatomical landmarks (see Figure 18-11).	Correct site avoids injury to underlying nerves, bone, or blood vessels.
10. Cleanse site with an antiseptic swab. Apply swab at center of site and rotate outward in circular direction for about 5 cm (2 inches) (see illustration).	Mechanical action removes microorganisms.
11. Hold swab or square of gauze between fingers of nondominant hand.	

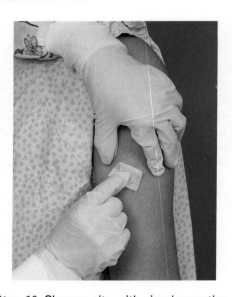

Step 10 Cleanse site with circular motion.

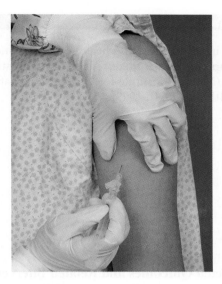

Step 13 Hold syringe as if grasping a dart.

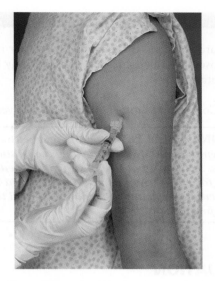

Step 14b Inject medication slowly.

Steps	Rationale
12. Remove needle cap or sheath from needle by pulling it straight off.	Prevents contamination of needle.
13. Hold syringe between thumb and forefinger of dominant hand as if grasping dart (see illustration), holding syringe across tops of fingertips.	Quick, smooth injection requires proper manipulation of syringe parts.
14. Administer injection:	
a. *Average-size client:* Spread skin tightly across injection site or pinch skin with nondominant hand, and inject needle quickly and firmly at 90-degree angle.	Needle penetrates tight skin easier than loose skin. Pinching skin elevates SQ tissue.
b. *Thin client or child:* Gently pinch skin, and inject needle quickly and firmly at 45-degree angle or use a ½- to ⁵⁄₁₆-inch needle (see illustration).	Angle ensures that medication reaches SQ tissue rather than muscle.
c. *Obese client:* Pinch skin at site, and inject needle at 90-degree angle below tissue fold.	Obese clients have fatty layer of tissue above SQ layer. Pinching elevates SQ tissue.
15. After needle enters site, grasp lower end of syringe barrel with nondominant hand. Move dominant hand to end of plunger. Avoid moving syringe.	Movement of syringe may displace needle and cause discomfort.

NURSE ALERT   *Do not aspirate medication.*

16. With dominant hand, inject medication slowly but smoothly.	Slow injection reduces pain and trauma.

NURSE ALERT   *Injecting SQ heparin over 30 seconds may create less pain and bruising (Chan, 2001).*

17. Withdraw needle quickly while placing antiseptic swab or sterile gauze gently above or over site.	Supporting tissues around injection site minimizes discomfort during needle withdrawal. Dry gauze may lessen discomfort associated with alcohol on nonintact skin.
18. Apply gentle pressure to site. Do *not* massage site. (If heparin is given, hold alcohol swab or gauze to site for 30 to 60 seconds.)	Aids absorption. Massage can injure underlying tissue.

Steps	Rationale
19. Discard sheathed or uncapped needle or needle enclosed in safety shield in appropriately labeled receptacle.	Prevents injury to client and health care personnel. Recapping needles increases risk of needle-stick injury (National Institute for Occupational Safety and Health [NIOSH], 1999).
20. See Completion Protocol (inside front cover).	

COMMUNICATION TIP *Use this time with client to ask if client has questions regarding medication and its effects. Explain what to expect from a medication. If caring for client who has self-administered injection, give immediate feedback regarding how well the injection was performed.*

• • • • • • • • • •

EVALUATION

1. Observe client's response to medication at times that correlate with the medication's onset, peak, and duration to determine effectiveness of drug and observe for adverse reactions.
2. Ask if client feels any acute pain, burning, numbness, or tingling at injection site.
3. Inspect and palpate injection site for lumps, tenderness, or swelling.
4. Have client describe purpose, dosage, intended effects, and side effects of medication.

For Insulin

5. Monitor blood glucose readings before meals, at bedtime, or as ordered and when possibility of hypoglycemia is evident.
6. Ask client to list symptoms and treatment of hypoglycemia and hyperglycemia, and have client describe blood glucose values and signs and symptoms that should be reported to health care provider.

For Heparin

7. Routinely monitor client for signs of thrombus formation and bleeding.
8. Have client describe symptoms of bleeding to report.

Unexpected Outcomes and Related Interventions

1. Client complains of localized pain or continued burning at injection site, possibly indicating potential injury to nerve or tissues.
   a. Assess injection site, and notify client's health care provider. Warm or cool compresses may be provided for comfort.
2. Client displays signs of urticaria, eczema, pruritus, wheezing, and dyspnea.
   a. Follow institutional policy or guidelines for appropriate response to allergic reactions, and notify client's health care provider immediately.

Recording and Reporting

- Document medication administration immediately after giving medication on MAR to record care provided and to prevent future drug administration errors.
- Record client's response to medication.
- Report undesirable effects from medication to client's health care provider, and document treatment of adverse effects according to institutional policy.

Sample Documentation

0900 Heparin injection given in RLQ of abdomen. Bruise (4 cm in diameter) noted on RLQ of abdomen, deep purple, soft and nontender. Urine clear; stool negative for occult blood.

SPECIAL CONSIDERATIONS

Pediatric Considerations
Only amounts up to 0.5 ml may be administered subcutaneously to small children (Hockenberry and others, 2003).

Geriatric Considerations
- Visual and dexterity impairment may make it difficult for an older adult to prepare and administer an injection. This can be aggravated during times of illness. A friend or family member may need to be taught how to administer injections. Assistive devices, such as magnifiers, are also available to help clients prepare their own injections.
- Jet injectors are available for insulin administration. These devices may improve accuracy of insulin administration in clients with visual impairment or dexterity problems. However, the cost of the injectors is

high and they may cause trauma to the skin if used incorrectly. Several penlike devices and insulin-containing cartridges are available that deliver insulin through a needle (ADA, 2001).

- Clients over the age of 60, especially women, are more susceptible to the hemorrhagic effects of heparin (McKenry and Salerno, 2001).

Home Care Considerations

- Instruction regarding site selection and site rotation is required for clients who must self-administer SQ medications at home (see Procedural Guideline 18-3).
- Clients should always have a spare bottle of each type of insulin used. A slight loss in potency may occur after the bottle has been in use for more than 30 days (ADA, 2001).
- Home care agencies can usually provide puncture-proof containers for needle and syringe disposal. Local trash-disposal authorities should be consulted to determine appropriate disposition of containers.

- It is safe and practical for clients to reuse syringes in the home. The syringe should be discarded when the needle becomes dull, has been bent, or has contacted any surface other than the client's skin (ADA, 2001).
- Clients with inadequate personal hygiene, an acute concurrent illness, open wounds on the hands, or decreased resistance to infection should not reuse a syringe (ADA, 2001).
- Family members, friends, and co-workers should be instructed in use of glucagon for situations when the individual cannot take carbohydrate orally for hypoglycemia.
- Clients on daily insulin or heparin doses at home should wear a medical alert bracelet.
- Instruct clients receiving heparin to read labels of over-the-counter (OTC) medications that may contain ibuprofen, aspirin, and other salicylates.
- Fall prevention is important for clients receiving heparin therapy.

Skill 18.2

Intramuscular Injections

An IM injection deposits medication into deep muscle tissue. The vascularity of muscle results in rapid drug absorption. An aqueous solution when given intramuscularly is absorbed in 10 to 30 minutes, as opposed to at least 30 minutes when given subcutaneously. A larger volume of drug (up to 5 ml) can be injected into the well-developed muscles of adults because fluid spreads rapidly through the muscle's elastic fibers (Rodger and King, 2000). A volume of 1 to 2 ml is generally recommended for individuals with less well developed muscles (Beyea and Nicoll, 1995). Older infants and children under the age of 2 years receiving IM injection should receive no more than 1 ml of medication (Hockenberry and others, 2003).

IM injections require a longer-gauge needle to penetrate deep muscle tissue. Generally, for the average adult a 21- to 25-gauge, 1½-inch needle inserted at a 90-degree angle will pass through SQ tissue and enter deep muscle. Older adults, cachetic clients, and children require shorter needles, whereas larger clients may need 2-inch or longer needles (Engstrom and others, 2000). The size of the syringe is determined by the volume of medication and should correspond as closely as possible to the amount to be administered. Volumes of less than 0.5 ml should be given with a low-dose syringe to ensure dosage accuracy.

The Z-track technique is recommended for all IM injections to reduce leakage of medication into SQ tissue and minimize pain (Beyea and Nicoll, 1995; Rodger and King, 2000). This technique leaves a zigzag path that seals the needle track, preventing the medication from escaping the muscle tissue.

INTRAMUSCULAR SITE SELECTION

When selecting an IM site, the nurse determines if the area is free of infection, necrosis, bruising, and abrasions. The location of underlying bones, nerves, and major blood vessels and the volume of medication to be given are also considered. Each site has certain advantages and disadvantages (Box 18-4). The dorsogluteal muscle has traditionally been a site recommended for injections. However, studies have demonstrated that the exact location of the sciatic nerve varies from one person to another. If a needle hits the sciatic nerve, the client may experience permanent or partial paralysis of the involved leg. Therefore this site should **not** be used (Beyea and Nicoll, 1995; Rodger and King, 2000). The preferred site for an IM injection for adults and children over 7 months old is the ventrogluteal site (Beyea and Nicoll, 1995). This site provides the greatest thickness of gluteal muscle, does not have nerves and blood vessels penetrating it, has the most consistent and thin layer of fat covering it, and has very few documented injuries associated with it (Rodger and King, 2000).

Location of an appropriate site for IM injection involves the ability to palpate anatomical landmarks accurately and knowledge of the location of underlying nerves and major blood vessels. Presence of excessive fatty tissue may make location of bony structures difficult; with experience, however, accurate site location is achieved. Correct techniques for locating standard IM sites for injection are described in Table 18-4.

At times the nurse must teach the client or a significant other how to administer an IM injection. Examples of medications administered via the IM route at home include vitamin B_{12} and epinephrine. Steps the nurse takes in teaching this skill to the client are provided in Procedural Guideline 18-3.

Box 18-4
Advantages and Disadvantages of Intramuscular Injection Sites

- *Ventrogluteal:* Muscle is situated deep and away from major nerves and blood vessels. Provides most consistent layer of adipose tissue. Preferred injection site for adults and children over 7 months of age (Beyea and Nicoll, 1995; Rodger and King, 2000). Is also safe for infants under 7 months of age (Hockenberry and others, 2003).
- *Vastus lateralis:* Muscle is thick and well developed and is not located near major nerves and blood vessels. Preferred site for infants under 7 months of age (Hockenberry and others, 2003). Has small nerve endings resulting in discomfort after injection.
- *Deltoid:* Easily accessible muscle. Used only for small medication volumes (0.5 to 1.0 ml) or when other sites are inaccessible because of dressings or casts. Muscle is not well developed in many adults. Hepatitis B vaccine should be given only in the deltoid (Beyea and Nicoll, 1995).

Table 18-4
Locating Sites for Intramuscular Injections

Site/Steps	Figure
Ventrogluteal Site 1. Position client on either side, with knee bent and upper leg slightly ahead of the bottom leg. Client may also remain supine or may be lying on abdomen. Instruct client to relax muscles to be injected. 2. Palpate the greater trochanter at the head of the femur and the anterior superior iliac spine. To locate the proper site, use the left hand when the client lies on the left side and the right hand when the client lies on the right side (see illustration). 3. Place the palm of the hand over the greater trochanter and index finger on the anterior superior iliac spine. Point the thumb toward the client's groin and fingers toward the client's head (see illustration). 4. Spread the middle finger back along the iliac crest toward the buttock as far as possible. 5. The injection site is the center of the triangle formed by the index and middle fingers. 6. Change hands as needed to spread skin taut to give injection. Use dominant hand to give injection (see illustration).	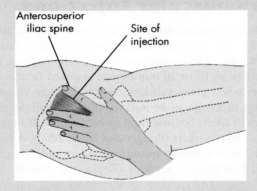 Step 2 Anatomical view of ventrogluteal muscle. 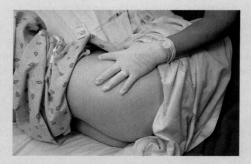 Step 3 Ventrogluteal injection site.

Table 18-4

Locating Sites for Intramuscular Injections—cont'd

Site/Steps	Figure

Ventrogluteal Site—cont'd

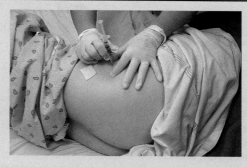

Step 6 Administering IM injection in ventrogluteal site.

Vastus Lateralis Site
1. Client may be lying supine or sitting with site well exposed. If supine, have client flex knee on side where medication will be given.
2. Place one hand above the knee and one hand below the greater trochanter of the femur (see illustration).
3. Locate the midline of the anterior thigh and the midline of the thigh's lateral (outer) side.
4. The injection site is located within a rectangle formed by these boundaries (see illustration).

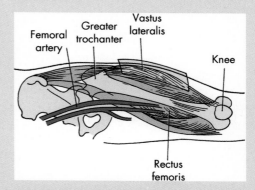

Step 2 Anatomical view of vastus lateralis muscle.

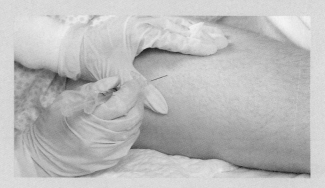

Step 4 Administering IM injection in vastus lateralis site.

Continued

Table 18-4

Locating Sites for Intramuscular Injections—cont'd

Site/Steps	Figure

Deltoid Site

1. Client may be sitting or lying down, exposing the upper arm and shoulder. A tight-fitting sleeve should be removed rather than rolled up.
2. Ask client to relax the arm at the side with the elbow flexed.
3. Palpate the lower edge of the acromion process, which forms the base of a triangle (see illustration).
4. Place four fingers across the deltoid muscle, with the top finger along the acromion process.
5. The injection site is in the center of the triangle, three finger widths or 2.5 to 5 cm (1 to 2 inches) below the acromion process (see illustration).

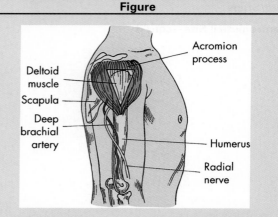

Step 3 Anatomical view of deltoid muscle.

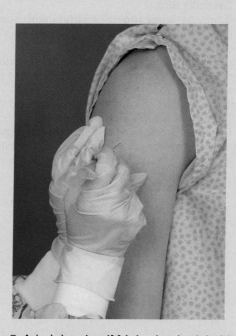

Step 5 Administering IM injection in deltoid site.

ASSESSMENT

1. Review physician's medication order for client's name, drug name, dose, time, and route of administration. *Rationale: Ensures safe and accurate drug administration.*
2. Review information pertinent to drug(s) ordered: action, purpose, appropriate route, time of onset and peak action, normal dose, common side effects, and nursing implications.
3. Check expiration date of medication.
4. Consider factors that may contraindicate IM injection (e.g., muscle atrophy, reduced blood flow, circulatory shock).
5. Assess client's medical history, history of allergies, and medication history.
6. Assess client's knowledge regarding medication and dosage schedule. *Rationale: Information may pose implications for client education.*
7. Observe client's verbal and nonverbal responses toward receiving injection. *Rationale: Injections can cause anxiety which may increase pain.*

PLANNING

Expected outcomes focus on safe, effective administration of injection with minimal anxiety and discomfort.

Expected Outcomes

1. Client demonstrates desired effect of medication without evidence of adverse effects.
2. Client experiences minimal pain or burning at the injection site.
3. Client understands purpose and desired effects of medication.

Equipment

- Syringe (1 to 5 ml)
- Needle (1 to 2 inch, 21 to 25 gauge)
- Medication ampule or vial
- Alcohol swab
- Dry sterile gauze
- Disposable gloves
- MAR or computer printout

Delegation Considerations

The skill of administering IM injections requires the critical thinking and knowledge application unique to a nurse. Delegation is inappropriate. Inform assistive personnel (AP) of possible side effects to report immediately to the nurse.

IMPLEMENTATION FOR INTRAMUSCULAR INJECTIONS

Steps	Rationale
1. See Standard Protocol (inside front cover).	
NURSE ALERT *Review the six rights for administration of medications.*	
2. Check expiration date of medication, prepare medication in syringe (see Tables 18-1 and 18-2 and Procedural Guidelines 18-1 and 18-2).	
3. Identify client by checking identification arm band and asking client's name. Compare with MAR.	Ensures right client receives right medication.
4. Explain procedure, location of injection site, and how positioning lessens discomfort. Proceed in calm manner.	Allows client to anticipate injection so as to lessen anxiety.
5. Choose appropriate IM injection site (ventrogluteal preferred) by assessing size and integrity of muscle. Palpate for areas of tenderness or hardness. Note presence of bruising or area of infection.	Muscle is soft when relaxed and firm when tense; absence of tenderness or bruising indicates healthy tissue.
6. Assist client to comfortable position, depending on site (see Table 18-4).	Minimizes discomfort of injection.
7. Relocate site using anatomical landmarks.	Injection into correct anatomical site prevents injury to nerves, bones, and blood vessels.
8. Carefully remove cap or sheath from needle.	
9. With nondominant hand, pull the skin 2.5 to 3.5 cm (1 to 1½ inches) laterally down so as to administer the injection in a Z-track manner. Hold the skin taut.	Z-track technique reduces discomfort and leakage of medication into SQ tissues (McConnell, 2000).
10. Cleanse site with an antiseptic swab beginning at the center of the site and moving outward in a circular direction for about 5 cm (2 inches). Allow alcohol to dry.	Cleansing reduces surface pathogens, reducing risk of infecting deep tissues.
11. Hold swab or gauze square between fingers of nondominant hand or place near site.	Swab remains accessible when needle is withdrawn.
12. Hold syringe between thumb and forefinger of dominant hand as if holding a dart, with palm down at 90-degree angle to client's skin.	Needle must be injected at 90-degree angle to enter muscle.

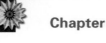

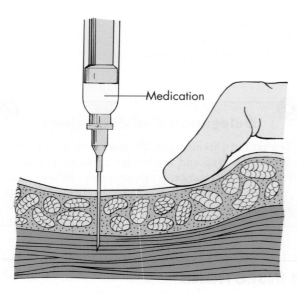

Step 13 Pull the skin laterally down and hold while administering injection.

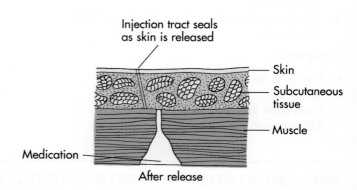

Step 15 The Z-track left after injection prevents the deposit of medication through sensitive tissue.

Steps	Rationale
13. Insert needle quickly at 90-degree angle into muscle (see illustration). Hold syringe, and aspirate with one hand for at least 5 to 10 seconds. If no blood appears in syringe, inject medication slowly at a rate of 1 ml every 10 seconds.	Aspirating for 5 to 10 seconds is adequate to ensure needle is not in a small blood vessel. A slow, steady injection rate promotes comfort and minimizes tissue damage (Rodger and King, 2000).

NURSE ALERT   *If blood appears in syringe, remove needle and dispose of medication and syringe properly. Prepare new syringe with medication.*

Steps	Rationale
14. Wait 10 seconds after injecting the medication before withdrawing the needle.	Allows medication to deposit into muscle and to begin to diffuse.
15. Smoothly and steadily withdraw the needle and release the skin (see illustration). Apply gentle pressure at site with dry sponge or swab.	Minimizes tissue injury. Leaves a zigzag path that seals the needle track where tissue planes slide across each other. Massaging site can cause tissue irritation (Beyea and Nicoll, 1995).
16. Place small adhesive bandage over puncture site if bleeding is noted.	
17. Discard sheathed or uncapped needle and attached syringe into appropriate receptacle. Discard gloves, and wash hands.	Prevents injury to client and health care personnel. Recapping needles increases risk of needle-stick injury (NIOSH, 1999).
18. See Completion Protocol (inside front cover).	

• • • • • • • • • •

EVALUATION

1. Observe client's response to medication at times that correlate with the medication's onset, peak, and duration to determine effectiveness of drug and observe for adverse reactions.
2. Assess the injection site 2 to 4 hours after injection for redness, swelling, pain, or other effects.
3. Have client verbalize desired effect and reason for medication.

Unexpected Outcomes and Related Interventions

1. Client develops signs and symptoms of allergy or side effects.
   a. Follow institutional guidelines for the appropriate response and reporting of adverse drug reactions, and notify client's health care provider immediately.
2. Client insists on selecting site using incorrect criteria.
   a. Educate client about need to identify site correctly.

3. Client continues to complain of localized pain, numbness, or tingling, indicating potential injury to nerves or tissues.
   a. Assess injection site and other involved areas, and notify client's health care provider.

Recording and Reporting

- Document medication administration immediately after giving medication on MAR to record care provided and to prevent future drug administration errors.
- Record client's response to medication.
- Report undesirable effects from medication to client's health care provider, and document treatment of adverse effects according to institutional policy.

Sample Documentation

1826 Rates incision pain as an 8 on 0-10 pain scale. 10 mg morphine sulfate IM administered as ordered in right ventrogluteal site.

SPECIAL CONSIDERATIONS

Pediatric Considerations

- The deltoid muscle is no longer recommended as an injection site in children.
- Children can be very anxious or fearful of needles. Assistance with proper positioning and holding of the child may be necessary. Distraction, such as bubble blowing and touch, can help alleviate the child's anxiety and pain perception (Sparks, 2001).
- If possible, apply EMLA cream to site and cover with an occlusive dressing at least 1 hour before IM injection or use a vapocoolant spray just before injection to decrease pain (Hockenberry and others, 2003).

Geriatric Considerations

Older adults are prone to muscle atrophy, requiring careful assessment and selection of injection sites. The muscle may have to be grasped between the thumb and fingers for injection.

Home Care Considerations

Clients requiring regular injections (e.g., vitamin B_{12}) should learn importance of rotating sites. Injections may be given by family members, client, or home health nurse. Instruction will be necessary in proper injection preparation and administration and disposal of syringes and needles (see Procedural Guideline 18-3).

Skill 18.3

Intradermal Injections

Intradermal injections are used for administering small amounts of local anesthetic and skin testing, such as in TB screening and allergy tests. Because these medications are potent, they are injected in small amounts into the dermis, where blood supply is reduced and drug absorption occurs slowly. A client may have an anaphylactic reaction if the medication enters the circulation too rapidly. For clients with a history of numerous allergies, the physician may perform skin testing.

Skin testing requires the identification of changes in color and tissue integrity. Therefore intradermal sites should be lightly pigmented, free of lesions, and relatively hairless. The inner forearm and upper back are ideal locations.

A TB or 1-ml syringe with a short ($\frac{1}{4}$- to $\frac{1}{2}$-inch), fine-gauge (26 or 27) needle is used for intradermal injections. Very small amounts of medication (0.01 to 0.1 ml) are injected. If a bleb does not appear or if the site bleeds after needle withdrawal, the medication may enter SQ tissues. In this case, skin test results will not be valid.

ASSESSMENT

1. Review physician's medication order for client's name, drug name, dose, time, and route of administration. *Rationale: Ensures safe and accurate drug administration.*
2. Review information regarding drug action, purpose, normal route, dosage, and expected reaction when testing skin with specific allergen or medication.
3. Assess client's history of allergies, substance to which client is allergic, and normal allergic reaction.
4. Determine if client has had previous reaction to skin testing. *Rationale: Can prevent a major allergic response.*
5. Check date of expiration for medication or test solution.
6. Assess client's knowledge of purpose and reactions of skin testing. *Rationale: Reveals need for client education.*

PLANNING

Expected outcomes focus on safe administration and the identification of allergies or exposure to tuberculosis.

Expected Outcomes

1. Desired effect of medication is achieved.
2. Client experiences very mild burning sensation during injection but no discomfort or adverse effects from the medication after the injection.
3. Small, light-colored bleb, approximately 6 mm (¼ inch) in diameter, forms at site and gradually disappears.
4. Client verbalizes and identifies signs of a skin reaction.

Equipment

- 1-ml TB syringe with 26- or 27-gauge (¼- to ½-inch) needle
- Alcohol swab
- Dry sterile gauze pad
- Vial or ampule of skin test solution
- Disposable gloves
- Skin pencil (optional)
- MAR or computer printout

Delegation Considerations

The skill of administering intradermal injections requires the critical thinking and knowledge application unique to a nurse. Delegation is inappropriate. Inform assistive personnel (AP) of possible allergic reactions to report immediately to the nurse.

IMPLEMENTATION FOR INTRADERMAL INJECTIONS

Steps	Rationale
1. See Standard Protocol (inside front cover).	

NURSE ALERT *Review the six rights for administration of medications.*

Steps	Rationale
2. Prepare medication or test solution in syringe (see Procedural Guidelines 18-1 and 18-2, p. 466).	
3. Identify client by checking identification arm band and asking client's name. Compare with MAR.	Ensures right client receives right medication.
4. Select appropriate injection site. Inspect skin surface for bruises, inflammation, or edema. If possible, select site three to four fingerwidths below antecubital space and one hand above wrist. If forearm cannot be used, inspect the upper back. If necessary, sites appropriate for SQ injections (see Figure 18-11) can be used (Workman, 1999).	Injection sites should be free of abnormalities that may interfere with drug absorption. An intradermal site should be clear so results of skin test can be seen and read correctly.
5. Assist client to comfortable position with elbow and forearm extended and supported on flat surface.	Stabilizes injection site for easiest accessibility.
6. Cleanse site with an antiseptic swab, beginning at center of the site and rotating outward in a circular direction for about 5 cm (2 inches). Allow to dry.	Mechanical action of swab removes secretions containing microorganisms. Drying prevents antiseptic from affecting test results.
7. Hold swab or square of sterile gauze between fingers of nondominant hand.	Swab or gauze remains readily accessible when needle is withdrawn.
8. Remove needle cap or sheath from needle by pulling it straight off.	Preventing needle from touching sides of cap prevents contamination.
9. Hold syringe between thumb and forefinger of dominant hand with bevel of needle pointing up.	Bevel up facilitates correct needle placement.
10. With nondominant hand, stretch skin over site with forefinger or thumb.	Needle pierces tight skin more easily.

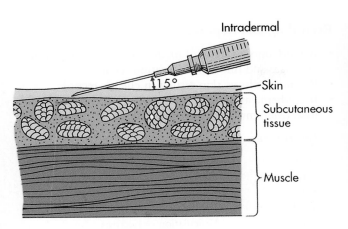

Step 11 Inject intradermal needle at a 5- to 15-degree angle.

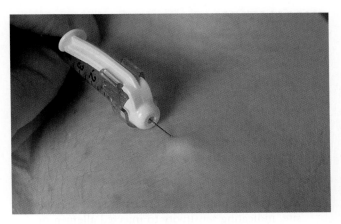

Step 13 Injection creates a small bleb.

Steps	**Rationale**
11. With needle almost against client's skin, insert it carefully at a 5- to 15-degree angle until resistance is felt (see illustration), and advance needle through epidermis to approximately 3 mm (⅛ inch) below skin surface. Needle tip can be seen through skin.	Ensures needle tip is in dermis.
12. Inject medication slowly. It is not necessary to aspirate, because dermis is relatively avascular. Normally resistance is felt. If not, needle is too deep; remove and begin again.	Slow injection minimizes discomfort at site. Dermal layer is tight and does not expand easily when solution is injected.
13. While injecting medication, a bleb resembling a mosquito bite approximately 6 mm (¼ inch) in diameter forms at site (see illustration).	Bleb indicates medication is in dermis.

COMMUNICATION TIP   *During this time, explain to client what the skin will look like: Normally the skin will remain clear, or you might notice a needle mark. If the test is positive, you will notice redness and a lump at the site.*

---

14. Withdraw needle while applying alcohol swab or gauze gently over site.	Support of tissue around injection site minimizes discomfort during needle withdrawal.
15. Do not massage site.	Massage may disperse medication into underlying tissue layers and alter test results.
16. Discard uncapped needle and syringe in appropriately labeled receptacle. Discard gloves, and wash hands.	Prevents injury to client and health care personnel.
17. If skin testing, read site within appropriate amount of time, designated by type of medication or skin test given. If client is tested in a clinic or other outpatient setting, have client call in results to health care provider's office.	There is a prescribed wait of 20 minutes to several days (depending on the antigen) before the local reaction should be evaluated for positive test. TB tests should be read in 48 to 72 hours (McKenry and Salerno, 2001).
18. See Completion Protocol (inside front cover).	

• • • • • • • • • •

EVALUATION

1. Evaluate for desired effect of medication. If medication is for skin testing, assess site at appropriate time for erythema and induration.
2. Assess for pain and any allergic reactions.
3. Inspect bleb. *Optional:* Use skin pencil and draw circle around perimeter of injection site. Tell client not to wash off markings around injection site.
4. Ask client to describe implications of skin testing and signs of expected skin reaction or hypersensitivity.

Unexpected Outcomes and Related Interventions

1. Erythema or induration appears around injection site, indicating sensitivity to injected allergen or positive test for tuberculin skin testing.
   a. Document results, and notify client's health care provider.
   b. Positive TB reaction is indicated by induration 9 mm or more of injection site. Five to 9 mm is a questionable result and should be investigated further (McKenry and Salerno, 2001). Explain that a positive tuberculin test indicates exposure, not active disease. A person who has contact with an individual with TB and whose initial TB reaction (induration) is more than 5 mm should have a chest x-ray film and be considered for preventive therapy. Contacts who initially have negative skin test results should receive a repeat skin test 10 to 12 weeks after the initial test.
2. Onset of anaphylactic response occurs within minutes.
   a. Follow institutional policy or guidelines for appropriate response to allergic reactions.
   b. Notify client's health care provider immediately.
   c. Anticipate administration of epinephrine and need for respiratory and circulatory support (McKenry and Salerno, 2001).
3. Occasionally a highly positive reaction will result in vesiculation and necrosis of overlying skin (McKenry and Salerno, 2001).
   a. Notify client's health care provider immediately. Anticipate order for corticosteroid.
4. Client is unable to explain purpose or reading of skin testing.
   a. Provide further instruction, or make alternative plans for reading of skin site if client is unable to learn at this time.

Recording and Reporting

- Record amount, type of medication, site of injection, and date and time on medication record.
- Record results of skin testing in client's record.
- If erythema and induration occur, record results as follows (McKenry and Salerno, 2001):

For erythema

Trace	Faint discoloration
+ (one plus)	Pink
++	Red
+++	Purplish red
++++	Vesiculation or necrosis

For induration

Trace	Barely palpable
+	Palpable, but not visible
++	Palpable and visible, indurated area buckles when squeezed gently
+++	Palpable and visible, but does not buckle when squeezed gently
++++	Vesiculation or necrosis

Sample Documentation

1000 PPD injection site in left lower forearm read at 72 hours; test site without redness or induration.

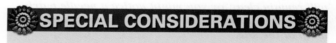

SPECIAL CONSIDERATIONS

Geriatric Considerations

- TB skin testing in older adults is an unreliable indicator of TB. Older adults often display a false-negative skin test as a result of reduced immune system activity.
- The skin becomes less elastic during physiological changes in the older adult. Therefore the skin must be held taut to ensure the intradermal injection is administered correctly.

Skill 18.4

Continuous Subcutaneous Medications

The continuous subcutaneous infusion (CSQI or CSCI) route of medication administration is often used as an alternative to IV, IM, or SQ injections of medication. CSQI is mainly used for the administration of medications for pain management (e.g., opioids) and insulin. It has also been used with medications that stop preterm labor. For optimal medication absorption, no more than 1 to 2 ml/hr should be administered using CSQI.

CSQI is used in many settings, including the home, because it enables clients to manage their illness and/or

pain without the risks and expenses involved with IV medication administration. When used for pain management, this route has been associated with better pain control and less sleep disturbance related to pain when compared with IV pain medications (Dawson and others, 1999). Box 18-5 summarizes indications for the use of CSQI in clients requiring pain management. Criteria for clients considering an insulin pump are listed in Box 18-6.

The procedure to initiate and discontinue CSQI therapy is similar regardless of the type of medication that is being delivered. However, nursing assessment and interventions vary depending on the medication being delivered. For example, if the medication is used for pain management, the nurse evaluates the effectiveness of the medication by assessing the client's pain. Alternatively, if the client is receiving insulin, the nurse assesses the client's blood glucose levels and occurrences of hypoglycemia and hyperglycemia.

A small-gauge (25 to 27) winged butterfly IV needle is used to deliver medications through CSQI (Figure 18-12). Alternatively, a special commercially prepared Teflon cannula may be used. Although Teflon cannulas are generally more expensive, they tend to be more comfortable for the client and have lower rates of complications when compared with winged IV needles. The needle used should be of the shortest length and the smallest gauge necessary to establish and maintain the infusion (Intravenous Nursing Society, 2000).

Anatomical sites for SQ injections (see Figure 18-11) and the upper chest may be used for CSQI. Site selection depends on the client's activity level and the type of medication delivered. For example, insulin is absorbed most consistently in the abdomen; thus a site in the abdomen, away from the waistline, is the preferred site for insulin administration. Sites should avoid scar tissue and areas of

Box 18-5

Common Characteristics of Clients Receiving Pain Medication by Continuous Subcutaneous Infusion

- Inability to tolerate oral medications (e.g., nausea and vomiting, dysphagia, malabsorption)
- Requires continuous or large amounts of medications to control pain
- Poor venous access
- Will require injections (e.g., SQ, IM) for more than 48 hours
- Is confused or drowsy or has altered level of consciousness
- Inability to afford IV therapy

Box 18-6

Selection Criteria for Clients Using Insulin Pumps

- Requires or desires improved control of blood glucose levels
- Daily routine requires greater flexibility than allowed by traditional insulin injection schedules
- Strong motivation and commitment to use diabetes management skills
- Acceptance of responsibilities associated with the self-management of diabetes
- Ability to perform self-monitoring of blood glucose levels and to operate the insulin pump
- Evidence of effective coping patterns
- Availability of support systems
- Availability of financial resources to cover costs associated with CSQI

Modified from American Association of Diabetes Educators: AADE position statement: education for continuous subcutaneous insulin infusion pump users, *Diabetes Educ* 23(4):397, 1997.

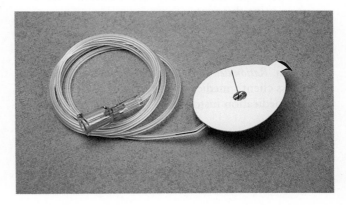

Figure 18-12 Small-gauge butterfly needle and tubing for CSQI therapy.

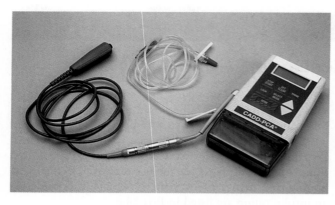

Figure 18-13 Medication pump.

hardened tissues. The nurse also should attempt to avoid sites where clothing could rub or constrict the pump's tubing. Sites should be free from irritation and away from bony prominences and the waistline. Sites should be rotated at least every 72 hours or whenever complications, such as leaking or infection, occur (Infusion Nursing Society, 2000).

This route requires the use of a computerized pump with safety features, including lockout intervals and warning alarms. A variety of medication pumps are currently available (Figure 18-13). Ideally medication pumps should be chosen for each individual, based on the medication being delivered and the client's needs. The availability and cost of the pump and its supplies should also be considered. When possible, clients should be allowed to select the pump that fits their needs the best and that is the easiest to use.

ASSESSMENT

1. Review physician's medication order for client's name, drug name, dose, time, and route of administration. *Rationale: Ensures safe and accurate drug administration.*
2. Review information pertinent to drug ordered: action, purpose, side effects, safe dosage range, and nursing implications. Verify that medication can be given using this route.
3. Check expiration date of medication.
4. Assess for factors that may contraindicate CSQI, such as circulatory shock or reduced local tissue perfusion. *Rationale: Conditions will reduce drug absorption.*
5. Assess client's medical history, history of allergies, and medication history.

6. Assess adequacy of client's adipose tissue. *Rationale: Determines appropriate site for needle insertion.*
7. Assess client's knowledge regarding medication to be received and use of the medication pump. *Rationale: Determines client's ability to problem-solve and manage pump.*

PLANNING

Expected outcomes focus on safe, effective administration of medication with minimal anxiety and discomfort.

Expected Outcomes

1. Needle insertion site remains free from infection.
2. Desired effect of medication is achieved with no signs of adverse reactions.
3. Client explains purpose, dosage, and effects of medication and verbalizes understanding of CSQI therapy.

Equipment

Initiation of CSQI

- Clean, nonsterile gloves
- Alcohol swab
- Povidone-iodine swab
- Small-gauge (25 to 27) winged IV catheter with attached tubing or catheter especially for CSQI (e.g., Sof-set)
- Infusion pump
- Occlusive, transparent dressing
- Tape
- Medication in appropriate syringe or container

Discontinuing CSQI

- Clean, nonsterile gloves
- Small, sterile gauze dressing and tape or adhesive bandage
- Alcohol swab and povidone-iodine swab (optional)

Delegation Considerations

The skill of administering continuous SQ medications requires the critical thinking and knowledge application unique to a nurse. Delegation is inappropriate. Inform assistive personnel (AP) of possible side effects to report immediately to the RN.

IMPLEMENTATION FOR CONTINUOUS SUBCUTANEOUS MEDICATIONS

Steps	Rationale
1. See Standard Protocol (inside front cover).	

NURSE ALERT   *Review the six rights for administration of medications.*

Steps	Rationale
2. **To initiate CSQI**	
a. Prepare correct medication dose from vial or ampule or check dose on prefilled syringe, and prime tubing with medication following manufacturer's directions.	
b. Obtain and program medication administration pump.	
c. Identify client by checking identification arm band and asking client's name. Compare with MAR.	
d. Explain procedure to client, and proceed in calm, confident manner.	Involves client in care and eases anxiety.
e. Select appropriate injection site. Most common sites used are subclavicular, abdominal, upper arms, or thighs (Infusion Nursing Society, 2000).	Site must be free from irritation and not over bony prominences.
f. Assist client to comfortable position.	Minimizes discomfort of insertion of needle.
g. Cleanse injection site with alcohol followed by povidone-iodine in a circular fashion. Allow both alcohol and povidone-iodine to dry	Reduces risk of infection at insertion site.

NURSE ALERT   *Clients allergic to povidone-iodine or managing CSQI at home may use an antibacterial soap (e.g. Hibiclens, pHisoHex) to cleanse insertion site (Frazzitta-Luersen, 1997).*

Steps	Rationale
h. Hold needle in dominant hand, and remove needle guard.	Prepares needle for insertion.

COMMUNICATION TIP   *Inserting this needle may feel like a mosquito bite. Tell client, "I am going to inject this now."*

Steps	Rationale
i. With nondominant hand, pinch or lift up skin and gently and firmly insert needle at a 45- to 90-degree angle (see illustration).	Ensures needle will enter SQ tissue.

NURSE ALERT   *Some prepackaged needles (e.g., Sof-Set, Sub-Q-Set) are inserted at a 90-degree angle because they are shorter than butterfly needles. Refer to manufacturer's directions.*

Steps	Rationale
j. Release skinfold, and apply tape over "wings" of needle.	Secures needle.

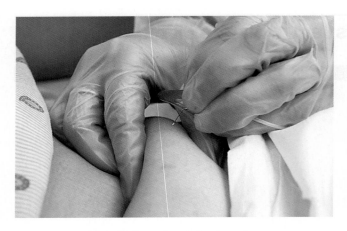

Step 2i Securing injection site.

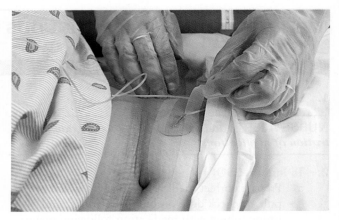

Step 2k Insertion of butterfly needle into SQ tissue of abdomen.

Steps	Rationale

NURSE ALERT *Some cannulas have a sharp needle with a plastic catheter covering the needle. In this case, remove the needle and leave the plastic catheter in the skin.*

k. Place occlusive, transparent dressing over insertion site (see illustration).

Protects site from infection and allows site to be inspected for signs of infection.

l. Attach tubing from needle to tubing from infusion pump, and turn pump on.

Allows medication to be administered.

NURSE ALERT *Some pumps require additional priming at this point to clear air from the dead space of the new infusion set. Refer to pump manufacturer's guidelines.*

COMMUNICATION TIP *Some medications (e.g., fentanyl) burn with initiation of medication pump. Tell client, "You may feel some burning with this medication, but this should go away as the medication infuses for a while. Please let me know if this medication makes you uncomfortable."*

m. Dispose of any sharps into appropriate receptacle. Discard gloves, and wash hands.

Prevents injury to clients and health care personnel.

n. Assess site before leaving client, and instruct client to inform nurse if site becomes red or begins to leak.

A new site with a new needle must be initiated whenever erythema or leaking occurs (Infusion Nursing Society, 2000).

3. **To discontinue CSQI**
   a. Verify order, and establish alternative method for medication administration if applicable.

If medication will be required after discontinuing CSQI, a different medication and/or route may be necessary to continue to manage client's illness or pain.

   b. Stop infusion pump.
   c. Remove dressing without dislodging or removing needle.

Exposes needle.

   d. Cleanse site with alcohol and then povidone-iodine if site is infected or if indicated by institutional policy.

Cleans insertion site.

Steps	Rationale
e. Remove tape from the wings of needle or cannula, and pull needle out at the same angle it was inserted.	Minimizes discomfort to client.
f. Apply gentle pressure at site until no fluid leaks out of skin.	
g. Apply small sterile gauze dressing or adhesive bandage to site.	Prevents bacterial entry into puncture site.
h. Discard used supplies, and perform hand hygiene.	
4. See Completion Protocol (inside front cover).	

• • • • • • • • • •

EVALUATION

1. Assess site at least every 4 hours for redness, pain, drainage, or swelling.
2. Evaluate client's response to medication.
3. Ask client to verbalize understanding of medication and CSQI therapy.

Unexpected Outcomes and Related Interventions

1. Client complains of localized pain or burning at needle's insertion site, or site appears red, swollen, or is leaking, indicating potential infection or dislodgement of needle.
   a. Remove needle, and place new needle in different site.
   b. Continue to monitor old site for signs of infection, and notify health care provider if infection is suspected.
   c. Assess client to determine potential effects of not receiving medication (e.g., assess pain level if client is receiving pain medication).
   d. Document nursing interventions in client's medical record. Complete incident report if necessary.
2. Client displays allergic symptoms to medication.
   a. Follow institutional policy or guidelines for appropriate response to allergic reactions, and notify client's health care provider immediately.
3. Desired effect of medication is not achieved.
   a. Follow established protocols for titration of medication, or notify client's health care provider for either change in dosage or medication.

Recording and Reporting

- Immediately after initiating CSQI, chart medication, dose, route, site, time, date, and type of medication pump in appropriate place in client's medical record.
- Record client's response to medication and appearance of site every 4 hours or according to institutional policy.
- Report any adverse effects from medication or infection at insertion site to client's health care provider, and document according to institutional policy. Client's condition may indicate need for additional or different medical therapy.

Sample Documentation

2210 Initiated CSQI site per institutional protocol. Client instructed on need to call if pain persists or if site becomes red or begins to drain.

❀ SPECIAL CONSIDERATIONS ❀

Pediatric Considerations

Despite the barriers to CSQI in adolescents with diabetes, insulin pumps offer more flexibility and insulin dosage can be quickly changed based on the client's current situation. To achieve successful diabetes management, intensive education is required both for the client and the family, especially during the first few weeks after starting CSQI. The nurse must ensure that clients and their families have all the information and skills necessary to use CSQI (Boland, Ahern, and Grey, 1998).

Geriatric Considerations

CSQI can be used to deliver isotonic IV solutions to dehydrated older adults. This is called hypodermoclysis therapy. This method of providing hydration avoids the need to transfer the client from home or long-term care facility to an acute care hospital. Fluids should infuse slowly (e.g., 30 ml/hr) during the first hour of therapy. If the client remains comfortable, the rate may be increased but should not exceed 80 ml/hr (Worobec and Brown, 1997). Fluids given this way should only be given for a short time. For long-term administration of fluids, IV access should be initiated.

Home Care Considerations

Clients at home with CSQI should identify an additional caregiver if possible. The nurse should educate the client and the caregiver about the desired effect of the medication, side effects and adverse effects of the medication, operation of the pump, when and how to assess and rotate injection sites, and when to call a health care provider for problems. They also will need to determine where and how to obtain required supplies.

CRITICAL THINKING EXERCISES

1. You are about to administer insulin to Mr. Pontiac, a 35-year-old man with type 1 diabetes, who will be going to physical therapy for arm and leg strengthening exercises in about an hour. Where will you inject the insulin? What factors helped you make your decision?

2. Mrs. Martin is scheduled to receive an IM injection of morphine. She fell and broke her hip earlier this morning and is in Buck's traction. Where will you give her injection and why?

3. Sally is about to go to college and needs a TB skin test. As you are assessing her forearms, you realize that both of her arms are sunburned. Where will you administer her skin test and why?

4. Jessica is receiving fentanyl through CSQI. Upon assessment, you notice the site is reddened and leaking. She is complaining of 6/10 pain, whereas 2 hours earlier she rated her pain as 0/10. What will you do about her infusion, and how will you manage her pain?

REFERENCES

American Association of Diabetes Educators: AADE position statement: education for continuous subcutaneous insulin infusion pump users, *Diabetes Educ* 23(4):397, 1997.

American Diabetes Association: Position statement: insulin administration, *Diabetes Care* 24(11):1984, 2001.

American Nurses Association: Nursing facts about needlestick injuries, http://www.nursingworld.org/readroom/fsneedle.htm, 1999, retrieved Jan 7, 2002.

American Nurses Association: 2001 legislation: needlestick injury prevention, http://www.nursingworld.org/gova/state/2001/2001maps/ganeedle.htm, 2001, retrieved Jan 7, 2002.

Beyea SC, Nicoll LH: Administration of medications via the intramuscular route: a integrative review of the literature and research-based protocol for the procedure, *Appl Nurs Res* 8(1):23, 1995.

Boland E, Ahern J, Grey M: A primer on the use of insulin pumps in adolescents, *Diabetes Educ* 24(1):78, 1998.

Chan H: Effects of injection duration on site-pain intensity and bruising associated with subcutaneous heparin, *J Adv Nurs* 35(6): 882, 2001.

Dawson L and others: Improving patients' postoperative sleep: a randomized control study comparing subcutaneous with intravenous patient-controlled analgesia, *J Adv Nurs* 30(4):875, 1999.

Engstrom J and others: Procedures used to prepare and administer intramuscular injections: a study of infertility nurses, *J Obstet Gynecol Neonatal Nurs* 29(2):159, 2000.

Frazzitta-Luerssen M: Infusion site do's and don'ts, *Diabetes Forecast* 50(2):45, 1997.

Hockenberry MJ and others: *Wong's nursing care of infants and children*, ed 7, St Louis, 2003, Mosby.

Infusion Nursing Society: Standards for continuous subcutaneous medication administration, *J Intraven Nurs* 23(65):S64, 2000.

McConnell, EA: Administering subcutaneous heparin, *Nursing* 30(6):17, 2000.

McKenry LM, Salerno E: *Pharmacology in nursing*, ed 21, St Louis, 2001, Mosby.

National Institute for Occupational Safety and Health (NIOSH): *NIOSH alert: preventing needlestick injuries in health care settings*, NISOH Publications Dissemination DHHS (NIOSH) Pub No. 2000-108, Nov 1999.

Occupational Safety and Health Administration (OSHA): Occupational exposure to bloodborne pathogens; needlestick and other sharps injuries; final rule, *Federal Register*, CFR 29, part 1910 (*Federal Register* 66:5317, Jan 18, 2001); also available at www.osha.gov/needlesticks.

Peragallo-Dittko V: Rethinking subcutaneous injection technique, *Am J Nurs* 97(5): 71, 1997.

Posey D, Long B: Always swab the stopper on vials before each use, *RN* 59(2):9, 1996.

Rodger MA, King, L: Drawing up and administering intramuscular injections: a review of the literature, *J Adv Nurs* 31(3):574, 2000.

Sparks L: Taking the "ouch" out of injections for children, *MCN Am J Matern Child Nurs* 26(2):72, 2001.

Workman B: Safe injection techniques, *Nurs Stand* 13(39):47, 1999.

Worobec F, Brown M: Hypodermoclysis therapy in a chronic care hospital setting, *J Gerontol Nurs* 23(6):23, 1997.

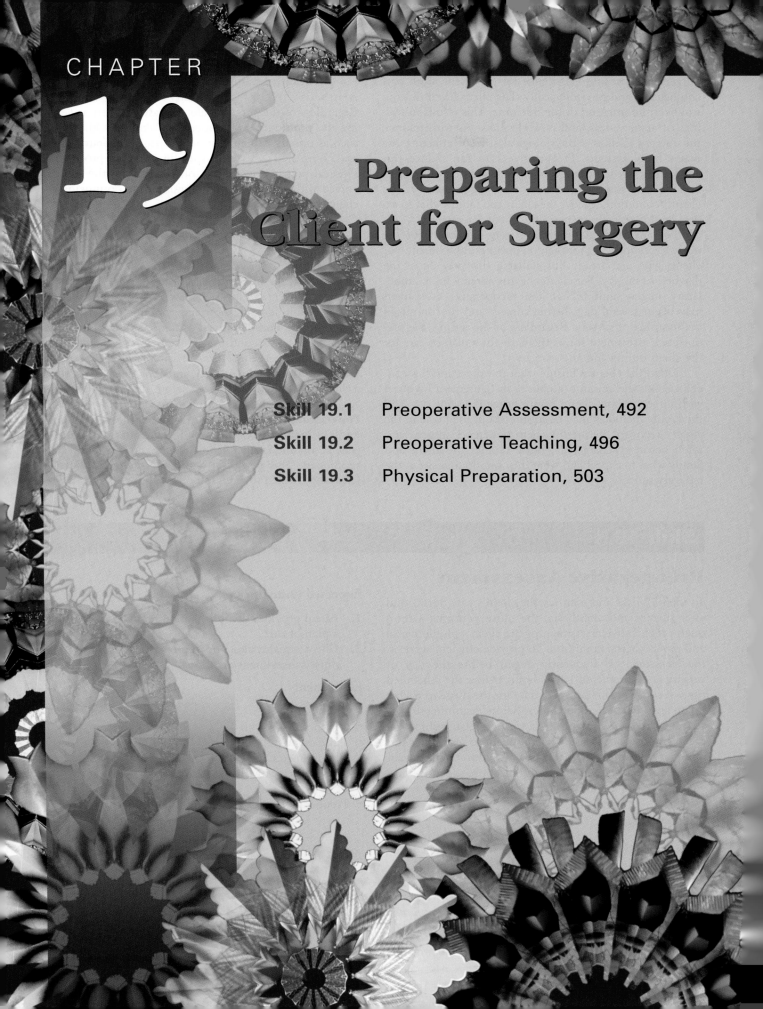

CHAPTER 19

Preparing the Client for Surgery

Surgery is a stressful experience for the client, both psychologically and physiologically. The client has little control over the situation or the outcome. This results in feelings of anxiety, fear, and powerlessness. As with trauma, the surgery itself is a physiological stressor affecting the major body systems. Preoperative care can reduce this stress and place the client in the best condition possible to undergo the surgery. The nurse thoroughly assesses the client's condition, teaches the client and family what to expect, and physically prepares the client for surgery.

For any surgical procedure, it is important for the nurse to complete a thorough preoperative assessment. For clients who are already hospitalized, this may occur the day before surgery. For clients having surgery in an ambulatory surgery unit (ASU), the preoperative assessment may begin several days before surgery and be completed the morning of surgery. Regardless of the setting, the preoperative assessment forms the basis for a plan of care for the client during and after surgery.

Often the client is unsure what to expect and has concerns about the amount of pain or disfigurement involved with surgery. Many clients return home the same day, and the family members may be unsure about their role in the client's recovery. Before the client undergoes surgery, and again before discharge, the nurse teaches the client and family what to expect and what they can do to assist in the recovery process.

Physically preparing the client to undergo surgery and anesthesia involves important skills for the nurse. Regardless of the surgery, safety measures, such as verifying the procedure and consent, are critical. Other steps, such as urinary catheterization or special laboratory tests, are completed only for specific surgical procedures. Physical preparation focuses on minimizing the risks involved with surgery and anesthesia, while optimizing the client's condition.

NURSING DIAGNOSES

Nursing diagnoses associated with the surgical experience include **Risk for Infection** related to the surgical incision, urinary catheter, and invasive lines, **Risk for Injury** related to inadequate identification and communication of risks, and **Risk for Perioperative-Positioning Injury** related to surgical positioning and placement of electrical equipment used in the operating room. Psychological states such as **Deficient Knowledge, Anxiety,** and **Fear** often result when a client is unsure what to expect before, during, and after the surgery. The inability to control the situation often results in **Powerlessness,** and the inability to accept the situation may result in **Ineffective Coping.** During and after surgery using general anesthesia, the client's cough and gag reflexes are suppressed. This results in a risk for **Ineffective Airway Clearance** related to retention of secretions.

Skill 19.1

Preoperative Assessment

To identify risks and plan for the client's care during and after surgery and anesthesia, the nurse performs a thorough preoperative assessment of the client's physiological and psychological condition. To provide efficient services, the assessment is frequently begun before the day of surgery and completed 1 to 2 hours before the scheduled time of surgery. This provides time for the nurse to follow up on any unexpected outcomes. Before beginning this assessment, the nurse establishes a trusting relationship with the client. It is not unusual for the client to remember and report at this time facts that were not told to the physician earlier. To encourage open communication, the nurse provides privacy and a location free of interruption.

PLANNING

Expected outcomes of the preoperative assessment focus on obtaining accurate information and identifying risk factors related to the intended surgery.

Expected Outcomes

1. Client provides the information required to establish a plan of care.
2. Client remains alert and appropriately responsive to nurse's assessment questions.

Equipment

- Stethoscope
- Blood pressure cuff
- Pulse oximeter
- Thermometer
- Watch or clock with a second hand
- Scale
- Preoperative assessment form (Figure 19-1)

A-1c4 NURSE'S DETAILED PERIOPERATIVE NOTE

	DATE
	HOSP. #
	NAME
	BIRTH DATE
	ADDRESS
	SS#

1. Place initials in the space preceding the appropriate response (YES/NO, MET/NOT MET, NOT APPLICABLE)
2. Explain any "NO" or "NOT MET" in the space provided adjacent to the item or in the comment section provided, except for * items.
3. Record additional information in the comment section.
4. Record initials immediately following narrative entry.

IF NOT IMPRINTED, PLEASE PRINT DATE, HOSP. #, NAME AND LOCATION

PERIOPERATIVE TRANSPORT BY:	METHOD:	PREOPERATIVE UNIT/AREA:
TIME RECEIVED IN PRESURGICAL CARE UNIT:		TIME RECEIVED IN OR:

PATIENT ASSESSMENT/PREPARATION	YES	NO	COMMENT
PATIENT IDENTIFIED			ID Band Location
BLOOD BAND PRESENT*			#/Location
ALLERGIES* (If yes, please list)			
LATEX PRECAUTIONS INDICATED*			
CONSENT			
NPO			
HEALTH CHANGED SINCE LAST APPT			If Yes, Specify: Physician Notified:
INFECTIONS, PROBLEMS WITH HEART OR LUNGS			If Yes, Specify: Physician Notified:
TAKING ANY NEW MEDICATIONS			If Yes, Specify: Physician Notified:
PREOPERATIVE ORDERS COMPLETED			
SKIN ASSESSMENT COMPLETED			
VITALS OBTAINED DAY OF SURGERY			
HISTORY AND PHYSICAL PRESENT			
LAB VALUES REVIEWED			
LEVEL OF CONSCIOUSNESS—Answers questions/responds appropriately for age			
IMPLANTS/PROSTHESIS* (If yes, please list)			

Preoperative pain score (0–10) _____
Surgical site verified and marked with patient ☐ _____
Patient voided @ _____ Belongings: _____
Nursing comments _____

NURSING DIAGNOSIS	NURSING ORDERS/INTERVENTIONS	EXPECTED PATIENT OUTCOMES
ANXIETY—Risk of, Related to Surgical Intervention and Outcomes	1. Psychologic & physiologic comfort measures are provided. ___ Yes ___ No	The patient reports and/or demonstrates a reduction in anxiety. ___ MET ___ NOT MET
KNOWLEDGE DEFICIT—Risk of, Related to Surgical Intervention	1. The patient's understanding is assessed and questions/concerns are addressed by the appropriate individuals. ___ Yes ___No	The patient's (guardian's) description of surgery corresponds with the Operative Consent (G-2d). ___ MET ___ NOT MET
INJURY—Risk for, Related to Tubes, Catheters, Lines ___ Not Applicable	1. Integrity of tubes, catheters, and lines is maintained. ___ Yes ___ No Catheters/Tubes/Drains/Lines: _____	The patient's risk for injury related to care and management of tubes, catheters, and lines is minimized. ___ MET ___ NOT MET

Initials	Standards Implemented By:	Initials	Standards Implemented By:

26304/9-01/MH05859   **UNIVERSITY OF IOWA HOSPITALS AND CLINICS**

Side tabs: A -1c4 | B CLIN. NOTES | C LABORATORY | D X-RAY EXAM | E CONSULTATION | F SPEC. EXAM | G THERAPY | H PATHOLOGY | I PT. QUES.

Figure 19-1   Preoperative assessment form. (Courtesy University of Iowa Hospitals and Clinics.)

Delegation Considerations

The skills of assessment that are part of preparing the client for surgery requires the critical thinking and knowledge application unique to a nurse. For these skills delegation is inappropriate. Assistive personnel (AP) may obtain vital signs and weight and height measurements. Instruct AP on proper precautions for these delegated procedures as needed.

IMPLEMENTATION FOR PREOPERATIVE ASSESSMENT

Steps	Rationale
1. See Standard Protocol (inside front cover).	
2. Determine if the client has any communication impairment (e.g., blindness, hearing loss), is able to understand English, and is mentally competent. For example, have the client read an instruction booklet.	Allows nurse to adapt instructional approach to ensure client understanding.
3. Assess the client's understanding of the intended surgery and anesthesia. Have the client describe in his or her own words.	Asking client to offer a description rather than asking a simple yes or no question (e.g., "Do you understand your surgery?") provides a better determination of level of understanding.
4. Obtain a nursing history:	
a. Condition leading to surgery.	Allows nurse to anticipate post-op needs and complications.
b. Chronic illnesses (e.g., hypertension—bleeding and stroke; asthma—impaired ventilation; hiatal hernia—aspiration; diabetes—poor wound healing).	Some chronic conditions increase the risk of complications from surgery and anesthesia.
c. Last menstrual period (for female clients in childbearing years).	Anesthetic agents and other medications could injure the fetus.
d. Previous hospitalizations.	Determines client's familiarity with hospital procedures.
e. Medication history, including prescription, over-the-counter (OTC), and herbal remedies and date/time of last doses.	Client may not report OTC medications and herbal remedies unless specifically asked. Herbal remedies can interact with anesthetic agents or other medications given during surgery. The client may be instructed to take any routine blood pressure, cardiac, or seizure medications. Changes in dosages of oral diabetic agents or insulin may be ordered.
f. Previous experience with surgery and anesthesia. Have client clarify if any undesirable outcomes occurred.	Information will assist in preventing recurrent problems with the planned surgery.
g. Family history of complications from surgery or anesthesia.	A family history of reactions to anesthetic agents may indicate a familial condition, malignant hyperthermia, which is life threatening.
h. Allergies to medications, food, or tape, including specific questions about natural rubber latex. Ask clients if they have had any problem with medication or anything placed on their skin.	Reactions to latex can be life threatening, and prevention in sensitized clients requires specific precautions. Many clients do not understand that rubber and latex are the same. Using both words will help obtain accurate information (Steelman, 1999).

Steps	Rationale

COMMUNICATION TIP *When asking the client about allergies, ask a specific question about reactions or problems the client might have had to natural rubber latex. Most clients do not know that rubber is latex. Using both words with the examples of balloons and gloves has been found to obtain otherwise missed information.*

Steps	Rationale
i. Physical impairment.	Physical impairments may cause limited mobility and situations that could lead to problems with positioning during surgery. This information should be communicated to the operating room nurse because these clients may need special positioning or considerations (Heizenroth, 1999).
j. Prostheses and implants (e.g., dentures, hearing aid, pacemaker, internal defibrillator, hip prosthesis).	These devices could become damaged or malfunction from electrical equipment used during surgery. This information should be communicated to the operating room nurse.
k. Smoking, alcohol, and drug use.	Increases risk of intra- and post-op complications.
l. Occupation.	Anticipates how post-op restrictions will affect a client's return to work.
5. Assess client's weight (see Procedural Guideline 8-1, p. 195), height, and vital signs (see Skill 12.1, p. 275).	Height and weight are used to calculate drug dosages.
6. Assess client's respiratory status, including character and rate of respirations, oxygen saturation, ability to breathe lying flat, and chest x-ray report.	Poor respiratory condition can affect the client's response to general anesthesia.
7. Evaluate client's circulatory status, including apical pulse, electrocardiogram (ECG) report, and peripheral pulses (see Skills 13.3, p. 319 and 15.4, p. 397).	Circulation may be a factor in positioning the client on the operating room table.
8. Determine client's neurological status, including level of consciousness (LOC) (see Skill 13.1, p. 301).	Client's neurologic status affects attentiveness to instruction. Offers important baseline for post-op evaluation.
9. Evaluate client's musculoskeletal system, including range of motion (ROM) of joints (see Skill 13.5, p. 335).	If the ROM is limited, extra care will be needed to prevent injury related to positioning in surgery.
10. Examine client's skin; identify any breaks in skin integrity and determine level of hydration (see Skill 13.1, p. 301). Pay particular attention to area of body in which client will be positioned.	If skin is thin, broken, or bruised, extra padding will be needed in surgery.
11. Evaluate client's emotional status, including level of anxiety, coping ability, and family support.	If client has high level of anxiety or fear, consultation with a social worker, pastoral care, or advanced practice nurse might be useful.
12. Review the results of laboratory tests, including complete blood count (CBC), electrolytes, urinalysis, and other diagnostic tests.	Laboratory work provides an assessment of major body systems.
13. Ask if client has an advance directive (see Chapter 39).	Advance directives protect client's rights by communicating client's desires.
14. Identify the time of client's last intake of food or drink.	With client under general anesthesia, the esophageal sphincter relaxes and the stomach contents can be aspirated.
15. See Completion Protocol (inside front cover).	

• • • • • • • • • •

EVALUATION

1. Determine if client information is complete so plan of care can be established.
2. Evaluate client's ability to cooperate (e.g., makes eye contact, answers appropriately).

Unexpected Outcomes and Related Interventions

1. The client does not understand English.
   a. Obtain an interpreter.
2. The client is not mentally competent.
   a. Determine who is legally authorized to consent to surgery (see agency policy).
3. Client does not understand what surgery will be performed.
   a. Notify the surgeon.
4. The client reports a condition that is a risk factor for surgery such as hiatal hernia, pregnancy, family history of complications associated with anesthesia, cold or upper respiratory infection, or recent chest pain.
   a. Notify the surgeon and anesthesiologist/nurse anesthetist.
5. The client has been taking anticoagulants.
   a. Notify the surgeon.
6. Client reports an allergy to latex.
   a. Remove all supplies containing latex from client's room.
   b. Post a latex precautions sign on the door or stretcher.
   c. Notify surgeon, anesthesiologist/nurse anesthetist, and operating room nurse (Steelman, 1999).
7. Appropriate laboratory tests were not ordered or completed.
   a. Notify surgeon and anesthesiologist/nurse anesthetist, and make arrangements for tests to be completed.
8. Chest x-ray report, ECG, or laboratory tests show abnormal findings.
   a. Notify surgeon and anesthesiologist/nurse anesthetist.
9. Client has a blister, abrasion, or boil near the incision site.
   a. Notify surgeon.

Recording and Reporting

- Document findings on the preoperative portion of the nurses' detailed preoperative notes (see Figure 19-1, p. 493) or other designated agency form.
- Report abnormal laboratory values or other concerns to the surgeon or anesthesiologist.

Sample Documentation

0830 Nursing history completed. Client states that "after her knee surgery last year she vomited for 6 hours." Anesthesiologist notified of client history of vomiting after surgery.

SPECIAL CONSIDERATIONS

Pediatric Considerations

- Young children fear parental separation during surgery and can view surgery as a form of punishment. Allowing children to handle the equipment and to keep a security item with them can decrease their fears (Maldonado and Nygren, 1999).
- Allow the parents to wait with the child until initial sedation begins to take effect. The child does not remember the parents leaving. Reunite parents with child postoperatively as soon as the child is waking in recovery.

Geriatric Considerations

The older adult client may have some limitation in ROM. If this limitation is significant, notify the operating room nurse so that surgical position can be modified.

Skill 19.2

Preoperative Teaching

Preoperative client teaching involves assisting a client with understanding and mentally preparing for the surgical experience (Iowa Intervention Project, 2000). Research has shown that preoperative teaching has a positive effect on postoperative outcomes in clients having a variety of surgeries (Shuldham, 2001). Based on the preoperative assessment, the nurse plans preoperative teaching. Every attempt should be made to ensure privacy for the client. The best learning method for the client should be selected. In many settings, videotape and written materials are available to assist the nurse. Whenever possible, the family members responsible for the client's care after surgery should be present. Later they serve as coaches and assist the client in performing exercises. Plan to have the client demonstrate expected postoperative skills to allow for practice and facilitate understanding.

Clients and their families are often very anxious about impending surgery. Learning can be impaired by anxiety. Speaking in a clear, slow voice helps reduce the client's anxiety. Extra time may be needed for teaching and reinforcement to ensure client understanding. This anxiety can also increase heart rate and blood pressure during and after surgery, which can contribute to bleeding and complications. Postoperatively, high anxiety can lead to negative psychological and physiological outcomes. Preoperative information about expected perioperative sensations has been shown to decrease the distress associated with surgery. By teaching the client preoperatively, the nurse can make a significant contribution to the success of surgery and to the client's postoperative recovery (Butcher, 1999).

ASSESSMENT

1. Ask about client's previous experiences with surgery and anesthesia. *Rationale: This provides information that the nurse may use to individualize teaching and address specific concerns of the client.*
2. Determine client and family's understanding of surgery. *Rationale: This information determines if correction of misunderstanding is necessary.*
3. Identify the client's cognitive level, language, and culture. *Rationale: These factors may alter the client's ability to understand the meaning of surgery.*
4. Assess client's anxiety related to surgery. *Rationale: This information directs the nurse to provide additional emotional support and indicates the client's readiness to learn.*

PLANNING

Expected outcomes of preoperative teaching focus on reducing the anxiety level of the client and family and having the client demonstrate understanding of key information and specific skills necessary to prevent complications.

Expected Outcomes

Expected outcomes focus on demonstrating an understanding of skills taught.

1. Client demonstrates eye contact and asks and answers questions appropriately.
2. Client correctly performs splinting, turning and sitting, breathing exercises, and leg exercises.
3. Family identifies the location of the waiting room.
4. Family verbalizes the ability to care for client at home.
5. Family provides emotional support for client preoperatively.
6. Client and family demonstrate appropriate coping skills.

Equipment

- Stretcher or bed
- Pillow
- Incentive spirometer
- Preoperative education flow sheet (Figure 19-2, p. 498)

Delegation Considerations

The skills of preoperative teaching require the critical thinking and knowledge application unique to a nurse. For this skill delegation is inappropriate. Assistive personnel (AP) can reinforce and assist clients in performing postoperative exercises.
- Review with AP any precautions unique for a particular client (e.g., turning method).
- Be sure staff know when to inform the nurse if the client is unable to perform the exercises correctly.

IMPLEMENTATION FOR PREOPERATIVE TEACHING

Steps	Rationale
1. See Standard Protocol (inside front cover).	
2. Inform client and family of date, time, and location of surgery; anticipated length of surgery; additional time in the postanesthesia recovery area; and where to wait.	Accurate information helps reduce the stress associated with surgery.
3. Answer questions client and family ask.	
4. Describe perioperative routines (e.g., intravenous [IV] therapy, urinary catheterization, enema, hair clipping or removal, laboratory tests, transport to operating room).	Allows client to anticipate and recognize routine procedures, reducing anxiety.

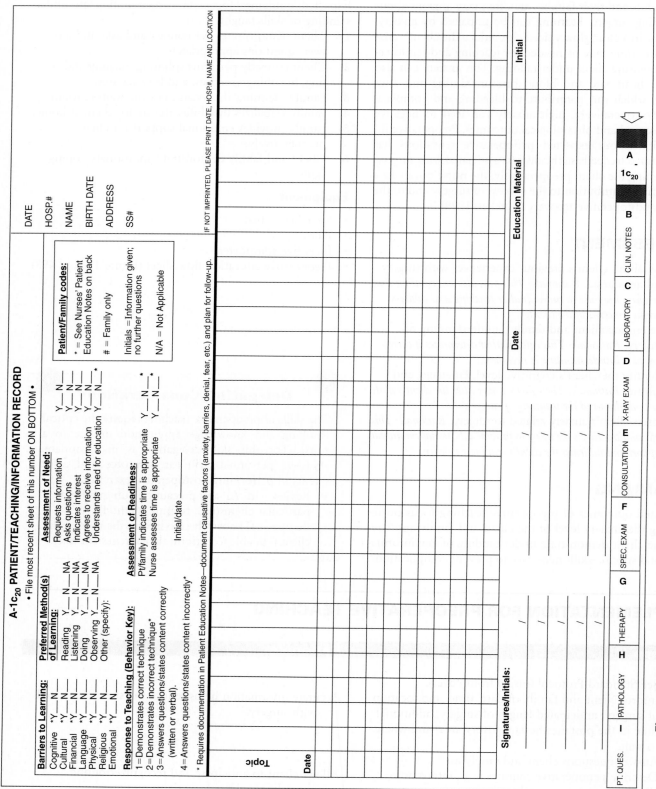

Figure 19-2 Preoperative education flow sheet. *TCDB*, Turn, cough, and deep breathe; *IS*, incentive spirometry. (Courtesy University of Iowa Hospitals and Clinics.)

Steps	**Rationale**

5. Describe planned effect of preoperative medications.

6. Review which routine medications are to be discontinued before surgery.

Some medications are discontinued before surgery. For example, anticoagulants may increase bleeding and are usually discontinued several days before surgery. Insulin dosages are usually adjusted because of the reduced intake of food preoperatively.

7. Describe perioperative sensations (e.g., blood pressure cuff tightening, ECG leads, cool room, beep of monitor).

Describing what sensations client will experience has been shown to reduce distress associated with the experience (Fox, 1999).

8. Describe pain-control methods. Many clients have a patient-controlled analgesia (PCA) pump (see Chapter 21).

Clients are fearful of postoperative pain. Explaining pain-management techniques will reduce this fear.

9. Describe what client will experience postoperatively (e.g., frequent vital signs, turning, catheters, drains, tubes).

Provides a concrete description of what the client can expect after surgery so that the client is prepared (Fox, 1999).

10. Instruct client in splinting incision following abdominal surgery. Hold pillow to abdomen for support while sitting up or coughing (see illustration).

Splinting the incision protects the abdominal incision and provides support for weakened muscles (Lewis and others, 2000).

11. Instruct client on turning and sitting up.

   a. Instruct client to flex knees while lying supine and move toward left side of bed.

Promotes circulation and ventilation.

   b. Have client splint incision with right arm and pillow. Have client keep right leg straight and flex left knee up. Have client grab right side rail with left hand, pull toward right and roll onto right side.

Supports incision and decreases discomfort while turning.

   c. To sit up on the right side of the bed, turn onto right side. While lying on the right side, push on the mattress with right arm and swing feet over the edge of the bed (see illustration). To sit up on the left side of the bed, reverse this process.

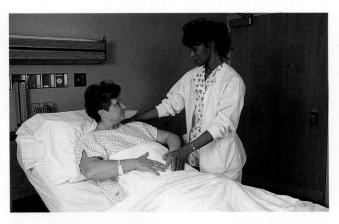

Step 10 Splinting the incision for coughing after abdominal surgery.

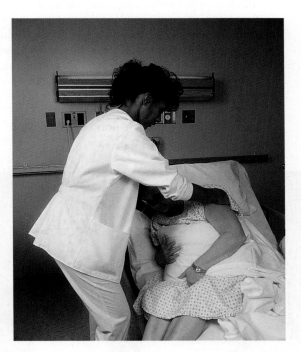

Step 11c Splinting the incision while sitting up after abdominal surgery.

Steps	Rationale
12. Instruct client in deep breathing and coughing (see illustration).	Client may be unable or reluctant to deep breathe because of weakness or pain, resulting in secretions remaining in the base of the lungs. This collection of secretions increases the risk of pulmonary complications such as pneumonia.
a. Assist client to sitting position.	Sitting position facilitates diaphragmatic expansion.
b. Instruct client to place palms of hands over the lower border of the rib cage with third fingers touching.	This allows the client to feel the rise and fall of the abdomen during deep breathing (Lewis and others, 2000).
c. Have client take slow, deep breaths, inhaling through the nose, and feel fingers separate.	This will help prevent hyperventilation or panting in the client.
d. Have client hold the breath for 3 seconds and exhale through the mouth slowly, as if blowing out a candle.	Resistance during exhalation helps to prevent alveolar collapse.
e. Splint abdominal incision with pillow.	This will help decrease discomfort during deep breathing and coughing.
f. Following four to six deep breaths, instruct client to cough forcefully.	Deep breathing can help move up secretions in the respiratory tract to stimulate the cough reflex without voluntary effort on the part of the client (Lewis and others, 2000).
g. Have the client practice several times.	Ensures mastery of technique.
h. Instruct client to perform turn, cough, and deep breathing every 2 hours.	Frequent pulmonary exercises will decrease risk of postoperative atelectasis and pulmonary complications (Richardson and Sabanathan, 1997).
13. Instruct client in use of an incentive spirometer (see illustration).	Encourages deep breathing and loosens secretions in lung bases.
a. Position in a setting or reclining position.	
b. Instruct client to exhale completely, then place mouthpiece so that lips completely cover it and inhale slowly, maintaining constant flow through unit.	Promotes complete inflation of lungs and minimizes atelectasis.
c. After maximum inspiration, client should hold breath for 2 to 3 seconds and then exhale slowly.	Promotes alveolar inflation.
d. Set marker on inspirometer at maximum inspiration point to establish postoperative target.	Establishes normal maximum breath for client. Provides an objective comparison of deep breathing postoperatively with the goal of returning to the preoperative volumes (Fink and Hunt, 1999).
e. Instruct client to breathe normally for a short period, and then repeat process.	Prevents hyperventilation and fatigue.

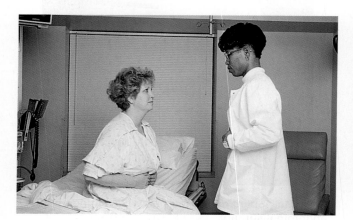

Step 12 Position for coughing and deep breathing after abdominal surgery.

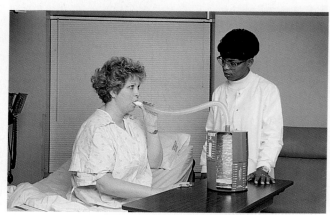

Step 13 Use of an incentive spirometer.

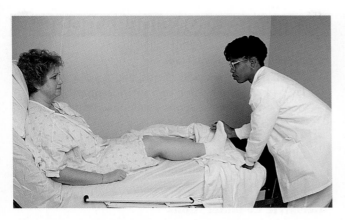

Step 14d   Dorisflexion and plantar flexion of foot.

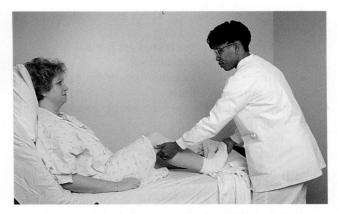

Step 14e   Flexion and extension of knees.

Steps	Rationale
14. Instruct client in leg exercises: ankle rotation, dorsiflexion and plantar flexion, leg extension and flexion, straight leg raises.	Leg exercises encourage circulation in the lower extremities and reduce the risk of circulatory complications such as a venous thrombus.
a. Position client supine.	
b. Rotate each ankle in a complete circle.	Promotes joint mobility.
c. Instruct client to draw imaginary circles with the big toe 5 times	
d. Alternate dorsiflexion and plantar flexion while instructing client to feel calf muscles tighten and relax. Repeat 5 times (see illustration).	Helps maintain joint mobility and promote venous return to prevent thrombus formation.
e. Instruct client to alternate flexing and extending knees one leg at a time. Repeat 5 times (see illustration).	Maintains knee joint mobility and contracts muscles of upper leg.
f. Instruct client to alternate raising leg straight up from bed surface. Leg should be kept straight. Repeat 5 times.	Causes quadriceps muscle contraction and relaxation that helps promote venous return (Lewis and others, 2000).
g. Instruct client to perform these four leg exercises 10 to 12 times every 1 to 2 hours while awake.	
15. Verify that client's expectations of surgery are realistic. Correct expectations as needed.	
16. Reinforce therapeutic coping strategies. If ineffective, encourage alternatives.	
17. See Completion Protocol (inside front cover).	

• • • • • • • • • •

EVALUATION

1. Ask client to repeat key information.
2. Ask client to demonstrate splinting, turning and sitting, deep breathing, and leg exercises.
3. Ask family to identify location of the waiting room.
4. Ask family if they are able to care for client at home after discharge.
5. Observe the level of emotional support family provides client.
6. Observe client and family coping strategies.

Unexpected Outcomes and Related Interventions

1. Client identifies an incorrect date, time, or location of surgery.
   a. Provide the correct information verbally and in writing for client and family.
2. Client questions the importance of not drinking the morning of surgery.
   a. Explain that under anesthesia, the fluid can come up from the stomach and go into the lung.
3. Client is withdrawn.
   a. Explain that it is normal to feel anxious about surgery.
   b. Ask how client feels about the surgery.
4. Client incorrectly performs breathing exercises.
   a. Explain the correct breathing technique.
   b. Explain the importance of postoperative breathing.
   c. Instruct client to repeat the demonstration.

5. Family verbalizes anxiety about care for client at home.
   a. Explain that these feelings are normal.
   b. Provide written instructions.
   c. Provide a telephone number for contact if there are further questions.
6. Family indicates that they are unable to care for client at home.
   a. Contact physician, and discuss the alternative of a home health care referral.

Recording and Reporting

• Record preoperative teaching on the preoperative education flow sheet (see Figure 19-2, p. 498) or designated agency form.

Sample Documentation

0940 Preoperative teaching completed. Client's daughter expressed concern about her mother being able to care for herself at home after surgery. Home health nurse contacted to see client before discharge.

SPECIAL CONSIDERATIONS

Pediatric Considerations

• When teaching pediatric clients, use an age-appropriate level of communication and provide simple explanations using familiar terms (Maldonado and Nygren, 1999).
• The use of pictures, models, equipment and play rather than verbal explanations increases preschool and school-aged children's learning (Maldonado and Nygren, 1999).

Geriatric Considerations

• Age-related changes in the central nervous system may inhibit short-term memory and make learning more difficult (Williams and Salisbury, 1999). Sensory deficits related to vision and hearing may affect learning (Meckes, 1999). The older adult client may retain verbal information better than nonverbal information.
• The room should be well lighted and free of distractions. Presenting one idea at a time and reinforcing information verbally will aid in learning (Daley, 1996).

Skill 19.3

Physical Preparation

Physical preparation of the client for surgery involves providing nursing care immediately before surgery, verifying required procedures and tests, and documenting care in the client's record (Iowa Intervention Project, 2000). Specific steps are taken to prepare every client. These steps depend on the type of surgery being performed and the risks involved. For example, antiembolism stockings and/or sequential compression stockings may be used for adult clients undergoing surgery that will last several hours and require a long period of immobilization afterward (Brenner, 1999). The bowel may need to be prepped with an enema or by taking a laxative or cathartic (this may be done at home by clients admitted the morning of surgery) even for abdominal surgery on or near the intestine. Hair near the incision site may need to be removed. It is important to check the physician's orders to determine what steps are needed for the surgical client. Regardless of the type of surgery, the goal of physical preparation is to place the client in the best condition possible to minimize the risks of the surgery that is planned.

ASSESSMENT

The preoperative assessment forms the basis for physical preparation of the client for surgery (see Skill 19.1).

PLANNING

Expected outcomes focus on the physical preparation of the client for surgery.

Expected Outcomes

1. Client cooperates during preparatory measures (e.g., starting an IV, laboratory tests).
2. Client undergoes measures to reduce the risk of infection (e.g., preoperative antibiotic, skin preparation).

Equipment

• Hospital gown
• IV solution, tubing, catheter, tourniquet, alcohol swab, and IV tape

- Skin cleansing solution (when ordered)
- Antiembolism stockings (when ordered)
- Sequential compression device (when ordered)
- Urinary catheterization kit (when ordered)
- Preoperative checklist

Delegation Considerations

Coordinating the client's preparation for surgery requires the critical thinking and knowledge application unique to a nurse. However, assistive personnel (AP) may administer an enema or a douche, obtain vital signs, apply antiembolic stockings, and assist client in removing clothing, jewelry, and prostheses.

- Instruct AP in proper precautions when preparing a client for surgery.
- Instruct AP in proper observations and precautions if the client has an IV catheter in place.

IMPLEMENTATION FOR PHYSICAL PREPARATION

Steps	Rationale
1. See Standard Protocol (inside front cover).	
2. Assist client with putting on hospital gown and removing personal items.	
3. Instruct client to remove makeup, nail polish, hairpins, and jewelry.	During and after surgery, the skin and nails are assessed to determine tissue perfusion. (In some settings, clients are allowed to have a ring taped and to remove polish from only one nail.)
4. Ensure that money and valuables have been locked up or given to a family member.	
5. Verify that client's identification and blood band are correct and legible.	In an ASU, these bands are applied at this time.
6. Ensure that client has had nothing to eat or drink during the past 8 hours.	Under general anesthesia, the sphincters in the stomach relax, and contents can reflux into the esophagus and into the trachea. (Some settings now use a shorter time frame.)
7. Verify that client has taken medications as instructed.	Missed or inaccurate dosage could precipitate complications.
8. Verify that a bowel preparation (e.g., laxative, cathartic, enema) has been completed if ordered.	For clients admitted the morning of surgery, this may have been performed at home.
9. Ensure that a medical history and physical examination results are in client's record.	
10. Verify that surgical consent is complete.	Ensuring that the client has consented to the intended procedure is essential. In most settings the surgeon obtains the consent and the nurse verifies that it is complete and consistent with the client's understanding (refer to agency policy).
11. Ensure that necessary laboratory work, ECG, and chest x-ray studies have been completed and results are on the chart.	
12. Check that type and crossmatch has been completed if ordered by the physician and that blood transfusions are available as needed.	In many cases, surgery cannot begin without availability of blood units.
13. Ask if client has an advance directive. If so, place it in client's record.	Document conveys client's wishes if life support measures are necessary.

Steps	Rationale
14. Assess and record client's heart rate, blood pressure, respiratory rate, oxygen saturation, and temperature.	Provides a baseline for client's preoperative status.
15. Administer purgatives or enemas if ordered (see Skill 9.4, p. 213).	Enemas are used when surgery is near the lower intestine.
16. Instruct client to void.	Prevents risk of bladder distention or rupture during surgery.
17. Start an IV line; refer to unit standards or physician's orders (see Skill 29.1, p. 676).	IV provides access for fluids and medications administered in OR.
18. Administer preoperative medications as ordered.	

NURSE ALERT *To be most effective, preoperative antibiotics should be administered within 2 hours preoperatively (Butts and Wolford, 1997).*

COMMUNICATION TIP *Clients are often anxious before surgery. Explaining how equipment will feel (e.g., cold, tight) before it will touch the client reduces anxiety.*

---

19. Apply antiembolism stockings.	Antiembolism stockings promote circulation during periods of immobilization, reducing the risk of an embolism.
a. Measure client while standing, from gluteal fold to the floor, circumference of largest part of the calf (refer to agency policy).	
b. With the client lying down, invert the stocking down over the heel, and then slip it over the foot (see illustration).	Facilitates ease of application.
c. Ease the stocking snugly up over the leg (see illustration). Be sure there are no folds in the stocking.	
20. Apply sequential compression stockings if ordered.	Sequential compression stockings promote circulation by sequentially compressing the legs from the ankle upward and thus promoting venous return.
a. Measure around the largest part of the thigh.	
b. Wrap stockings around the leg, starting at the ankle, with the opening over the patella (see illustration).	

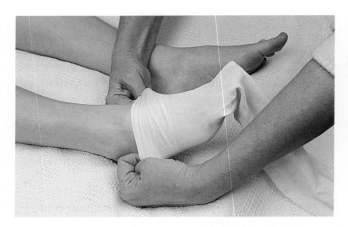

Step 19b Slip antiembolism stocking over foot.

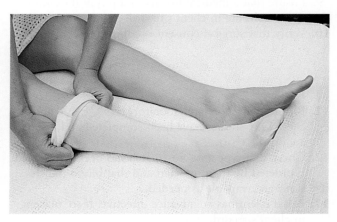

Step 19c Ease antiembolism stocking over the leg.

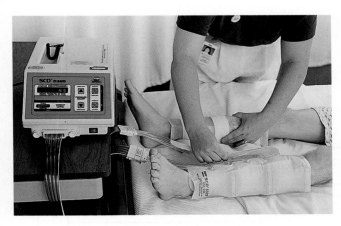

Step 20b   Wrap stocking around leg.

Steps	Rationale

c. Attach the stockings to the insufflator, and verify that the intermittent pressure is between 35 and 45 mm Hg.

21. Cleanse and prepare the surgical site if ordered.

Cleansing with an antimicrobial soap decreases bacterial flora on the skin.

22. Insert a urinary catheter if ordered (see Chapter 35).
23. Administer an enema if ordered (see Chapter 9).

Cleansing of the bowel may need to be done before surgery to reduce the risk of fecal contamination during surgery.

24. Allow the client to wear eyeglasses, dentures, or hearing aid as long as possible before surgery. Remove contact lenses, eyeglasses, hairpieces, and dentures just before surgery.

These aids facilitate client cooperation by ensuring that the client has clear vision and maximal auditory perception throughout the preoperative phase. In some settings, dentures are left in place.

25. Place a cap on client's head.

The cap contains the hair and minimizes operating room contamination during surgery. Plastic or reflective caps reduce heat loss during surgery.

26. Assist client onto stretcher for transport to operating room.

Some ambulatory surgery clients walk to operating room.

27. See Completion Protocol (inside front cover).

• • • • • • • • • •

EVALUATION

1. Observe client's level of cooperation during preparation.
2. Ask client to assist with measures to reduce the risk of infection (preoperative antibiotics, skin preparation).

Unexpected Outcomes and Related Interventions

1. Client reports having eaten breakfast or drinking fluids.
   a. Notify surgeon and anesthesiologist/nurse anesthetist.
2. Client refuses to go to surgery until contacting a family member.
   a. Notify surgeon.
   b. Assist client with contacting family member.
3. Consent is incomplete or incorrect.
   a. Notify surgeon and anesthesiologist/nurse anesthetist.

4. Client did not follow instructions regarding medications.
   a. Notify surgeon.
5. Client has a reaction to a preoperative medication.
   a. Discontinue the medication.
   b. Treat the reaction as per institutional policy.
   c. Notify surgeon.
6. Client is scheduled to be discharged postoperatively and does not have an accompanying adult.
   a. Notify surgeon and anesthesiologist/nurse anesthetist.
   b. Assist client in contacting someone to provide care at home.

A-1c PREOPERATIVE CHECKLIST

● File with other A-1c's of same date ●

1. Place initials in appropriate box: YES, NO. Each item must have an entry.
2. Explain any "No." This can be done in the space after the item or in the "Comments" section. Use back of form, if needed.
3. To give more information on any item, use the space after the item. If more space needed, use the "Comments" section on back of form.

DATE *8/1/XX*

HOSP. # *99-23764-1*

NAME *James Lee*

BIRTH DATE

ADDRESS

SS #

IF NOT IMPRINTED, PLEASE PRINT DATE, HOSP. #, NAME AND LOCATION

YES	NO	NA		A-1c
X/ML			**Special Information/Transport Needs** (e.g., blind, O$_2$, monitoring) *Mr. Lee is very hard of hearing*	
ML			Preoperative orders written.	
ML			Consent complete and in medical record.	
		ML	**Specify Allergies:** *N K A*	B
		ML	Allergies (or NKA) labeled on cover of medical record.	
		ML	Latex precautions indicated.	
		ML	Isolation label on cover of medical record. **Specify Type:**	CLIN. NOTES
		ML	Has health changed since last appt? **If Yes, Specify:**	
		ML	Infections, problems with heart or lungs? **If Yes, Specify:**	C
		ML	Taking any new medications? **If Yes, Specify:**	
ML			Teaching completed and documented.	
ML			Chest X-ray completed *7/30/XX* Ordered labs completed *7/30/XX* EKG completed *7/30/XX*	LABORATORY
ML			Forms completed and filed in medical record.	
ML			Anesthesia preop evaluation in medical record.	
ML			NPO since: *0015*	D
ML			Vitals (Obtain Day of Surgery) T *98⁶* P *100* R *24* BP *110* / *70*	
ML			Jewelry absent. Specify item(s) removed and disposition of jewelry/valuables. *valuables are at home*	X-RAY EXAM
		ML	Prostheses removed: hearing aid, eye glasses, contact lenses (circle).	
		ML	Other: Disposition:	
ML			Identification band on patient and legible. **Specify location:** (R) *wrist*	E
ML			(Type and cross) screen (circle) done. Date drawn: *7/30/XX*	
ML			Blood band on patient and legible. **Specify location:** (R) *wrist*	CONSULTATION
ML			Anti-embolism stockings with patient.	
		ML	Sequential compression device sleeve on per orders.	
ML			Preps/tests completed as ordered. **Specify:** *Routine LAB, EKG results in medical record*	F
ML			(Voided)/catheterized (circle). Time: *0730*	
ML			Level of consciousness—Answers questions/responds appropriately for age	SPEC. EXAM
ML			Medication(s) given.	
		ML	Medication(s) sent with patient. **Specify:**	
		ML	Article(s) sent with patient. **Specify:**	
ML			Addressograph plate with medical record. All volumes with patient.	G

COMMENTS:

Initials	Signature and Title of Individuals Filling Out Form	Initials	Signature and Title of Individuals Filling Out Form
ML	*Margaret Lenz*		

88574/10-98/MH07528

THE UNIVERSITY OF IOWA HOSPITALS AND CLINICS

(Right side vertical tabs: A-1c, B CLIN. NOTES, C LABORATORY, D X-RAY EXAM, E CONSULTATION, F SPEC. EXAM, G THERAPY, H PATHOLOGY, I DIAGNOSIS)

Figure 19-3 Preoperative checklist. (Courtesy University of Iowa Hospitals and Clinics.)

Recording and Reporting

- Preoperative physical preparation is frequently documented on a form called a preoperative checklist (Figure 19-3).

Sample Documentation

0850 client states that he did not take his morning dose of 20 units of NPH insulin. Dr. Thompson notified. Client given 10 units of NPH insulin subcutaneous per order. IV of 5% dextrose and ½ normal saline started in right hand per order.

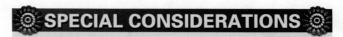

SPECIAL CONSIDERATIONS

Pediatric Considerations

Giving the child as many choices related to procedures as possible, such as which hand to put the IV in, can help decrease fears related to the procedures. Allowing parents to stay with the child as long as possible is helpful in decreasing anxiety and fear for both the child and the parents (Maldonado and Nygren, 1999).

Geriatric Considerations

Because of cognitive, sensory, or physical impairments, it may take the older client increased time to dress for surgery and complete needed physical preparation.

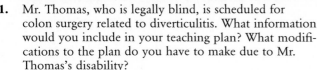

CRITICAL THINKING EXERCISES

1. Mr. Thomas, who is legally blind, is scheduled for colon surgery related to diverticulitis. What information would you include in your teaching plan? What modifications to the plan do you have to make due to Mr. Thomas's disability?
2. Mrs. Samson is scheduled for an elective cholecystectomy. During the preoperative nursing assessment, she reports that when her sister had surgery last year she had trouble during the surgery with a very high fever. As the nurse, how would you respond to Mrs. Samson's statement and what action (if any) do you need to take?
3. Sonya, age 4 years, is scheduled for a tonsillectomy and adenoidectomy. She arrives in the ambulatory surgery unit crying and clinging to her mother. Sonya's mother states that she is not sure about leaving Sonya as she goes to surgery. What actions can you take to help Sonya and her mother best prepare for the surgery?

REFERENCES

Brenner ZR: Preventing postoperative complications: what's old, what's new, what's tried-and-true, *Nursing* 29(10):34, 1999.
Butcher L: Teaching: preoperative. In Bulechek GM, McCloskey JC, editors: *Nursing interventions: effective nursing treatments,* ed 3, Philadelphia, 1999, WB Saunders.
Butts JD, Wolford ET: Timing of preoperative antibiotic administration, *AORN J* 65(10):109, 1997.
Daley K: Learning theory. In *Core curriculum for geriatric nurses,* Baltimore, 1996, Mosby.
Fink JB, Hunt GE: *Clinical practice in respiratory care,* Philadelphia, 1999, Lippincott Williams & Wilkins.
Fox VJ: Patient education and discharge planning. In Meeker MH, Rothrock JC, editors: *Alexander's care of the patient in surgery,* ed 11, St Louis, 1999, Mosby.
Heizenroth PA: Positioning the patient for surgery. In Meeker MH, Rothrock JC, editors: *Alexander's care of the patient in surgery,* ed 11, St Louis, 1999, Mosby.
Iowa Intervention Project: *Nursing interventions classification,* ed 3, St Louis, 2000, Mosby.
Lewis SM and others: *Medical-surgical nursing: assessment and management of clinical problems,* ed 5, St Louis, 2000, Mosby.
Maldonado SS, Nygren C: Pediatric surgery. In Meeker MH, Rothrock JC, editors: *Alexander's care of the patient in surgery,* ed 11, St Louis, 1999, Mosby.
Meckes PF: Geriatric surgery. In Meeker MH, Rothrock JC, editors: *Alexander's care of the patient in surgery,* ed 11, St Louis, 1999, Mosby.
Richardson J, Sabanathan S: Prevention of respiratory complications after abdominal surgery, *Thorax* 52(suppl): S35, 1997.
Shuldham CM: Preoperative education for the patient having coronary artery bypass surgery, *Patient Educ Couns* 43:129, 2001.
Steelman V: Latex precautions. In Bulechek GM, McCloskey JC, editors: *Nursing interventions: effective nursing treatments,* ed 3, Philadelphia, 1999, WB Saunders.
Williams MP, Salisbury SA: Cognitive assessment. In Stone JT, Wyman JF, Salisbury SA, editors: *Clinical gerontological nursing: a guide to advanced practice,* ed 2, Philadelphia, 1999, WB Saunders.

Intraoperative Techniques

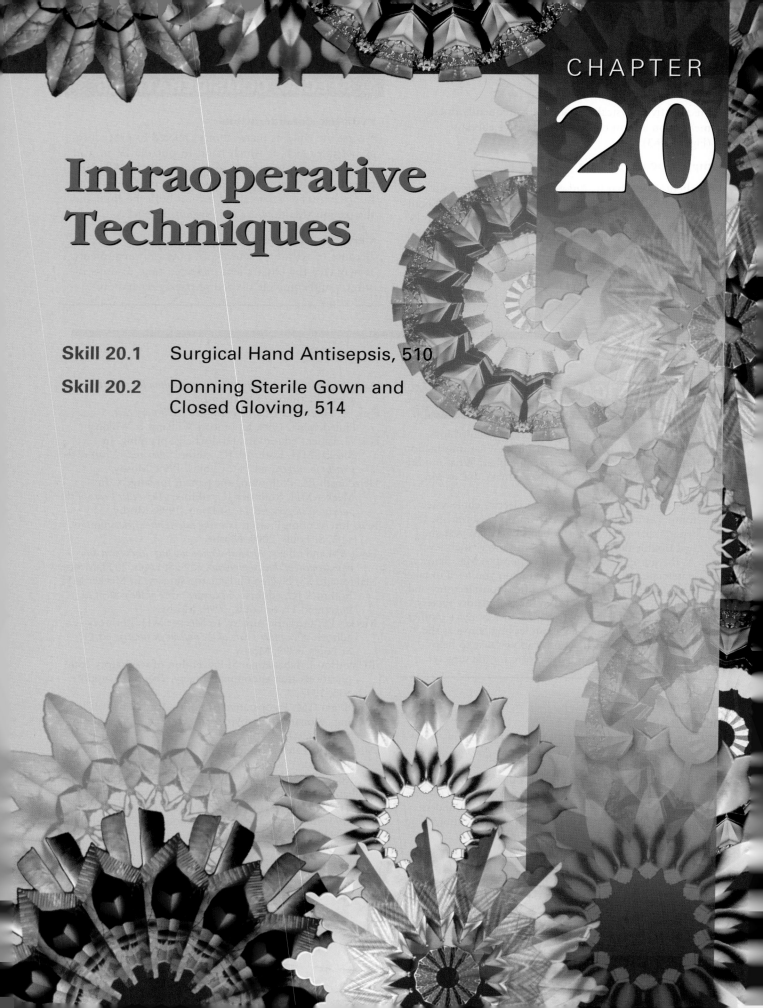

The intraoperative phase of surgical care starts when the client enters the operating room suite and ends with admission to the postanesthesia care unit (PACU). During this intraoperative phase, the perioperative nurse applies the nursing process to coordinate each client's care, keeping in mind safety, comfort, and support.

Members of the surgical team may include the surgeon, physician's assistant, registered nurse first assistant (RNFA), certified registered nurse anesthetist (CRNA) and/or physician anesthesiologist, circulating nurse, and scrub nurse or surgical technologist. A few examples of more specialized team members include a cardiopul-

monary perfusionist, blood (cell) saver technologist, or orthopedic technician. These team members collaborate to achieve an optimal level of care that ensures the client's safety and comfort.

The perioperative nurse assumes one of two roles in the operating room: the circulating nurse or the scrub nurse. The circulating nurse is always a registered nurse (RN) and is considered to be the charge nurse in the room (Association of Perioperative Nurses [AORN], 1998b). The circulator assists the scrubbed personnel by linking the team to the unsterile environment (e.g., continuously monitors operative procedure for breaks in aseptic technique, anticipates the needs of scrubbed personnel, opens additional sterile supplies for the scrub nurse). The circulator assumes responsibility and accountability for the delivery of safe, quality client care (Box 20-1).

The scrub nurse, who may be an RN, licensed practical nurse (LPN), or surgical technologist, passes sterile instruments and supplies to the surgeons and assistants and maintains the sterile field (Box 20-2). Both the circulating and the scrub nurses monitor for and enforce strict adherence to the principles of aseptic technique (see Chapter 4), ensuring optimum client protection against contamination of microorganisms during the surgical procedure.

It is essential that perioperative nurses fully understand and follow the principles of aseptic technique and are willing to develop a sterile conscience. A sterile conscience requires knowledge of the principles of aseptic technique; self-discipline; good communication skills to

---

Box 20-1

Role of the Circulating Nurse

- Organizes and prepares operating room before start of surgical procedure; checks to see equipment works properly
- Gathers supplies for surgical procedure and opens sterile supplies for scrub nurse
- Counts sponges, sharps, and instruments with scrub nurse before incision is made, at the beginning of wound closure, and at the end of the surgical procedure
- Sends for client at appropriate time
- Conducts preoperative client assessment, including:

  Explains role and identifies client
  Reviews medical record and verifies procedure and consents
  Confirms client's allergies, nothing by mouth (NPO) status, laboratory values, electrocardiogram (ECG), and x-ray studies

- Safely assists client to operating table and positions client according to surgeon's preference and procedure type, using safety precautions (e.g., safety belt, securing arms, padding bony prominences)
- Applies conductive pad to client if electrocautery used; may prepare client's skin; may apply ECG electrodes
- Explains briefly to the client what the circulating nurse and scrub nurse are doing
- Assists surgical team by tying gowns and arranging equipment
- Assists anesthesia personnel during induction and extubation
- Continuously monitors procedure for any breaks in aseptic technique and anticipates needs of the team; opens additional sterile supplies for scrub nurse
- Handles surgical specimens per institutional policy
- Documents on perioperative nurses' notes
- Communicates to family and recovery personnel during the surgical procedure

---

Box 20-2

Role of the Scrub Nurse

- Assists circulating nurse in preparing operating room
- Performs surgical hand scrub, dons sterile gown and gloves
- Prepares sterile field with procedure-appropriate supplies and instruments; checks to make sure all work properly
- Counts sponges, sharps, and instruments with circulating nurse before incision is made, at the beginning of wound closure, and at the end of the surgical procedure
- Gowns and gloves surgeons and assistants as they enter the operating room
- Assists surgical team with sterile draping of client
- Keeps sterile field orderly and monitors progress of procedure and any breaks in aseptic technique
- Passes sterile instruments and supplies to surgeons and assistants
- Handles surgical specimens per institutional policy
- Constantly monitors location of all sponges, sharps, and instruments in the sterile field

identify, address, and correct any breaks in sterile technique; and the maturity to overcome personal preferences.

If any question exists about sterility, the item must be considered to be unsterile. A sterile gown that touches the floor while being put on is discarded and exchanged for a new one; the surgeon who touches an unsterile area with a gloved hand changes the affected glove; the scrub nurse who accidentally touches the faucet with one hand while rinsing rescrubs. These are all examples of following one's sterile conscience and being committed to safe, quality client care.

Most clients who undergo surgery are unfamiliar with the operating room environment and what to expect. The perioperative nurse must assess and document the client's emotional status and understanding of the surgical procedure to be performed.

NURSING DIAGNOSES

Risk for Infection is the most appropriate nursing diagnosis for clients undergoing invasive procedures. When the surgical procedure involves an incision or entrance into a sterile body cavity, such as the abdomen or thorax, prevention of infection is a major nursing responsibility. Even when aseptic technique is followed, some clients will have a greater-than-average risk for infection (see Chapters 21 and 22).

Skill 20.1

Surgical Hand Antisepsis

In the operating room setting, it is imperative that surgical hand antisepsis be achieved through effective handwashing or hand rub (Boyce and Pittet, 2002). To reduce the risk that clients may acquire postoperative infections, use of an antimicrobial preparation for hand antisepsis is an integral part of the presurgical scrubbing procedure for operating room personnel. Although the skin cannot be sterilized, the number of microorganisms can be greatly reduced by chemical, physical, and mechanical means.

The surgical hand scrub has been the traditional method for surgical asepsis. Through the use of an antimicrobial agent and sterile brushes, the surgical hand scrub removes debris and transient microorganisms from the nails, hands, and forearms; reduces the resident microbial count to a minimum; and inhibits rapid/rebound growth of microorganisms (AORN, 2001). New evidence suggests that a brushless technique, with or without water, containing at least 60% alcohol, is an alternative to the traditional hand scrub with a brush with the same microbial efficacy (Gruendemann and Bjerke, 2001). Both hand antiseptic methods are currently used in operating room settings. This skill will address both techniques.

Surgical attire (i.e., scrubs) are worn in the operating room to reduce the chance for contamination from surgical personnel to clients, and vice versa. Fingernails should be short, clean, and healthy. If polish is worn, it should not be chipped or worn more than 4 days. Artificial nails should not be worn (AORN, 2001). All rings, watches, and bracelets are removed before the surgical scrub.

The Association of Operating Room Nurses (AORN) recommends a 2- to 3-minute hand and arm scrub with an approved antimicrobial agent for all surgical procedures. The institution should standardize the surgical hand scrub procedure for all staff using either the anatomical timed scrub or the counted stroke method (AORN, 2001) (see agency policy). Some procedures described as clean procedures require performing hand hygiene but not necessarily a surgical scrub. Some examples of clean procedures are laryngoscopy, esophagoscopy, and proctoscopy.

ASSESSMENT

1. Determine type and length of time for hand rub or scrub per agency policy.
2. Remove bracelets, rings, and watches. *Rationale: Items contain microorganisms.*
3. Inspect fingernails, which must be short, clean, and healthy. Artificial nails should be removed. Nail polish should be removed if chipped or worn longer than 4 days. *Rationale: Chipped or old polish increases number of bacteria residing on nails. Long fingernails can puncture gloves, causing contamination. Artificial nails are known to harbor gram-negative microorganisms and fungus (Atkinson and Fortunato, 1996).*
4. Inspect skin and cuticles of hands and arms for abrasions, cuts, or open lesions. *Rationale: These tend to ooze serum, which is a medium for prolific bacterial growth and can endanger the client by increasing the hazards of infection (Meeker and Rothrock, 1999).*

PLANNING

Expected outcomes should focus on prevention of infection resulting from breaks in aseptic technique.

Expected Outcome

Client does not develop signs of surgical wound infection.

Equipment

- Deep sink with foot or knee controls for dispensing water and soap
- Antimicrobial agent approved by agency
- Surgical scrub brush with plastic nail file
- Paper face mask, cap, or hood and surgical shoe covers
- Sterile towel
- Proper scrub attire
- Protective eyewear

Delegation Considerations

The role of the scrub nurse can be delegated to a surgical technologist or licensed practical nurse (LPN). Assistive personnel (AP) can assist the RN in the circulating role by opening sterile supplies, setting up sterile fields, and running errands under the direction of the RN.

IMPLEMENTATION FOR SURGICAL HAND ANTISEPSIS

Steps	Rationale
1. Put on surgical shoe covers, cap or hood, face mask, and protective eyewear.	Protective eyewear is mandated for reasons such as blood or body fluids splashing from the sterile field with the risk of infection (e.g., human immunodeficiency virus [HIV], hepatitis B virus [HBV]). Also, laser surgery requires the wearing of special protective eyewear to prevent damage to the eye by stray laser energy.
2. Turn water on using foot or knee control, and adjust to comfortable temperature.	
3. Prescub wash/rinse: Wet hands and arms under running lukewarm water, and lather with antimicrobial agent up to 2 inches above elbows.	A short prescrub wash/rinse removes gross debris and superficial microorganisms and is an essential step before surgical antisepsis.
4. Rinse hands and arms thoroughly under running water. Remember to keep hands above elbows.	Water runs from fingertips to elbows by gravity; hands are maintained as the cleanest part of the upper extremity.
5. Under running water, clean under nails of both hands with file; discard file (see illustration).	Removes dirt and organic materials that harbor a large number of microorganisms.
6. **Surgical hand scrub (with brush)** a. Wet brush, and apply antimicrobial agent. Scrub the nails of one hand with 15 strokes. Scrub the palm, each side of thumb and fingers, and the posterior side of the hand with 10 strokes each (see first illustration).	Ensures removal of resident microorganisms on all surfaces of hands and arms.

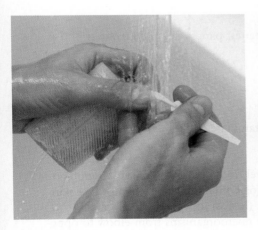

Step 5   Cleaning under fingernails.

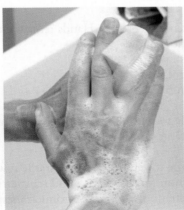

Step 6a   Scrubbing side of fingers.

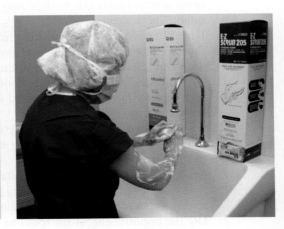

Step 6b   Scrubbing forearms.

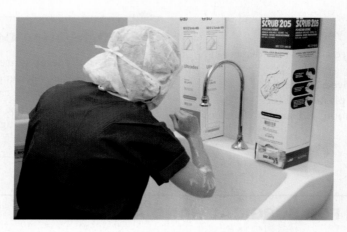

Step 6c   Rinsing arms.

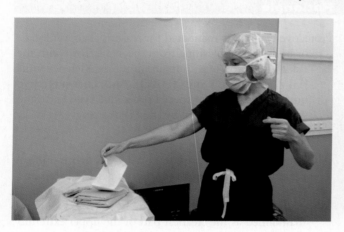

Step 6e   Grasping sterile towel.

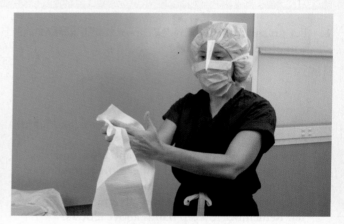

Step 6f   Drying sequence.

Steps	Rationale
b. Next, the arm is mentally divided into thirds, and each third is scrubbed 10 times (see second illustration) (Perry and Potter, 1998). Some agencies may scrub by time rather than 10 strokes. Rinse brush, and repeat the sequence for the other arm. A two-brush method may be substituted. Check agency policy.	Eliminates transient and reduces resident hand flora.
c. Discard brush; flex arms and rinse from fingertips to elbows in one continuous motion, allowing water to run off at elbow (see illustration).	Hands remain cleanest part of upper extremities.
d. Turn off water with foot or knee control, and back into room with hands elevated in front of and away from body.	
e. Approach sterile setup and grasp sterile towel, taking care not to drip water on the sterile field (see illustration).	Water would contaminate field.
f. Bending slightly at the waist, use a sterile towel to dry one hand thoroughly, moving from fingers to elbow in a rotating motion (see illustration).	Avoids sterile towel from contacting unsterile scrub attire and transferring contamination to hands. Dry skin from cleanest (hands) to least clean (elbows).
g. Use the opposite end of the towel to dry the other hand.	Avoids transfer of microorganisms from elbow to opposite hand.
h. Drop towel into linen hamper or into circulating nurse's hand.	

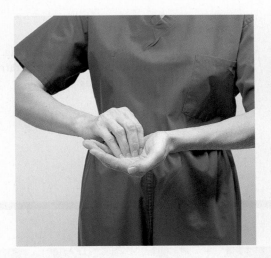 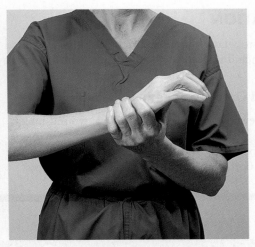

Step 7a   Application of antimicrobial agent for brushless hand scrub. Nurse using 3M Avagard (Chlorhexide Gluconate 1% Solution and Ethyl Alcohol 61% w/w) Surgical and Healthcare Personnel Hand Antiseptic With Moisturizers. (Photo courtesy of 3M Health Care.)

Steps	Rationale

7. **Option: brushless antiseptic hand rub**
  a. Dispense 2 ml of antimicrobial agent (hand prep) into the palm of one hand. Dip the fingertips of the opposite hand into the hand prep and work it under the nails (see illustration). Spread the remaining hand prep over the hand and up to just above the elbow, covering all surfaces (see illustration).
  b. Using another 2 ml of hand prep, repeat above procedure with the other hand.
	Ensures reduction in microorganisms on all surfaces of hands and arms.

NURSE ALERT   *This is an example of one particular brushless product. Please see manufacturer's instructions for application. There are many new products on the market, and strict adherence to their guidelines is essential to achieving surgical asepsis.*

  c. Dispense another 2 ml of hand prep into either hand, and reapply to all aspects of both hands up the wrist. Allow to dry before donning gloves.

• • • • • • • • • •

EVALUATION

Monitor postoperative client for signs of surgical wound infection, including redness, tenderness, and purulent drainage.

Unexpected Outcomes and Related Interventions

1. Client develops postoperative surgical wound infection.
   a. Interventions should be individualized to client situation (e.g., wound care, antibiotic therapy).

Recording and Reporting

- No recording is required for handwashing. Record area and description of surgical site postoperatively to provide baseline for monitoring wound.

Skill 20.2

Donning Sterile Gown and Closed Gloving

Immediately following surgical hand antisepsis, a sterile gown should be applied, followed by application of sterile gloves. All members of the surgical team must prepare in this manner before entering the sterile field. Once applied, the surgical gown is considered sterile in the front from chest to waist or table level. The sleeves are considered sterile from 5 cm (2 inches) above the elbow to fingertips. The back of the gown is not considered sterile when worn.

Surgical gowns should cover all garments worn underneath. All sterile gowns that are free of tears, punctures, strain, and abrasion provide an effective barrier against microorganisms passing between unsterile and sterile areas (AORN, 1998a).

The scrub nurse should use the closed-glove method when initially entering the sterile field. If a glove becomes contaminated during the surgery, the circulating nurse, wearing protective unsterile gloves, grasps the outside of the glove and pulls off the glove inside out, leaving the stockinette cuff of the gown in place. Another sterile team member assists in regloving, or the open-glove method can be used. If both the scrub nurse's gloves become contaminated, it is recommended to regown and reglove using the closed-glove method.

ASSESSMENT

1. Select proper size and type of sterile gloves. Latex-free gloves should be selected if latex sensitivity of client or any surgical personnel in the room is sus-

pected. *Rationale: Proper fit ensures ease of handling instruments and supplies. Prevents latex allergic response.*
2. Select proper size and type of sterile surgical gown.

PLANNING

Expected outcome should focus on prevention of infection resulting from breaks in aseptic technique.

Expected Outcome

Client does not develop signs of surgical wound infection.

Equipment

- Package of proper-size sterile gloves (latex-free if necessary)
- Sterile pack containing sterile gown
- Clean, flat, dry surface (table or Mayo stand) on which to open gown and gloves
- Paper face mask, cap or hood, surgical shoe covers
- Protective eyewear

Delegation Considerations

The skills of sterile gowning and gloving can be delegated to a surgical technologist or licensed practical nurse (LPN) who has received the proper training.

IMPLEMENTATION FOR DONNING STERILE GOWN AND CLOSED GLOVING

Steps	Rationale
1. Open sterile gown and glove package on a clean, dry, flat surface. This can be done by the scrub nurse (before scrubbing hands) or circulating nurse.	Preferably done on a small table separate from the sterile field containing the sterile instruments and supplies.
2. Perform surgical hand antisepsis (see Skill 20-1, p. 510).	
3. After drying hands, pick up gown (folded inside out) from sterile package, grasping the inside surface of gown at the collar.	The hands are not completely sterile. The inside surface of the gown will contact the skin's surface and is thus considered contaminated.
4. Lift folded gown directly upward, and step back, away from the table.	Prevents gown from touching contaminated object.
5. Locate neckband; with both hands, grasp the inside front of gown just below neckband.	Clean hands may touch inside of gown without contaminating outer surface.
6. Allow gown to unfold, keeping at arm's length away from body with the inside of gown toward body. Do not touch outside of gown or allow it to touch the floor.	Outside of gown remains sterile.
7. With hands at shoulder level, slip both arms into armholes simultaneously (see illustration). Do not allow hands to move through cuff opening. Have circulating nurse pull gown over shoulders by reaching inside arm seams. Gown is pulled on, leaving sleeves covering hands.	Careful application prevents contamination. Gown covers hands to prepare for closed gloving.
8. Have circulating nurse tie gown at neck and waist (see illustration). If gown is wraparound style, sterile front flap is not touched until the scrub nurse has gloved.	

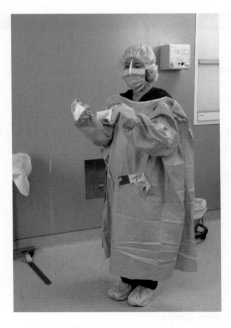

Step 7 Placing arms in sleeves.

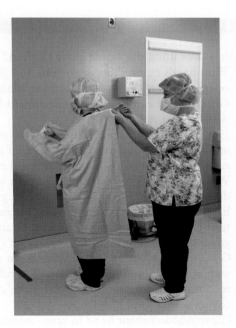

Step 8 Circulating nurse ties scrub gown.

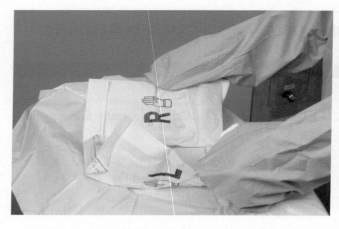

Step 9a Scrub nurse opens glove package.

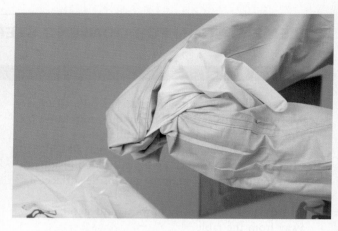

Step 9d Glove applied as hands remain inside cuff.

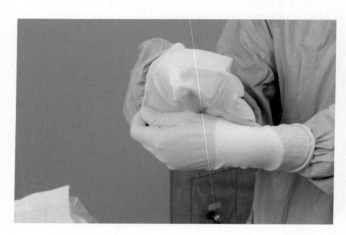

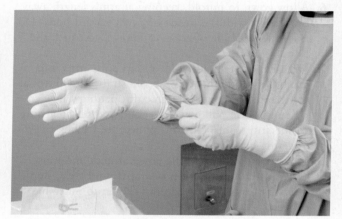

Step 9f Second glove applied.

Steps	Rationale

9. Apply gloves using the closed-glove method:

a. With hands covered by gown cuffs and sleeves, open inner sterile glove package (see illustration).

Sterile gown cuff will touch sterile glove surface.

b. Grasp folded cuff of glove for dominant hand with the nondominant hand.

Sterile gown touches sterile glove.

c. Extend dominant forearm forward with palm up, and place palm of glove against palm of dominant hand. Gloved fingers point toward elbow.

Positions glove for application over cuffed hand, keeping glove sterile.

d. While holding glove cuff through gown with dominant hand on which it was placed, grasp back of glove cuff with nondominant hand and turn glove cuff over end of dominant hand and gown cuff (see illustration).

Positions glove over gown for hand insertion.

e. Grasp top of glove and underlying gown sleeve with covered nondominant hand. Carefully extend fingers into glove, being sure glove's cuff covers gown's cuff.

f. Glove nondominant hand in same manner with gloved, dominant hand (see illustration). Keep hand inside sleeve. Be sure fingers are fully extended into both gloves (see illustration).

Gloves remain sterile.

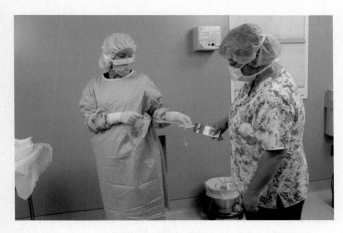

Step 10c   Disposable paper gown with paper tab.

10. *For wraparound gown:*
   a. Grasp sterile front flap/waist tie with gloved hands and untie.

   b. Pass tie to circulating nurse, who stands still as scrub nurse turns. This may also be held by another team member with sterile gloves. Keep gown tie in left hand.

   c. Allowing margin of safety, turn to the left one-half turn, covering back with extended gown flap. Retrieve tie only from team member, and secure both ties in place.
   NOTE: On disposable sterile gowns, there is often a paper tab attached to the tie that can be passed to a nonsterile team member for turning and then is pulled off and discarded (see illustration).

Front of gown is sterile.

Maneuver covers entire body with gown.

• • • • • • • • • •

EVALUATION

Monitor postoperative client for signs of surgical wound infection, including redness, tenderness, and purulent drainage.

Unexpected Outcomes and Related Interventions

1. Client develops postoperative surgical wound infection.
   a. Interventions should be individualized to client situation (e.g., wound care, antibiotic therapy).

Recording and Reporting

• No recording is required for sterile gowning and gloving. Record area and description of surgical site postoperatively to provide baseline for monitoring wound.

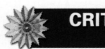

CRITICAL THINKING EXERCISES

1. You are the circulating nurse during an emergency appendectomy. While the scrub nurse, Sarah, is gowning and gloving the surgeon, you notice the sleeve of his sterile gown touches an IV pole. Sarah and the surgeon do not seem to notice. He starts to raise his voice at Sarah to hurry up and pass him the sterile drapes. What should you do?

2. James is a new scrub nurse on the heart team. He has been scrubbing by himself (without a preceptor) for only 1 week. When he entered the operating room after performing a surgical scrub, he notices he drips water on the sterile gown he is about to put on. The anesthesiologist just wheeled the client into the room, and no one saw James drip water onto the gown. He asks the circulating nurse to open him a new gown and gloves. What do James's actions demonstrate?

REFERENCES

Association of Operating Room Nurses: Recommended practices for protective barrier materials for surgical gowns and drapes. In *AORN standards and recommended practices for perioperative nursing,* Denver, 1998a, The Association.

Association of Operating Room Nurses: Statement on mandate for the registered nurse as circulator in the operating room. In *AORN standards and recommended practices for perioperative nursing,* Denver, 1998b, The Association.

Association of Operating Room Nurses: Recommended practices for surgical hand scrubs. In *AORN standards and recommended practices for perioperative nursing,* Denver, 2001, The Association.

Atkinson L, Fortunato N: *Berry and Kohn's operating room technique,* ed 8, St Louis, 1996, Mosby.

Boyce JM, Pittet D: Guidelines for hand hygiene in health care settings. *AJIC* 30(8):S1-S46, 2002.

Gruendemann BJ, Bjerke NB: Is it time for brushless scrubbing with an alcohol-based agent? *AORN J* 74(6):859, 2001.

Meeker MH, Rothrock JC: *Alexander's care of the patient in surgery,* ed 11, St Louis, 1999, Mosby.

Perry A, Potter P: *Clinical nursing skills and techniques,* ed 5, St Louis, 2002, Mosby.

Caring for the Postoperative Client

The care of postoperative clients may be divided into two phases: the immediate postanesthesia recovery and the convalescent phase. The first phase extends from the time the client leaves the operating room (OR) to the time of transfer from the postanesthesia care unit (PACU) to the nursing unit. This phase can require 2 or more hours. The early recovery phase involves several days followed by a convalescent phase for several additional days or weeks at home for the continued healing process. The client with a chronic medical condition, such as chronic respiratory disease or diabetes, may require even longer.

Cost containment measures and reimbursement policies have dramatically changed routines for surgical procedures. Many surgical procedures that once required an overnight hospital admission are not reimbursed by insurance for inpatient services. Newer technologies, such as laser and laparoscopy, are less invasive and also decrease the need for inpatient admission. Many clients are admitted the morning of surgery rather than receiving inpatient preparation for surgery. The current trend involves more ambulatory outpatient surgery and shorter hospitalizations to achieve cost containment. In addition, clients often recover better at home.

Table 21-1

Postanesthesia Monitoring

Condition	Interventions
Airway	
Mechanical obstruction: decreased level of consciousness and muscle relaxants resulting in flaccid muscles and tongue blocking airway	Hyperextend neck; pull mandible forward; use nasal or oral airway; encourage deep breathing.
Retained thick secretions: irritation from anesthesia; anticholinergic medications; history of smoking	Suction; encourage coughing.
Laryngospasm: stridor from excessive secretions or airway irritation	Encourage to relax and breathe through the mouth. If extreme may require positive-pressure ventilation with oxygen, small dose of muscle relaxant (ordered by anesthesiologist), and intubation.
Laryngeal edema: allergic reaction, irritation from endotracheal tube, fluid overload	Administer humidified oxygen, antihistamines, steroids, sedatives, and in some cases perform reintubation.
Bronchospasm: preexisting asthma, anesthetic irritation (expiratory wheeze)	Administer bronchodilators as ordered.
Aspiration: vomiting from hypotension, accumulated gastric secretions and delayed gastric emptying, pain, fear, position changes	Position on side; suction airway; administer antiemetic as ordered.
Breathing: Hypoventilation/Hypoxemia	
Central nervous system depression: anesthesia, analgesics, muscle relaxants (respiratory rate shallow)	Encourage to cough and deep breathe; use mechanical ventilator; administer narcotic antagonist, muscle relaxant reversal agent.
Mechanical restriction: obesity, pain, tight cast or dressings, abdominal distention	Reposition; give analgesic; loosen cast or dressings; implement measures to reduce gastric distention (e.g., nasogastric intubation, nasogastric suction).
Circulation	
Hypovolemia: blood loss, dehydration	Elevate legs; give oxygen, IV fluids, or blood replacement; administer vasopressors; monitor I&O, stimulation, hemoglobin, and hematocrit.
Hypotension: Anesthesia/drug effects, spinal anesthesia may cause vasodilation; narcotics	
Cardiac failure: preexisting cardiac disease; circulatory overload; excessive/too-rapid fluid replacement	Provide digitalization, diuretics; monitor ECG.
Cardiac arrhythmias: hypoxemia; myocardial infarct; hypothermia; imbalance of potassium, calcium, magnesium	Provide IV fluid replacement; monitor ECG, urine output; identify and treat cause.
Hypertension: pain; distended bladder; preexisting hypertension; vasopressor drugs	Compare to preoperative baseline; identify and determine cause.
Compartment syndrome: pressure from edema causing enough compression to obstruct arterial and venous circulation resulting in ischemia, permanent numbness, loss of function; forearm and lower leg most common sites	Elevate extremity no higher than heart level; remove or loosen bandage or cast to relieve compression; if left untreated, amputation may be required. Do not apply ice.

The PACU, once called the "recovery room," is in many respects a critical care unit. Staff in the PACU are professional nurses with specific education and experience to recognize and help manage anesthesia-related and surgery-related complications (American Society of Perianesthesia Nurses [ASPAN], 2000).

The client is accompanied to the PACU by a member of the anesthesia care team, who provides a verbal report, including preanesthesia status, medical history, and medications. Additional information includes (1) actual surgical procedure done; (2) postoperative status (e.g., vital signs, oxygen saturation, allergies); (3) length of anesthesia and technique (general, regional, or local); (4) anesthesia, muscle relaxant, narcotic, and reversal agents used; (5) current vital signs, intravenous (IV) fluids or blood products used in surgery; (6) presence of drains, estimated blood loss and replacement; and (7) complications that occurred during surgery (ASPAN, 2000).

Preoperative orders typically are canceled by surgery. Postoperative orders usually specify when any of the preoperative orders are to be continued. Postoperative orders also include frequency of vital signs and special assessments, types of IV fluids and infusion rate, postoperative medications, fluids or foods allowed by mouth, level of activity or type of positioning, intake and output (I&O), laboratory tests or x-ray studies to be done, and special interventions such as dressing changes, an immobilizing device, or an incentive spirometer. For ambulatory surgery clients, orders include discharge instructions, follow-up appointment, analgesic prescriptions, and activity limitations for 24 hours following anesthesia.

The immediate postoperative recovery phase requires frequent assessments for potentially life-threatening complications resulting from anesthesia or surgery. It is important to emphasize the ABCs: *A* is for airway, *B* is for breathing, and *C* is for circulation (Table 21-1). Postoperative clients still are sedated and easily become hypoxic. Oxygen saturation levels are routinely monitored, and supplemental oxygen is provided for as long as needed.

Size, location, and depth of a wound influence type and amount of drainage. It is important to know what type of drainage is expected (Table 21-2). Nurses can estimate drainage by counting the number of saturated gauze sponges. Drainage may be collected in wound drainage systems, such as chest tube, Hemovac, or bulb drainage (see Skill 22-2, p. 541). Some bloody drainage is expected through chest tubes. Bloody drainage must be reported if it exceeds 100 to 200 ml/hr for an adult. Hemorrhage is loss of large amounts of blood either externally or internally in a short time and will result in shock if uncontrolled. Arterial bleeding is bright red and gushes forth in waves related to heart rhythm. If a vessel is very deep, flow will be steady. Venous bleeding is dark red and flows smoothly. Capillary bleeding is oozing of dark red blood; self-sealing controls this bleeding. A hematoma can develop at the incision.

Some surgical wounds have gauze dressings or are covered with a clear, transparent dressing. Some are left

Table 21-2

Expected Drainage From Tubes and Catheters: Adults

Substance	Daily Amount	Color	Odor	Consistency
Indwelling Catheter Urine	500-700 ml, 1-2 days postoperatively; 1500-2500 ml thereafter	Clear, yellow	Ammonia	Watery
Nasogastric or Gastrostomy Tube Gastric contents	Up to 1500 ml/day	Pale, yellow-green Bloody following gastrointestinal (GI) surgery	Sour	Watery
Hemovac Wound drainage	Varies with procedure	Varies with procedure Usually serosanguineous	Same as wound dressing	Variable
T Tube Bile	500 ml	Bright yellow to dark green	Acid	Thick

Modified from Lewis SM and others: *Medical-surgical nursing: assessment and management of clinical problems,* ed 5, St Louis, 2000, Mosby.

open to air (OTA). Physician's orders will specify type and frequency of dressing changes. If excessive drainage is noted, the physician must be notified.

NURSING DIAGNOSES

Nursing diagnoses are identified based on assessment data and are related to the prevention of complications of surgery and anesthesia. Some incisional pain is expected and can increase the risk for postoperative complications; therefore **Acute Pain** related to inflammation or injury in the surgical area could be an appropriate nursing diagnosis. **Ineffective Airway Clearance** related to incisional pain and increased secretions secondary to general anesthesia and history of smoking could be appropriate if the client is unable to remove secretions from the airway due to pain. **Ineffective Breathing Pattern** related to sedation secondary to general anesthesia could be appropriate for clients who need stimulation to promote respiratory effort and tend to hypoventilate. **Risk for Aspiration** related to depressed cough/gag reflex secondary to anesthesia focuses interventions on prevention of airway obstruction. Nausea related to gastrointestinal distention or effects of medications and anesthesia may require treatment.

Decreased Cardiac Output may be used to identify hemorrhage caused by slipping of suture, inadequate clotting, or excessive blood or fluid loss for any reason. **Risk for Deficient Fluid Volume** is also related to excessive loss of fluid and blood from wound drainage or from inadequate fluid replacement. **Risk for Ineffective Tissue Perfusion** related to venous stasis or vessel trauma may be indicated after surgery of the legs, abdomen, pelvis, and major blood vessels. This is also appropriate when blood coagulation studies indicate increased coagulation and when clients are immobilized, have chronic hypoxia, or use oral contraceptives containing estrogen.

Risk for Imbalanced Body Temperature related to extremes of age, cool environment, or altered metabolic rate is appropriate when the client's body temperature drops below 96.8° F (36° C) or symptoms such as shivering occur. This problem may be seen more in infants and children due to immature thermoregulation centers. **Risk for Infection** related to surgical incision (specify location) is appropriate when the client has lowered resistance to infection for any reason, including conditions such as obesity, advanced age, impaired circulation, diabetes, immunosuppression, radiation, smoking, poor cellular nutrition, very deep wounds, or wounds healing by secondary intention. These conditions result in increased risk of infection. **Ineffective Health Maintenance** related to inadequate knowledge of postoperative self-care may be appropriate for clients who have not had surgery previously or who require an extended convalescence because of the nature of the surgery. Teaching needs should be considered for all postoperative clients.

Skill 21.1

Providing Immediate Postoperative Care in Postanesthesia Care Unit

The first phase of postoperative care takes place during the immediate recovery period, which extends from the time the client leaves the OR to the time the client has stabilized in the PACU, meets discharge criteria, and has been transferred to the nursing unit.

The first 1 to 2 hours are the most critical for assessing aftereffects of anesthesia, including airway clearance, cardiovascular complications, temperature control, and neurological function. The client's condition can change rapidly, and assessments must be timely, knowledgeable, and accurate. Quick judgment regarding the most appropriate interventions is essential. The client is usually considered ready for discharge to the general unit when specific standardized criteria are met. The Aldrete Score is one of several scoring systems for assessment (Table 21-3). It uses parameters of activity, respiration, circulation, consciousness and O_2 saturation. A score of 8 or less requires additional monitoring (Aldrete, 1998). A score of 10 indicates a fully recovered client.

Recovery from ambulatory surgery requires the same assessments; however, the depth of general anesthesia may be less because the surgery is less involved and of shorter duration. Some clients have only IV conscious sedation, for which intensive monitoring usually requires a shorter length of time. As soon as the client is stable and alert, instructions for home care are given to the client and caregiver. Demonstrations and written instructions are provided. Encourage the client not to drive, to avoid drugs and alcohol, and to postpone making important decisions for 24 hours. A ride home and adequate support for home care must be established.

ASSESSMENT

1. On client's arrival in PACU, obtain report from circulating nurse and anesthesiologist or nurse anesthetist that provides review of client's physiological status and baseline data to determine any change in condition.

Table 21-3

Aldrete Score for Postanesthesia Monitoring

			Admission	5 min	15 min	30 min	45 min	60 min	Discharge
Activity	Able to move four extremities voluntarily or on command	2							
	Able to move two extremities voluntarily or on command	1							
	Unable to move extremities voluntarily or on command	0							
Respiratory	Able to breathe deeply and cough freely	2							
	Dyspnea or limited breathing	1							
	Apneic	0							
Circulation	BP + 20% of preanesthetic level	2							
	BP + 20%-49% of preanesthetic level	1							
	BP + 50% of preanesthetic level	0							
Consciousness	Fully awake	2							
	Arousable on calling	1							
	Not responding	0							
O_2 saturation	Able to maintain O_2 Saturation >92% on room air	2							
	Needs O_2 inhalation to maintain O_2 saturation >92%	1							
	O_2 saturation <90% even with O_2 supplement	0							
Totals									

Aldrete, JA: Modification to the Postanesthesia Score for Use in Ambulatory Surgery. *J PeriAnesth Nurs.* 13(3):148, 1998.
BP, Blood pressure.

2. Review the client's preexisting conditions during operative procedure, including baseline and intraoperative vital signs, oxygen saturation, blood volume or fluid loss, fluid replacement, type of anesthesia, type of airway and size, and extent of surgical wound, including presence of surgical drains. *Rationale: This determines the client's general status and allows the nurse to anticipate the need for special equipment, nursing care, and activities in PACU.*

3. Consider the effects of the client's type of surgery and anesthesia and restrictions to movement. *Rationale: This information influences type of assessments nurse initiates, type of complications to observe for, and specific nursing interventions.*

PLANNING

Expected outcomes focus on early detection of complications from surgery or anesthesia and adequate pain control by the time of transfer (usually 1 to 2 hours).

Expected Outcomes

1. Client's airway remains clear, and respirations are deep, regular, and within normal limits by the time of transfer.
2. Client's blood pressure, pulse, and temperature remain within previous baseline or normal expected range by the time of transfer.
3. Dressings are clean, dry, and intact by discharge from recovery.

4. Intake and output are within expected parameters by discharge from recovery.
5. Client reports relief of discomfort after analgesia or other pain relief measures by the time of transfer from the immediate recovery area (usually 1 to 2 hours).
6. Client's postoperative assessments are within expected normal postoperative parameters.

Equipment

- Stethoscope, sphygmomanometer, pulse oximeter, cardiac monitor, thermometer
- Oxygen equipment such as mask, oxygen regulator and tubing, and positive-pressure delivery system
- Suction equipment
- Dressing supplies
- Warmed blanket or active rewarming device
- Emergency equipment
- Emergency medications

Delegation Considerations

The skill of initiating and managing postoperative care of the client requires the critical thinking and knowledge application unique to a nurse. Assistive personnel (AP) may obtain vital signs, apply nasal cannula or oxygen mask, and provide basic comfort and hygiene measures.

IMPLEMENTATION FOR PROVIDING IMMEDIATE POSTOPERATIVE CARE IN POSTANESTHESIA CARE UNIT

Steps	Rationale
1. See Standard Protocol (inside front cover).	
2. As client enters PACU on stretcher, immediately attach oxygen tubing to regulator and check IV flow rates.	Inhaled oxygen promotes tissue oxygenation during recovery from anesthesia. IV fluids maintain circulatory volume and provide route for emergency drugs.
3. Connect or secure drainage tubes to intermittent suction.	Drainage tubes must remain patent to prevent pressure within wound cavity.
4. Attach monitoring devices (e.g., blood pressure cuff, pulse oximeter, electrocardiogram (ECG), arterial lines).	Maintains continual assessment and monitoring of physiological parameters.
5. Compare vital signs with client's preoperative baseline. Continue assessing vital signs at least every 5 to 15 minutes until stable.	Vital signs can reveal respiratory depression, cardiac irregularity, hypotension, or hypothermia.
6. ✋ Maintain airway after general anesthesia. a. If client is supine, elevate head of bed slightly, pull jaw forward, or turn head to side unless contraindicated. Initially client may need to be reminded to breathe (see illustration).	Maintains opens airway by keeping tongue out of the way while client has decreased level of consciousness (LOC).

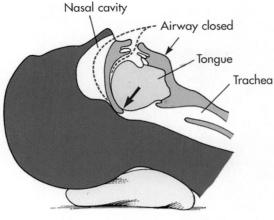

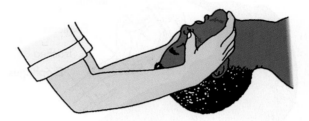

Step 6a   Head positioning for maintenance of airway.

Steps	Rationale

NURSE ALERT   *Always stay with the sedated client until respirations are well established. Clients with an artificial airway may gag and vomit, become restless, or stop breathing.*

    b. Suction artificial airway and oral cavity with Yankauer suction tip if secretions accumulate (see illustration on p. 526) (see Chapter 31). Assist client with spitting out oral airway as gag reflex returns.

Indicates client can clear airway independently.

7. Call client by name in normal tone of voice. If there is no response, attempt to arouse client by touching or gently moving a body part. Explain that surgery is over and client is in the recovery area.

Determines client's LOC and ability to follow commands. Assists client in being oriented to place.

8. Encourage client to cough and deep breathe every 15 minutes (see Chapter 19).

Promotes lung expansion, elimination of inhalation anesthetic, and expectoration of mucous secretions. A mucous plug will result in collapsed alveoli and atelectasis (see illustration in Step 6b, p. 526).

9. Inspect color of nail beds and skin. Palpate for skin temperature.

Indicators of peripheral tissue perfusion.

10. Assess closely for potential cardiovascular and pulmonary complications of general anesthesia (see Table 21-1, p. 520).

Postoperative clients may be sedated and can easily become hypoxic.

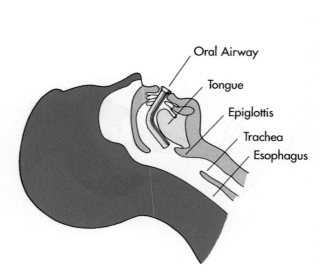

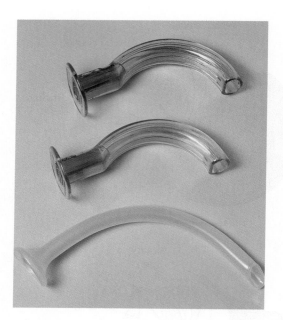

Step 6b Oral airways.

Steps	Rationale

11. Monitor sensory and circulatory and neurological responses after spinal or epidural anesthesia.

a. Monitor for hypotension, bradycardia, and nausea and vomiting.

Blockade of sympathetic nervous system may result in vasodilation of major vessels and systemic hypotension.

b. Maintain adequate IV infusion.

Maintains blood pressure by increasing fluid volume and fills temporarily expanded vascular space.

c. Keep client supine or with head slightly elevated, and maintain position.

Minimizes risk of post–spinal anesthesia headache from leakage of spinal fluid at injection site, with increased pressures induced by elevation of upper body. Headache is more common with spinal than epidural anesthesia. Incidence of headache is less with use of smaller-gauge spinal needles (Lewis and others, 2000).

d. Clients are observed in PACU until movement has been regained in extremities.

Clients may fear permanent loss of function.

e. Assess respiratory status, level of sensation, and mobility in lower extremities. Following IV sedation, drowsiness will be apparent. Level of anesthesia can be determined by location of sensation change using an alcohol wipe to elicit awareness of cold sensation (see illustration).

Spinal block is set within 20 minutes of onset. However, if level of anesthesia moves above sixth thoracic vertebra (T6), respiratory muscles may be affected. Client may feel short of breath and, if severe, may require mechanical ventilation.

COMMUNICATION TIP

- *If client had general anesthesia: As client arouses, introduce yourself and orient client to surroundings.*
- *If client has spinal anesthesia: Remind client that loss of extremity sensation and movements is normal and they will be restored in several hours.*

NURSE ALERT *In an emergency situation, document interventions and evaluation as reported to physician, including maintenance of airway and bleeding control, distal pulses, vital signs, IV line, LOC, oxygenation or hypoxia, and anxiety level.*

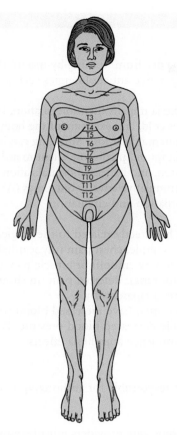

Step 11e   Assess level of spinal anesthesia.

Steps	Rationale

12.   Monitor drainage.

a. Observe dressing and drains for any evidence of bright red blood.

           Dressing maintains hemostasis and absorbs drainage. First dressing changes usually occur 24 hours postoperatively and are done by the surgeon unless otherwise ordered.

b. Inform physician of unexpected bloody drainage, and reinforce dressing as indicated. Apply direct pressure. Also, look underneath client for any pooling of bloody drainage. Monitor for decreased blood pressure and increased pulse.

           Hemorrhage from a surgical wound is most likely within first few hours, indicating inadequate hemostasis during surgery.

           As a dressing becomes saturated, blood may ooze down client's side and collect under client.

c. Inspect condition and contents of any drainage tubes and collecting devices. Note character and volume of drainage (see Chapter 22).

           Determines drainage tube patency and extent of wound drainage.

d. Observe amount, color, and appearance of urine from indwelling Foley catheter (if present).

           Urine output of less than 30 ml/hr may indicate decreased renal perfusion or altered renal function (see Table 21-2, p. 521).

e. If nasogastric (NG) tube is present, assess drainage. If not draining, check placement and irrigate if necessary with normal saline (see Chapter 32).

           Maintains patency of tube to ensure gastric decompression. Expected drainage may be dark or pale, yellow, green, and 100 to 200 ml/hr. Bloody drainage may be expected after some surgeries.

f. Monitor IV fluid rates. Observe IV site for signs of infiltration (see Chapter 29).

           Provides adequate hydration and circulatory function.

Steps	Rationale

13. Promote comfort.

a. Provide mouth care by placing moistened washcloth to lips, swabbing oral mucosa with dampened swab, or apply petrolatum to lips.

Mouth may be dry from nothing-by-mouth (NPO) status and preoperative anticholinergics such as atropine.

b. Provide a warm blanket or active rewarming therapy to promote warmth and minimize shivering.

General anesthesia impairs thermoregulation, the OR environment is cold, and exposure of the body cavity may result in internal heat loss. Shivering can increase oxygen consumption, predispose client to arrhythmias and hypertension, and increase hospitalization costs because of cumulative adverse outcomes (ASPAN, 2001).

c. Assist with position changes, and provide supportive pillows.

Improves ventilation and circulation.

14. Assess pain as client awakens, including quality, severity, and location. Do not assume that all postoperative pain is incisional pain.

Pain may not be directly related to the surgical procedure, for example, chest pain (myocardial infarction/pulmonary emboli) or muscle pain (trauma from positioning). Referred pain (in shoulder) often occurs after a laparoscopy.

15. Provide pain medication as ordered and when vital signs have stabilized.

Clients in pain often have increased blood pressure and occasionally decreased blood pressure. Pain medication can influence anesthesia effects.

16. Explain client's condition to client, and inform of plans for transfer to nursing unit or discharge.

17. When client's condition is stabilized, contact anesthesiologist to approve transfer to nursing unit or release to home (see Table 21-3, p. 523).

A physician is responsible for authorizing transfer or discharge.

18. Before discharge to home from the ambulatory surgery unit (ASU), provide verbal and written instructions.

Clients and home care providers must be aware of potential complications and follow-up care.

a. Signs and symptoms of possible complications.

b. Do not drive for 24 hours.

c. Avoid important legal decisions for 24 hours.

d. Surgical site care.

e. Activity restrictions.

f. Pain control.

g. Dietary modifications or restrictions.

h. Plan for follow-up visit.

i. Clarify reasons to call physician and number to call.

19. See Completion Protocol (inside front cover).

• • • • • • • • • •

EVALUATION

1. Observe respirations: rate, depth, and rhythm. Auscultate breath sounds.
2. Compare all blood pressure, pulse, and temperature readings with client's baseline and expected normal values.
3. Inspect dressings for drainage.
4. Measure I&O. Urine output is at least 30 to 50 ml/hr.
5. Ask client to rate pain on scale of 0 to 10, and determine location and characteristics.
6. Conduct complete physical assessments for all clients, with special attention to appropriate assessments according to client's unique type of surgery, for example:

    a. Craniotomy—neurological assessment
    b. Neck surgery—airway status
    c. Vascular surgery—circulation and bleeding
    d. Orthopedic surgery—immobility or positioning

Unexpected Outcomes and Related Interventions

These include alterations from effects of anesthesia or surgical complications.

1. Client exhibits respiratory depression (pulse oximetry less than 92%, respiratory rate less than 10 breaths per minute and/or shallow).

    a. Administer oxygen at 1 to 3 L/min by nasal cannula.
    b. Encourage deep breathing every 5 to 15 minutes.

c. Position to promote chest expansion (on side or semi-Fowler's).

d. Administer prescribed medications (epinephrine, muscle relaxant, or narcotic reversal agent).

2. Client exhibits respiratory obstruction (abnormal lung sounds, snoring, stridor or crowing sounds, wheezing).

a. Reposition head/jaw to open airway.

b. Administer oxygen at 6 to 10 L/min by mask

c. Encourage to cough and deep breathe.

d. Suction if needed.

e. Notify anesthesiologist if unresponsive to interventions; may need to be reintubated if severe.

3. Client exhibits signs of hypovolemia related to internal or incisional hemorrhage.

a. Client's legs should be elevated enough to maintain a downward slope toward the trunk of the body. The head should not be lowered past flat position, which would increase respiratory effort and potentially decrease cerebral perfusion.

b. Administer oxygen at 6 to 10 L/min by mask.

c. Increase rate of IV fluid, or administer blood products.

d. Monitor blood pressure and pulse every 5 to 15 minutes.

e. Apply pressure dressings as follows.

(1) *Abdominal dressing.* Cover bleeding area with several thicknesses of gauze compresses, and place tape 7 to 10 cm (3 to 4 inches) beyond width of dressing with firm even pressure on both sides close to bleeding source. Maintain pressure as entire dressing is taped to maximize pressure at the source of bleeding.

(2) *Dressing on extremity.* Apply rolled gauze, pressing gauze compress over bleeding site. Tape must not be continued around entire extremity.

NURSE ALERT   *Monitor to ensure adequate blood flow to distal tissues, and identify compartment syndrome resulting from edema that creates sufficient pressure to cause ischemia (see Unexpected Outcome 4).*

---

(3) *Dressing in neck region.* Assess every 5 to 15 minutes for evidence of airway obstruction.

f. Client should remain NPO, because it may be necessary to return to surgery for control of bleeding.

g. Promptly report to physician present status of client's bleeding control, time bleeding was discovered, estimated blood loss, nursing interven-

tions (including effectiveness of applied pressure bandage), apical and distal pulses, blood pressure, LOC, and signs of restlessness.

4. Client complains of severe incisional pain.

a. The earliest symptom of compartment syndrome in an extremity is pain unrelieved by analgesics. Other symptoms include numbness, tingling, pallor, coolness, and absent peripheral pulses. The physician *must* be notified. Do not elevate extremity above the level of the heart because this may raise venous pressure. Application of ice is contraindicated because vasoconstriction will occur (Lewis and others, 2000).

b. Nurse should administer analgesics before the pain is severe. It is not necessary to wait for client to request pain medication.

c. Pain can sometimes lower blood pressure; thus analgesia may restore vital signs to normal. Monitor vital signs carefully.

d. For clients with patient-controlled analgesia (PCA), be sure client is using device correctly.

5. Client has hypothermia (temperature less than 36° C [96.8° F]) resulting from effects of anesthesia or loss of body heat from surgical exposure. Shivering can increase oxygen consumption and predispose client to arrhythmias and hypertension.

a. Use warm blankets, socks, head coverings, or active rewarming device.

b. Monitor temperature and client's thermal comfort level every 30 minutes until normal is reached.

Recording and Reporting

• Document in progress notes the client's arrival time at PACU; include vital signs, LOC, and assessment findings. Also include the dressings, tubes, and drainage, and all nursing measures initiated.

• Record vital signs and I&O on appropriate flow sheets.

• Report any abnormal assessment findings and signs of complications to physician.

Sample Documentation

1000 Client received from OR via stretcher. Alert and oriented ×3. Oxygen administered at 3 L/nasal cannula. Abdominal dressing saturated with bright red blood and pad under client saturated, 12- × 20-cm area. Dressing reinforced with pressure dressing. IV infusing with lactated Ringer's at 150 ml/hr. Dr. J notified of excessive drainage and immediate interventions. Blood pressure 110/60, pulse 98, respirations 22, pulse ox. 96%. Client is NPO. Warm blanket applied.

SPECIAL CONSIDERATIONS

Pediatric Considerations
- Maintenance of body temperature in infants and children following surgery is a priority because of the immature temperature control mechanism in this group (Maldonado and Nygren, 1999).
- Infants and children normally have higher metabolic rates and differences in physiological makeup than adults, which are stressed more during surgery, resulting in greater oxygen, fluid, and calorie needs (Maldonado and Nygren, 1999).

Geriatric Considerations
- The ability of older adults to tolerate surgery depends on the extent of physiological changes that have occurred with aging, the presence of any chronic diseases, and the duration of the surgical procedure.

- When communicating with older adults, be aware of any auditory, visual, or cognitive impairment that may be present.

Home Care and Long-Term Care Considerations
- Teach primary caregiver about any postoperative exercises, home modifications, or activity limitations.
- If client is discharged with dressing changes, bedroom or bathroom is usually ideal for procedure. Have primary caregiver perform return demonstration of dressing change.

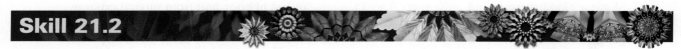

Skill 21.2

Providing Comfort Measures During Early Postoperative Recovery

Providing comfort measures is essential during the early postoperative recovery period, which extends from the time the client is discharged from the PACU to the time the client is discharged from the hospital. Clients who have outpatient surgery undergo convalescence at home. Nursing care must be individualized depending on the type of surgery, preexisting medical conditions, the risk or development of complications, and the rate of recovery. Teaching promotes the client's independence, educates the client about any limitations, and provides resources needed for the client to achieve an optimal state of wellness.

ASSESSMENT

1. Obtain phone report from nurse in PACU. *Rationale: A preliminary report allows nurse to prepare hospital room with necessary supplies and equipment for client's special needs.*
2. On arrival, assist with transfer and complete initial assessment. Review chart to identify type of surgery, preoperative medical risks, and baseline vital signs. *Rationale: Data provide baseline to detect any change in client's condition.*
3. Review surgeon's postoperative orders.

PLANNING

Expected outcomes focus on prevention of complications, maintenance of pain control adequate for recovery activities, and teaching to promote optimal wellness.

Expected Outcomes

1. Client's breath sounds remain clear.
2. Client's vital signs remain within normal limits compared with preoperative baseline.
3. Client describes pain as less than 3 (scale of 0 to 10) while engaged in moderate activity by discharge.
4. Fluid balance is evident by I&O records.
5. Normal bowel sounds present after bowel surgery or general anesthesia within 48 to 72 hours postoperatively.
6. Incision wound edges are well approximated; no drainage is noted.
7. Client (or caregiver) describes plans for coping with stress of surgery (altered function or body image).
8. Client (or caregiver) describes evidence of complications that should be reported to physician by discharge.

9.   Client (or caregiver) describes or demonstrates incision care, dietary modifications, activity restriction, and plans for follow-up visit.

Equipment

- Postoperative bed (recliner for day surgery recovery)
- Stethoscope, sphygmomanometer, thermometer
- IV fluid poles
- Emesis basin
- Washcloth and towel
- Waterproof pads
- Equipment for oral hygiene
- Pillows
- Facial tissue
- Oxygen equipment
- Oxygen mask, and provide basic comfort and hygiene measures
- Suction equipment (to suction airway)
- Dressing supplies
- Intermittent suction (to connect to NG or wound drainage tubes)
- Orthopedic appliances (if needed)

Delegation Considerations

The skill of initiating and managing postoperative care of the client requires the critical thinking and knowledge application unique to a nurse. Assistive personnel (AP) may obtain vital signs, apply nasal cannula or oxygen mask and provide hygiene or repositioning for comfort.

IMPLEMENTATION FOR PROVIDING COMFORT MEASURES DURING EARLY POSTOPERATIVE RECOVERY

Steps	Rationale
1. See Standard Protocol (inside front cover).	Initial postoperative care
2. Prepare bed in high position (level with the stretcher), with sheet folded to side and room for a stretcher to be easily placed beside bed (see illustration) (see Chapter 6).	Arrangement of equipment facilitates smooth transfer process.
3. Assist transport staff to move client from stretcher to bed (see Chapter 6).	
4. Attach any existing oxygen tubing, position IV fluids, check IV flow rate, and check drainage tubes (Foley catheter or wound drainage).	Maintains integrity of drainage tubings.
5. Maintain airway. If client remains sleepy or lethargic, keep head extended and support in side-lying position (see Skill 31.2, p. 755).	Minimizes chances of aspiration and obstruction of airway with tongue.

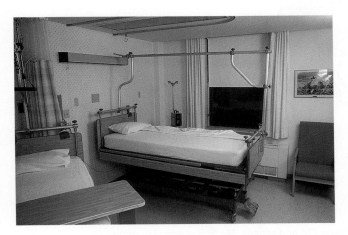

Step 2   Postoperative bed prepared for client.

Steps	Rationale
6. Take vital signs, and compare findings with vital signs in recovery area, as well as client's baseline values. Continue monitoring as ordered.	During transfer, client's status may change. Movement of client and pain level can influence stability of vital signs.
7. Encourage coughing and deep breathing (see Chapter 19) to prevent atelectasis (see illustration).	Anesthesia, medications, and intubation irritate airways, resulting in secretions and atelectasis.
8. If NG tube is present, check placement (see Chapter 32) and connect to proper drainage device. Connect all drainage tubes to appropriate suction device as indicated, and secure to prevent tension.	Transfer and movement may dislodge tube, which would interfere with drainage.
9. Assess client's surgical dressing for appearance and presence and character of drainage. Unless contraindicated by physician, outline drainage along the edges with a pen and reassess in 1 hour for increase. If no dressing present, inspect condition of wound (see Chapter 22).	Hemorrhage is most likely to occur on the day of surgery. Dressing should be clean, dry, and intact.
10. Assess client for bladder distention. If Foley catheter is present, check placement and be sure it is draining freely and is properly secured. Client may have continuous bladder irrigations or suprapubic catheter for urinary drainage (see Chapter 35).	
11. If no urinary drainage system is present, explain that voiding within 8 hours postoperatively is expected. Male clients may void successfully if allowed to stand.	After spinal or epidural anesthesia, risk for urinary retention is increased. Clients may be unable to feel the urge to void. If client is unable to void and bladder is distended, catheterization may be required.
12. Measure all sources of fluid I&O (including estimated blood loss during surgery). Remove and discard gloves, and perform hand hygiene.	Altered fluid and electrolyte balance is a potential complication of major surgery (see Chapter 30).
13. Describe the purpose of equipment and frequent observations to client and significant others.	Unfamiliar sights (equipment, client's appearance) can be anxiety provoking.

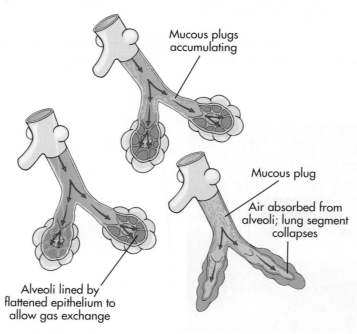

Step 7 Postoperative atelectasis. (From Lewis SM and others: *Medical-surgical nursing: assessment and management of clinical problems,* ed 5, St Louis, 2000, Mosby.)

Steps	Rationale
14. Position client for comfort, maintaining correct body alignment. Avoid tension on surgical wound site.	Reduces stress on suture line. Helps client relax and promotes comfort.
15. Place call light within reach, and raise side rail. Instruct client to call for assistance to get out of bed.	Promotes client's safety as effects of anesthesia continue to diminish.
16. Assess the need for pain medication based on client's level of discomfort and last time analgesic was given. PCA may be used for pain control (see Chapter 11).	Client should be medicated freely every 3 to 4 hours during the first 24 to 48 hours. Adequate pain control is needed to permit client to participate with breathing exercises, coughing, and ambulation.
Continued postoperative care	
17. Assess vital signs at least every 4 hours or as ordered.	Temperature above 38° C (100.4° F) in the first 48 hours may indicate atelectasis, the normal inflammatory response, or dehydration. Elevation above 37.7° C on the third day or after may indicate wound infection, pneumonia, or phlebitis (Lewis and others, 2000). Altered blood pressure and/or pulse may indicate cardiovascular complications (see Table 21-1, p. 520).
18. Provide oral care at least every 2 hours as needed. If permitted, offer ice chips.	Medication given preoperatively, such as atropine (anticholinergic), makes mouth dry. Oral care and ice chips promote comfort.
19. Encourage all clients to turn, cough, and deep breathe at least every 2 hours.	Promotes adequate ventilation and minimizes hypoventilation and atelectases. Especially necessary for clients with history of smoking or pneumonia along with chronic obstructive pulmonary disease (COPD), or confined to bed rest.
20. Encourage use of incentive spirometer as ordered (see Chapter 19).	Promotes adequate ventilation.
21. Promote ambulation and activity as ordered. Assess vital signs before and after activity to assess tolerance. Clients often are encouraged to be up in a chair the evening of surgery or the following morning and progress to walking in room or hallway.	Ambulation is the most significant nursing intervention to prevent postoperative complications. Mobility promotes circulation, lung expansion, and peristalsis. Sudden position changes can cause postural hypotension.
22. Progress from clear liquids to regular diet progressively as tolerated if nausea and vomiting do not occur.	Nausea and vomiting are associated with anesthesia and surgery. IV fluids are usually discontinued when oral intake is tolerated. Some clients must be NPO for several days until bowel sounds are heard.
23. If possible, include client and family in decision making and answer questions as they arise.	Promotes client's sense of control and independence and improves self-esteem.
24. Provide opportunity for clients who must adjust to a change in body appearance or function to verbalize feelings.	Radical surgery (mastectomy, colostomy), amputation, or inoperable cancer may result in anxiety and depression. The grief response to loss of a body organ (e.g., the uterus) is common and should be expected.
25. Discuss plans for discharge with client and caregivers, including dietary modifications or restrictions, wound care, medications, activity restrictions, and symptoms that should be reported to the physician. Clarify follow-up appointments, and encourage quick access to emergency telephone numbers. Provide answers to individual client questions or concerns.	Verifies client's and caregiver's level of knowledge and any additional teaching needs for discharge. Assists in promoting noncomplicated discharge.
26. See Completion Protocol (inside front cover).	

• • • • • • • • • •

EVALUATION

1. Auscultate breath sounds.
2. Obtain vital signs.
3. Ask client to describe pain (scale of 0 to 10) after moderate activity.
4. Evaluate I&O records.
5. Auscultate bowel sounds.
6. Inspect incision (wound edges well approximated, no drainage is noted).
7. Ask client to describe ability to cope with stress of surgery (altered function or body image).
8. Ask client (or caregiver) to indicate symptoms of complications that should be reported to the physician by discharge.
9. Have client (or caregiver) describe incision care, dietary modifications or restrictions, activity restrictions, and plans for follow-up visit.

Unexpected Outcomes and Related Interventions

1. Vital signs are above or below client's baseline or expected range. Initially this could be related to anesthesia efforts, pain, hypovolemic shock, airway obstruction, fluid and electrolyte imbalance, or hypothermia.
   a. Identify contributing factors.
   b. Notify the physician.
2. Bowel sounds are absent or decreased. Client experiences nausea and vomiting. Client is unable to pass flatus, and abdomen is hard and distended. Paralytic ileus is a common complication after bowel surgery. Intestinal motility may return slowly.
   a. Report to physician.
   b. Placement of an NG tube may be required (see Chapter 32).

Recording and Reporting

- Document client's arrival at nursing unit; describe vital signs, assessment findings, and all nursing measures initiated in progress note. Document every 4 hours or more frequently as client condition warrants.
- Record vital signs and I&O on appropriate flow sheet.
- Report any abnormal assessment findings and signs of complications to physician.

Sample Documentation

Third Postoperative Day After Abdominal Surgery

1800 Client vomited 300 ml dark green mucus. Abdomen firm and distended. No bowel sounds heard. Not passing flatus. Rates pain at 7 (scale 0 to 10). Morphine sulfate 10 mg IV. Instructed not to eat or drink anything.

1910 Vomited 200 ml dark green material and c/o being "very nauseated." Abdominal pain now rated at 6 (scale 0 to 10). Dr. K notified. NG tube inserted and connected to low intermittent suction as ordered with return of 400 ml dark green material within 15 minutes. Phenergan 5 mg given intramuscularly for nausea.

1950 Resting comfortably. Denies nausea. Pain now rated at 4 (scale 0 to 10). NG draining large amount of dark green drainage.

SPECIAL CONSIDERATIONS

Pediatric Considerations
An assessment of the child's perception of the surgical experience should be made during the recovery period to support or correct their perceptions about the surgical experience. Drawing and storytelling are effective methods that allow children to share their thoughts and feelings (Wong and others, 1999).

Geriatric Considerations
- Older adults may experience a longer and more difficult postoperative recovery. Assess carefully for the development of postoperative complications.
- Postoperative delirium and changes in mental status should be assessed for along with potential causes.
- Postoperative pain tends to be undertreated in older adults. Some clients fear "becoming addicted" or minimize pain because they are stoic. Assess for pain, and encourage use of pain medications (Lewis and others, 2000).

Home Care and Long-Term Care Considerations
- Teach client and primary caregiver about any postoperative exercises, home modifications, activity limitations, wound dressing care, medications, and nutritional needs.
- If client is discharged with dressing changes, the bedroom or bathroom is usually ideal for procedure. Have client and primary care giver perform return demonstration of dressing change.
- Make referral to home health services if client and caregiver will have difficulty providing the expected level of care needed.

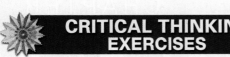

CRITICAL THINKING EXERCISES

1. Susan, age 1 year, is admitted to PACU following gastric surgery. Taking of her vital signs reveals her temperature to be 96.2° F, and she is shivering. What actions should the nurse take?
2. Mr. Dodd was admitted to the surgical floor following an open reduction and internal fixation of fractures in his right lower leg. Three hours after surgery, he is complaining of pain rated as 9 (scale 0 to 10) in his right leg an hour after receiving his pain medication. The leg is edematous and cool, and the pedal pulse is 1+.
   a. Explain the complication that Mr. Dodd may be developing.
   b. What actions should the nurse take and why?

REFERENCES

Aldrete JA: Modification to postanesthesia score for use in ambulatory surgery. *J Postanesth Nurse* 13(3):148, 1998.

American Society of Perianesthesia Nurses: *Standards of perianesthesia nursing practice,* Cherry Hill, NJ, 2000, The Society.

American Society of Perianesthesia Nurses: Hypothermia guidelines, http://www.aspan.org/Hypothermia.htm, retrieved 1/22/03.

Lewis SM and others: *Medical-surgical nursing: assessment and management of clinical problems,* ed 5, St Louis, 2000, Mosby.

Maldonado SS, Nygren C: Pediatric surgery. In Meeker MH, Rothrock JC, editors: *Alexander's care of the patient in surgery,* ed 11, St Louis, 1999, Mosby.

Wong DL and others: *Whaley and Wong's nursing care of infants and children,* ed 6, St Louis, 1999, Mosby.

Surgical Wound Care

Proper wound care is necessary to promote healing after a surgical incision. The expected goal or outcome for the surgical incision is healing but may be dependent upon the client and numerous other factors. Factors that influence wound healing include age, nutrition, circulation, smoking, chronic illness, drug therapy, infection, and the wound environment (Box 22-1).

The stages of healing and interventions related to dressings are described in Chapter 24. Types of healing include healing by primary intention and healing by secondary intention. Healing by primary intention is expected when the edges of a clean surgical incision are sutured or stapled together, tissue loss is minimal or absent, and the wound is not contaminated with microorganisms. Epidermal cells multiply, and there is reestablishment of the epidermal layers to restore the protective function of the skin. By the fifth postoperative day it is possible to palpate a "healing ridge" just under the intact incision. Absence of this healing ridge indicates improper wound healing, and the client may be at an increased risk of dehiscence (Waldrop and Doughty, 2000).

Box 22-1
Factors That Influence Healing of an Incision

1. With increasing age, the reproductive function of epidermal cells diminishes and replacement is slowed and the dermis atrophies, which slows wound contraction and increases risk of wound dehiscence (Sussman, 1998).
2. Inadequate nutrition, including proteins, carbohydrates, lipids, vitamins, and minerals, delays tissue repair and increases risk for infection.
3. The obese client is at risk for wound infection and dehiscence or evisceration. Fat tissue has less vascularization, which decreases transport of nutrients and cellular elements required for healing.
4. A hematocrit value below 20% and a hemoglobin value below 10 g/100 ml negatively influence tissue repair because of decreased oxygen delivery. Oxygen release to tissue is reduced in smokers.
5. Impaired wound healing in diabetic clients results from collagen synthesis reduction and deposition, decreased wound strength, and impaired leukocyte (white blood cell) function.
6. Wound infection prolongs the inflammatory response, and the microorganisms use nutrients and oxygen that are intended for repair.
7. Long-term steroid therapy may diminish the inflammatory response and reduce the healing potential.
8. An open wound must be maintained in a moist environment, and a closed wound must be protected from microorganisms and stress.

Healing by secondary intention often accompanies traumatic open wounds with tissue loss or wounds with a high microorganism count (high risk of infection). The wound is not sutured at the skin level. Wounds that heal by secondary intention go through a regeneration process involving scar tissue formation and heal slowly because of the volume of tissue needed to fill the defect. These wounds require ongoing wound care (a moist environment) to support healing.

Nutritional support of a client with a wound is fundamental to normal cellular integrity and tissue repair. The client with a surgical wound has an increase in caloric need and a greater need for protein. The increase in energy requirements for the client undergoing elective surgery is approximately 10% above the normal requirement. A thorough nutritional assessment should be done for all clients with a wound and an individualized nutritional plan of care developed (Stotts, 2000).

When drainage is expected within the wound, a Penrose drain (Figure 22-1) may be used to help prevent complications. This soft rubber drain is a soft tube that can be "advanced" or pulled out in stages as the wound heals from the inside out. A safety pin is inserted through this drain to prevent the tubing from migrating into the wound. Nursing interventions include protection of skin surfaces in direct contact with the drainage and dressing changes as indicated.

Meticulous hand-hygiene and infection-control procedures relating to wound care limit the risk of nosocomial infection. Antiseptic swabs are used to clean the skin around the wound, beginning at the cleanest area to avoid transmitting microorganisms from one area to another. The presence of some wound exudate is an expected stage of epithelial cell growth. After the third postoperative day, increasing inflammation and a temperature above 37.7° C (100° F) with or without apparent drainage indicate possible wound infection. Wound infection, particularly from aerobic organisms, is often accompanied by a fever that spikes in the afternoon or evening and returns to near-normal levels in the morning.

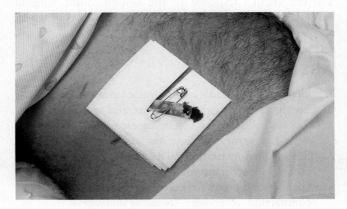

Figure 22-1 Penrose drain with dressing. (Modified from Lewis SM, Collier IC: *Medical-surgical nursing: assessment and management of clinical problems,* ed 4, St Louis, 1996, Mosby.)

Table 22-1

Some Common Pathologic Organisms That Cause Wound Infections

Microorganism	Possible Sources/Comments
Gram Positive	
Staphylococcus aureus	Skin infections, pneumonia, and urinary tract infections. Methicillin-resistant *S. aureus* (MRSA) is a common nosocomial infection resistant to many antibiotics and very difficult to treat.
Streptococcus faecalis	Genitourinary infection, common infection in surgical wounds.

Modified from Lewis SM and others: *Medical-surgical nursing: assessment and management of critical problems,* ed 4, St Louis, 1996, Mosby.

Intermittent high fever accompanied by shaking chills and diaphoresis suggests septicemia, a systemic infection with microorganisms in the bloodstream. The source of microorganisms may be the wound site, a urinary infection, phlebitis, or peritonitis (Table 22-1). Wound culture reveals the type of organisms causing infection. Sensitivity reports indicate which antibiotics will be effective for the specific microorganism present.

NURSING DIAGNOSES

Nursing diagnoses related to care of the client with a surgical wound might include **Impaired Tissue Integrity** related to the surgical incision. Rigorous wound care including ongoing assessment is necessary to promote healing. **Risk for Infection** related to the surgical incision is an appropriate diagnosis when the client has a lower resistance to microorganisms because of one or more of the following: increased age, obesity, poor nutrition, impaired circulation, chronic illness, immunosuppressive drug therapy, and wounds healing by secondary intention. **Acute Pain** related to the surgical incision may be appropriate for the first days after surgery. If the client is to be discharged with a surgical incision requiring home care management, **Deficient Knowledge** may be used to plan for the client's educational needs. **Disturbed Body Image** related to the surgical incision may apply if the client is concerned about disfigurement from the wound.

Skill 22.1

Providing Surgical Wound Care

The surgical wound healing by primary intention will require protection. The wound should be guarded against trauma (no pressure over the area and no heavy lifting by the client) and local infection. The dressing change allows the caregiver the opportunity to assess the wound, the sutures, the drain sites (if used), the skin around the wound, and the client's response to the wound. Some surgical wounds may have the dressings removed and left open to air 24 to 48 hours following surgery.

ASSESSMENT

1. Identify the wound's location, size (measure depth, length, width), presence of drains, and type of dressing. *Rationale: Assists nurse in planning for proper types and amount of supplies and marks progression toward healing.*
2. Review documentation related to incisional healing; include approximation of wound edges and drainage from wound (amount, color), to provide basis for comparison. *Rationale: Amount of drainage decreases as healing takes place; serous drainage is clear; presence of small amounts is normal; bright red drainage indicates fresh bleeding; purulent drainage is thick and yellow, pale green, or beige.*
3. Review culture reports (if ordered) to identify presence of pathogenic organisms (see Table 22-1).
4. Assess client's comfort level and identify symptoms of anxiety. Administer prescribed analgesic 30 to 45 minutes before changing dressing if appropriate. *Rationale: Discomfort may be related directly to wound or indirectly to muscle tension and immobility. Anxiety may result from outcome of surgery, awaiting pathology reports, anticipation of pain, or other factors.*
5. Identify client's history of allergies. *Rationale: Common allergens include tape and latex. This will require the nurse to use different cleansing agents, tape, or latex-free gloves. Known allergies suggest application of a sample of prescribed antiseptic as skin test and avoidance of certain types of tape.*

PLANNING

Expected outcomes focus on wound healing and prevention and early detection of infection.

Expected Outcomes

1. Client's incision displays wound edges that are well approximated.
2. Absence of drainage or drainage begins to lighten in color and amount from client's surgical site.
3. Wound drain, if present, is patent and intact. Skin around drain is free of irritation.
4. Client verbalizes pain at less than 4 (scale of 0 to 10).

Equipment

- Clean gloves
- Sterile gloves
- Waterproof underpad, if needed
- Dressing supplies (unless incision is open to air)
- Disposable waterproof bag
- Gown, if risk of spray
- Goggles, if risk of spray

 Delegation Considerations

Check institutional policy and the state's Nurse Practice Act regarding which wound care interventions can be delegated to assistive personnel (AP). In some states, aspects of wound care such as dressing change can be delegated. This may include the changing of dressings using clean technique for chronic wounds. In this situation instruct staff in what to report when a wound is cleansed. AP must also know how to use clean technique so as to avoid cross contamination. The care of acute new wounds and those that require sterile technique for dressing changes generally remains within the domain of professional nursing practice. The assessment of the wound requires the critical thinking and knowledge application unique to a nurse even when the dressing change is delegated to others.

IMPLEMENTATION FOR PROVIDING SURGICAL WOUND CARE

Steps	Rationale
1. See Standard Protocol (inside front cover).	
2. Form cuff on waterproof bag, and place near bed.	
3. Carefully remove dressing, release tape from skin toward suture line.	Prevents tension on suture line.
4. Inspect dressing for drainage. A small amount of serous drainage is normal. Discard soiled dressings and gloves directly into waterproof bag, perform hand hygiene.	
5. Assess incision for inflammation and signs of healing; describe appearance to client. Client may want to see incision. Provide a mirror if client wants to see incision.	Inflammation is evidenced by pink area and slight swelling, which confirms increased circulation to enhance healing. Incision edges should be well approximated and may be stapled or closed with visible or subcutaneous sutures (West and Gimbel, 2000).
6. Open supplies for dressing and antiseptic swabs using aseptic technique.	

COMMUNICATION TIP *Explain expected wound appearance and review how to provide wound care (if appropriate). Instruct client and primary caregiver in signs of improper wound healing, wound infection, and what should be reported.*

Steps	Rationale
7. **Put on sterile gloves.**	
8. Cleanse suture line from top to bottom (see illustration). Discard antiseptic swab.	Avoids introducing microorganisms from surrounding skin into the incision.
9. Cleanse skin along each side of incision using a single, sterile antiseptic swab for each stroke.	
10. To cleanse a drain site, use a circular stroke starting with the area immediately next to the drain and moving out from the drain (see illustration).	

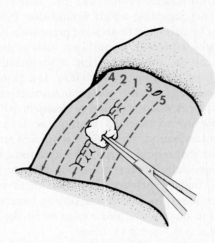

Step 8   Method of cleansing the suture line area.

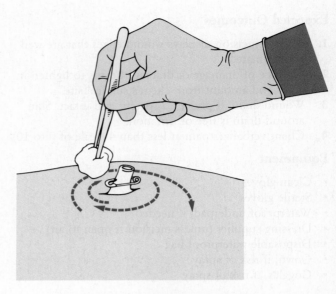

Step 10   Cleansing drain site.

Steps	Rationale

11. Apply dry, sterile dressing and secure with tape, ends folded under 0.5 cm (¼ inch). In pen, write on dressing or tape the date, time, and initials of person changing dressing.
12. See Completion Protocol (inside front cover).

• • • • • • • • • •

EVALUATION

1. Inspect incision with each dressing change.
2. Note amount, color, and consistency of drainage.
3. If drain is present, inspect skin integrity. Drainage may be irritating to skin.
4. Ask client to describe pain (scale of 0 to 10) and indicate quality, location, and factors that intensify or relieve pain.

Unexpected Outcomes and Related Interventions

1. Client develops increased tenderness and pain at wound site.
   a. Monitor for temperature above 37.7° C (100° F) and increased white blood cell count.
   b. Observe for purulent drainage; a culture and sensitivity test can identify infectious microorganisms and appropriate antibiotic therapy (see Chapter 15).
2. Client develops purulent drainage from wound site.
   a. Assess drainage for appearance and odor.
   b. Note approximate amount of drainage by documenting number of dressing changes.

Recording and Reporting

- Report and record in the progress notes:
  Appearance of wound and drainage (if present)
  Change in wound characteristics or wound drainage
  Type of dressing applied

- Record subjective data related to client's overall response to dressing change and level of discomfort.

Sample Documentation

0930 Abdominal dressing changed. Two 4 × 4s saturated with serosanguineous drainage at site of Penrose drain. Sutures intact, wound edges well approximated, no redness or swelling noted. Three 4 × 4s and abdominal dressing (ABD) applied and secured with paper tape. Client describes pain as 3 (scale of 0 to 10) and denies need for analgesic. Client observed dressing change and asked appropriate questions.

SPECIAL CONSIDERATIONS

Pediatric Considerations
- Avoid excessive amount of adhesive tape on young, immature skin.
- When removing the tape, press skin away from the tape, avoid pulling the tape.

Geriatric Considerations
- Prevent injury to older skin by avoiding skin tears from tape removal or products that can cause skin injury. Older skin is thinner and at greater risk for damage.
- Compensate for any auditory, visual, or cognitive impairment the client has when performing a dressing change.

Home Care Considerations
- If client is discharged with dressing changes, bedroom or bathroom is usually ideal for procedure. Have primary caregiver perform return demonstration of dressing change.
- Assess client's home environment to determine adequacy of facilities for performing wound care; check for adequate lighting, running water, dry area of storage for supplies, and disposal of dressings and used supplies.

Long-Term Care Considerations
- Include in transfer papers: dressing frequency, wound assessment, and participation level of client.
- Wound healing may be delayed because of inadequate nutritional stores, immobility, or medications.

Skill 22.2

Monitoring and Measuring Drainage Devices

When drainage may interfere with healing, the surgeon will insert a drain directly through a small stab wound near the suture line into the wound area. Two common types of drainage devices are portable, self-contained suction units that connect to drainage tubes within the wound and provide constant low-pressure suction to remove and collect drainage without wall suction. When the container is one-half to two-thirds full, it should be emptied and reset to apply suction. A Jackson-Pratt drain (Figure 22-2) is used when small amounts (100 to 200 ml) of drainage are anticipated. A Hemovac drainage system can be used for larger amounts (up to 500 ml) of drainage.

ASSESSMENT

1. Identify placement of closed wound drain or type of drainage system when client returns from surgery. System may include one straight tube or a Y-tube arrangement with two tube insertion sites and one drainage container. *Rationale: Awareness of drain placement is needed to plan skin care and identify quantity of dressing supplies required.*
2. Inspect for tube patency by observing drainage movement through tubing in direction of the reservoir, and look for intact connection sites. *Rationale: Properly functioning system maintains suction until reservoir is filled or drainage is no longer being produced or accumulated. Tension on drainage tubing increases injury to skin and underlying muscle.*

PLANNING

Expected outcomes focus on promoting wound healing and comfort by maintaining adequate suction and preventing infection.

Expected Outcomes

1. Quantity and appearance of wound drainage remain within expected guidelines based on type of surgery.
2. Client's drainage device is properly located and intact.

Equipment

- Measuring container (size varies)
- Alcohol sponge
- Gauze sponges
- Sterile specimen container, if needed
- Dressings, if needed
- Clean gloves
- Disposable drape
- Sterile forceps *(optional)*

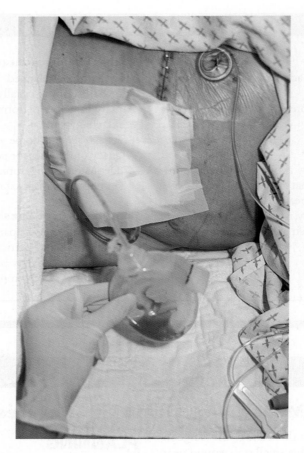

Figure 22-2 Jackson-Pratt drainage tube and reservoir.

Delegation Considerations

Assessment of wound drainage and maintenance of drains and the drainage system require the critical thinking and knowledge application unique to a nurse. However, delegation to assistive personnel (AP) may be appropriate for emptying a closed drainage container, measuring the amount of drainage, and reporting the amount on the client's intake and output (I&O) record.

IMPLEMENTATION FOR MONITORING AND MEASURING DRAINAGE DEVICES

Steps	Rationale

1. See Standard Protocol (inside front cover).
2. **Empty Hemovac, VacuDrain, or Constavac.**
   a. Open plug on port for emptying drainage reservoir. Slowly squeeze the two flat surfaces together, tilting container toward measuring container.

   Vacuum is broken, and reservoir pulls air in until chamber is fully expanded. Squeezing empties reservoir of drainage.

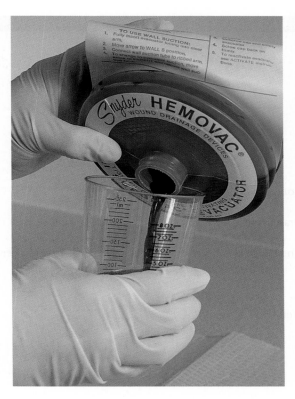

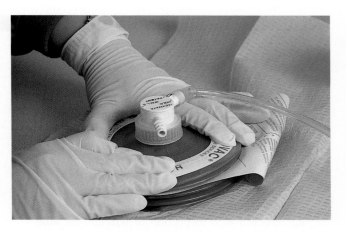

Step 2c Activating Hemovac suction.

Step 2b Emptying Hemovac contents into measuring container.

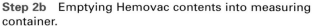

Steps	Rationale
b. Drain contents into measuring container (see illustration).	Contents counted as fluid output.
c. Place container on a flat surface, and press downward until bottom and top are in contact (see illustration).	Compression of surface of Hemovac creates vacuum.
d. Hold surfaces together with one hand, cleanse opening and plug with alcohol swab using other hand, immediately replace plug.	Cleansing of plug reduces transmission of microorganisms.
e. Check for patency of drainage tubing and absence of tension on tubing.	Facilitates wound drainage and prevents pressure and trauma to tissues.
f. Note characteristics of drainage; measure volume, discard by flushing in the commode.	

3.   **Empty Hemovac with wall suction.**
a. Turn suction off.
b. Disconnect suction tubing from Hemovac port.

COMMUNICATION TIP *Instruct client on anticipated postoperative drainage, expected progress of wound healing, drainage volume, and estimate of drainage removal. Remind client to keep drain lower than the wound level when ambulating, sitting, or lying down.*

---

c. Empty Hemovac as described in Step 2.	Re-establishes suction to wound bed.
d. Reconnect tubing with connection to open port of Hemovac. Tape securely, if needed.	
e. Set suction level as prescribed or on low if physician does not specify suction level.	

Steps	**Rationale**

4.   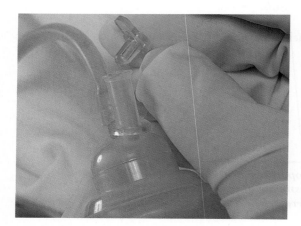 **Empty Jackson-Pratt drain.**

a. Open port on the end of bulb-shaped reservoir (see illustration).

b. Hold bulb over drainage container to empty drainage (see illustration). Cleanse end of emptying port with alcohol sponge.

c. Compress bulb to reestablish vacuum (see Figure 22-2, p. 542). Replace cap immediately.

d. Note characteristics of drainage; measure volume, and discard by flushing in the commode.

Contents counted as fluid output.

e. Proceed with inspection of skin and dressing change using drain sponges.

Drainage can be irritating to skin and may cause skin breakdown.

f. Instruct client in anticipated postoperative drainage, expected progress of wound healing and drainage volume, and estimated removal of drain as volume diminishes.

Unexplained bloody drainage is worrisome to any client. Knowing what to expect reduces anxiety.

g. Instruct client to keep drain lower than insertion site when ambulating, sitting, and lying.

Facilitates drainage.

h. Instruct client not to pull or tug on tubing; secure drain below incision to dressing with tape and safety pin.

NURSE ALERT   *Be sure there is slack in the tubing from the reservoir to the wound allowing client movement and no pulling at the insertion site.*

---

5.   **Remove drains (Penrose, Jackson-Pratt, Hemovac).**

a. Check physician's order for drain removal.

b. Remove dressings, discard in receptacle, and clean the area around the drain.

Step 4a   Opening port of Jackson-Pratt drain.

Step 4b   Emptying contents from Jackson-Pratt drainage device.

Steps	Rationale
c. If removing a Jackson-Pratt or Hemovac drain, release the suction on the drainage device by opening the drainage port.	Continued suction increases the tension required for drain removal and the risk of tissue damage and bleeding.
d. Inform client that there will be a pulling sensation as the drain is removed.	Gains cooperation and alleviates anxiety.
e. Place a disposable drape adjacent to the area to receive the drain after removal.	Allows immediate enclosure of drain and prevents spread of microorganisms.
f. Clip and remove the suture if present (see Skill 22-3, p. 546).	
g. Grasp the drain with sterile forceps or gloved fingers, and gently remove the drain. Inform client that momentary increased tension is felt just before completion of the removal.	Jackson-Pratt drains have a wide flat area that must be pulled through the stab wound with force.
h. Immediately cover the stab wound with a 4 × 4 dressing and tape in place.	Some drainage may continue for a few hours.
i. Instruct client to notify you if dressing becomes saturated with drainage.	Dressing may need to be changed.
6. See Completion Protocol (inside front cover).	

· · · · · · · · · ·

EVALUATION

1. Routinely empty container every 8 hours or sooner if half to two-thirds full. Compare amount and characteristics of drainage with what is expected to determine patency of tubing and functioning of drainage evacuator.
2. Inspect wound for drainage around the tubing, which may indicate obstruction of drainage system.
3. Ask client to describe level of comfort in relation to drainage tubing.

Unexpected Outcomes and Related Interventions

1. Drainage is not accumulating in drainage system.
   a. Position tubing to enhance gravity flow, and eliminate kinks or pressure on tubing.
   b. Gently "milk" tubing to release any clots that may block tubing.
2. Drainage containers expand rapidly:
   a. Check all connections for leakage.
   b. Tape or otherwise eliminate leaks in system.
3. Excessive amount of bright bloody drainage accumulates over a short time (e.g., 4 hours). Drainage that is bright red in large amounts may indicate hemorrhage.
   a. Report excessive bright red drainage to surgeon.

   b. Keep client on nothing-by-mouth (NPO) status, because it may be necessary to return to surgery for suturing of a bleeding vessel.
4. Wound infection develops as evidenced by unexpected purulence or foul odor.
   a. Collect diagnostic specimen for culture and sensitivity.
   b. Assess for additional indications of infection: fever, elevated white blood cell count, redness, swelling, and increasing pain.
   c. Report findings to physician.
5. Pain can result from manipulation of drainage device or accumulation of drainage within the wound. Infection accompanied by inflammation and edema may increase pain.
   a. Secure tubing to minimize irritation from moving or pulling at the insertion site.
   b. Report unrelieved increasing pain to the physician.

Recording and Reporting

Emptying Drain and Dressing Change

• Record results of emptying wound drainage system and dressing change in progress notes and I&O record. Note characteristics of insertion site and drainage; note volume.

- Record subjective data related to discomfort.
- Report presence of functioning drainage system and emptying frequency at end-of-shift report to nurse.

Drain Removal

- Record number and type of drain(s) removed from client in progress notes. Note characteristics of the insertion site and drainage. Note the type of dressing applied to the insertion site.
- Record subjective data related to discomfort.

Sample Documentation

Emptying Drain and Dressing Change

1300 Dark red drainage (700 ml) emptied from Hemovac. Dressing changed around insertion site. Site is pink. Quarter-size spot of serosanguineous drainage noted on dressing. Drain securely sutured with one suture. 4 × 4 drain dressings applied around drain site. Client reports no discomfort with dressing change.

Drain Removal

1020 Hemovac drain and 1 suture removed as ordered. Site pink (1 cm around perimeter), covered with 4 × 4. Client reports no discomfort. No drainage apparent on dressing.

SPECIAL CONSIDERATIONS

Pediatric Considerations

- Secure drain to prevent client from dislodging while active.
- Advise family members to keep drainage container less than one-third full to prevent tugging of drainage collector.

Geriatric Considerations

- Be aware that clients with large amounts of drainage will need additional fluid intake to prevent dehydration.
- Measures may need to be taken to prevent a confused client from pulling out drain.

Home Care Considerations

- Instruct primary caregiver and client in how to change dressings located over old drain site or stab wound. Have primary caregiver perform return demonstration of dressing change.
- Assess client's home environment to determine adequacy of facilities for performing wound care; check for adequate lighting, running water, and storage of supplies.
- Instruct caregiver to wear clean gloves and perform hand hygiene after procedure.

Skill 22.3

Removing Staples and Sutures (Including Applying Steri-Strips)

Sutures are used for closure of a surgical wound both within tissue layers in deep wounds and for the skin layer. The client's history of wound healing, site of wound, tissues involved, and the purpose of the sutures determines the closure material selected. Deep sutures may be a material that is absorbed or an inert wire that remains indefinitely. Sutures are available in silk, steel, cotton, linen, wire, nylon, and Dacron. Skin sutures that are removed may be interrupted or continuous. Interrupted sutures are separate stitches, each with its own knot (Figure 22-3, *A*). A continuous suture is one long "thread" that spirals along the entire suture line at evenly spaced intervals. The surface appearance is very similar to a line of interrupted sutures, except that each section crossing the incision line does not have a knot (Figure 22-3, *B*). Another type of continuous stitch is blanket continuous suture. This spirals along the incision with each turn pulled over to one side. The suture is looped around the thread of the previous stitch before making the next turn in spiral (Figure 22-3, *C*).

When appearance and minimal scarring are important, very fine Dacron or subcutaneous sutures beneath the skin are used. An obese client with abdominal surgery

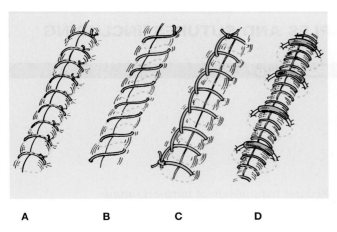

Figure 22-3   Sutures. **A,** Interrupted. **B,** Continuous. **C,** Blanket continuous. **D,** Retention.

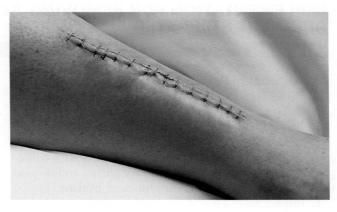

Figure 22-4   Suture line secured with staples.

may have retention sutures covered with rubber tubing to provide greater strength (Figure 22-3, *D*). Wire sutures are usually removed by the physician.

Staples are made of stainless steel wire, are quick to use, and provide ample strength. They are popular for skin closure of abdominal incisions and orthopedic surgery when appearance of the incision is not critical (Figure 22-4). The time of removal is based on the stage of incisional healing and extent of surgery. Sutures and staples are generally removed within 7 to 10 days after surgery if healing is adequate. Retention sutures are left in place longer (14 days or more). The physician determines the time for removal of sutures or staples.

Routinely, every other suture or staple is removed first, with the rest removed if the incision remains securely closed. If any sign of suture line separation is evident during the removal process, the remaining sutures are left in place and a description is documented and reported to the physician. In some cases, these sutures are removed several days to a week later.

ASSESSMENT

1. Review physician's orders for specific directions related to suture or staple removal, including which sutures to be removed. *Rationale: Indicates specifically which sutures are to be removed (e.g., every other suture).*
2. Check for allergies to antiseptic solution, tape, or latex.
3. Assess client's level of comfort on scale of 0 to 10. *Rationale: Provides baseline to determine tolerance of procedure.*
4. Inspect skin integrity of suture line for uniform closure of wound edges, normal color, and absence of drainage and inflammation. *Rationale: Adequate healing needs to take place before removal of sutures or staples.*

PLANNING

Expected outcomes focus on maintaining skin integrity, preventing infection, and promoting comfort.

Expected Outcomes

1. Client's incision is intact with edges well approximated after suture/staple removal.
2. Client describes pain as less than 2 (scale of 0 to 10) during suture removal.
3. Client demonstrates ability to perform self-care related to promoting wound healing by discharge.

Equipment

- Disposable waterproof bag
- Sterile suture removal set (forceps and scissors) or sterile staple remover
- Sterile applicators or antiseptic swabs
- Steri-Strips (optional)
- Clean gloves
- Sterile gloves (optional)
- Tincture of Benzoin

 Delegation Considerations

The skill of suture removal requires the critical thinking and knowledge application unique to an RN. For this skill, delegation is inappropriate.

IMPLEMENTATION FOR REMOVING STAPLES AND SUTURES (INCLUDING APPLYING STERI-STRIPS)

Steps	Rationale
1. See Standard Protocol (inside front cover).	
2. Check local Nurse Practice Act and agency policy to determine if RN may remove sutures.	
3. Prepare sterile field with supplies if required by agency.	
4. Remove dressing, and discard in disposable waterproof bag. Remove gloves, and dispose of in same receptacle. Perform hand hygiene.	Reduces transmission of microorganisms.
5. Inspect wound for approximation of wound edges and absence of drainage and inflammation (redness, warmth, and swelling).	Presence of these findings may indicate need for delay of suture/staple removal.
6. **Apply sterile gloves if required by policy.**	Reduces chance of contaminating wound during suture removal.
7. Cleanse sutures or staples and healed incision with antiseptic swabs.	Removes surface bacteria from incision and sutures or staples. Softens dry crusting and facilitates gentle removal.
8. **Remove staples.**	
a. Place lower tips of staple remover under first staple (see illustration).	
b. Squeeze handles together all the way (without lifting).	Releases the ends of staple from the skin with minimal suture line pressure and pain.

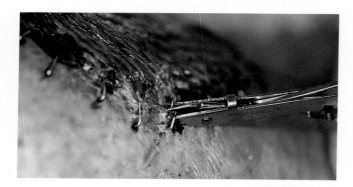

Step 8a Staple extractor placed under staple.

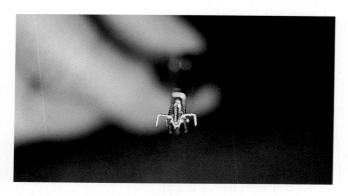

Step 8c Metal staple removed by extractor.

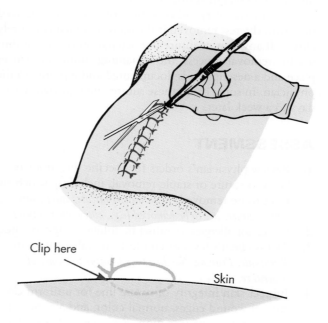

Clip here

Skin

Step 9b Removal of interrupted sutures. Cut suture away from knot as close to skin as possible.

Steps	Rationale

c. When both ends of staple are visible, gently lift from skin surface. If necessary, alter the angle and remove one end at a time (see illustration).

d. Release handles of staple remover over disposable waterproof bag.

Allows staple to drop into disposable waterproof bag.

e. Repeat steps for every other staple.

Minimizes risk of separation of wound edges.

f. Assess for healing ridge and secure approximation of incision edges before remaining staples are removed.

If edges separate, staple removal should be discontinued.

9. **Remove interrupted sutures.**

a. Hold scissors in dominant hand and forceps (clamp) in nondominant hand.

b. Grasp knot of suture with forceps, and gently pull while slipping tip of scissors under suture near skin (see illustrations).

c. Snip suture as close to skin as possible, and pull the suture through from the other side.

Portion of the suture on the skin's surface harbor microorganisms and debris, which could lead to infection if pulled through the underlying tissue.

d. Gently remove suture, and place on gauze.

e. Repeat steps until every other suture has been removed.

f. Assess for healing ridge and secure approximation of incision edges before remaining sutures are removed.

If edges separate, suture removal should be discontinued.

10. **Remove continuous sutures (see Figure 22-3, *B*, p. 547).**

a. Snip suture close to skin surface at end distal to knot.

b. Snip second "suture" on same side.

Avoids tension to suture line.
Technique prevents pulling contaminated portion of suture through skin.

c. Grasp knot, and gently pull with continuous smooth action, removing suture from beneath the skin. Place suture on gauze.

d. Grasp and lift next suture, and snip with tip of scissors close to skin.

e. Grasp suture, and gently remove loop of suture.

f. Repeat these steps until the end knot is reached. Cut the last one, and remove it by grasping and pulling the knot.

11. **Remove blanket continuous suture (see Figure 22-3, *C*, p. 547).**

a. Cut the suture opposite the looped blanket edge.

b. Remove each "suture" by grasping at the looped end.

12. **Apply Steri-Strips.**

a. Gently cleanse suture line with antiseptic swab.

b. Using a strong light, carefully inspect incision to be sure all sutures are removed.

c. Apply tincture of benzoin to the skin on each side of suture line. Allow to dry.

Assist Steri-Strips to adhere more securely.

d. Cut Steri-Strips to allow strips to extend 4 to 5 cm (1½ to 2 inches) on each side of the incision.

e. Remove backing, and apply across incision (see illustration).

f. Apply light dressing if drainage is apparent or if clothing may rub and irritate the suture line, or the incision may be left open to air.

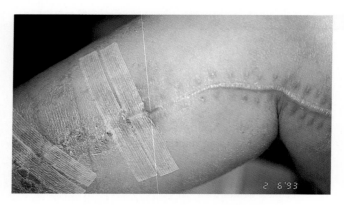

Step 12d Steri-Strips over incision.

Steps	Rationale
g. Inform client to take showers rather than soak in bathtub according to physician's preference.	Steri-Strips are not removed and are allowed to fall off gradually.

COMMUNICATION TIP

- *Teach client how to apply own dressing and inspect suture line for continued healing.*
- *Instruct client in adequate nutrition for wound healing (protein, vitamins).*

13. Review local and systemic indications of infection. Instruct client to notify physician if these occur after discharge.	Provides information to client for reporting wound infection to physician.
14. Inform client to minimize abdominal strain during defecation, and show how to support the incision with pillow or bath blanket.	Minimizes tension on incision and discomfort.
15. Encourage ambulation.	Promotes circulation and healing.
16. Follow physician's instructions for limiting activity.	Heavy lifting, driving, and stair climbing may need to be avoided for a time.
17. Provide written instructions, as well as verbal instructions, allowing opportunity to answer questions as they arise.	
18. See Completion Protocol (inside front cover).	

• • • • • • • • • •

EVALUATION

1. Inspect incision for approximation of wound edges.
2. Ask client to rate pain using a scale of 0 to 10.
3. Ask client to explain self-care guidelines before discharge.

Unexpected Outcomes and Related Interventions

Predisposition to delayed wound healing includes diabetes, immunosuppression, infection, inadequate nutrition and tissue oxygenation, obesity, and smoking.

1. Client exhibits wound dehiscence (separation of wound or incision edges).
   a. Client reports feeling something "gave way."
   b. Increased serosanguineous drainage is noted.
2. Evisceration is seen, involving protrusion of visceral organs through wound opening. This is a serious emergency because blood supply to tissues may be compromised when organs protrude.
   a. Organs must be kept moist by applying sterile towels that have been saturated in warm sterile saline solution.
   b. Immediately notify surgeon so that surgical intervention can be arranged.

Recording and Reporting

- Record number of sutures or staples removed in the client's progress note. Indicate that the entire suture was removed, if appropriate.
- Record time and client's response to suture removal.
- Notify physician immediately of any of the following findings: suture line separation, dehiscence, evisceration, bleeding, or purulent drainage.

Sample Documentation

1030 Wound edges well approximated. Healing ridge palpated. All sutures removed from abdominal incision, Steri-Strips applied and left open to air (OTA). No redness, swelling, or drainage. Client instructed to shower, avoid tension on incision, and avoid heavy lifting.

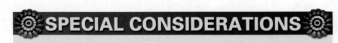

SPECIAL CONSIDERATIONS

Pediatric Considerations

- Young clients will need reassurance before suture removal. Involve parent; demonstrate removal technique before the actual removal.
- Talk to client as sutures are removed, reassuring client to remain inactive and calm.

Geriatric Considerations

- Older adults may need reassurance about the suture removal procedure. Assess mental status for comprehension of the procedure.
- Older skin may be at higher risk for dehiscence after sutures are removed.

Home Care Considerations

- Instruct primary caregiver and client in how to maintain clean technique when changing dressings.
- Wear clean gloves, and perform hand hygiene after procedure.

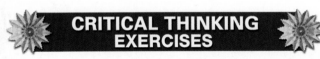

CRITICAL THINKING EXERCISES

1. Mr. Palmer is a 68-year-old retired banker who has just undergone a partial gastrectomy. On the third postoperative day the nurse notices the abdominal dressing saturated with beige foul-smelling drainage; the client has a Jackson-Pratt drain located next to the incision. Describe the actions the nurse should take, and include the rationalizations for those actions.
2. Mrs. Smith is a 64-year-old at 5 days after abdominal hysterectomy. She has abdominal staples that are ordered to be removed.
   a. What assessment should be made before removing the sutures and why?
   b. What supplies should the nurse prepare before starting the procedure?
3. Mr. Sellers is admitted to the general surgical unit after a right hemicolectomy. His Jackson-Pratt drain bulb collector is three-fourths full. The AP will be emptying the collector.
   a. What should the AP report to the nurse, and what charting on the emptying can the AP do?
   b. Mr. Sellers is now awake and preparing to ambulate. How should the Jackson-Pratt drain and bulb collector be secured?

REFERENCES

Lewis SM and others: *Medical-surgical nursing: assessment and management of clinical problems,* ed 5, St Louis, 2000, Mosby.

Stotts NA: Nutritional assessment and support. In Bryant RA, editor: *Acute and chronic wounds: nursing management,* St Louis, 2000, Mosby.

Sussman C: Wound healing biology and chronic wound healing. In Sussman C, Bates-Jensen BM: *Wound care,* Gaithersburg, Md, 1998, Aspen.

Waldrop J, Doughty D: Wound healing physiology. In Bryant RA, editor: *Acute and chronic wounds: nursing management,* St Louis, 2000, Mosby.

West J, Gimbel M: Acute surgical and traumatic wound healing. In Bryant RA, editor: *Acute and chronic wounds: nursing management,* St Louis, 2000, Mosby.

Pressure Ulcers

PRESSURE ULCERS

Pressure ulcers are defined as "localized areas of tissue necrosis that develop when soft tissue is compressed between a bony prominence and an external surface for a prolonged period of time" (National Pressure Ulcer Advisory Panel [NPUAP], 1992, 1998). The ulcers have also been called bedsores and decubitus ulcers; however, these terms are inaccurate because it is known that such ulcers result from positions other than the lying position. Pressure ulcers can occur when clients are in the sitting position and/or when an external source such as a cast edge applies unrelieved pressure to skin. Pressure points over bony prominences where pressure ulcers can develop in sitting and lying positions are shown in Figure 6-1, *A* and *B*, p. 113). Common sites for the development of pressure ulcers include the sacrum, heels, elbows, lateral malleoli, trochanters, and ischial tuberosities (Pieper, 2000). Three pressure-related forces contribute to the development of a pressure ulcer: (1) intensity of pressure (how much pressure is applied), (2) duration of pressure (how long the pressure is applied), and (3) tissue tolerance (the ability of the tissue to redistribute the weight). The intensity of the pressure must exceed capillary closure pressure, thus compressing the blood flow to the skin. Low pressure over a prolonged period of time, as well as high pressure over a short time period, can create a pressure ulcer. The third factor, tissue tolerance, refers to the ability of the tissue to react to the pressure; three extrinsic factors, shear, friction, and moisture, make the tissues less tolerant of pressure (Bates-Jensen, 1998).

Shear is a parallel force that acts to stretch tissue and blood vessels, such as when the client is in a semi-Fowler's position and begins to slide toward the foot of the bed. The skin over the sacrum sticks to the bed sheets, but the bony structure slides down, occluding the blood vessels, causing deep tissue destruction (see Figure 6-2, p. 113). Friction, the rubbing of the tissue against a surface, abrades the top layer of skin (epidermis), which can lead to tissue susceptibility to pressure injury. Skin moisture (most often from fecal and urinary incontinence) softens skin, making it vulnerable to skin breakdown. Other factors important in pressure ulcer development include poor nutrition, advanced age, medical conditions that support poor tissue perfusion (low blood pressure, smoking, elevated temperature, anemia), and psychosocial status, in particular stress-induced cortisol secretion (Pieper, 2000) (Table 23-1).

WOUND HEALING

Skin, the body's largest organ, protects the body from chemical and mechanical insults and bacterial and viral entry and regulates fluid loss and electrolytes. When wounded, the skin and tissue must go through a complex repair process. Nurses have an important role in wound healing, supporting the client by providing the appropriate wound-healing environment. The nurse makes a comprehensive wound assessment and using that information, plans wound care for the client. To provide appropriate wound care, the nurse must understand the process of wound healing. The physiology of wound healing occurs via two mechanisms: regeneration, replacement of damaged or lost tissue with more of the same, or connective tissue repair in wounds with tissue loss where scar formation replaces lost tissue (Waldrop and Doughty, 2000).

Types of healing include primary intention (partial-thickness wounds) and secondary intention (full-thickness wounds) (Figure 23-1). Healing by primary intention is expected when the edges of a clean surgical incision are sutured together, tissue loss is minimal or absent, and the wound is not contaminated with microorganisms. Epidermal cells regenerate, and there is reestablishment of the epidermal layers to restore the protective function of the skin. Examples of this type of wound include a partial-thickness wound such as an abrasion or skin tear (injury to the top layer on skin, the epidermis).

Table 23-1

Factor	Rationale
Factors That Delay Wound Healing	
Older adult	Physiological changes of aging alter the immune system, resulting in decreased resistance to pathogens and a slowed collagen deposition.
Obesity	Fatty subcutaneous tissue has diminished vascularity.
Diabetes	Associated vascular changes reduce blood flow to peripheral tissues; leukocyte malfunction results from hyperglycemia.
Compromised circulation	Vascular changes decrease the delivery of oxygen and nutrients.
Malnutrition	Inadequate nutrition slows healing because of the altered cellular metabolism.
Immunosuppressive therapy	Decreases inflammatory response and collagen synthesis.
Chemotherapy	Interferes with leukocyte (white blood cell) production and immune response.
High levels of stress	Increased cortisol levels reduce number of lymphocytes and decrease inflammatory response.

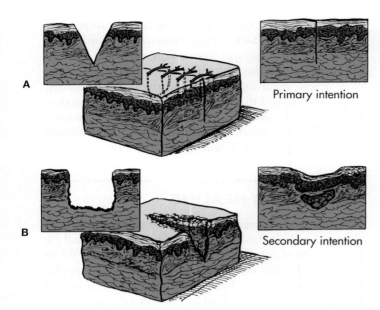

A

B

Primary intention

Secondary intention

Figure 23-1 **A,** Wound healing by primary intention, such as with a surgical incision *(left).* Wound edges are pulled together and approximated with sutures, staples, or adhesive tapes, and healing occurs mainly by connective tissue deposition. **B,** Wound healing by secondary intention. Wound edges are not approximated, and healing occurs by granulation tissue formation and contraction of the wound edges. (Redrawn from Trott AT: *Wounds and lacerations,* ed 2, 1997, Mosby.)

Box 23-1

Phases of Wound Healing

INFLAMMATORY PHASE
Starts when skin integrity is impaired and continues for 4 to 6 days (if healing is proceeding in a normal fashion).
- Hemostasis: Blood vessels constrict, platelets aggregate, and bleeding stops. Scab forms, preventing entry of infectious organisms.
- Inflammation: Increased blood flow to wound resulting in localized redness and edema, attracts white blood cells and wound growth factors.
- White blood cells arrive: Clean debris from wound.

PROLIFERATIVE PHASE
- Collagen synthesis: Base structural support to wound (provides wound strength).
- Establishment of new capillaries: To feed new tissue.
- Creation of granulation tissue: Provides surface for reepithelialization.
- Wound contraction: To decrease size of defect.
- Epithelialization: Resurfacing of wound, wound closure.

REMODELING PHASE
This final healing stage may continue for 1 year or more.
- Remodeling of the scar tissue to provide wound strength.

Partial-thickness wound repair regenerates the epidermis and dermis. The steps in partial-thickness wound healing include an initial inflammatory response, epithelial proliferation and migration, and the reestablishment of the epidermal layers. The new epidermal cells move from wound edges and from epidermal appendages. Epidermal cells only migrate across a moist surface; if the wound base is allowed to dry, the epidermal cells must tunnel down to a moist level to begin the migration process. Thus a moist wound environment supports rapid wound healing (Waldrop and Doughty, 2000).

Healing by secondary intention often accompanies traumatic open wounds with tissue loss or wounds with a high microorganism count (high risk of infection). Wounds that heal by secondary intention go through a process involving scar tissue formation and heal slowly because of the volume of tissue needed to fill the defect. Examples of this type of wound include a contaminated surgical wound or a full-thickness pressure ulcer.

Full-thickness repair is described as undergoing three phases: inflammatory, proliferative, and remodeling (Box 23-1). There is overlap between phases, and it is a complex process. In the inflammatory phase the key events are hemostasis (clotting off of the injured area to prevent excessive bleeding and to provide a barrier from bacteria) and inflammation (redness, edema, and warmth that bring white blood cells to the wound for clean up). In the proliferative phase the key events are the establishment of new capillaries, collagen synthesis (the wound's support matrix), the creation of granulation tissue, contraction, and epithelialization (new epidermis). In the remodeling phase the key events are wound matrix breakdown and the synthesis of new matrix, in which the scar tissue gains strength (Waldrop and Doughty, 2000). Full-thickness wounds, like partial-thickness wounds, heal more efficiently in a moist, protected environment.

Many factors influence wound healing. Some of these factors include nutritional status, infection, oxygenation, age, and medications. Nutrition is critical to healing because with injury more calories and substrates are needed for healing (Stotts, 2000). Malnutrition will delay wound healing. Infection prolongs the inflammatory phase, which prevents epithelialization. Oxygen fuels the cellular function essential to the repair process and is critical to wound healing (Waldrop and Doughty, 2000). Increased age slows the healing process, and older adults are plagued with chronic illness, which can slow healing. (Stotts and Wipke-

Tevis, 2001). Medications such as steroids slow the inflammatory process, making wounds more prone to infection and delayed healing (see Table 23-1).

NURSING DIAGNOSES

Nursing diagnoses that are associated with prevention of pressure ulcers might include **Risk for Impaired Skin Integrity** related to immobility, decreased sensation, inadequate nutrition, urinary or fecal incontinence, and/or altered perfusion. Related nursing diagnoses that contribute to the client's risk for pressure ulcers include **Bowel Incontinence** and/or **Functional Urinary Incontinence, Hyperthermia, Hypothermia, Impaired Physical Mobility, Imbalanced Nutrition: Less Than Body Requirements,** and **Disturbed Sensory Perception.**

Nursing diagnoses that are associated with treatment of pressure ulcer and wound management include **Impaired Skin Integrity** related to a partial-thickness ulcer or wound, **Impaired Tissue Integrity** related to a full-thickness ulcer or wound, and **Disturbed Body Image** related to the ulcer and the way that the client feels about the change in body image.

Skill 23.1

Pressure Ulcer Risk Assessment and Prevention Strategies

A comprehensive program to prevent pressure ulcers includes the use of a risk assessment tool to identify factors that may be present and allow the nurse to plan prevention interventions. In addition to the risk assessment tool, a daily skin inspection, including an examination of pressure points, is essential.

There are several risk assessment tools used to predict pressure ulcer formation. The tool utilized should be reliable, valid, and used by the registered nurse. There are several published pressure ulcer risk assessment tools, including the Braden scale. The Braden scale (Table 23-2) has six subscales that measure degrees of sensory perception, moisture, activity, mobility, nutrition, and friction and shear (Braden and Bergstrom, 1989). Each subscale is given a score, resulting in a total score indicative of the client's risk for pressure ulcer development. The scale is used upon admission to a health care facility and at periodic intervals.

All individuals at risk should have a systematic skin inspection at least once a day, paying particular attention to the bony prominences (Bergstrom and others, 1992). The skin can be inspected during routine care and the results documented.

ASSESSMENT

1. Select the pressure ulcer risk assessment tool used in your client's setting. *Rationale: A validated risk assessment tool is recommended by the Agency for Health Care Policy and Research (AHCPR) (Bergstrom and others, 1992) and the National Pressure Ulcer Advisory Panel (NPUAP) (1992).*

2. Identify client's risk for pressure ulcer formation by assessing each factor according to the selected tool. Determine the risk assessment score (e.g., Braden score: 10-12, high-risk; 13-14, moderate risk; 15-18, at risk), and compare the client's score with established scores that indicate high risk for skin breakdown. *Rationale: To prevent pressure ulcers, individuals at risk must be identified so that risk factors can be reduced through intervention (Bergstrom and others, 1992).*

3. Inspect the condition of the client's skin; pay particular attention to the bony prominences. If redness or discoloration is noted, this could be the first stage of skin breakdown. The discoloration may vary from pink to a deep red. In dark-skinned clients the discoloration appears as a deepening of normal ethnic color (Bennett, 1995; Bates-Jensen, 1998) or a persistent red, blue, or purple hue (NPUAP, 1998) (Box 23-2). *Rationale: Skin inspection is fundamental to risk assessment and developing a plan for preventing pressure ulcers (Bergstrom and others, 1992).*

4. Assess client for areas of potential pressure, other than bony prominences: nares (nasogastric [NG] tubes, oxygen cannula), tongue and lips (oral airway, endotracheal tube), skin next to drainage tubes or beneath orthopedic devices (braces, casts). *Rationale: Clients may have sites other than bony prominences related to pressure necrosis.*

5. Observe client for preferred positions when in bed or chair. *Rationale: Weight of body will be placed on certain bony prominences, and the client may resist repositioning off these areas.*

6. Observe ability of client to initiate and assist with position changes. *Rationale: Potential for friction and shear increases when client is completely dependent on others for position changes.*

7. Assess client and support person's understanding of risks for pressure ulcers and knowledge of preventative measures. *Rationale: Client and family are integral to prevention and management of pressure ulcers (Bergstrom and others, 1992).*

PLANNING

Expected outcomes focus on identifying clients at risk for skin breakdown and prevention of skin breakdown.

Table 23-2

Braden Scale for Predicting Pressure Sore Risk

Sensory Perception Ability to respond meaningfully to pressure-related discomfort	**1. Completely Limited** Unresponsive (does not moan, flinch, or grasp) to painful stimuli because of diminished level of consciousness or sedation. OR Limited ability to feel pain over most of body surface.	**2. Very Limited** Responds only to painful stimuli. Cannot communicate discomfort except by moaning or restlessness. OR Has a sensory impairment that limits the ability to feel pain or discomfort over ½ of body.	**3. Slightly Limited** Responds to verbal commands, but cannot always communicate discomfort or need to be turned. OR Has some sensory impairment that limits ability to feel pain or discomfort in one or two extremities.	**4. No Impairment** Responds to verbal commands. Has no sensory deficit that would limit ability to feel or voice pain or discomfort.
Moisture Degree to which skin is exposed to moisture	**1. Constantly Moist** Skin is kept moist almost constantly by perspiration, urine, etc. Dampness is detected every time client is moved or turned.	**2. Moist** Skin is often, but not always, moist. Linen must be changed at least once a shift.	**3. Occasionally Moist** Skin is occasionally moist, requiring an extra linen change approximately once a day.	**4. Rarely Moist** Skin is usually dry. Linen only requires changing at routine intervals.
Activity Degree of physical activity	**1. Bedfast** Confined to bed.	**2. Chairfast** Ability to walk severely limited or nonexistent. Cannot bear own weight and/or must be assisted into chair or wheelchair.	**3. Walks Occasionally** Walks occasionally during day, but for very short distances, with or without assistance. Spends majority of each shift in bed or chair.	**4. Walks Frequently** Walks outside the room at least twice a day and inside room at least once every 2 hours during waking hours.
Mobility Ability to change and control body position	**1. Completely Immobile** Does not make even slight changes in body or extremity position without assistance.	**2. Very Limited** Makes occasional slight changes in body or extremity position but unable to make frequent or significant changes independently.	**3. Slightly Limited** Makes frequent though slight changes in body or extremity position independently.	**4. No Limitations** Makes major and frequent changes in position without assistance.

Continued

Table 23-2

Braden Scale for Predicting Pressure Sore Risk—cont'd

Nutrition Usual food intake pattern	1. Very Poor	2. Probably Inadequate	3. Adequate	4. Excellent
	Never eats a complete meal. Rarely eats more than $\frac{1}{3}$ of any food offered. Eats 2 servings or less of protein (meat or dairy products) per day. Takes fluids poorly. Does not take a liquid dietary supplement. OR Is NPO and/or maintained on clear liquids or IVs for more than 5 days.	Rarely eats a complete meal and generally eats only about $\frac{1}{2}$ of any food offered. Protein intake includes only 3 servings of meat or dairy products per day. Occasionally will take a dietary supplement. OR Receives less than optimum amount of liquid diet or tube feeding.	Eats over half of most meals. Eats a total of 4 servings of protein (meat, dairy products) each day. Occasionally will refuse a meal, but will usually take a supplement if offered. OR Is on a tube feeding or TPN regimen that probably meets most of nutritional needs.	Eats most of every meal. Never refuses a meal. Usually eats a total of 4 or more servings of meat and dairy products. Occasionally eats between meals. Does not require supplementation.
Friction and Shear	1. Problem	2. Potential Problem	3. No Apparent Problem	
	Requires moderate to maximum assistance in moving. Complete lifting without sliding against sheets is impossible. Frequently slides down in bed or chair, requiring frequent repositioning with maximum assistance. Spasticity, contractures, or agitation leads to almost constant friction.	Moves feebly or requires minimum assistance. During a move skin probably slides to some extent against sheets, chair, restraints, or other devices. Maintains relatively good position in chair or bed most of the time but occasionally slides down.	Moves in bed and in chair independently and has sufficient muscle strength to lift up completely during move. Maintains good position in bed or chair at all times.	
TOTAL SCORE				

Instructions: Score client in each of the six subscales. Maximum score is 23, indicating little or no risk. A score of 18 indicates "at risk"; 9 indicates very high risk.

- 15-18 = at risk
- 13-14 = moderate risk
- 10-12 = high risk
- 9 or below = very high risk

Box 23-2

Cultural Considerations for Skin Assessment for Pressure Ulcers: The Client With Intact, Darkly Pigmented Skin

1. Assess localized skin color changes
   Any of the following may appear:
   - Skin color changes, different from usual skin tone
   - Color darker than surrounding skin, purplish, bluish, eggplant
   - Taut
   - Shiny
   - Indurated
2. Assess for edema
3. Obtain adequate lighting for skin assessment
   - Use natural or halogen light
   - Avoid fluorescent lamps, which can give the skin a bluish tone
4. Assess skin temperature
   - Initially may feel warmer than surrounding skin
   - Subsequently may feel cooler than surrounding skin
   - Use the back of your hand and fingers and, if client condition permits, no gloves when doing this assessment

Modified from Bennett MA: Report of the Task Force on the Implications for Darkly Pigmented Intact Skin in the Prediction and Prevention of Pressure Ulcers, *Adv Wound Care* 8(6):34, 1995.

Expected Outcomes

1. Client's skin remains intact and without discoloration.
2. Client has an acceptable level of comfort (4 on a scale of 0 to 10) in pressure reduction positions.
3. Client's risk assessment score on Braden scale remains above 17.

Equipment

- Risk assessment tool
- Client's documentation record

Delegation Considerations

This skill requires the critical thinking and knowledge application unique to a nurse. For this skill, delegation is inappropriate.

IMPLEMENTATION FOR PRESSURE ULCER RISK ASSESSMENT AND PREVENTION STRATEGIES

Steps	Rationale
1. See Standard Protocol (inside front cover).	
2. Inspect skin at least once a day.	Skin inspection provides the information essential for designing interventions to reduce risk and for evaluating the outcomes of those interventions (Bergstrom and others, 1992).
a. Examine all bony prominences, noting skin integrity. If redness is noted, use thumb to gently press on area of redness.	Nonblanchable erythema is the first indicator of skin injury (Pieper, 2000).
b. If client has darkly pigmented skin, look for color changes that differ from the client's normal skin color.	Darkly pigmented skin does not always show direct changes in color (Bennett, 1995; NPUAP, 1998).
3. Check all assistive devices (catheters, casts, braces) for potential pressure points.	
4. Review client's actual risk score for pressure ulcer.	By evaluating each risk factor and assigning a score, the interventions to lessen or eliminate the present risk factors will be identified (Pieper, 2000).

Steps	Rationale

COMMUNICATION TIP   *Assessment for pressure ulcer risk is a good time to discuss skin care with client and family.*
- *Inform client and family about risks for pressure ulcer development and alert family to manifestations of impaired skin integrity.*
- *Demonstrate to client and family how to correctly position client off pressure points.*
- *Discuss the impact of prolonged moisture exposure on the client's skin.*

5. If immobility, inactivity, or poor sensory perception are noted to be risk factor(s) for the client, consider one of the following interventions:
   a. Reposition client at least every 2 hours; use a written schedule (Bergstrom and others, 1992).
   b. When the client is in the side-lying position in bed, use the 30-degree lateral position (see Skill 6-1, Step 5d, p. 117).
   c. When needed, use pillow bridging (see illustration).

   d. Place client (when lying in bed) on a pressure-reducing support surface.
   e. Place client (when in a chair) on a pressure-reducing device, and shift the points under pressure at least every hour.
6. If friction and shear are identified as risk factors, consider the following interventions:
   a. Use a turning sheet to reposition the client.

   b. Moisturize areas that are prone to friction injuries (heels, elbows).

Reduces the duration and intensity of pressure.

Avoids direct contact of the trochanter with the support surface.

Use of pillows will prevent direct contact between bony prominences.
Reduces the amount of pressure exerted against the tissues.

Reduces the amount of pressure on the sacral tissues.

Proper repositioning of the client prevents dragging along the sheets.
Lubrication decreases friction between skin and bed linens (Colburn, 2001).

NURSE ALERT   *Do not massage reddened areas, because this may cause breakdown.*

   c. Maintain the head of the bed at 30 degrees.
7. If the client receives a low score on the moisture subscale, consider one or more of the following interventions:

Decreases potential for client to slide toward foot of bed and incur a shear injury.

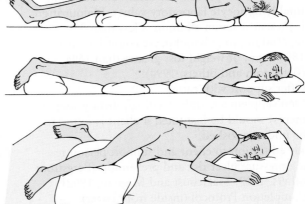
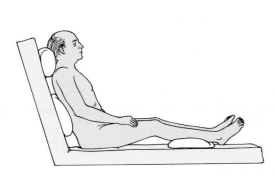

Step 5c   Pillow bridging.

Table 23-3

Measures to Reduce Risk of Pressure Ulcers: Practical Management of Loose Bowel Movements Related to Tube Feeding*

Possible Cause(s)	Treatment
Antibiotic use	Lactobacilli per feeding tube (2 packets tid × 3 doses)
Lactose intolerance	Use lactose-free liquid diet
Choleretic diarrhea	Questran, 1 g q6-8h and/or Titralac tabs, 2 q6-8h
Mild enterotoxigenic pathogens	Pepto-Bismol, 30 ml q6-8h
Severe enterotoxigenic pathogens with WBCs in stool on Gram stain	Selected antibiotic per stool culture and sensitivity testing
Insufficient fiber	Fiber supplement, 3 g q6-8h
Idiopathic	Lomotil, Imodium, paregoric (Warning: This may cause reactive constipation.)

From Bergstrom N and others: *Treatment of pressure ulcers,* Clinical practice guideline No.15, AHCPR Pub No. 95-0652, Rockville, Md, Dec 1994, Agency for Health Care Policy and Research, Public Health Service, U.S. Department of Health and Human Services.
*Any or all treatments may be indicated. *tid,* Three times daily; *q,* every; *h,* hours; *WBCs,* white blood cells.

Steps	Rationale
a. Use a moisture barrier ointment, applied after each incontinent episode.	Protects reddened intact skin from fecal or urinary incontinence.
b. If skin is denuded, use a protective barrier paste after each incontinent episode.	Provides a barrier between the skin and the stool/urine, allowing for healing.
c. If incontinence is ongoing, consider a collection device: fecal incontinence collector or in-dwelling urinary catheter. (Table 23-3 lists interventions designed to reduce the risk of pressure ulcer development resulting from tube-feeding–related diarrhea.)	Collection of the irritating substance may be appropriate if the cause of the incontinence cannot be controlled.
d. If source of moisture is from wound drainage, consider frequent dressing changes, skin protection with protective barriers, or collection devices.	
8. If the client scores low on the nutrition subscale of the risk assessment, consider the following interventions:	There is a strong relationship between nutrition and pressure ulcer development.
a. Assess client's nutritional status including fluid intake (see Chapter 8).	Dehydration can affect albumin levels and tissue integrity.
b. Review weight pattern and serum albumin and total lymphocyte laboratory values. Malnutrition is present if serum albumin is less than 3.5 mg/100 ml, total lymphocyte count less than 1800/mm³, or weight loss greater than 15% (Bergstrom and others, 1994).	Hypoalbuminemia may be associated with pressure ulceration (Bates-Jensen, 1998). Malnutrition inhibits cell regeneration.
c. Offer support with eating.	
d. Oral supplements (tube feedings, dietary supplements) should be instituted if client is found to be undernourished.	
9. Provide education to client and support person regarding pressure ulcer risk and prevention (Bergstrom and others, 1992; Maklebust and Magnan, 1992).	Assists in adhering to interventions to reduce pressure ulcer risk.
10. See Completion Protocol (inside front cover).	

• • • • • • • • • •

EVALUATION

1. Observe client's skin for areas at risk, noting change in color, appearance, or texture.
2. Observe tolerance of client for position change.
3. Compare subsequent risk assessment scores and skin assessments.

Unexpected Outcomes and Related Interventions

1. Skin does not blanch when firmly pressed, has a purple discoloration, or has significant color changes.
   a. These are early signs of pressure-related injury.
   b. Reassess frequency of turning schedule.
   c. Per agency's protocol, obtain order for a pressure reduction support surface.

Recording and Reporting

- Record client's risk score and skin assessment.
- Record turning intervals, pressure reduction support surface, and moisture protection interventions.
- Report need for additional consultations for the high-risk client.

Sample Documentation

1500 Braden scale assessment completed on admission. Client risk assessment score is 12; client determined to be at high risk for skin breakdown. Inspection of client's skin reveals intact skin, pressure ulcer prevention protocol implemented.

SPECIAL CONSIDERATIONS

Pediatric Considerations

- Immature skin in the young client is susceptible to skin tears.
- Moist skin covered with a diaper may soften skin, causing skin breakdown.

Geriatric Considerations

- A score of 17 or 18 (rather than the usual 16) on the Braden scale may be a more accurate predictor of pressure ulcer risk in older adults (Bergstrom and others, 1998).
- In the older adult the epidermal-dermal junction becomes flatter, putting the client at increased risk for epidermal damage.

Home Care Considerations

- The home environment should be evaluated for the use of a pressure reduction support surface.
- If the client shares a bed with a family member, consider obtaining a bed frame with the appropriate support surface.
- Evaluate the seating surface for an appropriate pressure reduction support surface.

Skill 23.2

Treatment of Pressure Ulcers and Wound Management

Treatment of the client with a pressure ulcer necessitates a holistic approach, supporting the client in a healing environment. The healing environment for a client with a pressure ulcer includes systematic support of the client, reduction or elimination of the cause of the skin breakdown, and wound management that provides an environment conducive to healing. Wound healing will not occur, or will occur slowly, in the malnourished client or the client with a poor cardiovascular status; thus measures must be instituted to systemically support the client. Other factors that impede wound healing include immunosuppressive therapy and uncontrolled diabetes mellitus.

The cause(s) of the wound must be addressed before wound therapy can be instituted. If the contributing cause(s) of the pressure ulcer (pressure, shear, friction, and/or moisture) are not addressed, the tissue damage continues; healing does not take place. A wound environment conducive to healing can be achieved by using topical therapy while employing the following principles: prevent and manage infection, cleanse the wound, remove nonviable tissue, manage exudate, eliminate dead space, control odor, and protect the wound (Rolstad, Ovington, and Harris, 2000). The choice of topical wound management (dressings and solutions) will be dictated by these principles.

The type of dressing that will support healing will be chosen after an assessment of the wound. Ongoing assessment will assist the nurse in evaluating the effectiveness of the wound care. Parameters to include in the wound assessment are summarized in Box 23-3.

ASSESSMENT

1. Assess client's level of comfort and need for pain management. *Rationale: Client should be as comfortable as possible during the dressing change.*
2. Determine if client is allergic to topical agents. *Rationale: Topical agents contain elements that may cause localized skin reactions.*
3. Determine reason that client has pressure ulcer, and control or eliminate the cause. *Rationale: Failure to address causative factors will result in a nonhealing wound (Rolstad, Ovington, and Harris, 2000).*
4. Review order for topical agent and/or dressings. *Rationale: Ensures that proper medication and treatment are administered.*
5. Assess the client's wounds using the following wound parameters, and continue ongoing wound assessment per agency's protocol. *Rationale: Ongoing assessment will assist the nurse in evaluating the effectiveness of the wound care and will drive the treatment plan of care.*
   a. *Wound location:* Describe the body site where the wound is located.
   b. *Stage of wound:* Describe the extent of tissue destruction (Table 23-4).
   c. *Phase of wound healing:* Describe the stage of healing.
   d. *Wound size:* Length, width, and depth of the wound is measured per the facility's protocol. A disposable measuring guide is used for length and width, and a cotton-tipped applicator is used for depth. Some facilities trace the wound

shape on an acetate sheet that is kept for comparison (Figure 23-2).
   e. *Presence of undermining, sinus tracts, or tunnels:* Use a clean cotton-tipped applicator to measure depth and if needed a gloved finger to examine the wound edges.
   f. *Condition of the wound bed:* Describe the type and percentage of tissue in the wound bed.
   g. *Volume of exudate:* Describe the amount and characteristics.
   h. *Condition of periwound skin:* Examine the skin for breaks, dryness, or the presence of a rash.
   i. *Presence of pain:* Note pain at or around the wounded area; have client rate pain on scale.
6. Assess factors that affect wound healing: poor perfusion, immunosuppression, or preexisting infection.
7. Assess the client's nutritional status. Clinically significant malnutrition is present if (a) serum albumin level is less than 3.5 g/dl, (b) lymphocyte count is less than 1800/mm³, or (c) body weight decreases more than 15% (Bergstrom and others, 1994). *Rationale: Delayed wound healing will occur in the poorly nourished client.*
8. Assess client's and support persons' understanding of pressure ulcer characteristics and purpose of treatment (Bergstrom and others, 1994). *Rationale: Explanations relieve anxiety and promote cooperation during procedure.*

PLANNING

Expected outcomes focus on healing of the ulcer and prevention of further skin breakdown.

Expected Outcomes

1. Reduction in wound dimensions in 2 weeks.
2. Reduction in the amount of wound drainage.
3. Skin surrounding ulcer remains intact.
4. The amount of red granular tissue in the wound base will increase by 20% in 2 weeks.
5. Client remains afebrile.
6. Pain level is at or below client's previously assessed level.

Equipment

- Clean gloves
- Plastic bag for dressing disposal
- Tracing film, wound measuring device, cotton-tipped applicators
- Normal saline or cleansing agent
- Gauze pads
- Dressings and topical agent as ordered
- Tape, if needed

Table 23-4

Staging of Pressure Ulcers

Definition

Stage I

An observable pressure-related alteration of intact skin whose indicators compared with the adjacent or opposite area on the body may include changes in one or more of the following: skin temperature (warmth or coolness), tissue consistency (firm or boggy feel), and/or sensation (pain/itching). The ulcer appears as a defined area of persistent redness in lightly pigmented skin, whereas in darker skin tones the ulcer may appear with persistent red, blue, or purple hues.

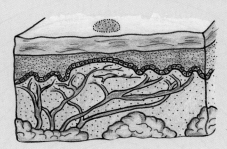 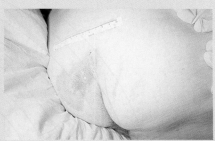

Stage II

Partial-thickness skin loss involving epidermis and/or dermis. The ulcer is superficial and presents clinically as an abrasion, blister, or shallow crater.

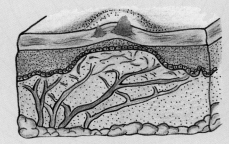 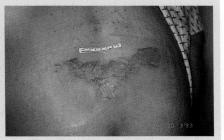

Stage III

Full-thickness skin loss involving damage or necrosis of subcutaneous tissue that may extend down to, but not through, underlying fascia. The ulcer presents clinically as a deep crater with or without undermining of adjacent tissue.

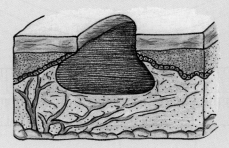 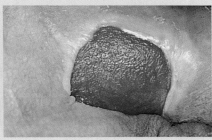

Stage IV

Full-thickness skin loss with extensive destruction, tissue necrosis, or damage to muscle, bone, or supporting structures, for example, tendon or joint capsule. (NOTE: Undermining and sinus tracts may also be associated with stage IV pressure ulcers.)

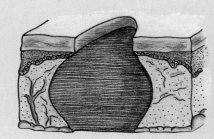 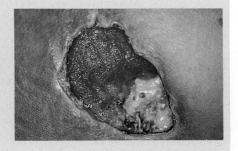

Staging definitions recognize these assessment limitations:
1. Identification of stage I pressure ulcers may be difficult in patients with darkly pigmented skin.
2. When eschar is present, accurate staging of the pressure ulcer is not possible until the eschar has sloughed or the wound has been debrided.

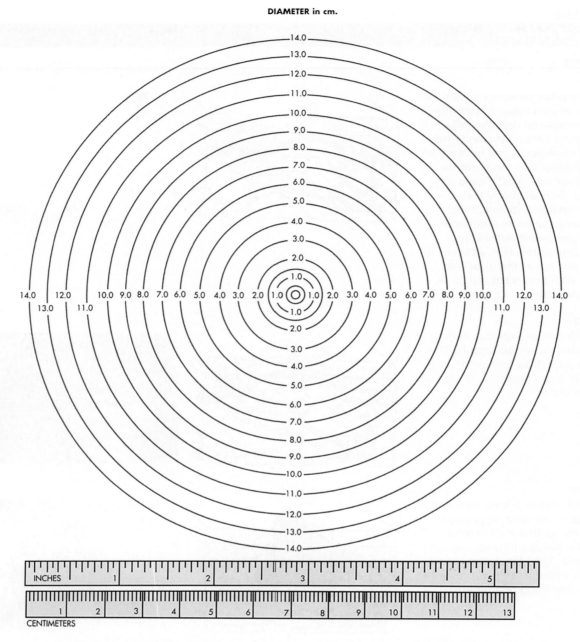

DIAMETER in cm.

Figure 23-2 Measuring guide. Center over wound to be measured. (Modified from Maklebust J, Sieggreen M: *Pressure ulcers: guidelines for prevention and nursing management,* ed 2, Springhouse, Pa, 1996, Springhouse Corp.)

Delegation Considerations

This skill requires the critical thinking and knowledge application unique to a nurse. For this skill, delegation is inappropriate. However, it is important to instruct assistive personnel (AP) to notify the nurse if wound drainage changes, when a wound odor is present, or if the client complains of increased wound discomfort.

IMPLEMENTATION FOR TREATMENT OF PRESSURE ULCERS AND WOUND MANAGEMENT

Steps	Rationale
1. See Standard Protocol (inside front cover).	
2. Select pressure ulcer management based on principles of local wound care:	
a. Prevent and manage infection.	Infected wounds do not heal.
b. Cleanse the wound.	Removes surface bacteria.
c. Remove nonviable tissue.	Nonviable tissue supports infection (Polynchuk, 2001).
d. Manage exudates.	Excessive wound exudate will macerate tissues.
e. Eliminate dead space.	Prevents exudate buildup.
f. Control odor.	Odor may indicate infection.
g. Provide a moist environment.	A moist environment supports wound healing.
3. Select an appropriate dressing (Table 23-5) based on the pressure ulcer assessment, principles of wound management, and client care setting. Dressing options include:	The dressing maintains an appropriate wound healing environment while keeping surrounding skin dry (AHCPR, 1994).
a. Gauze pads	Used for wicking, maintaining a moist environment, packing, and delivery of solutions to the wound.
b. Transparent film dressings	Used on partial-thickness wounds with minimal wound exudate.
c. Hydrogel	Used to provide moisture to the wound.
d. Hydrocolloid	Indicated on wounds with minimal to moderate exudate, maintains a moist environment, and can promote autolysis (Rolstad, Ovington, and Harris, 2000).
e. Alginate dressings	Absorbs moderate to heavy wound exudate and maintains a moist environment.
f. Foam dressings	Absorbent dressing used for wounds with moderate to heavy drainage, maintains a moist environment.

COMMUNICATION TIP *When caring for a wound or applying dressings, use the time to communicate to client:*

- *Progress of wound healing*
- *Changes in treatment regimen*
- *Role of nutrition in promoting wound healing*
- *How the client may independently manage the wound*
- *If possible, show client the wound*

Steps	Rationale
4. Open sterile packages and topical solution containers. (Goggles and moisture-proof cover gown should be worn if potential for contamination from spray exists when cleansing the wound.)	Supplies should be ready for easy application so that nurse can use supplies without contaminating them; reduces transmission of microorganisms.
5. Remove bed linen and client's gown to expose ulcer and surrounding skin. Keep remaining body parts draped.	Prevents unnecessary exposure of body parts.
6. Remove old dressings, and discard in plastic bag. Discard gloves, perform hand hygiene as per agency protocol, and put on fresh pair of gloves.	
7. Cleanse wound with prescribed solution.	Reduces surface bacteria, removes wound exudate and/or dressing residue.
a. Rinse with solution, gently wipe wound base and surrounding skin with moistened gauze.	
b. Pulsed lavage (delivery of solution under pressure) may be used to loosen necrotic tissue.	

Table 23-5

Dressing Selection Based on Phase of Wound Healing

Phase and Wound Description	Clinical Wound Needs	Approach and Dressings
Inflammatory Phase		
Necrotic tissue	Debridement	Autolysis alone or in combination with other methods of debridement
		Moisture-retentive dressings such as alginates, hydrogels, impregnated gauzes, hydrocolloids
		Enzyme debridement with gauze
Dry wound	Hydrate	Film, hydrogels
Moderate to heavy exudate	Absorption	Hydrocolloid, foam, absorbent impregnated gauze, alginate, hydrofiber, superabsorbent
May exhibit depth	Packing	*Shallow:* powder, paste, alginate
		Deep: impregnated gauze, alginate, cavity foam or sheet foam, strip packing
Erythema, warmth, edema, tenderness, pain	Managing infection	*Local:* antimicrobial dressings
		Systemic: systemic antibiotics/antimicrobial dressings or moisture-retentive dressings
Open wound	Protection	Film, hydrocolloid, foam, composite
Periwound skin	Protection	Skin sealant, barrier ointment
Granulation Phase (Proliferative)		
Red, granulating wound	Protection	Film, hydrocolloid, foam, composite
Minimal to moderate exudate	Absorption	*Minimal:* thin hydrocolloid, thin foam, absorbent powder/film, absorbent paste/composite
		Moderate: hydroclloid, foam, alginate/film
May exhibit depth	Packing	*Shallow:* powder, paste, alginate
		Deep: impregnated gauze, alginate, cavity foam or sheet foam, strip packing
Periwound skin	Protection	Skin sealant, barrier ointment
Remodeling/Maturation Phase		
Pink, resurfacing wound	Protection	Film, thin or traditional hydrocolloid, thin or traditional foam, composite

From Rolstad BS, Ovington LG, Harris A: Principles of wound management. In Bryant RA, editor: *Acute and chronic wounds: nursing management,* ed 2, St Louis, 2000, Mosby.

Steps	Rationale

   c. Whirlpool treatments can be used to loosen necrotic tissue on large wounds.

8. Apply prescribed wound dressing:

   a. Gauze

      (1) Apply solution to gauze, wring out excess. — Gauze should be damp, allowing the gauze to "wick" drainage.

      (2) Unfold gauze, and if wound has depth, pack the wound with the dressing; if shallow, lay gauze over wound. — Unfolded gauze allows for wicking of the drainage.

      (3) Cover with secondary dry dressing, tape.

   b. Transparent film dressings (see Chapter 24) — Applied over superficial ulcers and skin subjected to shear.

   c. Hydrogel (available as amorphous [in a tube], in sheets, or impregnated in gauze) — Hydrogel will maintain a moist environment to facilitate wound healing.

      (1) Cover wound base with a thick layer of the amorphous hydrogel, or cut a sheet to fit wound base.

Steps	Rationale
(2) Cover with secondary dressing, tape.	
(3) If using impregnated gauze, pack loosely into wound, cover with secondary dressing, tape.	
d. Hydrocolloid	
(1) Select proper size, allowing at least 1 inch to extend beyond the wound edges.	The hydrocolloid will form a gel over the wounded area; the outer edge will create the seal.
(2) Remove paper backing from adhesive side, and place over wound.	Hydrocolloids are most effective when at body temperature (Rolstad, Ovington, and Harris, 2000).
(3) Hold in place for 30 to 60 seconds.	
e. Alginate	
(1) Cut to the size of the wound, and loosely pack into wound.	The dressing will swell and increase in size; tightly packing the wound is not advised.
(2) Cover with a secondary dressing, tape.	
f. Foam dressings	
(1) Select a dressing that extends 1 inch onto intact surrounding skin.	Protective; will prevent wound dehydration; absorbs small to moderate amount of drainage.
(2) Apply over wound, and tape.	
9. If prescribed, apply topical agents as ordered.	
a. *Antibacterials:* Options include bacitracin, metronidazole, and silver sulfadiazine. Requires a physician's order.	Destroy or stop bacterial growth.
b. *Antiseptics:* Options include acetic acid, hypochlorite (Dakin's solution), hydrogen peroxide, and povidone-iodine (Betadine).	Used to reduce bacteria on the wound surface. Use is limited because of cell toxicity (Stotts, 2000).
c. *Enzyme debriding agents:* Cover wound with debriding agent, and use a moist dressing over wound. Options include Accuzyme, Elase, and Santyl.	Solutions remove dead tissue. The wound must be moist for the enzyme preparation to work.
10. Reposition client comfortably off wound.	
11. See Completion Protocol (inside front cover).	

• • • • • • • • • •

EVALUATION

1. Observe skin surrounding wound or ulcer for inflammation, edema, and tenderness.
2. Inspect dressings and exposed wounds, observing for drainage, foul odor, and tissue necrosis. Monitor client for signs and symptoms of infection, including fever and elevated white blood cell count.
3. Compare subsequent wound or ulcer measurements.
4. Ask client to rate pain on a 0 to 10 scale during and following pressure ulcer care.

Unexpected Outcomes and Related Interventions

1. Skin surrounding ulcer becomes macerated.
   a. Reduce exposure of surrounding skin to topical agents and moisture.
   b. Consider the use of a liquid skin barrier on peri-wound skin.
2. Ulcer becomes deeper with increased drainage and/or development of necrotic tissue.
   a. Notify physician for possible change in pressure ulcer status.

   b. Additional consults, for example, a wound care nurse specialist, may be indicated.
   c. Obtain necessary wound cultures.

Recording and Reporting

- Record assessment of ulcer in client's record.
- Describe type of topical agent and/or dressing used and client's response.
- Report any deterioration in ulcer appearance.

Sample Documentation

0900 Sacral pressure ulcer, stage II, 2 × 3 cm irregular shape. Base of wound is covered 100% by granulation tissue, no drainage present. Surrounding skin intact. Wound cleansed with normal saline and hydrocolloid dressing applied. On a low-air-loss overlay, repositioned every 2 hours. Nutritional supplements taken as offered. Client and family have read AHCPR booklets *Preventing Pressure Ulcers: A Patient's Guide* and *Pressure Sore Treatment* and are practicing positioning techniques.

SPECIAL CONSIDERATIONS

Pediatric Considerations
Wound dressings in the diaper zone should be reinforced with a water-resistant tape. This tape should be carefully removed to avoid skin stripping.

Geriatric Considerations
- Wound healing may be slower in the older adult.
- Skin in older adults has a slower and less intense inflammatory reaction; therefore older clients should be closely monitored.

Home Care Considerations
- The bed surface at home should have the appropriate type of support surface.
- Be sure that family and client are comfortable with the product chosen and know how to use it.

- Choose a dressing that does not require multiple dressing changes in a 24-hour period. This will decrease the amount of time that the family and/or staff members will need to pay to the wound management program, should increase compliance, and will make a good use of home care resources.

Long-Term Care Considerations
- Long-term care, rehabilitation units may use a variety of position-relief devices and beds.
- Clients may be discharged to long-term care facilities that specialize in pressure ulcer and wound care treatment.

CRITICAL THINKING EXERCISES

1. A client was admitted to the medical floor for treatment of poorly controlled diabetes mellitus. Your skin assessment notes a 3-cm round ulcer on the right heel and a black covered (6 × 7 cm) ulcer over the sacral area.
   a. What other assessments must you make of this client?
   b. What interventions will you plan for this client?
2. Name two types of dressings that would be appropriate for a client's wound with 100% granulation tissue in the wound base, no report of pain, intact surrounding skin, and no evidence of odor or exudates.
3. You have been providing wound care to a client with a stage III pressure ulcer. What indices will you use to determine if the wound is healing?

REFERENCES
Bates-Jensen BM: Pressure ulcers: pathophysiology and prevention. In Sussman C, Bates-Jensen BM: *Wound care,* Gaithersburg, Md, 1998, Aspen.

Bennett MA: Report of the task force on the implications for darkly pigmented intact skin in the prediction and prevention of pressure ulcers, *Adv Wound Care* 8(6):34, 1995.

Bergstrom N and others: *Pressure ulcers in adults: prediction and prevention,* Clinical practice guideline No. 3, AHCPR Pub No. 92-0047, Rockville, Md, May 1992, Agency for Health Care Policy and Research, Public Health Service, U.S. Department of Health and Human Services.

Bergstrom N and others: *Treatment of pressure ulcers,* Clinical practice guideline No.15, AHCPR Pub No. 95-0652, Rockville, Md, Dec 1994, Agency for Health Care Policy and Research, Public Health Service, U.S. Department of Health and Human Services.

Bergstrom N and others: Predicting pressure ulcer risk: a multisite study of the predictive validity of the Braden scale, *Nurs Res* 47(5):261, 1998.

Braden BJ, Bergstrom N: Clinical utility of the Braden scale for predicting pressure sore risk, *Decubitus* 2(3):441, 1989.

Colburn L: Prevention of chronic wounds. In Krasner DL, Rodheaver GT, Sibald RG, editors: *Chronic wound care: a clinical source book for healthcare professionals,* ed 3, Wayne, Pa, 2001, HMP Communications.

Maklebust J, Magnan MA: Approaches to patient and family education for pressure ulcer management, *Decubitus* 5(4):18, 1992.

Maklebust J, Sieggreen M: *Pressure ulcers: guidelines for prevention and nursing management,* ed 2, Springhouse, Pa, Springhouse Corp.

National Pressure Ulcer Advisory Panel: *Statement on pressure ulcer prevention,* 1992, available at http://www.NPUAP.org/position1/htm.

National Pressure Ulcer Advisory Panel: *Position statement on stage I assessment in darkly pigmented skin,* 1998, available at http://www.NPUAP.org/position4/htm.

Pieper B: Mechanical forces: pressure, shear, friction. In Bryant RA, editor: *Acute and chronic wounds: nursing management,* ed 2, St Louis, 2000, Mosby.

Polynchuk KN: Debridement. In Krasner DL, Rodheaver GT, Sibald RG, editors: *Chronic wound care: a clinical source book for healthcare professionals,* ed 3, Wayne, Pa, 2001, HMP Communications.

Rolstad BS, Ovington LG, Harris A: Principles of wound
management. In Bryant RA, editor: *Acute and chronic
wounds: nursing management,* ed 2, St Louis, 2000, Mosby.

Stotts NA: Wound infection: diagnosis and management. In
Bryant RA, editor: *Acute and chronic wounds: nursing
management,* ed 2, St Louis, 2000, Mosby.

Stotts NA, Wipke-Tevis DD: Co-factors in impaired wound
healing. In Krasner DL, Rodheaver GT, Sibbald RG, editors: *Chronic wound care: a clinical source book for healthcare professionals,* ed 3, Wayne, Pa, 2001, HMP
Communications.

Waldrop J, Doughty D: Wound-healing physiology. In
Bryant RA, editor: *Acute and chronic wounds: nursing
management,* ed 2, St Louis, 2000, Mosby.

CHAPTER 24

Dressings

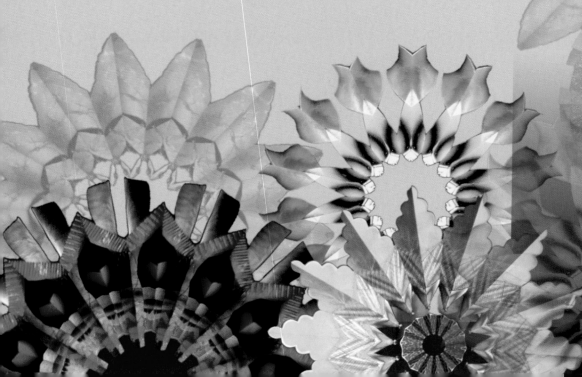

When a client has a wound, surgical or traumatic, a priority of care is to promote healing through meticulous wound care. Wound healing is a complex process. In addition, there are multiple factors that impede or promote healing (see Chapter 22).

Wounds heal best in a moist environment, and dressings help promote such an environment. In addition to maintaining a moist environment, dressings serve several functions, such as protection from outside contaminants, further tissue injury, and spread of microorganisms; in-

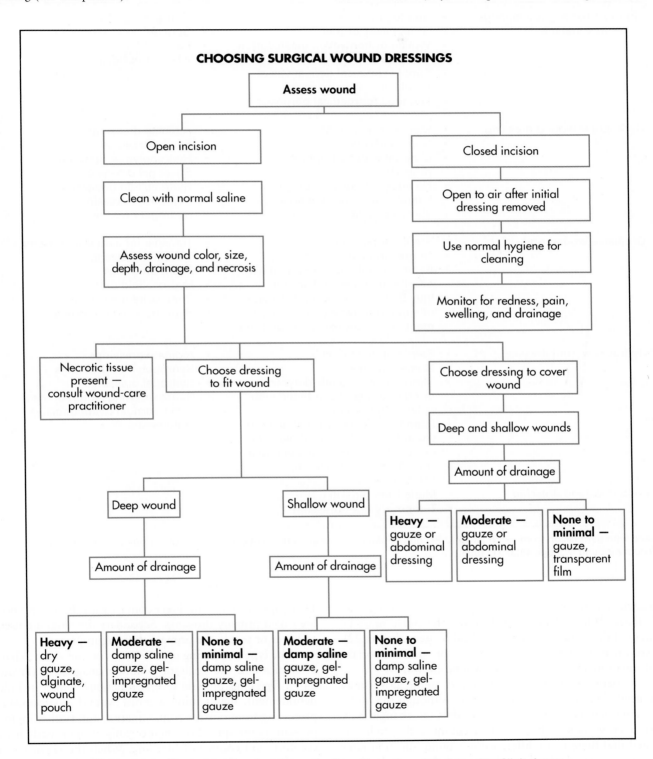

Figure 24-1   Flow chart for dressing selection. (From Perry AG, Potter PA: *Clinical nursing skills and techniques,* ed 5, St Louis, 2002, Mosby.)

Table 24-1

Dressing Category Definitions and Examples of Products as Presented by Health Industry Manufacturers Association (HIMA)

Category	Definition	Examples
Nonresorbable gauze/sponge for external use	• Sterile or nonsterile • Strip, piece, or pad • Woven or nonwoven mesh cotton cellulose • Simple chemical derivatives of cellulose • Intended for medical purposes	• Gauze • Sponge • Pads • Island dressings
Hydrophilic wound dressing	• Sterile or nonsterile • Nonresorbable • Material with hydrophilic properties • No added drugs or biologics • Intended to cover wound and absorb exudate	• Alginate dressings • Foam dressings • Hydropolymer dressings • Sheet gel dressings • Hydrocolloid dressings • Composite dressings • Hydrogel dressings
Occlusive wound dressing	• Sterile or nonsterile • Nonresorbable • Synthetic polymeric material with or without adhesive backing • Intended to cover wound, provide or support moist wound environment, and allow exchange of gases	• Transparent adhesive dressings • Thin film dressings • Foam dressings • Hydrocolloid dressings • Composite dressings • Hydropolymer dressings
Hydrogel wound dressing	• Sterile or nonsterile • Nonresorbable • Matrix of hydrophilic polymers or other material combined with at least 50% water • Intended to cover wound, absorb wound exudate, control bleeding or fluid loss, protect against abrasion, friction, dessication, contamination	• Alginate dressings • Hydropolymer dressings • Hydrogel dressings • Gauze dressings impregnated with hydrogel (without active ingredients)
Porcine wound dressing	• Made from pigskin • Temporary burn dressing	

Used with permission from van Rijswijk L: Recommendations to change the FDA classification of various wound dressings, *Ostomy Wound Manage* 45(3):31, 1999.

creased client comfort; and control of bleeding and drainage. When changing a dressing, the nurse must be aware of the principles of wound healing (see Chapter 22). Assessment of a wound and exudate provides important information about the status of wound healing.

Depending on the type of wound, sterile gloves may be needed to apply the new dressing. Although the initial dressing may be sterile, subsequent dressing changes may use a clean rather than sterile technique. Research has noted that there is no difference in wound infection rates when using sterile or clean gloves and there is a lowered cost for dressing supplies (Stotts and others, 1997).

Dressings that come in direct contact with the wound bed are called primary dressings. Secondary dressings are used to cover or secure the primary dressing in place.

The type of dressing used depends on the wound characteristics and the goals of wound management (Figure 24-1). Dressings provide several functions, which include debridement, maintaining a moist wound environment, protecting from outside contamination and further injury, preventing the spread of microorganisms, increased client comfort, and control of bleeding. When the client has a draining wound, the dressing must be highly absorbent. When control of bleeding is necessary, the dressing should

Box 24-1

AHCPR 1994 Pressure Ulcer Dressing Recommendations

- Use a dressing that keeps the ulcer bed continuously moist. Wet-to-dry dressings should be used only for debridement and are not considered continuously moist saline dressings.
- Use clinical judgment to select a type of moist wound dressing suitable for the ulcer. Studies of different types of moist wound dressings showed no differences in pressure ulcer healing outcomes.
- Choose a dressing that keeps the surrounding (periulcer) intact skin dry while keeping the ulcer bed moist.
- Choose a dressing that controls exudate but does not desiccate the ulcer bed.
- Consider caregiver time when selecting a dressing.
- Eliminate wound dead space by loosely filling all cavities with dressing material. Avoid overpacking the wound.
- Monitor dressings applied near the anus, because they are difficult to keep intact.

From Agency for Health Care Policy and Research: *Treatment of pressure ulcers,* Clinical practice guideline No.15, Rockville, Md, 1994, Agency for Health Care Policy and Research, Public Health Service, U.S. Department of Health and Human Services.

apply and maintain pressure on the site of bleeding. Other factors to consider are client comfort, dressing flexibility, ease of dressing application, and cost of supplies.

Various types of dressings can be applied to wounds; currently there is a U.S. Food and Drug Administration (FDA) classification for various wound dressings (Table 24-1). These products are grouped into functional categories in which one dressing may be classified in more than one category (van Rijswijk, 1999). When the wound is a pressure ulcer, the Agency for Health Care Policy and Research (AHCPR) (1994) has dressing recommendations (Box 24-1).

When providing dressing care, it is important to follow guidelines of care. Dressing changes are provided carefully so as not to injure the periwound skin and the wound base. Gloves are worn during the procedure, and to prevent cross contamination, clean, nonsterile gloves should be used to remove soiled dressings, and a new pair of gloves should be used to apply the new dressing (Stotts and others, 1997; Rolstad, Ovington, and Harris, 2000a).

NURSING DIAGNOSES

A nursing diagnosis that is appropriate for clients with wounds and related dressings is **Impaired Skin Integrity** related to trauma, surgical incision, and/or decreased circulation. Related nursing diagnoses that affect wound care and dressing applications might include **Risk for Impaired Skin Integrity** related to restricted movement; decreased strength, and endurance; **Acute Pain;** or **Deficient Knowledge Regarding Dressing Application.**

Skill 24.1

Applying Dressings

Dry dressings protect the wound from injury, prevent introduction and spread of bacteria, reduce discomfort, and speed healing. Drainage from surgical or traumatic wounds may be serous, sanguineous, or serosanguineous (Table 24-2). Dressings promote hemostasis by direct pressure and absorption of drainage. Dressings also may support or immobilize a body part. The ideal dressing is easy to apply, conforms to body contours, is durable but flexible, is able to absorb or contain exudate, is easily removed without damage to the healing surface, and is acceptable in appearance (Bolton, van Rijswijk, 1999).

Dry woven gauze dressings, the oldest and most common type, do not interact with wound tissues and cause little wound irritation. These are most often used for abrasions and postoperative incisions when minimal drainage is anticipated. Gauze dressings come in a variety of sizes,

such as 4 × 4 (16 inches square), 4 × 8 (rectangle), precut drain sponge, and rolls. Telfa gauze dressings contain a shiny, nonadherent surface on one side that does not stick to the wound. Drainage passes through the nonadherent surface to the outer gauze dressing (Figure 24-2). A dry dressing is not intended to debride the wound and should not be selected for wounds requiring debridement. On occasion a dry dressing may adhere to the wound, and in this case, the nurse should moisten the dressing with sterile normal saline or sterile water before removing the gauze to minimize trauma to the wound as it is removed. Moistening of the dressing is usually applied to dry dressings only and is not applicable to wet-to-dry dressings.

Moist dressings are often used for helping to heal full-thickness wounds that look like craters. Granulation tissue and new capillary networks must form to fill in the defect

Table 24-2

Types of Wound Drainage

Type	Appearance
A. Serous	Clear, watery plasma
B. Purulent	Thick, yellow, green, tan, or brown
C. Serosanguineous	Pale, red, watery: mixture of serous and sanguineous
D. Sanguineous	Bright red: indicates active bleeding

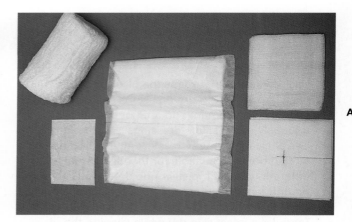

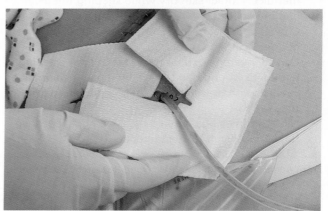

Figure 24-2 **A,** Types of gauze dressings. *Left to right:* Rolled gauze, Telfa, ABD, 4 × 4, and drain dressing. **B,** Applying a drain dressing.

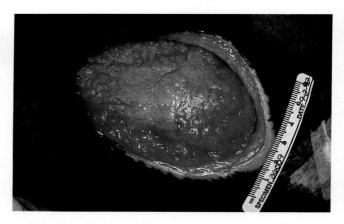

Figure 24-3 Granulation tissue in an open wound.

(Figure 24-3). Wet-to-dry dressings are used for wounds requiring debridement. The nurse moistens the contact dressing layer that touches the wound surface. The moistened gauze increases the absorptive ability of the dressing to collect exudate and wound debris. This layer dries and adheres to dead cells and debrides the wound when the dressing is removed. An outer absorbent layer is a dry dressing to protect the wound from invasive microorganisms.

A wet-to-dry dressing removes necrotic tissue and absorbs small amounts of exudates. However, this dressing is a nonselective method of debridement, and exposed healthy tissue in the wound bed may be damaged (Ramundo and Wells, 2000). This dressing is best used with heavily necrotic, infected wounds. Because granulation tissue is fragile and bleeds easily, damp dressings are less likely to result in tissue damage as old dressings are removed. The outermost layer is dry for this type of dressing as well (Ramundo and Wells, 2000).

Table 24-3

Principles for Wrapping an Extremity

Action	Rationale
Position body part in comfortable position of normal alignment.	Reduces risk of deformity or injury.
Prevent friction between and against skin surfaces by placing gauze or cotton padding (e.g., between toes).	Skin surfaces that touch may cause friction or skin breakdown.
Apply securely to prevent slipping, beginning at distal end and moving toward trunk.	Promotes venous return and minimizes edema or circulatory impairment.
Observe areas distal to bandage for signs of circulatory impairment (cool, pale, swollen, numbness, tingling, slow capillary refill).	Prompt attention to circulatory impairment prevents serious complications.
Avoid complete wrap at distal parts of extremities.	Provides exposure for assessment of peripheral circulation of extremity.

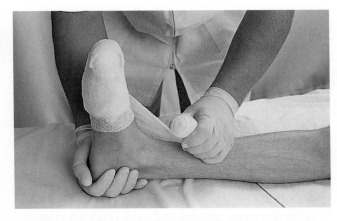

A

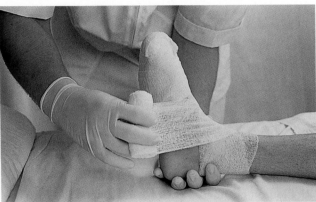

B

Figure 24-4   Applying circular dressings to an extremity.

Common wetting solutions for moistened dressings include normal saline and lactated Ringer's solution, which are isotonic solutions that aid in mechanical debridement and create an environment conducive to tissue growth.

Most dressings are secured with tape, which may be paper, plastic, woven, or elastic material with adhesive. Some clients are allergic to the adhesive. Frequent removal of tape for dressing changes is irritating to the skin. These dressings should be secured with Montgomery straps (see Skill 24-1, Step 14, p. 579). Montgomery straps are wide tapes with holes to use with ties that secure dressings and facilitate changes without removing the tape each time. Dressings on an extremity may be secured with rolls of gauze (Table 24-3). The dressing is secured by several turns around the extremity (Figure 24-4, *A*), continuing with a figure-eight method of application (Figure 24-4, *B*).

ASSESSMENT

1. Assess size and location of wound to be dressed. *Rationale: Assists nurse in planning for proper type and amount of supplies needed (see Skill 22.1, Assessment, p. 538).*
2. Ask client to rate pain using a scale of 0 to 10. *Rationale: Client may require pain medication before dressing change to allow drug's peak effect during procedure.*

3. Assess client's knowledge of purpose of dressing change. *Rationale: Determines level of support and explanation required.*
4. Determine the need for client or family member to participate in dressing wound. *Rationale: Prepares client or family member if dressing will be changed at home.*

PLANNING

Expected outcomes focus on preventing infection, promoting healing, pain control, and client and family education.

Expected Outcomes

1. Client's wound shows evidence of healing by smaller size and less drainage, redness, or swelling.
2. Client reports pain less than previously assessed level (scale of 0 to 10) during and after dressing change.
3. Dressing remains clean, dry, and intact.
4. Client or family demonstrates correct method of dressing changes.

Equipment

- Clean disposable gloves
- Sterile gloves

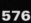

- Sterile dressing set (scissors and forceps)
- Sterile drape (optional)
- Sterile basin (optional)
- Necessary dressings: fine-mesh gauze, dressings, and/or abdominal (ABD) pads
- Tape or ties as needed, including nonallergic tape if necessary
- Sterile normal saline (or prescribed solution)
- Cleansing solution as prescribed
- Antiseptic ointment as prescribed
- Protective waterproof underpad
- Adhesive remover (optional)
- Waterproof bag
- Protective gown, goggles, and mask (used when spray from wound is a risk)
- Cleansing agents as ordered
- Measuring guide (optional)

 Delegation Considerations

The skill of applying certain dressings, such as a dry dressing, may be delegated to assistive personnel (AP) (check agency policy). AP may also be able to change dressings using clean technique for chronic wounds. All wound assessment, care of acute new wounds, and those that require sterile technique for dressing change require the critical thinking and knowledge application unique to the nurse and may not be delegated.

IMPLEMENTATION FOR APPLYING DRESSINGS

Steps	Rationale
1. See Standard Protocol (inside front cover).	
2. Position client comfortably, and drape to expose only wound site. Instruct client not to touch wound or sterile supplies.	Maintaining client comfort assists in completing skill smoothly. Draping provides access to wound while minimizing unnecessary exposure.

NURSE ALERT *If evidence of highly contagious infection is suspected, it may be necessary to place client in a private room (see Chapter 3). The physician often changes first postoperative dressings. If excessive drainage is noted, the dressing is reinforced (added to) without removing existing dressings (check agency policy). Staff does subsequent changes as ordered.*

3. Place disposable waterproof bag within reach of work area with top folded to make a cuff (see illustration).	Facilitates safe disposal of soiled dressings.
4. Remove tape: pull parallel to skin, toward dressing. If over hairy areas, remove in the direction of hair growth. Secure client permission to shave area (check agency policy).	Reduces stress on suture line or wound edges and reduces irritation and discomfort.
5. With clean gloves, remove dressings one layer at a time, observing appearance and drainage on dressing. Use caution to avoid tension on any drains that are present.	Determine dressings needed for replacement. Avoids accidental removal of drain because it may or may not be sutured in place.

NURSE ALERT *Moistening adherent dressings is no longer practiced. When moisture is applied to adherent dressings, the resultant removal of wound debris is reduced (Ramundo and Wells, 2000).*

6. Inspect wound for appearance, size, depth, drainage, approximation (wound edges are together), granulation tissue, or odor.	Provides assessment data for drainage and wound integrity. Monitors status of wound healing.

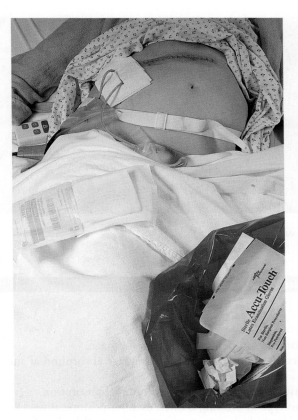

Step 3 Disposable waterproof bag placed near the dressing site.

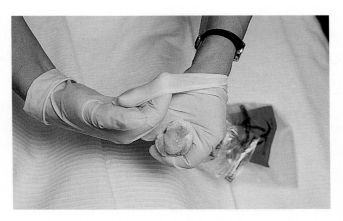

Step 7 Removal of disposable glove over contaminated dressing.

Steps	Rationale
7. Fold dressings with drainage contained inside, and remove gloves inside out. With small dressings, remove gloves inside out over dressing (see illustration). Dispose of gloves and soiled dressings in waterproof bag. Perform hand hygiene.	Provides containment of soiled dressings, prevents contact of nurse's hands with drainage, reduces transmission of cross-contamination microorganisms (Stotts and others, 1997).
8. Create a sterile field with a sterile dressing tray or individually wrapped sterile supplies on over-bed table (see Chapter 4). Pour necessary prescribed solution into sterile basin.	Sterile dressings remain sterile while on or within sterile area.
9. Apply sterile gloves or use no-touch technique with sterile forceps, which maintain sterility of all items in direct contact with the wound (Krasner and Kennedy, 1994).	Sterile gloves may be used for more complex situations with extensive drainage.

10. Cleanse wound.
  a. Use a separate swab for each cleansing stroke.
  b. Clean from least contaminated area to most contaminated (see illustrations).
  c. Cleanse around drain (if present), using a circular stroke starting near the drain and moving outward.
	Prevents transfer of organisms from previously cleaned area.

11. Use sterile dry gauze to blot in same manner as Step 10 to dry wound.	Drying reduces excess moisture, which could harbor microorganisms.
12. Apply prescribed antiseptic ointment using same technique as for cleansing, Step 10.	

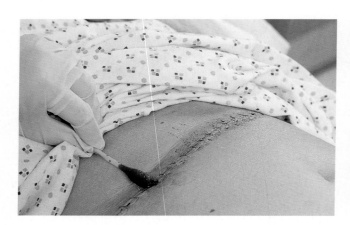
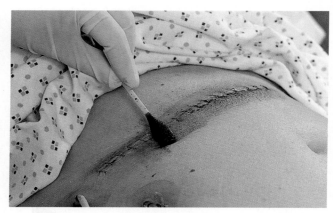

Step 10 Cleansing wound site.

Steps	Rationale

13. Apply dressing.
  a. Dry sterile dressing:
  (1) Apply loose, woven gauze as contact layer. — Promotes proper absorption of drainage.
  (2) Cut 4 × 4 gauze flat to fit around drain, if present. Precut gauze is also available. — Secures drain and promotes drainage absorption at site.
  (3) Apply additional layers of gauze as needed. — Ensures proper coverage and optimal absorption.
  (4) Apply thicker woven pad (e.g., ABD or Surgipad) — This type of dressing is often used for postoperative wounds. It is more effective in wound healing for postoperative cardiac and abdominal wounds (Wikblad and Anderson, 1995; Cannavo and others, 1998).

  b. Wet-to-dry dressing:
  (1) Place fine-mesh gauze in container of sterile solution. Wring out excess solution. — Moist gauze absorbs drainage and, when allowed to dry, traps debris (Ramundo and Wells, 2000).
  (2) Apply moist fine-mesh, open-weave gauze as a single layer directly onto wound surface. If wound is deep, gently pack gauze into wound with forceps until all wound surfaces are in contact with moist gauze. Be sure gauze does not touch surrounding skin (see illustration). — Inner gauze should be moist, not dripping wet, to absorb drainage and adhere to debris. Wound should be loosely packed to facilitate wicking of drainage into absorbent outer layer of dressing. Having inner gauze too wet (so it does not dry) is a common error in technique for this type of dressing (Barr, 1995).

NURSE ALERT *If wound is deep, gently lay gauze over wound surface with forceps until all surfaces are in contact with moist gauze and the wound is loosely filled with the moistened gauze. Fill the wound, but avoid packing the wound too tightly beyond the top of the wound.*

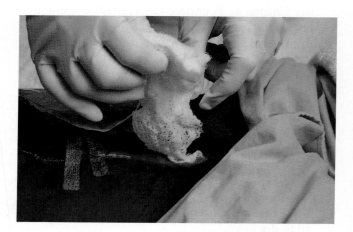

Step 13b(2) Packing wound with one layer of gauze.

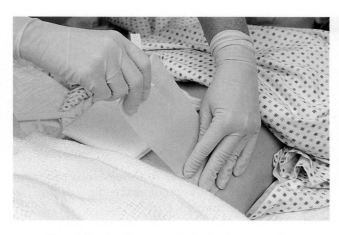

Step 14b(3) Placement of Montgomery ties.

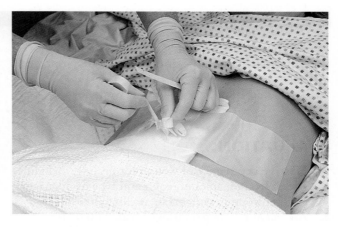

Step 14b(4) Securing Montgomery ties.

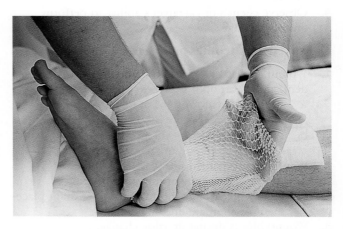

Step 14c Elastic net securing a lower extremity dressing.

Steps	Rationale
(3) Observe packing to ensure that any dead space from sinus tracts, undermining, or tunneling is loosely packed with gauze.	Do not overpack the wound; it can cause wound trauma when the dressing is removed (Cuzzell, 1997).
(4) Apply dry, sterile 4 × 4 gauze over moist gauze.	Pulls moisture from wound.
(5) Cover with ABD pad, Surgipad, or gauze.	Protects wound from the entrance of microorganisms.
14. Secure dressing.	
a. *Tape:* Apply tape to secure dressing. When necessary, use nonallergenic tape	
b. *Montgomery ties*	
(1) Be sure skin is clean. Application of a skin barrier is recommended.	Skin barrier (Stomahesive) protects intact skin from stretch and tension of adhesive tape.
(2) Expose adhesive surface of tape ends.	
(3) Place ties on opposite sides of the dressing over skin or skin barrier (see illustration).	
(4) Secure dressing by lacing ties across dressing snugly enough to hold dressing secure but without pressure on the skin (see illustration).	
c. For dressing on an extremity, dressing is secured with roller gauze (see Figure 24-4, p. 575) or Surgiflex elastic net (see illustration).	

Steps	Rationale
15. Remove cover gown and goggles, and remove gloves inside out and dispose of them in a waterproof container.	Reduces transmission of microorganisms.
16. See Completion Protocol (inside front cover).	

• • • • • • • • • •

EVALUATION

1. Observe appearance of wound for healing, including size of wound, amount, color and type of drainage, and periwound erythema or swelling.
2. Ask client to rate pain using a scale of 0 to 10.
3. Inspect status of dressing at least every shift or as ordered.
4. Observe client's or caregiver's ability to perform dressing change.

Unexpected Outcomes and Related Interventions

1. Wound appears inflamed and tender, drainage is evident, and/or an odor is present.
   a. Monitor client for signs of infection, for example, fever, increased white blood cell (WBC) count.
   b. Notify physician.
   c. Obtain wound cultures as ordered.
2. Wound drainage increases.
   a. Increase frequency of dressing changes.
   b. Notify physician, who may consider drain placement or alternate dressing method.
3. Wound bleeds during dressing change.
   a. Observe color and amount of drainage. If excessive, may need to apply direct pressure.
   b. Inspect area along dressing and directly underneath client to determine the amount of bleeding.
   c. Obtain vital signs as needed.
   d. Notify physician of findings.
4. Client reports a sensation that "something has given way under the dressing."
   a. Observe wound for increased drainage or dehiscence (partial or total separation of wound

layers) or evisceration (total separation of wound layers and protrusion of viscera through the wound opening).
   b. Protect wound. Cover wound with sterile moist dressing.
   c. Instruct client to lie still.
   d. Notify physician.
5. Client or caregiver is unable to perform dressing change.
   a. Provide additional teaching and support.
   b. Obtain services of home care agency as needed.

Recording and Reporting

• Record appearance of wound, color, characteristics of drainage, response to dressing change in nurses' notes.
• Note client's level of comfort during dressing change.
• Write date and time dressing applied in ink (not marker) on outer tape.
• Report brisk, bright bleeding or evidence of wound dehiscence or evisceration to physician immediately.

Sample Documentation

1000 Wet-to-dry dressing on right ankle changed using sterile technique. First layer of gauze had pea-sized spot of light-yellow drainage. Ulceration is 4 cm in diameter, 0.5 cm deep, with pinpoint spots of yellow drainage along the border; erythema noted on surrounding area. Used one moist and one dry 4 × 4 gauze and wrapped with Kling gauze. Client reported 0 pain on a scale of 0 to 10.

SPECIAL CONSIDERATIONS

Pediatric Considerations
• Check that dressing products are safe to use on pediatric clients, especially premature infants.
• Pediatric clients may be fearful of dressing changes. Use age-specific interventions such as having personnel available to keep child from moving during procedure, diversion such as music for older children, or letting children observe dressings before procedure (Wong and others, 2001).

Geriatric Considerations
• Adhesive tape may be too irritating to older adults' skin and cause skin tears. Use paper tape, nonallergic tape, or wraps or mesh without tape contacting client's skin.
• Normal changes associated with aging may delay wound healing (Lueckenotte, 2000).

Home Care Considerations

- Some wounds may be cleansed in the shower. Have client verify this practice with physician before discharge.
- Clean dressings may be used in the home environment.
- Disposal of contaminated dressings should be done in a manner consistent with local regulations (AHCPR, 1994). For adequate reimbursement, payers require a signed physician's order and treatment plan. Documentation of need for services and status of wound healing is needed for reimbursement or continuing professional wound care services in the home (Wright and McNichol, 2000).

Long-Term Care Considerations

- Centers with subacute care units often provide specialized wound care. Clients are admitted to the center for continued wound care management (Beshara, Jameson, and Barr, 2000).
- Be sure that wound care and dressing materials do not interfere with physical or occupational therapies.

Skill 24.2

Changing Transparent Dressings

A film dressing is a "clear, adherent, nonabsorptive polymer-based dressing that is permeable to oxygen and water vapor but not to water" (AHCPR, 1994). Polyurethane moisture- and vapor-permeable film dressings were developed to manage superficial wounds. They are often used following laparoscopic surgery, for small, superficial wounds, and as a dressing over an intravenous (IV) catheter site. These dressings are not appropriate for moist surfaces, such as a wound bed or moist periwound skin, because the adhesive will not stick (Rolstad, Ovington, and Harris, 2000b).

Transparent dressings are thin, self-adhesive elastic films (e.g., Op-Site or Tegaderm). This synthetic permeable membrane acts as a temporary second skin, adheres to undamaged skin to contain exudate and minimize wound contamination, and allows the wound surface to "breathe."

With the use of a transparent dressing, a moist exudate forms over the wound surface, which prevents tissue dehydration and allows for rapid, effective healing by speeding epithelial cell growth. Because these dressings are clear, the nurse is able to assess the wound without removing the film. This dressing conforms well to body contours with less restriction of movement.

For best results these dressings should be used on clean, debrided wounds that are not actively bleeding. The film should be applied wrinkle free but not stretched over the skin. Should fluid accumulation and a white, opaque appearance with erythema of the surrounding tissue develop, an infection may be present. Remove the dressing, and obtain a wound culture.

ASSESSMENT

1. Assess location, appearance, and size of wound (see Skill 22.1, p. 538) to be dressed. *Rationale: Provides information regarding status of wound healing, presence of complications, and the proper type of supplies and assistance needed to apply a new transparent dressing.*
2. Determine size of transparent dressing needed. *Rationale: Dressing should allow 2.5 cm (1 inch) overlap from wound margin to intact surrounding tissue (Rolstad, Ovington, and Harris, 2000b).*
3. Assess client's comfort level using a scale of 0 to 10. *Rationale: Data will determine effectiveness of comfort control interventions before, during, and after dressing change.*

PLANNING

Expected outcomes focus on promoting wound healing.

Expected Outcomes

1. Client's wound shows decrease or absence of drainage.
2. Skin surrounding the client's wound remains clean and intact.
3. Client reports less pain than previously assessed level (scale of 0 to 10) during and after dressing change.

Equipment

- Clean disposable gloves
- Waterproof bag for disposal

- Sterile gloves (optional)
- Sterile scissors and forceps (optional)
- Sterile saline or other wound cleanser (as ordered)
- Transparent dressing (size as needed)
- Sterile gauze pads (2 × 2, 4 × 4)
- Cotton swabs
- Skin prep materials
- Waterproof bag for disposal
- Moisture-proof gown, goggles, and mask (if risk of splashing is present)

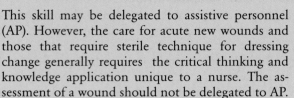

Delegation Considerations

This skill may be delegated to assistive personnel (AP). However, the care for acute new wounds and those that require sterile technique for dressing change generally requires the critical thinking and knowledge application unique to a nurse. The assessment of a wound should not be delegated to AP.

IMPLEMENTATION FOR CHANGING TRANSPARENT DRESSINGS

Steps	Rationale
1. See Standard Protocol (inside front cover).	
2. Cuff top of disposable waterproof bag to prevent contamination of outer bag. Place within easy reach of work area.	
3. Moisture-proof gown, mask, and eye goggles are worn when the risk of spray exist. Remove old dressing by pulling back slowly across dressing in direction of hair growth and toward the center.	Reduces excoriation, pain, and irritation of skin after dressing removal.
4. Dispose of soiled dressings, remove disposable gloves by pulling them inside out over soiled dressings, and dispose of them in waterproof bag.	Decreases risk of cross contamination (Stotts and others, 1997).
5. Prepare supplies; for some wounds sterile supplies are needed.	
6. Reapply sterile (or clean) gloves (check agency policy).	Prevents risk of exposure to body secretions if present.
7. Cleanse area gently, swabbing toward area of most exudate, or spray with cleanser (check agency policy and physician preference).	Reduces transmission of organisms from contaminated area to cleaner site. Transparent dressings adhere more readily to clean, dry skin.
8. Dry skin around wound thoroughly with sterile gauze. Make sure skin surface is dry.	Transparent dressing with adhesive backing will not adhere to damp surface. Nonadhesive transparent dressing will cling to moist wound surface (Rolstad, Ovington, and Harris, 2000b).
9. Inspect wound for color, odor, and drainage; measure if indicated.	Appearance indicates state of wound healing.
10. Apply transparent dressing according to manufacturer's directions.	
a. Remove paper backing, taking care not to allow adhesive areas to touch each other (see illustration).	Results in wrinkles and may be impossible to use.
b. Place film smoothly over wound without stretching (see illustration).	Wrinkles can provide tunnel for drainage.
c. Label with date, initials, and time if required by agency policy (see illustration).	
11. Remove gloves and discard in waterproof bag.	
12. See Completion Protocol (inside front cover).	

• • • • • • • • • •

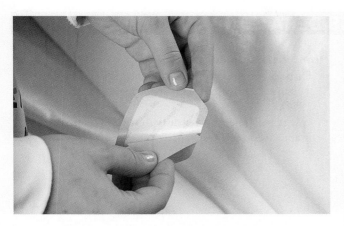

Step 10a   Removal of paper backing.

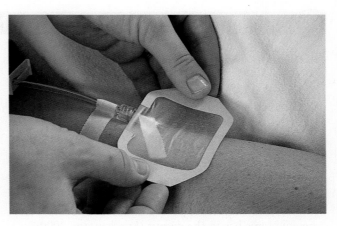

Step 10b   Transparent dressing placed smoothly over an IV site.

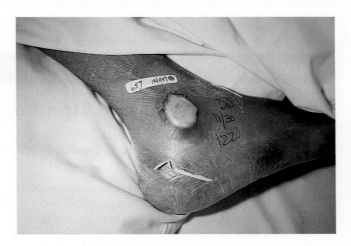

Step 10c   Labeled dressing covering leg ulcer.

EVALUATION

1. Inspect appearance of wound and amount of drainage, and compare with previous assessment.
2. Inspect condition of skin around the wound.
3. Ask client to rate pain using a scale of 0 to 10.

Unexpected Outcomes and Related Interventions

1. Wound appears inflamed and tender, drainage is evident, and/or an odor is present.
   a. Remove dressing, and obtain wound culture according to agency policy.
   b. A different type of dressing and more frequent dressing changes may be ordered.
2. Dressing does not stay in place.
   a. Evaluate size of dressing used for adequate (1 to 1½ inches) margin.
   b. Dry client's skin thoroughly before reapplication.
3. Outer layer of client's skin tears on removal of dressing.
   a. Adhesive backing may be too strong for fragile skin.
   b. Use non–adhesive-backed transparent dressing.

Recording and Reporting

- Record appearance of wound, color, characteristics of drainage, and response to dressing change.
- Write date and time dressing applied in ink (not marker) and nurse's initials on outer label.

Sample Documentation

1000 Transparent dressing changed. Wound on left thigh is 6 × 10 cm, with oozing serosanguineous drainage. Area erythematous, swollen, and very tender to touch. Client describes pain as 6 (on a scale of 0 to 10). Refusing medication at this time.

SPECIAL CONSIDERATIONS

Pediatric Considerations

- Adhesive backing may cause skin tears on babies' delicate skin (Wong and others, 2001).
- Children may tolerate a transparent dressing change better because they know the dressing can be left on for a longer period of time.

Geriatric Considerations

Adhesive backing may be too strong for the skin of older adults. Do not use a film dressing that has an adhesive backing that has a stronger bond to the epidermis than the epidermis has to the dermis (Lueckenotte, 2000).

Home Care Considerations

- Disposal of contaminated dressings should be done in a manner consistent with local regulations (AHCPR, 1994).
- Client may take shower or bath with dressing in place, if approved by physician.

Skill 24.3

Applying Binders and Bandages

Binder and bandages applied over or around dressings can provide extra protection and therapeutic benefits by the following:

1. Creating pressure over a body part (e.g., an elastic pressure bandage applied over an arterial puncture site)
2. Immobilizing a body part (e.g., an elastic bandage applied around a sprained ankle)
3. Supporting a wound (e.g., an abdominal binder applied over a large abdominal incision and dressing)
4. Reducing or preventing edema (e.g., a breast binder used to minimize swelling between skin and tissue layers after a mastectomy)
5. Securing a splint (e.g., a bandage applied around hand splints for correction of deformities)
6. Securing dressings (e.g., elastic webbing applied around leg dressings after a vein stripping)
7. Maintaining the position of special equipment for applying traction (e.g., Buck's extension)
8. Enabling the client to participate in effective respiratory functions of deep breathing, coughing, and clearing of airway secretions (e.g., a breast or abdominal binder that supports local incisions, reducing the pain from respiratory maneuvers)

Bandages are available in rolls of various widths and materials, including gauze, elasticized knit, elastic webbing, flannel, and muslin. Gauze bandages are lightweight and inexpensive, mold easily around contours of the body, and permit air circulation to prevent skin maceration. Elastic bandages conform well to body parts but can also be used to exert pressure over a body part. Elastic bandages are used to secure dressings on extremities, stumps, and the hand (Table 24-4). Flannel and muslin bandages are thicker than gauze and thus stronger for supporting or applying pressure. A flannel bandage also insulates to provide warmth.

Binders are bandages made of large pieces of material specially designed to fit a specific body part. Most binders are made of elastic, cotton, muslin, or flannel. The most common types of binders are the breast binder and the abdominal binder.

A breast binder looks like a tight-fitting sleeveless vest. It conforms to the shape of the chest wall and is available in different sizes. Breast binders can provide support after breast surgery.

An abdominal binder supports large abdominal incisions that are vulnerable to tension or stress as the client moves or coughs (Figure 24-5). The nurse secures a binder with Velcro strips, metal fasteners, or safety pins.

Correctly applied bandages and binders do not cause injury to underlying and nearby body parts or create discomfort for the client. For example, an abdominal binder must be applied correctly to allow for normal chest expansion.

ASSESSMENT

1. Observe client with need for support of thorax or abdomen. Observe ability to breathe deeply and cough effectively. *Rationale: Baseline assessment determines client's ability to breathe and cough. Impaired ventilation of lungs from a tight binder or bandage application can lead to alveolar collapse (atelectasis) and inadequate arterial oxygenation.*

Table 24-4

Types of Bandage Turns

Type	Description	Purpose or Use
Circular	Bandage turn overlapping previous turn completely	Anchors bandage at the first and final turn; covers small part (finger, toe)
Spiral	Bandage ascending body part, with each turn overlapping previous one by one-half or two-thirds width of bandage	Covers cylindrical body parts such as wrist or upper arm
Spiral–reverse	Turn requiring twist (reversal) of bandage halfway through each turn	Covers cone-shaped body parts such as the forearm, thigh, or calf; useful with nonstretching bandages such as gauze or flannel
Figure eight	Oblique overlapping turns alternately ascending and descending over bandaged part, each turn crossing previous one to form figure eight	Covers joints, such as to support the ankle or elbow; snug fit provides excellent immobilization
Recurrent	Bandage first secured with two circular turns around proximal end of body part; half turn made perpendicular up from bandage edge; body of bandage brought over distal end of body part to be covered with each turn folded back over on itself	Covers uneven body parts such as head or stump

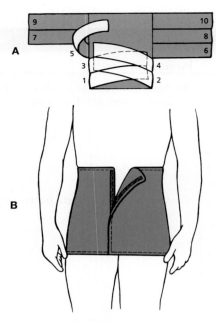

Figure 24-5 Abdominal binders. **A,** Sculteus. **B,** Straight.

PLANNING

Expected outcomes focus on improving client's comfort level, maintaining baseline respiratory functioning, securing underlying dressing, and maintaining underlying skin integrity.

Expected Outcomes

1. Client reports pain less than previously assessed level (scale of 0 to 10) during and after dressing change.
2. Client's respiratory rate remains within 3 breaths of baseline.
3. Client's underlying surgical dressing remains intact.
4. Client's skin is intact on tissue underneath and surrounding binder.

Equipment

- Clean gloves, if wound drainage is present
- Correct type and size of binder
- Safety pins (unless Velcro closure is available)

2. Review medical record for order of binder type. *Rationale: Application of supportive binders may be used based on a nursing judgment. In some situations a physician's order may be required (check agency policy).*
3. Inspect skin for actual or potential alterations in integrity. Observe for irritation, abrasion, skin surfaces that rub together, or allergic response to adhesive tape. *Rationale: Actual impairments in skin integrity can be worsened with the application of a binder. Binders can cause pressure and excoriation.*
4. Inspect surgical dressing. *Rationale: Dressing replacement or reinforcement precedes application of any binder.*
5. Assess client's comfort level, using a scale of 0 to 10 and noting any objective signs and symptoms. *Rationale: Data will determine need for analgesia before dressing change and effectiveness of binder placement to support underlying tissues.*

Delegation Considerations

The skills of applying a binder (abdominal or breast) can be delegated to assistive personnel (AP). However, it is the responsibility of the nurse to assess the client's ability to breathe deeply, cough effectively, and move independently before and after binder application. The nurse is also responsible for assessing the client's skin for irritation/abrasion, the underlying wound, and client's level of comfort.

IMPLEMENTATION FOR APPLYING BINDERS

Steps	Rationale

1. See Standard Protocol (inside front cover).

NURSE ALERT *Cover any exposed areas of incision or wound with sterile dressing.*

2. Apply gloves if there is likely contact with wound drainage

Steps	**Rationale**

3. Apply binder:

   a. Abdominal binder:

     (1) Position client in supine position with head slightly elevated and knees slightly flexed.

                              Minimizes muscular tension on abdominal organs.

     (2) Fanfold far side of binder toward midline of binder.

                              Facilitates placement of binder under client.

     (3) Instruct and assist client in rolling away from nurse toward raised side rail while firmly supporting abdominal incision and dressing with hands.

                              Reduces pain and discomfort.

     (4) Place fanfolded ends of binder under client.

                              Permits placement and centering of binder with minimal discomfort.

     (5) Instruct or assist client in rolling over folded ends.

     (6) Unfold and stretch ends out smoothly on far side of bed.

                              Maintains skin integrity and comfort.

     (7) Instruct client to roll back into supine position.

                              Facilitates chest expansion and adequate wound support when the binder is closed.

     (8) Adjust binder so that supine client is centered over binder using symphysis pubis and costal margins as lower and upper landmarks.

                              Centers support from binder over abdominal structures, which reduces incidence of decreased lung expansion.

     (9) Close binder. Pull one end of binder over center of client's abdomen. While maintaining tension on that end of binder, pull opposite end of binder over center and secure with Velcro closure tabs, metal fasteners, or horizontally placed safety pins.

                              Provides continuous wound support and comfort.

     (10) Assess client's comfort level.

                              Helps determine effectiveness of binder placement.

     (11) Adjust binder as necessary.

                              Promotes comfort and chest expansion.

   b. Breast binder:

     (1) Assist client to sit up and place arms through binder's armholes.

                              Eases binder placement process.

     (2) Assist client to supine position in bed.

                              Supine positioning facilitates normal anatomical position of breasts; facilitates healing and comfort.

     (3) Pad area under breasts if necessary.

                              Prevents skin contact with undersurface.

     (4) Using Velcro closure tabs, secure binder at nipple level first. Continue closure process above and then below nipple line until entire binder is closed.

                              Horizontal placement of pins may reduce risk of uneven pressure or localized irritation.

     (5) Make appropriate adjustments, including individualizing fit of shoulder straps and pinning waistline darts to reduce binder size.

                              Maintains support to client's breasts.

     (6) Instruct and observe skill development in self-care related to reapplying breast binder.

                              Self-care is integral aspect of discharge planning. Skin integrity and comfort level goals are ensured.

4. If gloves were applied, remove and dispose of properly

5. Remove binder at scheduled intervals to assess underlying skin integrity (check agency policy).

                              Promotes timely identification of impaired skin integrity.

6. See Completion Protocol (inside front cover).

• • • • • • • • •

EVALUATION

1. Ask client to rate pain on a scale of 0 to 10.
2. Observe client's respiratory status when using an abdominal binder.
3. Observe site to be sure underlying dressings are intact.
4. Remove binder, and observe underlying and surrounding skin.

Unexpected Outcomes and Related Interventions

1. Client's pain increases.
   a. Remove binder and assess wound site.
   b. Reapply binder using less pressure.
2. Client's respiratory rate decreases.
   a. Remove binder.
   b. Encourage client to cough and deep breathe.
   c. Reapply binder using less pressure
3. Client develops a break in the skin because of binder application.
   a. Remove binder.
   b. Initiate skin care measures to heal affected area.

Recording and Reporting

- Record baseline data about client's respiratory status, level of comfort, status of dressings, and skin integrity.
- Following use of binder, record information pertaining to client's level of comfort, respiratory status, tolerance to binder, and status of underlying wound and skin.
- Report client's tolerance to binder application and the prescribed duration of the application.

Sample Documentation

1000 Client complains of "pulling" sensation around abdominal incision line. Pulling sensation increases with ambulation. Vital signs stable. Dressings to abdominal wound dry and intact. Underlying skin intact. Abdominal binder applied. Client rates pain as 1 (scale of 0 to 10), able to ambulate with ease.

◉ SPECIAL CONSIDERATIONS ◉

Pediatric Considerations
Binders with Velcro closures are preferable. If these are not available, secure binder with adhesive tape. Avoid securing binder with clips or pins as they can become a choking hazard for clients.

Geriatric Considerations
The increased fragility of the skin of an older adult may contraindicate the use of a binder. Assess skin thoroughly before any binder application. May need to observe underlying skin more frequently for this population.

Home Care and Long-Term Care Considerations
Client are encouraged have two binders. Because binders are washable and need to be "line dried," the client has one to wear and one that is in the process of being washed or dried.

Skill 24.4

Wound Vacuum Assisted Closure

The wound Vacuum Assisted Closure (wound V.A.C.) is a device that assists in wound closure by applying localized negative pressure to draw the edges of a wound together (Figures 24-6 and 24-7). V.A.C. accelerates wound healing by promoting the formation of granulation tissue, collagen, fibroblasts, and inflammatory cells in order to completely close or improve the health of a wound in preparation for a skin graft. The use of negative pressure removes fluid from the area surrounding the wound, thus reducing local peripheral edema and improving circulation to the area (Chua and others, 2000) (Figure 24-8). In addition, after 3 to 4 days of therapy, bacterial counts in the wound drop (Argenta and Morykwas, 1997; Evans and Land, 2001).

Wound V.A.C. may be used to treat acute and chronic wounds. The schedule for changing Wound V.A.C. dressings vary. An infected wound may need a dressing change every 24 hours, whereas a clean wound can be changed 3 times a week (Mendez-Eastman, 1998; Chua, 2000). As the wound heals, the wound base becomes redder and granulation tissue will line the surface of the wound. The wound has a stippled or granulated appearance. Last, the surface area of the wound may increase or decrease depending on wound location and the amount of drainage removed by the Wound V.A.C. system. As the wound heals, paler areas in the wound may develop. This indicates an increase in fibrous tissue (Melendez-Eastman, 1998).

ASSESSMENT

1. Assess location, appearance, and size of wound (see Skill 22.1, p. 538) to be dressed. *Rationale: Provides in-*

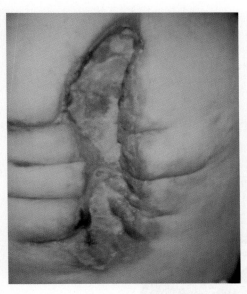

Figure 24-6   Dehisced wound before Wound V.A.C. therapy. (Courtesy Kinetic Concepts, Inc. [KCI], San Antonio, Tex.)

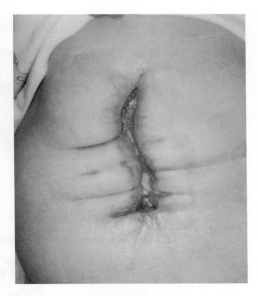

Figure 24-7   Dehisced wound after Wound V.A.C. therapy. (Courtesy Kinetic Concepts, Inc. [KCI], San Antonio, Tex.)

formation regarding status of wound healing, presence of complications, and the proper type of supplies and assistance needed to apply a new transparent dressing.

2. Assess client's comfort level using a scale of 0 to 10. *Rationale: Data will determine effectiveness of comfort control interventions before, during, and after dressing change.*

3. Assess client's knowledge of purpose of dressing change. *Rationale: Determines level of support and explanation required.*

4. Determine the need for client or family member to participate in dressing wound. *Rationale: Prepares client or family member if dressing will be changed at home.*

PLANNING

Expected outcomes focus on preventing infection, promoting healing, pain control, and client and family education.

Expected Outcomes

1. Client's wound shows evidence of healing by smaller size and less drainage, redness, or swelling.

2. Client reports pain less than previously assessed level (scale of 0 to 10) during and after dressing changes.

3. Dressing remains intact with airtight seal and prescribed negative pressure.

4. Client or family demonstrates correct method of dressing changes.

Equipment

- V.A.C. unit (requires physician order) (Figure 24-9)
- V.A.C. foam dressing
- Tubing for connection between V.A.C. unit and V.A.C. dressing

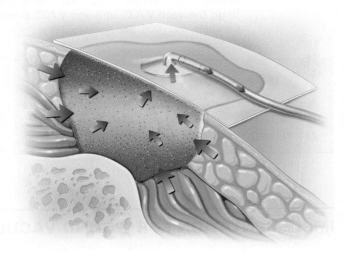

Figure 24-8   Wound V.A.C. system using negative pressure to remove fluid from area surrounding the wound, reducing edema, and improving circulation to area. (Courtesy Kinetic Concepts, Inc. [KCI], San Antonio, Tex.)

- Gloves, clean and sterile
- Scissors (sterile)
- Skin prep/skin barrier
- Moist washcloth
- Plastic trash bag
- Linen bag

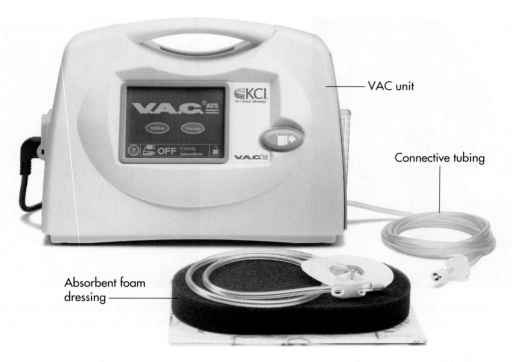

Figure 24-9 Wound V.A.C. unit: *Top* to *bottom:* V.A.C. unit itself, connector tubing to go between V.A.C. unit and V.A.C. dressing, absorbent foam. (Courtesy Kinetic Concepts, Inc. [KCI], San Antonio, Tex.)

Delegation Considerations

Application of this skill requires the critical thinking and knowledge application unique to an RN. Delegation is inappropriate.

IMPLEMENTATION FOR WOUND VACUUM ASSISTED CLOSURE

Steps	Rationale
1. See Standard Protocol (inside front cover).	
2. Position client comfortably, and drape to expose only wound site. Instruct client not to touch wound or sterile supplies.	Maintaining client comfort assists in completing skill smoothly. Draping provides access to wound while minimizing unnecessary exposure.
3. Place disposable waterproof bag within reach of work area with top folded to make a cuff.	Facilitates safe disposal of soiled dressings.
4. When V.A.C. is in place, begin by pushing therapy on/off button.	Deactivates therapy and allows for proper drainage of fluid in drainage tubing.
a. Keeping tube connectors with V.A.C. unit, disconnect tubes from each other to drain fluids into canister.	
b. Before lowering, tighten clamp on canister tube.	
5. With dressing tube unclamped, introduce 10 to 30 ml of normal saline, if ordered, into tubing to soak underneath foam.	Facilitates loosening of foam when tissue adheres to foam (Chua and others, 2000).

Steps	**Rationale**
6. Gently stretch transparent film horizontally, and slowly pull up from the skin.	Reduces stress on suture line or wound edges and reduces irritation and discomfort.
7. Remove old V.A.C. dressing, observing appearance and drainage on dressing. Use caution to avoid tension on any drains that are present. Discard dressing, and remove gloves. Perform hand hygiene.	Determine dressings needed for replacement. Avoids accidental removal of drains because they may or may not be sutured in place.
8. Apply sterile or clean gloves. Irrigate the wound with normal saline or other solution ordered by the physician. Gently blot to dry.	Irrigation removes wound debris.

NURSE ALERT *If this is a new surgical wound, sterile technique may be ordered. Chronic wounds may use clean technique.*

9. Measure wound as ordered: at baseline, first dressing change, weekly, and discharge from therapy. Remove and discard gloves.	Objectively documents wound healing process in response to negative pressure, wound therapy (Banwell, Holten, and Martin, 1998).

NURSE ALERT *Wound cultures may be ordered on a routine basis. However, when drainage looks purulent, there is change in amount or color, or drainage has a foul odor, wound cultures should be obtained even when they are not ordered for that particular dressing change (Banwell, Holten, and Martin, 1998; Chua and others, 2000).*

10. Depending on the type of wound, apply sterile gloves or new clean gloves.	Fresh sterile wounds require sterile gloves. Chronic wounds may require clean technique. However, do not use the same gloves worn to remove old dressing because cross contamination may occur (Stotts and others, 1997; Mendez-Eastman, 1998).

11. Prepare V.A.C. foam.
  a. Select appropriate foam.
  b. Using sterile scissors, cut foam to wound size. Proper size of foam dressing helps maintain negative pressure to entire wound. Dressing must be cut to fit the size and shape of the wound, including tunnels and undermined areas.
	Black polyurethane (PU) foam has larger pores and is most effective in stimulating granulation tissue and wound contraction. White polyvinyl alcohol (PVA) soft foam is denser with smaller pores and is used when the growth of granulation tissue needs to be restricted (KCI, 1999).

NURSE ALERT *Clients may experience more pain with the black foam because of excessive wound contraction. For this reason they may need to be switched to the PVA soft foam.*

12. Gently place foam in wound, being sure that the foam is in contact with entire wound base and margins and tunneled and undermined areas.	Maintains negative pressure to entire wound. Edges of the foam dressing must be in direct contact with the client's skin (Broussard, Mendez-Eastman, and Frantz, 2000).
13. Apply tubing to foam in the wound (see illustration).	Connects the negative pressure from the V.A.C. unit to the wound foam.

NURSE ALERT *For deep wounds regularly reposition tubing to minimize pressure on wound edges. In addition, clients with restricted mobility or sensation must be repositioned frequently so that they do not lie on the tubing and cause further skin damage (KCI, 1999).*

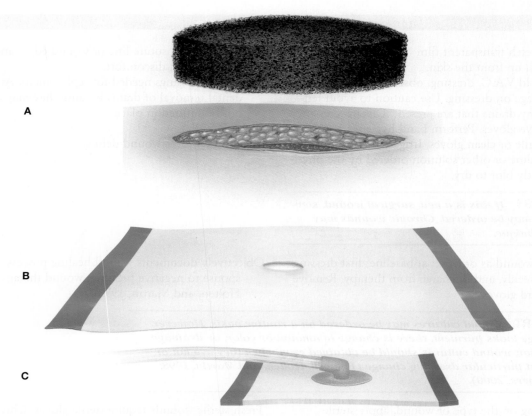

Step 13 Dressing application. From *bottom* to *top:* **A,** Properly sized foam to cover wound. **B,** Wrinkle-free transparent dressing applied over foam. **C,** Secure tubing to the foam and transparent dressing unit (step 14). (Courtesy Kinetic Concepts, Inc. [KCI], San Antonio, Tex.)

Steps	Rationale
14. Apply skin protectant, such as skin prep or Stomahesive wafer, to skin around the wound.	Protects periwound skin from injury that may result from the occlusive dressing
15. Apply Wound V.A.C. dressing.	Ensures that the wound is properly covered and a negative pressure seal can be achieved (Box 24-2).
a. Cover the V.A.C. foam, 3 to 5 cm of surrounding healthy tissue.	
b. Apply wrinkle-free transparent dressing.	Excessive tension may compress foam dressing and impede wound healing. Excessive tension also produces a shear force on periwound area (KCI, 1999).
c. Secure tubing to transparent film, aligning drainage holes to ensure an occlusive seal (see illustration). **Do not apply tension to drape and tubing.**	
16. Secure tubing several cemtimeters away from the dressing.	Prevents pull on the primary dressing, which can cause leaks in the negative pressure system (KCI, 1999; Chua and others, 2000).
17. Once wound is completely covered, connect the tubing from the dressing to the tubing from the canister and V.A.C. unit.	Intermittent or continuous negative pressure can be administered at 50 mm Hg to 200 mm Hg, according to physician order and client comfort. The average is 125 mm Hg (Baxandall, 1996; Chua and others, 2000).
a. Remove canister from sterile packaging, and push into V.A.C. unit until a click is heard. **NOTE: An alarm will sound if the canister is not properly engaged.**	

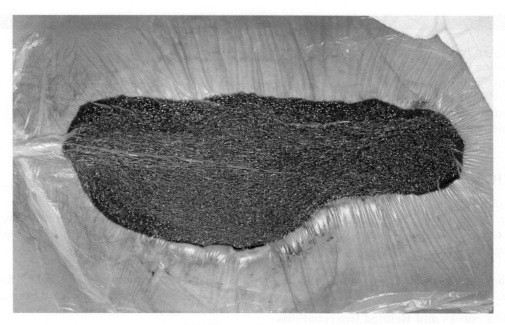

Step 15 Foam dressing, transparent dressing, and Wound V.A.C. tubing secured over existing wound. (Courtesy KCI, San Antonio, Tex.)

Box 24-2

Maintaining an Airtight Seal

To avoid wound desiccation, the wound must stay sealed once therapy is initiated. Problem seal areas include wounds around joints and near the sacrum. The following points may assist in maintaining an airtight seal:

- Shave hair around wound.
- Cut transparent film to extend 3 to 5 cm beyond wound parameter.

- Avoid wrinkles in transparent film.
- Patch leaks with transparent film.
- Use multiple small strips of transparent film to hold dressing in place before covering dressing with large piece of transparent film.
- Avoid adhesive remover because it leaves a residue that hinders film adherence.

From Chua PC and others: Vacuum-assisted wound closure, *Am J Nurs* 100(12):45, 2000.

Steps	Rationale
b. Connect the dressing tubing to the canister tubing. Make sure both clamps are open.	
c. Place V.A.C. unit on a level surface, or hang from the foot of the bed. **NOTE: The V.A.C. unit will alarm and deactivate therapy if the unit is tilted beyond 45 degrees.**	
d. Press in green-lit power button, and set pressure as ordered.	
18. Discard old dressing materials, remove gloves, and perform hand hygiene.	Reduces transmission of microorganisms.
19. Inspect wound V.A.C. system to verify that negative pressure is achieved.	Negative pressure is achieved when an airtight seal is achieved (see Box 24-2).
a. Verify that display screen reads THERAPY ON.	
b. Be sure clamps are open and tubing is patent.	

Steps	Rationale

c. Identify air leaks by listening with stethoscope or by moving hand around edges of wound while applying light pressure.

d. If a leak is present, use strips of transparent film to patch areas around the edges of the wound.

20. See Completion Protocol (inside front cover).

• • • • • • • • • •

EVALUATION

1. Compare appearance of wound with previous assessment.
2. Ask client to rate pain using a scale of 0 to 10.
3. Verify airtight dressing seal and proper negative pressure.
4. Observe client or caregiver's ability to perform dressing change.

Unexpected Outcomes and Related Interventions

1. Wound appears inflamed and tender, drainage has increased, and an odor is present.
   a. Notify physician.
   b. Obtain wound culture.
   c. Increase frequency of dressing changes.
2. Client reports increase in pain.
   a. If using black foam, switch to the PVA foam product.
   b. Client may need more analgesic support when V.A.C. is first initiated.
   c. Negative pressure may need to be reduced.
3. Negative pressure seal has broken.
   a. Take preventive measures (see Box 24-2, p. 593).
   b. Shave surrounding skin.

4. Client or caregiver is unable to perform dressing change.
   a. Provide additional teaching and support.
   b. Obtain services of home care agency.

Recording and Reporting

- Record appearance of wound, color, characteristics of any drainage, presence of wound healing augmentation, such as wound V.A.C., and response to dressing change.
- Record date and time of dressing change on new dressing.
- Report brisk, bright bleeding, evidence of poor wound healing, evisceration or dehiscence, and possible wound infection to physician.

Sample Documentation

1100 Client and wife in wound clinic for V.A.C. dressing change. Wound on lower abdomen is pink, moist, and without edema in periwound region. Size decreased to 2 × 2.2 cm. Client states that there is less pain in wound area. Comfort achieved by 600 mg Motrin. Dressing is still changed every 48 hours. Wife correctly performed dressing change and activated wound V.A.C. to 125 mm Hg; continue with dressing changes every 48 hours.

 SPECIAL CONSIDERATIONS

Pediatric Considerations
- This wound application is not appropriate for fragile neonatal skin.
- Parents need to actively participate in wound V.A.C. treatment.

Geriatric Considerations
- Use skin care practices to protect periwound tissue. Transparent film may be irritating to fragile skin. Skin protectant is one method to reduce the risk of tissue injury.

- Visual impairment may prevent self-care and require home care services.

Home Care Considerations
- When wound V.A.C. is used in the home, the client and caregiver may benefit from initial visits with home care agency to monitor initial treatments.
- Provide information to family and caregiver regarding proper disposal of contaminated product.

CRITICAL THINKING EXERCISES

1. Compare and contrast techniques for securing dressings for the following clients:
   a. Client with an open wound on the anterior aspect of leg
   b. Client with an abdominal wound
   c. Client with a scalp wound
2. A client with a left trochanter wound was just admitted to a chronic wound service. The wound is 2 × 3 cm; edges are red; yellow, foul-smelling drainage is present; and the periwound area is swollen and tender to the touch. Wound V.A.C. is ordered. List, in order of priority, your nursing actions.
3. Mr. Bennet has a large stasis ulcer on his left lower leg. He requires wet-to-dry dressing changes every 8 hours. What aspect of his wound care must you do, and what can you delegate?

REFERENCES

Agency for Health Care Policy and Research: *Treatment of pressure ulcers*, Clinical practice guideline No.15, Rockville, Md, 1994, Agency for Health Care Policy and Research, Public Health Service, U.S. Department of Health and Human Services.

Argenta LC, Morykwas MJ: Vacuum-assisted closure: a new method for wound control and treatment–clinical experience, *Ann Plast Surg* 38(6):563, 1997.

Banwell PE, Holten IW, Martin DL: A new concept in wound healing: the management of wounds with negative pressure therapy, *Br J Surg* 82(suppl 2):149, 1998.

Barr JE: Physiology of healing: the basis for the principles of wound management, *Medsurg Nurs* 4(5):387, 1995.

Baxandall T: Healing cavity wounds with negative pressure, *Nurs Stand* 11(6):49, 1996.

Beshara M, Jameson G, Barr B: Practice development in acute and long-term care settings. In Bryant RA, editor: *Acute and chronic wounds: nursing management*, ed 2, St Louis, 2000, Mosby.

Bolton L, van Rijswijk L: Cost effective wound care, *Caet J,* 18(1):23.

Broussard CL, Menendez-Eastman S, Frantz R: Adjuvant wound therapies. In Bryant RA, editor: *Acute and chronic wounds: nursing management,* ed 2, St Louis, 2000, Mosby.

Cannavo M and others: A comparison of dressings in the management of surgical abdominal wounds, *J Wound Care* 7(2):57, 1998.

Chua PC and others: Vacuum-assisted wound closure, *Am J Nurs* 100(12):45, 2000.

Cuzzell J: Choosing a wound dressing, *Geriatr Nurs* 18(6): 269, 1997.

Evans L, Land L: Topical negative pressure for treating chronic wounds: a systematic review, *Br J Plast Surg* 54(3):238, 2001.

KCI USA: *The V.A.C.: Vacuum Assisted Closure: guidelines for use—physician and caregiver reference manual,* product information, San Antonio, Tex, 1999.

Krasner D, Kennedy KL: Using the no touch technique to change a dressing, *Nursing* 24(9):50, 1994.

Lueckenotte A: *Gerontologic Nursing,* ed 2, St Louis, 2000, Mosby.

Mendez-Eastman S: When wounds won't heal, *RN* 61(10): 20, 1998.

Perry AG, Potter PA: *Clinical nursing skills and techniques,* ed 5, St Louis, 2002, Mosby.

Ramundo J, Wells J: Wound debridement. In Bryant RA, editor: *Acute and chronic wounds: nursing management,* ed 2, St Louis, 2000, Mosby.

Rolstad BS, Ovington LG, Harris A: Principles of wound management. In Bryant RA, editor: *Acute and chronic wounds: nursing management,* ed 2, St Louis, 2000a, Mosby.

Rolstad BS, Ovington LG, Harris A: Wound care product formulary. In Bryant RA, editor: *Acute and chronic wounds: nursing management,* ed 2, St Louis, 2000b, Mosby.

Stotts NA and others: Sterile versus clean technique in postoperative wound care of patients with open surgical wounds: a pilot study, *J Wound Ostomy Continence Nurs* 24:10, 1997.

Van Rijswijk L: Recommendations to change the FDA classification of various wound dressings, *Ostomy Wound Manage* 45(3):31, 1999.

Wikblad K, Anderson B: A comparison of three wound dressings in patients undergoing heart surgery, *Nurs Res* 44(5):312, 1995.

Wong D and others: *Wong's essentials of pediatric nursing,* ed 6, St Louis, 2001, Mosby.

Wright K, McNichol LL: Home environment: implications for wound care practice development. In Bryant RA, editor: *Acute and chronic wounds: nursing management,* ed 2, St Louis, 2000, Mosby.

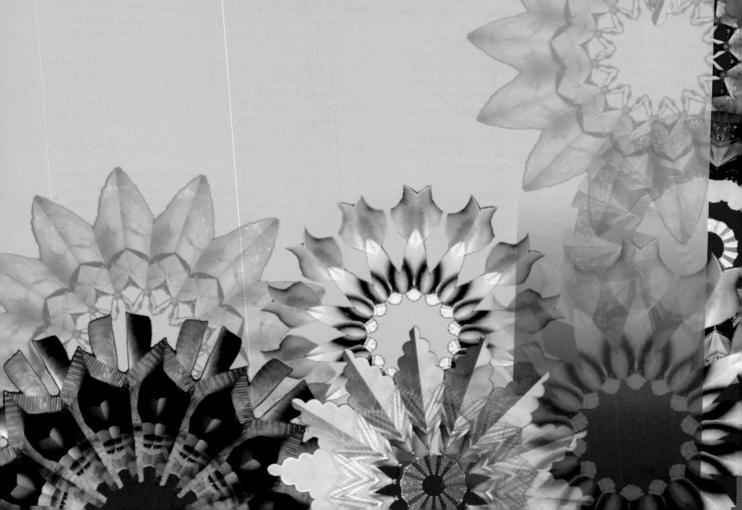

Therapeutic Use of Heat and Cold

There are benefits to the therapeutic application of heat and cold. The use of local heat produces vasodilation and a subsequent decrease in tissue congestion. Vasodilation leads to improved circulation at the capillary level. Kloth and others (2000) demonstrated an acceleration in wound healing with the use of noncontact radiant heat therapy. Additional benefits of the application of heat include analgesia, a decrease in muscle spasm, decreased muscle stiffness, and a decreased sensitivity to stretching (Stitik and Nadler, 1999). Risks associated with the application of heat are burns, bleeding, dehydration, maceration, and edema.

Local cold application produces vasoconstriction. Vasoconstriction results in decreased blood flow, relieving edema and soft tissue bleeding. Additional benefits include slowed nerve conduction and analgesia (Stitik and Nadler, 1998) (Table 25-1). Potential risks include chilling, ischemia, and frostbite.

Clients at greatest risk for adverse reactions to local heat and cold therapies are those with circulatory problems and sensory deficits (Lindsey, 1990). This would include clients with peripheral vascular disease, diabetes, and Raynaud's phenomenon. Other contraindications would be a known sensitivity to heat or cold, a concurrent health condition as with delayed wound healing or altered level of consciousness (Stitik and Nadler, 1998, 1999)

Normally sensory receptors adapt to changes in temperature, preventing awareness of changes before damage occurs. It is imperative to verify the temperature of hot and cold treatments before application and to assess the client's condition frequently (Table 25-2).

Table 25-1

Therapeutic Effects of Heat and Cold Applications

Therapy	Physiological Response	Therapeutic Benefit	Examples of Conditions Treated
Heat	Vasodilation	Improves blood flow to injured body part, promotes delivery of nutrients and removal of wastes, lessens venous congestion in injured tissues.	Inflamed or edematous body part; new surgical wound; infected wound; arthritis, degenerative joint disease; localized joint pain; muscle strains; low back pain; menstrual cramping; hemorrhoidal, perianal, and vaginal inflammation; local abscesses.
	Reduced blood viscosity	Improves delivery of leukocytes and antibiotics to wound site.	
	Reduced muscle tension	Promotes muscle relaxation and reduces pain from spasm or stiffness.	
	Increased tissue metabolism	Increases blood flow; provides local warmth.	
	Increased capillary permeability	Promotes movement of waste products and nutrients.	
Cold	Vasoconstriction	Reduces blood flow to injured body part, prevents edema formation, reduces inflammation	Immediately after direct trauma such as musculoskeletal sprains, or strains, fractures, muscle spasms; after superficial laceration or puncture wound; after minor burn; when malignancy is suspected in area of injury or pain; after injections; for arthritis, joint trauma.
	Local anesthesia	Reduces localized pain.	
	Reduced cell metabolism	Reduces oxygen needs of tissues.	
	Increased blood viscosity	Promotes blood coagulation at injury site.	
	Decreased muscle tension	Relieves pain.	

Table 25-2

Temperature	Centigrade Range	Fahrenheit Range
Very hot	41° to 46° C	105° to 115° F
Hot	37° to 41° C	98° to 105° F
Warm	34° to 37° C	93° to 98° F
Tepid	26° to 34° C	80° to 93° F
Cool	18° to 26° C	65° to 80° F
Cold	10° to 18° C	50° to 65° F

NURSING DIAGNOSES

Reasons for implementing hot and cold therapies can include **Acute Pain, Chronic Pain, Impaired Skin Integrity, Impaired Tissue Integrity,** and **Impaired Physical Mobility** related to inflammation or injury. Risks associated with these therapies include **Risk for Injury** and **Risk for Impaired Skin Integrity.** Each of these risks is greatest for clients with **Ineffective Tissue Perfusion, Disturbed Sensory Perception,** and **Acute Confusion** or **Chronic Confusion.** The nurse has an opportunity to teach about these therapies if the client has **Deficient Knowledge,** especially if use in the home is required.

Skill 25.1

Moist Heat

The application of moist heat refers to the process of applying a compress moistened with warmed solution to an affected area. The compress can be a clean cloth or sterile gauze if the integrity of the skin has been compromised. Compresses can be warmed and replaced intermittently or heated continuously if a temperature-controlled aquathermia pad (Figure 25-1) is placed over the compress (Stitik and Nadler, 1999). The affected area may also be fully immersed in warm water. This may be done with a basin, with a whirlpool treatment (Figure 25-2), or a sitz bath.

Moist heat penetrates quickly and deeply. Heat effectively increases the temperature of subcutaneous tissue. Care to prevent burns must be taken because heat application may raise the temperature of the skin significantly (Brandt, 1998). If unchecked, maceration due to moist heat application may occur. Never use a microwave to heat a compress. The temperatures achieved are often unreliable, increasing the risk of burn.

Always make the client as comfortable as possible during an application. The use of a blanket or the client's clothing may aid in the prevention of chilling.

ASSESSMENT

1. Inspect wound for, size, color, drainage volume and character, presence of pain (rate on 0 to 10 scale), and odor. *Rationale: Provides a baseline to determine changes in wound following heat application.*
2. Assess skin around wound for integrity, color, temperature, edema, pain, and sensitivity. *Rationale: This provides a baseline to determine changes in skin following heat application.*
3. Measure affected joint range of motion. *Rationale: This provides baseline to determine changes in joint mobility.*

4. Assess client for altered perception of heat (e.g., diabetic neuropathy, victims of stroke, spinal cord injury).
5. Assess blood pressure and heart rate for client using moist heat. *Rationale: Client may become hypotensive during procedures. Helps to identify risks.*

PLANNING

Expected outcomes focus on increasing mobility, decreasing pain, and decreasing signs and symptoms of inflammation while preventing burns.

Expected Outcomes

1. Client's wound size and character are improved after multiple treatments.
2. Client's skin remains intact, and skin color, temperature, edema, pain, and sensitivity to touch improve after multiple treatments (client's skin may be slightly red and warm after treatment).
3. Client's joint mobility will improve.

Equipment

All Moist Heat

- Bath blanket
- Warmed prescribed solution
- Dry bath towel.

Compresses

- Waterproof pad
- Ties or cloth tape
- Aquathermia pad

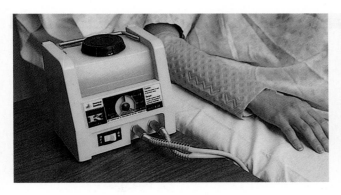

Figure 25-1   Aquathermia pad.

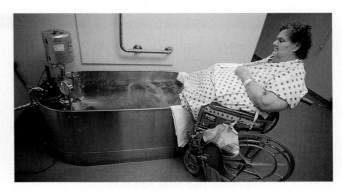

Figure 25-2   Whirlpool moist heat therapy.

Clean Compress

- Clean basin
- Clean gauze or towel

Sterile Compress

- Sterile basin
- Clean gloves
- Sterile gloves
- Biohazard waste bag

Soak or Sitz Bath

- Clean or sterile basin or sitz bath
- Biohazard waste bag

Delegation Considerations

The application of heat to intact skin may be delegated to assistive personnel (AP). The skill of moist heat application requires the critical thinking and knowledge application unique to nurse to assess and evaluate the condition of the client's skin.

- Caution AP to maintain proper temperature of the application.
- Instruct AP on skin changes to immediately report to nurse.

IMPLEMENTATION FOR MOIST HEAT

Steps	Rationale
1. See Standard Protocol (inside front cover).	
2. Provide warmth for client, and position for comfort.	Prevents chilling by preventing heat loss.
3. Place waterproof pad under client (except for sitz bath).	Protects bed linen from moisture.
4. Apply moist compress.	
a. Clean moist compress to intact skin	
(1) Heat prescribed solution to desired temperature by immersing closed bottle in warm water.	
(2) Test temperature of solution by pouring small amount over forearm.	Prevents burns by ensuring proper temperature.
(3) Pour solution into clean basin.	
(4) Place gauze or towel into solution.	
(5) Remove gauze or towel from basin.	

NURSE ALERT   *If there is bleeding, redness, underlying inflammation, or elevated body temperature, do not apply heat because it may exacerbate the problem (Perry and Potter, 2002).*

Steps	Rationale
b. Sterile moist compress to open skin	Ensures gauze remains sterile.
(1) Heat prescribed solution to desired temperature by immersing closed bottle in warm water.	
(2) Test temperature of solution by pouring small amount over forearm. Solution should feel warm but not uncomfortably so.	Prevents burns by ensuring proper temperature.
(3) Open package of sterile gauze. Pour solution onto gauze. *Option:* Place gauze in sterile basin and pour solution.	
(4) Remove dressing, inspect wound, dispose of old dressing and gloves.	

COMMUNICATION TIP   *Tell the client that the treatment should feel warm but that the nurse should be informed if any discomfort develops, requiring termination of the treatment.*

---

(5) **Don sterile gloves.**	Allows for manipulation of gauze without contaminating it.
(6) Remove sterile gauze from basin or waterproof package.	
5. Wring excess moisture from compress, and place lightly on area.	Excessive moisture causes skin maceration and increases potential for skin breakdown.
6. Assess the area for tolerance to application of the compress (redness, discomfort).	Increased redness may indicate burn.
7. Cover with clean or sterile dry dressing and then a dry bath towel.	Encloses gauze to prevent rapid cooling.
8. Secure with ties if necessary.	
9. Repeat Steps 1 to 8 every 5 minutes or as ordered.	Prevents cooling and maintains therapeutic benefit of compress.
10. If desired, apply aquathermia pad over compress for the desired time or as ordered. (see Skill 25.2, p. 602).	Maintains constant temperature to compress.

NURSE ALERT   *Local application of heat greater than 20 to 30 minutes without interruption may result in changes to the microcirculation, such as vasoconstriction (Stitik and Nadler, 1999).*

---

11. Provide warm soak to intact or open skin.	Cleansing area prevents transfer of microorganisms.
a. Cleanse intact skin around open area with clean cloth and soap and water or sterile gauze (sterile gloves needed) and sterile water.	
b. Pour heated solution into clean or sterile basin (see agency policy). Test temperature as described in Step 4b(2).	
c. Remove dressing, and dispose of it and gloves.	
d. Immerse affected area into solution.	Immersion needed for full therapeutic benefit.
e. Every 10 minutes empty solution and replace with new.	Ensures proper temperature and prevents the transfer of microorganisms.
12. Provide sitz bath to intact or open skin.	Sitz bath may be disposable (see illustration) or special device with circulating water and temperature.
a. Set disposable sitz bath under toilet seat, hang bag above the level of the toilet seat, and connect tubing into sitz bath.	Establishes route for stream of water.
b. Pour heated solution into bag. Test temperature of solution as in Step 4b(2).	Prevents burning of client's skin.
c. Fill sitz bath one-third full of solution from the bag by opening the clamp on the tubing.	Allows for immersion of perineal area when client sits in sitz bath.

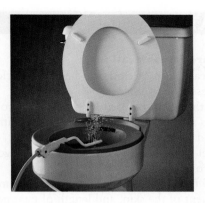

Step 12 Disposable sitz bath. (Courtesy Andermac, Inc. Yuba City, California.)

Steps	Rationale

d. If there is a dressing, remove it and dispose of it and gloves.

e. Assist client with sitting in solution.

f. Loosen clamp to regulate flow of warmed water.

NURSE ALERT *Clients with a history of cardiac difficulty may develop hypotension. Be alert for dizziness and light-headedness. Monitor blood pressure.*

---

g. Every 5 to 10 minutes assess client's vital signs and level of comfort.

Determines tolerance of treatment.

h. Remove treatment after a total of 20 minutes. For positive therapeutic effects, the sitz bath may be repeated after the client has been out of the bath for 15 minutes.

Allows for assessment of affected area and tolerance for the procedure.

13. See Completion Protocol (inside front cover).

• • • • • • • • • •

EVALUATION

1. Assess wound for size, color, drainage volume and character, and odor.
2. Ask client to rate pain on 0 to 10 or other appropriate scale.
3. Assess skin around wound and in area for integrity, color, temperature, edema, pain, and sensitivity.
4. Measure affected joint range of motion.

Unexpected Outcomes and Related Interventions

1. Client's wound remains the same size or is larger, has the same or increased amount of drainage of the same or different color, consistency, and amount.
   a. Report to physician.
   b. In collaboration with other health care team members, evaluate effectiveness of concurrent therapies and plan alternative treatments.
2. Client's skin area is broken, erythematous and warm, hypersensitive to touch, and blistered either during treatment or up to 30 minutes after treatment.
   a. Stop treatment.

   b. Report to physician.
   c. Ensure proper temperatures, or check equipment for proper functioning.
   d. Collaborate with physician to treat complications.

Recording and Reporting

• Describe in Nurse's Notes condition of surrounding skin and affected area, type of therapy, time of application, and client's response.

Sample Documentation

0930 Warm moist compress applied for complaint of pain (rating 5 on 0 to 10 scale) at discontinued intravenous (IV) site left (L) forearm. Area red, edematous, 6 cm long, 3 cm wide, slightly raised, tender to touch, and warm. States has been worsening since IV discontinued early AM.

   0950 Moist compress discontinued. No drainage noted, area pink, 4.5 cm long, 2.5 cm wide, pain rated 2 on 0 to 10 scale. Client reports "feels much better."

   1020 L forearm swelling 3 cm long, 2 cm wide, pain 1 on 0 to 10 scale.

SPECIAL CONSIDERATIONS

Pediatric Considerations

- Discourage parents from using heat-producing creams before examination.
- Perform frequent neurovascular evaluations to ensure adequate blood flow.

Geriatric Considerations

- Older clients have thinner, more fragile skin, especially those undergoing long-term steroid therapy.
- Check skin after 2 minutes and every 5 minutes thereafter.
- Ask for client's subjective pain assessment whenever assessing skin.

Home Care Considerations

- Any clean basin or cloth can be used for clean moist compresses or soaks.
- The bathtub can be used for sitz baths, provided the client is safe and the tub is cleaned with antiseptic before and after each treatment.
- A towel immersed in warmed water is a good clean warm compress.
- Careful teaching is needed about temperature control, assessment of the skin, and length of treatment.
- Remind clients to never use a microwave oven to heat compresses. Burns can easily result.

Long-Term Care Considerations

A warm gentle shower substitutes for a warm soak if not contraindicated.

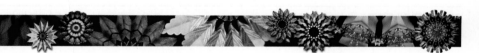

Skill 25.2

Dry Heat

Dry heat can be applied directly to the skin with an aquathermia pad, an electric heating pad, or a commercial heat pack. Dry heat treatments penetrate superficially but maintain temperature changes longer than moist heat treatments. This superficial heating is not effective in penetrating deep joints such as the knee or hip (Brandt, 1998). The temperature and duration of these treatments must be controlled carefully. It is important to protect the client from burns, skin dryness, and loss of body fluids through diaphoresis. Special consideration must be given to clients returning home with this therapy. A review of appropriate use and safety should be completed to decrease any risk of injury.

ASSESSMENT

1. Ask the client to report pain on scale of 0 to 10 or other appropriate scale. *Rationale: This provides baseline to determine if pain relief is achieved.*
2. Assess range of motion of body part. *Rationale: This provides baseline to determine changes in joint mobility.*
3. Assess client's skin for integrity, color, temperature, sensitivity to touch, blistering, and excessive dryness. *Rationale: Establishes baseline for condition of skin.*
4. Check temperature level of external heating device, to make sure it functions properly.

PLANNING

Expected outcomes focus on decreasing pain and improving mobility while preventing burns and dehydration.

Expected Outcomes

1. Client reports decreased level of pain.
2. Client's range of motion increases.
3. Client's skin remains intact, pink, warm, and sensitive to touch, with no excessive dryness and no blisters. Immediately after treatment, skin may be pink to red and warm.

Equipment

- Aquathermia pad, electric heating pad, or commercial chemical heat pack
- Bath towel
- Ties or tape

Delegation Considerations

Application of heat can be delegated to assistive personnel (AP). The skill of dry heat application requires the critical thinking and knowledge application unique to a nurse to assess and evaluate the condition of the client's skin.

- Caution AP to maintain proper temperature of the application.
- Caution AP to maintain application for only the length of time ordered by the physician.
- Caution AP to check client's skin for excessive redness and pain during application and to report any such adverse reactions to the nurse.
- Ask AP to report to the nurse when the treatment is completed so that the evaluation of the client's response can be made.

IMPLEMENTATION FOR DRY HEAT

Steps	Rationale
1. See Standard Protocol (inside front cover).	

COMMUNICATION TIP *Tell client that it is normal for treatment to feel warm, but that if it feels uncomfortably so, the nurse should be notified so the treatment can be evaluated.*

Steps	Rationale
2. Prepare heat application.	
a. Aquathermia pad	Ensures safe temperature application.
(1) Turn aquathermia unit on. Most units are preset to 105° F, or 40.5° C to 43° C (Perry and Potter, 2002).	
(2) If uncovered, wrap pad with towel.	Prevents heated surface from touching client's skin.
b. Electric heating pad	
(1) Turn pad on. Set temperature to low or medium.	

NURSE ALERT *A higher setting, over 105° F, should never be used (Perry and Potter, 2002). Avoid placing heat source under body part. Never position the client directly on pad.*

Steps	Rationale
(2) If uncovered, wrap pad with towel.	Prevents heated surface fom touching client's skin.
c. Commercial heat pack	
(1) Break pouch inside larger packet (follow manufacturer's instructions for use).	

NURSE ALERT *Do not puncture outer pack. Do not allow chemicals to come in contact with the skin or eyes.*

Steps	Rationale
(2) Knead chemicals.	Promotes release of heat.
(3) Wrap pack in washcloth or soft cloth.	Prevents direct exposure to the skin, reducing risk of burns.
3. Place heat application on intact skin.	Applications deliver warm heat to injured tissues.
4. Secure with cloth tape or ties.	

NURSE ALERT *To prevent electrical shock, never use pins to secure aquathermia or electric heating pad. A chemical heat pack will leak and cause burns if a pin is used to secure it.*

---

5. Monitor condition of site every 5 minutes, assessing client's tolerance of treatment.	Determines if heat exposure is resulting in burn.
6. Remove treatment after 20 minutes (or time ordered by physician).	Local application of heat greater than 20 minutes without interruption may result in changes to the microcirculation, such as vasoconstriction (Stitik & Nadler, 1989).
7. See Completion Protocol (inside front cover).	

• • • • • • • • • •

EVALUATION

1. Ask client to rate pain level on scale of 0 to 10 or other appropriate scale.
2. Measure client's range of motion.
3. Assess client's skin for integrity, color, temperature, dryness, and blistering. Evaluate again after 30 minutes.
4. Assess client's skin turgor to determine hydration status.

Unexpected Outcomes and Related Interventions

1. Client reports increased pain.
   a. Stop treatment.
   b. Assess skin for signs of burns.
   c. Report to physician.
   d. Reduce temperatures for susceptible client.
   e. Check for proper function of equipment.
2. Client's range of motion is decreased.
   a. Report to physician.
   b. In collaboration with other health care team members, evaluate effectiveness of concurrent therapies and plan new treatments.
3. Client's skin is broken, red, excessively warm, dry, and blistered.
   a. Stop treatment.
   b. Report to physician.
   c. In collaboration with physician, begin treatment of complications.

4. Client's skin turgor is inelastic.
   a. Assess client's vital signs and fluid intake and output (I&O).
   b. Begin measuring I&O if not ordered.
   c. Report vital signs, I&O, and skin turgor to physician.
   d. Prepare to encourage fluids or administer IV fluids as ordered by physician.

Recording and Reporting

• Record pain level.
• Record range of motion of body part.
• Record skin integrity, color, temperature, sensitivity to touch, dryness, and blistering.
• Record skin turgor.
• Record temperature and duration of treatment.
• Record client tolerance of treatment.

Sample Documentation

1000 Heating pad set on low, applied to right bicep for complaint of pain with motion. Pain severity 6 on 0 to 10 scale. Flexion 140 degrees and extension 20 degrees. Skin intact, pink, warm, turgor elastic.

1020 Heating pad removed. Right bicep pink to red and warm. No blisters, turgor elastic. States feels light touch to affected area. States pain 2 on 0 to 10 scale. Flexion 145 degrees, extension 20 degrees.

1050 Left bicep pink and warm.

SPECIAL CONSIDERATIONS

Pediatric Considerations

- Discourage parents from using heat-producing creams before examination.
- Teach parents home and activity safety to prevent recurrent soft tissue and musculoskeletal injuries.
- Further assessment in children with frequent soft tissue or musculoskeletal injuries may be necessary.
- Assess body temperature gain and loss, which occur more readily in pediatric clients.

Geriatric Considerations

- Older clients have thinner, more fragile skin that is more susceptible to burns.
- Ask for client's subjective pain assessment whenever assessing the skin.
- Use extreme caution with electric heating pads in older clients.

Home Care Considerations

- Client teaching is very important to prevent burns. Teaching should emphasize the purpose of the treatment, the temperature setting and duration of treatment, demonstration of treatment, and the importance of frequent skin assessments.
- Assess client's use of alternative treatments at home (e.g., use of rice socks or herb packs). Educate clients in proper use of such treatments.
- Remind clients that the microwave oven must never be used to heat chemical heat packs. Burns can easily result.

Long-Term Care Considerations

- Check skin after 2 minutes of beginning therapy and every 5 minutes thereafter.
- Older clients are less sensitive to pain.
- Use sterile materials when used with open skin.
- The safest dry heat treatment for older clients is one with good temperature control such as an aquathermia pad with the temperature set lower than 100° F.

Skill 25.3

Cold Compresses and Ice Bags

Cold treatment has long been accepted as the treatment of choice for acute soft tissue injuries (MacAuley, 2001). Pasero (1999) indicates that the use of cold therapy for pain relief is indicated in the presence of swelling, bleeding, trauma, and acute soft tissue injury.

Rest, compression bandages, such as snug elastic wraps, and elevation of the injured area are all adjunct therapies to the vasoconstriction provided by ice. All contribute to decreased blood flow, which prevents bruising, edema, and pain. RECIPE has become the acronym of choice to include all aspects of the healing of musculoskeletal injuries (Lindsey, 1990) (Box 25-1). The acronym RICE (Box 25-2) is also an effective tool in managing musculoskeletal injuries (Stitik and Nadler, 1998).

To deliver cold treatments, simple ice bags or compresses work well. Commercial reusable gel packs and instant disposable chemical ice bags are available, as are electronically controlled cooling devices.

ASSESSMENT

1. Assess client's pain on scale of 0 to 10. *Rationale: Provides baseline to determine pain relief.*

2. Assess area of injury for edema and bleeding. *Rationale: Provides baseline to determine changes in soft tissue following treatment.*

3. Assess surrounding skin for integrity, color, temperature, and sensitivity to touch. *Rationale: This provides baseline for determining change in condition of injured tissues.*

PLANNING

Expected outcomes focus on decreasing pain, edema, bleeding, and bruising while preventing ischemia.

Expected Outcomes

1. Client will report decreased pain.
2. Client's skin or area of injury will have less edema and bleeding.
3. Client's surrounding skin will remain intact, be pink and warm, and remain sensitive to touch. Immediately after treatment the client's skin may be pale, cool, and less sensitive to touch.

Box 25-1

RECIPE Acronym

Rest
Elevation
Compression
Ice
Proper
Exercise

Box 25-2

RICE Acronym

Rest
Ice
Compression
Elevation

Equipment

All Compresses, Bags, and Packs

- Soft cloth covering, stockinette, towel, or pillowcase
- Cloth tapes or ties
- Bath towel
- Bath blanket for warmth

Cold Compress

- Towel or gauze
- Prescribed solution, ice
- Basin

Ice Bag

- Ice bag
- Ice chips and water
- Reusable commercial gel pack (cold pack)
- Disposable commercial chemical cold pack
- Electrically controlled cooling device (cooling blanket)
- Gauze roll or elastic wrap

Delegation Considerations

The application of cold therapy to intact skin may be delegated to assistive personnel (AP). The skill of cold application requires the critical thinking and knowledge unique to a nurse to assess and evaluate the condition of the client's skin.

- Caution AP to maintain proper temperature of the application.
- Caution AP to maintain application for only the length of time ordered by the physician.
- Caution AP to check client's skin for excessive redness or pain and immediately report any such adverse reactions to the nurse.
- Ask AP to report to the nurse when the treatment is complete so that the evaluation of the client can be made.

IMPLEMENTATION FOR COLD COMPRESSES AND ICE BAGS

Steps	Rationale
1. See Standard Protocol (inside front cover).	
2. Provide warm covering for client.	To prevent chilling.
3. Position client carefully, keeping affected body part in proper alignment and exposing only the area to be treated.	Prevents further injury to area. Avoids unnecessary exposure of body parts, maintaining client's warmth, comfort, and privacy.

4. Prepare cold application.
  a. Cold compress
    (1) Place ice and water into basin.
    (2) Test temperature of solution by pouring small amount over forearm.
    (3) Place gauze or towel into solution.
    (4) Wring excess solution from compress.
	Prevents injury to client's skin

Steps	**Rationale**

COMMUNICATION TIP   *Tell client that there is a normal progression of sensation changes during cold therapy: cold, then pain relief followed by burning skin pain, and finally numbness.*

---

b. Ice pack or bag

    (1) Fill bag with water, then empty.

Prevents skin maceration by testing for leaks.

    (2) Fill bag two-thirds full with ice and water.

    (3) Express air from bag.

Allows ice bag to conform to area and promotes maximum contact.

    (4) Secure closure and wipe bag dry.

    (5) Place in second bag if desired.

Reduces risk of spillage from ice pack.

    (6) Wrap pack with towel, stockinette, or pillowcase or cover client's skin with towel.

NURSE ALERT   *Sterile supplies must be used with open wounds.*

---

c. Commercial gel pack

    (1) Remove pack from freezer.

    (2) Wrap pack in towel, stockinette, or pillowcase (optional if client's skin is covered).

Prevents direct exposure of skin to cold application.

    (3) Cover client's skin with towel if pack is uncovered (see illustration).

Covering prevents direct exposure of cold application to the skin, reducing risk of tissue injury.

d. Electrically or gravity controlled cooling device (see illustration)

    (1) Make sure all connections are intact and temperature (if adjustable) is set. (See agency policy, physician's order, and manufacturer's directions.)

Ensures safe temperature for application.

    (2) Cover cool water flow pad with towel .

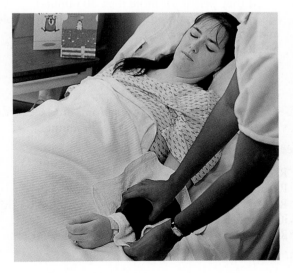

Step 4c(3)   Protecting client's skin.

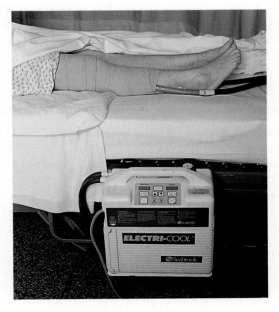

Step 4d   Electric cooling device.

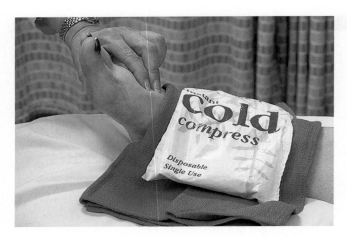

Step 5 Applying a cold compress.

Steps	Rationale
5. Apply cold application to skin (see illustration).	Direct cold applications should never be placed directly on the skin because damage can occur to underlying tissues from direct exposure to cold.
6. Secure with gauze roll, cloth tape, or ties.	Ensures even application of cold therapy.
7. Remove treatment when client reports numbness (Maher and others, 1998). The actual duration of treatment may vary but generally ranges from 20 to 30 minutes every 2 hours (Stitik and Nadler, 1998). Stop treatment if client reports the area being cooled feels "hot."	Indicates that vasodilation from the application of cold may be occurring (Stitik and Nadler, 1998), increasing edema.
8. See Completion Protocol (inside front cover).	

• • • • • • • • • •

EVALUATION

1. Ask client to report pain level on scale of 0 to 10.
2. Inspect tissue or wound for edema, bruising, and bleeding.
3. Assess surrounding tissues for integrity, color, temperature, and sensitivity to touch. Reevaluate after 30 minutes.

Unexpected Outcomes and Related Interventions

1. Client expresses increased pain in tissues.
   a. Remove treatment.
   b. Maintain immobility and good alignment.
   c. Report to physician.
   d. Collaborate with other health care team members to determine effectiveness of concurrent therapies and diagnostic tests. Together plan revised diagnostics and care.
2. Client has increased bleeding, bruising, and edema.
   a. Remove treatment.
   b. Apply compress for bleeding or bruising.
   c. Elevate edematous area if not contraindicated.
   d. Report to physician if symptoms are excessive or if they persist for more than 30 minutes.
3. Client's skin is mottled, reddened, or bluish-purple and cold with breaks.
   a. Remove treatment.
   b. Position tissues in dependent manner if not contraindicated.
   c. Apply warm blanket.
   d. Report to physician if symptoms are excessive or if they persist for more than 30 minutes.

Recording and Reporting

- Record pain level.
- Record bleeding, bruising, and edema.
- Record skin integrity, color, temperature, and sensitivity to touch.
- Record temperature and duration of treatment.

Sample Documentation

0930 Left ankle edematous following twisting injury. Ankle measures 32 cm at medial malleolus and 31 cm across metatarsal region of foot. Pain reported at 7 on 0 to 10 scale. Ecchymosis present, extending 8 cm on medial aspect with surrounding skin warm, pink. Dorsalis pedis and posterior tibialis pulses present and strong. Left extremity elevated with ice pack applied to ankle.

0950 Ice pack removed from ankle. Ankle measures 32 cm. Pain reported at 2 on 0 to 10 scale. Ecchymosis 8 cm on medial aspect of ankle. Skin pink and cool; states numbness upon palpation.

1020 Ankle measures 32 cm. Pain reported at 2 on 0 to 10 scale. Skin pink, warm, client denies numbness or tingling. Pedal pulses present unchanged. Client medicated with hydrocodone 5/500 1 tab.

 ## SPECIAL CONSIDERATIONS

Pediatric Considerations
- Discourage parents from using heat-producing creams before examination.
- Teach parents home and activity safety to prevent recurrent soft tissue and musculoskeletal injuries.
- Further assessment in children with frequent soft tissue or musculoskeletal injuries may be necessary.

Geriatric Considerations
- Older clients are more sensitive to cold.
- Stay with client for first 5 minutes of treatment to assess subjective response.
- Anticipate shortening duration of treatment.
- Assess skin every 2 to 3 minutes after the first 10 minutes of treatment.
- Older clients may require more covering for warmth.

Home Care Considerations
- Gel packs kept in the freezer at home make easy cold treatments.
- Avoid leaving extremity dependent when applying cold treatments (Stitik and Nadler, 1998).
- A Styrofoam cup of ice may be used to treat a sprain.
- A bag of frozen vegetables or snow conforms nicely to an affected area and is effective for brief periods of treatment (Wong and others, 2001).

CRITICAL THINKING EXERCISES

1. Allen has been a nurse on the medical/surgical floor for 3 months. He works nights. One of his geriatric clients has been admitted to the unit following a slip and fall on the ice outside his home. The client's physician has ordered ice packs 20 minutes on and 30 minutes off to the right ankle. What pretreatment assessments should Allen make? If delegated to AP, what are Allen's responsibilities in this case? What special considerations should Allen make with regard to this particular client?

2. Your 21-year-old client in the clinic has an inflamed and painful right elbow from a fall sustained 3 hours earlier while skateboarding. He has been diagnosed with a sprain of his elbow. He states he has used both heat and cold treatments on various injuries in the past and he is not sure which would be best. The physician has told the client to use whichever works best for him. Based on your knowledge of cold and heat therapy, what criteria would you use to determine which therapy would work best?

3. Your client is status 1-day post hemorrhoidectomy. You have completed your assessment, and she has requested that you set up her sitz bath in the bathroom. She was medicated 45 minutes ago with hydrocodone 5/500 1 tab. She has been out of bed to a bedside commode but has not ventured to the bathroom. Her vital signs are temperature, 37.2° C oral; pulse, 105 beats per minute; respirations, 20 breaths per minute; and blood pressure, 90/58 mm Hg. She reports she is drowsy. The AP assigned to work with you indicates he will be happy to handle the sitz bath with this client. How would you proceed in this instance?

REFERENCES

Brandt K: The importance of nonpharmacologic approaches in management of osteoarthritis, *Am J Med* 105(1B): 39S, 1998.

Kloth LC and others.: Effects of a normothermic dressing on pressure ulcer healing, *Adv Skin Wound Care* 13(2):69, 2000.

Lindsey B: Client care guidelines: cold and heat application in musculoskeletal injury, *J Emerg Nurs* 16(1):54, 1990.

MacAuley D: Do textbooks agree on their advice on ice? *Clin J Sports Med* 11:67, 2001.

Maher AB and others: *Orthopaedic Nursing*, ed 7, Philadelphia, 1998, Saunders.

Pasero C: Using superficial cooling for pain control, *Am J Nurs* 99(3):24, 1999.

Perry A, Potter P: *Clinical nursing skills and techniques*, ed 5, St Louis, 2002, Mosby.

Stitik T, Nadler S: When—and how—to use cold most effectively, *Consultant* 38(12):2881, 1998.

Stitik T, Nadler S: When—and how—to apply the heat, *Consultant* 39(1):144, 1999.

Wong DL and others: *Wong's essentials of pediatric nursing*, ed 6, St Louis, 2001.

CHAPTER

26

Special Mattresses and Beds

There are a variety of special mattresses and beds to reduce the client's risk of skin breakdown and other risks associated with decreased mobility. These should be used in conjunction with other risk reduction interventions (Agency for Health Care Policy and Research [AHCPR], 1992, 1994; Maklebust, 1999). These support surfaces can be categorized as mattress overlays, replacement mattresses, and specialty beds. They have differing purposes, including pressure reduction, pressure relief, shear and friction reduction, moisture control, repositioning, and support of the morbidly obese client. These beds are used in acute, rehabilitative, long-term, and home care settings. Although they are designed to reduce the hazards of immobility to the skin and musculoskeletal system, no bed or mattress totally eliminates the need for meticulous nursing care.

Tissue damage occurs when the pressure exerted on the capillaries is high enough to close the capillaries. The normal capillary pressure (the amount of pressure that keeps vessels open) is considered to be 12 to 32 mm Hg (Pieper, 2000). When the capillary closing pressure is exceeded (for example, when pressure above 32 mm Hg is applied over the vessels), the capillaries begin to collapse. In a normal healthy adult, high capillary pressures stimulate a shifting of body weight to relieve pressure on the affected tissue. Repositioning helps to avoid tissue compression and subsequent ischemia. When immobility prevents these natural shifts in weight, tissue is compressed between the skeletal structure and the mattress, resulting in tissue damage (see Chapter 23).

For clients with restricted mobility, chronic diseases or disabilities, and older adults, pressure management on tissue is a significant nursing concern because these clients lack the ability to reposition themselves. Special support mattresses and beds are frequently used to reduce or relieve pressure on tissues (Wind, Tomaselli, and Goldberg, 1993). According to Fletcher (1997), pressure-relieving devices consistently maintain external skin pressure at below 32 mm Hg, whereas a pressure-reducing device maintains external skin pressures at lower than a standard hospital mattress, but does not consistently reduce pressure to less than capillary closing pressure.

Several support surfaces reduce friction, shear, and moisture. Mattresses or beds with a slick surface help decrease friction and shear. Surfaces with porous covers allow airflow, which reduces moisture, resulting in less chance of skin maceration.

Support surfaces designed for pressure management may also incorporate lateral rotation therapy, percussion, or vibration to aid in pulmonary management, or pulsation to improve cutaneous circulation. The Rotokinetic bed provides skeletal alignment with constant side-to-side rotation up to 90 degrees (Tomaselli, Goldberg, and Wind, 2001). The bariatric bed, also called an obesity bed, is wider and sturdier than standard hospital beds. It is useful in the care of the morbidly obese client.

Static devices (pressure-reducing) are nonpowered. Examples are mattress overlays made of foam, gel, and water and some air mattresses. The Agency for Health Care Policy and Research (AHCPR) (1994) recommends use of a static support surface if the client cannot assume a variety of positions without bearing weight on a pressure ulcer. For clients with stage III or IV pressure ulcers on multiple turning surfaces of the body, a low-air-loss or air-fluidized bed may be indicated.

Dynamic devices (pressure-relieving) have moving parts. Examples are alternating air mattresses, air-fluidized beds, low-air-loss beds or overlays, Rotokinetic beds, and some bariatric beds. The AHCPR (1994) recommends the use of a dynamic support surface if a client cannot assume a variety of positions and if the client fully compresses a static device.

NURSING DIAGNOSES

Multiple conditions (e.g., cerebrovascular accident, head injury, multiple sclerosis, spinal cord injury) may limit mobility and necessitate the use of specialty beds. When a client has **Impaired Physical Mobility** or **Impaired Bed Mobility,** pressure reduction/relief or rotational beds may lessen the effects of immobility. Clients with actual or risk for **Impaired Skin Integrity** or **Impaired Tissue Integrity** may benefit from the use of pressure reduction/relief surfaces to counteract the combined effects of immobility, pressure friction, shear, and moisture.

The client may experience **Anxiety** and **Fear,** especially with the use of kinetic beds. The constant turning and rigid structure may contribute to sympathetic stimulation, restlessness, increased tension, and apprehension.

With air-fluidized beds, diaphoresis may go undetected. Therefore the client may experience **Risk for Deficient Fluid Volume.**

The client may also have **Deficient Knowledge** related to the effects of tissue compression. An explanation of the rationale for the use of the device may affect cooperation and acceptance of the therapy.

Skill 26.1

Using a Support Surface Overlay or Mattress

An overlay rests on top of the hospital mattress and uses foam, air, water, gel, or combinations of these products to reduce or relieve pressure. Other surfaces actually replace the standard hospital mattress.

A 4-inch dense foam mattress overlay is a static, pressure-reducing device with head, trunk, and foot sections with varying degrees of foam density and contours that reduce pressure in these areas (Figure 26-1). An optional protective film sleeve is available to protect the foam from soiling and to decrease heat and moisture. These overlays can be used for prevention of pressure ulcers or for clients with existing pressure ulcers who can be turned and repositioned on at least two intact skin surfaces. It is important to note that the 2-inch convoluted foam pads are for comfort only and do not reduce pressure (Whittemore, 1998) .

Air mattress overlays can be static or dynamic and consist of interconnected air cells or cushions inflated once by the use of a blower (Figure 26-2). These mattresses use a pressure-cycling device to intermittently inflate and deflate or to maintain constant inflation and slight air movement in the mattress.

Replacement mattresses are denser, thicker, and more resilient to weight and actually decrease pressure to a greater degree than some overlays (Vyhlidal and others, 1997). Replacement mattresses have built-in foam, gel, air, or fluid sections that can be customized to the needs of a specific client with moderate to high risk for skin breakdown (Figure 26-3). Another available option is an air mattress that replaces the conventional mattress. These mattresses may also be fully integrated into the bed. Air mattresses can be used for clients with moderate to high risk for skin breakdown. Air mattresses must be deflated before initiating cardiopulmonary resuscitation (CPR). Most units have instant-deflate mechanisms to provide a hard surface for chest compressions.

Use of support surfaces simply aids in pressure reduction or relief. Clients still must be repositioned regularly and have meticulous skin care and range-of-joint-motion exercises to reduce complications of immobility such as pressure ulcers, pulmonary congestion, and contractures.

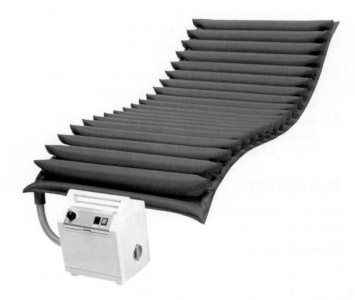

Figure 26-2   Dynamic air mattress overlay. (© 2002 Hill-Rom Services, Inc. Reprinted with permission—All rights reserved.)

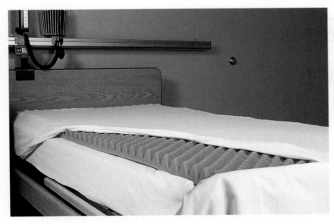

Figure 26-1   "Egg-crate" foam overlay is primarily for comfort.

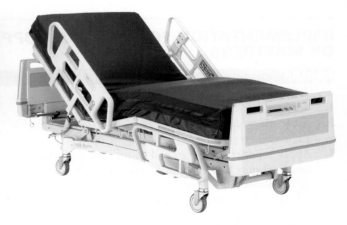

Figure 26-3   Air-integrated replacement mattress. (© 2002 Hill-Rom Services, Inc. Reprinted with permission— All rights reserved.)

ASSESSMENT

1. Determine client's risk for pressure ulcer formation using a validated risk assessment tool such as the Braden scale. *Rationale: Risk assessment tools as suggested by the AHCPR (e.g., Braden scale) provide an objective measure of risk consistent between evaluators over time.*

2. Perform routine skin assessment, especially over dependent sites and bony prominences. Look for changes in color (erythema or pallor), texture (edema or induration), temperature (warmth or coolness), blistering, or ulceration. *Rationale: Provides baseline on ongoing data to determine change in skin integrity or change in existing pressure ulcer.*

3. Assess client's level of comfort and using a 0 to 10 scale of pain. *Rationale: Client may require pain medication to tolerate movement to another bed/mattress surface. Inadequate pain control may limit client's tolerance of position changes.*

4. Assess client's understanding of purposes of support surfaces. *Rationale: Misconceptions can affect client's cooperation in use of support surface.*

5. Verify physician's order for surface. *Rationale: A physician's order is usually required for third-party payment of the support surface.*

PLANNING

Expected outcomes focus on maintenance of skin integrity and client comfort.

Expected Outcomes

1. Client's skin remains intact without evidence of abnormal reactive hyperemia or mottling.
2. Existing pressure ulcers show evidence of healing by formation of granulation tissue.
3. Client rates comfort no greater than a 4 (on a scale of 0 to 10).

Equipment

- Risk assessment tool (see Chapter 23)
- Foam overlay (see Figure 26-1, p. 613)
- Air mattress overlay (see Figure 26-2, p. 613)
- Replacement mattress (see Figure 26-3, p. 613)
- Sheet(s)
- Disposable gloves (if soiled linen is being handled)
- Standard bed frame (with mattress if overlay is to be used)

Delegation Considerations

The skills of applying support surface mattresses or preparation of an alternative bed can be delegated to assistive personnel (AP); however, assessment of the need for a special support surface, choice of type to use, client teaching, and evaluation of effectiveness requires critical thinking and knowledge application unique to a nurse. Inform and assist the care provider in proper method of applying support surface to bed. Encourage the care provider to obtain assistance when positioning the client to reduce risk of friction and shear and to prevent self-injury. Explain to the care provider the rationale for the client to be routinely repositioned even though the client is on the support surface. Caution the care provider to routinely inspect the skin, bony prominences, and heels for signs of pressure and to notify the nurse to conduct assessment when abnormalities are noted.

IMPLEMENTATION FOR USING A SUPPORT SURFACE OVERLAY OR MATTRESS

Steps	Rationale
1. See Standard Protocol (inside front cover).	
2. Close room door or bedside curtain. Assist client to a chair when possible.	Provides client privacy during application of overlay or mattress. Eases application of device.
3. Apply support surface to bed or prepare alternate bed (bed may be occupied or unoccupied).	
a. *Replacement mattresses:*	
(1) Apply mattress to bed frame after removing standard hospital mattress.	Hospital mattress needs to be stored, or mattress replacements may be used instead of hospital mattresses.
(2) Apply sheet over mattress. Keep layers between client and surface to a minimum.	Sheet reduces soiling. Manufacturer's instructions may state that excessive layers of linen decrease the effectiveness of the support surface.

Steps	Rationale

b. *Air mattress/overlay:*
   (1) Apply deflated mattress over surface of bed mattress. (There may be directions on pad indicating which side to place up.)

Provides smooth, even surface.

NURSE ALERT *Avoid use of sharp objects near mattress.*

COMMUNICATION TIP *Tell client that the mattress may inflate and deflate periodically, may feel cool, and may require a period of adjustment.*

---

   (2) Bring plastic strips or flaps around corners of bed mattress.

Secures air mattress in place.

   (3) Attach connector on air mattress to inflation device. Inflate mattress to proper air pressure determined by air pump or blower.

Mattresses vary as to requiring one-time or continuous inflation cycle (Pieper, 2000). Manufacturer's directions indicate desired air pressure designed to distribute client's body weight evenly. Directions are included with each mattress (Pieper, 2000).

   (4) Place sheet over air mattress. Do not tighten sheet; however, be sure sheet is free of wrinkles.

Prevents soiling of mattress and reduces direct contact of skin against plastic surface.

   (5) Check air pump to be sure pressure cycle alternates if alternating air is used.

Alternating airflow mattress produces intermittent cycling, inflating only parts of mattress at any one time. Intermittent cycle continually alternates pressure against skin and soft tissue (Whittemore, 1998).

c. *Air-surface bed:*
   (1) Obtain and make bed.

Bed may be available in all client rooms; if not, see agency policy for ordering one.

   (2) Place switch in the "Prevention" mode.

In the "Prevention" mode, surface pressures change automatically with client position to equalize pressure and eliminate points of pressure.

NURSE ALERT *This and other support beds are equipped with a CPR switch to instantly lower head section from an elevated position and to deflate the mattress to provide a firm surface for chest compressions.*

---

4. Position client comfortably as desired over support surface. Reposition routinely.
5. Reassess client's level of risk for skin breakdown.

Location of existing pressure sore might influence type of positioning (AHCPR, 1994; Pieper, 2000).
Verifies if support surface is still appropriate and necessary.

6. Instruct client to call for assistance to get in and out of bed.

Height of the bed may be increased with overlay, making getting in and out of bed difficult (Pieper, 2000).

7. See Completion Protocol (inside front cover).

• • • • • • • • • •

EVALUATION

1. Inspect condition of skin every 8 hours to determine changes in skin and effectiveness of support mattress.
2. Assess existing pressure ulcers for evidence of healing.
3. Ask client to rate comfort on a 0 to 10 scale.

Unexpected Outcomes and Related Interventions

1. Client develops localized areas of abnormal reactive hyperemia for longer than 30 minutes, mottling, swelling, and tenderness with evidence of breakdown. Existing pressure ulcers fail to demonstrate signs of healing.

a. Revise turning schedule for more frequent position changes.

b. Avoid prolonged exposure on any one side.

c. Keep skin clean and dry.

d. Notify physician. Advancement of existing pressure ulcers may be related to infection, nutritional deficiencies, or an exacerbation of other systemic factors.

e. Evaluate need for alternative surface.

2. Client expresses discomfort.

a. Evaluate air level of surface.

b. Evaluate need for alternative surface.

c. Reposition client more frequently.

d. Unless contraindicated, provide back massage. Do not massage reddened areas, because this contributes to skin breakdown.

3. Support surface develops a leak.

a. Take corrective action in accordance with institutional policies.

Recording and Reporting

- Record type of support surface applied, extent to which client tolerated procedure, and condition of client's skin in nurses' notes or skin assessment flow sheet.

- Report evidence of pressure ulcer formation to nurse in charge or to physician.

Sample Documentation

1000 Air mattress overlay applied to bed. Client's skin dry and intact without erythema. Client comfortable and tolerating support surface well.

SPECIAL CONSIDERATIONS

Pediatric Considerations

Parents can be helpful in assisting children with treatment preferences.

Geriatric Considerations

- Implement preventive measures for older adults because the aging process causes their skin to become drier, thinner, and less pressure sensitive, increasing the risk of skin breakdown.

- Adding a mattress overlay changes bed height. Care should be taken when transferring client in and out of bed.

Home Care Considerations

- Most of the devices covered in this section may be adapted for home use on a standard twin or hospital bed.

- Selection should be based on client needs and environmental audit. For example, the client on total bed rest who smokes would not be an ideal candidate for a foam mattress because of the flammability of foam products.

- The client with pets that sleep in bed may not be suited for a water- or air-filled mattress because of puncture risk.

- Reimbursement varies by surface type and payer source (Weaver and McCausland, 1998).

Long-Term Care Considerations

- Many clients are at risk for pressure ulcer development in this setting.

- A client may be admitted from home or another facility with pressure ulcers.

Skill 26.2

Using a Low-Air-Loss Bed

Low-air-loss beds are dynamic devices used to promote skin integrity in the immobile or bedridden client (Figure 26-4). They reduce and/or relieve the effects of shear, friction, maceration, and pressure. Air-filled cushions mounted on a standard hospital bed frame are divided into four or five sections for support and relief of pressure.

A controlled amount of air is continually lost through the surface of the bed cushions. This air loss has a drying effect on the skin, which decreases the effects of maceration without dehydrating the client. Maximum client weight ranges from 300 to 500 pounds depending on the

low-air-loss model. Special high-air-loss cushions may also be used to draw moisture from a certain area. In addition, there are split or U-shaped cushions to enhance pressure relief for the head, sacrum, and heel areas; proning cushions; extended height cushions; foot and lateral arm supports; and heavy-duty cushions. Drawsheets are made of the same material as the cushions for those clients who are incontinent.

These beds have CPR switches for immediate deflation to provide a hard surface for chest compressions (Figure 26-5). Scales may be built into the bed for ease in

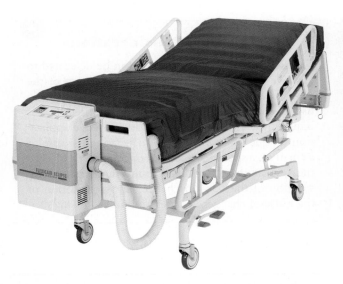

Figure 26-4 Low-air-loss bed. (© 2002 Hill-Rom Services, Inc. Reprinted with permission—All rights reserved.)

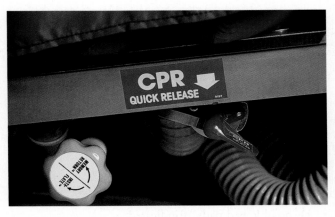

Figure 26-5 Cardiopulmonary resuscitation switch deflates low-air-loss bed to provide hard surface.

weighing. A battery system is necessary to maintain inflation during interruptions of power or during transport.

Other adaptations of the low-air-loss bed for pulmonary care are lateral rotation or kinetic therapy, pulsation, percussion, and vibration (Figure 26-6). This surface should not be used with a client who has an unstable spinal cord or who is in traction. A pediatric version also exists. These beds are marketed widely to intensive care areas, and one has the ability to transform to a full chair position.

Low-air-loss overlays can be placed over a regular mattress and have a motorized pump that maintains constant inflation and slight air movement to prevent moisture buildup on the client's skin. The fabric covering is air- and bacteria-permeable, waterproof, and reduces friction and shear. Some low-air-loss overlays have kinetic features.

ASSESSMENT

1. Determine client's risk for pressure ulcer formation using a validated risk assessment tool such as the Braden scale. *Rationale: Risk assessment tools as suggested by the AHCPR (e.g., Braden scale) provide an objective measure of risk consistent between evaluators over time (see Chapter 23).*

2. Perform routine skin assessment, especially over dependent sites and bony prominences. Look for changes in color (erythema or pallor), texture (edema or induration), temperature (warmth or coolness), blistering, or ulceration. *Rationale: Provides baseline on ongoing data to determine change in skin integrity or change in existing pressure ulcer.*

3. Assess client's level of comfort and pain using a 0 to 10 scale. *Rationale: Client may require pain medication to tolerate movement to another bed/mattress surface.*

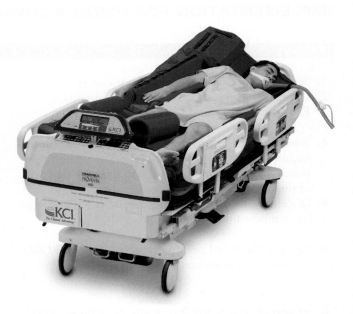

Figure 26-6 Lateral rotation bed. (TriaDyne® Proventa™ Bed. Courtesy Kinetic Concepts [KCI], Inc, San Antonio, Texas.)

Inadequate pain control may limit client's tolerance of position changes.

4. Assess client's understanding of purposes of support surfaces. *Rationale: Misconceptions can affect client's cooperation in use of support surface.*

5. Review client's medical orders. *Rationale: A physician's order is required to obtain reimbursement in the United States.*

PLANNING

Expected outcomes focus on the maintenance of skin integrity and client comfort.

Expected Outcomes

1. Client's skin remains intact without evidence of abnormal reactive hyperemia or mottling.
2. Existing pressure ulcers show evidence of healing by formation of granulation tissue.
3. Client rates comfort no greater than a 4 (on a scale of 0 to 10).
4. Client remains alert and oriented.

Equipment

- Low-air-loss bed (see Figure 26-4, p. 617)
- Sheet (supplied by distributor)
- Disposable bed pads, if indicated
- Disposable gloves (optional)

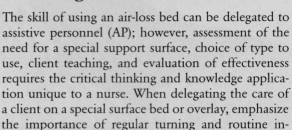

Delegation Considerations

The skill of using an air-loss bed can be delegated to assistive personnel (AP); however, assessment of the need for a special support surface, choice of type to use, client teaching, and evaluation of effectiveness requires the critical thinking and knowledge application unique to a nurse. When delegating the care of a client on a special surface bed or overlay, emphasize the importance of regular turning and routine inspection of the skin for changes and notification of the nurse of changes in skin condition.

IMPLEMENTATION FOR USING A LOW-AIR-LOSS BED

Steps	Rationale
1. See Standard Protocol (inside front cover).	
2. Close client's room door or bedside curtain.	Maintains client's privacy during transfer.
3. Explain steps of transfer.	Reduces anxiety and helps client be a part of decision making during maneuvering.
4. Transfer client to bed using appropriate transfer techniques (see Chapter 6). Turn bed on by depressing switch. Set Instaflate to allow safe and easy transfer of the client onto the surface.	Appropriate transfer techniques maintain alignment and reduce risk of injury during procedure. Company representative will adjust bed to client's height and weight.
5. Once the client is transferred, release Instaflate; regulate temperature.	Pressure cushions will adjust automatically to preset optimal levels to minimize pressure, friction, and shear (Pieper, 2000).
6. Position client and perform range-of-motion (ROM) exercises as appropriate.	Promotes comfort and reduces contracture formation. The bed relieves pressure on skin, but clients must still be turned and exercised to avoid joint deformity or contractures (AHCPR, 1994).
7. To turn clients, position bedpans, or perform other therapies, set Instaflate. Once procedure is completed, release Instaflate.	According to the manufacturer's instructions, Instaflate firms the bed surface to facilitate turning and handling client.

NURSE ALERT *Client will not receive pressure relief when bed is firm for procedures. Activate CPR switch to quickly deflate the bed in an emergency (see Figure 26-5, p. 617).*

---

8. There are a number of special features listed below. Specify what special features may be required.	
a. Scales for client weight.	
b. Portable transport units to maintain inflation when primary power source is interrupted.	Provides continuous pressure relief.
c. Specialty cushions for proning, pressure relief, reducing moisture, preventing sliding down in bed, relieving heavy weight from orthopedic devices.	Helps prevent friction and shearing forces.
d. Lateral rotation features that allow approximately 30 degrees of turning.	Helps prevent pulmonary complications.

Steps	Rationale

9. Provide adequate fluid intake.

10. See Completion Protocol (inside front cover).

Bed surface may be drying and contributes to dehydration.

• • • • • • • • • •

EVALUATION

1. Inspect condition of skin periodically to determine changes in skin and effectiveness of low-air-loss therapy.
2. Inspect client's pressure ulcers for evidence of healing.
3. Ask client to rate comfort on a 0 to 10 scale.
4. Observe client's level of consciousness and orientation.

Unexpected Outcomes and Related Interventions

1. Client develops areas of breakdown, or existing areas of breakdown worsen.
   a. Evaluate and revise turning schedule as needed.
   b. Avoid prolonged exposure on any one side.
   c. Keep skin clean and dry.
   d. Notify physician. Advancement of existing pressure ulcer may be related to tissue necrosis, infection, nutritional deficiencies, or exacerbation of other systemic factors. Surgical debridement may be required.
   e. Evaluate need for alternative therapy.
2. Client experiences restlessness or nausea or becomes disoriented because of constant flotation.
   a. Reposition client for comfort.
   b. Notify physician. Symptomatic treatment may be required while adjusting to the bed.
   c. Evaluate the need for alternative support mattress.
3. Bed malfunctions.
   a. Follow institutional policies to obtain replacement. Client may need to be transferred to hospital bed in interim.

Recording and Reporting

• Record transfer of client to low-air-loss bed or overlay, tolerance of procedure, and condition of skin in nurses' notes or skin assessment flow sheet.

• Report changes in condition of skin to physician.
• Report restlessness or change in orientation.

Sample Documentation

1000 Client transferred onto low-air-loss bed without injury. Skin warm, dry, and intact without erythema or breakdown. Denies dizziness. Rates comfort as an 8 on a scale of 0 to 10.

❀ SPECIAL CONSIDERATIONS ❀

Pediatric Considerations
Parents can help with explaining the necessity for a special bed.

Geriatric Considerations
When hospitalized, older adult clients may experience significant misperceptions of their environment. This type of sensory perceptual change may be intensified by the constant flotation of the low-air-loss bed or overlay.

Home Care Considerations
• A version of the bed is available for rent or purchase.
• Instruct family in importance of maintaining client hydration.
• Instruct family regarding the need to provide client's skin care.

Skill 26.3

Using an Air-Fluidized Bed

An air-fluidized bed is a dynamic device designed to distribute a client's weight evenly over the support surface (Figure 26-7). The bed minimizes pressure and reduces shear force and friction through the principle of fluidization. Fluidization is created by forcing a gentle flow of temperature-controlled air upward through a mass of fine ceramic microspheres. The client lies directly on a polyester filter sheet that allows air to pass through but does not allow the microspheres to escape. Clients feel as though they are floating on a surface like a warm waterbed. The contact pressure of the client's body against the filter sheet stays at 11 to 16 mm Hg.

Air-fluidized beds are useful in the care of clients who require minimal movement to prevent skin damage by shearing force and for clients who experience significant pain when being turned or positioned such as those with

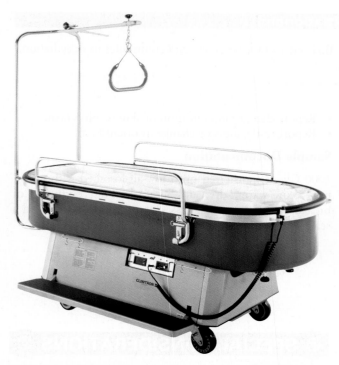

Figure 26-7 Air fluidized bed. (© 2002 Hill-Rom Services, Inc. Reprinted with permission—All rights reserved.)

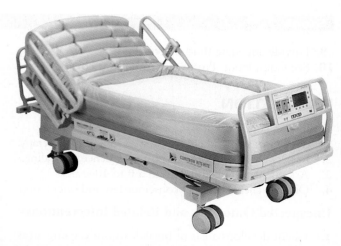

Figure 26-8 Combination air-fluidized therapy and low-air-loss bed. (© 2002 Hill-Rom Services, Inc. Reprinted with permission—All rights reserved.)

burns, skin grafts, pressure ulcers, or trauma. The surface of the filter sheet warms, clients perspire, and moisture is quickly absorbed into the circulating microspheres. Diaphoresis can go undetected, and thus insensible fluid loss may not be noticed until a client develops fluid and electrolyte imbalances. This surface should not be used with a client who has an unstable spinal cord or severe pulmonary problems. Clients may also experiences agitation, restlessness, or disorientation related to flotation.

Conventional fluidized beds do not allow for head-of-bed position changes. Foam wedges are used to elevate the head. There are also combination fluidized–low-air-loss beds that allow head-of-bed elevation (Figure 26-8). These beds use air to lift the upper body, while the lower body stays in a fluidized bed surface. The weight of the bed structure makes transport extremely difficult.

ASSESSMENT

1. Determine client's risk for pressure ulcer formation using a validated risk assessment tool such as the Braden scale. *Rationale: Risk assessment tools as suggested by the AHCPR (e.g., Braden scale) provide an objective measure of risk consistent between evaluators over time. Immobilized clients are particularly vulnerable to pressure ulcer formation (AHCPR, 1994).*
2. Carefully inspect the skin for evidence of pressure and impending breakdown. *Rationale: These data provide a baseline to determine changes in client's skin.*

3. Review client's temperature and serum electrolyte levels. *Rationale: Body fluids may be lost through diaphoresis.*
4. Assess client's emotional response and level of orientation. *Rationale: Flotation effect may cause altered sensory perceptions.*
5. Identify clients at risk for complications of air-fluidized therapy:
   a. Older adult clients may become dehydrated from the airflow, increasing insensible fluid losses.
   b. Clients receiving enteric tube feedings are at risk for aspiration from the inability to elevate head of bed other than with foam wedges under their back and shoulders.
   c. Clients who have limited ability to change positions and who are susceptible to dehydration may have tenacious pulmonary secretions that are difficult to remove.
6. Review client's medical orders. *Rationale: A physician's order may be required to obtain reimbursement.*

PLANNING

Expected outcomes focus on maintenance of skin integrity, comfort, and adequate fluid and electrolyte balance and the client's comfort.

Expected Outcomes

1. Client's skin remains warm, clean, and intact, and/or there is evidence of healing of pressure ulcers.
2. Client rates comfort no greater than a 4 (on a scale of 0 to 10).
3. Client's skin remains well hydrated, with good turgor; mucous membranes are moist; and electrolyte levels are in normal range.
4. Client remains alert and oriented or shows no change in level of consciousness.

Equipment

- Air-fluidized bed (see Figure 26-7).
- Foam positioning wedges, if indicated
- Filter sheet (supplied by the distributor)
- Disposable gloves (if contacting body fluids)

Delegation Considerations

The skill of applying an air-fluidized bed can be delegated to assistive personnel (AP); however, assessment of the need for a an air-fluidized bed, choice of type to use, client education, and evaluation of effectiveness requires the critical thinking and knowledge application unique to a nurse. Inform caregiver of the need to get help when changing client positions and to report any observed changes in client's skin and if client becomes disoriented, restless, or complains of nausea. Either of these requires further nursing assessment.

IMPLEMENTATION FOR USING AN AIR-FLUIDIZED BED

Steps	Rationale
1. See Standard Protocol (inside front cover).	
2. Review manufacturer's instructions. Company representative may be in attendance. Premedicate client 30 minutes before transfer if needed. Obtain additional personnel as needed.	Ensures proper and safe use of bed. Promotes comfort during transfer for those clients in moderate to severe pain. Aids in ensuring client's safety. Company representatives ensure proper functioning of bed.
3. Transfer client onto air-fluidized bed using appropriate transfer techniques (see Chapter 6). A slide or lift may be used.	A slide or lift is needed to maneuver client over the rigid sides of the bed.

COMMUNICATION TIP   *Tell client that there may be a sensation of floating or nausea when first placed on the bed. Encourage client to move and use upper extremities and participate in ROM exercise because fluidization accelerates muscle weakness.*

Steps	Rationale
4. Depress the "on" switch to begin fluidization; regulate temperature.	Fluidization relieves pressure on the skin (Pieper, 2000).
5. Position client and perform ROM exercises routinely. Foam wedges may be needed to place client in Fowler's position.	Positioning and ROM exercises are necessary to prevent pulmonary complications and contractures (Pieper, 2000).
6. Use fluidization switch to provide hard surface for turning, positioning bedpans, and other procedures. Remember to reactivate fluidization after procedure.	According to manufacturer's instructions, when fluidization is stopped, the bed becomes firm, allowing for ease in positioning. Reactivation of fluidization is necessary to minimize pressure.

NURSE ALERT   *Activate CPR switch when resuscitation is necessary to provide hard surface for performing manual chest compressions.*

Steps	Rationale
7. Obtain assistance when positioning client.	Reduces risk of friction and shear forces, as well as preventing self-injury.
8. Use of a foam wedge facilitates elevating the head of the client for position changes. Areas supported by wedge do not benefit from bed surface.	Air-fluidized bed does not have capacity to raise head of bed.

Steps	**Rationale**

9. Inspect bony prominences and heels for signs of pressure every 8 to 12 hours. Avoid use of under pads.

10. 🕊️ Replace soiled sheets as needed; soiled sheets are sent to the rental company for cleaning.

11. Maintain adequate nutritional and fluid intake.

12. See Completion Protocol (inside front cover).

According to manufacturer's instructions, under pads interfere with the therapeutic effects of the bed.

Promotes tissue healing and helps prevent skin breakdown (see Chapter 23).

• • • • • • • • • • •

EVALUATION

1. Inspect condition of skin periodically to determine changes in skin and effectiveness of air-fluidized therapy.
2. Ask client to rate level of comfort on a scale of 0 to 10.
3. Observe moisture of client's skin and mucous membranes and skin turgor. Monitor client's temperature and laboratory serum electrolyte levels.
4. Evaluate client's emotional response and orientation to flotation. Assess client's level of orientation.

Unexpected Outcomes and Related Interventions

1. Client develops areas of breakdown, or existing areas of breakdown worsen.
   a. Evaluate and revise turning schedule as needed.
   b. Keep skin clean and dry.
   c. Reevaluate the client's risk factors affecting wound healing.
   d. Notify physician. Advancement of existing pressure ulcer may be related to tissue necrosis, infection, nutritional deficiencies, or other systemic factors.
2. Client experiences agitation, restlessness, or disorientation related to flotation.
   a. Reposition for comfort.
   b. Provide reassurance and emotional support. Encourage client to verbalize concerns.
   c. Notify physician. Symptomatic treatment may be necessary while adjusting to constant flotation.
   d. If unable to adjust to flotation, evaluate the need for alternative measures.
3. Client's skin and mucous membranes are dehydrated and serum electrolyte levels are abnormal related to the temperature and evaporative effects of the bed.
   a. Evaluate nutritional and fluid status, including intake and output.
   b. Increase fluid intake unless contraindicated.
   c. Collaborate with physician for other treatment modalities.

4. The filter sheet tears, expelling small sandlike particles in the air.
   a. Cover the puncture site to prevent particles from getting on client and wounds.
   b. Promptly follow the institution's policy to obtain a replacement. Client may need to be transferred to another bed in the interim.

Recording and Reporting

- Record transfer of client to bed, tolerance to procedure, and condition of skin in nurses' notes or skin assessment flow sheet.
- Report changes in condition of skin and electrolyte levels to nurse in charge or to physician.
- Report change in orientation.

Sample Documentation

1600 Client transferred onto air-fluidized bed without incident. Skin warm, dry, and intact. Mucous membranes moist. A 3-cm reddened area noted to sacrum with brisk capillary refill. Client oriented to person, place, and time. Rates comfort as 6 on a scale of 0 to 10.

❈ SPECIAL CONSIDERATIONS ❈

Geriatric Considerations
- Older adult clients are at increased risk for dehydration.
- When hospitalized, older adult clients may experience intensified flotation of the air-fluidized bed.

Home Care Considerations
- Beds weigh between 1700 and 2100 pounds; therefore the rental company leasing the bed needs to inspect the home for accessibility and structural support.
- Rental company is responsible for cleaning the tank of microspheres at regular intervals, usually every 1 to 4 weeks, depending on need as body fluids drain into bed.

Skill 26.4

Using a Rotokinetic Bed

The Rotokinetic bed is a dynamic device used to maintain skeletal alignment while providing constant rotation (Figure 26-9). It is used in the care of spinal cord–injured and multitrauma clients. The support structure of the bed maintains proper alignment when secured properly. The bed rotates from side to side at a 60- to 90-degree angle every 7 minutes. Turning angles may be adjusted to meet the client's needs. Constant rotation reduces pressure ulcer development and stimulates body systems. It is recommended that the bed stay in the rotation mode for at least 20 hours a day. There is an emergency gatch that can quickly interrupt rotation when needed. To initiate CPR, the bed is returned to the horizontal position and locked in place.

The constant motion may lead to sensory distress for the client, especially older adults. This may be associated with the constant kinetic stimulation, the limited visual field, and inner ear disequilibrium. The nurse must be mindful of these complications and provide necessary emotional support.

ASSESSMENT

1. Determine client's risk for pressure ulcer formation using a validated risk assessment tool such as the Braden scale. *Rationale: Provides an objective measure of risk consistent between evaluators and over time.*

2. Identify clients who require complete immobilization and continuous skeletal alignment.

3. Carefully inspect the skin for evidence of pressure. *Rationale: Proper position is critical to stabilize client in proper alignment and prevent pressure and shear.*

4. Assess the client's level of consciousness, inner ear equilibrium, orientation, and anxiety. *Rationale: Establishes a baseline assessment to detect any change while client is on the bed. Constant motion may lead to sensory distress.*

5. Assess client's breath sounds, blood pressure, height, and weight before placement on bed. *Rationale: Provides baseline data before using Rotokinetic bed.*

6. Assess the client's and family members' understanding of and response to the Rotokinetic bed.

7. Review client's medical orders. *Rationale: A physician's order is required to obtain reimbursement in the United States.*

PLANNING

Expected outcomes focus on maintaining skin integrity and proper body alignment, promoting client comfort, decreasing client's anxiety, preventing pulmonary congestion, and maintaining skin integrity.

Expected Outcomes

1. Client's skin remains intact without evidence of abnormal reactive hyperemia or mottling.
2. Client's existing pressure ulcers show evidence of healing.
3. Client's musculoskeletal system is properly aligned and free of contractures.
4. Client's breath sounds improve or remain clear to auscultation.
5. Client remains alert, oriented, and cooperative.
6. Client denies inner ear disequilibrium or other sensory distress.
7. Client's blood pressure remains consistent with baseline vital signs.

Equipment

- Rotokinetic bed with support packs, bolsters, and safety straps (see Figure 26-9)
- Top sheet
- Pillowcases for bolsters

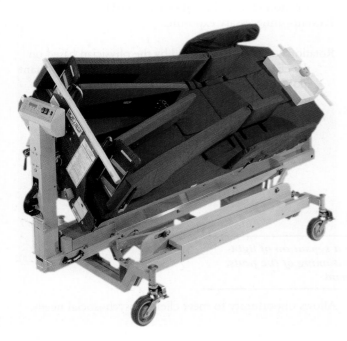

Figure 26-9   Rotokinetic bed. (RotoRest® Delta Bed. Courtesy Kinetic Concepts, Inc., [KCI], San Antonio, Tex.)

Delegation Considerations

The skill of preparation of a Rotokinetic bed can be delegated to assistive personnel (AP); however, assessment of the need for a Rotokinetic bed, client teaching, and evaluation of effectiveness requires the critical thinking and knowledge application unique to a nurse. When delegating the care of a client on a Rotokinetic bed, stress the importance of maintaining bed rotation and routine inspection of the skin for tissue trauma. The AP need to notify the nurse of changes in skin condition and concerns expressed by the client.

IMPLEMENTATION FOR USING A ROTOKINETIC BED

Steps	Rationale
1. See Standard Protocol (inside front cover) and review manufacturer's instructions.	
2. Premedicate client 30 minutes before transfer if needed.	Promotes comfort during transfer.
3. Place Rotokinetic bed in horizontal position, and remove all bolsters, straps, and supports. Close posterior hatches.	
4. Unplug electrical cord. Lock gatch.	Prevents accidental rotation during transfer.
5. Maintaining proper alignment, transfer client to Rotokinetic bed (see Chapter 6).	Reduces risk of further tissue injury during transfer. May need physician available to assist in transfer.
6. Secure thoracic panels, bolsters, head and knee packs, and safety straps.	Maintains proper alignment and prevents sliding during rotation (Tomaselli and others, 2001).
7. Cover client with top sheet.	Prevents unnecessary exposure.
8. Plug bed in.	
9. Have company representative set rotational angle as ordered by the physician. May gradually increase rotation. Monitor client's BP.	Rotational angle is determined by the physician based on the client's overall condition and tolerance to constant motion. Gradually increasing rotation may prevent nausea, dizziness, and orthostatic hypotension (Tomaselli and others, 2001).
10. Increase degree of rotation gradually according to client's tolerance.	

NURSE ALERT *The bed must be stopped for CPR and bedside procedures (e.g., portable chest x-ray examination, dressing changes).*

COMMUNICATION TIP *Tell the client that there may be a sensation of light-headedness or falling, which will not occur because of positioning of the pads, which are checked by two people to ensure proper placement.*

11. It is difficult to maintain eye contact when talking with clients during rotation. Provide adequate space for caregivers and family to move around the bed to facilitate communication.	Allows opportunity to meet client's psychosocial needs.

Steps	Rationale

12. The bed may be stopped for assessment and procedures. To stop the bed, permit bed to rotate to the desired position, turn the motor off, and push knob into a lock position. If necessary, the bed can be manually repositioned.

NURSE ALERT   *Manual rotation may cause nausea or dizziness if done too rapidly. Keep bed stopped no longer than 30 minutes at a time.*

---

13. See Completion Protocol (inside front cover).

• • • • • • • • • •

EVALUATION

1. Inspect condition of skin (occiput, ears, axillae, elbows, sacrum, groin, and heels) and musculoskeletal alignment every 2 hours to determine changes in skin and effectiveness of Rotokinetic therapy.
2. Inspect client's pressure ulcers for evidence of healing.
3. Observe alignment and ROM of all joints.
4. Auscultate lung sounds every shift, and compare with baseline.
5. Determine client's level of orientation at least once per shift.
6. Ask whether client is experiencing nausea or dizziness.
7. Monitor blood pressure.

Unexpected Outcomes and Related Interventions

1. Client develops areas of breakdown, or existing areas of breakdown worsen.
   a. Evaluate rotation schedule; bed should stay in rotation for 20 hours a day to prevent breakdown.
   b. Keep skin clean and dry. Change linen on bolsters as needed.
2. Client experiences hypotension.
   a. If severe drop in blood pressure, stop rotation. Notify physician. Monitor vital signs every 5 minutes.
   b. For less severe blood pressure changes, decrease the rotational angle. Gradually increase the rotational angle as client adjusts to rotation.
3. Client becomes disoriented, confused, or uncooperative related to sensory/perceptual distortion.
   a. Reorient client to person, place, and time.
   b. Provide audio stimulation via radio or tape recorder.
   c. Provide TV secured to bed frame (available from manufacturer).
   d. Hang mirror on ceiling so that client may view surroundings.
   e. Notify physician. Symptomatic treatment for motion sickness may be helpful.
4. Client develops crackles in lung fields.
   a. Have client cough and deep breathe every 2 hours.

   b. Notify physician. Incentive spirometry or other treatment measures may be warranted.
5. Bed malfunctions or fails to rotate.
   a. Ensure safety of client.
   b. Follow institutional policies to correct situation. Client may need to be transferred to conventional hospital bed in the interim.

Recording and Reporting

- Describe the condition of skin before placement on the Rotokinetic bed. A photograph may be taken to document skin condition and provide a baseline for later assessments for progress in healing.
- Record time of transfer to Rotokinetic bed and the degree of rotation.
- Record and report subjective data indicating response to the constant rotation and presence/absence of dizziness, nausea, or blood pressure changes.
- A flow sheet may be used to document routine assessment and care, including the length of time the bed rotation is stopped. The bed needs to be rotating at least 20 hours out of every 24 hours and stopped for no more than 30 minutes at a time.

Sample Documentation

0930 Client transferred to a Rotokinetic bed to maintain proper skeletal alignment and prevent skin breakdown. Skin intact. An area of redness noted on sacrum 4 inches in diameter, and both heels are reddened. Initial rotation begun at 30 degrees without c/o nausea or dizziness. BP stable at 130/74.

❀ SPECIAL CONSIDERATIONS ❀

Geriatric Considerations
Older adults may have an increased sensation of lightheadedness or dizziness.

Skill 26.5

Using a Bariatric Bed

A morbidly obese client may benefit from a bariatric bed, which is capable of allowing upright or sitting positioning, client transport, and in-bed scales (Figure 26-10). The bed is capable of supporting weights up to 850 pounds, providing a stable, balanced surface.

The nurse can change the bed position to move the client to reduce risk of staff injury. The in-bed scale provides the nurse with a means of obtaining accurate weights, which is frequently a problem with the obese client. The bed is slightly wider than a standard hospital bed, yet it fits through the standard door width.

The at-risk obese client should have some type of pressure-relief mattress placed on the bariatric bed. Choices for pressure relief may include static air or gel type of mattresses. Several manufacturers have low-air-loss mattress replacement systems for the bariatric bed. These beds have CPR switches, which permit immediate deflation to provide a hard surface for chest compressions.

Another type of bed for the bariatric client is a full or double-wide bed. These beds are equipped to accommodate a client weighing up to 1000 pounds. Because this bed will not move through a doorway, another means of moving the client from the room must be available.

ASSESSMENT

1. Determine client's need for bed based on height and weight. *Rationale: A bariatric bed provides a safe surface. Standard hospital bed frames are not designed to support obese clients safely.*
2. Assess condition of skin. Note condition of skin between skinfolds. Note potential pressure sites. *Rationale: Determines need for client to have a low-air-loss or other pressure-relieving surface on the bed.*
3. Assess client's and family members' understanding of purpose of bed.
4. Review client's medical orders. *Rationale: A physician's order is required to obtain reimbursement in the United States.*

PLANNING

Expected outcomes focus on safety, maximum independence, and maintaining skin integrity.

Expected Outcomes

1. Client is able to reposition independently for comfort.
2. Client remains free of injury.
3. Client's skin remains intact without abnormal reactive hyperemia.

Equipment

- Bariatric bed (see Figure 26-10)
- Sheets
- Overhead frame (optional)
- Heavy-duty lift (optional)

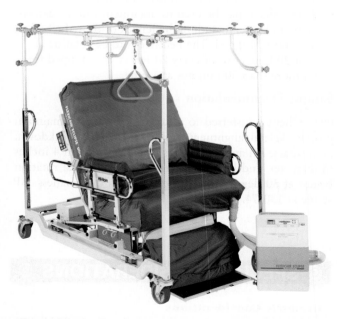

Figure 26-10   Bariatric bed with low-air-loss mattress replacement. (© 2002 Hill-Rom Services, Inc. Reprinted with permission—All rights reserved.)

Delegation Considerations

The skill of preparation for a bariatric bed may be delegated to assistive personnel (AP); however, assessment of the need for a bariatric bed, choice of type to use, client teaching, and evaluation of effectiveness requires the critical thinking and knowledge application unique to the nurse. Be sure adequate assistance is available to reduce risk of friction and shearing forces and to prevent injury to client and caregivers.

IMPLEMENTATION FOR USING A BARIATRIC BED

Steps	Rationale
1. See Standard Protocol (inside front cover).	
2. Position four to six persons around stretcher or bed to allow a distribution of client's weight during the lift.	Appropriate transfer techniques provide for smooth transfer to the bed and reduce the risk of injury to client and health care personnel.

NURSE ALERT *Consider the use of a heavy-duty lift.*

Steps	Rationale
3. Place pull sheet, side board, or other assistance device under the client, and transfer safely.	Minimizes trauma to client's skin from shearing forces as client is moved.
4. Position client for comfort with hand controls and trapeze bar within reach. Be sure that out-of-bed alarm is on if needed.	Encourages maximum independence and mobility. Alarm alerts the caregiver that client is out of bed.
5. Encourage client to initiate frequent position changes and move in the bed as much as possible.	Promotes client independence and reduces risks of reduced mobility
6. See Completion Protocol (inside front cover).	

• • • • • • • • • •

EVALUATION

1. Observe client's ability to operate the bed and change positions independently for comfort.
2. Assess client's risk for injury.
3. Inspect client's skin every 8 hours for evidence of breakdown.

Unexpected Outcomes and Related Interventions

1. Client is unable to operate bed independently.
   a. Assist client as needed.
   b. Consult physician regarding physical therapy or occupational therapy evaluation to increase mobility or to provide facilitative devices.
2. Client develops areas of skin breakdown, or existing areas worsen.
   a. Reevaluate need for support surface in use.
   b. Evaluate turning schedule. May need to change or shift position more frequently than every 2 hours.

Recording and Reporting

- Record transfer of client to bed, subjective response, and condition of skin in nurses' notes or skin assessment flow sheet.
- Report changes in condition of skin.

Sample Documentation

1000 Transferred to bariatric bed. Client demonstrated use of hand controls and trapeze bar. Skin without erythema or evidence of breakdown.

❊ SPECIAL CONSIDERATIONS ❊

Home Care Considerations

- Full-size bariatric (e.g., Size-Wise, Equitron) beds are available for rental or purchase.
- Persons of extreme obesity who are immobile should alert their local emergency service personnel; ensures availability of adequate equipment and personnel.

CRITICAL THINKING EXERCISES

1. You have determined that a client is at moderate risk for skin breakdown and plan to use an air mattress overlay.
   a. To whom could you delegate the application of the mattress overlay?
   b. What information should you relay to the AP before placing the client on the mattress overlay?
2. Mr. L. is a morbidly obese, 75-year-old client admitted today from home. He has difficulty getting out of bed because of his obesity and multiple medical problems. He has a sacral pressure ulcer and multiple areas of skin breakdown on his hips and lower extremities from friction and shear. Prioritize the following nursing assessments from the most important to the least important.
   a. Assess the need for a heavy-duty lift and a larger wheelchair.
   b. Perform a risk assessment to determine the need for a pressure-relief overlay.
   c. Determine the need for bariatric devices at home.
   d. Assess the need for a physical therapy evaluation to increase mobility.
   e. Assess the client's ability to operate the bed and change positions independently.
3. In addition to skin assessment, what information should you gather when caring for a client placed on an air-fluidized bed?
4. You are caring for a 17-year-old client who sustained a cervical spine injury after diving into a shallow stream. He is on a Rotokinetic bed. What can you do to facilitate his adjustment to the bed and provide some distraction?

REFERENCES

Agency for Health Care Policy and Research, Panel for the Prediction and Prevention of Pressure Ulcers: *Pressure ulcers in adults: prediction and prevention*, Clinical practice guideline No. 3, AHCPR Pub No. 92-0047, Rockville, Md, 1992, Agency for Health Care Policy and Research, Public Health Service, U.S. Department of Health and Human Services.

Agency for Health Care Policy and Research, Panel for the Treatment of Pressure Ulcers: *Treatment of pressure ulcers*, Clinical practice guideline No. 15, AHCPR Pub No. 95-0652, Rockville, Md, 1994, Agency for Health Care Policy and Research, Public Health Service, U.S. Department of Heath and Human Services.

Fletcher J: Pressure-relieving equipment: criteria and selection, *Br J Nurs* 6(6):323, 1997.

Maklebust J: An update on horizontal patient support surfaces, *Ostomy Wound Manage* 45(1A Suppl):70S, 1999.

Pieper B: Mechanical forces: pressure, shear, and friction. In Bryant RA, editor: *Acute and chronic wounds: nursing management*, ed 2, St Louis, 2000, Mosby.

Tomaselli N, Goldberg ME, Wind S: Pressure-reducing devices: lateral rotation therapy. In Lynn-McHale DJ, Carlson KK, editors: *AACN procedure manual for critical care*, ed 4, Philadelphia, 2001, WB Saunders.

Vyhlidal S and others: Mattress replacement or foam overlay: a prospective study on the incidence of pressure ulcers, *Appl Nurs Res* 10(3):111, 1997.

Weaver V, McCausland D: Revised Medicare policies for support surfaces: a review, *J Wound Ostomy Continence Nurs* 25(1):26, 1998.

Whittemore R: Pressure-reduction support surfaces: a review of the literature, *J Wound Ostomy Continence Nurs* 25(1):6, 1998.

Wind S, Tomaselli N, Goldberg ME: Pressure-relieving and pressure-reducing devices. In Boggs RL, Wooldridge-King M, editors: *AACN procedure manual for critical care*, ed 3, Philadelphia, 1993, WB Saunders.

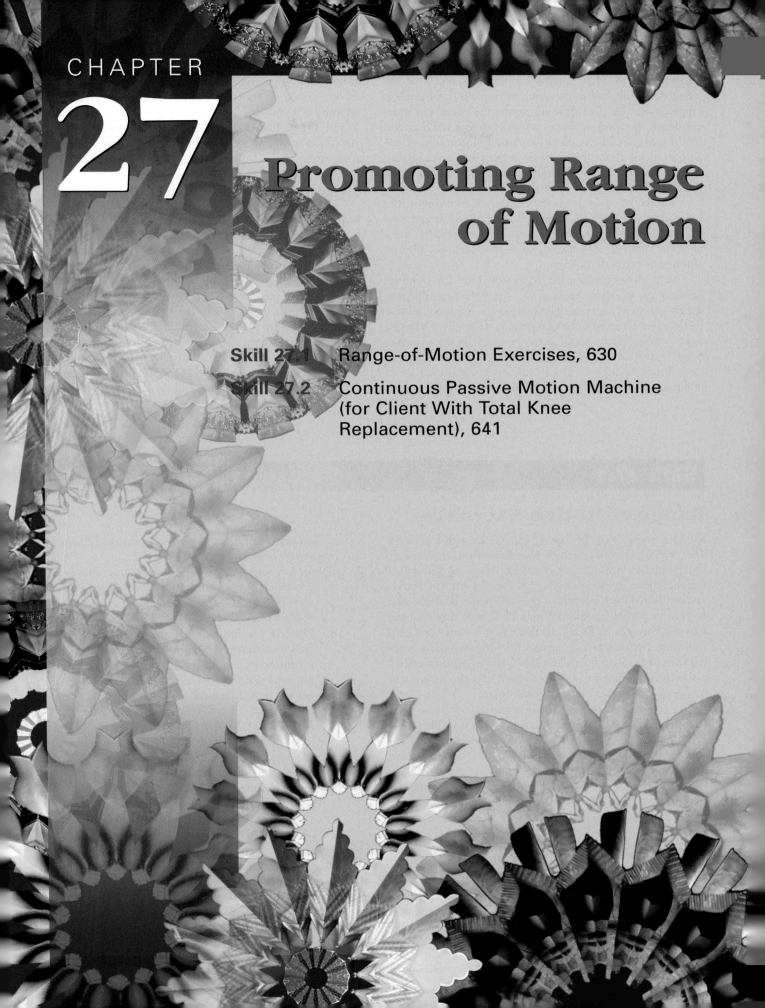

Promoting Range of Motion

Nurses need to assess clients for mobility levels. If the client is mobile, can move about freely, and has complete range of motion (ROM) in all joints, the client can independently perform activities of daily living (ADLs) and ROM exercises. If the client is partially immobile or unable to move about freely (hemiplegic, paraplegic, quadriplegic), the nurse or a mechanical device is needed to assist the client with ROM exercises.

The ROM of a joint is the maximum movement that is possible for that joint. Each person's range is determined by genetic inheritance, developmental patterns, the presence or absence of disease, and the person's normal amount of physical activity.

Motions involved in ROM exercises are the same regardless of whether one can do the exercises independently or some degree of assistance is required. Active ROM exercises need to be encouraged if the client's health status allows. Active and active-assisted ROM exercises help (1) to restore or maintain strength of the muscles; (2) to maintain or increase the flexibility of the joints; (3) to maintain or promote the growth of bones through application of physical stressors; (4) to improve the functioning of other body systems, such as the cardiovascular and gastrointestinal systems, and (5) to prevent contractures. When clients have limited mobility, passive ROM exercises help to maintain joint function but do not result in sufficient muscle tension to maintain muscle tone.

NURSING DIAGNOSES

Impaired Physical Mobility is appropriate when the inability to move a joint independently could result in the development of contractures or decreased strength and endurance. **Ineffective Health Maintenance** may be related to lack of knowledge or difficulty following through with prescribed ROM exercises. When clients are unable to independently move a joint, **Risk for Disuse Syndrome** is appropriate, and in some cases this results in further joint limitations. Anytime a client's ability to move is restricted by joint mobility or deformity or impaired extremity functioning there is the potential for **Self-Care Deficit,** which can affect hygiene, toileting, feeding, and dressing and grooming.

Skill 27.1

Range-of-Motion Exercises

ROM exercises may be active, passive, or active assisted. They are active if the client is able to perform the exercise independently and passive if the exercises are performed for the client by the caregiver. A client performs active-assisted ROM exercises with some assistance. A client who is weak or partially paralyzed may be able to move a limb partially through its ROM. In this case the nurse can help the client perform active-assisted ROM exercises by helping the client finish the full ROM. Another form of active-assisted ROM exercise is when a client uses the strong arm to exercise the weaker or paralyzed arm.

In every aspect of daily living activities, the nurse must encourage the client to be as independent as possible (Table 27-1). Active ROM and/or passive ROM exercises are encouraged and supervised every day by the nurse. Active ROM exercises can be incorporated into the client's ADLs. Passive ROM can easily be incorporated into bathing and feeding activities. The nurse, in collaboration with the client, needs to develop a schedule for ROM activities.

ASSESSMENT

1. Review client's chart for physical assessment, findings, physician orders, medical diagnosis, medical history, and progress. *Rationale: Nursing judgment is needed before beginning exercises for clients with joint pain or limitations or cardiac conditions aggravated by energy expenditure or exercise.*

2. Obtain data on client's baseline joint function.
   a. Observe client's ability to perform ROM exercises during ADLs. *Rationale: Provides observation of client's functional abilities.*
   b. Observe for limitations in joint mobility, redness or warmth over joints, joint tenderness, deformities, or crepitus produced by joint motion. *Rationale: May contraindicate ROM. Limitations in motion, redness, warmth, and/or pain may indicate an inflammatory process in the joint (McCance and Huether, 2002). Crepitus, a crunching or grating sensation that is audible or palpable during joint motion indicates presence of pathology within the joint (Ignatavicius and Workman, 2002).*

3. Determine client's or caregiver's readiness to learn. Explain all rationales for the ROM exercises, and describe and demonstrate exercises to be performed. *Rationale: Readiness to learn affects ability to independently perform activities. Relieves client/caregiver anxiety and encourages cooperation and participation.*

4. Assess client's level of comfort (on a scale of 0 to 10) before exercises. *Rationale: Determines if client will need an analgesic before exercising.*

Table 27-1

Incorporating Active ROM Exercises Into Activities of Daily Living

Joint Exercised	Activity of Daily Living	Movement
Neck	Nodding head yes	Flexion
	Shaking head no	Rotation
	Moving right ear to right shoulder	Lateral flexion
	Moving left ear to left shoulder	Lateral flexion
Shoulder	Reaching to turn on overhead light	Flexion
	Reaching to bedside stand for book	Extension
	Applying deodorant	Abduction
	Combing hair	Flexion
Elbow	Eating, bathing, shaving, grooming	Flexion, extension
Wrist	Eating, bathing, shaving, grooming	Flexion, extension, abduction, adduction
Fingers and thumb	All activities requiring fine motor coordination (e.g., writing, eating, hobbies)	Flexion, extension, abduction, adduction, opposition
Hip	Walking	Flexion, extension
	Moving to side-lying position	Flexion, extension, abduction
	Moving from side-lying position	Extension, adduction
	Rolling feet inward	Internal rotation
	Rolling feet outward	External rotation
Knee	Walking	Flexion, extension
	Moving to and from side-lying position	Flexion, extension
Ankle	Walking	Dorisflexion, plantar flexion
	Moving toe toward head of bed	Dorsiflexion
	Moving toe toward foot of bed	Plantar flexion
Toes	Walking	Extension, flexion
	Wiggling toes	Abduction, adduction
		Extension, flexion

PLANNING

Expected outcomes focus on maintaining joint ROM and client's physical and emotional ability to perform exercises.

Expected Outcomes

1. Client performs ROM according to prescribed routine.
2. Client's range of joint motion remains within normal range or maintains baseline range.
3. Client denies discomfort during exercises.
4. Client or caregiver correctly demonstrates ROM by discharge.

Equipment

No mechanical or physical equipment is needed.

Delegation Considerations

The skill of performing ROM exercises can be delegated to assistive personnel (AP). Clients with spinal cord or orthopedic trauma or surgery usually require exercise by nurses or physical therapists. When delegating this skill, instruct caregiver to perform exercises slowly and provide adequate support to joint being exercised. In addition, caregivers need to be reminded not to exercise joints beyond the point of resistance or to the point of fatigue or pain. In addition, if muscle spasms occur, stop exercise until the spasms have subsided.

IMPLEMENTATION FOR RANGE-OF-MOTION EXERCISES

Steps	Rationale

1. See Standard Protocol (inside front cover).
2. Wear gloves (only if there is wound drainage or skin lesions).

Steps	Rationale
3. Assist the client to a comfortable position, preferably sitting or lying down.	
4. When performing active-assisted or passive ROM exercises, support joint by holding distal and proximal areas adjacent to joint (see illustrations), by cradling distal portion of extremity, or by using cupped hand to support joint.	Provides physical support to joint while exercises are performed.

COMMUNICATION TIP

- *When chronic mobility problems exist, discuss with client which exercises need to be performed and the limitation of joint mobility for the affected area.*
- *If client has had recent orthopedic injury or surgery, reinforce how the ROM should feel and how the ROM for the affected joint(s) should progress.*

Steps	Rationale
5. Complete exercises in head-to-toe sequence. Each movement should be repeated 5 times during exercise period. Inform client how these exercises are done and how they can be incorporated into ADLs.	An orderly, well-explained sequence of exercises assists in client cooperation, and, when possible, independence in performing exercises.

NURSE ALERT *Discontinue exercise if client complains of discomfort or if there is resistance or muscle spasm.*

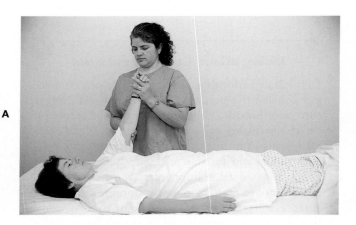

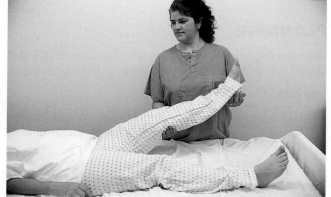

Step 4 A, Support joint by holding distal and proximal areas adjacent to joint. **B,** Support joint by cradling distal portion of extremity. **C,** Support joint by using cupped hand to support joint.

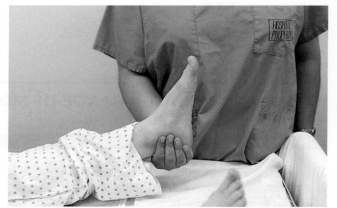

Steps	**Rationale**

a. Neck

(1) *Flexion:* Bring chin to rest on chest (ROM: 45 degrees) (see illustration).

(2) *Extension:* Return head to erect position (ROM: 45 degrees).

(3) *Hyperextension:* Gently bend head back (ROM: 10 degrees) (see illustration).

(4) *Lateral flexion:* Tilt head toward each shoulder (ROM: 40 to 45 degrees) (see illustration).

(5) *Rotation:* Rotate head in circular motion (ROM: 360 degrees) (best done in sitting position) (see illustration).

(6) Turn head side to side (see illustration).

Complete range of neck motion is necessary for independent functioning.

If flexion contracture of neck occurs, client's neck is permanently flexed with chin toward or actually touching chest. Ultimately, client's total body alignment is altered, visual field is changed, and overall level of independent functioning is decreased (Phipps, Sands, and Marek, 1999).

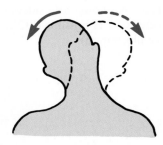

Step 5a(4)   Lateral flexion of neck.

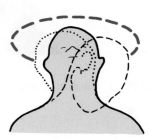

Step 5a(5)   Rotation of neck in circular motion.

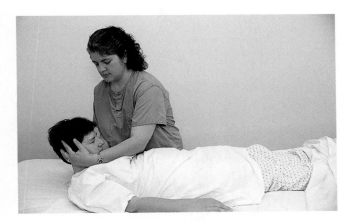

Step 5a(1)   Flexion of neck.

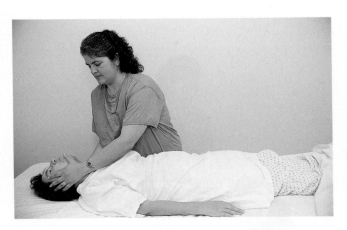

Step 5a(3)   Hyperextension of neck.

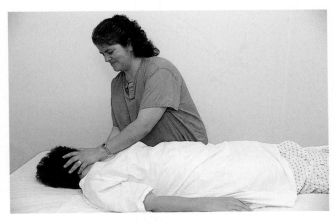

Step 5a(6)   Turning of head with client in supine position.

Steps	**Rationale**

b. Shoulder

   (1) *Flexion:* Raise arm from side position forward to above head (ROM: 180 degrees) (see illustration).

   (2) *Extension:* Return arm to position at side of body (ROM: 180 degrees).

   (3) *Hyperextension:* In standing position, move arm behind body, keeping elbow straight (ROM: 45 to 60 degrees) (see illustration).

   (4) *Abduction:* Raise arm from side to position above head with palm away from head (ROM: 180 degrees) (see illustration).

   (5) *Adduction:* Lower arm sideways and across body as far as possible (ROM: 320 degrees) (see illustration).

Exercising shoulder actively increases power of deltoid muscle and facilitates use of crutches or a walker.

Promotes reaching activities and maintains mobility. A frozen shoulder makes it impossible to reach overhead and makes dressing difficult.

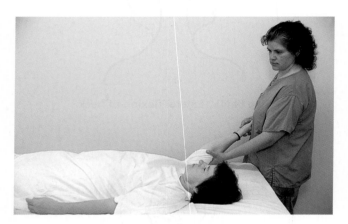

Step 5b(1)   Flexion of shoulder.

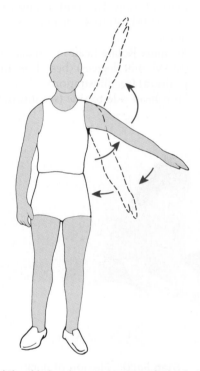

Step 5b(4)   Abduction and adduction of shoulder.

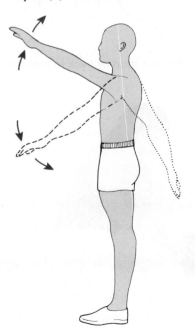

Step 5b(3)   Hyperextension of shoulder.

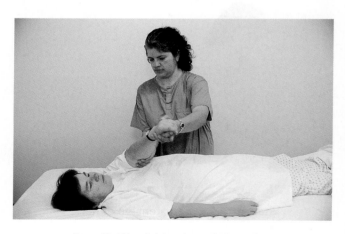

Step 5b(5)   Adduction of shoulder.

Steps	**Rationale**

(6) *External rotation:* With elbow flexed, move arm until thumb is upward and lateral to head (ROM: 90 degrees) (see illustration).

(7) *Internal rotation:* With elbow flexed, rotate shoulder by moving arm until thumb is turned inward and toward back (ROM: 90 degrees) (see illustration).

(8) *Circumduction:* Move arm in full circle. Circumduction is a combination of all movements of ball-and-socket joint (ROM: 360 degrees) (see illustration).

c. Elbow

(1) *Flexion:* Bend elbow so that lower arm moves toward its shoulder joint and hand is level with shoulder (ROM: 150 degrees) (see illustration).

(2) *Extension:* Straighten elbow by lowering hand (ROM: 150 degrees) (see illustration).

(3) *Hyperextension:* With arm extended, bend lower arm back (ROM: 10 to 20 degrees).

Elbow fixed in full extension or full flexion is very disabling and limits client's independence. For optimal functioning, elbow must be able to fully extend and flex.

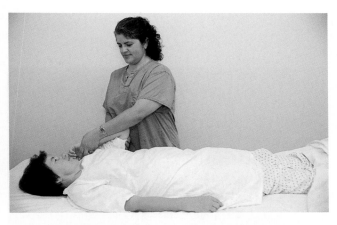

Step 5b(6) External rotation of shoulder.

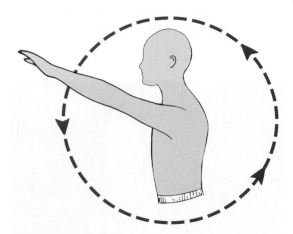

Step 5b(8) Circumduction of shoulder.

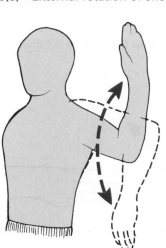

Step 5b(7) Internal rotation of shoulder.

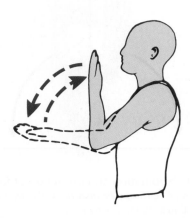

Step 5c(1,2) Flexion and extension of elbow.

Steps	Rationale

d. Forearm
   (1) *Supination:* Turn lower arm and hand so that palm is up (ROM: 70 to 90 degrees) (see illustration).
   (2) *Pronation:* Turn lower arm so that palm is down (ROM: 70 to 90 degrees) (see illustration).

For optimal functioning forearm must rotate from supination to pronation.

e. Wrist
   (1) *Flexion:* Move palm toward inner aspect of forearm (ROM: 80 to 90 degrees) (see illustration).
   (2) *Extension:* Move palm so fingers, hands, and forearm are in the same plane (ROM: 80 to 90 degrees).
   (3) *Hyperextension:* Gently bring dorsal surface of hand back (ROM: 80 to 90 degrees) (see illustration).
   (4) *Abduction (radial flexion):* Bend wrist medially toward thumb (ROM: up to 30 degrees) (see illustration).
   (5) *Adduction (ulnar flexion):* Bend wrist laterally toward fifth finger (ROM: 30 to 50 degrees) (see illustration).

If wrist becomes fixed in even slightly flexed position, client's grasp is weakened. Wrist strength is necessary to be able to use crutches.

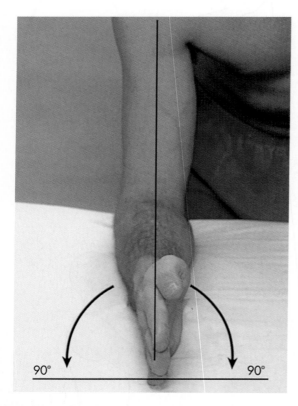

Step 5d(1,2) Supination and pronation of forearm.
(From Mourad LA: *Orthopedic disorders,* Mosby's clinical nursing series, St Louis, 1991, Mosby.)

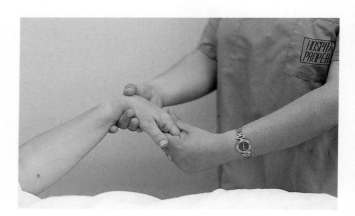

Step 5e(1) Flexion of wrist.

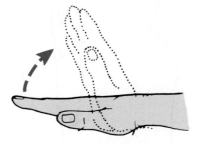

Step 5e(3) Hyperextension of wrist.

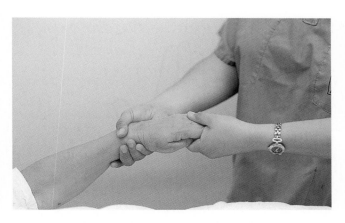

Step 5e(4)   Abduction (radial flexion) of wrist.

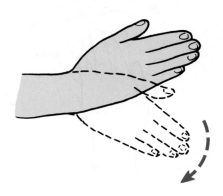

Step 5e(5)   Adduction (ulnar flexion) of wrist.

Steps	Rationale
f. Fingers (1) *Flexion:* Make fist (ROM: 90 degrees) (see illustration).	Flexibility of fingers and thumb is necessary to grasp items (e.g., holding onto a crutch, using feeding utensils).
(2) *Extension:* Straighten fingers (ROM: 90 degrees).	If not stretched into extension, natural tendency is for flexion. (In between ROM sessions, client with cerebrovascular accident [CVA] may need a firm device placed in hand to prevent full flexion.)

(3) *Hyperextension:* Gently bend fingers back (ROM: 30 to 60 degrees) (see illustration).
    (4) *Abduction:* Spread fingers apart (ROM: 30 degrees) (see illustration).
    (5) *Adduction:* Bring fingers together (ROM: 30 degrees) (see illustration).	

g. Thumb (1) *Flexion:* Move thumb across palmar surface of hand (ROM: 90 degrees) (see illustration).	Flexibility of thumb maintains coordination for fine motor activities.
(2) *Extension:* Move thumb straight away from hand (ROM: 90 degrees). (3) *Abduction:* Extend thumb laterally (usually done when placing fingers in abduction and adduction) (ROM: 30 degrees).	

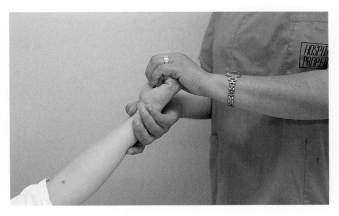

Step 5f(1)   Flexion of fingers.

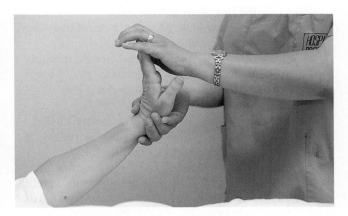

Step 5f(3)   Hyperextension of fingers.

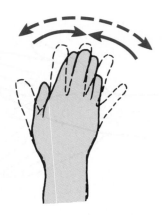

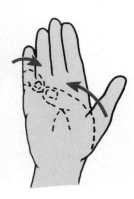

Step 5f(4,5)   Abduction and adduction of fingers.

Step 5g(5)   Opposition of thumb.

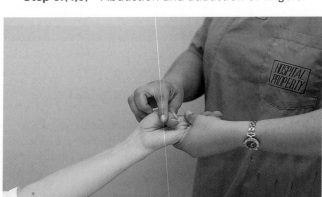

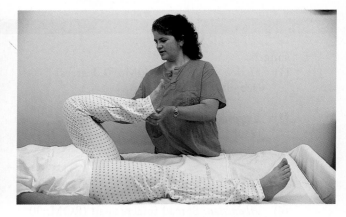

Step 5g(1)   Flexion of thumb.

Step 5h(1)   Flexion of hip with client supine.

Steps	Rationale

(4) *Adduction:* Move thumb back toward hand (ROM: 30 degrees).

(5) *Opposition:* Touch thumb to each finger of same hand (see illustration).

h. Hip

(1) *Flexion:* Move leg forward and up (ROM: 90 to 120 degrees) (see illustration).

(2) *Extension:* Move leg back beside other leg (ROM: 90 to 120 degrees).

(3) *Hyperextension:* Move leg behind body (best done standing or lying on abdomen) (ROM: 30 to 50 degrees) (see illustration).

(4) *Abduction:* Move leg laterally away from body (ROM: 30 to 50 degrees) (see illustration).

(5) *Adduction:* Move leg back toward medial position and beyond if possible (ROM: 30 to 50 degrees) (see illustration).

(6) *Internal rotation:* Turn foot and leg toward other leg (ROM: 90 degrees) (see illustration).

(7) *External rotation:* Turn foot and leg away from other leg (ROM: 90 degrees).

(8) *Circumduction:* Move leg in circle (ROM: 360 degrees) (see illustration).

Adequate ROM in lower extremities (i.e., hip, knee, ankle, foot) allows client to walk with stable gait.

Contracture of hip can cause unsteady gait or difficulty ambulating.

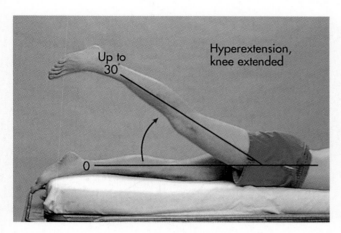

Step 5h(3) Hyperextension of hip. (From Mourad LA: *Orthopedic disorders,* Mosby's clinical nursing series, St Louis, 1991, Mosby.)

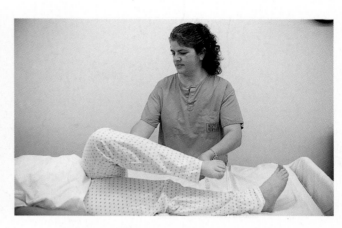

Step 5h(6) Internal rotation of hip.

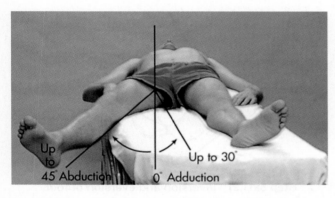

Step 5h(4,5) Abduction and adduction of hip. (From Mourad LA: *Orthopedic disorders,* Mosby's clinical nursing series, St Louis, 1991, Mosby.)

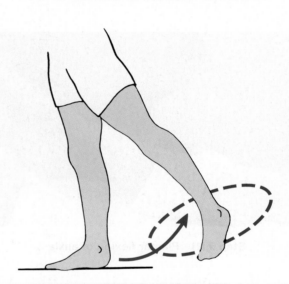

Step 5h(8) Circumduction of hip.

Steps	Rationale
i. Knee	Flexibility of the knee is essential to lift objects and to ambulate (Solomon, 1997). Severity of disability depends on the position in which knee is stiffened. If knee is fixed in full extension, client must sit with leg thrust straight out in front. If knee is fixed in any flexed position, client limps when walking or may be unable to "touch down" with foot.
(1) *Flexion:* Bring heel toward back of thigh (done with hip flexion) (ROM: 120 to 130 degrees) (see illustration).	
(2) *Extension:* Return leg to straight position on bed (ROM: 120 to 130 degrees) (see illustration).	
j. Ankle	
(1) *Plantar flexion:* Move foot so toes are pointed downward (ROM: 45 to 50 degrees) (see illustration).	Deformity of ankle can impair client's ability to walk. When footdrop occurs, the foot is permanently fixed in plantar flexion.

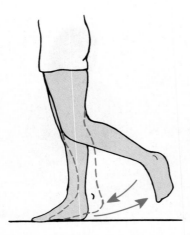

Step 5i(1,2)   Flexion and extension of knee.

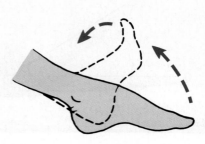

Step 5j(2)   Dorsiflexion and plantar flexion of ankle.

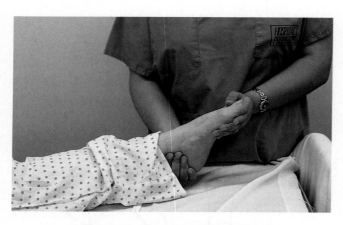

Step 5j(1)   Plantar flexion of ankle.

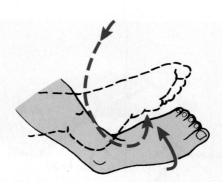

Step 5k(1,2)   Inversion and eversion of foot.

Steps	Rationale

(2) *Dorsal flexion:* Move foot so toes are pointed upward (ROM: 20 to 30 degrees) (see illustration).

k. Foot

Adequate ROM of foot permits steady gait and stable base of support.

(1) *Inversion:* Turn sole of foot medially (ROM: 10 degrees or less) (see illustration).

(2) *Eversion:* Turn sole of foot laterally (ROM: 10 degrees or less) (see illustration).

(3) *Flexion:* Curl toes downward (ROM: 30 to 60 degrees).

(4) *Extension:* Straighten toes (ROM: 30 to 60 degrees).

(5) *Abduction:* Spread toes apart (ROM: 15 degrees or less).

(6) *Adduction:* Bring toes together (ROM: 15 degrees or less).

6. See Completion Protocol (inside front cover).

• • • • • • • • • • •

EVALUATION

1. Observe client performing ROM activities; measure ROM as needed.
2. Measure joint motion, measured in degrees (e.g., elbow flexion/extension 150 degrees)
3. Ask client to rate any discomfort on a scale of 0 to 10.
4. Observe client/caregiver performing ROM exercises.

Unexpected Outcomes and Related Interventions

1. Client experiences discomfort with ROM exercises.
   a. Stop exercises.
   b. Reposition client to a comfortable position.
   c. Consider premedicating client 30 minutes before ROM exercises begin, if necessary.
2. New resistance in joint is encountered.
   a. Do not force joint motion.
   b. Consult with physical therapist or physician for necessary exercise plan changes.
3. Client or caregiver cannot perform ROM exercises correctly.
   a. Assess joint ROM, and note any limitations.
   b. Demonstrate and observe return demonstration of specific exercises to client/caregiver.

Recording and Reporting

- Record joints exercised, type of exercise, degree of joint motion, any joint abnormalities, and client's activity tolerance.
- Report immediately any resistance to range of joint motion; pain on ROM; swelling, heat, or redness in joint.

Sample Documentation

0900 Client able to correctly perform hip flexion greater than 90 degrees, 5 times without sign of fatigue. Client demonstrated this correctly and verbalized willingness to perform these exercises independently.

1300 Client reported that he forgot to do exercises. Discussed activities to trigger memory, including before/after meals, before/after sleep, and visitors.

SPECIAL CONSIDERATIONS

Pediatric Considerations

Incorporating ROM into play activities promotes exercise and improves joint mobility (Wong and others, 1999). These activities may include coloring (hands, fingers), musical chairs (legs, hips), etc.

Geriatric Considerations

- Older adults who have chronic illnesses may need ROM exercises in two or more sessions to control fatigue (Lueckenotte, 2002).
- Inadequate intake of calcium or exposure to sunlight increases older adults' risk of bone loss and increases their need for ROM and weight-bearing exercises, such as walking (Ignatavicius and Workman, 2002).

Home Care Considerations

- Assess family member or primary caregiver's ability, availability, and motivation to assist client with exercises client is unable to perform independently.
- Assist family or primary caregiver to arrange home environment to promote exercise program (e.g., space allocation, lighting, temperature, safety precautions).

Long-Term Care Considerations

- Consult physical therapist for additional assistance or exercises and client's response to exercise program.
- Group activities (e.g., simple games, walking, tossing a ball in a large circle) can assist in maintaining ROM.

Skill 27.2

Continuous Passive Motion Machine (for Client With Total Knee Replacement)

The continuous passive motion (CPM) machines are designed to exercise many different joints, including the hip, ankle, shoulder, wrist, and fingers. Orthopedic surgeons routinely order a knee CPM machine postoperatively for a total knee arthroplasty (replacement). Continuous passive motion may be initiated on the day of surgery or on the first postoperative day, according to the individual surgeon's preference. CPM machines are also used often in outpatient physical therapy or home health settings. The most common CPM machine used is the knee CPM (Lawrence, 1996).

The purpose of the CPM machine is to mobilize the knee joint to prevent contracture, muscle atrophy, venous stasis, and thromboembolism. Passive movement of the joint can replace more strenuous exercises during the first few postoperative days. Properly used, the CPM can decrease complications and shorten a client's hospital stay (Babis and others, 2001). If initiated on the day of surgery, heavier wound drainage should be expected (Montgomery and Eliasson, 1996).

The electronically controlled CPM machine flexes and extends the knee to a prescribed degree and at a set speed as ordered by the physician. A typical initial setting is 20 to 30 degrees of flexion and full extension (0 degrees) at 2 cycles per minute; however, this setting varies according to the client's condition and surgeon's preference (Ignatavicius and Workman, 2002). There are many different brands and models. They differ slightly, but each includes a full-length leg cradle hinged at the knee and ankle, a foot support, a motor controller, an electric plug, and an on/off switch. The foot support and the cradle frame adjust to fit the length of the client's thigh and calf. The frame is metal or plastic. Sheepskin or liners are available from most manufacturers. Velcro straps attached to the liner loosely secure the leg to the cradle. When the device is turned on, the frame slides slowly back and forth, gently moving the joint through a preset ROM (Birdsall, 1986).

Before the CPM can be adjusted, it is applied to the client's affected lower extremity. This process will take two hospital personnel because the CPM is heavy and weighs approximately 20 to 25 pounds. Using two hospital personnel will (1) prevent damage to the client's knee and (2) prevent unnecessary strain on the staff's backs.

ASSESSMENT

1. Check the machine for electrical safety. *Rationale: All electrical equipment in health care settings is routinely checked for safety. Routine observation of electrical cord and functioning of equipment each time it is used further monitor safety.*
2. Assess the setup of the machine before placing on bed: Check the stability of the frame, the flexion/extension controls, speed controls, and the on/off switch. *Rationale: Ensures that all pieces of the equipment are operational and will prevent damage to the client's knee.*
3. Assess the client's comfort on a scale of 0 to 10 before and during use. *Rationale: Determines if the client will be able to tolerate the CPM at the ordered flexion and extension.*
4. Assess client's baseline HR and BP. *Rationale: Provides baseline to measure exercise tolerance.*
5. Assess the client's ability and willingness to learn about the CPM machine. *Rationale: Determines readiness to learn effects, reduces anxiety, and promotes client participation.*
6. Assess client's ROM before therapy begins (see Skill 27-1, Assessment, p. 630). *Rationale: Provides baseline to use as a measure for evaluation of effect of CPM.*

PLANNING

Expected outcomes focus on improving joint ROM, maintaining physical mobility, and skin integrity.

Expected Outcomes

1. Client increases length of time in CPM machine as ordered with no evidence of increased heart rate or increased blood pressure.
2. Client denies discomfort during or after CPM exercise.
3. Client increases flexion 6 to 7 degrees daily (Chiarello, Gunderson, and O'Halloran, 1997).
4. Client maintains intact skin throughout use of CPM.

Equipment

- CPM machine and sheepskin that is applied to the CPM (Figure 27-1).

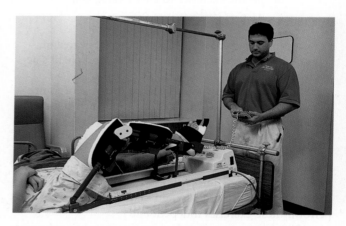

Figure 27-1 Use of CPM for continuous passive motion of knee.

 Delegation Considerations

The skill of using the CPM machine requires the critical thinking and knowledge application unique to a nurse and should not be delegated. The nurse may delegate aspects of care, such as hygiene. The RN should instruct the assistive personnel (AP) to immediately report increased pain, skin breakdown, or joint inflammation.

IMPLEMENTATION FOR CONTINUOUS PASSIVE MOTION MACHINE (FOR CLIENT WITH TOTAL KNEE REPLACEMENT)

Steps	Rationale
1. See Standard Protocol (inside front cover).	
2. Provide analgesia as ordered 20 to 30 minutes before CPM is needed.	Assists client in tolerating exercise.
3. ✋ Wear gloves (if wound drainage is present).	
4. Test all CPM controls to make sure they are functional.	Testing equipment first saves time for nurse and client. This machine must function properly to maintain safety, promote joint mobility, and prevent injury and unnecessary pain.
5. Demonstrate machine functioning before placing client's leg into the device.	Reduces anxiety and increases client cooperation.
6. Stop the machine in full extension.	This position allows correct fit of client's leg.

COMMUNICATION TIP *Discuss diversional activities with client that may be used during CPM.*

Steps	Rationale
7. Place client's leg in the machine, being sure to support above, below, and at knee.	Two nurses perform this step to prevent damage or injury to client or nurse.
8. Fit CPM machine to client by lengthening and shortening appropriate section of the CPM frame.	Ensures a proper fit.
9. Align client's knee joint (bend of the knee) with the machine knee hinge, then position the client's knee 2 cm below knee joint line of the CPM.	This is extremely important because if the client's new knee is not properly aligned, the knee may be damaged (Babis and others, 2001).
10. Center client's leg in the machine.	Avoids pressure on the lateral and medial aspects of the knee joint.
11. Adjust the foot support to approximately 20 degrees of dorsiflexion to prevent footdrop.	Footdrop is an abnormal condition caused by damage of the perineal nerve and can cause abnormal gait.
12. When client's leg is in correct position, secure the Velcro straps across lower extremity (thigh) and top of foot (see illustration).	Correct placement of the thigh and foot straps prevents friction and skin breakdown.
13. Start CPM machine. Watch at least two full cycles of prescribed flexion and extension. Remove and discard gloves, if worn, and perform hand hygiene.	Ensures that CPM machine is fully operational at the preset flexion and extension modes (Sheppard, Westlake, and McQuarrie, 1995).
14. Make sure client is comfortable. Provide client with the on/off switch. Instruct to use only if CPM seems to be malfunctioning.	Allows client to stop the machine if the degree of flexion/extension or speed changes, creating intolerable discomfort.
15. See Completion Protocol (inside front cover).	
16. Periodically reassess client's comfort level and proper function of the machine.	CPM exercises are ordered intermittently and are generally used for 8 to 12 hours per day. Clients may need analgesia during CPM activity (Ignatavicius and Workman, 2002).

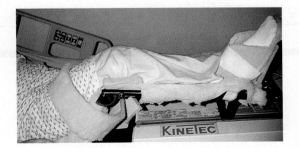

Step 12 Client's extremity correctly placed and secured to CPM.

EVALUATION

1. Ask client to keep a log of when the CPM machine is in use, with times and dates.
2. Observe client at the initial onset of an increase in the flexion of the machine.
3. Routinely ask client to rate comfort level on a scale of 0 to 10.
4. Measure joint ROM achieved with CPM machine.
5. Observe skin every 2 hours for signs of breakdown.

Unexpected Outcomes and Related Interventions

1. Client cannot increase flexion.
   a. Increase activities throughout the day to improve muscle strength (e.g., ambulation, physical therapy exercises).
   b. Give "time out" periods throughout the day to rest the leg.
   c. Consider need for analgesia before CPM
   d. Sit client in chair, and have gravity assist with increasing knee flexion.
2. Client experiences increased pain when in CPM machine.
   a. Reassess efficacy of current analgesia, and obtain new orders.
   b. Release leg out of CPM until pain subsides.
   c. Determine cause of increased pain.
3. Client develops reddened areas on heel from foot support.
   a. Readjust foot in CPM machine at least every 2 hours.
   b. Pad the foot support more.

Recording and Reporting

- Record joint exercised, degree of joint motion, time of CPM use, pain and need for analgesia, any joint abnormalities, and client's activity tolerance.
- Report immediately any resistance to range of joint motion; increased pain with CPM; swelling, heat, or redness in joint.

Sample Documentation

1000 medicated with 2 Tylenol with codeine #3 tabs 30 minutes before initiation of CPM. Functional CPM applied to client's left leg. Client able to tolerate 0 degrees extension and 40 degrees flexion at slow speed. Skin dry and intact, without evidence of breakdown.

1200 Client tolerating CPM well at 0 to 40 degrees. Stated the Tylenol with codeine tablets reduced pain to a rating of 2 (scale of 0 to 10) in the left knee. Skin assessed for breakdown, top of left foot slightly red under CPM foot strap. Foot repositioned in CPM and strap readjusted to a secure but loose position. Reassessment will be done in 1 hour.

SPECIAL CONSIDERATIONS

Geriatric Considerations

- Older adults who have chronic illnesses may need rehabilitation care to continue CPM because they are not able to manage the equipment in their home.
- Older adults have increased risk of skin breakdown because of decreased elasticity and increased fragility of the skin. Pressure from the CPM increases the risk of pressure ulcer development on the pressure points, especially the heel (Lueckenotte, 2002).

Home Care Considerations

- Home care physical therapist may assist client/family in continuing CPM in the home.
- Be sure client/family have specific instructions regarding use of the CPM device, length of time for each session, expected outcomes, and what to do if the client experiences increased pain, the client is unable to tolerate the CPM sessions, or the equipment malfunctions (Branson and Goldstein, 2001).

Long-Term Care Considerations

- Because of insurance guidelines regarding length of stay in the hospital, most clients are discharged after a relatively short period. If the client needs additional physical therapy to maintain function of the new knee replacement and to increase flexion, client may be placed in a temporary rehabilitation, short- or long-term facility.
- Instruct client that CPM in extended care setting is needed to increase joint mobility and client needs to actively participate in care.
- Additional physical therapy may be used in combination with CPM.

CRITICAL THINKING EXERCISES

1. Mr. Kline is a 58-year-old who has left hemiplegia following a stroke. His affected extremities are flaccid; however, when he gets nervous or excited, his extremities do have some spasticity. He has a prescription for ROM to the affected side. You will be delegating ROM for Mr. Kline to Kathryn Clark, the nurse assistant. What do you need to tell Kathryn about this skill?

2. Ms. Isaac is a 50-year-old independent single woman who is having decreased ROM in her hands and fingers as a result of arthritis. When you see her in a clinic setting, Ms. Isaac feels that the doctor's prescription for pain is sufficient, but she wants to increase her ROM in her hands so that she can quilt and sew. How would you assess her ROM in relation to these activities?

3. You are caring for Jim Butler, a 23-year-old athlete who has had a knee replacement procedure. He receives CPM to increase mobility of the joint. As an RN you are responsible for the CPM activities, but the caregiver is responsible for Mr. Butler's hygiene and skin care. What information is needed by the caregiver about the CPM?

REFERENCES

Babis G and others: Poor outcomes of isolated tibial insert exchange and arthrolysis for the management of stiffness following knee arthroplasty, *J Bone Joint Surg* 83-A(10):1534, 2001.

Birdsall C: How do you use the continuous passive motion device. *AJN* 86(6):657, 1986.

Branson JJ, Goldstein WM: Sequential bilateral total knee arthroplasty, *AORN J* 73(3):608, 2001.

Chiarello CM, Gunderson L, O'Halloran T: The effect of continuous passive motion duration and increment on ROM in total knee arthroplasty patients, *J Orthop Sports Phys Ther* 25(2):119, 1997.

Ignatavicius DD, Workman ML: *Medical surgical nursing: critical thinking for collaborative care*, ed 4, Philadelphia, 2002, WB Saunders.

Lawrence BR: The dose effect of continuous passive motion in postoperative rehabilitation of the first metatarsophalangeal joint, *J Foot Ankle Surg* 35(2):155, 1996.

Lueckenotte A: *Gerontologic nursing*, ed 2, St Louis, 2002, Mosby.

McCance K, Huether S: *Pathophysiology: the biologic basis for disease in adults and children*, ed 4, St Louis, 2002, Mosby.

Montgomery F, Eliasson M: Continuous passive motion compared to active physical therapy after knee arthroplasty: similar hospitalization times in a randomized study of 68 patients, *Acta Orthop Scand* 67(1):7, 1996.

Mourad LA: *Orthopedic disorders*, Mosby's clinical nursing series, St Louis, 1991, Mosby.

Phipps W, Sands JK, Marek JF: *Medical-surgical nursing: concepts and clinical practice*, ed 6, St Louis, 1999, Mosby.

Sheppard MS, Westlake SM, McQuarrie A: Continuous passive motion—where are we now? *Physiotherapy Canada* 47(1):36, 1995.

Solomon L: Clinical features of osteoarthritis. In Kelley WN and others, editors: *Textbook of rheumatology*, ed 5, Philadelphia, 1997, WB Saunders.

Wong DL and others: *Wong's essentials of pediatrics*, ed 6, St Louis, 2001, Mosby.

Traction, Cast Care, and Immobilization Devices

Trauma or disease affecting the musculoskeletal system requires immobilization, stabilization, and support to the involved body part. Traction, casts, and immobilization devices are examples of methods used to accomplish these purposes which enhance the healing process.

Traction is prescribed for one or more of the following general uses: (1) correction of deformities, (2) gradual correction or improvement of a joint contracture, (3) treatment of a joint dislocation, (4) reduction, immobilization, and alignment of a fracture (Box 28-1), (5) prevention and management of muscle spasms, (6) prevention of further soft tissue damage, (7) preoperative and postoperative positioning and alignment, (8) maintenance of skeletal length and alignment, and (9) rest of a diseased joint (Schoen, 2000).

Traction involves a pulling force applied through weights to a part of the body while a second force, called countertraction, pulls in the opposite direction. Age, condition of the client, and purpose of the traction determine the amount of the weights for the pulling force. A system of pulleys, ropes, and weights attached to the client provides this pulling force of traction. The client's body provides countertraction by elevating the foot or head of the bed. In straight or running traction, the traction force pulls against the long axis of the body while the client's body supplies the countertraction. In balanced traction, the amount of force in the traction is equal to the amount of force in the countertraction. A suspension is a mechanism that suspends a body part by using traction equipment, but it does not involve a pulling force. However, traction may be added to a suspension. In balanced suspension traction, a sling or hammock and a system of weights attached to an over-bed frame support the affected part while weight is attached to the pin or wire traversing the bone (Perry and Potter, 2002).

Although there are many types of traction for different parts of the body, five general principles apply: (1) maintain the established line of pull, (2) prevent friction on the skin, (3) maintain countertraction, (4) maintain continuous traction unless ordered otherwise, and (5) maintain correct body alignment (Beare and Myers, 1998).

The two main types of traction are skin traction and skeletal traction. Skin traction noninvasively applies pull to an affected body structure by straps attached to the skin around the structure. Skeletal traction is a type of traction applied by a physician under sterile conditions and used for treatment of fractures. It involves placement of a pin or wire through the bone. Weights are then attached to the device using ropes and pulleys. The entry through the skin provides a site for microorganisms to enter the soft tissues and bone. Meticulous skin care prevents the development of infection at these sites.

A second treatment method for immobilization involves the use of a cast. Applied externally, a cast immobilizes injured or deformed musculoskeletal tissues in proper position to promote healing. A cast prevents movement of injured tissues. Therefore correct application of the cast, with tissue structures in optimal position for healing, is imperative. An advantage of using a cast is that it permits early ambulation and, in some cases, weight bearing.

A third treatment device used with musculoskeletal injury or disorder is the orthotic device. These devices immobilize a body part, prevent deformity, protect against injury, relieve pain and muscle spasm, maintain position until healing is complete, or assist with function. Immobilization devices are applied externally to the body. They are available in many variations ranging from arm slings to back braces and finger splints. They are made from a variety of materials such as rubber, leather, metal, and plastics.

Swelling from soft tissue trauma in the presence of a fracture can create pressure that affects circulation and neurological function. In addition, pressure exerted from tightly applied circumferential bandages, casts, or braces may result in neurovascular deficits. Cool skin temperature, pale skin color, diminished pulses, and increased capillary refill are evidence of decreased perfusion. Sensory complaints such as pain, numbness, and tingling and motor changes such as weakness or inability to move the extremity distal to the pressure may indicate a developing neurovascular problem (Box 28-2). Development of compromised circulation must be reported to the physician promptly.

Box 28-1

Types of Fractures

Closed fracture—skin intact over fracture

Open or compound fracture—skin punctured by bone ends

Comminuted—having three or more bone fragments

Compression—bone that is crushed (e.g., vertebra)

Depressed—bone fragments pushed inward

Displaced—two edges of fracture have moved out of alignment

Impacted—bone ends pushed into each other

Longitudinal—fracture runs parallel with bone

Oblique—fracture slants across bone

Pathologic—results from minor stress applied to pathologically weakened bone

Segmental—segment of bone fractured and detached

Spiral—around the bone

Transverse—across the bone

Box 28-2

Assessment of Neurovascular Function (The Five *P's*)

Pain	Paresthesia
Pallor	Paralysis
Pulselessness	

NURSING DIAGNOSES

Nursing diagnoses for clients in immobilization devices focus on comfort and prevention of complications. **Anxiety** related to pain and/or immobility is appropriate when the immobilization results in muscle spasms or if it creates feelings of isolation, apprehension, and helplessness. **Bathing/Hygiene Self-Care Deficit, Dressing/Grooming Self-Care Deficit,** and **Toileting Self-Care Deficit** are appropriate when the client is learning to adapt to limitations; **Risk for Impaired Skin Integrity** and **Impaired Physical Mobility** are appropriate if immobilization is maintained continuously for days to weeks. **Risk for Peripheral Neurovascular Dysfunction** is appropriate when there is soft tissue swelling and/or the devices themselves put pressure on tissues. **Risk for Infection** is related to pin sites for the client having skeletal traction, external fixation, or halo traction or the client with an open wound. **Impaired Home Maintenance** is a possibility for the client going home with a cast or immobilization device.

Deficient Knowledge is appropriate because clients require information regarding care of the cast or immobilization device and cast removal. Instruction provides information regarding contact with water, restrictions in activity and positioning, and expectations regarding cast removal. Clients must know to report the development of numbness or tingling to the physician. Teaching includes application, removal, and schedule of wearing of immobilization devices.

Skill 28.1

Care of the Client in Skin Traction

Skin traction is the application of a pulling force directly to the skin and soft tissue that indirectly pulls on the skeletal system. Skin traction immobilizes a fracture and relieves muscle spasms and pain, requiring continuous application to achieve that goal. Skin traction usually provides temporary immobilization until open reduction and internal fixation (ORIF) or skeletal traction can be implemented. Furthermore, skin traction maintains alignment and reduces contractures and dislocations. Clients need written physician orders for specific traction weights, bed position, and turning regimen.

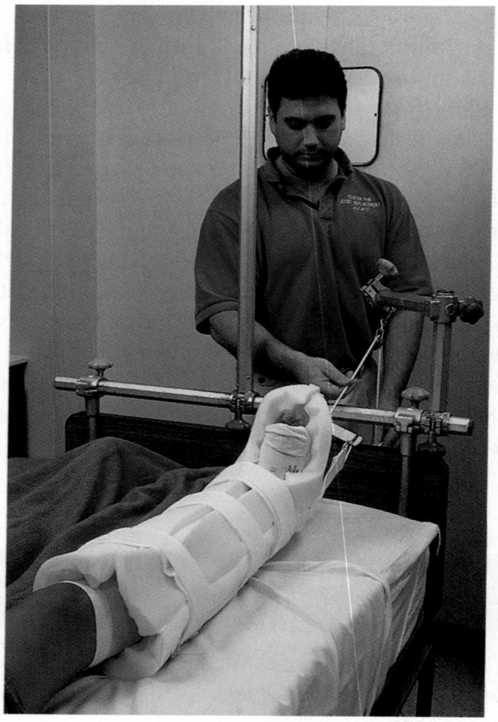

There are several types of skin traction. The most common type of adult skin traction is Buck's extension. It is applied to one or both legs using straps or a commercially prepared foam boot with Velcro straps (Figure 28-1). Dunlop's traction is another form of Buck's extension applied to the forearm to treat fractures of the humerus (Figure 28-2).

Cervical traction using a head halter involves a halter with a cutout for the ears and face (Figure 28-3). The halter cradles the chin and has straps leading to a bar attached to ropes, pulleys, and weights. Cervical traction immobilizes arthritic conditions of the cervical vertebrae, not fractures. It can be removed periodically.

Bryant's traction is skin traction used to immobilize infants with congenital hip dislocation and fractures of the femur for children weighing less than 40 pounds (Figure 28-4). Traction to both legs maintains immobilization in a vertical position for 7 to 10 days followed by a spica cast to continue recovery.

The more weight applied to the traction, the greater the chance of skin breakdown. No more than 7 pounds is used for Buck's traction. Cervical traction may use 7 to 10 pounds. Skin problems such as ulcers, dermatitis, burns, or abrasions prevent the use of skin traction because of the danger of exacerbation. Older clients and clients with diabetes are also at increased risk of skin breakdown.

When caring for a client in traction, personnel initially and regularly monitor correct maintenance of the traction device. Hospital policy may specify a frequency of checks, which needs to be at least every 4 to 8 hours. Traction maintenance involves monitoring the weights,

Figure 28-1 Buck's extension.

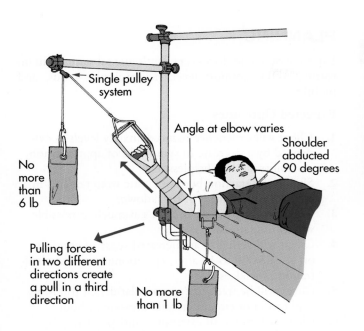

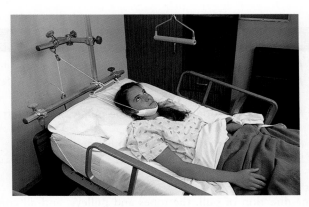

Figure 28-3 Cervical traction.

Figure 28-2 Dunlop's traction. (From Folcik MA, Carini-Garcia G, Birmingham JJ: *Traction: assessment and management,* St Louis, 1994, Mosby.)

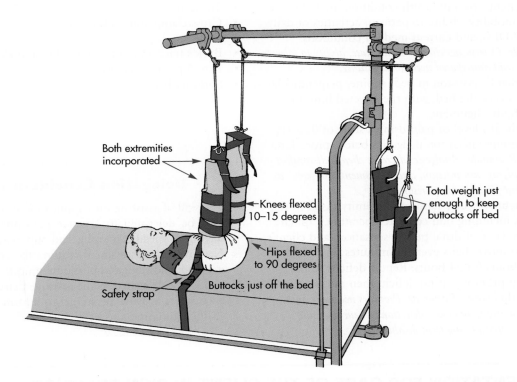

Figure 28-4 Bryant's traction. (From Folcik MA, Carini-Garcia G, Birmingham JJ: *Traction: assessment and management,* St Louis, 1994, Mosby.)

Box 28-3
Traction Assessment (The Four P's)

Pounds: Is the correct weight in place?
Pull: Is the direction of pull aligned with the long axis of the bone?
Pulleys: Is the rope riding over the pulley and gliding smoothly?
Pressure: Is each clamp and connection tight?

the direction of pull, the ropes and pulleys, and all connections (Box 28-3).

ASSESSMENT

1. Assess client's knowledge of the reason for traction. *Rationale: Determines concerns, fears, and need for further teaching.*
2. Assess integrity and condition of skin to be placed in traction. *Rationale: Determines ability of local tissues to tolerate traction's pulling forces. Skin traction is not placed over irritated, damaged, or broken skin.*
3. Assess client's overall health condition, including degree of mobility, ability to perform activities of daily living (ADLs), and current medical conditions. *Rationale: Determines client's health state, ability to tolerate traction, and anticipated need for assistance.*
4. Assess client's position in bed: supine, perpendicular to the ends of the bed, with the affected limb in proper body alignment.
5. Assess client's level of pain using a scale of 0 to 10, and determine need for analgesics before procedure begins. *Rationale: Analgesics decrease client's discomfort while applying skin traction, and assessment also serves as the baseline for later comparison.*
6. Assess neurovascular status of extremity distal to the traction, including skin color, temperature, capillary refill, presence of distal pulses, sensation, and client's ability to move digits every 30 minutes times 2, then every 2 hours for 24 hours. Report deficits to the physician promptly. If no deficit, then assess every 4 hours thereafter. *Rationale: Provides necessary baseline information, and early detection of neurovascular deficit can prevent long-term disabilities.*

PLANNING

Expected outcomes focus on client's mental status, skin integrity, ADLs, comfort level, neurovascular status, and mobility.

Expected Outcomes

1. Client will experience reduced anxiety levels as evidenced by a decrease in symptoms of apprehension, irritability, and/or helplessness.
2. Skin under traction boot or elastic wrap remains intact, without redness or breakdown.
3. Client will participate in ADLs as much as possible within limitations.
4. Client will verbalize an increased sense of comfort on a scale of 0 to 10 after repositioning and administration of analgesics.
5. Client will be free of neurovascular deficit following application of circumferential dressing or boot.
6. Client will move all extremities independently by date of discharge.

Equipment for Buck's Extension

- Overhead frame
- Traction bar
- Cross clamp and pulley
- Rope
- Buck's traction boot or moleskin and elastic bandages
- 1- to 5-pound weights
- Spreader bar

 Delegation Considerations

The skill of assisting with application of skin traction may be delegated to assistive personnel (AP) who have had specific training and supervised practice. Neurovascular assessment requires the critical thinking and knowledge application unique to the RN and is not delegated to the assistive personnel.

- Instruct assistive personnel to inform the nurse if client complains of discomfort.

IMPLEMENTATION FOR CARE OF THE CLIENT IN SKIN TRACTION

Steps	Rationale
1. See Standard Protocol (inside front cover).	
2. Position client supine and nearly flat with no more than 30 degrees elevation, with the affected leg halfway between the edge of the bed and middle of the bed.	

Steps	Rationale

COMMUNICATION TIP *Tell the client, "I will hold your extremity using slight tension." This will minimize any discomfort as traction is applied.*

Steps	Rationale
3. Wash affected leg (or legs) gently, and pat dry. 4. Apply foam boot, moleskin, or elastic bandages to affected leg, proceeding from distal to the proximal.	Application distal to proximal enhances circulation.

NURSE ALERT *Skin traction that is too tight puts pressure on nerves and vascular structures that could result in an irreversible neurovascular deficit. Skin traction that is too loose will slip.*

5. Attach weight to boot gradually and gently at the end of the bed.

NURSE ALERT *When applying Buck's extension, avoid pressure to the peroneal nerve at the neck of the fibula. Decreased sensation in the web space between the great toe and second toe, as well as inability to dorsiflex the foot and extend the toes, may indicate pressure to the nerve. Be alert to pressure over bony prominences about the ankle or the back of the heel.*

Steps	Rationale
6. Inspect traction setup: knots secure; ropes in pulleys; weights hanging freely, not caught on bed or resting on floor; and bedclothes not interfering with traction apparatus. Check the four *P*'s of traction maintenance (see Box 28-3, on facing page).	Routine observation of these checkpoints is necessary to maintain appropriate amount of tension and effective immobilization.
7. Assess neurovascular status of extremity distal to the traction, including skin color and temperature, capillary refill, presence of distal pulses, sensation, and client's ability to move digits every 30 minutes times 2, and every 4 hours while traction is in place.	Altered circulation, sensation, or motion can indicate potential problems that can result in permanent neurovascular damage.

NURSE ALERT *If tissues distal to skin traction are cold or cool, or if capillary refill is greater than 3 seconds, then compare with unaffected extremity. If deficit is related to traction wrap. Remove traction, and report neurovascular compromise.*

8. Release traction boot every 4 to 8 hours, and provide skin care according to physician's orders.
9. See Completion Protocol (inside front cover).

• • • • • • • • • •

EVALUATION

1. Evaluate traction setup: knots tied, not frayed, ropes in pulleys, weights hanging freely.
2. Inspect skin tissues for signs of pressure, color changes, edema, or tenderness.
3. Evaluate client's ability to perform ADLs.
4. Ask client to rate discomfort on a scale of 0 to 10 and to report muscle spasms.
5. Evaluate neurovascular status, and report deficits.
6. Observe client's use of trapeze and unaffected limbs to reposition self correctly.

Unexpected Outcomes and Related Interventions

1. Client complains of increased pain after Buck's extension is applied.
   a. Take the traction off (if allowed by physician), reposition client, and then reapply the traction. If not allowed, loosen traction slightly and reassess neurovascular status.

b. Administer analgesics as prescribed.
c. Realign body and/or limb.
d. If increased pain continues or pain occurs upon passive motion, then notify physician of possible neurovascular deficit.

2. Client has reddened areas on leg or heel under Buck's traction boot.
   a. Obtain physician order to remove foam boot for 1 hour to relieve pressure.
   b. Apply foam boot securely (nurse is able to insert one finger between client's skin and Buck's traction boot). Recheck correct tightness frequently.
   c. Increase skin checks to every hour.
   d. Apply protective barrier agent (e.g., Aloe Vista or Sween cream) to affected limb for protection against skin breakdown.
   e. Ensure heels do not rest on bed or pillow.

Recording and Reporting

- Record assessment of skin integrity beneath traction and nursing interventions implemented to maintain skin integrity.
- Record neurovascular assessment every 2 hours for the first 24 hours and, if no deficit, then every 4 hours thereafter.
- Report any neurovascular deficits to physician immediately.
- Record length of time client is in or out of specific traction.

Sample Documentation

0900 Buck's traction applied to client's left leg using a 5-pound weight. No c/o pain, tingling, or numbness. Capillary refill 3 seconds in nail beds of toes bilaterally; able to wiggle toes; skin warm, dry, and pink to lower left leg. Side rails up, bed down, 5-pound weights hanging freely. Knots tied, rope in pulley. Client in supine position with left leg in proper alignment.

1100 Client assessed for comfort. States he is "hurting a lot"—an 8 on a 0 to 10 scale. Medicated with 5 mg morphine sulfate IV push. Buck's boot removed. Skin assessed, and no breakdown evident. Buck's reapplied. Client repositioned. No skin breakdown noted to heel, malleolus, coccyx, or back.

1200 Client reassessed for comfort. Verbalized that pain medication helped and that pain is a 2 and reports feeling relaxed and comfortable.

SPECIAL CONSIDERATIONS

Pediatric Considerations

- Babies and young children are unable to remain still and in alignment.
- Bryant's traction is rarely used in children because of the risk for altered peripheral perfusion. Gravitational forces and circumferential wraps increase the risk for vasospasm and avascular necrosis (Wong and others, 1999).
- Bryant's traction is not removed for sleep. The elastic wraps are only loosened when there is marked edema of feet.

Geriatric Considerations

- Older clients may have keratoses, rashes, or other lesions that could become irritated in skin traction.
- Older clients may have long-standing conditions of musculoskeletal tissues such as arthritis or gout that could lead to inflamed tissues and skin breakdown.
- Older and chronically ill clients may have increased need for position changes resulting from limitations from osteoporosis, osteomalacia, weakened muscles, or increased risk of skin breakdown.
- Older clients' skin heals more slowly, is more fragile, less elastic, and thinner than when they were younger (Ebersole and Hess, 1998). Devices such as alternating air pressure mattresses or foam overlays decrease the risk of impaired skin integrity (see Chapter 26).

Home Care Considerations

- If client is to be discharged to home, relatives or caregivers are instructed in care needs (including home traction) and mode of ambulation.
- Teach family how to maintain integrity of traction by inspecting daily: weights hang freely, traction ropes rest in groove of pulley and hang freely, not caught on bed or resting on floor.

Skill 28.2

Care of the Client in Skeletal Traction and Pin Site Care

Skeletal traction immobilizes fractures of the femur below the trochanter, fractures of the cervical spine, and some fractures of the bones of the arm or ankle. Slow healing requires longer periods of traction (6 to 8 weeks) to promote bone repair. Skeletal traction is being used less frequently as a result of new surgical repair procedures. Skeletal traction involves puncturing the skin at the site where the pin enters and exits. In the case of external fixation or halo traction, the device attaches to the bone through the skin. Skeletal traction often immobilizes clients for weeks or sometimes months until healing occurs. Prolonged immobilization influences nursing care. This care focuses on supporting ADLs, maintenance of the traction, and prevention of fat emboli and complications of immobility, such as skin breakdown and pulmonary emboli.

A common form of skeletal traction is balanced-suspension skeletal traction (BSST), usually used for a fractured femur (Figure 28-5). Balanced suspension brings relief of muscle spasms, realignment of the fracture fragments, and callus formation. Callus formation is the development of new supportive bone around the injured site. BSST temporarily stabilizes the client's condition while waiting for

surgical insertion of an internal fixation device such as a plate or nail. Balanced suspension involves a sling attached to splints around the leg and a Steinmann pin or Kirschner wire supplying the traction (Figure 28-6). Sufficient weight to overcome the quadriceps and hamstring muscle spasms may be 30 to 40 pounds.

Other common forms of skeletal traction are side-arm traction (with a pin drilled through the lower humerus [Figure 28-7]), external fixation (used for comminuted fractures with soft tissue injury, skull and facial fractures, and pelvic bones [Figure 28-8]). For cervical spine fractures, Crutchfield or Gardner-Wells tongs are inserted into the skull. Halo traction is frequently used for neurologically intact clients, preventing further injury to the spinal cord (Figure 28-9).

External fixation is a form of skeletal traction that consists of a frame or apparatus to hold pins placed into or through bones above and below a fracture site. External fixation devices promote early ambulation and use of other joints while maintaining immobilization of affected bones. A variety of external fixation frames are used for skull and facial fractures, ribs, bones of the extremities, and pelvic bones (Perry and Potter, 2002).

All skeletal traction involves placement of a device through the skin, called a pin site. Procedures for pin site care must be kept current with infection-control guidelines established by the Centers for Disease Control and Prevention (CDC). Some institutions have policies outlining pin site care, such as cleanse site with Betadine swab every 4 hours. Some agencies require specific physician's orders to specify frequency of pin site care and cleansing agent to use. Clients discharged with an external fixation device are given specific guidelines for con-

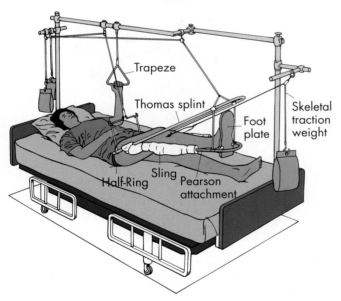

Figure 28-5 Balanced-suspension skeletal traction. Traction in long axis of right thigh is applied by means of Kirschner wire through proximal portion of tibia. Limb is supported by Thomas splint beneath thigh and Pearson attachment beneath leg. Footplate attachment prevents footdrop. Weights apply countertraction to upper end of Thomas splint and suspend its lower end. By using the left arm and leg as shown, client can shift position of the hips without change in amount of traction.

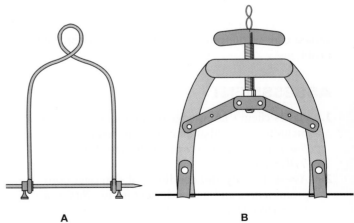

Figure 28-6 **A,** Kirschner wire and tractor. **B,** Steinmann pin and holder.

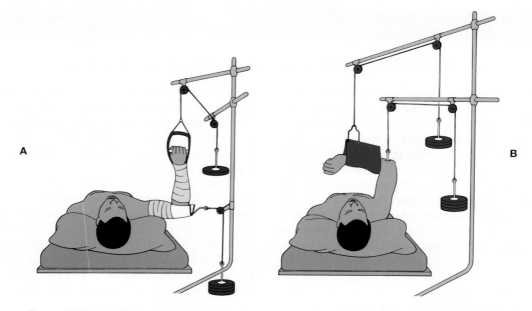

Figure 28-7 **A,** Side-arm traction (skin/skeletal). **B,** Overhead 90-90 traction (skeletal). (Redrawn from Beare PG, Myers JL: *Principles and practice of adult health nursing,* ed 3, St Louis, 1998, Mosby.)

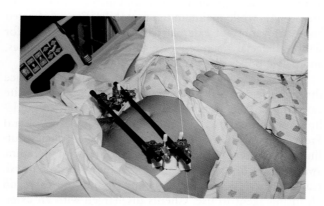

Figure 28-8 Pelvic AO fixator.

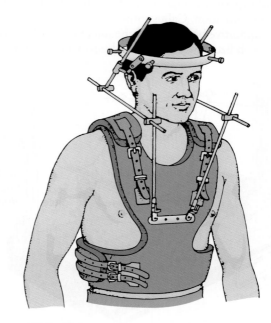

Figure 28-9 Halo vest. (From Beare PG, Myers JL: *Principles and practice of adult health nursing,* ed 3, St Louis, 1998, Mosby.)

tinued care of the pin sites and assessment for potential problems.

ASSESSMENT

1. Assess client's knowledge of the reason for traction, including nonverbal behavior and responses. *Rationale: Determines concerns, anxiety, and need for further teaching.*
2. Assess integrity and condition of skin over bony prominences and under devices in use. *Rationale: Determines baseline status of local tissues at risk for pressure ischemia.*
3. Assess client's overall health condition, including degree of mobility, ability to perform ADLs, and current medical conditions. *Rationale: Determines client's health state and serves as baseline for further reference.*
4. Assess client's level of pain using a scale of 0 to 10, and determine the need for analgesics before procedure begins. *Rationale: Decreases client's discomfort while applying traction and serves as baseline for later comparison.*
5. Following application, assess traction setup: weights hanging freely, ordered amount of weight applied,

ropes moving freely through pulleys, all knots tight in ropes and away from pulleys. *Rationale: Ensures accurate function of traction.*

6. Assess neurovascular status of extremity distal to the traction, including skin color, temperature, capillary refill, presence of distal pulses, sensation, and client's ability to move digits. *Rationale: Provides necessary baseline information and detects neurovascular deficits.*
7. Assess client's mobility. *Rationale: Determines client's ability to participate in repositioning and ADLs.*
8. Assess pin sites for redness, edema, discharge, or odor. *Rationale: Determines presence of infection.*
9. Assess for respiratory dysfunction. *Rationale: Pulmonary embolus can occur with the client who has associated spinal cord injury or who is on prolonged bed rest. Halo vests are not recommended for clients with respiratory insufficiency because of the restricted chest expansion.*

PLANNING

Expected outcomes focus on client's anxiety level, skin integrity, self-care abilities, comfort and mobility level, neurovascular status, infection risks, and pulmonary status.

Expected Outcomes

1. Skeletal deformity is reduced, alignment is maintained, and injury is healed.
2. Client will verbalize decreased anxiety, irritability, and/or helplessness.
3. Skin over bony prominences or under halo vest remains intact, without redness or breakdown.
4. Client performs ADLs independently to all unaffected areas.
5. Client verbalizes a sense of comfort (2 or below on a scale of 0 to 10) after repositioning and administration of analgesics.
6. Client is free of neurovascular deficit following application of traction.
7. Skin around pin sites remains free of redness, swelling, or drainage.

Equipment

Balanced-suspension Skeletal Traction (BSST) (see Figure 28-5, p. 653)

- Ropes, pulleys, weights
- Thomas splint
- Pearson attachment with sheepskin padding
- Footplate
- Trapeze

Halo Traction (see Figure 28-9, p. 654)

- Halo ring with four pins
- Molded vest jacket
- Vertical metal bars connecting ring to jacket
- Tracheostomy tray (for emergency resuscitation)
- Allen wrench (allows removal of screws for resuscitation)

Pin Site Care Supplies

- Sterile cotton-tipped applicators
- Sterile normal saline
- Prescribed cleansing agent
- Antiseptic ointment
- Split 2 × 2 dressings
- Disposable gloves

Delegation Considerations

Skeletal traction is applied by the physician. The skill of assisting with insertion of skeletal pins and pin site care may be delegated to assistive personnel (AP) who are adequately trained in principles of surgical asepsis. Assessment for complications, including infection or inflammation at pin insertion site, requires the critical thinking and knowledge application unique to the nurse and cannot be delegated.

IMPLEMENTATION FOR CARE OF THE CLIENT IN SKELETAL TRACTION AND PIN SITE CARE

Steps	Rationale
1. See Standard Protocol (inside front cover).	
2. Inspect traction setup: knots secure; ropes in pulleys; weights hanging freely, not caught on bed or resting on floor; and bedclothes not interfering with traction apparatus. (see Box 28-3, p. 650).	Routine observation of these checkpoints is necessary to maintain appropriate amount of tension and effective immobilization.

NURSE ALERT *Irreversible tissue death occurs within 4 to 12 hours.*

Steps	Rationale

3. Monitor neurovascular status of distal aspects of involved extremities in comparison with corresponding body part every 2 hours for the first 24 hours and every 4 to 12 hours thereafter (according to agency policy):

   a. Inspect color and temperature.

Pink, warm tissues are adequately oxygenated. Whitish tissue indicates decreased arterial supply, and bluish color signifies venous stasis.

   b. Monitor for edema.

May result from tissue trauma or venous stasis.

   c. Assess capillary refill by pressing on toe or fingernail, releasing, and noting "pinking" on nail within 3 seconds.

4. Provide pin site care according to hospital policy or physician's orders.

   a. Remove gauze dressings from around pins, and discard in receptacle.

   b. Inspect sites for drainage or inflammation.

Signs indicative of infection.

   c. Prepare supplies, and apply new disposable gloves.

   d. Clean each pin site with prescribed solution by placing sterile applicator close to the pin and cleaning away from the insertion site. Dispose of applicator.

NURSE ALERT *Touching one pin site with material used on another increases risk of transmission of microorganisms.*

---

   e. Repeat the process for each pin site.

   f. Using a sterile applicator, apply a small amount of topical antibiotic ointment to pin site (check for physician's orders or hospital policy).

   g. Cover with a sterile 2 × 2 split gauze dressing, or leave site open to air (OTA) as prescribed or according to hospital policy. Remove and discard gloves, and perform hand hygiene.

5. Inspect skin (bony prominences, heels, elbows, sacrum, and areas under appliances) for signs of pressure, and lightly massage pressure areas every 2 hours unless evidence of beginning skin breakdown is evident (tenderness, reactive hyperemia).

Light massage increases circulation to area. Firm massage to compromised tissues increases tissue breakdown.

6. Assess risk for pressure ulcers (e.g., use Braden scale), and consider need for special bed or mattress (see Chapter 25).

Clients at risk for pressure formation will require placement on pressure-relieving mattress.

7. Monitor respiratory status every shift (see Chapter 13). Assess for possible fat embolism syndrome, including hypoxia, restlessness, mental changes, tachycardia, tachypnea, dyspnea, low blood pressure, and petechial rash over upper chest and neck.

Clients with fractures of long bones are at especially high risk for fat embolism. All immobilized clients are at high risk for atelectasis and pulmonary emboli.

8. Assess level of discomfort, and provide nonpharmacological and pharmacological relief as indicated (see Chapter 11).

Pain may result from the traumatic injury and muscle spasms.

NURSE ALERT *Never ignore a client's complaint. Follow through and check it out.*

Steps	Rationale

9. Encourage the use of unaffected extremities for ADLs and active and passive exercises (see Chapter 27). Encourage use of trapeze bar for repositioning in bed.

Prevents muscle atrophy and maintains muscle tone for later ambulation.

10. For elimination provide a fracture pan (see Chapter 9).

Smaller bedpan is more comfortable for the client and easier to place under client.

11. See Completion Protocol (inside front cover).

• • • • • • • • • •

EVALUATION

1. Determine client's anxiety level in response to traction and immobilization.
2. Inspect skin for evidence of breakdown.
3. Observe participation in ADLs and use of unaffected extremities.
4. Evaluate level of pain and discomfort from muscle spasms.
5. Evaluate neurovascular status and peripheral tissue perfusion.
6. Evaluate for local and systemic indications of infection, including drainage and inflammation at pin sites, fever, elevated white blood cell count, continuous dull aching pain, redness, or warmth in extremity (possible osteomyelitis [i.e., bone infection]).

Unexpected Outcomes and Related Interventions

1. Client has severe edema, marked increase in pain, inability to actively move joint or increased pain on passive movement, indicating compartment syndrome, which leads to decreased venous perfusion and increased venous stasis; tissue anoxia may be developing with the potential for loss of function.
   a. Prompt management is critical. Notify physician.
   b. Apply cold compress and elevate to heart level if possible.
   c. Reduce or eliminate compression caused by therapeutic devices.
2. Redness, increased swelling, and drainage develop at pin site(s) or fracture site (osteomyelitis).
   a. Cultures of drainage may be indicated to identify infecting organism. (Physician's order is not usually required, see agency policy.) (See Chapter 14.)
   b. Notify physician for antibiotic orders.
3. Signs of osteomyelitis or systemic infection develop, including fever, elevated white blood cell count, general malaise. This is especially a concern with open fractures and extensive soft tissue injury.
   a. Notify physician. Orders may include irrigation of the site with antibiotic solution and/or intravenous (IV) antibiotics.
   b. Encourage fluid intake, and provide comfort measures for fever.
4. Evidence of nerve damage develops from pressure or trauma to nerves, depending upon type of traction in

place. For example, peroneal nerve: footdrop may develop with inability to evert and dorsiflex foot; radial or median nerve at wrist: inability to approximate thumb and fingers (radial) and numbness and tingling of thumb, index, middle fingers (medial) with wrist drop.
   a. Eliminate pressure if possible according to type of traction in place.
   b. Notify physician.
5. Client experiences fat embolism (more common in fractures of long bones) with symptoms of hypoxia, restlessness, mental changes, tachycardia, tachypnea, dyspnea, low blood pressure, and occasionally petechial rash over upper chest and neck.
   a. This is a life-threatening emergency—50% of persons with fat emboli die.
   b. Notify physician, and initiate major resuscitation efforts.

Recording and Reporting

- Record in nurses' notes type of traction, site to which traction is applied, amount of weights, and client's response.
- Often a flow sheet is used that specifies specific routine assessments and frequency of assessment.

Sample Documentation

0700 BSST in place with 20-pound weight to left femur. Knots secure, ropes in pulleys, weights hanging freely. Neurovascular assessment to left foot—color pink, temperature warm, no numbness or tingling, wiggles toes on command, capillary refill 2 seconds. Reports pain at 2 on scale of 0 to 10. Lateral pin site dry, medial pin site draining small amount clear fluid ($\frac{1}{4}$-inch diameter circle). No odor. No redness.

0900 Medial pin site drainage changed to yellow drainage ($\frac{1}{2}$-inch diameter circle). Pin site cultured. Reports pain of 6 on 0 to 10 scale. Dr. Morrison notified of pin site drainage.

0915 Tylenol 3 tabs 2 administered PO. Medial and lateral pin sites cleansed with Betadine, and triple antibiotic applied. Antibiotic started per order.

1000 Reports pain decreased to a 2. No drainage visible on medial or lateral pin site split dressing.

SPECIAL CONSIDERATIONS

Pediatric Considerations

- Blood loss from a fracture in a child poses a greater danger because the blood volume in a child is 70% to 85% of total body weight and only about 60% in the adult (Wong and others, 1999)
- Caregivers and parents work together to develop strategies to combat boredom of child in traction. Counseling regarding possibility of regressive type behaviors lessens the parents' anxiety. Interference with schoolwork is remedied by obtaining work from school as soon as the child is able to perform tasks.
- Children are assured that someone will be there to assist them while they are in traction.

Geriatric Considerations

- Older clients are particularly prone to the development of altered skin integrity when they are immobilized and not repositioned frequently. This tendency results from a decreased amount of subcutaneous fat and skin that is less elastic, thinner, drier, and more fragile than that of a younger adult.
- Older clients may have long-standing conditions of musculoskeletal tissues such as arthritis or gout that could lead to inflamed tissues and skin breakdown.
- Older and chronically ill clients may have increased need for position changes to prevent the complications of immobility and those resulting from limitations imposed by osteoporosis, osteomalacia, or weakened muscles.

- Severe varicose veins will prevent the use of skin traction in the older client because of the risk of skin breakdown.

Home Care Considerations

- Following removal of skeletal traction, client is taught to ambulate slowly within medical guidelines, gradually increasing length of time out of bed and distance walked.
- Client is taught to notify physician of undesirable signs, such as marked increase in pain, muscle spasms, and increased numbness. These symptoms may indicate reinjury or insufficient healing.
- Family members are taught to apply skin traction correctly if it is prescribed for home use following the removal of the skeletal traction.
- Client and family members are taught the use of muscle relaxants and analgesics if prescribed for home use.

Long-Term Care Considerations

- Clients are instructed in home safety methods to prevent further injuries.
- Clients are instructed in dosage of vitamin D and the minimum amount of calcium needed in diet to promote strong bones.

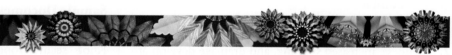

Skill 28.3

Care of the Client During Cast Application

A cast provides immobilization for an injured extremity to protect it from further injury, provides alignment of a fracture by holding the bone fragments in reduction and alignment during the healing process, and promotes comfort. In addition, it maintains a limb in alignment to prevent or correct structural abnormalities. Casts are used in many different ways (Figure 28-10). The use and application materials required depends on the anatomical area of injury.

One of two types of cast materials, plaster of Paris or synthetic, may be used. The type of cast material selected depends on the number of cast changes anticipated and the type of musculoskeletal injury. Plaster of Paris is composed of open-weave cotton roll or strip covered with calcium sulfate crystals. When moistened with water, this material molds easily during application, but drying may

require (1) 24 hours for a regular arm cast, (2) up to 48 hours before weight bearing or external pressure can be applied, and (3) 36 to 72 hours for large body casts (Schoen, 2000). During the period of drying, the cast must be exposed to air to dry, be well supported on firm surfaces, and handled with palms (not fingertips) to avoid indentations such as fingerprints, and turned regularly so that it will dry evenly. Lifting the cast by supporting the joints above and below the casted area prevents injury to underlying soft tissues. This type of cast is heavier than a synthetic cast.

Synthetic casting materials are composed of open-weave fiberglass tape covered with a polyurethane resin that is activated by water. This cast sets very quickly, in approximately 15 minutes, and can withstand pressure or weight bearing after 20 minutes (Table 28-1). It forms a light-

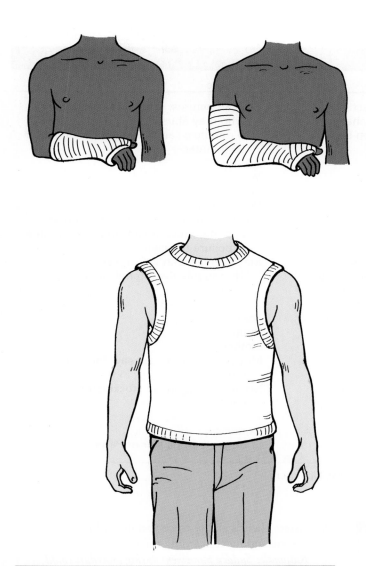

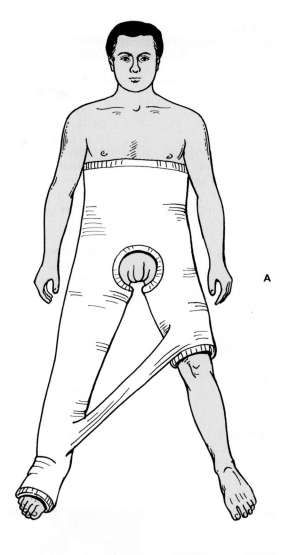

A

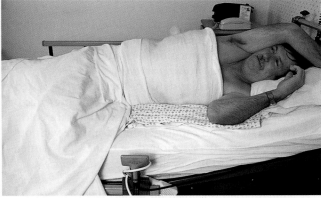

B

Figure 28-10   A, Types of casts. *Top left,* short arm cast; *top center,* long arm cast; *bottom left,* plaster body jacket cast; *far right,* one and one-half hip spica cast. **B,** Client in body cast.

weight, sturdy cast that is both radiolucent and waterproof. Different colors of this casting material are also available, ranging from fluorescent pink and green to navy blue and purple. Colors are often more appealing to children and aid in maintaining the appearance of the cast (Figure 28-11). These casts are more expensive than plaster casts.

This skill includes assessment parameters before, during, and after cast application, including peripheral neurovascular status. Assisting with the application of the cast is also discussed. It is important to follow guidelines for care after application with respect to pressure against cast and weight bearing.

Table 28-1

Comparison of Casting Materials

	Plaster of Paris	Synthetic
Indications	Unstable or displaced fractures, edema, frequent cast changes	Stable fractures, long-term cast, clients who may abuse cast
Drying time	24-72 hours depending on size of cast	7-15 minutes; can be weight bearing after 20 minutes
Drying method	Air dry	Air dry
Radiolucent	Minimal	Yes
Weight of cast	Heavy	Lightweight
Durability	May crumble and flake	Very sturdy
Bathing/immersibility	Must be kept dry	Can be immersed, as in swimming and bathing; must be thoroughly dried after exposure to water
Cleaning cast	Prevention of soiling is best approach. May use damp cloth and mild cleanser for slight soiling (do not wet cast)	May cleanse with warm water. Thoroughly dry after cleaning.
Choice of colors	No	Yes
Surface area	Smooth	Rough
Molding	Easy	Limited
Special equipment	None	May need special cast saw for cast removal
Padding	Cotton sheet wadding or Webril, stockinette	Nonabsorbent nylon stockinette and padding
Cost	Inexpensive	Expensive
Strength	Strong	Stronger than plaster of Paris

Data from Schoen DC: *Adult orthopaedic nursing*, Philadelphia, 2000, Lippincott.

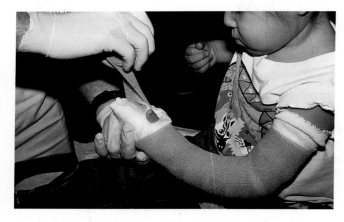

Figure 28-11 Synthetic casting materials are available in different colors that are appealing to children.

ASSESSMENT

1. Assess client's health status, focusing on factors that may affect wound healing, such as diabetes, poor nutritional status, or steroid medication use. *Rationale: Healing of the injured tissues may be slower in these clients, or additional nutritional supplements may be required.*

2. Assess client's ability to cooperate and level of understanding concerning the casting procedure. *Rationale: Sudden movement during procedure could cause injury.*

3. Assess condition of the skin that will be under the cast. Specifically, note any areas of skin breakdown, rashes present, or incisional wound. *Rationale: Provides baseline for skin condition..*

4. Assess neurovascular status of the area to be casted (see Box 28-2, p. 647). Specifically, note presence or absence of motor and sensory function, skin color, temperature, and capillary refill. Compare with opposite extremity or surrounding tissues. Pay particular attention to tissues distal to cast. *Rationale: Changes in neurovascular status may occur after casting, possibly further compromising already injured tissues. It is important to note the baseline neurovascular status so that these changes, if they occur, can be accurately assessed.*

5. Assess client's pain status using a scale of 0 to 10.

6. Consult with physician to determine the extent to which client will be able to use the casted body part. *Rationale: Determines extent to which self-care will be impaired.*

PLANNING

Expected outcomes focus on skin integrity, comfort, self-care, mobility, prevention of neurovascular complications, and maintenance of cast integrity.

Expected Outcomes

1. Client's exposed skin distal to cast is warm and pink, with capillary refill less than 3 seconds.
2. Pulses distal to the cast are palpable, strong, and regular.
3. Cast remains clean, without indentions or fraying, until removal.
4. Client has edema of 1+ or less and demonstrates less than 25% decrease in active range of motion (ROM) of affected extremity after cast application.
5. Client verbalizes pain less than 3 (scale of 0 to 10) after analgesic administration 20 to 30 minutes before the procedure.
6. Client requires minimal assistance with ADLs after an extremity is casted.
7. Client demonstrates proper cast care.

Equipment (may be on cast cart) (Figure 28-12)

- Plaster cast
- Plaster rolls: sizes 2, 3, 4, or 6 inch
- Padding material (felt, sheet wadding, Webril, stockinette, or gore lining)
- Disposable gloves, apron, or protective cover
- Plastic-lined bucket or basin
- Water warmed at time of application
- Cart, chair, and fracture table scissors
- Paper or plastic sheets
- Synthetic cast

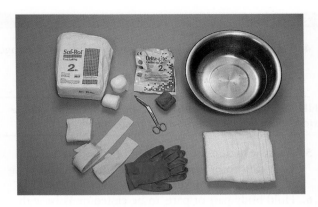

Figure 28-12   Casting materials.

- Synthetic rolls: 2, 3, or 4 inch
- Pail with water to dampen rolls
- Padding materials (nylon stockinette and synthetic padding)
- Cast cutter (to trim edge of cast, if needed)

Delegation Considerations

A complete assessment of the client before cast applications requires the knowledge application and critical thinking skills unique to an RN. The skill of assisting with cast application may be delegated to assistive personnel (AP).
- Inform AP in method to assist in positioning for specific client with mobility restrictions.

IMPLEMENTATION FOR CARE OF THE CLIENT DURING CAST APPLICATION

Steps	Rationale
1. See Standard Protocol (inside front cover).	
2. Administer analgesic before cast application: orally (PO), 30 to 40 minutes before; intramuscularly (IM), 20 to 30 minutes before; IV, 2 to 5 minutes before.	Reduces pain during cast application. Provides optimal analgesic effect.
3. Assist physician or certified technician in positioning client and injured extremity as desired, depending on type of cast to be used and area to be casted.	The parts to be casted must be supported and in optimal alignment.

COMMUNICATION TIP *Explain procedure to client, including how client can help, position, and how it will feel. "You may experience dampness and warmth under the cast during the cast application process and heat as it dries. This is normal and expected."*

Steps	Rationale
4. Prepare skin that will be enclosed in the cast. Change any dressing (if present), and cleanse the skin with mild soap and water.	Assists in maintaining skin integrity.

NURSE ALERT *Clients with skin damage or skin lesions may not be candidates for casting.*

Steps	Rationale
5. Assist with application of padding material around body part to be casted (see illustration). Avoid wrinkles or uneven thicknesses.	Decreases complications to the skin and prevents pressure points under the cast. Plaster gives off heat from a chemical reaction when drying.
6. Hold body part or parts to be casted or assist with preparation of casting materials.	Support of body part may require application of slight manual traction.
a. *Plaster cast:* Mark the end of the roll by folding one corner of the material under itself. Hold plaster roll under water in a plastic-lined bucket or basin until bubbles stop, then squeeze slightly and hand roll to person applying the cast.	Once dampened, the end of the casting tape may be difficult to find. Dampened plaster rolls are unrolled and molded to fit the extremity or body part to be casted.
b. *Synthetic cast:* Submerge cast roll in lukewarm water for 10 to 15 seconds. Squeeze to remove excess water.	Submersion in water initiates the chemical reaction, which will eventually result in hardening of the cast.
7. Continue to hold the body parts as necessary as the cast is applied (see illustration), or supply additional rolls of casting tape as needed.	Thickness of the plaster cast determines strength of the cast.
8. Provide walking heel, brace, bar, or other material to stabilize the cast as requested by the physician. An abduction bar or wooden post may be used to stabilize a spica cast.	Ambulation may be permitted with partial weight bearing on the affected extremity after cast has dried. Braces may be incorporated into a cast to assist in joint motion and mobility.

NURSE ALERT *Do not use abduction bar as a handle for positioning the client.*

Steps	Rationale
9. Assist with "finishing" the cast by folding the edge of the stockinette down over the cast to provide a smooth edge. A dampened plaster roll is unrolled over the stockinette to hold it in place.	Smooth edges decrease the chance for skin irritation or tissue injury.
10. Using scissors, trim the cast around fingers, toes, or the thumb as necessary. Remove and discard gloves, and perform hand hygiene.	The cast should not restrict joint movement or constrict circulation.
11. Elevate the casted tissues on cloth-covered pillows or in a sling. Avoid complete encasing of the cast. Air dry.	Pillows or other soft areas prevent indentation or other undesirable hardening of the cast. Covering of the cast delays drying.

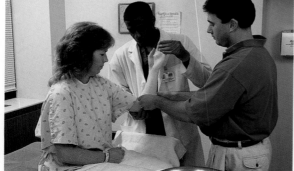

Step 5 Padding under cast is smooth.

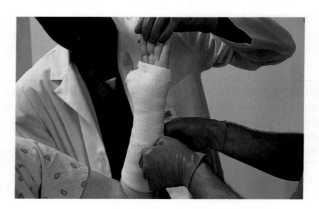

Step 7 Support extremity during cast application.

Steps	Rationale
12. Inform client to notify caregiver of any alteration in sensation, numbness, tingling, unusual pain, or inability to move fingers or toes in affected extremity.	Edema within a casted extremity causes pressure on nerves, blood vessel, and muscle tissues. This leads to neurovascular deficit, compartment syndrome, and necrosis of tissues.
13. Using palms of hands to support casted areas, assist client with transfer to stretcher or wheelchair for return to unit, or prepare for discharge.	Avoids indentations in cast that could cause pressure areas on underlying skin. Additional personnel may be required to transfer client safely, especially with client in a spica or other large body cast. Pillows, restraints, and side rails may also be needed to maintain principles of safe transport.

NURSE ALERT   *Client with wet large-limb or wet spica cast requires three people to assist in turning and transfer. Proper assistance prevents undue pressure on cast and prevents client injury.*

---

14. Review all home care instructions with client and significant other (Box 28-4).

Box 28-4

Cast Care Instructions

THE FIRST 24 HOURS
- Follow the physician's instructions.
- Keep the cast and extremity above the level of the heart for at least 48 hours by propping your cast up on firm pillows.
- Put ice directly over the fractured area for 24 hours, but be sure to enclose the ice in a plastic bag to keep the cast dry.
- Move the parts of your body above and below the cast regularly to aid circulation and relieve stiffness. Massaging the joints and extremities around the cast will also improve circulation.
- Your cast needs at least 24 hours to dry if it is plaster. Avoid handling it as much as possible. When you do have to move the cast, such as when you change your body position, use only the palms of your hands and support the cast under your joints. You want to avoid putting indentations in the cast that will put pressure on the skin inside.
- Use a fan placed 18 to 24 inches from the cast to aid its drying in the first 24 hours. Be sure to expose the whole cast for drying, and do not cover it with linen for the first 24 hours.
- Never insert any object into your cast for any purpose; for example, do not try to scratch under cast when it itches.

HOW TO CARE FOR YOUR CAST
Plaster
- Do not get the cast wet because it will lose its strength. If cast does become wet, dry immediately. Use a towel to blot moisture off the cast, then dry it

with a hair dryer set on low. When your cast does not feel cold and damp, it is dry.
- To keep the cast clean and dry, cover it with plastic when bathing, using the toilet (if it is a spica cast), or going out in rain or snow.
- Use a damp cloth and scouring powder to clean soiled spots on the cast. Be sure to brush away plaster crumbs or other objects from the edges of the cast, but do not remove or rearrange any padding. Do not break off or trim cast edges.

Synthetic
- If you have a fiberglass cast without wounds or incisions under it, you may be able to continue a more normal lifestyle, for example, bathing or swimming, if your doctor approves. A fiberglass cast can become wet.
- If you swim in a pool or a lake, be sure to rinse both the inside and outside of the cast to flush out any dirt and chemicals. You should use only a small amount of mild soap around your cast and should rinse under your cast thoroughly.
- Washing or rinsing inside your fiberglass cast may reduce odor and irritation and improve the overall skin condition of the cast area. You may use a spray nozzle at a sink or a flexible shower head to rinse inside your cast with warm water.
- You must thoroughly dry the cast after wetting. Lightly towel off excess water and use a hair dryer on cool or low setting to dry inside cast. Do not cover the cast while it is drying.

Continued

Box 28-4

Cast Care Instructions—cont'd

SKIN CARE

- Skin care is very important during the time a cast is worn. Routinely inspect the skin condition around the cast.
- Do not insert objects under the cast because you could scrape the skin or add pressure and cause an infection or sore under the cast.
- You may use powders and lotions only outside the cast so that the skin stays clean and soft. Powder inside a cast can cake and cause sore areas.

ACTIVITY

Do not walk on a leg cast for the first 48 hours. If you are allowed to walk on it, be sure to walk on the walking heel. If your arm is in a cast, be sure to use your sling for support and comfort.

CONTACT YOUR DOCTOR IF

- You have pain, burning, or swelling
- You feel a blister or sore developing inside the cast
- You notice an unusual odor coming from the cast
- You experience numbness or persistent tingling
- Your cast becomes badly soiled
- Your cast breaks, cracks, or develops soft spots
- Your cast becomes too loose
- You develop skin problems at the cast edges
- You develop a fever or foul odor under cast
- You have any questions regarding your treatment

Steps	Rationale
15. Clean used equipment, and return to usual storage area.	Expedites use of equipment for the next client and maintains principles of infection control.
16. Explain to client the need to keep cast exposed until drying is complete and the use of elevation or ice.	Casts must dry from the inside out for thorough drying. Elevation and application of ice assist in decreasing edema formation.
17. Have client turn every 2 to 3 hours when a body jacket or a hip spica cast is applied.	Avoids indentation and prevents continuous pressure to one area.
18. See Completion Protocol (inside front cover).	

• • • • • • • • • •

EVALUATION

1. Inspect exposed skin, and assess capillary refill by pressing on toe or finger if the cast is on an extremity (Figure 28-13).

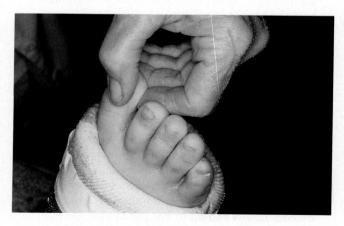

Figure 28-13   Inspecting toe to assess capillary refill.

2. Palpate the temperature of tissues around the casted area for warmth, and assess for hot spots, which could indicate underlying localized infection.
3. Palpate any accessible pulses distal to the cast.
4. Inspect condition of the cast.
5. Observe for edema of tissues distal to the cast for signs of vascular compromise (whitish or bluish coloration).
6. Observe client for signs of pain or anxiety (hyperventilation, tachycardia, blood pressure elevation).
7. Observe client performing ADLs and ROM.
8. Ask client to describe cast care.
9. Observe client perform cast care.

Unexpected Outcomes and Related Interventions

1. Client experiences impaired physical mobility related to the cast.
   a. Assist client with ROM exercises every 3 to 4 hours.
   b. Teach isometric exercises.

2. Client complains of pain after application of the cast.
   a. Assess description, amount, type, and severity (using a scale of 0 to 10).
   b. Reposition casted extremity or client. Adjust elevation of pillows as necessary.
   c. Apply ice bags along sides of cast as needed. Do not place heavy ice bags on top of damp cast because of risk of indentation.
   d. Administer analgesics as ordered to maintain client's comfort level.
   e. Perform neurovascular checks.
   f. Assess tightness of the cast by checking with fingers around the edges and checking with client. Cast should be snug but not tight.
   g. If pain continues, notify physician.
3. Client develops compartment syndrome, a condition in which increased pressure within a limited space severely compromises the circulation and function of tissues within that space.
   a. Assess for severe pain unrelieved by analgesics. Pain is usually more severe than expected with the particular injury.
   b. Assess change in neurovascular status, such as numbness, tingling, or decreased movement in distal skin and tissues.
   c. Assess for pulse in area distal to casted extremity (pulselessness develops late in the syndrome) or capillary refill over 3 seconds.
   d. Notify physician.
   e. Prepare to bivalve cast using a cast cutter.
4. Client reports a sensation of heat beneath the cast.
   a. Assess for indications of localized and systemic infection.
   b. Notify physician.

Recording and Reporting

- Record application of cast.
- Record condition of skin.
- Record circulation, temperature, sensation, and motion of distal part.
- Record instructions given to client and family.
- Report abnormal or untoward findings from neurovascular checks; report the following immediately: bluish color to distal parts, marked increase in edema or pain, delayed capillary refill (longer than 3 seconds), inability to palpate distal peripheral pulses if originally palpable, increased numbness or tingling, cold tissues, and inability to move tissues actively.

Sample Documentation

0900 Left long arm synthetic cast applied and left arm placed in shoulder sling by Dr. Melancon. Capillary refill of left index finger is 2 seconds. Client able to move all fingers of left hand, fingers warm to touch, nail beds pink, no swelling noted. Complains of pain at 5 (scale of 0 to 10).

0910 Tylox 1 tab administered PO. Left long arm cast and sling readjusted.

0945 Left long arm cast intact with sling. Capillary refill of left index finger unchanged. Client moves all fingers of left hand, fingers warm to touch, denies any numbness or tingling present. No edema noted. Reports pain decreased to 1 (scale of 0 to 10).

SPECIAL CONSIDERATIONS

Pediatric Considerations

- Allow the child to choose the color of a synthetic cast.
- Teach caregivers to protect plaster cast from moisture. Teach caregivers to ensure that synthetic casts are dried thoroughly if damp. Lower-extremity casts are protected with plastic wrap during urination or defecation.
- Monitor children closely to ensure that objects are not placed beneath cast to scratch. Antihistamines and a hair dryer set to cool setting can be used to control itching (Hart and Kester, 1999).
- Recognize that babies and young children demonstrate pain by restlessness and crying.
- Provide child with doll that has cast similar to child's cast to reduce anxiety and to use as a teaching tool.

Geriatric Considerations

- Lightweight, synthetic casts are better for older clients. Cast is less restrictive, and light weight helps clients maintain better balance.
- Plaster of Paris casts on older clients may have less plaster, to aid in moving or lifting.
- Older clients may have reduced sensation and be less able to detect compression (Ebersole and Hess, 1998).
- Older clients may take longer for bone healing than younger clients.
- Older clients may experience age-related decrease in muscle strength. This may cause difficulty in ambulating with a cast.

Home Care Considerations

- Reinforce cast care instruction (see Box 28-4, p. 663).
- Instruct to elevate affected extremity when sitting to help reduce swelling.
- Remind to inspect cast daily for foul odor, which indicates skin excoriation or infection under cast.
- Remind to inspect skin daily for pressure or friction areas.
- Remind to inspect cast daily for cracks or changes in alignment.

Skill 28.4

Care of the Client During Cast Removal

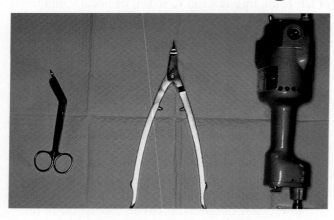

Figure 28-14 Cast saw and equipment.

When caring for clients with casts, it is also important to understand the techniques for cast removal, which consist of removing the cast and padding, followed by skin care to the affected area. The cast is removed by use of a cast saw (Figure 28-14). The saw is noisy, but the procedure is painless because the saw vibrates and thus will not cut the skin. It is necessary, however, to prepare the client adequately for cast removal. A small child or confused adult may require gentle restraint during removal to avoid any injury. Careful removal of a synthetic cast (with gore lining) is important to prevent burns which may result from the heat generated by the vibrating saw.

This skill includes gathering the equipment necessary for cast removal, adequate client preparation, and providing skin care to the casted area after cast removal. After cast removal, the client may experience tenderness, soreness, or muscle weakness.

ASSESSMENT

1. Assess client's understanding and ability to cooperate with cast removal. *Rationale: Cast removal may require a cast saw. Client needs to understand that the saw is noisy but does not cut skin.*

2. Assess client's readiness for cast removal (physician's orders, x-ray examination results, physical findings).
3. Ask if client feels itching or burning under the cast. *Rationale: Skin dryness or irritation may be present.*

PLANNING

Expected outcomes focus on skin integrity of the underlying skin and client understanding of the cast removal procedure.

Expected Outcomes

1. Client is able to describe and demonstrate levels of activity and weight-bearing limitations.
2. There is no underlying tissue damage after cast removal.
3. Client can describe skin care measures and perform ADLs as appropriate.

Equipment

- Cast saw
- Plastic sheets or paper
- Cold water enzyme wash
- Skin lotion
- Basin, water, washcloth, towels
- Scissors

Delegation Considerations

The skill of assisting with cast removal may be delegated to assistive personnel (AP) who have had specific training and supervised practice.
- Review with care provider proper method of cast removal.

IMPLEMENTATION FOR CARE OF THE CLIENT DURING CAST REMOVAL

Steps	Rationale
1. See Standard Protocol (inside cover).	
2. Assist with positioning of client.	Prevents accidental injury to skin during cast removal.
3. Describe the physical sensations to expect during cast removal (vibration of cast saw and generation of heat) (see illustration).	Knowledge of the procedure decreases level of anxiety.

COMMUNICATION TIP   *Tell client, "You may feel warmth from the vibration of the saw, but the saw doesn't cut your skin. Here, let me demonstrate on my thumb."*

Steps	Rationale
4. Describe the expected appearance of the extremity.	Skin under cast becomes scaly, and dead cells that normally slough off accumulate.
5. Describe and demonstrate the loud noise of the cast saw.	
6. Stay with client, and explain progress of procedure as cast is removed (see illustration).	
7. Inspect tissues underlying the cast after removal. Note areas of irritation or breakdown may require treatment.	
8. If skin is intact, apply cold water enzyme wash (if available) to skin, and leave on for 15 to 20 minutes. Oil may be used to soften crust. Mild soap and water may also be used. Do not scrub the skin.	Enzyme wash assists in dissolving dead cells and fatty deposits. Vigorous scrubbing damages delicate tissues.
9. Gently wash off enzyme wash. Immerse tissues in basin or tub, if possible, to assist in dead cell removal.	
10. Pat extremity dry, remove and discard gloves, perform hand hygiene, and apply thin coat of skin lotion.	Rubbing may further traumatize the tissues.
11. After cast removal, explain and write out skin care procedures for client (Box 28-5).	Provides ongoing home care instruction for client and family.
12. Obtain physician's order to perform active and passive ROM, and clarify level of activity allowed.	After immobilization, the involved joints and muscles will be weak and ROM may be limited. Activity is resumed slowly.

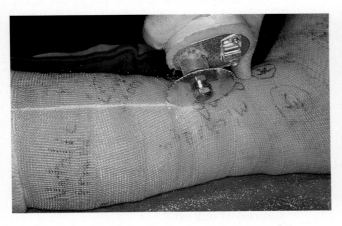

Step 3   Vibration of cast cutter generates heat.

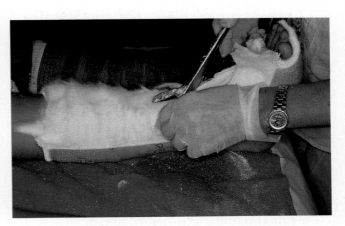

Step 6   Removing padding beneath cast.

Box 28-5
Care After Cast Removal

SKIN CARE

Provide client written instructions concerning general care before discharge.

- Apply enzyme wash solution such as Woolite or Delicare, and leave in place for at least 20 minutes. The enzymes in the solution loosen dead cells and help emulsify fatty or crusty lesions but cause no skin irritation.
- After 20 minutes, immerse the area in warm water and gently wash away the debris. Do not rub or scrub the skin areas, but gently swab the areas with a soft cloth.
- Rinse with clear warm water, and pat dry.
- Apply a moisturizing skin lotion or apply a little oil, gently massaging it in to help maintain the integrity of the cells.
- Repeat the above steps in 24 to 48 hours, after which the area should need no special care.

RELIEVING EDEMA

- Apply cloth-covered ice bags if the edema is marked. Do not place ice directly on skin.
- Elevate the affected tissues for the next 24 hours or when swelling occurs.

MANAGING TENDERNESS, WEAKNESS, DISCOMFORT

- Take prescribed nonnarcotic analgesic every 3 to 4 hours to build a therapeutic blood level, and continue the medication for 24 to 48 hours.
- Immerse the part or entire body in warm water, and gently exercise muscles under water.
- Wrap an elastic bandage from distal to proximal area if extra support is needed.
- Begin to reuse affected tissues and muscles slowly to avoid pain. Explain that usually it takes twice as long a time as the part was in a cast to regain full function.
- Perform prescribed muscle exercises with 5 to 10 repetitions every 4 hours to aid in regaining muscle strength. If muscle soreness persists, continue intake of prescribed nonnarcotic analgesic. Soak in warm water before exercise. Soreness should lessen as the muscle regains strength. Consult with therapist to prescribe appropriate exercises to increase mobility and strength.

Steps	Rationale
13. Assist in transfer of client for return to unit or discharge.	
14. Clean all equipment. Dispose of cast and materials according to standard precautions.	Prevents spread of infection.
15. See Completion Protocol (inside cover).	

• • • • • • • • • •

EVALUATION

1. Ask client to explain and demonstrate activity level and ROM exercises prescribed.
2. Inspect underlying skin for pressure areas, erythema (redness), or other signs of irritation or trauma.
3. Observe client perform skin care.

Unexpected Outcomes and Related Interventions

1. Client becomes very tense and is unable to cooperate during the cast removal.
   a. Offer reassurance and support.
   b. Reexplain the cast removal procedure and expected sensations during removal.
2. Client experiences edema, pain, and difficulty moving affected tissues after removal of cast.
   a. Assess neurovascular status of involved tissues.
   b. Assess the type, length, site, amount, and severity of the pain, including onset.

   c. Assess ability to perform active and passive ROM.
   d. Contact physician with findings.
3. Client has scratch on underlying skin.
   a. Inspect skin edges and severity of scratch.
   b. Cleanse area and apply water-soluble lotion or ointment as ordered.
4. Client is unable to explain self-care measures or skin care.
   a. Reassure client as necessary.
   b. Reinstruct client in self-care after cast removal.
   c. Instruct client in skin care measures, including gentle cleansing of the casted area (avoid scrubbing) and patting the area dry (avoid rubbing). Apply a water-soluble lotion or ointment to any scratches as ordered.

Recording and Reporting

- Record cast removal.
- Record condition of tissues formerly in cast.
- Record person removing cast.
- Record instructions given to client and family.

Sample Documentation

1000 Attempted to remove left long arm cast. Client began crying. Reexplained procedure and action of cast saw. Demonstrated vibration action.

 1015 Left long arm cast removed without difficulty. Left arm soaking in basin of enzyme wash, rinsed. Skin intact.

 1045 Skin on left arm remains dry, lotion applied.

SPECIAL CONSIDERATIONS

Pediatric Considerations

Demonstrate the cast saw on your own skin and on a doll before using on child. Allow the child to see that it does not cut to decrease anxiety.

Geriatric Considerations

- Older clients may experience marked stiffness or weakened muscles, depending on length of time in cast.
- Older client's skin is drier, thinner, and more fragile than that of a baby, child, or younger adult.

Home Care Considerations

- Elevate extremity with intermittent edema by using chair or bed with pillows.
- Suggest regular use of moisturizers for dry, scaly skin of casted extremity. Instruct client not to attempt to remove scaly skin.
- Teach client to ambulate slowly and carefully until muscle strength is regained in affected extremity.
- Assess client's environment for potential safety risks.

Skill 28.5

Care of the Client With an Immobilization Device (Brace, Splint, Sling)

Immobilization devices increase stability, support a weak extremity, or reduce the load on weight-bearing structures such as hips, knees, or ankles. A splint immobilizes and protects a body part. Temporary splints reduce pain and prevent tissue damage from further motion immediately after an injury such as a fracture or sprain. Air splints, Thomas splints, and improvised splints from material on hand are examples of temporary splints applied in emergency situations. Upper extremity fractures are sometimes managed using splints such as hand and digital splints or sugar-tong splints. Slings are used to support splints, casts, or injured upper extremities (Figure 28-15). They are commercially available or can be made for almost any body part (see Procedural Guideline 28-1, p. 672). Velcro or buckle closures permit these devices to be adjusted to fit a body part of almost any size and shape. The abduction splint, used after hip replacement surgery, maintains the client's legs in an abducted position. This permits the client to be turned without changing the healing limb's position and prevents dislocation of the hip prosthesis. The device is easily removed for nursing care such as skin care, dressing changes, or neurovascular assessments. A posterior splint with elastic wraps is sometimes used to support an extremity.

Cloth and foam splints, known as immobilizers, provide long-term immobilization (Figure 28-16). Immobilizers treat sprains and dislocations that do not require complete and continuous immobilization in a cast or traction. Immobilizers are often used following orthopedic surgery. Other common types of immobilizers include cervical collars (soft or hard), belt type of shoulder immobilizers, and vinyl wrist forearm splints. Molded splints, made of plastic, provide support to clients with chronic injuries or diseases such as arthritis. They maintain the body part in a functional position to prevent contractures and muscle atrophy during the period of disuse. A splint goes into place and removes quickly and easily when assessing skin or a wound.

Braces support weakened structures during weight bearing. For this reason, they are made of sturdy materials such as leather, metal, and molded plastic. Chest and abdominal braces, such as the Milwaukee and Boston braces, immobilize the thoracic and lumbar vertebral column to treat scoliosis (curvature of the spine). The brace does not

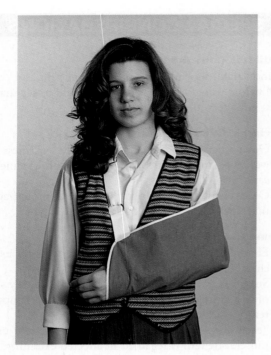

Figure 28-15   Sling for shoulder/arm immobilization. (From Beare PG, Meyers JL: *Principles and practice of adult health nursing,* ed 3, 1998, Mosby.)

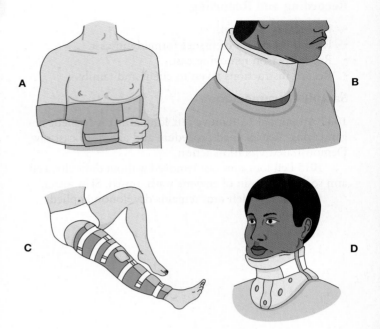

Figure 28-16   Examples of immobilizers. **A,** Shoulder immobilizer. **B,** Soft cervical collar. **C,** Knee immobilizer. **D,** Hard cervical collar. (From Beare PG, Meyers JL: *Principles and practice of adult health nursing,* ed 3, 1998, Mosby.)

correct the curve but instead prevents its progression. Lumbar braces support lumbar and sacral tissues after spinal surgery or fusion. Leg braces hold the thigh, leg, and foot in functional positions for weight bearing and ambulation (Figure 28-17). Both short leg and long leg braces support weak leg muscles, aid in control of involuntary muscle movement, or maintain surgical correction during the postoperative healing process. They are commonly used for clients with cerebral palsy, muscular dystrophy, multiple sclerosis, after polio, and fractures (Bakker and others, 2000).

ASSESSMENT

1. Review client's chart, including medical history, previous and current activity level, and description of the condition requiring bracing or splinting. *Rationale: Reveals client's current and previous health status and purpose for the brace/splint.*
2. Assess client's previous experience with braces or splints. *Rationale: Reveals client's baseline knowledge and need for instruction.*
3. Assess client's understanding of reason for brace/splint and its care, application, and schedule of wear.
4. Assess client's risk for skin breakdown because of bracing/splinting or immobilization. Look at area of skin to be in contact with support device. *Rationale: Immobile and older clients are particularly vulnerable.*

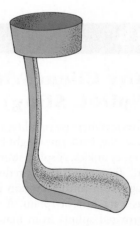

Figure 28-17   Ankle-foot orthosis (AFO). (Modified from Sorrentino SA: *Assisting with patient care,* St Louis, 1999, Mosby.)

5. Assess client's level of pain on a scale of 0 to 10. *Rationale: Provides baseline to determine if immobilization device affects comfort.*
6. Refer to occupational or physical therapy consult to determine type of brace to be used, desired position, and amount of activity and movement permitted.
7. Assess client's additional need for an assistive device such as a cane, walker, or crutches. *Rationale: An assistive device may be needed to provide support and promote balance during ambulation.*

PLANNING

Expected outcomes focus on maintaining skin integrity, improving client's knowledge, and preventing risk for injury.

Expected Outcomes

1. Client's skin remains in good condition without circulatory impairment.
2. Client/significant other verbalizes purpose, correct application, and care of the device.
3. Client does not experience an increase in pain during device application.
4. Circulation and sensation distal to brace/splint is maintained.
5. Client uses the device correctly, including schedule of wear, activity limitations, and positioning.

Equipment

- Brace/splint
- Cotton shirt or gown

Delegation Considerations

The skill of caring for the client wearing a brace, splint, or sling may be delegated to assistive personnel (AP) but assessment cannot. The following information is needed when delegating this skill to nursing staff or family members:

- Review the purpose of the brace/splint/sling.
- Review correct application of the brace/splint and positioning of any ties or straps.
- Review prescribed schedule of wear and activities permitted while in the brace.
- Instruct AP to alert the nurse if client complains of pain, rubbing, or pressure from the brace or splint or if a change occurs in client's skin condition.

IMPLEMENTATION FOR CARE OF THE CLIENT WITH AN IMMOBILIZATION DEVICE (BRACE, SPLINT)

Steps	Rationale
1. See Standard Protocol (inside front cover).	
2. Explain reasons for the brace or splint, and demonstrate how the device works.	Teaching and demonstration enhance learning, reduce anxiety, and encourage cooperation.
3. Assist the client to a comfortable position, preferably sitting or lying down.	Client's position will depend on the type of brace/splint being used. Upper-extremity braces/splints are applied best with the client sitting upright. Lower-extremity braces are applied best with the client lying down.
4. Prepare the skin that will be enclosed in the brace/splint by cleaning the skin with soap and water; rinse, pat dry, and change any dressings (if present). If applying a back brace, put a thin cotton shirt or gown on the client. Ensure that there are no wrinkles causing pressure.	This protects the skin, absorbs moisture, and keeps the brace clean.

COMMUNICATION TIP *Tell the client, "Be sure to let me know if you feel pressure, pain, numbness, rubbing, or if the skin becomes reddened."*

Steps	Rationale
5. Inspect the device for wear, damage, or rough edges.	Potential for skin breakdown is decreased, and correct alignment is maintained.
6. Apply the brace/splint as directed by physician, orthotist, physical therapist, or occupational therapist. If securing splint with elastic bandage: a. Apply even tension as bandage is wrapped from distal to proximal. b. Prevent padding from gathering or bunching.	Proper application of the brace/splint is important to avoid skin breakdown, pressure ulcers, neurovascular compromise, calluses, or worsening of the deformity. Promotes venous blood return from the peripheral circulation to the central circulation.
7. Teach the client the prescribed schedule of wear and allowed activities while in the brace/splint as directed by physician, physical therapist, or occupational therapist.	Proper use of the brace/splint will facilitate healing and mobility and reduce pain and stress.

Steps	Rationale
8. Reinforce the signs of skin breakdown, pressure, or rubbing to report.	Brace/splint may need to be adjusted. Changes may also be required because of growth or atrophy, when muscles regain or lose strength, or after reconstructive surgery.
9. Teach the client how to care for the brace/splint.	Metal braces should be stored upright. Splints of molded materials should be stored away from heat. Leather materials should be treated with a leather preservative to prevent drying or cracking.
a. When not in use, store brace/splint in a safe but easily accessible location. b. Keep the brace clean, dry, and in good working order.	Plastic parts are cleaned with a damp cloth and thoroughly dried. Metal joints are cleaned with a pipe cleaner and oiled weekly. Remove rust with steel wool, and clean metal parts with a solvent.
10. Assist client in ambulating with brace/splint in place.	Determines if client is able to ambulate safely.
11. Have the client apply and remove the brace/splint. Promotes client independence; demonstration confirms level of learning skill.	

COMMUNICATION TIP *Let the client know that the brace/splint may seem awkward at first. Tell the client, "After you have had practice in using it you will feel more comfortable and better able to move about." Also let the client know that assistance may be needed to apply and remove the brace/splint.*

12. See Completion Protocol (inside front cover).

• • • • • • • • • •

Procedural Guideline 28-1

Sling Application

Equipment: Commercially prepared sling or triangular bandage and safety pin.
1. See Standard Protocol (inside front cover).
2. If commercial sling is used, follow directions on package for correct application.
3. If triangular bandage is used, position one end of the bandage over the shoulder of the unaffected arm.
4. Take the remaining bandage and place the material against the chest, then under and over the affected arm, cradling the arm.
5. Position the pointed end of the triangle toward the elbow.

6. Tie the two ends of the triangle at the side of the neck.
7. Fold the pointed end of the sling at the elbow in the front and secure with a safety pin, closing the end of the sling.
8. Adjust the length of the sling by adjusting the amount of material in the knot.
9. Ensure the sling supports the limb comfortably without interfering with circulation.
10. Assess neurovascular status (Box 28-2) after 20 to 30 minutes. Continue to monitor every 4 hours. Readjust sling as necessary.
11. See Completion Protocol (inside front cover).

EVALUATION

1. Inspect areas of the skin underneath the brace/splint for signs of pressure, including redness or breakdown.
2. Observe the client using the brace/splint.
3. Ask the client to rate level of comfort on scale of 0 to 10 while the brace/splint is in place.

4. Palpate pulse and test sensation of extremity distal to position of brace/splint.
5. Observe client while ADLs are performed while wearing the brace/splint.

Unexpected Outcomes and Related Interventions

1. Client is unable to use the brace/splint correctly.
   a. Reassess client for correct fit.
   b. Assess level of comfort.
   c. Assess muscle strength in uninvolved extremities.
   d. Obtain referral for physical or occupational therapy.
2. Client develops areas of pressure, redness, or skin breakdown.
   a. Assess device for proper fit and positioning.
   b. Observe client's ability to apply brace correctly.
   c. Inspect brace/splint for damage, wear, or rough edges.
   d. Inform the physician.
   e. Inform the orthotist, physical therapist, or occupational therapist so that adjustments to brace/splint can be made.
   f. Do not allow the client to use the brace/splint until adjustments are made.
   g. If necessary, temporarily pad the area of incorrect fit rather than the reddened or irritated area.
3. Circulation to the affected extremity is altered because of improper fit.
   a. Remove the device immediately.
   b. Notify physician.

Recording and Reporting

- Record the following:
  Type of brace/splint applied
  Schedule of wear
  Activity level
  Movement permitted
  Tolerance of procedure
  Specific assessments related to skin integrity and neurovascular status
  Instructions given to client and family.
  Observations regarding client's ability to apply, ambulate with, and remove the brace/splint.
- Immediately report any injury sustained while using the brace/splint.

Sample Documentation

0900 Knee immobilizer placed on client's right lower extremity. Client instructed in proper application and positioning of the device. Instructed to keep immobilizer on at all times when ambulating with crutches and to maintain partial weight-bearing status on the right leg. No signs of redness or skin breakdown. Skin dry and intact. Dorsalis pedis pulse present. Brisk capillary refill in all toes. Positive sensation and movement of right foot. No complaints of pain or discomfort at this time.

1100 Velcro straps readjusted to a secure but loose position after client complained of slight pressure on the knee. No redness and skin breakdown evident. Toes warm to touch; client denies any numbness, tingling, or pain.

SPECIAL CONSIDERATIONS

Pediatric Considerations

- For children immobilized in traction, extending the environment can be helpful by moving the bed into other areas (e.g., the playroom, the hallway, or outside if possible). Imaginative play can also offer distraction (e.g., making the bed into a boat or airplane using decorations) (Wong and others, 1999).
- Teach parents to apply and maintain the brace/sling.
- Place cotton T-shirt under upper extremity brace and long, cotton tube socks under lower extremity brace.
- Avoid lotions or powders that may irritate skin.
- Teach family exercises to perform when child is out of brace (e.g., Boston brace).
- Recognize that bracing in an adolescent often affects body image and self-esteem.

Geriatric Considerations

- Monitor integrity of the older client's skin closely.
- Assess for stiffness or weakened muscles of older client. This depends on length of time in the immobilization device.
- Assist older clients with limited mobility in applying the brace/splint.

Home Care Considerations

- Recognize that prolonged immobility in a brace/splint may cause decreased ROM or contractures.
- Assess the ability and willingness of the client and primary caregiver regarding care required for the brace/splint.
- Remove the brace/splint when bathing or showering.
- Assess for environmental factors in the home that may interfere with safe ambulation.
- Advise client and caregiver of signs and symptoms of impaired skin integrity to report.

Long-Term Care Considerations

- Inspect and clean braces/splints weekly.
- Assist clients with adapting clothing so that an acceptable appearance can be maintained.
- Teach client appropriate ROM exercises within limitation of device.
- Assist client or parents with developing plan to manage ADLs while braced. If child, base plan on developmental skills and abilities.
- Enlist occupational therapist in helping client develop the highest quality of life possible.

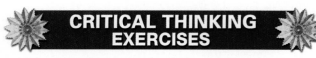

CRITICAL THINKING EXERCISES

1. Mrs. Edna Wenger has just had a cast placed on her lower leg for a closed tibial/fibula (tib/fib) fracture. She is scheduled to be discharged from the emergency department within the next hour. Her husband tells the nurse that the narcotic she was given an hour ago has not relieved her pain. What would be the nurse's priority for this client?

2. Jewell Cleveland, age 76 years, fell at home and broke her left hip. She has been admitted to the nursing unit to await hip pinning and is in Buck's skin traction. The nurse performs a baseline assessment and finds cold left toes, capillary refill of 5 seconds, and weak dorsalis pedis pulse.
   a. What should the nurse do?
   b. Following ORIF, Mrs. Cleveland is experiencing muscle spasms. Dr. Morrison orders a muscle relaxant and reapplication of the Buck's traction. Mrs. Cleveland tells you she does not understand why.
   c. In assessing her skin, the nurse notices a small reddened area on her left heel. What does the nurse do?

3. Mr. Limon had a long leg cast applied 2 hours ago. During your rounds on the orthopedic unit, you assess Mr. Limon's skin condition and neurovascular status. The skin of the feet is warm and pink, with capillary refill of less than 3 seconds. You can palpate a strong dorsalis pedis pulse. Mr. Limon complains of some swelling in the foot, but denies burning or discomfort. When you check the sensation of both lower extremities, Mr. Limon is able to distinguish a pin prick. What do your findings indicate?

4. Mr. Wang's cast of the lower leg has been on for approximately 2 weeks. During your assessment, you notice a foul odor coming from the cast. What might this indicate?

REFERENCES

Bakker JPJ and others: The effects of knee-ankle-foot orthoses in the treatment of Duchenne muscular dystrophy: review of the literature, *Clin Rehabil* 14(4):343, 2000.

Beare PG, Myers JL: *Principles and practice of adult health nursing,* ed 3, St Louis, 1998, Mosby.

Ebersole P, Hess P: *Toward healthy aging; human needs and nursing response,* ed 5, St Louis, 1998, Mosby.

Folcik MA, Carini-Garcia G, Birmingham JJ: *Traction: assessment and management,* St Louis, 1994, Mosby.

Hart KM, Kester K: Supracondylar fractures in children, *Orthop Nurs* 18(3):23, 1999.

Perry A, Potter P: *Clinical nursing skills and techniques* ed 5, St Louis, 2002, Mosby.

Schoen DC: *Adult orthopaedic nursing,* Philadelphia, 2000, Lippincott.

Sorrentino SA: *Assisting with patient care,* 1999, Mosby.

Wong DL and others: *Whaley and Wong's nursing care of infants and children,* ed 6, St Louis, 1999, Mosby.

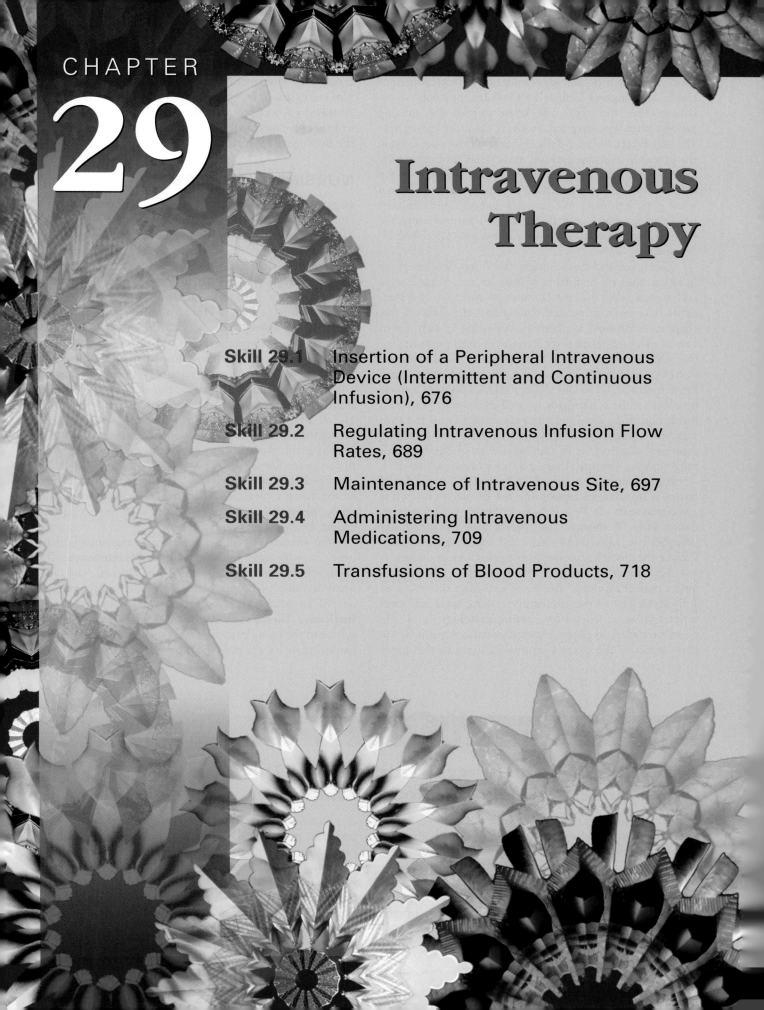

Intravenous Therapy

Delivery of infusion therapy is essential in the treatment of clients and requires a nurse's knowledge, professional accountability, and skill. The nurse applies the nursing process when assessing and choosing the most appropriate vascular access site and device, preparing the client, using the proper insertion technique, and closely monitoring the infusion until the completion of therapy. Because of the extensive use of intravenous (IV) therapy, the professional nurse plays a primary role in safely and efficiently delivering IV medications and fluids, as well as protecting the client from the potential complications associated with IV therapy.

The Infusion Nurses Society (INS) has developed the Infusion Nursing Standards of Practice to protect clients and nurses who administer infusion therapy. The standards have been integrated throughout the skills of this chapter. Additional guidelines supporting quality client care in this high-technology arena have been published by the Occupational Safety and Health Administration (OSHA) and the Centers for Disease Control and Prevention (CDC) (CDC, 2001; OSHA, 2001). As a nurse be aware of these standards, as well as those of your own institution. Individual practitioners should know the various Nurse Practice Act regulations in their state regarding care and insertion of IV devices for short-duration and long-duration therapy. These may vary from state to state.

A nurse must be highly skilled with IV therapy. An IV device is invasive, increasing the risk of infection. Pain is associated with any IV insertion. A client's previous experience with IV therapy also affects how the nurse approaches care. The nurse's skill and expertise directly influence the client's response to the initiation of therapy.

Assessment of a client who requires IV therapy requires critical thinking. The nurse considers the anatomy and physiology of the circulatory system, fluid and electrolyte balance, chemistry, pathophysiology, and the client's response to illness. Assessment also extends to the observation of the client's venous anatomy of the upper extremities, assessment of mobility or immobility, and previous attempts or experiences of IV therapy. The goal of all IV therapy is to restore, prevent, or correct fluid and electrolyte imbalance without complications associated with the delivery of IV medications or fluids.

NURSING DIAGNOSES

Nursing diagnoses for clients receiving IV therapy may include **Risk for Infection** related to an invasive procedure. The client with an IV line may also have the diagnosis **Risk for Impaired Skin Integrity.** For the client receiving IV therapy for correction of fluid and electrolyte imbalance or with potential or existing alterations in regulatory mechanisms of hydration, actual or risk for **Deficient Fluid Volume** or **Excess Fluid Volume** may be appropriate. **Risk for Injury** is created by the presence of an IV catheter acting as a foreign body and adverse events related to IV medications. **Deficient Knowledge** is a diagnosis that applies in most clients receiving IV therapy because of a lack of experience with this type of therapy. In addition, home care clients may misinterpret or have a lack of interest in information pertaining to care of IV devices. Noncompliance, especially in home care, is seen with failure to comply with medication administration or home infusion procedures.

Psychological factors such as **Fear** or **Anxiety** related to the client's previous experience with IV therapy may apply. **Acute Pain** is often associated with the actual procedure or IV-related complications.

For clients receiving care in the home, nursing diagnoses may include **Impaired Home Maintenance.** The client's home could be insufficiently cleaned, lack adequate lighting or proper medication and supply storage, or fail to have a telephone for emergency situations. **Ineffective Therapeutic Regimen Management** could result from the complexity of the IV therapy or excessive demands made on the individual or family.

Skill 29.1

Insertion of a Peripheral Intravenous Device (Intermittent and Continuous Infusion)

To maintain fluid and electrolyte balance, isotonic, hypotonic, or hypertonic fluids are delivered through a variety of methods using continuous and/or intermittent infusion. Infusion therapy also provides access to the venous system to deliver various medications in emergent and nonemergent situations and to infuse blood or blood products. Reliable access for IV administration is one of the most essential features of current medical care.

Successful delivery of peripheral IV therapy depends on client preparation, vein selection, selection of an appropriate catheter, and skilled catheter insertion. Several vascular access devices are available for use in peripheral veins (Table 29-1). Because potential for exposure to blood-borne pathogens is high during insertion and care of IV devices, adherence to asepsis and standard precautions is required (see Chapters 3 and 4).

Table 29-1

IV Access Device Options

Type	Use
Winged infusion butterfly needle	One-time infusion, IV push administration
Short, over-the-needle catheter (ONC) (less than 3 inches [7.5 cm])	Continuous infusion, intermittent infusion, short-term duration (less than 1 week)
Short, over-the-needle catheter (ONC) (less than 3 inches [7.5 cm])	Continuous infusion, intermittent infusion, short-term duration (less than 1 week)
Midline peripheral catheters (3- to 8-inch [7.5 to 20 cm])	Continuous infusion and intermittent infusion (7 to 14 days).

Recent studies support the use of needleless safety devices in infusion therapy. One study has shown as many as 83% of injuries caused by hollow-bore needles can be prevented, whereas others demonstrate that needleless and needle protector IV systems may reduce occupational needle-stick exposures by 50% to 94% (Orenstein, 1999). In April 2001 the U.S. Congress passed the Needlestick Safety and Prevention Act (OSHA, 2001), requiring health care employers to identify and make use of effective and safer medical devices. Safer medical devices, such as sharps with engineered sharps-injury protections (e.g., sliding sheaths that cover needles after use, needles that retract into syringes) and needleless systems (e.g., IV medication systems with nonneedle connections and ports), must be used when feasible. In addition, the INS recommends peripheral short catheters be equipped with a safety device with engineered sharps-injury protection (INS, 2000).

ASSESSMENT

1. Assess client's previous experience with IV therapy and arm placement preference. *Rationale: Determines level of emotional support and instruction necessary.*
2. Determine if client is to undergo any planned surgeries or procedures. *Rationale: Allows nurse to place an adequate-size catheter (i.e., 18 or 16 gauge for surgery) and avoids placement in an area that will interfere with medical procedures.*
3. Assess client's activities of daily living (ADLs). *Rationale: Ensures placement will not impair therapy or interfere with mobility and improves client's comfort and tolerance of IV therapy.*
4. Assess the type and duration of IV therapy as ordered by the physician or licensed independent practitioner. *Rationale: Assists in selection of an appropriate access device and early placement of longer-term infusion devices and minimizes multiple venipunctures.*
5. Assess laboratory data and client's history of allergies. *Rationale: May reveal information that affects insertion of devices, such as fluid volume deficit or anemia. Prepping agents, gloves, and plastic catheters may create serious problem for clients with allergies to iodine, adhesive, or latex.*

6. Assess client's medical history for chronic illnesses and all medications. *Rationale: Chronic cardiac or renal diseases and subsequent medications (e.g., diuretics) indicate the need for electronic control of the infusion (see Skill 29.2, p. 689).*

PLANNING

Expected outcomes focus on minimal complications from IV therapy, minimal discomfort to the client, restoration of normal fluid and electrolyte balance, and client's ability to verbalize complications that require immediate nursing intervention.

Expected Outcomes

1. Client remains free of vasovagal reaction during the procedure.
2. Client's fluid volume status is balanced, without fluid volume excess or deficit.
3. Client remains free of complications associated with the presence of the catheter, including absence of pain, swelling, or redness.
4. Client verbalizes comfort and minimal restrictions to ADLs immediately after catheter insertion.
5. Client identifies one symptom of infiltration (e.g., swelling), phlebitis (e.g., redness), and occlusion (e.g., stoppage of flow).
6. Client notifies the health care provider when symptoms are found.

Equipment

- IV Start kit (if available)—contains sterile tourniquet, sterile tape, sterile drape, antiseptic preps (Figure 29-1)
- Tourniquets (single client use or disinfected after each use) or blood pressure cuff
- Disposable gloves
- Antiseptic prepping agent(s) (70% alcohol, chlorhexidine, or per agency policy)
- IV fluids with time tape attached (if applicable)
- Administration set with tubing (for continuous infusion)
- prn adapter (intermittent infusion injection cap)

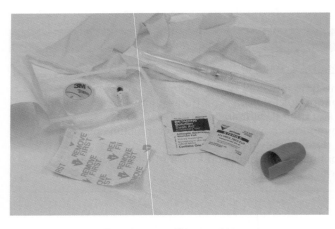

Figure 29-1   IV start kit.

- Appropriate IV catheter (gauge appropriate to type of solution infused) (see Table 29-1, p. 677)
- 5-ml syringe
- Sterile tape, 1 inch and ½ inch wide
- Flush solution (e.g., sterile normal saline [NS] or heparin flush solution)
- Transparent membrane dressing or sterile 2 × 2 gauze
- IV pole

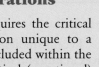

Delegation Considerations

The skill of basic IV insertion requires the critical thinking and knowledge application unique to a nurse. In many states this skill is included within the scope of practice for licensed practical (vocational) nurses (LPN/LVN). For this skill, delegation to assistive personnel (AP) is inappropriate.

IMPLEMENTATION FOR INSERTION OF A PERIPHERAL INTRAVENOUS DEVICE (INTERMITTENT AND CONTINUOUS INFUSION)

Steps	Rationale

1. See Standard Protocol (inside front cover).
2. Prepare equipment for insertion and prime IV tubing, maintaining sterility of closed system (see Skill 29.2, p. 689).
3. Place client in a comfortable supine position so you can extend the arm. Raise bed to nurse's level, and provide adequate lighting.

   Provides proper body mechanics and aids in successful vein location.

4. Assist client in techniques to minimize anxiety: visual imagery, deep breathing, and not looking at the site. Explain steps of procedure.

   Assists in minimizing apprehension, sympathetic nervous system stimulation, and possible vasovagal reaction to venipuncture.

5. (NOTE: Gloves can be left off to locate vein but must be applied before prepping site). Apply tourniquet 4 to 6 inches (10 to 15 cm) above the proposed insertion site (see illustration). Check for presence of radial pulse. Option: Apply blood pressure cuff instead of tourniquet. Inflate to a level just below client's normal diastolic pressure. Maintain inflation at that pressure until venipuncture is completed.

   Tourniquet should be tight enough to impede venous return but not occlude arterial flow.

COMMUNICATION TIP *Encourage client to ask questions. Provide honest answers with a calm and reassuring manner. Tell client, "The stick will hurt some but will be less painful if you can hold still. It's OK to move the other arm." After site preparation and just before puncturing the skin, say, "There is going to be a stick now," then proceed immediately with venipuncture. Keep reminding client to take slow, deep breaths, especially if you have difficulty entering vein. Distract client by discussing other topics.*

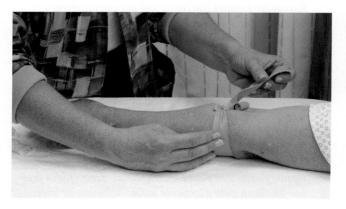

Step 5   Apply tourniquet.

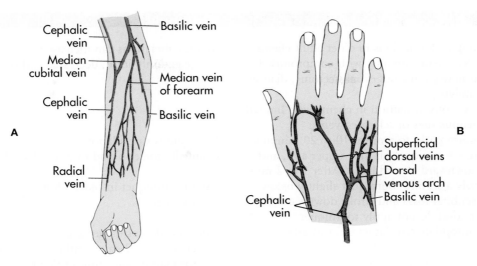

Step 6a   Common IV sites. **A,** Inner arm. **B,** Dorsal surface of hand.

Steps	Rationale
6. Select the vein.	
a. Use the most distal site in the nondominant arm, if possible (see illustrations).	Venipuncture should be performed distal to proximal, which increases the availability of other sites for future IV therapy.
b. Avoid areas that are painful to palpation.	May indicate inflamed vein.
c. Select a vein large enough for catheter placement.	Prevents interruption of venous flow while allowing adequate blood flow around the catheter.
d. Choose a site that will not interfere with client's ADLs or planned procedures.	
e. Use the fingers of your nondominant hand to palpate the vein by pressing downward and noting the resilient, soft, bouncy feeling as the pressure is released. Always use the same fingers to palpate (see illustration).	Use of the same fingers causes a development of sensitivity to better assess the vein condition. Fingers on nondominant hand tend to be more sensitive (Ellenberger, 1999).
f. Place the client's arm in a dependent position, asking the client to open and close the fist several times, and rubbing or stroking the client's arm.	Promotes venous distention.
g. Avoid sites distal to previous venipuncture site, veins in the antecubital fossa or inner wrist, sclerosed or hardened cordlike veins, infiltrated site or phlebotic vessels, bruised areas, and areas of venous valves or bifurcation.	Such sites increase risk of infiltration of newly placed IV line and excessive vessel damage. Veins in antecubital fossa are used for blood draws, and placement here limits mobility (Ellenberger, 1999). Inner wrist has numerous tendons that could easily be damaged.

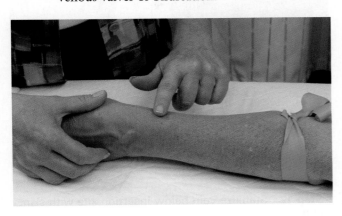

Step 6e   Palpate vein for resilience.

Steps	Rationale
h. Avoid fragile dorsal veins in older adult clients and vessels in an extremity with compromised circulation (e.g., in cases of mastectomy, dialysis graft, paralysis).	Venous alterations can increase risk of complications (e.g., infiltration, decreased catheter dwell time).
7. Options for venous distention in clients with limited peripheral venous sites or sclerosed veins:	
a. Apply warm packs to arm for 10 to 20 minutes.	Heat causes vasodilation.
b. Apply one tourniquet on mid–upper arm, and stroke downward toward hand. After 1 to 2 minutes, apply a second tourniquet slightly below the antecubital fossa and stroke downward. For an older adult do not apply tourniquet	Gradually forces blood to distend smaller veins.

Use of tourniquet in older adult raises venous pressure too high. |
| **8.** Select the appropriate size catheter for insertion. | Smaller catheters (larger gauge) are less traumatizing. In an adult a 22-gauge catheter is an appropriate choice for maintenance fluids (Ellenberger, 1999). |

NURSE ALERT   *The catheter selected shall be the smallest size (largest gauge) and shortest length that will accommodate prescribed therapy (INS, 2000). Large catheters, which occlude more of the vein lumen, impede blood flow around the catheter and can cause vessel wall damage from irritating medications.*

---

9. Release tourniquet temporarily and carefully. Clip arm hair with scissors. Avoid shaving the area.	Hair impedes venipuncture or adherence of the dressing. Shaving can cause microabrasions and predispose client to infection.
10. Cleanse the insertion site using friction and a circular motion moving from the insertion site outward in concentric circles, 2 to 3 inches from insertion site (see illustration). Use antiseptic prep as single agent or in combination. Allow to dry between agents, if agents used in combination. Reprep the skin if touched after preparation.	Drying prevents chemical reactions between agents and allows time for maximum microbicidal activity of agents (INS, 2000). Chlorhexidine has recently been shown to be an effective agent (Raad, 1998).

Touching cleansed area would introduce organisms from nurse's hand to site. |
| **11.** Reapply tourniquet. | |
| **12.** Stabilize the vein below the proposed insertion site. Pull the skin taut opposite the direction of the venipuncture (see illustration). Instruct client to relax hand. Avoid placing fingers above site. | Stabilization below site reduces risk of needle stick. |

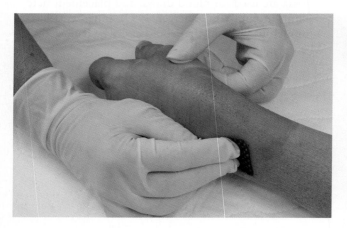

Step 10   Cleanse site chosen for insertion.

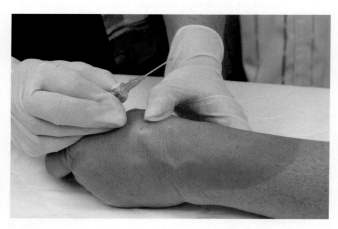

Step 12   Stabilize vein below insertion site with skin taut.

Steps	Rationale
13. Warn client of a sharp, quick stick. Puncture the skin and vein, holding the catheter at a 10- to 30-degree angle (see illustration).	Superficial veins require a smaller angle. Deeper veins require a greater angle.
14. Observe for a "flashback" of blood in the catheter's flashback chamber, lower the catheter until almost flush with the skin (see illustration), and slowly advance another $\frac{1}{8}$ to $\frac{1}{4}$ inch.	Allows for full penetration of the vein wall, placement of the catheter in the vein's inner lumen, and easy advancement of the catheter off the stylet.
15. Advance the catheter off the stylet until the catheter hub rests at venipuncture site. Continue to hold skin taut (see illustration). (If used, advance the safety device on catheter by using push-tab to thread the catheter.)	Reduces risk of introduction of infectious microorganisms along catheter length.
16. Stabilize catheter, and release tourniquet or blood pressure cuff.	Restores blood flow to arm.
17. After catheter is fully advanced, apply gentle but firm pressure with index finger of nondominant hand $1\frac{1}{4}$ inches (3 cm) above the insertion site (see illustration). Retract the stylet by pushing the safety tab (see illustration 1, p. 682). For the other safety devices, slide the catheter off the stylet while gliding the protective guard over the stylet (see illustration 2, p. 682). A click indicates device is locked over stylet.	Obstructs venous flow, minimizing blood loss.

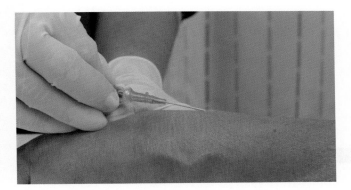

Step 13 Puncture skin with catheter at 10- to 30-degree angle. Catheter enters vein.

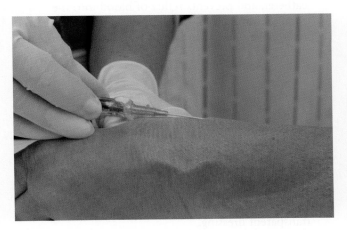

Step 14 Blood return in flashback chamber, catheter lowered flush with skin.

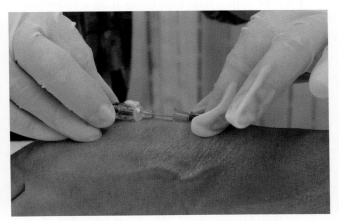

Step 15 Advance catheter into vein; use safety device push-tab.

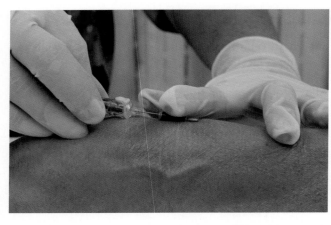

Step 17(1) Apply pressure above insertion site with index finger of dominant hand.

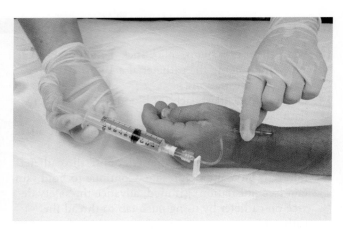

Step 18 Flush injection cap slowly.

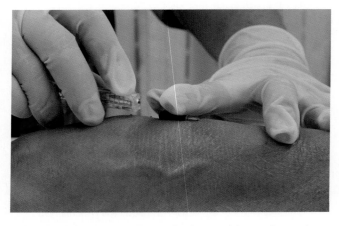

Step 17(2) Retract the stylet by pushing safety tab.

Steps	Rationale
18. **Intermittent infusion** Hold the catheter firmly with nondominant hand, and attach sterile injection cap of prn adapter. Insert prefilled 5-ml syringe containing flush solution into injection cap. Flush injection cap slowly with flush solution (see illustration). Withdraw the syringe, while still flushing, or close the slide clamp on extension tubing of injection cap while still flushing last 0.2 to 0.4 ml of flush.	"Positive pressure flushing" allows fluid to displace the removed needle, creates positive pressure in the catheter, and prevents reflux of blood into the catheter lumen (Phillips, 2001). Stabilizing the cannula prevents accident withdrawal or dislodgement.
19. **Continuous infusion** Connect end of IV tubing (see illustration) primed with fluid to catheter hub. Maintain sterile technique. Be sure connection is secure (see illustration). Begin the infusion by slowly opening the slide clamp or adjusting the roller clamp of the IV tubing.	Initiates flow of fluid through IV catheter, preventing clotting.
20. Tape or secure catheter. a. If applying transparent dressing, secure catheter with nondominant hand while preparing to apply dressing.	Do not tape because this will interfere with adherence of transparent dressing.

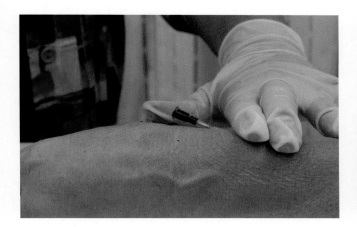

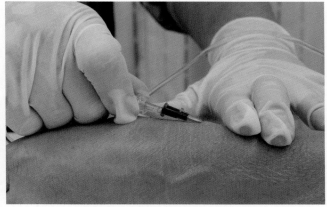

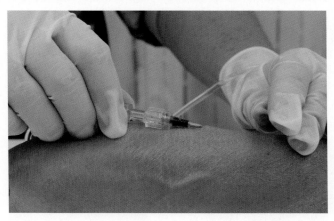

Step 19   Connect end of IV tubing to catheter tubing. Secure connector.

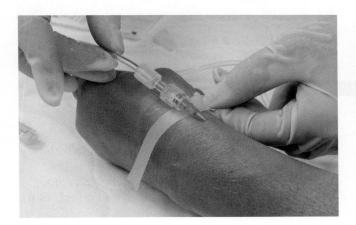

Step 20b(1)   Place tape under catheter hub.

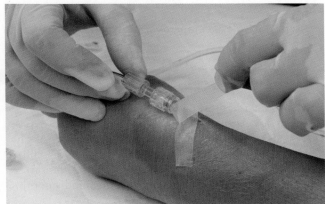

Step 20b(2)   Criss-cross ends of tape over hub.

Steps	Rationale
b. If applying a gauze dressing, tape the IV catheter. Prepare a ½-inch-wide piece of sterile tape, about 4 inches long. Place the sterile tape carefully under the hub of catheter with adhesive side up (see illustration). Criss-cross ends of tape over hub (see illustration) to make a chevron.	Securing the catheter and tubing prevents movement and tension on the device, reducing mechanical irritation and possible phlebitis or infection. Regular adhesive tape is potential source of pathogenic bacteria (Redelmeier and Livesley, 1999).
c. Place tape only on the catheter, *never* over the insertion site. Avoid applying tape around the extremity.	Allows easy visual inspection and recognition of complications. Taping around extremity could result in a "tourniquet effect" and impede venous return.

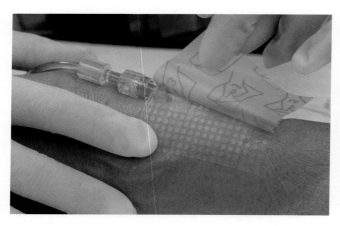

Step 21a(1)   Apply transparent dressing.

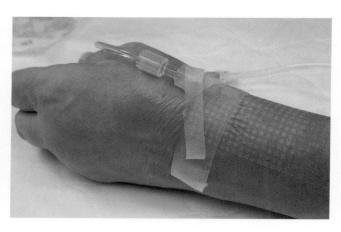

Step 21a(3)   Apply chevron over tape.

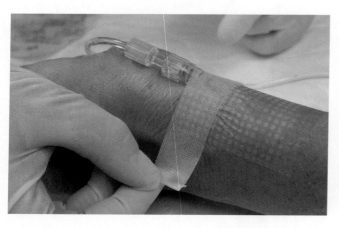

Step 21a(2)   Place tape over transparent dressing.

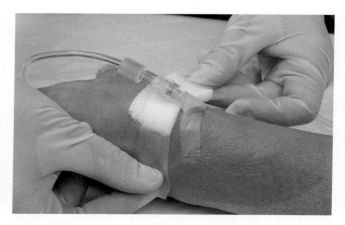

Step 21b(1)   Fold 2 × 2 gauze in half, cover with 1-inch tape, and place under catheter hub.

Steps	Rationale

21. Apply sterile dressing over site.
   a. *Transparent dressing:*
      (1) Carefully remove adherent backing. Apply edge of dressing over IV site, leaving end of catheter hub uncovered (see illustration). Then remove outer covering, and smooth dressing gently over site.
      (2) Take a 1-inch piece of tape, and place it from end of hub of catheter to insertion site, over transparent dressing (see illustration).

Transparent dressing allows continuous inspection of site, is more comfortable, and permits clients to bathe and shower without saturating dressing (Phillips, 2001). Transparent dressings are occlusive to moisture and microorganisms (Hankins and others, 2001).

NURSE ALERT   *Insertion site should still remain visible.*

---

      (3) Then apply chevron and place only over tape, not the transparent dressing (see illustration).
   b. *Sterile gauze dressing:*
      (1) *Optional:* Fold a 2 × 2 gauze in half and cover with a 1-inch-wide piece of tape extending about an inch from each side. Place under the tubing/catheter hub junction (see illustration).

Tape on top of tape makes it easier to access hub/tubing junction. Securing loop of tubing reduces risk of dislodging catheter from accidental pull.

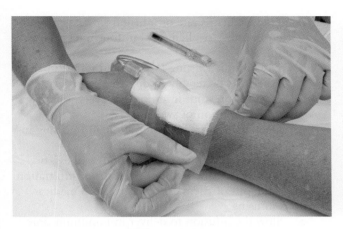

Step 21b(2)   Apply 2 × 2 gauze.

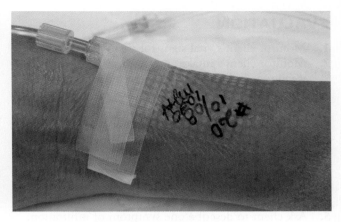

Step 23   Label dressing.

Steps	Rationale
(2) Place 2 × 2 gauze pad over venipuncture site and catheter hub. Secure all edges with tape. Do not cover connection between IV tubing and catheter hub (see illustration). (3) Curl a loop of tubing alongside the arm, and place a second piece of tape directly over the tubing and padded 2 × 2 (see illustration).	Gauze is less expensive than transparent dressing; may also be useful if there is bleeding from insertion site. All edges must be secured with tape to occlude air flow (Hankins and others, 2001).
22. Remove and dispose of gloves.	
23. Label the dressing, including the date, time, catheter gauge size and length, and nurse's initials (see illustration).	Allows for easy recognition of type of device and time interval for site rotation. INS standard for site rotation of peripheral IV access devices is every 72 hours (INS, 2000). CDC (2001) allows for replacement every 96 hours as supported by research of Lai (1998) and Bregenzer and others (1998) (check agency policy).
24. Instruct client in how to move about in and out of bed without dislodging IV line. Also instruct in signs and symptoms of complications to report (e.g., pain, swelling, moisture on arm)	
25. Dispose of sheathed stylet and any uncapped sharps(s) in appropriate sharps container as soon as device is secured.	
26. See Completion Protocol (inside front cover).	

NURSE ALERT *If venipuncture is unsuccessful, always obtain a new catheter before second attempt. Never reinsert stylet (needle) into catheter because this may damage catheter and cause catheter embolism. When the catheter is partially withdrawn through the stylet and/or reinserted, the damage can range from a small nick in the catheter to complete severing of distal tip (Hadaway, 1998). After second unsuccessful attempt, ask another practitioner to perform venipuncture.*

• • • • • • • • • •

EVALUATION

1. Monitor client's vital signs for vasovagal response.
2. Monitor client's intake and output (I&O), daily weights as indicated, skin turgor, mucous membranes, and vital signs for evidence of normal fluid volume.
3. Inspect client's IV site and extremity every 2 to 4 hours for the absence of pain, swelling, heat, or redness during the infusion.
4. On completion of IV insertion and during IV infusion, ask if client is comfortable. Observe client during activity for restrictions to mobility.
5. Ask client to describe one symptom of infiltration, phlebitis, and occluded infusion device complications (e.g., swelling, pain, tenderness, reduced flow).
6. Ask client to explain the action to take if symptoms of complications develop.

Unexpected Outcomes and Related Interventions

1. *Phlebitis:* Client complains of pain and tenderness at IV site with erythema at site or along path of vein. Insertion site is warm to touch, and rate of infusion may stop.
   a. Discontinue existing IV and restart in another site, preferably in opposite extremity, with new IV tubing and fluids.
   b. Monitor previous site every 4 hours.
   c. Document degree of phlebitis and nursing interventions per agency policy and procedure (Table 29-2).

2. *Infiltration:* Client's rate of infusion slows; site of insertion becomes swollen, cool to touch, pale, and painful.
   a. Discontinue existing IV line, and restart in another site, preferably in opposite extremity.
   b. Monitor previous insertion site every 4 hours until resolution of swelling.
   c. Document degree of infiltration and nursing intervention (Table 29-3).

3. Client experiences burning, irritation, redness, or pain during infusion without phlebitis or infiltration. May be result of chemical phlebitis from medications infusing.
   a. Slow the infusion to deliver in minimum time for best therapeutic response.
   b. Assess client's tolerance to prescribed therapy. Discuss with client and physician insertion of midline or peripherally inserted central catheter as an option if duration of therapy and venous access permit.

4. Infusion is completed before or after appropriate time frame.
   a. Evaluate access device for position and patency, and restart as necessary.

Table 29-2

Phlebitis Scale	
Score	**Clinical Signs**
0	No symptoms
1	Erythema at access site with or without pain
2	Pain at access site with erythema and/or edema.
3	Pain at access site with erythema and/or edema Streak formation Palpable venous cord
4	Pain at access site with erythema and/or edema Streak formation Palpable venous cord >1 inch in length Purulent drainage

From Intraveous Nurses Society: Infusion nursing standards of practice, *J Intraven Nurs* 23(6S):S1, 2000

Table 29-3

Infiltration Scale	
Grade	**Clinical Criteria**
0	No symptoms
1	Skin blanched Edema <1 inch in any direction Cool to touch With or without pain
2	Skin blanched Edema 1 to 6 inches on skin surface in any direction Cool to touch With or without pain
3	Skin blanched, translucent Gross edema >6 inches in any direction Cool to touch Mild to moderate pain Possible numbness
4	Skin blanched, translucent Skin tight, leaking Skin discolored, bruised, swollen Gross edema >6 inches in any direction Deep pitting tissue edema Circulatory impairment Moderate to severe pain Infiltration of any amount of blood product, irritant, or vesicant

Intravenous Nurses Society: Infusion nursing standards of practice, *J Intraven Nurs* 23(6S):S1, 2000.

b. Monitor client for too-rapid infusion or fluid overload. Check vital signs, respiratory status, and I&O.

c. Monitor client for signs and symptoms of drug toxicity.

d. Notify physician.

e. Reregulate remainder of infusion to infuse over prescribed time. Assess need for electronic flow-control device.

5. *Positional IV infusion:* Client's flow rate is altered and changes with position of extremity.

   a. Apply arm board or commercial protective device to protect the site (Figure 29-2).

   b. Remove dressing, apply additional prepping agents, and resecure devices.

   c. If catheter device has been withdrawn from vessel, do not reinsert exposed portion of catheter.

   d. Continue hourly monitoring for proper rate of infusion. Restart in another site, as needed.

6. *Infection:* Client complains of chills, fever, and malaise; IV site may show purulent drainage.

   a. Discontinue IV (see Skill 29-3, p. 697).

   b. Retain previous IV catheter for possible culture (follow agency policy), and notify physician.

   c. Document nursing intervention as delineated in agency policy and procedure.

Recording and Reporting

- Record in nurses' notes number of attempts for insertion, type of fluid, insertion site by vessel, flow rate, size and type catheter or needle, and when infusion was begun. A special parenteral therapy flow sheet may be used (Figure 29-3).
- Record client's response to IV fluid, amount infused, and integrity and patency of system every 1 to 2 hours or according to agency policy.
- Report to oncoming nursing staff: location of site, type of fluid, flow rate, status of venipuncture site, amount of fluid remaining in present solution, expected time to hang next IV bag or bottle, and any side effects.
- Report to physician immediately any adverse reactions such as pulmonary congestion, shock, or thrombophlebitis.

Sample Documentation

1500 After procedure explained and site prepped with alcohol and Betadine, left cephalic vein accessed with 20-gauge 1¼-inch Insyte catheter. Positive blood return after full advancement. Catheter flushed with 1 ml NS, and saline lock attached for IV antibiotics. Client stated insertion was nonpainful and "felt fine" after insertion.

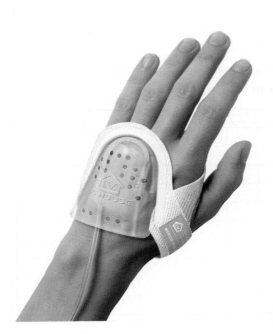

Figure 29-2 I.V. House Protective Device. (Courtesy I.V. House.)

ST. JOHN'S HOSPITAL
Springfield, Illinois
I.V. MAINTENANCE RECORD

I.V. FLUID & I.V. MEDICATION	

Site Code:
R.J. or L.J. – Right or Left Jugular
R.S.V. or L.S.V. – Right or Left Subclavian Vein
R.L.L. or L.L.L. – Right or Left Lower Leg
R.H. or L.H. – Right or Left Hand
R.F.A. or L.F.A. – Right or Left Forearm
R.U.A. or L.U.A. – Right or Left Upperarm
R.F. or L.F. – Right or Left Foot
R.S., L.S. or M.S. – Right, Left or Mid Scalp
R.F.V. or L.F.V. – Right or Left Femoral Vein
R.A.C. or L.A.C. – Right or Left Antecubital
R.W. or L.W. – Right or Left Wrist

K.V.O. – Keep Vein Open
H.L. – Heparin Lock
P.B. – Piggyback
P. – Push

Triple Lumen Catheter:
Proximal - 18 gauge (White) Draw blood, Blood Adm, Medications
Middle - 18 gauge (Blue) TPN, Medications
Distal - 16 gauge (Brown) Blood Adm., Colloids, Viscous Fluids, CVP Monitoring, Medications

Signature:

	DATE		
Allergy:	Night Nurse		
No. of last I.V. _____ Letter of last expander _____	Day Nurse		
No. of last Blood/Component _____	Evening Nurse		

Order Date	Amount, Solution, Infusing Time or Rate, Medication, Dose, Time	Site(s)	Pump	Time	Time
	One Time I.V. Meds.				
No.	I.V. Fluids				

I.V. SITE ASSESSMENT	

SITE CODE

R.J. or L.J. – Right or Left Jugular
R.S.V or L.S.V. – Right or Left Subclavian Vein
R.L.L. or L.L.L. – Right or Left Lower Leg
R.H. or L.H. – Right or Left Hand
R.F.A. or L.F.A. – Right or Left Forearm
R.U.A. or L.U.A. – Right or Left Upperarm
R.F. or L.F. – Right or Left Foot
R.S., L.S. or M.S. – Right, Left or Mid Scalp
R.F.V. or L.F.V. – Right or Left Femoral Vein
R.A.C. or L.A.C. – Right or Left Antecubital
R.W. or L.W. – Right or Left Wrist

K.V.O. – Keep Vein Open
H.L. – Heparin Lock
P.B. – Piggyback
P. – Push
Cath – Catheter

NA – Not Applicable

TYPE CODE

M.C. – Medicut
A.C. – Angiocath
S.V. – Scalpvein
A.S. – Angio-set
C.D. – Cutdown
I.C. – Intracath
I.P. – Infuse A Port

H.C. – Hickman Catheter
B.C. – Broviac Catheter
M.L.C. – Multi-lumen Catheter
M.L.P. – Multi-lumen Proximal
M.L.M. – Multi-lumen Middle
M.L.D. – Multi-lumen Distal
I. – Introducer

Document on each site once each shift & P.R.N.   No space is to be left blank.   Place "NA" in spaces which do not apply.

Date	Time	I.V. Site Start	d/c	Site Code	Cath Size	Type Code	Site Day	Cap Change	Dressing Change	I.V. Site: s̄ tenderness redness, edema, drainage	Signature

Figure 29-3 IV maintenance record. (Courtesy St. John's Hospital, Springfield, Ill.)

SPECIAL CONSIDERATIONS

Pediatric Considerations

- Know a child's cognitive and emotional stage of development and related approaches in handling insertion procedure.
- Consider having extra help when starting an IV on a child. AP can help with positioning.
- In addition to usual venipuncture sites, the four scalp veins and the dorsum of the foot are used in infants.
- A rubber band may be used to dilate scalp veins. In accessing scalp veins, aim the catheter downward, toward the heart, so the flow of infusion can follow venous return (Hankins and others, 2001).
- Needle selection is based on age: 26 to 24 gauge for neonates; 24 to 22 gauge for children.
- There is no recommendation for the use of chlorhexidine as a prepping agent in infants less than 2 months of age (CDC, 2001).
- Pediatric veins are very fragile. Use commercial protective device to cover area.

Geriatric Considerations

- Older adult clients have fragile veins. Consider eliminating use of tourniquet, apply very loosely, or reduce tourniquet time to avoid damaging vein during insertion (Ellenberger, 1999). After a tourniquet is applied, venous pressure goes up sharply, the vein is overstretched, and puncture with even a thin needle can rupture wall of vein (Chukhraev and Grekov, 2000).
- Place tourniquet, if used, over the client's sleeve to decrease shearing on fragile skin.
- Avoid veins that are easily moved or bumped, because there is less subcutaneous support of tissue. Dorsal metacarpal veins may not be the best choice. Use a commercial protective device to protect the site (see Figure 29-2).

- Selecting the smallest-sized catheter needed for therapy is even more important in the older adult client to minimize trauma to veins.
- With loss of supportive tissue, veins tend to lie more superficially. Lower insertion angle for venipuncture to 5 to 15 degrees.

Home Care Considerations

- Ensure that the client/caregiver is able and willing to administer IV therapy in the home. Determine if client or caregiver has the manual dexterity and cognitive ability to manage the infusion.
- Assess client's ability to obtain help (availability of caregiver, telephone, emergency access).
- Ensure that all devices (e.g., open needles, sheathed needles) are disposed of in puncture-resistant containers with lids: plastic milk cartons or coffee cans.

Long-Term Care Considerations

- If client is highly active or has been in physical restraints, application of an arm board may be useful in preventing dislodgement of catheter. Ensure that arm board does not restrict client's movement or impair circulation.
- Nosocomial infections are prevalent in long-term care facilities (Hankins and others, 2001). Use meticulous aseptic technique.
- Long-term care nurses should be skilled in the placement of peripheral IV catheters and be particularly aware of considerations given to catheter placement in older adults.

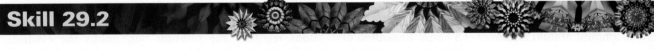

Skill 29.2

Regulating Intravenous Infusion Flow Rates

The ability to establish accurate infusion rates in IV therapy is essential to delivering prescribed infusion volumes and medications. Complications associated with IV therapy (e.g., infiltration, phlebitis, clotting of device, or circulatory overload) can be reduced or eliminated with a properly regulated IV infusion. Various factors can interfere with infusion rates (Table 29-4). Observation of the flow rate and IV system should occur hourly to achieve the desired therapeutic response.

Numerous methods are used to ensure an accurate hourly infusion rate for IV therapy. Fluids that run by gravity are adjusted through use of a flow control/regulator clamp. Fluids infused by an electronic infusion device or rate controller are regulated by a mechanical pump set at the prescribed rate. Physicians or licensed independent practitioners usually order the volume of fluid a client is to receive within a specific time frame. For example, "Administer 1 liter of D_5NS over 8 hours." The nurse must

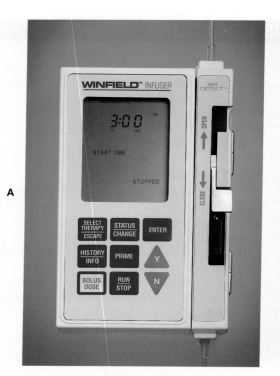
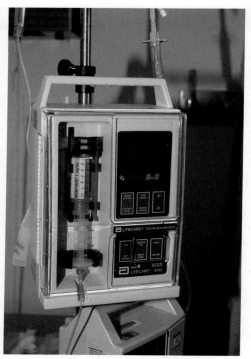

Figure 29-4 **A,** Electronic infusion device. **B,** Ambulatory infusion pump.

Table 29-4

Factors That Alter IV Flow Rates

Client Factors	Mechanical Factors
Change in client position	Height of parenteral container (should be higher than 36 inches [90 cm] above heart)
Flexion of involved extremity	Positional access device
Partial or complete occlusion of IV device	Viscosity or temperature of IV solution
	Occluded air vent
Venous spasm	Occluded in-line filter
Vein trauma (phlebitis)	Improperly placed restraints
Manipulated by client or visitor	Crimped administration set tubing
	Tubing dangling below bed
	Low battery of an electronic device

be able to calculate hourly flow rates to ensure the prescribed amount of fluid infuses over 8 hours. Regardless of whether gravity infusion or infusion via an electronic device is used, the nurse must assess infusion rates hourly.

Infusion pumps are necessary when administering low hourly volumes (e.g., 5 ml/hr or less, 20 ml/hr) to neonatal or pediatric clients or clients who are at risk for volume overload. In addition, when infusing high volumes of IV fluids (more than 150 ml/hr) to clients with impaired renal clearance, older adults, or pediatric clients, or when infusing drugs or IV fluids that require specific hourly volumes, electronic infusion pumps permit accurate, on-time infusion. Electronic infusion devices deliver the infusion via

positive pressure. A rate controller used on gravity infusions regulates the infusion but, unlike the electronic pump, can be affected by many mechanical and client factors. Recent advances in infusion technology have resulted in a variety of devices available for use to ensure accurate delivery.

Many devices have operating and programming capabilities that allow for single- and multiple-solution infusions at different rates (Figure 29-4, *A*). A variety of detectors and alarms respond to air in IV lines, completion of infusion, high and low pressure, low battery power, occlusion, and the inability to deliver at a preset rate. An anti–free flow safeguard (preventing bolus infusion in the event of machine malfunction) is an important element of an electronic infusion pump. Most pumps may be used for IV infusions. Manufacturer's recommendations for specific device features should always be checked.

Clients in alternative care settings achieve infusion accuracy with ambulatory infusion pumps. Most pumps weigh less than 6 pounds and range from palm size to backpack size. They function on battery power, allowing the client freedom to return to normal life. Programming capabilities include automatic rate adjustments, remote site adjustments via a telephone modem, and therapy-specific settings such as patient-controlled analgesia (PCA) (Figure 29-4, *B*). Follow the manufacturer's recommendations for specific device features.

ASSESSMENT

1. Review client's medical record for physician's order, stating type, amount, and rate or duration of IV fluid order or IV medications. *Rationale: Ensures right IV fluid is administered.*
2. Assess client's understanding of purpose of therapy and knowledge of how positioning affects flow rate.
3. Identify client's risk for fluid imbalance (e.g., child, older adult, history of heart failure or renal failure). *Rationale: Strict control of infusion volumes may be required.*
4. Determine the presence of any client or mechanical factor that may alter ordered fluid rates (e.g., client confusion, ability of client to cooperate, diuretic therapy, electrolyte imbalance). *Rationale: Decreases the risk of IV infusion complications.*
5. Obtain information from pharmacology references about specific infusion requirements of IV medication, admixture, or device. *Rationale: Reinforces Six Rights of Medication Administration; determines length of infusion time.*
6. Assess patency of IV device. *Rationale: Patency necessary for correct infusion flow.*

PLANNING

Expected outcomes focus on normal fluid and electrolyte balance and administration of IV fluids at the prescribed rate and correct dosage.

Expected Outcomes

1. Client receives prescribed volume of fluid within appropriate time frame, as evidenced by moist mucous membranes, adequate skin turgor, and balanced I&O.
2. Client's medications are administered over appropriate time frame with achievement of therapeutic response.
3. Client remains free of complications at IV site.

Equipment

- Watch with a second hand
- Paper and pencil (or calculator)
- IV tubing, macrodrip or microdrip, depending on rate ordered by physician and manufacturer specifications (some machines only use microdrip)
- Electronic infusion control device (optional)
- Volume control device (optional)
- Tape
- Label

Delegation Considerations

The skill of regulating IV flow rates requires the critical thinking and knowledge application unique to a nurse. In many states this skill is included within the scope of practice for licensed practical (vocational) nurses (LPN/LVN). Calculating and adjusting flow rates on gravity or electronic controlling devices is inappropriate for assistive personnel (AP) to perform. However, AP can be delegated to inform the nurse when a fluid container is almost empty, when the client complains of any discomfort, and when an electronic controlling device sounds an alarm.

IMPLEMENTATION FOR REGULATING INTRAVENOUS INFUSION FLOW RATES

Steps	Rationale
1. See Standard Protocol (inside front cover).	
2. Obtain IV fluid and appropriate tubing.	Use of correct tubing ensures more accurate infusion delivery. Macrodrip tubing allows for higher infusion volumes.
a. *Macrodrip:* Used to deliver rate *greater than* 100 ml/hr. (Drip factor is 10 to 15 gtt/ml depending on equipment used. Drop factor is printed on box.) Travenol Laboratories: 10 gtt/ml Abbott Laboratories: 15 gtt/ml McGraw Laboratories: 15 gtt/ml	

Steps	Rationale

b. *Microdrip:* Used to deliver rates *less than* 100 ml/hr.
Microdrip: 60 gtt/ml

Microdrip tubing is used for slow delivery and smaller volumes.

3. Calculate desired flow rate (hourly volume) of prescribed infusion:_____

Flow rate (ml/hr) = $\dfrac{\text{Total infusion (volume in ml)}}{\text{Hours of infusion (time to be infused)}}$

Example: $\dfrac{1000 \text{ ml}}{8 \text{ hr}} = \dfrac{125 \text{ ml}}{1 \text{ hr}}$

4. Calculate the drop rate based on drops per minute.

$$\dfrac{\text{gtt factor}}{60} \times \dfrac{\text{Flow rate}}{1} = \text{Drop rate}$$

Examples: Infuse 120 ml/hr via 10 gtt/ml drop factor:

$$\dfrac{10}{60} \times \dfrac{120}{1} = 20 \text{ gtt/min}$$

Via 15 gtt/ml:

$$\dfrac{15}{60} \times \dfrac{120}{1} = 30 \text{ gtt/min}$$

Via 20 gtt/ml:

$$\dfrac{20}{60} \times \dfrac{120}{1} = 40 \text{ gtt/min}$$

Via 60 gtt/ml (microgtt):

$$\dfrac{60}{60} \times \dfrac{120}{1} = 120 \text{ gtt/ml}$$

5. *Optional method for calculation:*
   If drop factor is 10 gtt/ml, take ordered rate per hour and divide by 6.
   If drop factor is 15 gtt/ml, take ordered rate per hour and divide by 4.
   If drop factor is 20 gtt/ml, take ordered rate per hour and divide by 3.
   If drop factor is 60 gtt/ml, take ordered rate per hour and divide by 1.

6. Time-tape the IV bottle or bag by securing adhesive tape or fluid indicator tape along side of fluid container (see illustration). Document each IV fluid bag sequentially, and note type of fluid, client's name, infusion span, and beginning and expected end of infusion.

Gives a visual scale to assess progress of infusion hourly. Avoid use of felt-tip pens or permanent markers on plastic bag; these can contaminate IV solutions. In some agencies all fluids, including those on pumps, should be labeled and time-taped (check agency policy).

7. Close rate-controlling clamp on IV tubing.

8. To insert infusion set into fluid bag, remove protective cover from IV bag port without touching opening. Remove cap from spike, and insert spike into port of IV bag, being careful not to puncture side of opening (see illustration). Hang bag from IV pole.

Maintains sterility of solution.

9. Fill drip chamber of tubing until half full by gently squeezing and releasing (see illustration).

Creates vacuum, allowing fluid to enter drip chamber.

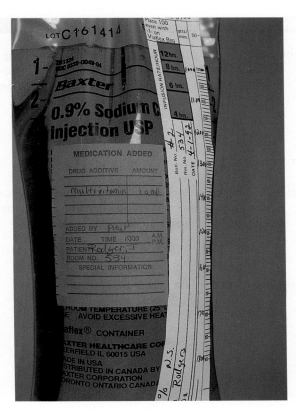

Step 6   IV bag with time tape.

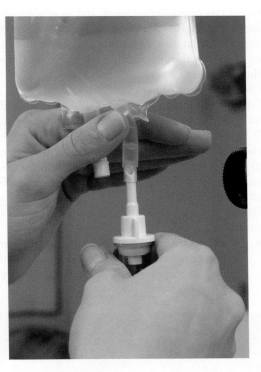

Step 8   Insert spike into IV bag port.

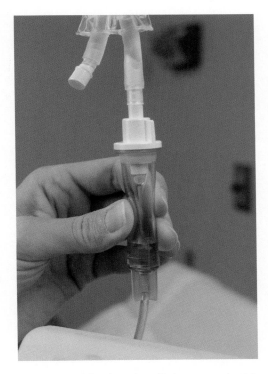

Step 9   Squeeze drip chamber. Release as chamber fills.

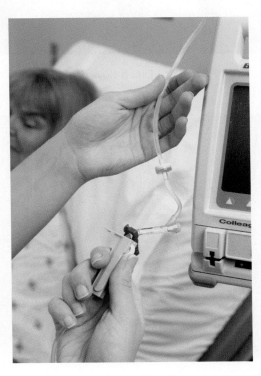

Step 10   Open rate-controlling clamp to fill tubing.

Steps	Rationale

10. Open rate-controlling clamp, and slowly fill remainder of tubing (see illustration). Invert Y connector sites to displace air. Most tubings can be fully filled or primed without removing the cover on the end of the IV tubing.

    Tubing must be fully filled with fluid before connecting to client to avoid air embolus. Too rapid filling promotes development of tiny air bubbles within tubing.

11. Close rate-controlling clamp on tubing.

12. Perform venipuncture (see Skill 29.1, p. 676), and attach catheter to end of IV tubing, maintaining sterility.

13. With IV fluid bag a minimum of 36 inches (90 cm) above IV insertion site, adjust rate-controlling clamp to deliver drops per minute. *Option:* a dial-a-flow device may be attached to IV tubing to regulate flow rate (see illustration).

    Fluid container heights of 36 to 48 inches usually are sufficient to overcome venous pressure and other resistance from tubing and catheter (Hadaway, 1998).

14. *Option:* Attach to electronic infusion device or rate controller.

    a. Place electronic eye on half-filled drip chamber below origin of drop and above fluid line if required (see illustration). NOTE: Some devices do not use electronic eye.

    Positioning necessary for accurate drip count.

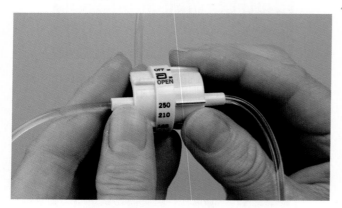

Step 13   Dial-a-flow device.

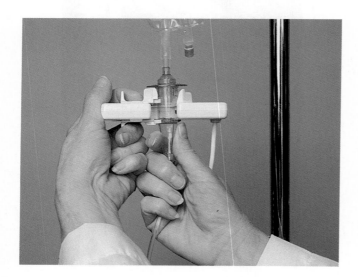

Step 14a   Electronic eye placed over drip chamber.

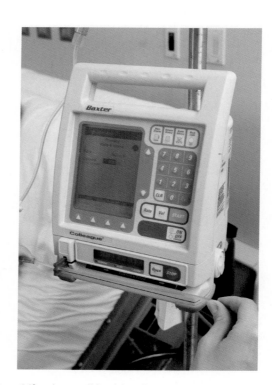

Step 14b   Insert IV tubing into chamber of control mechanism.

Steps	Rationale
b. Insert IV tubing into chamber of control mechanism (see illustration). (Consult manufacturer's instructions for use of pump.)	Pump chamber moves fluid through IV tubing.
c. Secure portion of IV tubing through "air in line" alarm system.	Allows for detection of air in tubing, which can enter vascular system, causing an embolus.
d. Close door to control chamber. Turn on pump, and select rate per hour and total volume to be infused (VTBI) (see illustration).	Ensures correct volume will be administered.
e. Open rate-controlling clamp on tubing if closed, and press start button (see illustration).	Rate control clamp should be open completely while infusion controller or pump is in use, to ensure accurate volume of infusion.
f. Monitor infusion hourly to assess patency of system when in alarm mode, and monitor for proper infusion rate and infiltration.	
15. *Option:* Attach IV tubing to volume control device.	
a. Place volume control device between IV bag and insertion spike of infusion set using sterile technique (see illustration).	Delivers small volume but must be refilled as it empties.
b. Fill IV tubing with fluid by opening regulator clamp.	
c. Place 2 hours of fluid allotment in chamber device.	This prevents infusion from running dry if 60 minutes elapses before nurse returns. Should infusion rate accidentally increase, will only allow 2 hours of fluids to infuse.

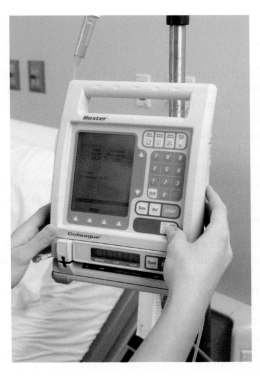

Step 14d   Select rate and volume to be infused.

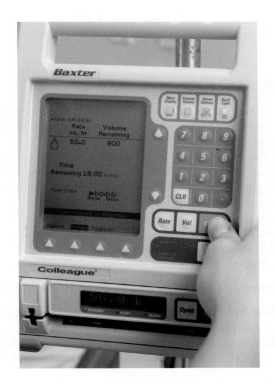

Step 14e   Press start button.

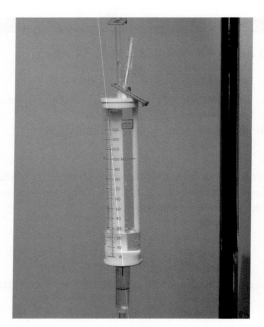

Step 15a   Volume control device positioned between IV bag and infusion tubing.

Steps	Rationale

16. Instruct client about the following:
   a.   To avoid raising hand or arm to a position that will affect flow rate
   b.   To avoid manipulation of rate control clamp
   c.   Purpose and significance of alarms

Instruction informs client on how to protect IV site and importance of not altering rate control.

17. See Completion Protocol (inside front cover).

• • • • • • • • • •

EVALUATION

1. Monitor client's IV infusion hourly for proper rate of infusion, and monitor I&O. Palpate skin for turgor and dryness.

2. Observe client and client's laboratory values for signs and symptoms of overhydration or dehydration during infusion, observing for restoration of fluid and electrolyte balance and therapeutic response.

3. Observe client for therapeutic response to fluids/medication(s).

4. Monitor client's IV site for signs of infiltration, phlebitis, kink or knot in tubing.

Unexpected Outcomes and Related Interventions

1. During hourly check, infusion is found to be behind.
   a.   Evaluate reason for delay in fluids.
   b.   Recalculate remainder of infusion, and confer with physician or licensed independent practitioner before reregulating.

2. Client experiences sudden onset of shortness of breath, tachycardia, restlessness, and confusion. Assessment of lung sounds reveals inspiratory crackles. Client has received more than prescribed infusion volume.
   a.   Evaluate for proper function of IV access device.
   b.   Slow rate to keep vein open (KVO).
   c.   Place client in high-Fowler's position, and notify physician or licensed independent practitioner.

Recording and Reporting

• Record rate of infusion, drops per minute, and milliliters per hour in nurses' notes every 4 hours or according to agency policy.

• Immediately record in nurses' notes any new IV fluid rates.

• Document use of any electronic infusion device or controlling device and number on that device.

• At change of shift or when leaving on break, report rate of infusion to nurse in charge or next nurse assigned to care for client.

Sample Documentation

Routine documentation is included on the IV mainte-nance record (see Figure 29-3, p. 688).

1700 Client complaining of SOB. Lungs auscultated with inspiratory crackles in right lower lobe. Dr. Lee noti-fied. Order noted to decrease IV to 25 ml/hr. Positive blood return noted via 20-gauge IV right cephalic vein. Changed to IMED Gemini infusion at 25 ml/hr via pump. Purpose of fluid restriction and symptoms of pul-monary edema reviewed with client and wife with verbal-ized understanding.

SPECIAL CONSIDERATIONS

Pediatric Considerations

- Children are not small adults. Physiological differences must be remembered, particularly focusing on total body weight (85% to 90% water). Dehydration is a common cause of fluid and electrolyte imbalance; as-sessment of fluid needs includes meter square weight or caloric method (Phillips, 2001).
- Use only small-volume containers for infusions (250 ml for children younger than 12 months, 500 ml for older children). Microdrip tubing is recommended for children.

Geriatric Considerations

- Renal changes in older adults may reduce the kidney's ability to concentrate and dilute urine in response to water or salt excess. Combined with cardiac deficiencies and decreased blood flow to organs, the older client is precariously balanced between dehydration and fluid overload. Use an electronic infusion pump and micro-drip. Monitor levels of electrolytes, blood urea nitrogen (BUN), and creatinine, urine output, and daily weight (Powers, 1999).

- Dextrose infused too rapidly may cause cerebral edema more readily in older clients. Normal saline, given to an older client with impaired renal function, can cause hypernatremia (Powers, 1999).

Home Care Considerations

- Ensure that client is able and willing to operate the electronic infusion device (if applicable). Assess any physical or visual limitations.
- The nurse should be in the home during initiation of IV therapy to assess proper functioning of equipment.
- Ensure that electrical outlets are functioning properly, grounded, and infusion device has backup power, if re-quired by type of infusate.
- Teach client and primary caregiver to time drops per minute using watch with second hand.

Long-Term Care Considerations

Careful monitoring of infusion rate is particularly impor-tant in the long-term care setting, noting the vulnerability of geriatric clients to complications.

Skill 29.3

Maintenance of Intravenous Site

Peripheral IV catheters and the therapy being infused are frequently associated with complications such as local or systemic infections, phlebitis, and infiltration. Appropriate management of IV sites will prevent or minimize these complications.

The skin insertion site is the most common source of colonization and infection for vascular catheters (Raad, 1998). Therefore catheter dressings must be securely ap-plied and must be changed when loose, wet, or soiled. A transparent membrane dressing or sterile gauze secured with tape is used to cover the site. A transparent dressing should be changed with catheter site rotation and imme-diately if integrity of dressing is compromised. Gauze dressings should be changed routinely every 48 hours and immediately if integrity is compromised. Gauze used in conjunction with transparent dressing should be consid-ered a gauze dressing and changed every 48 hours (INS, 2000; CDC, 2001) (check agency policy).

Fluid containers include plastic bags, plastic bottles, and glass bottles. These containers may be changed frequently depending on the rate of infusion and the volume in the container. The CDC (2001) does not make a recommenda-tion for the hang time of IV fluids, but the INS recommends that each container be changed within 24 hours after the administration set is added (INS, 2000). Fluid containers on ambulatory infusion devices may remain longer than 24 hours if aseptic technique is used, the system remains closed without injection ports or add-on tubing, and the medication is stable for the anticipated infusion time (Hankins and others, 2001; INS, 2001). The nurse must allow adequate time for this procedure, follow proper technique to prevent infection, and adhere to the specific agency policy.

Changing infusion tubing is much simpler and more efficient if changed when hanging a new fluid container. The CDC (2001) recommends changing tubing no more frequently than every 96 hours. The INS (2000) recommends 72-hour intervals for continuous tubing changes, adding that 48-hour tubing changes may be considered if the rate of catheter-related infection and phlebitis in an institution exceeds 5%. Several studies have shown the safety of 72-hour tubing changes (Lai, 1998). The INS also states that tubing used for intermittent infusion through an injection/access port should be changed every 24 hours because both ends of this tubing are manipulated more frequently than tubing used for continuous infusion. The CDC has no recommendation for changing of intermittent tubing.

An injection cap or prn adapter on a peripheral catheter is used to administer IV fluids or medications intermittently. The injection cap is changed when the catheter is changed. A short extension tubing or loop may be placed between the catheter hub and injection cap. This allows manipulation of the injection cap without movement of the catheter. This tubing remains attached to the peripheral catheter and is changed when the catheter is changed. For midline and central venous catheters, these caps should be changed at least every 7 days (INS, 2000). The fluid pathway and capped ends on all infusion tubing, stopcocks, extension tubing, and injection caps are sterile. The nurse must exercise caution to prevent contamination of these surfaces during changes.

The nurse must be prepared to assist the client with many aspects of hygiene, such as gown changes, while the client is receiving IV therapy (see Chapter 7). Gowns with snaps across the shoulders are best, especially for multiple infusions. When using a regular gown or the client's clothing, the nurse must thread the fluid container and tubing through the sleeve of the gown in the same manner as the client's arm. Infusion tubing should not be disconnected to change a gown or any article of clothing. Care can be coordinated so that bathing or hygiene activities are done after removal of an old infusion site and before another venipuncture is made.

ASSESSMENT

1. Changing a peripheral IV dressing:
    a. Determine when the dressing was last changed by checking the dressing label. *Rationale: This labeling provides instant identification for assessing and determining status of the site.*
    b. Observe present dressing for moisture and occlusiveness. Determine if moisture is from leakage from the puncture site or from an external source. *Rationale: Soiled dressing should be changed immediately.*
    c. Observe IV system for proper functioning or complications (tubing or catheter kinks).
    d. Palpate the catheter site through the intact dressing for complaints of tenderness, pain, or burning. *Rationale: Signs indicative of phlebitis.*
    e. Inspect exposed catheter site for swelling, redness, drainage, or blanching. *Rationale: Signs indicative of phlebitis or infiltration.*
    f. Monitor body temperature.
    g. Determine client's understanding of the need for continued IV infusion.

2. Changing infusion tubing:
    a. Determine when new infusion set is needed (e.g., according to agency policy, or after contamination or puncture of infusion tubing).
    b. Observe for occlusions in tubing such as kinking, drug or mineral precipitate, and blood. *Rationale: Infusion of incompatible medications can lead to precipitate formation. Blood may flow retrograde from vein and adhere to tubing. Infusion of viscous blood components may cause adherence to walls of tubing and decrease size of lumen.*
    c. Determine client's understanding of the need for continued IV infusions.

3. Changing fluid container:
    a. Check physician's or licensed independent practitioner's orders. *Rationale: Ensures that correct solution will be used and that the order is complete.*
    b. If order is written for KVO, contact physician or licensed independent practitioner for clarification of the rate of infusion. Note date and time when solution was last changed. *Rationale: Orders for KVO do not provide complete information and can result in fluid overload or deficit and electrolyte imbalance. A KVO order shall contain a specific infusion rate (INS, 2000) (check agency policy).*
    c. Verify client's identification. *Rationale: Ensures right client receives ordered IV fluid.*
    d. Determine the compatibility of all IV fluids and additives by consulting appropriate literature or the pharmacy. *Rationale: Patency of the inside of catheter depends on prevention of chemical interactions. Precipitation can occur because of concentration of drugs in solution. When pH changes by contact between solutions or medications, a precipitate can occur (Hadaway, 1998).*
    e. Determine client's understanding of need for continuing IV therapy.
    f. Assess patency of current IV access site. Check for blood return and/or free flow of infusion.

4. Discontinuing IV medications:
   a. Observe fluid container for complete infusion of all medication.
   b. Review care plan for any blood samples required after medication infusion. *Rationale: Monitoring of serum concentrations of some IV medications is required to avoid reaching toxic levels. Dosage adjustments or alterations of timing for next dose may be required (check agency policy).*
   c. Continue to monitor client's response to medications. *Rationale: Evaluates medication effects.*
5. Discontinuing peripheral IV access:
   a. Observe existing IV site for signs and symptoms of infection, infiltration, or phlebitis. *Rationale: Indications for discontinuing IV.*
   b. Review physician's order for discontinuation of IV therapy. *Rationale: Physician's or licensed independent practitioner's order is required to discontinue IV therapy. The specific wording may not include removal of the catheter, but this is implied.*
   c. Determine client's understanding of the need for removal of peripheral IV catheter.

PLANNING

Expected outcomes focus on reducing the risk of infection and phlebitis, minimizing client discomfort, reducing risk of overhydration, and maintaining a patent IV catheter.

Expected Outcomes

1. Client will have IV that flows freely without infiltration, phlebitis, or clot.
2. Client's temperature will remain normal.
3. Client will continue to receive the prescribed fluid infusion and/or medication as ordered.
4. Client's serum electrolyte levels remain or return to normal.

Equipment

Changing a Peripheral IV Dressing

- Antiseptic swabs (alcohol, povidone-iodine, chlorhexidine)
- Skin protectant solution
- Adhesive remover (optional)
- Strips of sterile, precut tape (or 36-inch roll of tape)
- Clean gloves
- Transparent dressing or sterile 2 × 2 gauze pads and tape
- Arm board or housing device (optional)

Changing Infusion Tubing

Continuous infusion:
- Microdrip or macrodrip infusion tubing, as appropriate
- 0.22-μ filter and extension tubing if necessary
- Tubing label

Intermittent saline/heparin lock:
- Injection cap or prn adapter
- Loop or short extension tubing (if necessary)
- Sterile 2 × 2 gauze pads
- 5-ml syringe filled with normal saline or heparin flush solution (check agency policy)
- Clean gloves
- If a new IV dressing must be applied, assemble additional equipment (see Skill 29.2, p. 689).

Changing Infusion Container

- Bottle/bag of IV solution as ordered by physician or appropriate prescriber
- Time tape
- Pen

Discontinuing IV Medications

- Clean gloves
- Sterile cap or cover for infusion tubing
- 5-ml syringe filled with normal saline or heparin flush solution (check agency policy)
- 10-ml syringe filled with normal saline or heparin flush solution (check agency policy)
- Antiseptic swabs
- Injection cap replacement (if needed)

Discontinuing Peripheral IV Access

- Clean gloves
- Sterile 2 × 2 or 4 × 4 gauze pad
- Tape
- Antiseptic swab

Delegation Considerations

These skills require the critical thinking and knowledge application unique to a nurse. In many states, these skills are included within the scope of practice for licensed practical (vocational) nurses (LPN/LVN). Assistive personnel (AP) may be delegated the task of collecting supplies, assisting with comfort measures, and distracting the client during the procedure.

IMPLEMENTATION FOR MAINTENANCE OF INTRAVENOUS SITE

Steps	Rationale

1. See Standard Protocol (inside front cover).

2. **Changing peripheral IV dressing**

a. Remove any overlying tape. Then remove transparent membrane dressing by picking up one corner and pulling the side laterally while holding catheter hub (see illustration). Repeat for other side. *or*

Technique minimizes discomfort during removal.

b. Remove gauze dressing and tape from old dressing one layer at a time by pulling toward the insertion site. Leave chevron tape securing catheter to skin. Check agency procedure.

Catheter moved during dressing change could accidentally dislodge and puncture blood vessel.

c. Observe insertion site for redness, swelling, drainage, pallor, or pain. If present, discontinue infusion (see Step 6, p. 706).

d. If IV is infusing properly, gently remove tape securing catheter. Stabilize catheter with one finger. Remove adhesive residue with adhesive remover, if necessary.

Prevents catheter from dislodging.

e. Using circular motion, cleanse peripheral insertion site with antiseptic swab (see illustration), starting at insertion site and working outward, creating concentric circles. Allow antiseptic solution to dry completely.

Antimicrobial solutions should be allowed to air-dry completely to effectively reduce microbial counts (INS, 2000). If antiseptic agents are used in combination, allow each to air-dry separately.

f. *Option:* Apply skin protectant solution (SkinPrep or No Sting Barrier Film) to the area where the tape or dressing will be applied. Allow to dry.

Coats the skin with protective solution to maintain skin integrity, prevent irritation from the adhesive, and promote adhesion of the dressing.

g. *Transparent dressing:*

(1) Place transparent dressing over venipuncture site by smoothing dressing over IV site and catheter, up to the hub (refer to manufacturer's directions). Do not cover the catheter hub/tubing junction with the dressing.

Transparent dressing allows inspection of site.

Access to catheter hub is needed in times of emergency and when changing tubing.

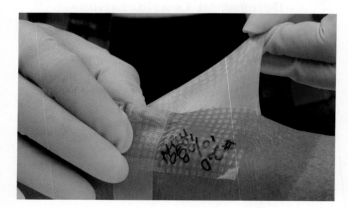

Step 2a Remove transparent dressing by pulling side laterally.

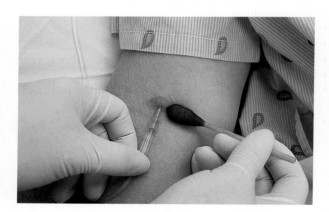

Step 2e Cleanse peripheral insertion site with antiseptic swab.

Steps	**Rationale**

(2) Take a 1-inch piece of tape and place it from end of hub of catheter to insertion site, over transparent dressing (see Skill 29-1, Step 21).

(3) The apply chevron and place only over tape, not over transparent dressing.

h. *Gauze dressing:*

(1) Place single 4-inch strip of sterile ½-inch nonallergenic tape under peripheral catheter hub with sticky side up. Criss-cross tape over catheter hub to anchor it to skin. Do not cover insertion site. If desired, place a second piece of sterile tape across catheter at hub.

Chevron secures catheter to skin.

(2) Place a 2 × 2 gauze over venipuncture site, and catheter hub. Secure all edges with tape. Do not cover the connection between IV tubing and catheter hub with the dressing.

Gauze dressings must be occlusive to prevent air flow (Hankins and others, 2001). Access to catheter hub is needed in times of emergency and when changing tubing.

i. Fold a 2 × 2 gauze in half, and cover with 1-inch-wide tape extending about an inch from each side of gauze. Place under the tubing/catheter hub junction. Curl a loop of tubing alongside the outside of the arm, and place a second piece of tape directly over the tubing and 2 × 2, securing the tubing in two places. When using a transparent dressing, avoid placing tape directly over dressing.

Securing the tubing at two places prevents catheter movement and dislodgement that increase the risk of phlebitis and infiltration. Placing tape on tape makes tubing removal easier and decreases the skin irritation.

Tape application loosens transparent dressings.

j. Label the dressing with date and time of insertion, date and time of dressing change, gauge and length of catheter, and identification of nurse.

Allows easy recognition of type of device and time interval for site rotation.

k. *Option:* Apply hand board or commercial housing device if venipuncture site or dressing is affected by the motion of the wrist.

Reduces the risk of phlebitis and infiltration from motion of the joint.

l. Discard used supplies, remove gloves, and perform hand hygiene.

3. Changing infusion tubing

a. Open new infusion set, and connect add-on pieces such as filters or extension tubing. Keep protective covering over spike and distal adapter. Secure all junctions with Luer-Loks, clasping devices, or threaded devices. Avoid the use of tape.

Separation of infusion tubing increases the risk of air emboli, hemorrhage, and infection.
Protective covers reduce entrance of microorganisms.

b. If catheter hub is not visible, remove IV dressing as directed in Steps 2a. and 2b. Do not remove tape securing catheter to skin (if gauze dressing was used). If transparent dressing has to be removed, place small piece of sterile tape across hub to temporarily anchor catheter during disconnection.

Movement of catheter may cause it to dislodge.

c. For existing continuous infusion:

(1) Close roller clamp on new tubing.

(2) Slow rate of infusion to KVO on existing IV by regulating roller clamp on old tubing.

(3) Compress and fill drip chamber of old tubing.

Steps	Rationale
(4) Remove IV container from pole, invert container, and remove old tubing from solution. Carefully hold container while hanging or taping the drip chamber on IV pole 36 inches above IV site.	Fluid in drip chamber will run slowly to keep catheter patent.
(5) Place insertion spike of new tubing into old fluid container opening. Hang container on IV pole, compress and release drip chamber on new tubing, and fill drip chamber one-third to one-half full (see illustration).	
(6) Slowly open roller clamp, remove protective cap from adapter (if necessary), and flush new tubing with solution. Stop infusion, and replace cap.	Slow flush of solution into tubing reduces formation of air bubbles in tubing.
(7) Turn roller clamp on old tubing to "off" position.	
d. *Option:* Place 2 × 2 gauze under catheter hub.	Prevents tubing from accidentally contacting skin and collects blood that may leak from catheter hub.
e. Stabilize hub of catheter, and apply pressure over vein just above catheter tip (at least 1½ inches above insertion site). Gently disconnect old tubing from catheter hub, and quickly insert adapter of new tubing into catheter hub (see illustrations).	Minimizes loss of blood as tubing is changed.

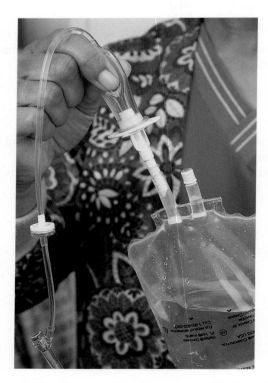

Step 3c(5) Squeeze drip chamber to fill with fluid.

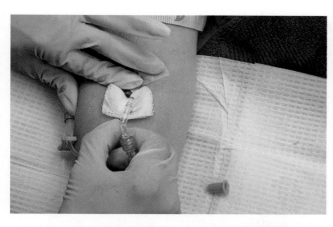

A

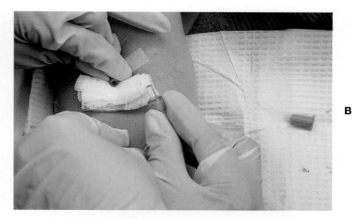

B

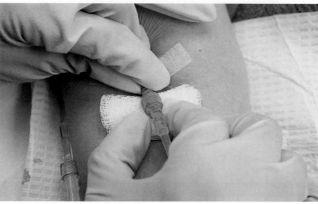

C

Step 3e   **A,** Disconnect old tubing. **B,** While compressing vein, attach end of new tubing. **C,** Make sure connection is secure.

Steps	Rationale
f. Open roller clamp on new tubing, allowing solution to run rapidly for 30 to 60 seconds, then regulate IV drip according to physician's or licensed independent practitioner's orders and monitor rate hourly (see illustration).	Clears catheter of any blood in lumen, preventing occlusion.
g. Attach a piece of tape or a preprinted label with date and time of tubing change onto tubing below the drip chamber.	Provides reference to determine next time for tubing change.
h. Remove and discard 2 × 2 gauze (if used) and old IV tubing. If necessary, apply new dressing (see Step 2, p. 700). Dispose of gloves.	
i. Form a loop of tubing, and secure it to client's arm with a strip of tape.	Avoids accidental pulling against site and catheter movement.
4. **Changing fluid container**	
a. Prepare next solution at least 1 hour before needed. If prepared in pharmacy, be sure it has been delivered to the client's location. Check that the solution is correct and properly labeled. Check solution expiration date. Observe for precipitate and discoloration.	Ensures no disruption in fluid therapy to client.
b. Change solution when fluid remains only in neck of container or when new type of solution has been ordered.	Prevents waste of solution.
c. Move roller clamp to stop flow rate, and remove old IV fluid container from IV pole.	

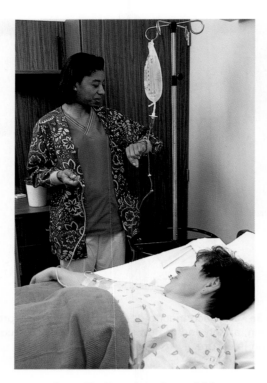

Step 3f   Regulate flow of IV.

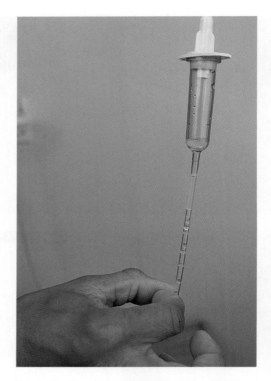

Step 4f   Remove air bubbles from tubing.

Steps	Rationale
d. Quickly remove spike from old container, keeping it sterile. Remove protective cover from new fluid container. Without touching tip of spike, insert it into new bag or bottle.	Ensures sterility of solution.
e. Hang new bag or bottle of solution on IV pole.	
f. Check for air in tubing. If bubbles form, they can be removed by closing the roller clamp, stretching the tubing downward, and tapping the tubing with the finger (the bubbles rise in the tubing to the drip chamber) (see illustration). For larger amounts of air, swab port with antiseptic swab, allow to dry, and connect a syringe to an injection port below the air and aspirate the air into the syringe.	Infusion of air in tubing can result in air embolus, which can be fatal to client.

COMMUNICATION TIP   *Tell client the "champagne type of bubbles" inside the tubing are not a problem. They will be removed by the filter in the line.*

Steps	Rationale
g. Make sure drip chamber is one-third to one-half full. If drip chamber is too full, pinch off tubing below the drip chamber, invert the container, squeeze the drip chamber, hang container, and release the tubing.	If chamber is completely filled, nurse cannot observe drip rate.
h. Regulate flow to prescribed rate.	
i. Place time label on the side of container, and label with the time hung, the time of completion, and appropriate interval. If using plastic bags, mark only on the label and not the container.	

Steps	Rationale

5. Discontinuing IV medications

a. 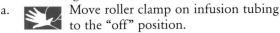 Move roller clamp on infusion tubing to the "off" position.

b. Remove any clasping devices, and disconnect medication delivery tubing from injection port.

NURSE ALERT *If the tubing spike, connector end, fluid pathway, or fluid container is contaminated, a new tubing set or fluid container is required.*

---

c. Remove the needle or needleless adapter on the infusion tubing; discard appropriately in receptacle, and replace with a sterile cap or cover, as required.

  Infusion tubing can be reused with next ordered medication.

d. Swab injection port or prn adapter on main IV tubing with antiseptic swab (see illustration).

  Ensures sterility of port.

e. For intermittent medication piggybacked into a continuous infusion, attach 5-ml saline-filled syringe to injection port, and flush the line gently. Regulate fluid flow of the continuous infusion as ordered.

  Saline flush prevents incompatible medications from coming into contact in the infusion tubing. There is no way to know how much pressure is exerted inside catheter lumen (Hadaway, 1998). A 5-ml syringe generates less pressure than a 3-ml syringe. Do not force irrigation if resistance is felt.

f. For intermittent medications through a saline or heparin lock, attach saline-filled 5- to 10-ml syringe to injection port and flush catheter gently, or attach heparin flush solution-filled syringe to injection port and flush gently, if necessary (check agency policy). Attach sterile injection port cover, if necessary.

  Flushing with 3 to 10 ml of saline after each medication is crucial. Volume of flush depends on lumen size, catheter length, and medication infused (Hadaway, 1998).

NURSE ALERT *Flushing of any IV catheter must be approached carefully. If resistance is met, first assess mechanical causes (e.g., closed clamps, kinked tubing, position of extremity). Never forcefully attempt to flush. Fibrin formation, drug precipitates, and blood clots can occlude catheter lumen. Forceful flush against these occlusions can cause fracture of catheter and possible embolization. Size of syringe used for flushing should be in accordance with manufacturer's guidelines for pounds per square inch (PSI) (INS, 2000).*

---

g. Prepare client for obtaining blood samples after medication infusion, if necessary.

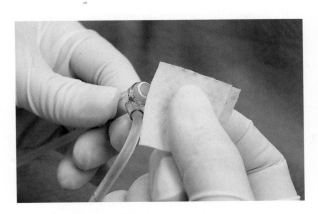

Step 5d   Cleanse injection port.

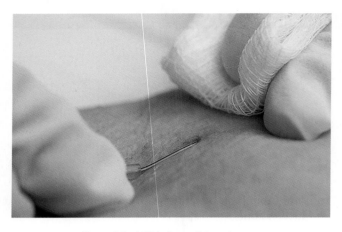

Step 6d Withdraw IV catheter.

Steps	Rationale

6. **Discontinuing peripheral IV access**
   a. Explain procedure to client. Explain that affected extremity must be held still and how long procedure will take.

   Minimizes client's anxiety and discomfort.

   b. Turn IV tubing roller clamp to "off" position. Remove tape securing tubing.

   c. Remove IV site dressing and tape while stabilizing catheter.

   Movement of catheter will cause discomfort.

NURSE ALERT *Never use scissors to remove the tape or dressing because the catheter could accidentally be cut.*

---

   d. With dry gauze or alcohol swab held over site, apply light pressure and withdraw the catheter, using a slow steady movement, keeping the hub parallel to the skin (see illustration).

   Changing the angle of the catheter inside the vein could cause additional vein irritation, increasing the risk of postinfusion phlebitis.

   e. Apply pressure to the site for 2 to 3 minutes, using a dry, sterile gauze pad. Secure with tape.

   Dry pad causes less irritation to the puncture site. Subcutaneous hematoma is common complication. When needle is removed, vein wall contracts to stop bleeding. Contraction is enhanced by pressure to site for at least 2 to 3 minutes (Chukhraev and Grekov, 2000).

   f. Inspect the catheter for intactness, noting tip integrity and length.

   Tips of catheter can break off, causing an embolus, and emergency situation. Notify MD if tip broken.

   g. Discard used supplies.
   h. Remove and discard gloves, and perform hand hygiene.
   i. Instruct client to report any redness, pain, drainage, or swelling that may occur after catheter removal.

   Postinfusion phlebitis may occur within 48 to 96 hours after catheter removal.

7. See Completion Protocol (inside front cover).

• • • • • • • • • •

EVALUATION

Changing Peripheral IV Dressing

1. Observe functioning, patency of IV system, and flow rate after changing dressing.
2. Inspect condition of IV site, noting color. Palpate for skin temperature, edema, and tenderness.
3. Monitor client's body temperature.

Changing Infusion Tubing

1. Evaluate flow rate of flush, and observe connection site for leakage.

Changing Fluid Container

1. Observe client for signs of fluid volume excess or deficit to determine response to IV fluid therapy.
2. Monitor electrolyte values and I&O.

Discontinuing IV Medications

1. Observe site for redness, pain, drainage, or swelling.
2. Observe continuous infusion for correct rate.
3. Observe tubing for leaking.

Discontinuing Peripheral IV Access

1. Observe site for evidence of bleeding.
2. Observe site for redness, pain, drainage, or swelling.

Unexpected Outcomes and Related Interventions

Changing Peripheral IV Dressing

1. IV catheter is infiltrated, as evidenced by edema, pallor, leakage from puncture site, or decreased skin temperature around insertion site.
2. Phlebitis is present, as evidenced by redness and tenderness along vein pathway.
3. IV catheter is accidentally dislodged.
4. Catheter is infected, as evidenced by redness, swelling, pain, and/or exudate.
   NOTE:
   a. For all of the above, temporarily discontinue infusion and remove catheter.
   b. Insert another catheter, preferably on the opposite extremity. Check agency policy for complication management.
5. Client has an elevated temperature, but the insertion site is free of signs and symptoms of infection.
   a. Assess all vital signs, and inform the physician or licensed independent practitioner of the client's condition.

Changing Infusion Tubing

1. Decreased or absent flow of IV fluid indicated by a slowed or obstructed flow.
   a. Open roller clamp, slide clamps, and recalibrate drip rate. Check for kinks in tubing.

b. Evaluate any pain or discomfort at the site for infiltration or temporary venous spasm.

Changing Fluid Container

1. Flow rate is incorrect; client receives too little or too much fluid.
   a. Regulate to the correct rate.
   b. Determine and correct the cause of the incorrect flow rate (e.g., change in client position, change in catheter position, kinked tubing).
   c. Use electronic infusion device when accurate flow rate is critical.
   d. Notify physician or licensed practitioner if client's anticipated infusion is less than or greater than 100 to 200 ml as expected (check agency policy).

Discontinuing IV Medications

1. Solution in tubing below piggyback site turns cloudy because of precipitate formation, indicating medication incompatibility.
   a. Stop all infusions.
   b. Change tubing on continuous infusion.

Discontinuing Peripheral IV Access

1. Hematoma formation.
   a. Apply a pressure dressing to the site.
   b. Apply ice to slow or stop bleeding.
   c. Monitor for additional bleeding.
   d. Assess circulatory, motor, and neurological function of the extremity.
2. Site is reddened and tender.
   a. Notify physician or licensed independent practitioner.

Recording and Reporting

- Record time peripheral dressing was changed, reason for dressing change, type of dressing material used, patency of system, and observation of venipuncture site.
- Record changing tubing on client's record, including the rate of infusion. A special IV flow sheet may be used.
- Record amount and type of fluid infused and amount and type of new fluid according to agency policy. A special flow sheet may be used for parenteral fluids.
- Record time of discontinuing medication and flushing infusion tubing/catheter, including amount and type of flush solution and condition of site.
- Record time peripheral IV was discontinued. Include site assessment information and gauge and length of catheter removed.
- Report to nurse in charge or oncoming nurse that the dressing was changed, any significant information about IV site or IV system, the time the medication or IV was discontinued, and the time of obtaining any blood samples.

Sample Documentation

1300 IV dressing became wet during shower; applied transparent membrane dressing; insertion site without redness, edema, or drainage. Infusing at 125 ml/hr. Client states there is no discomfort or tenderness in the hand or extremity.

1700 Gentamicin infusion complete; line flushed with 5 ml NS and 5% dextrose and water with multivitamins infusing at 125 ml/hr. IV site without redness or edema; client states there is no pain or discomfort at the site. Laboratory notified to obtain blood sample at 1745.

2100 20-g IV catheter removed from right hand. Site without redness, drainage, or swelling. Client states, "My hand feels good with the IV out." Removed catheter length is 1 inch; catheter tip intact.

 SPECIAL CONSIDERATIONS

Pediatric Considerations

- Because children many not be fully able to comprehend instructions, presence of a parent or use of a security toy during procedures may reduce fear and promote cooperation.
- Because of use of smaller gauge catheters, children's smaller vessels, and slow rates of infusion, clotting can occur more often. Also, due to small vessel size and greater physical activity, infiltration may be more likely. Phlebitis is seen less often in children until after the age of 10 years, when incidence approaches adult rates (Hankins and others, 2001).

Geriatric Considerations

- Infiltration in older adults may go unnoticed because of the skin's decreased integrity and loose skin folds.
- Because of decreased tactile sensation, a large amount of fluid may infiltrate before client experiences pain (Powers, 1999).
- Phlebitis may develop without pain but with significant inflammation resulting from the decreased sensitivity of the skin's nerve endings (Hankins and others, 2001).
- To avoid skin tears to thin, fragile skin, minimize the use of tape directly on the skin.
- Avoid use of arm boards because they restrict movement of arthritic joints or limit motion that increases circulation.
- Skin surface may have lost some of its moisture and excessive use of alcohol may contribute to skin dryness (Hankins and others, 2001).

Home Care and Long-Term Care Considerations

- Ensure that the client or caregiver is able and willing to provide the care needed for the IV site.
- If the client is unable to provide the needed care because of loss of vision, explore alterations in the delivery methods used. Medications can be admixed for multiple doses to be delivered through an ambulatory infusion pump, decreasing the need for repeated flushing and tubing changes.
- Assess support from caregiver to assist with providing care.
- Ensure that the client has adequate facilities for storing supplies and medications that need refrigeration.
- Ensure that the long-term care facility is capable of managing a client with peripheral IV therapy.

Home Care Considerations

- Teach client and caregiver about performing hand hygiene, aseptic technique, and signs and symptoms of complications.
- Instruct caregiver to apply pressure with gauze if catheter falls out. Apply clean dressing after bleeding stops.
- Teach client to keep site dry during bath (preferred) or shower by wrapping in plastic bag and taping occlusively. Unplug pump, if one is used, before bathing.
- Instruct client to wear garments with sleeves that do not interfere with catheter function.
- Discuss activity restrictions such as strenuous exercise of the affected arm.
- Discuss troubleshooting and emergency care routines with client and caregiver. Provide written instructions and 24-hour phone numbers for support (Hankins and others, 2001).
- Assess home environment to assess most suitable area for dressing changes and other procedures.

Long-Term Care Considerations

- Nursing staff must possess the necessary knowledge base and skills required for maintaining vascular access sites.
- Experienced IV nurses often provide "back-up call" to these facilities.

Skill 29.4

Administering Intravenous Medications

Technological advances have resulted in the increase of drug delivery by the IV route. IV administration of medications is often preferred to oral or parenteral injections because of efficacy of concentration, absorption, and rapid onset. The IV route is often required if the client is unable to take oral medications. Some drugs can be administered only by the IV route. Because of the principles that make IV administration the preferred route (rapid onset, improved serum drug concentrations), it also requires greater knowledge and skill by the nurse to prevent potentially dangerous complications when administering any IV medication. Parenteral administration of any drug is invasive and poses greater risk to the client.

When administering IV medications, the principles associated with delivery of any medication remain the same. The nurse should ensure it is the right client, right drug, right dose, right time, and right route. Drugs are documented immediately after administration. In addition to these basic rights, the nurse must also apply principles of IV therapy. Physical incompatibilities of IV medications, osmolality of drug admixtures, and potential for IV therapy–related complications must be considered before administering any medication intravenously.

A variety of methods are available for IV medication delivery. Dosages and admixtures vary and are usually calculated based on the client's weight, drug distribution and absorption, safety of administration, excretion, and solubility in solution. IV medications can be mixed in large admixture volumes (e.g., addition of 40 mEq KCl to 1000 ml IV fluid), by piggyback infusion (e.g., administration of an antibiotic concurrently with an IV infusion), or by bolus injection (delivery of an admixture or IV push medications through an existing IV access device). In all three methods of IV medication administration, the client is required to have an IV access device, either a continuous infusion or an access site such as a saline lock.

The nurse also must know the absorption, metabolism, and excretion rate and route of IV medications. Because the liver and kidneys metabolize and excrete byproducts of the IV drug, systemic diseases such as liver and renal impairment affect absorption. Older adults usually have diminished renal and liver function and are more likely to experience toxicity related to IV drug administration than individuals with normal liver and kidney function. Clients with lower plasma proteins have more adverse effects when receiving IV medications, because therapeutic response to the drug is related to the amount of drug not bound to a plasma protein or tissue. Drug binding influences both the effectiveness of the drug given and the duration of the effect.

Some drugs such as heparin are required to be given by continuous infusion to maintain a therapeutic action. The efficacy of other drugs (e.g., antibiotics) and their therapeutic response are determined by therapeutic drug monitoring. Serum drug levels such as peak and trough levels of aminoglycosides (e.g., gentamicin, tobramycin, amikacin and vancomycin) are performed at specific intervals during IV medication therapy to monitor response and to protect the client from adverse effects if excretion of the metabolized drug is reduced. Serum drug levels reveal if drug doses are too high or low. Dosages are adjusted by increasing or decreasing the time between administration or by increasing or decreasing the drug amount to provide therapeutic levels within a narrow range. Monitoring therapeutic drug levels is an additional responsibility of the nurse when administrating IV medications and is crucial in safe and effective delivery of care to the client.

When giving IV medications, the nurse also assesses clients for hypersensitivity (allergic) reactions. The rapid absorption of IV medications, if the client has an allergic response or delayed hypersensitivity, occurs quickly and can be exhibited by reactions ranging from a mild skin rash to anaphylaxis. The extent of the reaction is related to the hypersensitivity to the drug and the amount actually infused. If an allergic reaction occurs, the nurse should stop the medication, keep the IV line open with a plain fluid infusion, monitor the client for respiratory distress and changes in vital signs, notify the physician or licensed independent practitioner, and be prepared to administer emergency medications and resuscitative measures if necessary.

The Needle Safety and Prevention Act of 2001 has resulted in more institutions using manufactured needleless systems or use of a system with catheter ports or Y connector sites designed to contain a needle housed in a protective covering. Needleless infusion lines allow a direct connection with the IV line via a recessed connection port or a blunt-ended cannula or shielded needle device (Figure 29-5).

ASSESSMENT

1. Check physician's or licensed independent practitioner's orders to determine type of IV solution, medication, dose, and route and frequency of administration. *Rationale: Ensures right solution is administered correctly.*
2. Review client's history for presence of diseases or conditions that might impair drug absorption, metabolism, or excretion.
3. Review information about drug, including action, purpose, peak onset, normal dose, side effects, and nursing implications. Note appropriate time for infusion (e.g., mg/min).

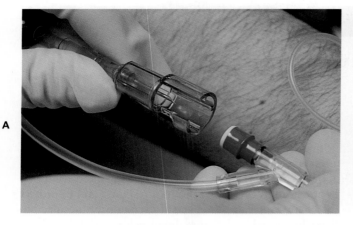
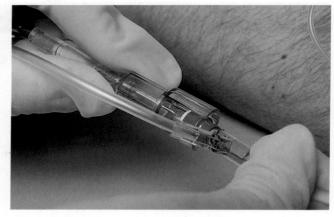

Figure 29-5 **A**, A needleless infusion system. **B**, Connection into an injection port.

4. When more than one medication is added to the IV solution, assess for compatibility. Check institutional reference or pharmacy for drug compatibility list.

5. Assess appropriate laboratory values (e.g., creatinine, peak and trough levels). *Rationale: Determines drug efficacy and toxicity.*

6. Assess existing IV line for patency and note rate of main IV line. *Rationale: Patent line necessary for medication administration.*

7. Assess IV insertion site for signs of infiltration or phlebitis (pain, tenderness, redness, swelling, heat on palpation). *Rationale: Administration of hyperosmolar drugs by IV route increases risk of phlebitis.*

8. Assess client's history of drug allergies. *Rationale: Ensures a contraindicated medication is not administered.*

9. Assess client's understanding of purpose for drug therapy.

PLANNING

Expected outcomes of IV medication administration focus on ensuring therapeutic response of drug with minimum adverse reactions.

Expected Outcomes

1. Drug infuses within desired period.
2. Client's IV site remains free of phlebitis or infiltration.
3. Client's laboratory values of therapeutic drug monitoring reveal desired response without renal toxicity.
4. Client does not show evidence of hypersensitivity, allergic reaction, or other side effects to IV medication.
5. Client or family is able to explain drug's purpose, action, side effects, and dosage.

Equipment

- IV medication

  Vial or ampule of prescribed medication
  Small-volume admixture (normal saline, dextrose and water, sterile water) in either syringe or 50- to 250-ml IV fluid bag

- Container for admixture diluent (Volutrol)
- Sterile 19- to 21-gauge needle, 1 inch in length (20-gauge, 1-inch needle typically used) if system is not needleless
- Label, if needed (Many small-volume admixtures are premixed and dispensed from pharmacy.)
- Syringe pump, if applicable
- Secondary administration set (needleless system preferred)
- Disposable gloves
- 2.5 ml syringes
- NS or 0.9% solution in vial for injection
- One 3-ml syringe filled with heparin flush solution (10 U/ml) (optional)
- Antiseptic swabs
- Tape (optional)
- IV pole
- Medication administration record or computer printout

Delegation Considerations

This skill requires the critical thinking and knowledge application unique to a nurse. In many states, the administration of certain IV medications is included within the scope of practice for a licensed practical or vocational nurse (LPN/LVN). Follow agency policy for the specific medications that may be administered by LPN/LVN. Delegation of this skill to assistive personnel (AP) is inappropriate.

IMPLEMENTATION FOR ADMINISTERING INTRAVENOUS MEDICATIONS

Steps	Rationale
1. See Standard Protocol (inside front cover).	
2. Assemble medications in medication room using aseptic technique (see Chapter 3).	
3. Check client identification, look at arm band, and ask client to state name.	Identification of client is required before any medication administration.
4. Explain procedure, and encourage client to report any symptoms of discomfort at IV site during infusion.	Keeps client informed.
5. **IV push (bolus) (through existing continuous infusion line)**	
a. Prepare medication from ampule or vial (Chapter 16).	
b. 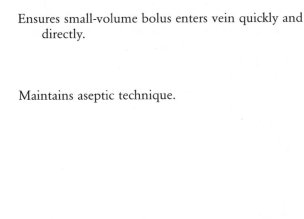 Select injection port closest to client. If add-on 0.22-μ filter is used, give IV push medications below the filter next to client, preventing medication from being absorbed in filter.	Ensures small-volume bolus enters vein quickly and directly.
c. Prepare injection site, or cleanse connection port with antiseptic swab. Allow to dry.	Maintains aseptic technique.
d. Connect syringe of medication to IV line. (1) *Needleless system:* Remove cap of needleless injection port, if present. Connect tip of syringe directly. *or* Insert blunt cannula through appropriate injection cap (see illustration). (2) *Needle system:* Insert short, small-gauge needle through center of injection port.	
e. Occlude IV system by pinching tubing above injection port (see illustration).	Prevents reflux of medication up tubing and inadvertent bolus when infusion is resumed.

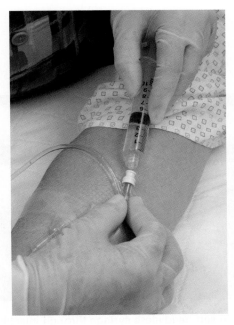

Step 5d Insert syringe with blunt cannula tip into injection cap on existing infusion line.

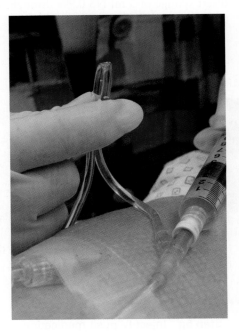

Step 5e Pinch IV tubing above injection port.

Steps	Rationale

f. Aspirate gently on syringe plunger, observing for blood return.

In some cases, blood return may not be aspirated, even with patent IV. If IV is infusing well and has no signs of infiltration, proceed with medication administration.

> **NURSE ALERT** *Checking for a blood return is not a reliable method of determining catheter patency (Phillips, 2001). Absence of a positive blood return does not always indicate infiltration. There may be no blood return because fibrin is occluding catheter tip or tip is pressed against vein wall. Likewise, a positive blood return does not always ensure the catheter is in correct position, because blood return may be present even when there is infiltration. This may occur when catheter tip has eroded through vein, yet tip remains partially inside lumen of vessel (Hadaway, 1999). Absence of blood return requires further assessment before proceeding with therapy.*

g. After observing for blood return, continue to occlude IV tubing and inject medication slowly over appropriate time (see illustration). Note if client reports any discomfort; if so, it may be necessary to stop administration. Use watch to time administration.

IV medications must be delivered at rate recommended by manufacturer. Discomfort indicates chemical phlebitis.

h. Release tubing, withdraw syringe, and recheck fluid infusion rate.

Fluid infusion may need to be readjusted if injection changed drip rate.

i. If using a needleless system with injection caps, replace injection port cap with new sterile cap.

j. Dispose of needles and syringes in appropriate container. Do not recap needles. Remove gloves.

Prevents contamination from needle-stick injury.

6. **IV push (through saline/heparin flush IV lock)**

a. Fill syringes with NS 0.9% (one containing 3 ml, the other containing 5 ml). Attach blunt cannula, or remove needle from syringe as indicated by the type of needleless system.

Flush will be used to clear lock before medication administration.

b. Cleanse injection port of IV lock with antiseptic swab after removing cap if present.

Ensures aseptic technique.

c. Insert syringe of 3 ml NS 0.9% through injection port of IV lock (see illustration).

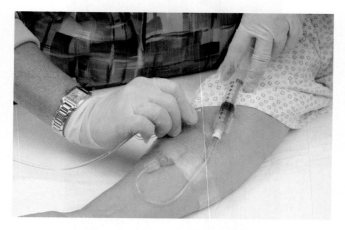

Step 5g   Inject IV push medication.

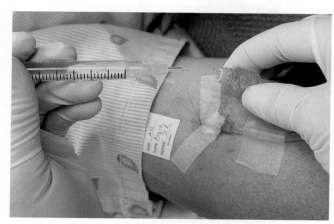

Step 6c   Insert needleless syringe through injection port.

Steps	Rationale
d. Aspirate gently, and observe for blood return.	In some cases, blood return may not be aspirated. In this case assess carefully for infiltration.
e. If lock is considered intact and patent, flush gently with NS while assessing for resistance. If resistance is felt, never continue to apply force. Stop and evaluate cause.	Ensures catheter patency and prevents dislodging blood clot or drug precipitate into bloodstream. If resistance is felt and if more pressure is applied to overcome it, catheter fracture could result (Hadaway, 1998). Amount of flush should be equal to at least twice the volume capacity of the catheter and any add-on device (INS, 2000). For short peripheral catheters, 1 ml of flush is adequate.
f. Detach NS syringe, repeat cleansing of port with antiseptic swab, and attach syringe filled with medication.	
g. Inject medication slowly over appropriate time, using a watch to ensure proper time of delivery.	IV medication must be delivered at rate recommended by manufacturer.
h. Remove medication syringe.	
i. Recleanse cap or port with antiseptic swab, and attach syringe with 5 ml 0.9% NS. Inject NS flush at same rate IV medication was delivered.	Irrigation with NS prevents occlusion of IV access device. Flushing at same rate as medication ensures that any medication remaining within IV is delivered at correct rate. Flushing with 3 to 10 ml of saline after each medication is crucial (Hadaway, 1998).
j. *Option* (if agency protocol): Inject syringe with heparin flush solution, maintaining positive pressure in IV access device. *Using SASH method:* Saline Administration Saline Heparin	Prevents incompatibility of heparin with drug administered because 0.9% NS is isotonic.
k. Dispose of all needles and syringes in proper container. Do not recap needle. Remove gloves.	Prevents accidental needle-stick injury with contaminated needle.

NURSE ALERT *Studies that have compared the use of saline versus heparin flush solutions in maintaining patency recommend saline for use with peripheral venous access devices (Hankins and others, 2001). The INS (2000) recommends flushing intermittently used peripheral catheters with 0.9% saline at established intervals. Use of heparin flush solution is more costly, requires an additional step with line manipulation, and carries potential for bioincompatibilities, alteration in clotting factors, and allergic reactions (Phillips, 2001) (check agency policy).*

---

7. **IV piggyback (IVPB) or syringe pump through existing line**
    a. Attach tubing of administration set to prepared admixture container.
       (1) *Piggyback infusion:* Small-volume admixture (50 to 250 ml) in a minibag that dilutes and administers drug. Insert spike of tubing into port of minibag (see illustration).
       (2) *Syringe pump:* Small-volume admixture in a syringe (10 to 60 ml) to dilute and administer drug. Place prefilled syringe into mini-infusor pump (see illustration) follow manufacturer's directions. Attach tubing to end of syringe.

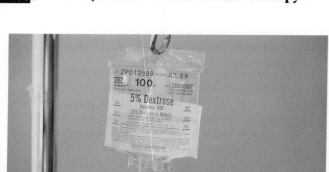

Step 7a(1) Small volume minibag for piggyback infusion.

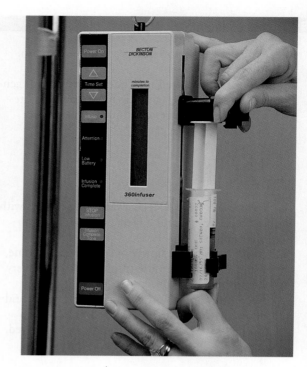

Step 7a(2) Syringe inserted into syringe pump.

Steps	Rationale

b. Fill tubing with IV fluid.
  (1) *Piggyback infusion:* Close roller clamp, squeeze chamber, and fill half full. Open roller clamp, and prime remaining tubing.
  (2) *Syringe pump:* Gently push plunger of syringe to fill tubing completely.
	Infusion tubing should be fluid filled and free of air bubbles to prevent air embolism.

c. Administer IVPB.
  (1) Attach needle to end of IV minibag tubing and insert into injection port at upper end of tubing after cleansing port with antiseptic swab, or, for needleless system, attach tubing to recessed connection port above backcheck valve (see illustration).
  (2) Lower primary IV line. (Hook may be used to lower primary IV line.)
  (3) Open regulator or clamp on minibag infusion.
  (4) Regulate flow rate of infusion with roller clamp on primary tubing to deliver medication over 20 to 90 minutes (see agency policy or pharmacy instruction).
	Use of injection port closest to drip chamber of primary IV line allows piggyback to infuse while stopping the flow of primary IV line through backcheck valve.
	
	Allows infusion of minibag and prevents infusion of primary line.

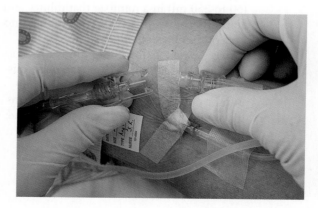

Step 7c Attach tubing to recessed connection port.

Steps	Rationale
(5) After medication has infused, check flow rate of primary infusion.	Backcheck valve prevents infusion of primary line while medication is infusing. Primary infusion will automatically begin to flow when tandem (piggyback) infusion is empty.

COMMUNICATION TIP   *If client complains of burning or stinging during infusion of hyperosmolar drugs (e.g., erythromycin, vancomycin) or highly alkaline drugs, assess IV site for symptoms of chemical phlebitis. IV infusion of drug greater than 650 mOsm/L is known to cause chemical phlebitis. If client has no signs of phlebitis, slow infusion and decrease rate to infuse over maximum time allowed. Consider option of further dilution of medication (confer with physician or practitioner). Continue vigilance in assessing IV. Discuss with client importance of communicating further symptoms.*

Steps	Rationale
(6) Reregulate primary infusion to desired IV rate.	Prevents infusion of excess fluid.
(7) Leave secondary bag and tubing in place for future drug administration, or discard in appropriate container. Discard needle in sharps container. Remove gloves.	Establishment of secondary line produces route for microorganisms to enter main line. Repeated changes in tubing increase risk of infection. Check agency policy and procedure for frequency of administration set tubing change.
d. Administer mini-infusion or syringe pump.	
(1) Attach blunt end of tubing to designated needleless port, or insert sterile needle into injection port of existing IV line after cleansing injection port with antiseptic swab.	Maintains aseptic technique.
(2) Hang mini-infusor pump with syringe on IV pole with primary IV line. If required by type of syringe pump, set pump to deliver medication within time recommended by policy, pharmacist, or medication reference manual. Press button to "on" position. The infusion-complete alarm in "on" position should be used if available and if infusing via saline/heparin lock.	Prevents delay in flushing after completion of infusion, maintaining patency of access device.
(3) After medication infuses, turn off pump. Check flow rate of primary IV infusion, and regulate to desired rate. (If stopcock is used, turn to "off" position after infusion is complete, and cap.)	Prevents infusion of excess fluid. Maintains sterility of system.
(4) Leave infuser tubing attached to primary line. Disconnect and cover end with sterile cap, or disconnect and discard in appropriate container. Remove gloves.	Tubing can be safely reused.
8. **IVPB: saline or heparin lock**	
a. Take minidrip (60 gtt/ml) IV tubing and insert spike into minibag.	Minidrip used to regulate small-volume infusion.
b. Close roller clamp, and squeeze drip chamber to fill half full.	
c. Open roller clamp, and fill remaining tubing.	Flushes air from tubing.
d. Attach sterile needle (e.g., 20 gauge, 1 inch) to tubing *or* attach sterile cap to end of primed tubing if using needleless system.	Needle should be changed with each administration. Keep end of tubing sterile.

Steps	Rationale
e. Prepare injection port of needleless system or the heparin stopper with antiseptic swab.	In some cases blood return may not be aspirated. Assess lock carefully. Symptoms may suggest phlebitis or infiltration and the need to restart peripheral IV line.
f. Insert 5-ml syringe filled with NS 0.9%, and gently aspirate. Check for blood return, then flush NS slowly. Note any pain, swelling, or burning at IV site.	
g. Recleanse port or stopper with antiseptic swab. Attach end of tubing to port (needleless system), or insert sterile needle.	Ensures safe medication delivery.
h. Open flow clamp, and regulate IV medication to infuse 20 to 90 minutes. (Refer to agency policy or pharmacy instructions.)	
i. Continue to observe infusion periodically until complete. When complete, disconnect, maintaining aseptic technique.	Always flush port and to prevent drug incompatibilities (see Step 6j). Flushing with 3 to 10 ml of saline after each medication is crucial. Volume of flush depends on lumen size and catheter length (Hadaway, 1998).
j. Prepare injection port with antiseptic swab, insert syringe with 5 ml NS, and gently flush, maintaining positive pressure in IV access device.	Use of heparin may be recommended by agency.
k. *Option:* Recleanse port, and inject heparin flush solution (per agency and procedure), repeating procedure and using positive pressure.	Maintains sterility of IV tubing for future reuse.
l. Apply new sterile needle and cap to minibag tubing, and retain for next administration.	
m. Dispose of syringe and needles in appropriate container. Remove gloves.	

9. See Completion Protocol (inside front cover).

NURSE ALERT *In instances of both phlebitis and infiltration, prompt removal of catheter is indicated. The duration and severity of phlebitis depends on how long catheter remains in place after first symptoms appear (Bregenzer and others, 1998). Treatment standard for phlebitis includes application of warm or cold compresses to affected site. Use of warm compresses to treat infiltration has become controversial. Cold may be better for some infusates, and warm may be more effective for others (Phillips, 2001). Recent research has brought into question the tradition of elevating the extremity as an intervention for infiltration, noting no difference in the rate of fluid reabsorption (Hadaway, 1999). Check agency policy for treatment options.*

• • • • • • • • • •

EVALUATION

1. Observe client's infusion for proper rate of administration, and note time of completion.
2. Inspect client's IV site and tubing for symptoms of IV complications (e.g., swelling, pain, tenderness, redness at site).
3. Monitor therapeutic drug levels (e.g., aminoglycosides, vancomycin, aminophylline, phenytoin).
4. Monitor client during infusion for allergic response or adverse reaction (e.g., urticaria, respiratory distress, tachycardia, hypotension).
5. Ask client to name IV medication, purpose, side effects, dosage, and frequency.

Unexpected Outcomes and Related Interventions

1. Client experiences burning, irritation, redness, or pain during infusion.
   a. Reinspect site, and check for blood return.
   b. If phlebitis is present, discontinue infusion and reinsert another catheter, preferably in the opposite extremity, if IV therapy is still necessary.
2. Client experiences adverse reaction or allergic reaction during infusion of drug.
   a. Stop the infusion.
   b. Maintain existing IV line with NS 0.9% or ordered solution.

c. Notify physician or licensed independent practitioner.

d. Monitor vital signs and respiratory status.

e. Administer medications as ordered.

f. Be prepared to perform cardiac or respiratory resuscitation.

g. After acute episode subsides, advise client of allergy and necessity for future reporting to health care personnel; advise client of significance of allergy; advise client as to the availability of medical alert identification tags.

3. Client is unable to state purpose of drug, significance to treatment of current illness, side effects, or health management related to drug.

a. Reinforce information, giving simple instructions, written if necessary.

b. Communicate to other health personnel, particularly if client is to continue IV therapy in home setting.

c. Include family or care provider during instruction.

Recording and Reporting

• Record drug dose, route, amount and type of diluent (e.g., 1 g in 50 ml D$_5$W), and time of administration on medication administration record or computer printout.

• Record volume of fluid on client's I&O record.

Sample Documentation

0810 During first 5 minutes of infusion of 100 ml NS and 1 g ampicillin, client complained of sudden onset of "can't catch my breath," clutching at throat; high-pitched inspiratory stridor noted. Macular rash generalized over face and upper extremities noted. Ampicillin stopped immediately, and IV fluids maintained at 125 ml/hr. VS 98/60, 120, 26. Physician notified. Epinephrine 0.5 mg IV push given, with inspiratory distress subsiding within 30 seconds of administration. Allergy band applied.

0830 VS 120/84, 96, 18. Client states breathing is normal. Expressing some fear over "how fast it came on." Significance of allergy, implications for future administration, and notification of dentists, physicians, and other health care providers discussed. Aware that vital signs will continue to be monitored and to notify nurse immediately for any signs of respiratory distress.

 ## SPECIAL CONSIDERATIONS

Pediatric Considerations

• Understand drug calculations with reference to age, height, weight or body surface area, dosage, and volume limitations (INS, 2000).

• Calculation of medication administration in children is most often based on body weight and body surface area, by use of a nomogram (Hankins and others, 2001).

• A syringe pump connected via an extension set directly into an intermittent infusion device (saline lock) or piggybacked into the primary line is a very accurate method of IV medication administration in children.

Geriatric Considerations

• Therapeutic and toxic ranges of medications in older adults are very close, partially due to impaired renal function. Monitor serum drug levels carefully (Powers, 1999).

• Due to the concurrent use of multiple medications in the geriatric population, it is important to realize the potential for drug interactions (INS, 2000).

• The older adult may not be aware of his or her surroundings and may be slower to report symptoms of infiltration and phlebitis.

• Minimize excessive use of extension tubing and use Luer-Lok connections to avoid mishaps with an older client who might become confused or hyperactive.

Home Care Considerations

• Premixed medications should be used in the home setting.

• Ensure that client has adequate facilities for storing supplies and medications that may require refrigeration. Be sure client is aware of those medications that need to be protected from light.

• Instruct client and caregiver to keep all medications out of the reach of children.

• Instruct client and caregiver of medication side effects and IV site complications. Discuss what should be reported to health care provider.

Long-Term Care Considerations

• Long-term care facilities are useful for infusion therapy in clients with physical or mental limitations or those insured by third-party payers who do not allow payment for in-home infusion therapy (Hankins and others, 2001).

• Antimicrobials are among the most commonly prescribed agents in long-term care (Hankins and others, 2001).

• An adverse outcome of inappropriate IV antimicrobial use in long-term care is the promotion of antimicrobial resistance and transmission of resistant microorganisms to other high-risk clients (Hankins and others, 2001).

Skill 29.5

Transfusions of Blood Products

Blood and blood component transfusion is a major factor in restoring and maintaining quality of life for the client with hematological disorders, cancer, injury, or surgical intervention. Caring for the client receiving blood or blood components may be a routine nursing responsibility, but overlooking a minor detail could be dangerous to the client.

Transfusions of blood and blood products are closely regulated and monitored. Standards of operations for all blood bank centers are set by the American Association of Blood Banks (AABB), OSHA, the U.S. Food and Drug Administration (FDA), and the American Red Cross. These standards include the collection of donor blood, distribution of the product, and standards for transfusion. Always verify specific agency or institutional policy regarding specific procedural requirements before any transfusion.

Blood and blood component therapies treat and restore hemodynamic homeostasis. A written physician's or licensed independent practitioner's order to transfuse should always include which component to transfuse and the duration of the transfusion. A single unit of whole blood or blood components should be infused within a 4-hour period (INS, 2000). If more than one blood product is to be given, the sequence or order of transfusion should be specified. Any additional medications, such as antihistamine (given when history shows previous allergic response), antipyretics (given when history shows previous febrile nonhemolytic response), or diuretics (given when history shows potential for congestive heart failure) or other special treatment of the components should also be included in the written order for the transfusion (Phillips, 2001).

Three blood typing systems, ABO, Rh, and most recently HLA typing, are used to ensure transfusion products match the recipient's blood as closely as possible (Table 29-5). Before transfusion in nonemergent situations, the client's blood type and Rh factor must always be verified to be compatible with the donor transfusion.

There is increasing public awareness of the possible transmission of infectious diseases through transfusion of blood products. Because of improved testing of donor blood, the risk of the blood recipient developing an infectious disease is lower than ever before. However, viral, bacterial, and parasitic diseases can still be transmitted through blood. Screening of blood donors is one of the most important steps to identify persons with a medical history, behavior, or events that put them at risk of transmissible disease. All donor blood is tested for syphilis, hepatitis B, and the presence of antibodies to hepatitis C, human immunodeficiency virus (HIV) 1 and 2, and human T-cell lymphotropic virus type I (Hankins and others, 2001).

Nurses and physicians must be prepared to inform the client thoroughly about the options, benefits, and risks of transfusion and must reassure the client that every effort has been taken to ensure a safe blood supply. Clients should know that there is never a completely risk-free transfusion.

One avenue for preventing the transmission of infectious diseases during blood transfusion is the use of autologous blood (i.e., the client's own blood). This can be done in several ways; however, the most frequent method is preoperative collection from the client. AABB standards establish the process for determining client eligibility, collecting, testing, and labeling the unit. Before transfusion, ABO and Rh typing of the client are performed. Autologous units must be used before units from the general blood supply. Identification and checking processes and methods of administration for autologous units are the same as those used for other units of blood.

The skill of transfusing blood or blood products requires the nurse to know thoroughly the policy and procedure of the agency or institution. The nurse must ensure the safe administration of the product and closely monitor before, during, and after the transfusion.

ASSESSMENT

1. Assess written order for type of blood product, length of transfusion (up to 4 hours for whole blood or red blood cells), and pretransfusion or posttransfusion medications to be given. *Rationale: Correct identification of ordered blood product is first step to ensure safe administration.*

2. Assess client's transfusion history, including previous transfusion reaction. Verify that type and crossmatch

Table 29-5

Blood Type Identification	
Client	**Compatible Transfusion**
Type A	A or AB plasma
	A or O RBCs
Type B	B or AB plasma
	B or O RBCs
Type AB	AB plasma
	A, B, AB, or O RBCs
Type O	A, B, AB, or O plasma
	O RBCs
Rh−	Must receive Rh− blood
Rh+	Can receive Rh− or Rh blood
O−	Universal donor for RBCs
AB+	Universal donor for plasma

RBCs, red blood cells.

has been completed within 72 hours of transfusion and, if applicable, that consent for transfusion is signed. *Rationale: Clients with recent transfusion, pregnancy (within 3 months), or uncertain history are at high risk because of potential antibody response.*

3. Establish that client has a large-bore IV catheter that is patent and without signs of infiltration or phlebitis. Standard catheter size for blood transfusions in adults is 18 gauge. Use of 22 gauge may be considered in client whose veins are inaccessible. *Rationale: Catheters used for blood transfusion should be large enough to accommodate the appropriate flow rate, but not large enough to damage the vein. Major concern is completing transfusion within recommended 4 hour time frame. If a smaller gauge catheter is used, consider requesting split blood units to ensure timely administration.*

4. Assess pretransfusion baseline vital signs (blood pressure, pulse, respiration, temperature). If client is febrile (temperature greater than 100° F [37.8° C]), notify physician or licensed independent practitioner before initiating transfusion (check agency policy). *Rationale: This provides comparison to detect change in client's condition during transfusion.*

5. Assess client's medication schedule. *Rationale: Allows nurse to plan time for blood administration without interrupting medication schedule.*

PLANNING

Expected outcomes focus on safe, complication-free transfusion therapy, restoration of normal cell count, and improvement in oxygenation and tissue perfusion.

Expected Outcomes

1. Client is free of signs and symptoms of transfusion reaction or fluid volume overload, evidenced by normal temperature and blood pressure and absence of chest pain, dyspnea, dizziness, or tachydysrhythmias.

2. Client demonstrates normal fluid balance, evidenced by normal urine output, improved hemoglobin

(Hgb) and hematocrit (Hct) levels, and normal red blood cell indices.

3. Client does not experience signs and symptoms of blood or blood product infiltrate or phlebitis.

4. Client lists two benefits and risks of transfusion therapy.

5. Client experiences lessened stress or fear, evidenced by verbalized understanding and acceptance of transfusion therapy.

Equipment

- Blood administration set with standard 170-µ filter
- Ordered blood product
- IV solution: NS 0.9%
- Disposable gloves
- Tape

Optional equipment

- Infusion pump (Verify that infusion pump can be used to deliver blood or blood products.)
- Leukocyte-depleting filter
- Blood warmer (used mainly when large volumes or rapid transfusion is needed)
- Pressure bag (used for rapid infusion in acute blood loss)

Delegation Considerations

This skill requires the critical thinking and knowledge application unique to a nurse. In some states the administration of blood and blood components is included within the scope of practice for licensed practical (vocational) nurses (LPN/LVNs). Follow agency policy. Delegation to assistive personnel (AP) may include obtaining vital signs, collecting equipment, transporting units from the blood bank, and instituting client comfort measures. However, the primary responsibility for donor and recipient identification, infusing the unit within the required time, and assessing outcomes remains with the nurse-transfusionist.

IMPLEMENTATION FOR TRANSFUSIONS OF BLOOD PRODUCTS

Steps	Rationale
1. See Standard Protocol (inside front cover).	
2. Obtain blood bag from laboratory following agency protocol. Blood transfusions must be initiated within 30 minutes after release from laboratory, blood bank, or controlled environment (INS, 2000).	Agencies differ as to personnel who can release a blood bag from a blood bank, but they always require two witnesses and some form of client identification. Only one unit is usually released at a time.

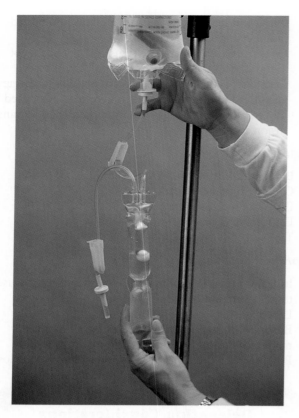

Step 3 Blood administration set primed with normal saline.

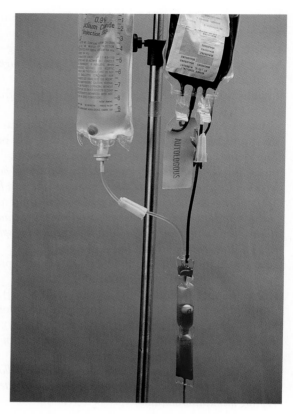

Step 7 Unit of blood connected to Y tubing setup.

Steps	Rationale
3. Open blood administration set, and prime the tubing with NS 0.9% (see illustration), completely filling filter with saline. Maintain sterility of system and close lower clamp.	If filter is not completely primed with saline, transfusion will slow because of collection of debris in partially primed filter. Saline is used to wet the filter, dilute red blood cells to reduce their viscosity if necessary, and flush blood components from the tubing. If a reaction occurs, a separate bag of saline with a separate infusion tubing must be hung to decrease the amount of blood given to the client.

NURSE ALERT *IV medications cannot be added to a blood bag or infused through a transfusion administration set. An additional IV site may be required if IV medications cannot be delayed or adjusted during blood transfusion(s).*

COMMUNICATION TIP *While preparing for blood administration, explain to client, "I will be staying with you for the first few minutes of the transfusion. We will be checking with you frequently while the blood is infusing, and taking your blood pressure and temperature frequently. If you feel discomfort of any type while the blood is infusing, please let me know immediately.*

4. Have client void or empty urinary drainage collection container.	If transfusion reaction occurs, urine specimen obtained must be recent and preferably taken after transfusion is initiated to assess for presence of red blood cells from a hemolytic reaction.

Steps	Rationale

5. With another registered nurse or licensed practical nurse, correctly verify blood product and identify client (check agency policy):
  a. Client's full name, identification number, and date of birth
  b. Client's full name, identification number, and date of birth with forms from blood bank and with written order in client's record
	If possible, have client identify self. Correct product must be administered to right client to avoid transfusion reaction.

NURSE ALERT *Because most severe transfusion reactions occur from identification error, mislabeled blood samples, and mislabeled units (Hankins and others, 2001), verification of client, product, product type, and crossmatch may be the most important step of the entire procedure.*

Steps	Rationale

c. Client's blood group and Rh type
  d. Crossmatch compatibility
  e. Donor's blood group and Rh type
  f. Unit and hospital number
  g. Expiration date and time on blood unit
  h. Type of blood component is correct component ordered by physician/licensed independent practitioner	

6. Inspect blood product for signs of leakage or unusual appearance, including clots, bubbles, or purplish color. Gently invert bag 2 to 3 times.	If signs of contamination are present, return blood product to laboratory. Inversion equally distributes cells throughout preservative solution.
7. Attach blood product to IV administration set by inserting spike of Y tubing located next to NS 0.9% tubing (see illustration). Close NS clamp above filter, and open clamp above filter to blood product.	Prevents blood product from entering normal saline bag.
8. Review with client the purpose of transfusion. Ask client to report immediately any signs and symptoms (during or after transfusion), including chills, low back pain, shortness of breath, nausea, excessive perspiration, rash, itching, or even a vague sense of uneasiness.	Once transfusion reaction occurs, staff must respond immediately with treatment.

NURSE ALERT *A transfusion reaction is an emergency.*

Steps	Rationale
9. Turn off existing IV. Disconnect and cap tubing. Then quickly connect NS-primed blood administration tubing directly to client's IV site.	Ensures aseptic technique.
10. Open lower clamp, and regulate blood infusion to allow only 10 to 24 ml to infuse in the first 15 minutes. Remain with client. Remove and discard gloves. Perform hand hygiene.	If a reaction occurs, infusion of this amount minimizes the amount of incompatible blood transfused.
11. Obtain vital signs (temperature, pulse, respiration, blood pressure) 15 minutes after initiation of transfusion.	Change from baseline vital signs may indicate transfusion reaction.
12. Reregulate flow clamp if there is no transfusion reaction, and infuse the remaining volume of blood as ordered. Packed red blood cells are usually infused over 2 hours and whole blood over 3 to 4 hours. Check blood tubing package for correct drop factor.	Careful regulation prevents adverse response. Client's condition and physician's or independent practitioner's orders dictate rate of blood infusion.

Steps	Rationale

NURSE ALERT *Blood must be transfused within 4 hours of spiking the blood bag. Even if infusion is not complete, blood must be discontinued. This reduces the potential for exposure to bacterial infection from blood. Blood bank can split blood units if client is at risk for fluid overload.*

Steps	Rationale
13. Continue to monitor vital signs per agency policy and procedure during transfusion.	Ensures early identification of adverse response.
14. After blood has infused, close roller clamp above filter to blood and open NS.	NS infusion clears IV catheter of blood product.
15. Infuse NS until blood administration is completely clear.	Ensures all blood cells infused.
16. Discontinue transfusion and blood administration set.	
17. Follow standard precautions and agency protocol for disposal of old blood bags and tubing. Remove and discard gloves, and perform hand hygiene.	Prevents transmission of microorganisms.
18. Blood transfusion increases risk of phlebitis. Apply injection cap and flush existing IV line with 5 to 10 ml normal saline, or restart primary IV fluids as ordered only after assessing IV site for patency and signs and symptoms of phlebitis. If transfusing more than one unit of blood or blood product, maintain NS via blood administration set at KVO rate until second unit is started. Because of the risk of bacterial growth, blood administration sets and add-on filters should be changed after each unit or at the end of 4 hours, whichever comes first (INS 2000). CDC (2001) recommends replacing tubing used to administer blood and blood products within 24 hours of completing infusion.	Maintains patency and integrity of existing IV line.
19. See Completion Protocol (inside front cover).	

• • • • • • • • • •

EVALUATION

1. Observe for chills, flushing, itching, hives, dyspnea, tachycardia, drop in blood pressure, or any sign of transfusion reaction.
2. Monitor I&O and laboratory values (Hgb, Hct, prothrombin time [PT], partial thromboplastin time [PTT], platelet count) after transfusion. (In the hematologically stable adult, one unit of packed red blood cells (PRBCs) should increase the Hgb by 1 g/100 ml and Hct by 3%. A unit of platelet concentrate prepared from a single unit of whole blood should increase the client's platelet count by 5000 to 10,000/ml) (Monahan and Neighbors, 1998).
3. Observe that client's behavior or appearance does not demonstrate signs of physical or emotional stress during the transfusion and that client can verbalize understanding of the need for transfusion.
4. Monitor IV site and status of infusion every time vital signs are taken.
5. Ask client to describe purpose, benefit, and risk of transfusion.

Unexpected Outcomes and Related Interventions

1. Client experiences pain, swelling, or discoloration at IV site.
   a. Stop the transfusion, and discontinue the IV infusion and catheter.
   b. Reinsert a new IV catheter in another site.
2. Client complains of pain at infusion site when blood is first initiated, but IV site is patent and not infiltrated.
   a. Apply warm pack to arm to prevent venous spasm from infusion of cold blood products.
3. Transfusion slows, and client is not receiving proper volume.
   a. Check patency of set.
   b. Ensure blood bag is elevated to proper height.
   c. Verify that all clamps and stopcocks are open.
   d. Ensure filter is completely primed.

e. Gently agitate blood bag.

f. Close primary clamp (below the filter). Lower blood bag, and open NS roller clamp. Dilute blood with 25 to 50 ml NS to facilitate infusion.

g. Place unit to be infused in an electronic infusion device that permits blood transfusion.

h. Apply pressure bag, and inflate to a maximum of 300 mm Hg.

i. Restart IV infusion with a large-gauge catheter.

Recording and Reporting

- Record pretransfusion medications, vital signs, and location and condition of IV catheter.
- Record type of blood component, recipient and unit identification, compatibility, and expiration date according to agency policy.
- Record volume of NS and blood component infused.
- Record vital signs taken during transfusion.
- Report signs and symptoms of a transfusion reaction immediately.

Sample Documentation

1000 Early AM CBC noted. Physician aware of Hct 22. Type and crossmatch drawn with two witnesses per phlebotomy.

1230 Voided 320 ml clear, amber urine. 18 angiocath inserted left cephalic vein. NS 0.9% initiated at KVO. 1 unit PRBCs started at 40 ml/hr, after witnessed by J. Doe, RN.

 ## SPECIAL CONSIDERATIONS

Pediatric Considerations

- Twenty-seven-gauge catheters can be used to infuse packed red cells without significant hemolysis (Hankins and others, 2001).
- Smaller aliquots of blood may be useful to infuse in children.
- Run the first 50 ml of a transfusion very slowly in a pediatric client, during which time the nurse should stay with the child.
- Autologous transfusions are not typical in children.

Geriatric Considerations

- Older adults may have compromised cardiac function, requiring slower infusion time. Split units may be helpful if the client cannot tolerate the volume of an entire unit of blood.
- Vigilance in monitoring an access site during transfusion is vital in an older adult who may be less sensitive to the symptoms of infiltration, as well as the generalized symptoms of a transfusion reaction.

Home Care Considerations

- Pretransfusion assessment and identification are the same as in an acute setting.
- Whole blood is not an alternative in the home setting (Phillips, 2001).
- Blood and blood products must be transported in a container with appropriate coolant. Check and record the temperature at the time of delivery.
- Clients who have had prior transfusion reactions, acute angina, or congestive heart failure are not good candidates for home transfusion.
- Plan for home health nurse to be present during entire transfusion process and 30 to 60 minutes afterwards.
- Inform client and caregiver of signs and symptoms of a delayed transfusion reaction (unexplained fever, malaise, jaundice). Complications may occur days to weeks after transfusion.
- A biohazard bag should be used to dispose of all contaminated equipment.

CRITICAL THINKING EXERCISES

1. You enter Mr. Rich's room and prepare to administer an IV bolus of Lasix. Mr. Rich has an existing IV line. After positioning Mr. Rich and making sure there is nothing interfering with the IV line, you cleanse the port and insert the syringe containing the Lasix. As you aspirate the syringe you fail to observe a blood return. What does this indicate? What should you do?

2. What is the most appropriate action to take for each of the following situations?
   a. The IV site is located slightly above the client's wrist in the cephalic vein. When the client moves his arm, the infusion rate slows down dramatically.
   b. The client complains of pain at the site of the IV catheter. On examination, no redness, edema, or skin temperature changes are found.
   c. While flushing an intermittent IV lock after a dose of medication has been infused, you notice clear liquid leaking from under the transparent dressing.

3. Mrs. Wilke is 82 years old and just returning from surgery to repair a large abdominal hernia. Her IV is ordered to be running at 100 ml/hr. You make a routine assessment of her IV for signs of phlebitis and infiltration. You palpate the IV site, and Mrs. Wilke denies discomfort. However, you notice that the area around the site appears inflamed. What might this indicate and why?

4. You have hung a dose of vancomycin to the client's intermittent IV lock. After 15 minutes of infusion, you learn that the client is complaining of feeling flushed and itching.
   a. What is the first action to take?
   b. What other signs or symptoms should be assessed?
   c. What information should be conveyed to the physician?

5. You enter a client's room to assist a colleague in starting a peripheral IV. As you observe the procedure, you see your colleague do the following: Prep the skin, allowing the povidone iodine to dry; stabilize the vein by pulling the skin taut and downward; insert the catheter at a 30- to 45-degree angle; and advance the catheter almost to the hub. What if anything was done incorrectly during the venipuncture?

REFERENCES

Bregenzer T and others: Is routine replacement of peripheral intravenous catheters necessary? *Arch Intern Med* 158:151, 1998.

Centers for Disease Control and Prevention: Guidelines for prevention of intravascular device-related infections, *Infect Control Hosp Epidemiol* 17(7):438, 2001.

Chukhraev AM, Grekov IG: Local complications of nursing interventions on peripheral veins, *J Intraven Nurs* 23(3): 167, 2000.

Ellenberger A: Starting an IV line, *Nursing* 99(3):56, 1999.

Hadaway LC: Major thrombotic and nonthrombotic complications, *J Intraven Nurs* 21(5S):S143, 1998.

Hadaway LC: IV infiltration: not just a peripheral problem, *Nursing* 99(9):41, 1999.

Hankins J and others: *Infusion therapy in clinical practice,* Philadelphia, 2001, WB Saunders.

Infusion Nurses Society: Infusion nursing standards of practice, *J Intraven Nurs* 23(6S):S1, 2000.

Lai KK: Safety of prolonging peripheral cannula and IV tubing use from 72 hours to 97 hours, *Am J Infect Control* 26(1):66, 1998.

Monahan FD, Neighbors M: *Medical-surgical nursing: foundations for clinical practice,* Philadelphia, 1998, WB Saunders.

Occupational Safety and Health Administration: Revision to OSHA's bloodborne pathogen standard, April 2001, http://www.osha-sic.gov/needlesticks/needlefact.html.

Orenstein R: The benefits and limitations of needle protectors and needleless intravenous systems, *J Intraven Nurs* 22(3):122, 1999.

Phillips D: *Manual of IV therapeutics,* ed 3, Philadelphia, 2001, FA Davis.

Powers FA: Your elderly patient needs IV therapy . . . can you keep her safe? *Nursing* 99(7):54, 1999.

Raad I: Intravascular-catheter-related infections, *Lancet* 351:893, 1998.

Redelmeier DA, Livesley NJ: Adhesive tape and intravascular-catheter-associated infections, *J Gen Intern Med* 14:373, 1999.

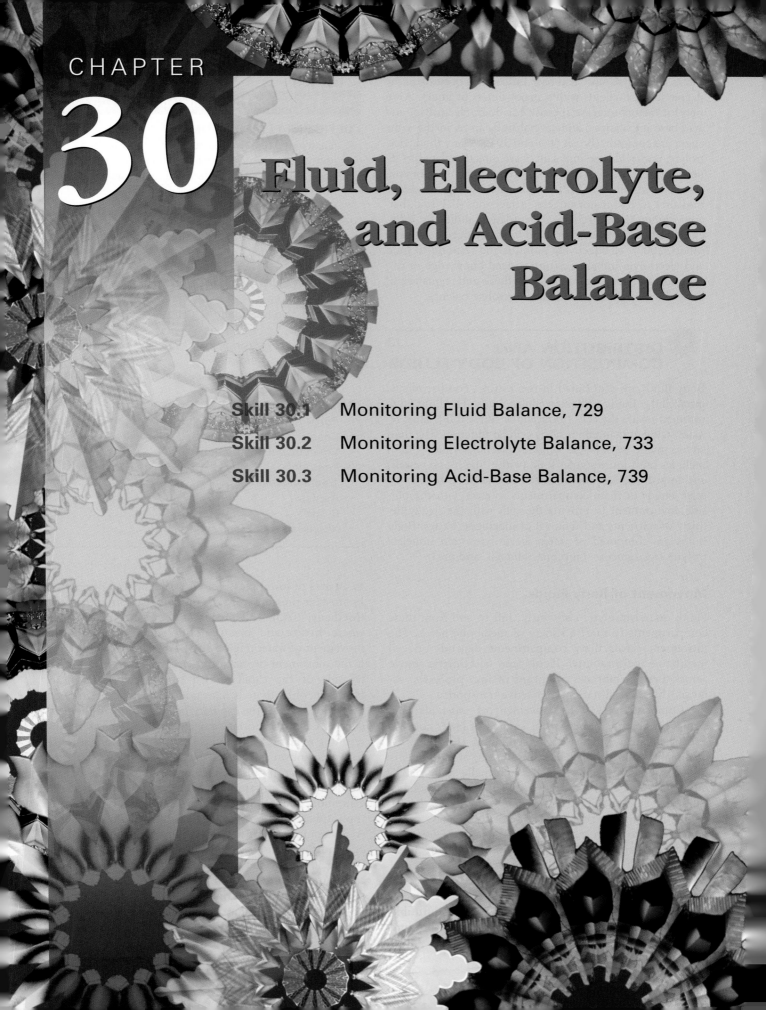

CHAPTER
30
Fluid, Electrolyte, and Acid-Base Balance

Fluid, electrolyte, and acid-base imbalances occur to some degree in most clients with a major illness or injury. A variety of factors increase the risk for fluid, electrolyte, and acid-base imbalances, and several imbalances in the same client are common (Boxes 30-1 and 30-2). Many fluid, electrolyte, and acid-base imbalances are directly related to illness or disease such as diabetes, burns, renal failure, or congestive heart failure (CHF). In other situations, therapeutic measures such as major surgery, intravenous (IV) fluid therapy, diuretics, or mechanical ventilation indirectly influence fluid, electrolyte, and acid-base balance (Lewis and others, 2000). To effectively monitor and respond to fluid and electrolyte imbalances nurses need knowledge of distribution and composition of body fluids and regulation of body fluids, as well as fluid and electrolyte balance.

DISTRIBUTION AND COMPOSITION OF BODY FLUIDS

Body fluids are distributed in two distinct compartments: intracellular fluids and extracellular fluids. The fluid environment inside the cells (intracellular fluid [ICF]) must remain stable to maintain healthy cellular function. The fluid environment outside the cells (extracellular fluid [ECF]) includes both intravascular fluid (within the blood vessels) and interstitial fluid (between the cells and the blood vessels). Fluids in these compartments interact with the outside environment to provide the cells with the steady delivery of nutrients and removal of metabolic wastes. Body fluids are composed of water, electrolytes, and nonelectrolytes (e.g., glucose, bilirubin, minerals, and urea).

Movement of Body Fluids

Fluids and electrolytes constantly shift to and from these compartments to meet a variety of metabolic needs. The movement across these compartments depends on cell membrane permeability. Fluids and electrolytes move across these membranes by means of four processes: osmosis, diffusion, filtration, and active transport.

Osmosis involves the movement of water across a semipermeable membrane from an area of lesser concentration to areas of greater concentration (Figure 30-1). Osmolality (number of solutes in solution) of serum refers to its osmotic pressure, which is normally 280 to 295 mOsm/kg. For example, an increase in ECF osmolality will cause fluid to shift from the ICF to the ECF.

Diffusion is the process in which a solute (gas or substance) in a solution moves from an area of higher concentration to an area of lower concentration (Figure 30-2). An example of diffusion is the movement of oxygen and carbon dioxide between the alveoli and the blood vessels in the lungs.

Filtration is the process by which water and diffusible substances move together from an area of higher pressure

---

---

to an area of lower pressure. The force behind filtration is hydrostatic pressure from the pumping action of the heart (Metheny, 2000). This process is active in capillary beds, where hydrostatic pressure differences determine the movement of water (Figure 30-3). An example of filtration is the movement of water and electrolytes from the arterial side of the capillary bed to the interstitial fluid. However, when there is increased hydrostatic pressure on the venous side of the capillary bed, as occurs in the presence of CHF, the normal movement of water is reversed, resulting in an accumulation of excess fluid in the interstitial space known as edema.

Active transport is the movement of molecules or ions "uphill" against an osmotic pressure to areas of higher concentration, and it requires energy in the form of adenosine triphosphate (ATP). An example is the sodium-potassium-ATPase pump, which moves sodium to the outside of the cell and then returns potassium to the inside of the cell (Figure 30-4). The sodium-potassium pump keeps a higher concentration of potassium in the ICF and a higher concentration of sodium in the ECF.

When illness or injury disrupts fluid and electrolyte imbalances, medical treatment may involve administration of

Box 30-2

Clinical Applications of Alterations in Fluid Balance

SURGERY

Because of the stress response to surgical trauma, 24 to 48 hours after surgery aldosterone and glucocorticoid hormones are increased, resulting in sodium, chloride, and fluid retention and potassium excretion. An increase in ADH secretion results in decreased urinary output, which helps maintain blood volume and blood pressure. After the second postoperative day, a diuretic phase begins as hormone levels return to normal and excess sodium and water are excreted.

BURNS

In clients with severe burns, the body loses fluids in several ways. The greater the body surface burned, the greater the fluid loss. Plasma leaves the intravascular space and enters the interstitial fluid as trapped edema. This phenomena is also called "third-spacing." Plasma and fluids are lost as burn exudate (weeping tissues). Sodium and water shift into the cells, depleting ECF volume.

CONGESTIVE HEART FAILURE

In CHF, decreased cardiac output results in less perfusion to the kidneys and decreased urine output. The client retains sodium and water, resulting in circulatory overload that may lead to pulmonary edema and peripheral edema.

CHRONIC OBSTRUCTIVE PULMONARY DISEASE

Alterations in respiratory function may interfere with the elimination of carbon dioxide to the extent that exceeds the buffers' ability to manage, resulting in a chronic acidosis and decreased pH. In chronic conditions the kidneys conserve bicarbonate to achieve compensation. When assessing levels of arterial blood gases (ABGs) with chronic obstructive pulmonary disease (COPD), it is important to compare present values with a previous baseline reflection of what is normal for the client.

KIDNEY FAILURE

Kidney failure results in abnormal retention of sodium, chloride, potassium, and water in the ECF and increased plasma levels of waste products such as blood urea nitrogen (BUN) and creatinine. Hydrogen ions are retained, resulting in metabolic acidosis. Because of the disease process, compensation by bicarbonate reabsorption in the kidneys is not possible.

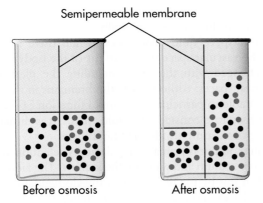

Figure 30-1   Osmosis through a semipermeable membrane. (From Lewis SM and others: *Medical-surgical nursing: assessment and management of clinical problems,* ed 5, St Louis, 2000, Mosby.)

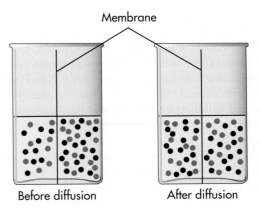

Figure 30-2   Diffusion. (From Lewis SM and others: *Medical surgical nursing: assessment and management of clinical problems,* ed 5, St Louis, 2000, Mosby.)

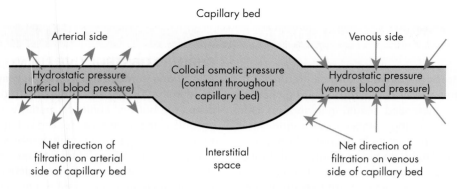

Figure 30-3 Filtration and hydrostatic pressure.

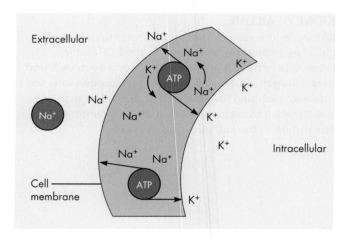

Figure 30-4 Sodium-potassium pump. (From Lewis SM and others: *Medical-surgical nursing: assessment and management of clinical problems,* ed 5, St Louis, 2000, Mosby.)

IV fluids (see Chapter 29). Nurses implement physician's orders through administering IV fluids and monitoring the client's response to fluid therapy. Nurses need to be aware of the contents of IV fluids, the intended purposes, and related contraindications and complications. An *isotonic* IV solution such as 0.9% normal saline has the same osmolality as blood plasma and will increase intravascular fluid volume without a fluid shift to other compartments. A *hypotonic* IV solution such as 0.45% saline has a lesser concentration of solutes than plasma and will move water into the cells. *Hypertonic* solutions such as those containing 3% saline have a greater concentration of solutes than plasma and will move water out of the cells and into the blood vessels.

Regulation of Body Fluids

Fluid imbalances may relate to excess loss of fluids or dehydration, excess fluid volume or retention of fluids, or third-space syndrome, when fluids are held within the body but are not accessible for normal body function (see Boxes 30-1, p. 726, and 30-2, p. 727).

Fluid intake is regulated primarily through the thirst mechanism, controlled by the hypothalamus in the brain. The thirst mechanism is affected by increased plasma osmolality, decreased plasma volume, dry mucous membranes, and other factors (Potter and Perry, 2001). Clients who are unable to perceive or respond to the thirst mechanism are at risk for dehydration. This includes infants, clients with neurological impairment or who are unconscious for any reason, and clients who are immobilized or restrained.

The average daily fluid gains and losses in adults are 2200 to 2700 ml (Table 30-1). In adults the kidneys produce about 60 ml/hr and about 1.5 L of urine per day. Insensible water losses are not perceptible to the person and total about 400 ml/day. For example, water loss from the skin occurs in the form of sweat, which is increased with exercise, exposure to a warm environment, and fever. Excessive perspiration or diaphoresis may result in losses of 1000 ml or more in 24 hours. Insensible fluid losses are also increased substantially with an increased respiratory rate and depth. Normal fluid loss via the gastrointestinal tract is 100 ml/day. Vomiting or diarrhea increases gastrointestinal fluid loss substantially.

Third-space fluid losses occur when there is a shift from the vascular space into portions of the body not easily exchanged with the ECF, including the pleural and peritoneal spaces. Although the fluid remains in the body, it is not able to participate in normal function of the ECF and is therefore considered a fluid "loss." It is difficult to observe or measure third-space fluid losses.

Fluid output is primarily regulated by retention and excretion of sodium and water by the kidneys. The kidneys accomplish this by the regulation of the glomerular filtration rate (GFR) and hormonal factors including the antidiuretic hormone (ADH), the renin-angiotensin-aldosterone (RAA) system, and the atrial natriuretic hormone (Cooper and Moore, 1999).

Hormone Regulation

ADH is released by the posterior pituitary gland and decreases the production of urine by reabsorption of water

Table 30-1

Adult Average Daily Fluid Gains and Losses				
Fluid Gains			**Fluid Losses**	
Oral fluids	1100-1400 ml		Kidneys	1200-1500 ml
Solid foods	800-1000 ml		Skin	500-600 ml
Metabolism	300 ml		Lungs	400 ml
			Gastrointestinal	100-200 ml
TOTAL GAINS	2200-2700 ml		TOTAL LOSSES	2200-2700 ml

by the kidney tubules. ADH helps the body retain water and is sometimes referred to as the "water conserving" hormone (Metheny, 2000). In the presence of deficient fluid volume, as with vomiting and diarrhea, ADH levels increase, resulting in conservation of water.

Aldosterone, which is part of the RAA system, is a hormone produced by the adrenal cortex that regulates sodium and thus potassium and water balance. The RAA system stimulates secretion of aldosterone when there is decreased blood flow to the kidneys as in CHF. In response to the presence of aldosterone, the kidneys excrete potassium and reabsorb sodium, and as a result, water is retained. Fluid deficits such as those produced by hemorrhage or gastrointestinal losses can increase aldosterone levels. The result of excessive aldosterone secretion is fluid volume overload due to excessive sodium retention. In the event of acute losses it often takes 2 or 3 days for both ADH and aldosterone to make corrective changes.

Another hormone, atrial natriuretic peptide (ANP), is released in the right atrium in the presence of atrial distention of the heart and acts on the kidney to initiate a diuresis of sodium and water. The result is a decrease in intravascular volume. The diuretic effect of ANP may be beneficial to the client in acute heart failure and fluid volume overload. Box 30-2 gives examples of changes in fluid balance related to several clinical situations.

NURSING DIAGNOSES

Nursing diagnoses relating to fluid and electrolyte imbalance include two major categories: **Deficient Fluid Volume** and **Excess Fluid Volume. Deficient Fluid Volume** occurs when there is prolonged or high decreased intake or prolonged or excessive fluid loss with high fever, sweating, diarrhea, vomiting, or third-space fluid losses. **Hyperthermia** (associated with systemic infection, septicemia, or draining wounds) and **Impaired Skin Integrity** (associated with burns) also contribute to fluid loss and electrolyte imbalance.

Excess Fluid Volume may be related to excessive intake of fluids, especially rapid IV infusion and excess sodium intake. **Excess Fluid Volume** may also occur from retention of fluids as a result of decreased circulation and/or redistribution within the compartments and compromised regulatory mechanisms as occurs with CHF and renal failure.

Skill 30.1

Monitoring Fluid Balance

Many variables can change the distribution of fluids in the body. Nurses monitor clients for actual and potential fluid and electrolyte imbalances. During assessment the nurse considers variables influencing the fluid status and whether the change is normal and adaptive or the result of a pathological process.

ASSESSMENT

1. Consult the medical record, or complete a nursing history with the client and family to identify risk factors for fluid volume imbalances (see Box 30-1). *Rationale: Current illness or disease processes, medications,*

treatments, and dietary restrictions can disrupt fluid and electrolyte balance.

2. Monitor cardiovascular status for the following changes at least every 4 hours.
   a. Assessments indicating hypovolemia (decreased circulating volume)
      (1) Falling blood pressure, especially orthostatic hypotension. Compare blood pressure lying, sitting, and standing. *Rationale: In the presence of decreased circulating blood volume, there is a drop in blood pressure and a compensatory rise in pulse rate when changing from a recumbent to sitting or standing positions.*

    (2) Increased pulse rate, weak pulse, and capillary filling time longer than 3 seconds.

    (3) Flat neck veins when supine.

    (4) Slow venous filling of dependent hands (longer than 3 to 4 seconds).

  b. Assessments indicating increased venous pressure or fluid excess

    (1) Assess for bounding pulse and inspect for jugular venous distention (JVD) when client is sitting upright (see Chapter 13). *Rationale: Indicates compromised ability of the right atrium to receive blood and pump it throughout the circulatory system.*

    (2) Monitor for increased respiratory rate, orthopnea, shortness of breath, or cough. Auscultate lungs for crackles (rales) and rhonchi. *Rationale: Indicates fluid buildup in the lung interstitial tissue (pulmonary edema), which requires immediate medical intervention.*

3. Check daily weights for changes (see Procedural Guideline 8-1). *Rationale: Daily weight is the most effective way to evaluate fluid balance. Rapid weight loss or gain of 5% to 10% of body weight suggests moderate imbalance; greater than 10% alteration suggests severe fluid imbalance. Each kg of loss equals 1 L fluid loss (Potter and Perry, 2001).*

  a. Compare fluid intake and output (I&O) over 24 to 48 hours (see Skill 9.1, p. 200). Monitor for intake significantly greater or less than output. *Rationale: In the presence of fluid excess and normal kidney function, urine will be pale and dilute and output will be increased. In the presence of kidney failure, oliguria intensifies the accumulation of fluids in the body.*

  b. Intake includes *all* liquids taken by mouth including ice chips, fluids given through nasogastric or jejunostomy feeding tubes, IV fluids, IV piggyback medications, and blood or blood components. *Rationale: Intake includes all sources of fluid; when intake exceeds output over time, it may result in fluid excess.*

  c. Output includes urine, diarrhea, vomitus, diaphoresis (excessive sweating), gastric suction, and drainage from surgical tubes. Observe urine for oliguria, dark, concentrated (tea-colored) appearance. *Rationale: Output greater than intake over time results in fluid deficit in which the body conserves water. Concentrated urine is apparent.*

4. Inspect oral mucous membranes. *Rationale: Sticky, dry membranes; dry, cracked lips; and decreased saliva production suggest dehydration.*

5. Inspect skin for temperature and moisture. *Rationale: Dryness and flushed appearance suggest dehydration. Cool, clammy skin suggests hypovolemia.*

  a. Palpate skin for inelastic turgor (tenting) over the sternum in adults or the abdomen in infants. *Rationale: Tenting indicates significant fluid deficit re-lated to dehydration. The back of the hand is not a reliable place to test skin turgor because of loose, thin skin, especially in older adults.*

  b. Assess for peripheral or central edema, periorbital edema, and blurred vision. Palpate dependent body parts such as feet/ankles for pitting edema +1 to +4). Palpate the abdomen for ascites, an accumulation of fluid in the abdomen. Measure abdominal girth every 12 to 24 hours. *Rationale: Presence of edema indicates fluid excess. Pitting edema indicates fluid excess of 10 pounds (20 L) or more. Clients on bed rest develop edema in sacral area when supine. Edema may shift from side to side as the client is turned.*

6. Assess mental status and level of consciousness (LOC). *Rationale: Dizziness, restlessness, confusion, lethargy, and coma may be related to dehydration or decreased cardiac output with hypovolemia.*

7. Monitor laboratory values for increased hematocrit (Hct), blood urea nitrogen (BUN), and urine specific gravity. *Rationale: Increased Hct suggests hemoconcentration caused by fluid loss. Increased BUN suggests hemoconcentration in the presence of normal kidney function. Increased urine specific gravity indicates concentrated urine. Decreased Hct suggests hemodilution caused by fluid retention. Decreased urine specific gravity indicates dilute urine.*

8. Assess client's and family's understanding of fluid imbalances and the importance of accurate assessment data.

PLANNING

Expected outcomes focus on identifying fluid imbalances. Treatment often needs to begin quickly to avoid potentially life-threatening complications.

Expected Outcomes

1. Client will achieve or maintain normal fluid balance.

2. Causes of imbalance are identified and corrected.

3. Complications will be prevented or detected and managed promptly.

Delegation Considerations

Monitoring and evaluating fluid balance requires the critical thinking and knowledge application unique to a nurse. The skill of measuring and recording oral intake and urinary output can be delegated to assistive personnel (AP). Emphasize the importance of standard precautions relating to body fluids and accuracy in measuring and recording I&O. All monitoring data must be reported to the nurse.

IMPLEMENTATION FOR MONITORING FLUID BALANCE

Steps	Rationale
1. See Standard Protocol (inside front cover).	
2. Provide oral hygiene every 2 to 4 hours, and keep lips moist with petrolatum jelly (see Skill 7.2, p. 158).	Fluid and electrolyte imbalances, especially FVD, result in dry, cracked oral mucosa. Frequent oral hygiene increases client comfort and helps to maintain integrity of oral membranes.
3. Monitor daily weights for trends toward normal.	Changes in body weight can be a valuable indicator of fluid changes in the presence of edema and fluid imbalance.
4. Provide careful skin care for comfort and to prevent tissue damage.	Dry or edematous skin is easily injured, which can lead to other impaired skin integrity problems (e.g., pressure ulcers).
5. Provide client safety and position changes.	Clients with fluid deficit are at risk of orthostatic hypotension and subsequent falls.
6. Implement specific interventions to improve fluid status.	
a. Deficient fluid volume	
(1) If oral intake is not restricted, encourage fluids. If client is allowed nothing by mouth (NPO) or unable to tolerate oral fluids, parenteral fluid administration is indicated (see Chapter 29).	
(2) During IV therapy, monitor carefully for fluid overload, including daily weights, I&O, vital signs, orthopnea, shortness of breath or cough, associated with crackles (rales) and rhonchi, JVD, and hyponatremia (decreased serum sodium).	Too rapid infusion can result in overhydration and sodium imbalance manifested by increased respiratory distress and cardiovascular changes.

NURSE ALERT *When clients require rapid rates of infusion, they must be assessed frequently for FVE, especially in the presence of cardiac, renal, or neurological problems. An inappropriate composition or rate of administration can be life threatening.*

Steps	Rationale
b. Excess fluid volume	
(1) Monitor IV therapy for appropriate rate of administration and effectiveness.	IV fluids can assist in the fluid shift and transport.
(2) In the presence of circulatory or respiratory changes elevate the head of the bed. Oxygen therapy may be indicated (see Skill 31.1, p. 748).	
(3) Administer medications such as diuretics as prescribed.	Diuretic medications act on the renal tubules to assist in excretion of excess fluid and electrolytes.
(4) Restrict fluids to 1200 to 1500 ml/day as prescribed.	Clients with renal and cardiovascular diseases may have impaired renal clearance and therefore retain fluid; restricting fluid intake is necessary to optimize physiological functioning.
7. Monitor output for trends toward normal fluid balance.	In fluid deficit the body will conserve fluids initially. Once cellular hydration occurs, urine output will trend toward normal. In fluid excess, output should increase following administration of diuretic therapy.

Steps	**Rationale**
8. Monitor appropriate laboratory values (e.g., electrolytes, hematocrit, urine specific gravity).	As fluid imbalances are corrected, these values should return to normal or client's baseline. For example, in fluid excess the client's hematocrit is decreased due to hemodilution.
9. See Completion Protocol (inside front cover).	

• • • • • • • • • •

EVALUATION

1. Conduct ongoing assessment to determine whether the fluid imbalance has been corrected.
2. Evaluate effectiveness of corrective action based on identified cause(s).
3. Evaluate for possible complications of overcorrection of the original problem. For example, if the client is treated for fluid deficit, observe for fluid excess.

Unexpected Outcomes and Related Interventions

1. After IV therapy for fluid deficit, client remains either hypovolemic or dehydrated.
    a. Analyze the data supporting the persistent fluid imbalance (excess loss or inadequate intake).
    b. In collaboration with other health care team members, increase volume or rate of ordered fluids either orally or intravenously, or seek orders for appropriate medications such as antiemetics to decrease losses.
2. After IV therapy for fluid deficit, client has evidence of fluid excess.
    a. Analyze the data to determine extent of overload.
    b. Decrease the infusion rate of parenteral fluids, and administer diuretics as ordered.

Recording and Reporting

*   Describe assessment data that indicate the extent of fluid excess.
*   Report significant alterations in vital signs, oliguria, laboratory results, and mental status to the physician promptly.
*   Record independent and collaborative nursing interventions implemented, including oral or IV fluids, medications, and comfort measures.

Sample Documentation

1000 States nausea, vomiting ×3 days at home. Vital signs: temperature 98.4° F, pulse 100 beats per minute, respirations 12 breaths per minute, supine blood pressure (BP) 118/80 mm Hg, standing BP 90/60 mm Hg. Alert; oriented to person, place, time. Complains of dizziness, thirst, nausea. Oral mucous membranes dry, jugular veins flat with head of bed flat, inelastic skin turgor, capillary refill longer than 5 seconds. Urine output 240 ml in 8 hr IV of D_5 LR infusing at 125 ml/hr via infusion pump left forearm. Antiemetic given as ordered.

 ## SPECIAL CONSIDERATIONS

Pediatric Considerations

*   Infants and small children are at greater risk for fluid deficit because of their relatively greater surface area, their high rate of metabolism, and their immature kidney function (Wong and others, 1999). As much as 80% of an infant's body weight is water.
*   When measuring output in infants, diapers may be weighed in grams. One gram of wet diaper weight equals 1 ml of urine.
*   Children frequently respond to illness with fevers of higher temperature or longer duration than adults, resulting in increased insensible water losses (Wong and others, 1999).
*   In the presence of fluid deficit in infants, inspection will reveal depressed or sunken fontanels, and in fluid excess bulging fontanels are apparent.

*   When a child is dehydrated nursing assessment needs to include the possibility of impending shock (Wong and others, 1999).
*   Young children who need encouragement to increase oral fluid intake require creative tactics. This could include freezer pops made from juice, gelatin in fun shapes, small medicine cups, or decorated cups, a tea party, a crazy straw, or sticker rewards for drinking a certain amount (Wong and others, 1999).

Geriatric Considerations

*   The amount of fluid in the body decreases with age. A person over 70 years of age may have as little as 45% to 50% of body fluid.
*   Older adults tend to have decreased thirst sensation or may have altered ability to request or obtain needed fluids.

- After age 65 years the kidneys lose nephrons and therefore the ability to concentrate urine.
- Atrophy of adrenal glands results in altered regulation of sodium and potassium and predisposes the client to fluid and electrolyte imbalance.

Home Care Considerations

If clients or families are required to monitor I&O at home, they may use household measures and calculate totals accordingly.

Skill 30.2

Monitoring Electrolyte Balance

Disturbances in electrolyte balance seldom occur alone and often are related to fluid imbalances. The basic types of electrolyte imbalances include sodium, potassium, calcium, and magnesium imbalances. Various risk factors are associated with electrolyte imbalances (Table 30-2). Electrolytes are substances that separate in solution into negatively charged ions (anions) and positively charged ions (cations) that conduct electrical currents. The numbers of positive and negative charges must be equal in body fluids. Electrolytes are vital to many body functions, including neuromuscular function, cardiac rhythm and contractility, mental processes, and gastrointestinal function. Most serum electrolytes are measured in milliequivalents (mEq) per liter.

Sodium is the most abundant cation in the ECF. Water follows sodium so that when sodium is excreted by the kidneys, water is also excreted. (This is the mechanism of action for some diuretics.) Hyponatremia is a low serum sodium level, associated with many conditions, including kidney disease, gastrointestinal losses, increased sweating, and certain diuretics to name a few. Severe hyponatremia can result in seizures, vascular collapse, and shock. Dilutional hyponatremia occurs in the presence of water excess. Hypernatremia is caused by extreme water loss or overall sodium excess (Schmidt, 2000).

Potassium is the predominant intracellular cation, which regulates neuromuscular excitability and muscle contraction and is primarily regulated by the kidneys. Because the normal range for serum potassium is a narrow one (3.5 to 5 mEq/L), relatively small deviations from normal can be very serious. Hyperkalemia is an elevated serum potassium level, which may be caused by altered kidney function because any condition that decreases urine output also decreases potassium excretion. Hyperkalemia is also related to massive cell damage such as from burns, myocardial infarction, crushing injuries, and cell destruction after chemotherapy and radiation therapy. Hypokalemia (low serum potassium level) is commonly from excessive losses related to potassium-wasting diuretics (Schmidt, 2000). Hypokalemia can also result from inadequate intake; malnutrition; gastrointestinal losses with vomiting, diarrhea, or gastric suctioning; kidney disease; and diabetic ketoacidosis.

Calcium contributes to the transmission of nerve impulses, cardiac contractions, blood clotting, and formation of teeth and bone (Lewis and others, 2000). Hypocalcemia (low serum calcium level) causes altered blood clotting and a tendency toward tetany. Hypocalcemia is associated with surgical removal of the parathyroid glands, acute pancreatitis, renal failure, decreased dietary intake, and excess loss with laxative abuse. Hypercalcemia is an increase in the total serum calcium level and frequently is a symptom of an underlying disease resulting in excess bone resorption with release of calcium (Potter and Perry, 2001). The most common cause of hypercalcemia is malignancy. Other causes include parathyroid disease, vitamin D overdose, thiazide diuretics, and prolonged immobilization.

Magnesium imbalances directly influence neuromuscular function and cardiovascular tone. Hypomagnesemia increases neuromuscular and central nervous system (CNS) activity. Hypermagnesemia diminishes the excitability of muscle cells and contributes to hypertension, cardiac dysrhythmias, ischemic heart disease, and sudden cardiac death. Magnesium deficit may be caused by excess losses via vomiting and diarrhea; large urine output; nasogastric suction; and decreased dietary intake because of chronic alcoholism, malnutrition, or inadequate absorption. Elevated magnesium levels are associated with renal failure, adrenal insufficiency, and overdose associated with IV administration for the prevention of seizures in toxemia of pregnancy.

ASSESSMENT

1. Consult the medical record, or complete a nursing history with the client and family to identify risk factors for electrolyte imbalances (see Table 30-2, p. 734). *Rationale: Electrolyte imbalances frequently occur with un-*

Table 30-2

Risk Factors for Electrolyte Imbalances

Electrolyte Deficit	Electrolyte Excess
Hyponatremia Renal disease Adrenal insufficiency Gastrointestinal losses Excessive sweating Use of thiazide diuretics (especially along with low-sodium diet) Interruption of sodium-potassium pump with decreased cell potassium and decreased serum sodium Metabolic acidosis	**Hypernatremia** Water deprivation Increased insensible water loss (e.g., burns, hyperventilation) Ingestion of large amounts of concentrated salt solution Iatrogenic administration of hypertonic saline IV solution Excess aldosterone secretion
Hypokalemia Use of potassium-wasting diuretics Diarrhea, vomiting, or other gastrointestinal losses Alkalosis Cushing's syndrome or adrenal hormone–producing tumors Polyuria Excessive sweating Excessive use of potassium-free IVs	**Hypercalcemia** Hyperparathyroidism Malignancies Metastatic bone tumors Paget's disease Osteoporosis Prolonged immobilization
Hypocalcemia Excessive administration of blood containing citrate Hypoalbuminemia Hypoparathyroidism Vitamin D deficiency Neoplastic diseases Sepsis Pancreatitis	**Hyperkalemia** Renal failure and oliguria Hypertonic dehydration Massive cellular damage (burns, trauma) Iatrogenic administration of large amounts of potassium IV Adrenal insufficiency Acidosis Rapid infusion of stored blood Use of potassium-retaining diuretics
	Hypomagnesemia Malnutrition/alcoholism Inadequate absorption: diarrhea, vomiting, nasogastric drainage, fistulas, excessive dietary calcium (competes with magnesium for transport sites), small intestine diseases Hypoparathyroidism Excessive loss resulting from thiazide diuretics Aldosterone excess Polyuria
	Hypermagnesemia Renal failure Excessive parenteral administration of magnesium

derlying diseases and require anticipatory nursing interventions. *For example, the client with CHF is at risk for sodium retention. An anticipatory intervention is a reduction in dietary sodium.*

2. Consider current illness or disease processes, health practices, medications, treatments, and dietary restrictions, which can disrupt electrolyte balance.

3. Check laboratory results to identify abnormal electrolyte levels. *Rationale: Provides current and/or baseline laboratory data from which to measure the success of interventions aimed at restoring electrolyte balance.*

4. Assess client and family's understanding of the risk for electrolyte imbalances. *Rationale: Helps to determine prior client experience and adherence to interventions to maintain electrolyte balance.*

PLANNING

Expected outcomes focus on identifying a high risk for or actual electrolyte imbalance. Treatment should begin quickly because complications can be life threatening.

Expected Outcomes

1. Client will have normal serum electrolyte levels.
2. There will be no evidence of complications of electrolyte imbalance.

Delegation Considerations

Monitoring electrolyte balance requires the critical thinking and knowledge application unique to a nurse. Assistive personnel (AP) may monitor assessment data (e.g., daily weight, I&O, vital signs) and report a client's mental status (sudden confusion), changes in strength (weakness or muscle rigidity), and subjective symptoms. All monitoring data must be reported to the nurse.

IMPLEMENTATION FOR MONITORING ELECTROLYTE BALANCE

Steps	Rationale
1. See Standard Protocol (inside front cover).	
2. *Sodium balance:* Identify conditions that contribute to sodium imbalance, including loss of sodium-containing fluids or water excess (see Table 30-2).	
a. *Hyponatremia:* Assess for evidence of hyponatremia (serum sodium level less than 135 mEq/L):	Hyponatremia causes hypoosmolality with a shift of water into cells (Lewis and others, 2000).
(1) Assess for abdominal cramps, nausea, and vomiting.	Early manifestations of hyponatremia.
(2) Assess mental status for personality change, irritability, apprehension, anxiety, convulsions, or coma.	Neurological symptoms are caused by fluid shift into brain cells (Lewis and others, 2000). Severe hyponatremia (less than 120 mEq/L) can result in neurological changes and irreversible neurological alterations or death at 110 mEq/L (Potter and Perry, 2001).
(3) Monitor vital signs for weak, rapid pulse and hypotension and orthostatic hypotension.	Severity of symptoms with hyponatremia depend on the magnitude, rapid onset, and cause (Metheny, 2000).
b. *Hypernatremia:* Assess for evidence of hypernatremia (serum sodium level greater than 145 mEq/L):	Hypernatremia causes hyperosmolality with a shift of water out of the cells into the hypertonic ECF, cellular dehydration in brain cells, and potential changes including tissue trauma or hemorrhage to cerebral vessels.
(1) Assess for thirst, lethargy, weakness, and irritability.	Early signs of hypernatremia. Severe hypernatremia (concentrations greater than 160 mEq/L) may lead to seizures or coma (Metheny, 2000).
(2) Inspect mouth for dry tongue and mucous membranes.	
(3) Assess for dry, flushed skin.	
(4) Monitor urine output for oliguria or anuria.	
c. Provide comfort and safety measures, including preparation for potential convulsions in severe cases (see Skill 5.4, p. 103).	
d. Refer to a dietician when a low-sodium diet is prescribed. Help client learn ways to consume less salt and sodium.	
(1) Read the nutrition labels, and minimize the use of processed foods containing high levels of sodium. Look for canned foods with reduced or no sodium.	
(2) Use fresh and plain frozen vegetables.	

Steps	Rationale

(3) Request no added salt when eating out or traveling.

(4) Use spices and herbs rather than salt to enhance the flavor of food.

(5) Avoid condiments such as pickles, olives, soy sauces, and other sauces high in sodium.

(6) Choose fresh fruits and vegetables as snacks rather than salted chips, nuts, or popcorn.

(7) Avoid over-the-counter medications that contain sodium (Na).

3. *Potassium balance:* Identify conditions that contribute to changes in potassium levels (see Table 30-1, p. 729).

a. *Hypokalemia:* Assess for evidence of hypokalemia (serum potassium level less than 3.5 mEq/L):

The most common cause of hypokalemia is the use of potassium-wasting diuretics such as thiazides and loop diuretics. Alkalosis may cause a temporary hypokalemia by a shift of serum potassium into the cells (Metheny, 2000).

(1) Assess vital signs for a weak, irregular pulse; shallow respirations; and hypotension.

(2) Assess electrocardiogram (ECG) changes (depressed ST, T wave inversion or flattening, and U waves), and ventricular arrhythmias.

NURSE ALERT *Severe hypokalemia (less than 2.5 mEq/L) can result in death from cardiac or respiratory arrest (Methany, 2000).*

(3) Assess for generalized fatigue, weakness, decreased muscle tone, or decreased reflexes.

(4) Assess abdomen for decreased bowel sounds and abdominal distention.

(5) Assess extremities for muscle cramps and paresthesias.

b. Maintain adequate dietary intake of potassium (potatoes, spinach, broccoli, winter squash, dates, bananas, cantaloupes, dried apricots, orange and grapefruit juice, dry beans, milk, and yogurt).

c. Administer IV fluids with KCl as ordered.

NURSE ALERT *The rate of administration of IV fluids containing KCl should not exceed 20 mEq of potassium per hour.*

d. *Hyperkalemia:* Assess for evidence of hyperkalemia (serum potassium level greater than 5.5 mEq/L):

(1) Assess ECG changes, including peaked T waves, prolonged PR interval, widening of QRS, complete heart block, ectopic beats, and ventricular fibrillation leading to cardiac arrest.

Hyperkalemia can be caused by renal failure, which leads to decreased excretion of potassium, massive tissue damage, or acidemia, which causes a shift of potassium out of the cells into the plasma. It can also be caused by rapid IV administration or massive oral ingestion.

Steps	Rationale

(2) Assess for nausea, vomiting, diarrhea, and cramping pain.

(3) Assess for muscle twitching, paresthesias or paralysis, or seizures.

e. In the presence of hyperkalemia, collaborate with the physician to prescribe Kayexalate or consider the possibility of renal dialysis.

4. *Calcium balance:* Identify conditions that contribute to calcium imbalance.

a. *Hypocalcemia:* Assess laboratory reports for hypocalcemia (total serum calcium level less than 8.5 mg/dl).

(1) Assess for muscle cramps, numbness, and tingling circumorally and in fingers and toes.

(2) Assess for ECG changes, including prolonged QT interval, bradycardia, ventricular tachycardia, or asystole.

(3) Observe for laryngeal spasm, and prepare for possible respiratory arrest.

NURSE ALERT *Severe hypocalcemia is a medical emergency, particularly if laryngeal spasms and respiratory arrest are imminent. It is treated with IV calcium gluconate.*

---

(4) Assess for colicky discomfort or diarrhea.

(5) Assess for Chvostek's sign, a contraction of facial muscles in response to a light tap over the facial nerve in front of the ear (see illustration).

(6) Assess for Trousseau's sign, carpal spasm induced by inflating a blood pressure cuff above the systolic pressure for as long as 3 minutes (see illustration).

(7) Prepare for possible seizures and tetany (see Skill 5.4, p. 103).

b. *Hypercalcemia:* Assess laboratory reports for hypercalcemia (total serum calcium level greater than 11 mg/dl):

(1) Assess for decreased gastrointestinal motility, including nausea, vomiting, constipation.

(2) Assess for lethargy, fatigue, malaise, and muscle weakness.

(3) Assess for confusion, impaired memory, sudden psychosis, or coma.

(4) Monitor for weight loss, dehydration, increased thirst, and polyuria.

(5) Assess for hypertension or ECG changes.

(6) Assess for decreased muscle strength, hypoventilation, and depressed deep tendon reflexes (DTR).

(7) Assess abdomen for hypoactive bowel sounds or paralytic ileus.

Kayexalate exchanges sodium for potassium, and potassium is excreted in stool. The excretion of potassium is achieved rapidly with dialysis.

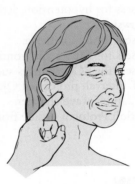

Step 4a(5) Chvostek's sign. (From Lewis SM and others: *Medical-surgical nursing: assessment and management of clinical problems,* ed 5, St Louis, 2000, Mosby.)

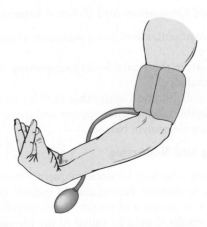

Step 4a(6) Trousseau's sign. (From Lewis SM and others: *Medical-surgical nursing: assessment and management of clinical problems,* ed 5, St Louis, 2000, Mosby.)

Steps	Rationale

c. Promote the excretion of calcium in urine by increasing fluid intake to 3000 to 4000 ml of fluid daily or administration of a loop diuretic as ordered.

5. *Magnesium balance:* Identify factors that contribute to magnesium imbalance.

     a. *Hypomagnesemia:* Assess for evidence of magnesium level less than 1.5 mEq/L or 1.8 mg/dl.

Hypomagnesemia may occur with and contribute to the persistence of hypokalemia and hypophosphatemia (Metheny, 2000).

         (1) Assess for hyperexcitability with muscular weakness or tremors, tetany, seizures, positive Chvostek's or Trousseau's sign (see illustrations for Steps 4a(4) and 4a(5)).

         (2) Assess mental status for sudden changes, including confusion, ataxia, vertigo, depression, and psychosis.

         (3) Monitor for cardiac dysrhythmias, which can be life threatening.

     b. *Hypermagnesemia:* Assess for evidence of magnesium level greater than 2.5 mEq/L.

         (1) Assess for hypotension, lethargy and drowsiness.

         (2) Assess for hyporeflexia.

         (3) Assess for nausea and vomiting.

         (4) Assess for ECG changes such as shortening QT interval, prolonged QRS and PR interval, and T wave changes.

6. See Completion Protocol (inside front cover).

• • • • • • • • • •

EVALUATION

1. Check laboratory values and physical signs to identify trends in response to medical treatment.
2. Monitor for evidence of complications related to treatment resulting in the opposite imbalance (e.g., treatment for hypokalemia may result in hyperkalemia).

Unexpected Outcomes and Related Interventions

1. After treatment, client has a persistent electrolyte imbalance.
   a. Analyze the available data supporting the imbalance.
   b. In collaboration with other health care team members, administer appropriate therapies to restore electrolyte balance.

Recording and Reporting

• Laboratory tests may be done frequently to monitor response to therapy. Report should include time electrolytes were drawn and results. When significantly abnormal, results should be called to the physician immediately for appropriate management.

• Documentation should include positive and negative assessment data related to abnormal electrolyte laboratory results and action taken, including notification of the physician.

Sample Documentation

1100 Serum Na 135 and K 3.0. Pulse 110 beats per minute, weak and irregular, respirations 28 breaths per minute. Client reports weakness, fatigue, nausea, and anorexia. Dozing and arouses easily. States, "My legs have been aching since yesterday." Client instructed to stay in bed. Dr. Johnson notified. Orders received.

SPECIAL CONSIDERATIONS

Pediatric Considerations

- Infants are at risk for hypocalcemia at birth due to termination of calcium transport across the placenta and are vulnerable to hypocalcemic tetany. Other risk factors for hypocalcemia in infants are low birth weight, intrauterine growth retardation, and feeding with cow's milk (Metheny, 2000).
- Particularly for premature infants, sodium is an important nutrient. It is associated with protein synthesis, bone mineralization, and maintenance of ECF volume.
- Infants of diabetic mothers are at risk of hypomagnesemia.
- If the mother was treated with magnesium sulfate for eclampsia or preterm labor, the infant is at risk for hypermagnesemia.
- Hyperkalemia may occur in premature infants because of a shift of potassium from the cells to the extracellular space.

Geriatric Considerations

- Atrophy of adrenal glands results in altered regulation of sodium and potassium and predisposes the client to fluid and electrolyte imbalance.
- It is now recognized that older adults have different norms than younger adults as well as complex health histories that can effect the overall responses of their bodies to fluid and electrolyte alterations. Laboratory tests and their results need to be considered within context and not in isolation from the overall clinical picture (Lueckenotte, 2000).

Long-Term Care Considerations

Monitoring for alterations in electrolyte imbalance is similar in long-term care as in the gerontologic population in the acute care setting.

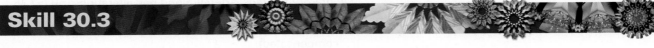

Skill 30.3

Monitoring Acid-Base Balance

Regardless of the client's age, injury, or illness, optimal cellular function depends upon adequate oxygenation and a balanced acid-base ratio, which can be monitored by measuring levels of arterial blood gases (ABGs) (Horne and Derrico, 1999). A disturbance of acid-base balance can come about in a variety of ways (Table 30-3). Simply stated, acidosis results from either accumulation of acid or loss of base, and alkalosis results from either accumulation of base or loss of acid.

The body's metabolic processes constantly produce acids, which are neutralized and excreted to maintain acid-base balance. Normally the body maintains an arterial pH between 7.35 and 7.45. The pH represents the concentration of hydrogen (H^+) in solution and indicates whether the imbalance is more acidic or more alkaline. It does not reflect the nature of the imbalance. Normally the ratio is 1 part acid to 20 parts base (Figure 30-5). The three regulatory mechanisms that act to protect the body against fluctuations in pH are the buffer mechanism, the respiratory system, and the renal system. The buffer mechanism reacts immediately to absorb or release hydrogen ions to maintain acid-base balance. The respiratory system responds within minutes, and the renal system takes 2 to 3 days to respond.

The respiratory system functions to excrete carbon dioxide (CO_2) and water. The amount of CO_2 in the blood is directly related to the carbonic acid concentration. With increased respirations, more CO_2 is eliminated at the alveolar level, which results in less carbonic acid. With decreased respirations, more CO_2 remains in the blood, which results in more carbonic acid.

The alkaline portion of the balance is maintained under normal conditions because the kidneys reabsorb and conserve bicarbonate. The kidneys can generate additional bicarbonate and eliminate excess hydrogen ions as compensation for acidosis. The body normally excretes acidic urine to help maintain acid-base balance. An acid-base imbalance is produced when the ratio between acid and base content of the blood is altered.

The primary types of acid-base imbalance are (1) respiratory acidosis related to carbon dioxide excess, (2) respiratory alkalosis related to carbon dioxide deficit, (3) metabolic acidosis related to bicarbonate deficit, and (4) metabolic alkalosis related to bicarbonate excess. To assess acid-base balance, a specimen of arterial blood is analyzed to determine the pH, the amount of carbon dioxide, and the amount of bicarbonate. This test, called an ABG, gives some information about the cause of acid-base imbalances (respiratory or metabolic) and whether the imbalance is being compensated for by the respiratory or renal system. ABG values also include the oxygenation status of the arterial blood. Normal ABG values are listed in Table 30-4.

Table 30-3

Acid-Base Imbalances

Causes	Signs and Symptoms
Respiratory Acidosis	
Hypoventilation Resulting From Primary Respiratory Problems	
Atelectasis (obstruction of small airways often caused by retained mucus) Pneumonia Cystic fibrosis Respiratory failure Airway obstruction Chest wall injury	*Physical examinations:* confusion, dizziness, lethargy, headache, ventricular dysrhythmias, warm and flushed skin, muscular twitching, convulsions, and coma *Laboratory findings:* arterial blood gas alterations: pH <7.35, partial pressure of carbon dioxide in arterial blood ($PaCO_2$) >45 mm Hg, arterial partial pressure of oxygen (PaO_2) <80 mm Hg, and bicarbonate level normal (if uncompensated) or >26 mEq/L (if compensated)
Hypoventilation Resulting From Factors Outside of the Respiratory System	
Drug overdose with a respiratory depressant Paralysis of respiratory muscles caused by various neurological alterations Head injury Obesity	
Respiratory Alkalosis	
Hyperventilation Resulting From Primary Respiratory Problems	
Asthma Pneumonia Inappropriate mechanical ventilator settings	*Physical examinations:* dizziness, confusion, dysrhythmias, tachypnea, numbness and tingling of extremities, convulsions, and coma *Laboratory findings:* arterial blood gas alterations: pH >7.45, $PaCO_2$ <35 mm Hg, PaO_2 normal, and bicarbonate level normal (if short lived or uncompensated) or <22 mEq/L (if compensated)
Hyperventilation Resulting From Factors Outside of the Respiratory System	
Anxiety Hypermetabolic states Disorders of the central nervous system (head injuries, infections) Salicylate overdose	
Metabolic Acidosis	
High Anion Gap	
Starvation Diabetic ketoacidosis Renal failure Lactic acidosis from heavy exercise Use of drugs (methanol, ethanol, formic acid, paraldehyde, aspirin)	*Physical examination:* headache, lethargy, confusion, dysrhythmias, tachypnea with deep respirations, abdominal cramps, and flushed skin *Laboratory findings:* arterial blood gas alterations: pH <7.35, $PaCO_2$ normal (if uncompensated) or <35 mm Hg (if compensated), PaO_2 normal or increased (with rapid, deep respirations), bicarbonate level <22 mEq/L, and oxygen saturation normal
Normal Anion Gap	
Renal tubular acidosis Diarrhea	
Metabolic Alkalosis	
Excessive vomiting Prolonged gastric suctioning Hypokalemia or hypercalcemia Excess aldosterone Use of drugs (steroids, sodium bicarbonate, diuretics)	*Physical examination:* dizziness; dysrhythmias; numbness and tingling of fingers, toes, and circumoral region; muscle cramps; tetany *Laboratory findings:* arterial blood gas alterations: pH >7.45, $PaCO_2$ normal (if uncompensated) or >45 mm Hg (if compensated), PaO_2 normal, and bicarbonate level >26 mEq/L

ASSESSMENT

1. Assess client's risk factors for acid-base imbalances (see Table 30-3).
2. Assess factors that influence ABG measurements.
   a. Suctioning. *Rationale: During suctioning a short-term oxygen desaturation may occur; wait until client's pulse oximetry reading returns to baseline status.*
   b. Oxygen therapy. *Rationale: The percentage of inspired oxygen concentration should be included in the client's laboratory requisition information. This value is taken into account when evaluating ABG results.*
   c. Ventilator setting change. *Rationale: Ventilator changes are done to improve the client's oxygenation status. However, ABG levels obtained immediately after a ventilator change may be false. Allow the client's physiology to compensate for these changes, and wait 20 to 30 minutes following ventilator changes before obtaining a new series of ABGs.*
   d. Body temperature. *Rationale: Body temperature affects the affinity of oxygen for hemoglobin and subsequently affects tissue oxygenation.*

3. Identify medications that may affect acid-base balance. *Rationale: Certain medications increase client's risk for acid-base imbalances, especially in the presence of other acute or chronic illnesses.*

PLANNING

Expected outcomes focus on identifying risks for or actual acid-base imbalance. Treatment should begin quickly to avoid any life-threatening complications.

Expected Outcomes

1. Client's extremity distal to puncture site remains warm, pink, has adequate capillary refill, and is free of pain.
2. Client will maintain or achieve normal acid-base balance.
3. Complications will be prevented or minimized.

Equipment

- 3-ml heparinized syringe
- 23 to 25 gauge needle
- Syringe cap
- Alcohol swabs (2)
- 2 × 2 gauze pad
- Tape
- Cup or plastic bag with crushed ice
- Label with client information
- Laboratory requisition
- Disposable gloves
- Protective eyewear
  NOTE: Commercial blood gas kits may be available.

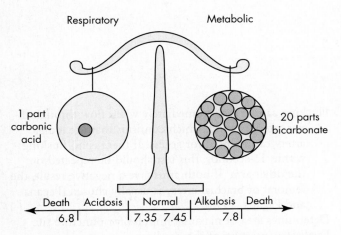

Figure 30-5   Carbonic acid/bicarbonate ratio and pH.

Table 30-4

Normal Arterial Blood Gas Values		
Component	**Normal Value**	**Significance**
pH	7.35-7.45	Indicates acid-base status of the body
PaCO₂	35-45 mm Hg	Pressure exerted by dissolved CO_2 in the blood
		Under control of the lungs
		Respiratory component
HCO₃	22-26 mEq/L	Buffers' effect of acid in the blood
		Under control of kidneys
		Metabolic component
Base excess (BE)	+/−2	Reflects status of all bases in blood
PaO₂	90-100 mm Hg	Pressure exerted by dissolved O_2 in blood
		Indicates effectiveness of oxygenation by lungs

Delegation Considerations

The skills of drawing arterial blood samples and monitoring acid-base balance require the critical thinking and knowledge application unique to a nurse. In some agencies specially trained laboratory technicians may draw arterial blood samples. Assistive personnel (AP) may monitor vital signs and report a client's subjective symptoms.

IMPLEMENTATION FOR MONITORING ACID-BASE BALANCE

Steps	Rationale
1. See Standard Protocol (inside front cover).	
2. Collect ABG sample by arterial puncture.	Blood can be collected through an existing arterial line or multilumen catheter if present.
a. Select an appropriate site. The radial, femoral, or brachial arteries are commonly used.	Factors that contraindicate use of arterial site include amputation, contractures, localized infection, dressings or cast, mastectomy, or arteriovenous shunts.
b. Assess collateral blood flow to the hand using Allen's test:	
(1) Have client make a tight fist and raise hand above heart.	
(2) Apply direct pressure to both radial and ulnar arteries.	
(3) Have client lower hand and open hand.	
(4) Release pressure over ulnar artery; observe color of fingers, thumbs, and hand.	Flushing can be seen immediately when flow through ulnar artery is good, which confirms that the radial artery can be used for access. If there is no flushing within 15 seconds, this test should be repeated on the other arm. If both arms give a negative result, the femoral or brachial artery is usually chosen (Pagana and Pagana, 1998).
c. Palpate selected site with fingertips.	Determines area of maximal impulse for puncture site.
d. Stabilize artery by hyperextending wrist slightly.	Facilitates insertion of the needle.
e. Clean area of maximal impulse with alcohol swab, wiping in circular motion.	

COMMUNICATION TIP *Tell client when you will insert the needle and that it will be painful for a short time.*

f. Hold needle bevel up, and insert at 45-degree angle, observing for blood return.	
g. Stop advancing needle when blood is observed, and allow arterial pulsations to pump 2 to 3 ml of blood into the heparinized syringe.	
h. When sampling is complete, hold 2 × 2 gauze pad over puncture site and quickly withdraw needle, applying pressure over and just proximal to puncture site.	
i. Maintain continuous pressure on and proximal to site for 3 to 5 minutes or longer.	Avoids hematoma formation.

Steps	Rationale
j. Inspect site for signs of bleeding or hematoma formation.	If client is receiving anticoagulant therapy or has bleeding disorder, pressure may be needed for up to 15 minutes.
k. Palpate artery distal to puncture site.	Verifies that arterial circulation to the hand has not been compromised.
l. Expel air bubbles from syringe.	Maintains accurate results.
m. Place identification label on syringe, place syringe in ice, and attach appropriate laboratory requisition. If the client is receiving supplemental oxygen, note this on the requisition. Indicate client's body temperature.	Supplemental oxygen influences results of testing. Elevated body temperature decreases the oxygen saturation results
n. Transport specimen to the laboratory immediately.	
3. Interpret ABG report using a systematic approach: Check the PaO_2 (normal is 80 to 100 mm Hg) and the SaO_2 (normal is 95% to 100%).	PaO_2 has no bearing on acid-base balance. Laboratory report includes whether supplementary oxygen was being administered when blood sample was drawn. Hypoxemia refers to low levels of oxygen in the arterial blood, whereas hypoxia refers to low tissue oxygenation. Hypoxia can exist with normal ABG levels when the oxygen-carrying capacity of the blood is compromised (low hemoglobin) or there is low cardiac output and inadequate perfusion.

4. Check the pH to determine the presence of alkalosis (greater than 7.45) or acidosis (less than 7.35).
5. Determine the primary cause of the change in the pH. Check the $PaCO_2$ to determine if it is high, within normal limits (WNL), or low (normal is 35 to 45 mm Hg).
   a. If the $PaCO_2$ is high, the client is hypoventilating and retaining carbonic acid, resulting in respiratory acidosis (see illustration). In collaboration with other health care team members, determine ways to improve the client's ventilation to eliminate excess CO_2 (e.g., deep breathing, pursed-lip breathing, bronchodilators).
   b. If the $PaCO_2$ is low, the client is hyperventilating and too much CO_2 is eliminated, resulting in respiratory alkalosis (see illustration). In collaboration with other health care team members, determine ways to promote retention of CO_2 (e.g., minimize anxiety, slow rate of breathing and breathe less deeply, breathe into a paper bag).
   c. If the $PaCO_2$ is WNL, the client is ventilating adequately.
6. Check the HCO_3 to determine if it is high, WNL, or low (normal is 22 to 26 mEq/L)
   a. If the HCO_3 is high, there is a bicarbonate excess, which can result from retention of bicarbonate or a metabolic loss of acids (see illustration). For example, prolonged vomiting or gastric suction can result in metabolic alkalosis. In collaboration with other health care team members, determine ways to minimize the metabolic loss of acids.

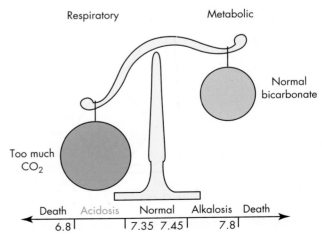

Step 5a   Uncompensated respiratory acidosis.

Steps	Rationale

b. If the HCO_3 is low and the CO_2 is normal, there is most likely a bicarbonate deficit from an accumulation of acids caused by a metabolic process (see illustration). Examples include such conditions as diabetic ketoacidosis and shock (with accumulation of lactic acid). With physician's orders, sodium bicarbonate may be given intravenously as an emergency measure. It is important to correct the condition that is causing abnormal production of acids, thereby decreasing acid production.
NOTE: Acidosis can be caused by carbon dioxide excess or by a bicarbonate deficit, and alkalosis can be caused by a carbon dioxide deficit or bicarbonate excess.

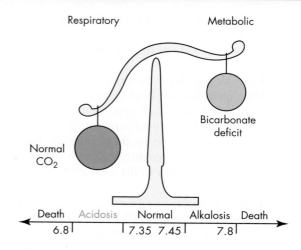

Step 6b   Uncompensated metabolic acidosis.

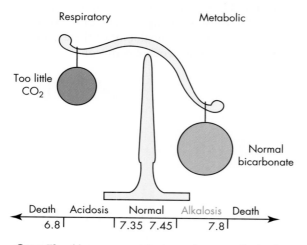

Step 5b   Uncompensated respiratory alkalosis.

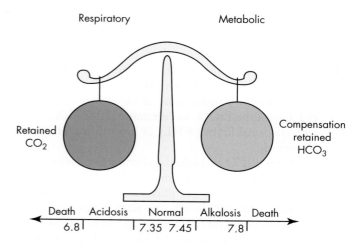

Step 7a   Compensated respiratory alkalosis.

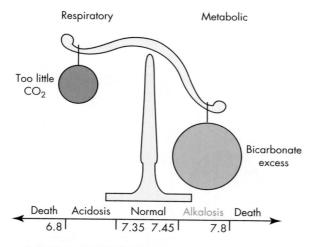

Step 6a   Uncompensated metabolic alkalosis.

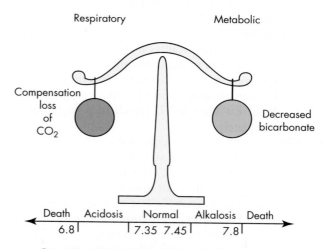

Step 7b   Compensated metabolic acidosis.

Steps	Rationale

7. Determine if there is evidence of the body attempting to compensate for the pH change.

   a. If the primary problem is respiratory acidosis (pH less than 7.4 with an elevated $PaCO_2$), the kidneys may compensate by retaining bicarbonate, which will cause the pH to trend toward the normal range (7.35 to 7.39). This process may take hours or days (see illustration).

   b. If the primary problem is metabolic acidosis (pH less than 7.4 with a bicarbonate deficit), the body may compensate by hyperventilating immediately and eliminating carbon dioxide, causing the pH to trend toward the normal range (7.35 to 7.39) (see illustration).

   c. If the primary problem is respiratory alkalosis (pH greater than 7.4 with low CO_2), the body may compensate by decreasing renal absorption of bicarbonate. The pH trends toward the normal range (less than 7.45). This begins in 8 hours and is maximal in 3 to 5 days (see illustration).

   d. If the primary problem is metabolic alkalosis (pH greater than 7.4 with bicarbonate excess), the body may compensate immediately with hypoventilation to promote retention of carbonic acid. The pH trends toward the normal range (less than 7.45) (see illustration).

8. See Completion Protocol (inside front cover).

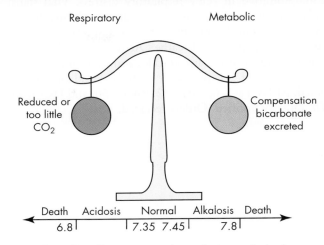

Step 7c   Compensated respiratory alkalosis.

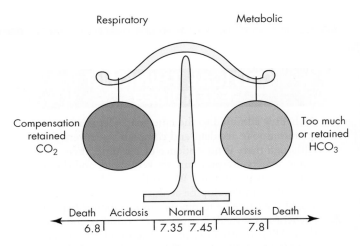

Step 7d   Compensated metabolic alkalosis.

• • • • • • • • • •

EVALUATION

1. Observe the puncture site for bleeding, and verify intact circulation to distal extremity.
2. Analyze the ABG to determine if acid-base imbalance has been corrected as a result of medical and nursing interventions. (Correction is evident by pH, CO_2, and HCO_3 levels all WNL.)
3. Assess for evidence of complications.

Unexpected Outcomes and Related Interventions

1. After treatment the client continues to have persistent acid-base imbalance.
   a. Analyze the available data to determine confounding factors.
   b. In collaboration with other health care team members, identify ways to correct imbalance.

Recording and Reporting

• Clients with acid-base imbalances are usually critically ill and may require frequent ABG analysis and prompt medical and nursing interventions.
• Often blood samples are drawn in emergency situations and sent to the laboratory stat. Results must be reported to the physician as soon as available.
• Documentation includes assessments related to client status, interventions used, and evaluation of client response.

Sample Documentation

2300 Admitted in acute respiratory distress. Vital signs: pulse 112 beats per minute, respirations 36 breaths per minute, BP 148/84 mm Hg. Reports dyspnea at rest and speech interrupted to breathe. Alert and oriented ×3. Lung sounds reveal coarse crackles and wheezing throughout. Oxygen at 2 L per nasal cannula. Head of bed elevated. ABGs: PaO_2 68, pH 7.32, $PaCO_2$ 50, and HCO_3 24. Dr. Lindsay notified. Orders received.

SPECIAL CONSIDERATIONS

Geriatric Considerations

The complex health histories presented by older adults can affect the overall responses of their bodies to acid-base imbalance. Laboratory tests and their results need to be considered within context and not in isolation from the overall clinical picture (Lueckenotte, 2000).

Home Care Considerations

Clients and caregivers need to recognize risk factors, implement appropriate prevention, and seek health care in a timely fashion.

Long-Term Care Considerations

Alterations in acid-base balance, similar in long-term care as in the gerontologic population, may require transport to acute care setting.

CRITICAL THINKING EXERCISES

1. A client is admitted to the emergency department after an automobile accident and complains of severe pain. Although there is no evidence of bleeding, there is extreme anxiety. Respirations are very rapid, and the pulse is 110 beats per minute. Would the acid-base balance most likely to develop be acidosis or alkalosis, and would the cause be respiratory or metabolic? Explain.

2. A client has several days of severe vomiting and diarrhea. ABGs reveal a pH of 7.3, $PaCO_2$ of 35 mm Hg, and HCO_3 of 20 mEq/L. What acid-base imbalance is present? What assessments could you make to detect compensation efforts by the body?

3. An older adult client has been living alone in an apartment. During your home health visit, the client demonstrates the following: weight loss of 5 pounds in 3 days; weak pulse; blood pressure 90/50 mm Hg (baseline 115/80 mm Hg); oliguria with dark, tea-colored urine; weakness; and dry lips and mucous membranes. What additional data would you need to determine if the condition is caused by decreased intake, excessive losses, or both?

4. A client with a known history of CHF becomes very short of breath, anxious, and diaphoretic. Blood pressure is 130/70 mm Hg; pulse is 114 beats per minute; respirations, 36 breaths per minute; temperature is 99° F. What fluid and electrolyte disturbance would be most likely, and what are the complications to anticipate? What other assessment data is needed? What aspects of nursing care, if any, could be delegated to AP?

REFERENCES

Beck L: The aging kidney: defending a delicate balance of fluid and electrolytes, *Geriatrics* 55(4):26, 2000.

Cooper A, Moore M: IV fluid therapy. I. Water balance and hydration assessment, *Aust Nurs J* 7(5):1, 1999.

Fann B: Fluid and electrolyte balance in the pediatric patient, *J Intraven Nurs* 21(3):153, 1998.

Horne D, Derrico D: Mastering ABG's: the art of arterial blood gas measurement, *Am J Nurs* 99(8):26, 1999.

Lewis SM and others: *Medical-surgical nursing: assessment and management of clinical problems*, ed 5, St Louis, 2000, Mosby.

Lueckenotte AG: *Gerontologic nursing*, ed 2, St Louis, 2000, Mosby.

McKenry LM, Salerno E: *Mosby's pharmacology in nursing*, ed 20, St Louis, 1998, Mosby.

Metheny N: *Fluid and electrolyte balance*, ed 4, Philadelphia, 2000, Lippincott.

Pagana KD and Pagana TJ: *Mosby's diagnostic and laboratory test reference*, ed 5, St Louis, 2001, Mosby.

Perry AG, Potter PA: *Clinical nursing skills and techniques*, ed 5, St Louis, 2002, Mosby.

Potter PA, Perry AG: *Fundamentals of nursing*, ed 5, St Louis, 2001, Mosby.

Schmidt TC: Assessing sodium and fluid imbalance. *Nursing 2000*, Jan, 30(1):18, 2000.

Wong DL and others: *Whaley and Wong's nursing care of infants and children*, ed 6, St Louis, 1999, Mosby.

Young A: A closer look at IV fluids, *Nursing* 28(10):52, 1998.

CHAPTER

31

Promoting Oxygenation

Physiological needs, such as food, water, and air, are the primary stimulus for behavior according to Maslow's hierarchy of human needs. It is only when these needs are met that humans may attempt to reach higher levels of needs, such as safety, intimacy, and the need for knowledge and understanding. Ineffective respirations are a cause of distress that will not allow humans to focus on any other event.

Respirations are effective when sufficient oxygenation is obtained at the cellular level and when cellular waste and carbon dioxide are adequately removed via the bloodstream and lungs. When this system is interrupted, such as by lung tissue damage, obstruction of airways by inflammation and excess mucus, or impairment of the mechanics of ventilation, intervention is required to support the client or death may occur.

NURSING DIAGNOSES

A variety of nursing diagnoses may apply to clients requiring promotion of oxygenation. Nursing diagnoses directly related to problems affecting optimum oxygenation include **Ineffective Airway Clearance** resulting from an ineffective cough or excessive secretions and **Ineffective Breathing Pattern** exhibited by clients with respiratory muscle weakness and fatigue or abnormal breathing pattern. In addition, **Impaired Gas Exchange** resulting from altered oxygen supply or alveolar hypoventilation and **Impaired Spontaneous Ventilation** may be present for those clients who exhibit an imbalance between ventilatory capacity and increased ventilatory demand. Last, **Dysfunctional Ventilatory Weaning Response (DVWR)** is an appropriate nursing diagnosis for those clients who are physically or psychologically unable to wean from mechanical ventilation. **Risk for Infection** is present in these clients due to the damaged defense systems of the lungs.

Clients with breathing problems may also be at risk for **Disturbed Thought Processes** from inadequate oxygenation and carbon dioxide retention. **Activity Intolerance** related to imbalance between oxygen supply and demand may lead to a **Self-Care Deficit.** Psychosocial nursing diagnoses such as **Anxiety, Fear,** and **Hopelessness** may be related to dyspnea and feelings of suffocation, as well as the fear of dying. **Ineffective Coping** may be related to the chronicity of many pulmonary diseases. **Impaired Verbal Communication** is an appropriate diagnosis when the client is severely dyspneic or has an artificial airway, such as a tracheostomy or endotracheal tube.

Skill 31.1

Oxygen Administration

Oxygen therapy refers to the administration of oxygen to a client to prevent or relieve hypoxia. Hypoxia is a condition in which insufficient oxygen is available to meet the metabolic needs of tissues and cells. Hypoxia results from hypoxemia, which is a deficiency of oxygen in the arterial blood. Supplemental oxygen for the relief of hypoxemia may be temporary, until the cause of the problem is corrected, or long term, when it is required for a chronic condition.

Room air has an oxygen concentration, or fraction of inspired oxygen (FiO_2), of 21%. Supplemental oxygen delivery is based on the FiO_2 required to maintain adequate oxygenation (Table 31-1), whether hospital or home use, and the portability desired (see Chapter 40).

ASSESSMENT

1. Perform a complete assessment of the respiratory system (see Chapter 13). Assess for impaired gas exchange (hypoxia or hypercapnea), with both rest and activity, including:
   a. Behavioral changes, apprehension, anxiety, decreased ability to concentrate, decreased level of consciousness, fatigue, and dizziness. *Rationale: Decreased levels of oxygen (hypoxia) or increased levels of carbon dioxide (hypercapnea) affect a person's cognitive abilities, interpersonal interactions, and mood. These changes might be slight; however, they can be early indicators of problems with oxygenation.*
   b. Assess vital signs, including rhythm and depth of respirations. *Rationale: Provides baseline of oxygenation status and enables early detection of hypoxia. Untreated hypoxia is life threatening.*
   c. Assess SpO_2 via pulse oximetry. *Rationale: Oxygen saturation monitors the percentage of hemoglobin fully saturated with oxygen. In the presence of hypoxemia, the percent of hemoglobin saturated with oxygen declines and the client's pulse oximetry level declines.*

Table 31-1

Oxygen Delivery Systems

Delivery System	FiO$_2$* Delivered	Advantages	Disadvantages
Nasal cannula	1-6 L/min: 24%-44%	Safe and simple Easily tolerated Effective for low concentrations Does not impede eating or talking Inexpensive, disposable	Unable to use with nasal obstruction. Drying to mucous membranes. Can dislodge easily. May cause skin irritation or breakdown. Client's breathing pattern will affect exact FiO$_2$.
Oxymizer	1-15 L/min: 24%-60%	Higher concentrations without mask Releases O$_2$ only on inhalation Conserves O$_2$, increased portability Does not require humidification	Nasal reservoir may interfere with drinking from cup. May be cosmetically unappealing. Potential reservoir membrane failure. Client's breathing pattern will affect exact FiO$_2$.
Venturi mask	4-10 L/min: 24%-50%	Delivers exact preset FiO$_2$ despite client's breathing pattern Does not dry mucous membranes Can be used to deliver humidity	Hot and confining, mask may irritate skin. FiO$_2$ may be lowered if mask does not fit snugly. Interferes with eating and talking.
Partial rebreathing mask	6-15 L/min: 35%-60%	Delivers increased FiO$_2$ Easily humidifies O$_2$ Does not dry mucous membranes	Hot and confining, may irritate skin, tight seal necessary. Interferes with eating and talking. Bag may twist or kink; should not totally deflate.
Nonrebreathing mask	6-15 L/min: 60%-100%	Delivers highest possible FiO$_2$ without intubation Does not dry mucous membranes	Requires tight seal, difficult to maintain and uncomfortable. May irritate skin. Bag should not totally deflate.

*FiO$_2$, Fraction of inspired oxygen concentration.

d. Assess skin and mucosa for changes in color: pallor, cyanosis, or flushing. *Rationale: Pallor may occur when client's oxygen levels decline. Cyanosis is a late sign of hypoxia. Flushing may be noted when hypercapnea is present.*

2. Check arterial blood gas (ABG) results. *Rationale: Objectively quantifies changes in oxygen and carbon dioxide that affect acid-base balance (see Chapter 30).*

PLANNING

Expected outcomes focus on optimum oxygenation, safe application of oxygen therapy, and an understanding of and compliance with the oxygen prescription.

Expected Outcomes

1. Client's oxygen saturation and ABGs return to or remain within normal limits or baseline levels.
2. Client verbalizes improved comfort and does not exhibit symptoms of hypoxemia.
3. Client's pulse; respirations; color; and subjective experiences of anxiety, fatigue, and decreased oxygenation status return to normal for client.
4. Client is able to state the indications for supplemental oxygen by discharge.
5. Client follows safety guidelines for supplemental oxygen therapy by discharge.
6. Client uses supplemental oxygen as prescribed by discharge.

Equipment

- Delivery device ordered by physician
- Oxygen tubing (consider extension tubing)
- Humidifier, if indicated
- Sterile water for humidifier
- Oxygen source
- Oxygen flow meter
- "Oxygen in use" sign (Figure 31-1)

Delegation Considerations

The skill of oxygen administration by nasal cannula or mask requires the critical thinking application unique to a nurse. The nurse is responsible for correct administration of oxygen including adjustment of oxygen flow rate and assessment of client response to oxygen therapy. Correct placement and adjustment of oxygen devices can be delegated to assistive personnel (AP). Instruct the care provider in possible unexpected outcomes associated with oxygen delivery and the need to report these to the nurse if they occur.

Table 31-2

Oxygen Safety Guidelines

Guideline	Explanation
"Oxygen in use" sign is on client's door (Figure 31-1). Make sure oxygen is set at prescribed rate.	Notifies all personnel of oxygen in client's room. Oxygen is a medication and should not be adjusted without a physician's order.
Smoking is not permitted. Avoid electrical equipment that may result in sparks.	Oxygen supports combustion. Delivery systems must be kept 10 feet from open flames and at least 5 feet from electrical equipment.
Store oxygen cylinders upright. Secure with chain or holder.	Prevents tipping and falling while stationary or when client is being transported.
Check oxygen available in portable cylinders before transporting or ambulating clients.	Gauge on cylinder should register in green range, indicating oxygen is available for transport and ambulation. Have backup supply available if level is low (Figure 31-2).

Figure 31-1   Proper display for "oxygen in use" sign.

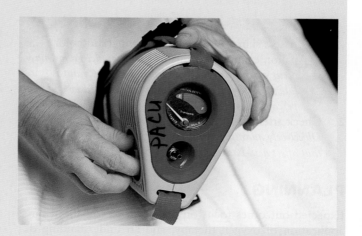

Figure 31-2   Gauge on portable oxygen system.

IMPLEMENTATION FOR OXYGEN ADMINISTRATION

Steps	Rationale

1. See Standard Protocol (inside front cover).

COMMUNICATION TIP *Explain to client the purpose of oxygen administration, and safety precautions (Table 31-2). Also explain to the client the possibility of continued dyspnea because of the etiology of the breathing problem (e.g., narrowed airways, fever).*

---

2. Attach delivery device to oxygen tubing. Consider extension tubing for clients who are not confined to bed.

   Extension tubing increases client's ability to move about and assists in avoiding complications of bed rest.

3. Attach appropriate flow meter to oxygen source, and attach oxygen tubing.

   Flow meters with smaller calibrations may be safer for clients requiring low-dose oxygen when larger doses may be harmful, as in clients with chronic obstructive pulmonary disease (COPD).

4. Adjust oxygen flow rate to prescribed dosage (see illustration). If a humidifier is used, verify that water is bubbling.

   Oxygen is a medication; correct dose is required.

5. Observe for proper fit, function, and FiO_2 of delivery device.

   a. *Nasal cannula:* Place tips of cannula into client's nares, and adjust headband or plastic slide until cannula fits snugly and comfortably (see illustration).

   Effective mechanism of oxygen delivery up to 6 L/min.

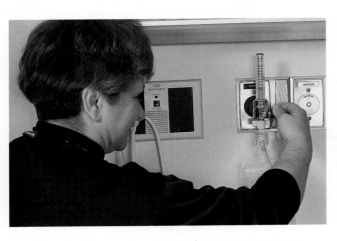

Step 4   Flow meter attached to oxygen source.

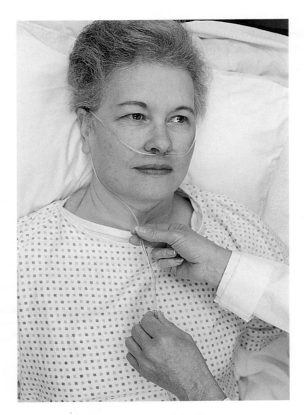

Step 5a   Nasal cannula is useful for low oxygen concentration (2 L/min) for clients with chronic lung disease.

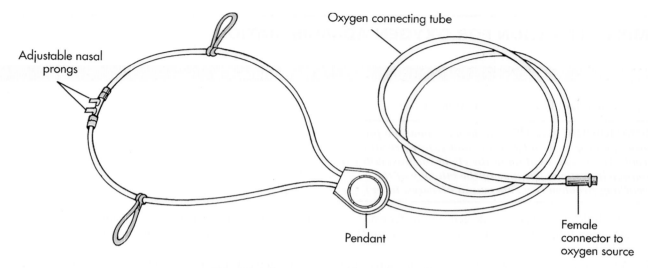

Adjustable nasal prongs

Oxygen connecting tube

Pendant

Female connector to oxygen source

Step 5b   Components of nasal cannula.

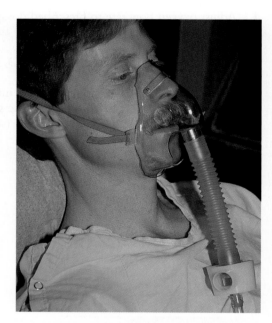

Step 5c   Venturi mask, 24% to 50% oxygen delivered by turning barrel to preset intervals.

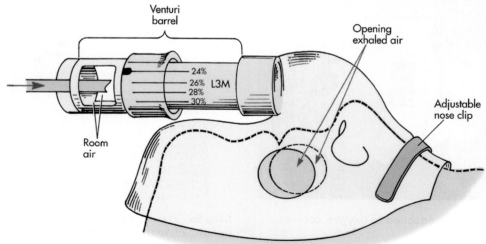

Venturi barrel

Opening exhaled air

Room air

24%
26% L3M
28%
30%

Adjustable nose clip

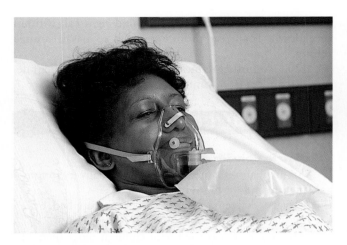

Step 5d Partial rebreathing mask can deliver concentrations of 60% to 90% using flow rates of 6 to 10 L/min.

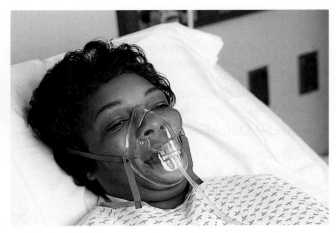

Step 5f Simple face mask can deliver concentrations of 35% to 50% using flow rates of 6 to 10 L/min.

Steps	Rationale
b. *Reservoir nasal cannula (Oxymizer):* Fit as for nasal cannula. Reservoir is located under nose or as a pendant (see illustration).	Able to deliver higher flow of oxygen than cannula without changing to a mask, which is claustrophobic for some clients. Delivers approximately a 2:1 ratio (e.g., 6-L nasal cannula is approximately equivalent to 3-L reservoir device or Oxymizer).
c. *Venturi mask:* Rate set on flow meter will determine FiO_2. Low- and high-concentration adapters are available. Setting should correlate with prescribed dosage (see illustration).	Delivers exact oxygen concentration despite respiratory pattern. Can also be attached to a tracheostomy collar for administration.
d. *Partial rebreathing mask:* Reservoir should fill on exhalation and almost collapse on inhalation (see illustration).	Effectively delivers higher oxygen concentrations.

NURSE ALERT *To ensure the client's inspiratory demands are being met, observe the reservoir bag; it should not completely collapse on inspiration.*

---

e. *Nonrebreathing mask:* Delivers highest possible oxygen concentration for nonintubated clients.	
f. *Simple face mask:* Place securely over client's nose and mouth (see illustration).	
6. Obtain an order for ABGs or pulse oximetry 10 to 15 minutes after initiation of therapy or change in oxygen concentration.	ABGs provide objective data regarding blood oxygenation and acid-base status (see Chapter 30).
7. Consult with physician regarding the need for continuous pulse oximetry if client's oxygen level is not stable.	Oximetry provides objective data regarding blood oxygenation and is used for trending (see Chapter 12).
8. See Completion Protocol (inside front cover).	

• • • • • • • • • •

EVALUATION

1. Observe repeat ABGs and/or pulse oximetry for objective measurement of improvement after initiation or change in therapy. Response must be evaluated both at rest and with activity to determine adequate oxygenation.

2. Observe client for improved oxygen saturation, as demonstrated by decreased anxiety, improved level of consciousness and cognitive abilities, decreased fatigue, and absence of dizziness.

3. Assess pulse and respirations, expect a decreased pulse with regular rhythm, decreased respiratory rate, and improved color. These are signs that oxygenation is improving.

4. Ask client to verbalize indications for supplemental oxygen.
5. Observe if client follows safety guidelines in present setting, and ask client to verbalize safety guidelines for home use.
6. Observe client or caregiver demonstrate use of supplemental oxygen.

Unexpected Outcomes and Related Interventions

1. Client experiences nasal irritation, drying of nasal mucosa, sinus pain, or epistaxis.
   a. Apply a water-soluble lubricant to areas of irritation around nares.
   b. Recommend use of an isotonic saline nasal spray.
   c. Determine if a reservoir cannula is appropriate (decreased liter flow without reducing FiO_2, oxygen delivery on inspiration only); if so, obtain order.
   d. Consider humidification.
2. Client develops irritation of the face or posterior surfaces of the ear.
   a. Apply ear protectors, or reposition nasal cannula so that it does not come into contact with irritated areas.
3. Client has continued hypoxia: increased and/or irregular heart rate, SpO_2 declines.
   a. Monitor ABGs and/or pulse oximetry.
   b. Perform a complete respiratory assessment.
   c. Notify physician.
   d. Identify methods to decrease oxygen demand (e.g., total bed rest, positioning).
4. Client develops carbon dioxide retention, as demonstrated by confusion, headache, decreased level of consciousness, flushing, somnolence, carbon dioxide narcosis, or respiratory arrest.
   a. Monitor ABGs.
   b. Notify physician of symptoms.
   c. Attempt to maintain oxygen pressure (PaO_2) at 55 mm Hg. Hypoxia must be treated, but PaO_2 levels that exceed 60 to 70 mm Hg may worsen hypoventilation.

Recording and Reporting

- Record and report the respiratory assessment findings.
- Record and report method of oxygen delivery, flow rate.
- Record and report client's response and any adverse reactions.

Sample Documentation

0800 Client alert and oriented. Respirations even and easy. Color pink. O_2 4-L nasal cannula. Productive cough of yellow sputum. Fluids encouraged.

1000 Reddened area noted behind right ear, without breakdown. Foam ear protector added to nasal cannula tubing.

1200 No further redness noted behind ears. Client denies discomfort from cannula.

SPECIAL CONSIDERATIONS

Pediatric Considerations

- An incubator is a method for oxygen delivery for premature and newborn infants.
- Oxygen delivered to infants is best supplied by a plastic oxygen hood (Wong and others, 1999).
- An oxygen tent is used with children older than 12 months. Oxygen concentration is difficult to control and maintain above 30% to 50% because room air is drawn into the tent whenever it is entered. The tent is a clear plastic shell wrapped around the bed but limits access to the child (Wong and others, 1999).

Geriatric Considerations

- Normal aging may decrease arterial oxygen levels. A 70-year-old may have a normal arterial PaO_2 between 75 and 80 mm Hg. Lung disease may further decrease the base PaO_2 to 50 to 60 mm Hg (Lueckenotte, 2000).
- The drive to breathe in clients who have chronically increased CO_2 levels is based on their oxygen status. Oxygen flow rates greater than 2 L/min are given with great caution in these individuals.
- The older adult may be at increased risk for skin breakdown. Frequent monitoring for redness is necessary. Early interventions such as loosening the straps, repositioning, or adding padding may prevent breakdown (Lueckenotte, 2000).

Home Care Considerations

- The client and family must be taught how to correctly administer oxygen based on which system is used and the safety measures to be followed (see Chapter 40).
- The dangers of changing the oxygen flow rate from the prescribed flow should be stressed.
- Emphasize that the client may be short of breath because of reasons other than hypoxemia and to contact the physician if increased shortness of breath occurs.
- The client and family must be taught the signs and symptoms for which to call the physician.

Long-Term Care Considerations

Oximetry may be used to monitor clients during rehabilitation services, requiring different flow rates and/or delivery systems for activity versus at rest.

Skill 31.2

Airway Management: Noninvasive Interventions

The respiratory system comprises a system of airways that must remain open and free of obstruction to decrease resistance of airflow to and from the lung. Interventions to maintain the airways depend on the pathophysiology responsible. Positioning, controlled cough, medications, hydration, and suctioning may be considered. Postoperative noninvasive procedures are addressed in Chapter 21.

Positioning and coughing are noninvasive techniques that may assist in improving airway patency. (Suctioning is discussed in Skill 31.3. p. 760.) Positioning to enhance airway patency should be considered with all clients. The goal is to position the client to allow the greatest chest expansion with the least amount of effort. Generally, if a client is short of breath, this position will be semi-Fowler's or Fowler's position. Controlled coughing is used to clear secretions that may obstruct the airway. It should be used frequently following thoracic or abdominal surgery. Repeated coughing that does not mobilize secretions is tiring and ineffective and should be prevented.

Medications such as bronchodilators can be used to dilate airways with some disease processes of the respiratory system. The purpose of hydration, through the oral route if possible, is to thin pulmonary secretions so that they can be expectorated more easily. Clients with certain disorders such as obstructive sleep apnea (OSA) may be unable to maintain a patent airway. In OSA, nasopharyngeal abnormalities that cause narrowing of the upper airway produce repetitive airway obstruction during sleep with the potential for periods of apnea and hypoxemia. Pressure can be delivered during the inspiratory and expiratory phases of the respiratory cycle by mask to maintain airway patency during sleep, but the process requires consideration of each individual's needs to obtain compliance. Pressure applied during the expiratory phase alone is administered by continuous positive airway pressure (CPAP) and during both inspiration and expiration by bilevel positive airway pressure (BiPAP) (Kryger, 1994). CPAP has been used in the client with congestive heart failure (CHF) with hypercapnea presenting in acute distress but remains controversial.

For clients who have measurable changes in the flow of their airways, such as clients with asthma or reactive airways disease, peak expiratory flow rate (PEFR) measurements may be useful. The PEFR is the maximum flow that a client can force out during one quick forced expiration, measured in liters. The client or nurse can use these measurements as an objective indicator of the client's current status and effectiveness of treatment. Decreased peak flow rates may indicate the need for further treatment such as bronchodila-

tors or antiinflammatory medications (National Asthma Education and Prevention Program, 1997).

ASSESSMENT

1. Assess work of breathing and ability to clear copious or tenacious secretions by coughing. *Rationale: Indicates risk of possible impairment of airway clearance. Secretions can plug the airway, decreasing the amount of oxygen available for gas exchange in the lung.*
2. Assess for shortness of breath, wheezing, use of accessory muscles of respiration, pallor or cyanosis. *Rationale: Signs of airway obstruction. Indicates client is in distress. Can range from mild to life threatening.*
3. Assess client's SpO_2 with oximetry or collect baseline ABG.
4. Assess for interrupted sleep, snoring respirations. Ask client about history of sleep apnea. *Rationale: Indications for use of CPAP or BiPAP.*
5. Monitor PEFR initially and with changes in therapy. Assess client's baseline knowledge of when and how to use PEFR and correct response to results. *Rationale: Client may monitor PEFR for early detection of problems after discharge.*

PLANNING

Expected outcomes focus on client's airway patency, comfort, and ability for self-care.

Expected Outcomes

1. Client maintains a position that promotes maximum lung expansion and comfort.
2. Client's airways are cleared of retained secretions.
3. Client's periods of sleep apnea are reduced to fewer than two episodes in 6 hours.
4. Client's objective measures of oxygenation improve or remain normal (ABGs, pulse oximetry).
5. Client and family demonstrate correct use of CPAP/BiPAP and express comfort using equipment by discharge.
6. Client and family demonstrate correct technique and verbalize an appropriate action plan based on PEFR values obtained, by discharge.
7. Client will maintain within prescribed parameters of personal best.
8. Client verbalizes the benefits of positioning, CPAP, and/or PEFR by discharge.

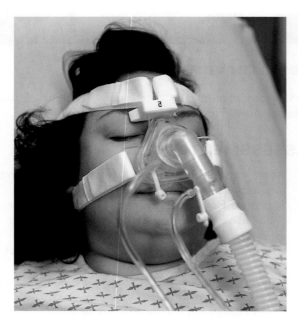

Figure 31-3   CPAP or BiPAP mask.

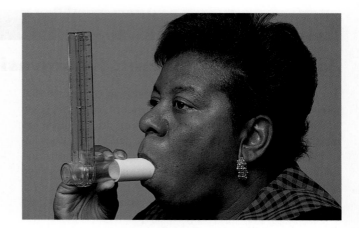

Figure 31-4   PEFR measurement.

Equipment

CPAP/BiPAP

- CPAP or BiPAP mask (Figure 31-3)
- Mask straps (face or nasal)
- Valve (CPAP or BiPAP)
- Oxygen source
- Generator (CPAP or BiPAP)
- Appropriate signs

PEFR

- Peak flow meter (Figure 31-4)
- Client diary/action plan, if appropriate

Delegation Considerations

The skills of positioning, therapeutic coughing, CPAP/ BiPAP mask application, and follow-up PEFR measurements can be delegated to appropriately trained assistive personnel (AP). The nurse is responsible for the initial PEFR measurement, correct application of CPAP/BiPAP, client instruction for CPAP/BIPAP and PEFR, and assessment of client response to CPAP/BIPAP and use of PEFR. Have AP report to nurse any signs of client distress.

IMPLEMENTATION FOR AIRWAY MANAGEMENT: NONINVASIVE INTERVENTIONS

Steps	Rationale

1.   See Standard Protocol (inside front cover).

COMMUNICATION TIP   *Explain to client that you are aware of the discomfort he or she is experiencing (i.e., breathlessness, pain) and that correct positioning will aid in the relief of this discomfort.*

2.   **Correct positioning of client**

    a.   *Sitting:* Semi-Fowler's or high Fowler's, sitting on side of bed, or in chair with elbows resting on knees. Clients with COPD may benefit from leaning over table with arms propped up (see illustrations).

       Promotes optimum lung expansion and maximizes use of accessory muscles. Decreases client's work of breathing.

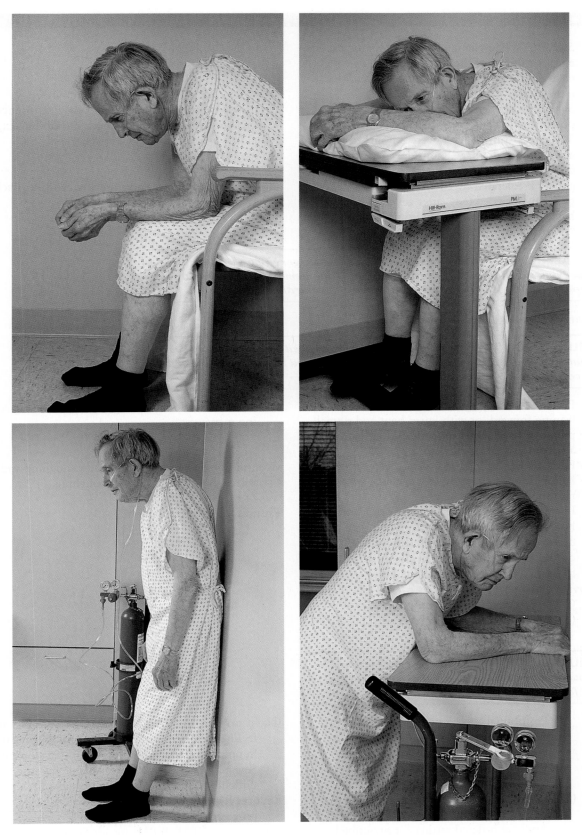

Step 2a and 2b   Positioning is a noninvasive technique used by COPD clients to optimize chest expansion and reduce work of breathing.

Steps	Rationale
b. *Standing:* When client who is ambulating experiences shortness of breath or the need to cough, encourage a position that supports client (see illustration).	
c. *Supine:* Most clients are more comfortable supported by two pillows or head of bed up at least 30 degrees. Turn at least every 2 hours to encourage secretion drainage. Consider maneuvers to drain areas of lungs with retained secretions by gravity if tolerated by client. If unilateral reexpansion is needed (e.g., after general surgery), have client lie with side requiring expansion up: "good side down, affected lung up."	Decreases orthopnea. Obese clients may experience decreased abdominal interference of full lung expansion when lying flat. Promotes lung expansion on the affected side. Exchange of respiratory gases is improved.

NURSE ALERT *Following some types of thoracic surgery (e.g. lobectomy), specific side-lying positions may be ordered to facilitate hemostasis and intrathoracic wound healing and certain positions may be contraindicated.*

3. Controlled coughing

COMMUNICATION TIP *Explain to client that controlled coughing clears secretions that may obstruct the airway by allowing air behind the mucus to move during the cough.*

a. Place client in upright position. High-Fowler's, leaning forward, or with knees bent and a small pillow or hand to support the abdomen may augment expiratory pressure.	Facilitates inhalation and lung expansion during coughing maneuver.
b. Instruct client to take two slow, deep breaths, inhaling through the nose and exhaling out the mouth.	Control of respiratory rate facilitates coughing and minimizes risk of paroxysms of coughing.
c. Instruct client to inhale deeply a third time, hold this breath, and count to three; then cough deeply for two or three consecutive coughs without inhaling between coughs. Instruct the client to push air forcefully out of the lungs.	Ensures full effective cough.

4. Provide assistive equipment
   a. CPAP/BiPAP administration
      (1) Position client comfortably with head elevated.

COMMUNICATION TIP *Before placing CPAP or BiPAP mask on the client explain that tight seal around face is needed.*

(2) Position face mask or nasal mask tightly, and adjust head strap until seal is maintained and client is able to tolerate (see Figure 31-3, p. 756).	Client may experience claustrophobic sensations and feelings of discomfort from continuous pressure. Support and education help client develop tolerance. Several types of masks are available because of the difficulties in achieving a comfortable fit.
(3) Instruct client to breathe normally.	Reduces hyperventilation and fatigue. Promotes optimum lung expansion.
(4) Apply at ordered setting for prescribed length of time.	Like oxygen, CPAP/BiPAP are administered at prescribed level.

Steps	Rationale

b. PEFR measurements
   (1) Instruct client about purpose and rationale.
   (2) Place client in an upright position.

Promotes optimum lung expansion.
Enables client to objectively monitor airway improvements during expiration.

   (3) Slide mouthpiece into base of the numbered scale.
   (4) Instruct client to take a deep breath.
   (5) Have client place meter mouthpiece in the mouth and close lips, making a firm seal (see Figure 31-4, p. 756).

Tight seal ensures all expired breath will be measured for accurate reading.

   (6) Have client blow out as hard and fast as possible through the mouth only.

Maximum effort is required for an accurate reading. Air expelled through nares will not be measured and will decrease PEFR readings.

   (7) This maneuver should be repeated 2 additional times, with the highest number recorded.
   (8) If client is to record PEFR at home, have client demonstrate PEFR technique independently and assess ability to record PEFR accurately in a diary.

Return demonstration is an effective method to evaluate learning.

COMMUNICATION TIP *Help client implement an appropriate action plan as prescribed by physician. Explain that PEFR is just one objective measure that can be used to judge symptom severity.*

---

5. See Completion Protocol (inside front cover).

• • • • • • • • • •

EVALUATION

1. Observe client's body alignment and position whenever in visual contact with client. Assist with repositioning as needed.
2. Auscultate lung fields for adventitious lung sounds
3. Assess client's respiratory status during sleep to determine response to CPAP. Ask if client subjectively feels more rested after arising.
4. Review repeat ABGs and/or pulse oximetry.
5. Observe client and caregiver use of CPAP/BiPAP mask and compliance with therapy.
6. Observe a return demonstration by client or family to determine if correct technique is being used with PEFR.
7. Determine client's PEFR, and compare with the client's personal best.
8. Ask client to explain purpose and benefits of positioning and CPAP/BiPAP or PEFR.

Unexpected Outcomes and Related Interventions

1. Client is unable to maintain a patent airway.
   a. Evaluate positioning. Consider suctioning.
   b. Monitor ABGs/pulse oximetry.
   c. An artificial airway may be considered, if not present.
2. Client experiences worsening dyspnea with bronchospasm and hypoxemia.
   a. Notify physician.
   b. Monitor ABGs/pulse oximetry.

   c. Medicate as ordered.
   d. Evaluate for methods to decrease oxygen demand.
3. Client is unable to tolerate CPAP/BiPAP.
   a. Mask fit: Check fit of delivery device. Consider alternative (alternate type of mask, nasal pillows) if difficulties continue. If skin breakdown occurs across bridge of nose, a Band-Aid may be applied until skin becomes adjusted to the pressure. If generalized breakdown occurs, consider a reaction to the mask material (i.e., latex).
   b. Pressure: Feelings of suffocation, shortness of breath, and discomfort related to pressure applied during CPAP/BiPAP. Determine if another pressure setting will give similar results with more comfort or if BiPAP is required. If client is able to continue trying, he or she usually can adapt to these feelings over time.
   c. Dryness: If a saline nasal spray is not effective, consider obtaining an order for a humidifier. Heated humidifiers are generally more effective than passover humidifiers but also more expensive.
4. Client is unable or unwilling to give maximum effort for PEFR.
   a. Provide client with encouragement and education.
   b. If unable to achieve adequate readings, contact physician immediately, medicate as ordered, and give support.

Recording and Reporting

- Record activity level, including assistance with positioning, if needed.
- Record cough effectiveness and respiratory assessment.
- For CPAP/BiPAP, record client compliance and tolerance, mask fit and skin assessment beneath mask, effectiveness of therapy, witnessed periods of apnea, and status of daytime hypersomnolence.
- For PEFR, record measurement before and after therapy and client's ability and effort to perform PEFR.

Sample Documentation

2400 Appears to sleep restfully. Respirations even and easy without snoring. No jerking movements noted. CPAP continues per face mask with good seal at 7.5 cm H$_2$O.

 0800 No change noted in assessment during night. CPAP applied for 10 hours. No areas of irritation noted from mask. States he slept well without awakening.

SPECIAL CONSIDERATIONS

Pediatric Considerations

- PEFR is a very effective assessment for assisting the school-aged children through adolescents in management of their asthma. Instruct parents and child to notify school nurse of use of PEFR and any related action plans (National Asthma Education and Prevention Program, 1997).
- Adolescents need a private area to obtain PEFR measurements during school, social events, or part-time jobs (Wong, and others, 1999).

Home Care Considerations

- Frequent follow-up may be necessary to enhance CPAP/BiPAP compliance and address unexpected outcomes promptly.
- PEFR may be incorporated into an "action plan" for the client at home as an objective measure of when a change in therapy is required.

Skill 31.3

Airway Management: Suctioning

For some clients, use of noninvasive techniques, along with medications, is not sufficient to maintain a patent airway. In these cases, suctioning is considered. The method of suctioning used depends on the level of the secretions to be removed, the presence of an artificial airway, and the client's condition. Oropharyngeal (Yankauer) suctioning is performed by using a rigid plastic catheter with one large and several small eyelets (Figure 31-5) through which mucus enters when suction is applied. Alert clients can easily be taught this suction method to control the secretions in the oral cavity.

 Nasotracheal suctioning is used to clear secretions from the trachea. This type of suctioning is used when secretions cannot be completely expectorated from the trachea, thus requiring sterile technique (Brooks and others, 2001).

 Endotracheal (ET) (Figure 31-6) and tracheostomy (Figure 31-7) tubes allow direct access to the lower airways for suctioning. These artificial airways may be inserted to create a route for mechanical ventilation, allow easy access of suctioning, relieve mechanical airway obstruction, or protect the airway from aspiration because of impaired cough or gag reflexes.

ASSESSMENT

1. Observe for signs and symptoms of excess pulmonary secretions requiring suctioning: abnormal lung sounds, productive coughing, ineffective cough, secretions in the airway, increased work of breathing, restlessness or irritability, unilateral breath sounds, cyanosis, decreased oxygen saturations or level of consciousness, or ineffective cough before deflation of an ET tube or tracheostomy cuff. *Rationale: Physical signs and symptoms result from airway obstruction and decreased oxygen to tissues.*

Figure 31-5   Oropharyngeal suctioning.

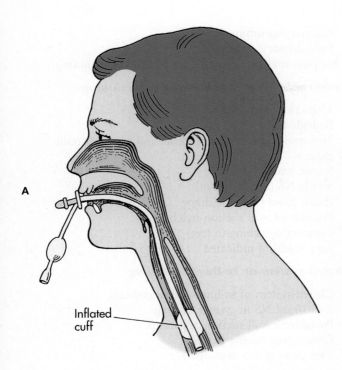

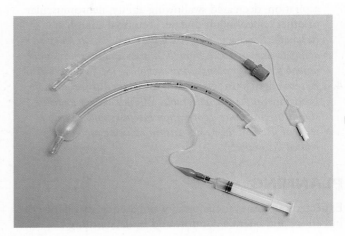

Inflated cuff

Figure 31-6   A, Endotracheal (ET) tube with inflated cuff. **B,** ET tubes with unin-flated and inflated cuffs and syringe for inflation. Client is unable to speak while tube is in place because air cannot flow through the vocal cords.

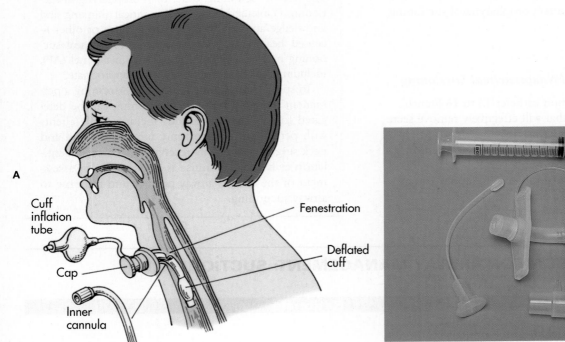

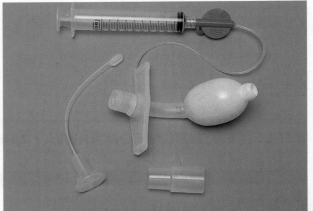

Cuff inflation tube

Cap

Inner cannula

Fenestration

Deflated cuff

Figure 31-7   Tracheostomy tube with obturator for insertion and syringe for infla-tion of cuff.

2. Assess upper airway: Assess nasal and oral cavity: gurgling on inspiration or expiration, obvious nasal or oral secretions, drooling, gastric secretions or vomitus in mouth. *Rationale: Removal of oral secretions prevents aspiration (Brooks and others, 2001).*

3. Assess for risk factors for the need for suctioning: post-operative decreased level of consciousness, history of aspiration, decreased swallowing ability, neuromuscular or other concomitant disease, abnormal anatomy. *Rationale: Presence of these risk factors may impair the client's ability to clear secretions from the airway and may necessitate nasopharyngeal or nasotracheal suctioning (St. John, 1999).*

4. Assess client's understanding of procedure. *Rationale: Procedure can be uncomfortable. When the client understands the procedure, cooperation increases and anxiety is reduced. Both of these can assist in reducing procedure-related discomfort.*

PLANNING

Expected outcomes focus on airway patency, avoidance of infection, and client's comfort and understanding.

Expected Outcomes

1. Client's airways are cleared of secretions. No sounds of congestion can be detected, and lung sounds are improved.
2. Client indicates easier breathing and decreased congestion.
3. Client performs correct oropharyngeal suctioning technique.

Equipment

Oropharyngeal and Nasotracheal Suctioning

- Oropharyngeal suction catheter 12 to 16 French (smallest diameter that will effectively remove secretions) or Yankauer suction tip*
- Sterile gloves or one sterile and one nonsterile
- Sterile basin (e.g., disposable cup)
- Sterile water or normal saline (NS) (about 100 ml)
- Clean towel or paper drape
- Portable or wall suction

- Connecting tubing (6 feet)
- Face shield, if indicated
* Supplies may be nonsterile for Yankauer suctioning.

Endotracheal or Tracheostomy Suctioning

- 12 to 16 French catheter (adult)
- Bedside table
- Two sterile gloves or one sterile and one nonsterile glove
- Sterile basin
- Sterile NS (about 100 ml)
- Clean towel or sterile drape
- Portable or wall suction machine
- Connecting tubing (6 feet)
- Face shield, if indicated

Closed-system or In-line Suctioning

- Closed-system or in-line suction catheter
- 5 to 10 ml NS in syringe or vials
- Portable or wall suction apparatus
- Connecting tubing (6 feet)
- Two clean gloves (optional)

 Delegation Considerations

The skill of suctioning, other than oropharyngeal suctioning (Yankauer), requires the critical thinking and knowledge application unique to a nurse or other licensed health care professional. Oropharyngeal suctioning may be delegated to assistive personnel (AP), including the client and family when appropriate.

In special situations the skill of performing a permanent tracheostomy tube suctioning can be delegated to AP. These situations include stable clients with permanent tracheostomy tubes after head and neck surgery and clients receiving mechanical ventilation at home. The nurse is responsible for assessment of the client's airway patency and response to airway suctioning.

IMPLEMENTATION FOR AIRWAY MANAGEMENT: SUCTIONING

Steps	Rationale
1. See Standard Protocol (inside front cover).	
2. Position client in semi-Fowler's or Fowler's position.	
3. Preparation for all types of suctioning	
a. Open suction kit or catheter using aseptic technique. If sterile drape is available, place it across client's chest. Do not allow suction catheter to touch any nonsterile surfaces.	Prepares catheter and prevents transmission of microorganisms.

Steps	Rationale
b. Fill basin or cup with approximately 100 ml of water (see illustration).	Unwrap or open sterile cup/basin. Place on bedside table.
c. Connect one end of connecting tubing to suction machine. Check that equipment is functioning properly by suctioning a small amount of water from basin.	
d. Turn on suction device. Set regulator to appropriate negative pressure: wall suction, 80 to 120 mm Hg; portable suction, 7 to 15 mm Hg for adults.	Elevated pressure settings increase risk of trauma to mucosa (Brooks and others, 2001).

4. 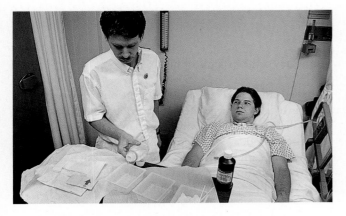 **Oropharyngeal suctioning**

Steps	Rationale
a. Consider applying mask or face shield. Attach suction catheter to connecting tubing. Remove oxygen mask if present.	Suction may cause splashing of body fluids.
b. Insert catheter into client's mouth. With suction applied, move catheter around mouth, including pharynx and gum line, until secretions are cleared.	If catheter does not have a suction control to apply intermittent suction, take care not to allow suction tip to invaginate oral mucosal surfaces with continuous suction (St. John, 1999).
c. Encourage client to cough, and repeat suctioning if needed. Replace oxygen mask if used.	Coughing moves secretions from lower and upper airways into mouth.
d. Suction water from basin through catheter until catheter is cleared of secretions.	Clearing secretions before they dry reduces probability of transmission of microorganisms and enhances delivery of preset suction pressures.
e. Place catheter in a clean, dry area for reuse with suction turned off or within client's reach, with suction on, if client is capable of suctioning self.	Facilitates prompt removal of airway secretions when suctioning is needed in the future.
f. Discard water if not used by client. Clean basin, or dispose of cup. Remove gloves and dispose.	

5. **Nasotracheal suctioning**

Steps	Rationale
a. Apply one sterile glove to each hand, or apply nonsterile glove to nondominant hand and sterile glove to dominant hand. Attach nonsterile suction tubing to sterile catheter, keeping hand holding catheter sterile.	Reduces transmission of microorganisms and allows nurse to maintain sterility of suction catheter.

Step 3b   Pouring sterile saline into tray.

Steps	Rationale
b. Secure catheter to tubing aseptically. Coat distal 6 to 8 cm (2 to 3 inches) of catheter with water-soluble lubricant.	Eases passage of catheter through nasotracheal tube.
c. Remove oxygen delivery device, if present, with nondominant hand. Ask client to extend neck slightly (if not contraindicated). Using dominant hand, gently insert catheter as client inhales. Do not apply suction. Do not force catheter through naris.	Forcing of the catheter causes trauma to the airway tissues. Extending of the client's neck may facilitate passage of the catheter.

NURSE ALERT   *Keep oxygen delivery device readily available in case the client exhibits symptoms of hypoxemia.*

Steps	Rationale
d. Advance catheter to just above entrance into trachea. Allow client to take a breath. Quickly insert catheter approximately 16 to 20 cm (6 to 8 inches in adults) into trachea. Client will begin to cough. One method of approximating the correct length of catheter to insert is to use the distance from the client's nose to the base of the earlobe as a guide.	Ensures proper placement of catheter in airway to remove secretions.
e. Advance catheter until resistance is felt as client coughs. Apply intermittent suction by placing and releasing nondominant thumb over vent of catheter. Slowly withdraw catheter while rotating it back and forth with suction on for no more than 10 seconds. Replace oxygen device, if applicable.	Intermittent suction and rotation of catheter prevents injury to tracheal mucosa. Suctioning longer than 10 seconds can cause worsen existing hypoxemia.

NURSE ALERT   *If catheter "grabs" mucosa, remove thumb to release suction.*

Steps	Rationale
f. Rinse catheter and connecting tubing by suctioning NS from the basin until tubing is clear. Dispose of catheter, gloves, and remaining saline in basin. Turn off suction device.	
6. Endotracheal or tracheostomy tube suctioning	
a. Prepare suction catheter. (See Step 2 for all types of suctioning.)	Reduces transmission of microorganisms and allows nurse to maintain sterility of suction catheter.
b. Apply one sterile glove to each hand, or apply nonsterile glove to nondominant hand and sterile glove to dominant hand. Attach nonsterile suction tubing to sterile catheter, keeping hand holding catheter sterile (see illustration, p. 765).	
c. Check that equipment is functioning properly by suctioning small amounts of saline from basin.	Lubricates catheter and tubing.
d. Hyperoxygenate client before suctioning, using manual resuscitation bag, increasing FiO_2 for a minute or 2, or using the sigh mechanism on mechanical ventilator.	Preoxygenation converts large proportion of resident lung gas to 100% oxygen to offset amount used in metabolic consumption while ventilator or oxygenation is interrupted, as well as to offset volume lost out of suction catheter (Brooks and others, 2001). Manual hyperinflation and installation of saline are not effective and potentially harmful (McKelvie, 1998).

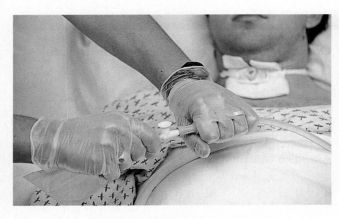

Step 6b   Attaching catheter to suction.

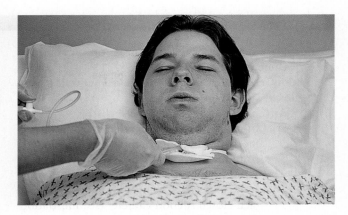

Step 5f   Suctioning tracheostomy.

Steps	Rationale
e. Open swivel adapter or tracheostomy or endotracheal tube or if necessary, remove oxygen or humidity delivery device with nondominant hand.	Exposes artificial airway.
f. Without applying suction and using dominant thumb and forefinger, gently but quickly insert catheter into artificial airway (best to time catheter insertion with inspiration) until resistance is met or client coughs, then pull back 1 cm (see illustration).	Application of suction pressure while introducing catheter into trachea increases risk of damage to tracheal mucosa. Stimulates cough and removes catheter from mucosal wall.
g. Apply intermittent suction by placing and releasing nondominant thumb over vent of catheter, and slowly withdraw catheter while rotating it back and forth between dominant thumb and forefinger. The maximum time catheter may remain in airway is 10 seconds. Encourage client to cough.	Intermittent suction and rotation of catheter prevent injury to tracheal mucosal lining. If catheter "grabs" mucosa, remove thumb to release suction. Increased hypoxia related to removal of oxygen in airways and blockage of airways will occur during suctioning procedure.
h. Close swivel adapter, or replace oxygen delivery device. Encourage client to deep breathe. Some clients respond well to several manual breaths from the mechanical ventilator or resuscitation bag.	Reoxygenates and reexpands alveoli. Suctioning can cause hypoxemia and atelectasis.
i. Rinse catheter and connecting tube with NS until clear. Use continuous suction.	Removes catheter secretions. Secretions left in tubing decrease suction and provide environment for growth of microorganisms.
j. Assess client's cardiopulmonary status for secretion clearance and complications. Repeat Steps d through i once or twice more to clear secretions. Allow adequate time (at least 1 full minute) between suction passes for ventilation and reoxygenation.	Suctioning can induce irregular heartbeats, hypoxia, and bronchospasms. Repeated passes with suction catheter clear airway of excessive secretions and promote improved oxygenation (Brooks and others, 2001).
k. Perform nasopharyngeal and oropharyngeal suctioning to clear upper airway of secretions. After these suctionings are performed, catheter is contaminated; do not reinsert into ET or tracheostomy tube.	Removes upper airway secretions. Upper airway is considered "clean," whereas lower airway is considered "sterile." Therefore same catheter can be used to suction from sterile to clean areas, but not from clean to sterile areas.
l. Disconnect catheter from connecting tube. Roll catheter around fingers of dominant hand. Pull glove off inside out so that catheter remains in glove. Pull off other glove in same way. Discard into appropriate receptacle. Perform hand hygiene. Turn off suction device.	Reduces transmission of microorganisms. Clean equipment should not be touched with contaminated gloves.

Steps	**Rationale**
m. Place new, unopened suction kit on suction machine or at head of bed.	Provides immediate access to suction catheter when needed.
7. Endotracheal or tracheostomy tube suctioning with a closed-system (in-line) catheter	
a. Attach suction.	
(1) In many institutions, catheter is attached to mechanical ventilator circuit by personnel from respiratory therapy (see illustration *A*). If not already in place, open suction catheter package using aseptic technique, attach closed-suction catheter (see illustration *B*) to ventilator circuit by removing swivel adapter and placing closed-suction catheter apparatus on ET or tracheostomy tube, and connect Y on mechanical ventilator circuit to closed-suction catheter with flex tubing.	Catheter becomes part of the circuit and is often changed by respiratory therapist with each circuit change, when contaminated, or per agency policy.
(2) Connect one end of connecting tube to suction machine, and connect other to end of closed-system or in-line suction catheter if not already done. Turn suction device on, and set vacuum regulator to appropriate negative pressure (80 to 120 mm Hg for adults).	Prepares suction apparatus. Excessive negative pressure damages tracheal mucosa and can induce greater hypoxia.
b. Hyperinflate and/or hyperoxygenate client using resuscitation bag or manual breathing mechanism on mechanical ventilator according to institution protocol and clinical status (usually 100% oxygen).	Decreases atelectasis caused by negative pressure and increases oxygen available to tissues during suctioning.
c. Unlock suction control mechanism if required by manufacturer. Open saline port, and attach saline syringe or vial.	
d. Pick up suction catheter enclosed in plastic sleeve with dominant hand.	

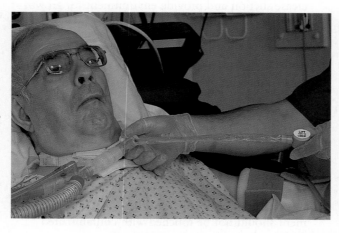
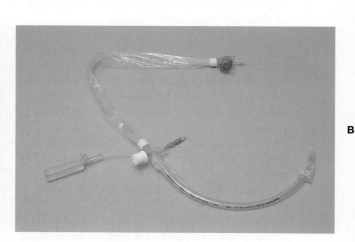

Step 7a(1)   **A,** Suctioning tracheostomy with closed-system suction catheter. **B,** Closed-system suction catheter attached to ET tube.

Steps	Rationale
e. Wait until client inhales NS or mechanical ventilator delivers a breath to dispense saline, then quickly but gently insert catheter on next inhalation. To insert catheter, use a repeating maneuver of pushing catheter and sliding (or pulling) plastic back between thumb and forefinger until resistance is felt or client coughs. (NOTE: Some catheters contain depth markings that are useful in positioning catheter.)	Catheter sterility and secretion containment are provided by plastic sheath. Mechanical ventilator breaths, oxygen, and positive end-expiratory pressure (PEEP) are not interrupted during suctioning. Catheter slides within plastic sheath. Coughing occurs or resistance is felt when catheter touches carina.
f. Encourage client to cough, and apply suction while withdrawing. Be sure to withdraw catheter completely into plastic sheath so it does not obstruct airflow.	Removes secretions from airway. Catheter left in ET or tracheostomy tube limits airflow.
g. Reassess cardiopulmonary status, including pulse oximetry, to determine need for subsequent suctioning or complications. If cardiac monitoring is available, observe rhythm during suctioning. Repeat Steps b through f 1 or 2 more times to clear secretions. Allow adequate time (at least 1 full minute) between suction passes for ventilation and reoxygenation.	Repeated passes clear airway of secretions to promote ventilation and oxygenation. Suctioning can cause complications such as irregular heartbeats, hypoxia, and bronchospasm.
h. When airway is clear, withdraw catheter completely into sheath. Be sure black line on catheter is visible in sheath. Squeeze vial or push syringe while applying suction to rinse inner lumen of catheter. Use at least 5 to 10 ml of NS. Lock suction mechanism, if applicable, and turn off suction.	Black line is reference point to determine correct position of catheter when not in use. Inability to see black line suggests catheter is in airway and may be impeding airflow. Interior of catheter must be rinsed to prevent bacterial growth. Failure to lock mechanism can result in inadvertent continuous suction and serious complications.
i. Client may require suctioning of oral cavity.	Catheter is continuously connected to ET or tracheostomy tube. Separate suction catheter is necessary for oral cavity.

8. See Completion Protocol (inside front cover).

· · · · · · · · · ·

EVALUATION

1. Auscultate lung fields, and compare client's respiratory assessments before and after suctioning.
2. Ask client if breathing is easier and if congestion is decreased.
3. Observe client's respirations.
4. Observe client's oropharyngeal suctioning technique.

Unexpected Outcomes and Related Interventions

1. Client becomes cyanotic or restless or develops tachycardia, bradycardia, or other abnormal heart rhythm.
   a. Discontinue attempt at suctioning until stabilized, unless client's condition is deteriorating because of secretions in airway.
   b. Monitor vital signs and pulse oximetry.
   c. Preoxygenate for repeated attempts.
2. Bloody secretions are returned, which may indicate trauma.
   a. Evaluate technique and frequency of suctioning.

   b. If bleeding continues, notify physician of potential hemorrhage and monitor vital signs.
3. Client has paroxysms of coughing.
   a. Reassure client.
   b. Instruct client about relaxation techniques.
   c. Medicate as needed.
4. No secretions are obtained.
   a. Reassess respiratory system for presence of secretions.
   b. Stimulate client's cough.
   c. Check that suction system is functioning.
5. Thick secretions are present and difficult to suction.
   a. Stimulate client's cough.
   b. Notify physician if signs and symptoms of infection are present.
   c. Provide increased fluids if not contraindicated. Inadequately hydrated clients may have thick secretions.

Recording and Reporting

- Record respiratory assessments before and after suctioning; size of catheter used; route; amount, consistency, and color of secretions obtained; frequency of suctioning.
- Record client's tolerance of procedure.

Sample Documentation

1200 Occasional productive cough. Client requires hourly suctioning per ET tube of moderate amount (5 ml or less) of thick yellow sputum. Able to use Yankauer catheter to suction mouth with good technique. Lungs clear after cough and suctioning. O_2 saturation 92% to 94%. Respirations nonlabored.

SPECIAL CONSIDERATIONS

Pediatric Considerations

- Diameter of suction catheter should be one-half the diameter of the child's tracheostomy or other artificial airway (Wong and others, 1999).
- Vacuum pressure should range from 40 to 60 mm Hg for preterm infants (Wong and others, 1999).
- Vacuum pressure should range from 60 to 100 mm Hg for infants and children (Wong and others, 1999).
- Closed suction systems are only used on older children. Care must be used so that the weight of the closed system does not displace the child's ET tube.

Geriatric Considerations

- Older adults with ischemic cardiac or obstructive pulmonary disease may benefit from maintenance of oxygen supply during suctioning in order to reduce the risk of irregular heartbeats.
- Due to increased fragility of tissues, older adults may have bloody suction returns. If this occurs, monitor the suction return for clearing and avoid unnecessary suctioning.

Home Care Considerations

- In the home it is necessary to adhere to best practices for infection control while weighing the necessity of cost-effectiveness in a chronic situation. For example, clean suctioning techniques may be acceptable, and the secretion collection container may be cleaned and disinfected every 24 hours.
- Assess the knowledge level of the client and caregivers to determine the amount of instruction and frequency of visits required for safe, effective practices.
- Portable suction machines are more common in the home or long-term care settings; with these suction machines, as the secretion jar fills, efficiency of the suction decreases.

Skill 31.4

Airway Management: Endotracheal Tube and Tracheostomy Care

The presence of an artificial airway places the client at high risk for infection. Correct care of the artificial airway will help to prevent infection from occurring. Artificial airways also make the client susceptible to airway injury. When artificial airways are used, it is essential that they be maintained in the correct position or damage may occur.

ET tubes are used as short-term artificial airways to administer mechanical ventilation, relieve upper airway obstruction, protect against aspiration, or clear secretions (see Figure 31-6, p. 761). ET tubes are generally removed within 14 days. If the client requires continued assistance from an artificial airway, a tracheostomy is considered for long-term use. A surgical incision is made into the trachea, and a short artificial airway (a tracheostomy tube) is inserted (see Figure 31-7, *A*, p. 761).

ASSESSMENT

1. Observe condition of tube and inspect around mouth/skin. ET tube: soiled or loose tape; pressure sores on nares, lip, or corner of mouth; nonstable tube; excessive secretions. Tracheostomy tube: soiled or loose ties or dressing; nonstable tube; excessive secretions. *Rationale: A client with an artificial airway is at increased risk due to an inability or difficulty controlling secretions and due to pressure points of the artificial airway.*

2. Identify factors that increase risk of complications from ET tubes: type and size of tube, movement of tube up and down trachea, depth of tube cuff size, and duration of placement. *Rationale: Tube moving up and down trachea disposes client to tracheal trauma or dislodgement. Cuff underinflation may allow aspiration, whereas overinflation may cause ischemia or necrosis of tracheal tissue. Longer duration increases risk of lower airway complications such as pneumonia (Perry and Potter, 2002).*
3. Auscultate lungs bilaterally. *Rationale: Provides baseline confirming bilateral lung inflation.*
4. Assess client's knowledge and comfort with procedure. *Rationale: Facilitates client's learning and participation in care.*
5. If applicable, assess client's understanding of and ability to perform own tracheostomy care. *Rationale: Increases client's feeling of autonomy and decreases feelings of lack of control over condition/secretions.*

PLANNING

Expected outcomes focus on the prevention of infection and breakdown around the artificial airway.

Expected Outcomes

1. Client's artificial airway/tube is in correct position and properly secured.
2. Client remains afebrile without signs and symptoms of infection.
3. Client's oral mucous membrane/stoma remains free of breakdown or accumulation of secretions.
4. Client's artificial airway is intact without persistent dried secretions.
5. Client understands purpose and is cooperative with care.
6. Client is able to demonstrate correct technique of tracheostomy care when appropriate.

Equipment

Endotracheal Tube Care

- Towel
- ET and oropharyngeal suction equipment
- 1 to 1½-inch adhesive or waterproof tape (not paper tape) or commercial ET stabilizer (follow manufacturer's instructions for securing)

- Two pairs of nonsterile gloves
- Adhesive remover swab or acetone on a cotton ball
- Mouth care supplies (e.g., toothbrush, toothpaste, mouth swabs)
- Face cleanser (e.g., wet washcloth, towel, soap, shaving supplies)
- Clean 2 × 2 gauze
- Tincture of benzoin or liquid adhesive
- Face shield (if indicated)

Tracheostomy Care

- Bedside table
- Towel
- Tracheostomy suction supplies
- Sterile tracheostomy care kit, if available, or

> Three sterile 4 × 4 gauze pads
> Sterile cotton-tipped applicators
> Sterile tracheostomy dressing
> Sterile basin
> Small sterile brush (or disposable cannula)
> Tracheostomy ties (e.g., twill tape, manufactured tracheostomy ties, Velcro tracheostomy ties)

- Hydrogen peroxide
- Normal saline (NS)
- Scissors
- Two sterile gloves
- Face shield, if indicated

Delegation Considerations

The skill of ET tube care requires the critical thinking and knowledge application unique to a nurse. The skill of tracheostomy care can be delegated to assistive personnel (AP) when a permanent or long-term tracheostomy is in place. In critically ill clients receiving mechanical ventilation this skill should not be delegated. Teach care provider emergency procedures in case the tracheostomy tube inadvertently becomes dislodged when ties are changed.

IMPLEMENTATION FOR AIRWAY MANAGEMENT: ENDOTRACHEAL TUBE AND TRACHEOSTOMY CARE

Steps	Rationale
1. See Standard Protocol (inside front cover).	
2. **Endotracheal tube care** a. Initiate endotracheal suction.	Removes secretions. Diminishes client's need to cough during procedure.

Steps	**Rationale**

NURSE ALERT *An oral airway should be immediately accessible in the event that the client bites down and obstructs the ET tube.*

COMMUNICATION TIP *Instruct client not to bite or move ET tube with tongue or pull on tubing; removal of tape can be uncomfortable.*

Steps	**Rationale**
b. Leave Yankauer suction catheter connected to suction source.	Prepares for oropharyngeal suctioning.
c. Prepare tape. Cut piece of tape long enough to go completely around client's head from naris to naris plus 15 cm (6 inches): adult, about 30 to 60 cm (1 to 2 feet). Lay adhesive side up on bedside table. Cut and lay 8 to 16 cm (3 to 6 inches) of tape, adhesive side down, in center of long strip to prevent tape from sticking to hair.	Adhesive tape must be placed around head from cheek to cheek below ears.
d. Have an assistant also apply a pair of gloves and hold ET tube firmly so that tube does not move.	Reduces transmission of microorganisms. Maintains proper tube position and prevents accidental extubation.
e. Carefully remove tape from ET tube and client's face. If tape is difficult to remove, moisten with water or adhesive tape remover. Discard tape in appropriate receptacle if nearby. If not, place soiled tape on bedside table or on distant end of towel.	Provides nurse with access to skin under tape for assessment and hygiene. Reduces transmission of microorganisms.
f. Use adhesive remover swab to remove excess adhesive left on face after tape removal.	Promotes hygiene. Unremoved adhesive can cause damage to skin and prevent poor adhesion of new tape.
g. Remove oral airway or bite block if present.	Provides access to and complete observation of client's oral cavity.
h. Clean mouth, gums, and teeth opposite ET tube with mouthwash solution and 4 × 4 gauze, sponge-tipped applicators, or saline swabs. Brush teeth as indicated. If necessary, administer oropharyngeal suctioning with Yankauer catheter.	Care must be taken to not allow aspiration to occur.
i. *Oral ET tube only:* Note "cm" ET tube marking at lips or gums. With help of assistant, move ET tube to opposite side or center of mouth. Do not change tube depth.	Prevents pressure sore formation at sides of client's mouth. Ensures correct position of tube.
j. Repeat oral cleaning as in Step h on opposite side of mouth.	Removes secretions from mouth and oropharynx.
k. Clean face and neck with soapy washcloth; rinse and dry. Shave male client as necessary.	Moisture and beard growth prevent adhesive tape adherence.
l. Pour small amount of tincture of benzoin on clean 2 × 2 gauze, and dot on upper lip (oral ET tube) or across nose (nasal ET tube) and cheeks to ear. Allow to dry completely.	Protects and makes skin more receptive to tape.
m. Slip tape under client's head and neck, adhesive side down. Take care not to twist tape or catch hair. Do not allow tape to stick to itself. It helps to stick tape gently to tongue blade, which serves as a guide. Then slide tongue blade under client's neck. Center tape so that double-faced tape extends around back of neck from ear to ear.	Positions tape to secure ET tube in proper position.

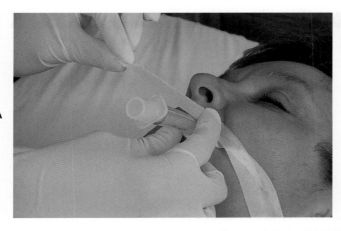

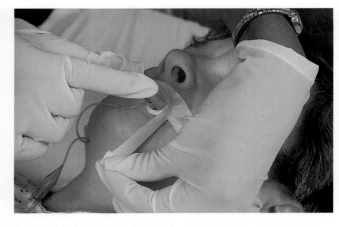

A B

Step 2n **A,** Securing bottom half of tape across client's upper lip. **B,** Securing top half of tape around tube.

Steps	Rationale
n. On one side of face, secure tape from ear to naris (nasal ET tube) or edge of mouth (oral ET tube). Tear remaining tape in half lengthwise, forming two pieces that are $\frac{1}{2}$- to $\frac{3}{4}$-inch wide. Secure bottom half of tape across upper lip (oral ET tube) or across top of nose (nasal ET tube) (see illustration *A*). Wrap top half of tape around tube (see illustration *B*).	Secures tape to face. Using top tape to wrap prevents downward drag on ET tube.
o. Gently pull other side of tape firmly to pick up slack, and secure to remaining side of face (see illustration). Assistant can release hold when tube is secure. Nurse may want assistant to help reinsert oral airway.	Secures tape to face and tube. ET tube should be at same depth at the lips. Check earlier assessment for verification of tube depth in centimeters.
p. Clean oral airway in warm soapy water, and rinse well. Hydrogen peroxide can aid in removal of crusted secretions. Shake excess water from oral airway.	Promotes hygiene. Reduces transmission of microorganisms.
q. Reinsert oral airway without pushing tongue into oropharynx.	Prevents client from biting ET tube and allows access for oropharyngeal suctioning.

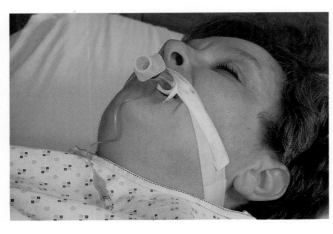

Step 2o Tape securing ET tube.

Steps	Rationale

3. **Tracheostomy care**

a. Suction tracheostomy (see Skill 31.3, p. 764). Before removing gloves, remove soiled tracheostomy dressing, discard in glove with coiled catheter, and perform hand hygiene.

Removes secretions so as not to occlude outer cannula while inner cannula is removed. Reduces need for client to cough.

b. While client is replenishing oxygen stores, prepare equipment on bedside table. Open sterile tracheostomy kit. Open three 4 × 4 gauze packages using aseptic technique, and pour NS on one package and hydrogen peroxide on another. Leave third package dry.

Allows for smooth, organized completion of tracheostomy care.

COMMUNICATION TIP   *Explain the importance of routine tracheostomy care to prevent infections or crusting and blockage. Explain that the procedure is not painful but that movement of the tracheostomy may promote coughing.*

---

c. Open two packages of cotton-tipped swabs, and pour NS on one package and hydrogen peroxide on the other.

Preparation and organization of equipment allows the nurse to complete tracheostomy care procedure efficiently and then reconnect client to oxygen source in a timely manner.

d. Open sterile tracheostomy package. Unwrap sterile basin, and pour about 2 cm (¾ inch) hydrogen peroxide into it. Open small sterile brush package, and place aseptically into sterile basin.

e. If using large roll of twill tape, cut appropriate length of tape (see Step 2c) and lay aside in dry area. Do not recap hydrogen peroxide and NS.

f. Apply sterile gloves. Keep dominant hand sterile throughout procedure.

Reduces transmission of microorganisms.

g. Remove oxygen source.

NURSE ALERT   *It is important to stabilize the tracheostomy tube at all times during tracheostomy care to prevent injury and unnecessary discomfort.*

---

h. If a nondisposable inner cannula is used:

(1) While touching only the outer aspect of the tube, remove the inner cannula with nondominant hand. Drop inner cannula into hydrogen peroxide basin.

Removes inner cannula for cleaning. Hydrogen peroxide loosens secretions from inner cannula.

(2) Place tracheostomy collar or T tube and ventilator oxygen source over or near outer cannula. (NOTE: T tube and ventilator oxygen devices cannot be attached to all outer cannulas when inner cannula is removed.)

Maintains supply of oxygen to client.

(3) To prevent oxygen desaturation in affected clients, quickly pick up inner cannula and use small brush to remove secretions inside and outside cannula (see illustration).

Tracheostomy brush provides mechanical force to remove thick or dried secretions.

(4) Hold inner cannula over basin, and rinse with NS, using nondominant hand to pour.

Removes secretions and hydrogen peroxide from inner cannula.

(5) Replace inner cannula, and secure "locking" mechanism (see illustration). Reapply ventilator or oxygen sources.

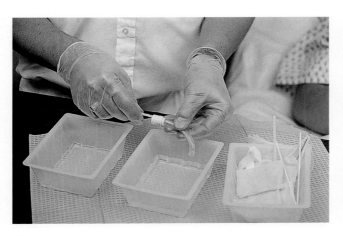

Step 3h(3)   Cleansing the tracheostomy inner cannula.

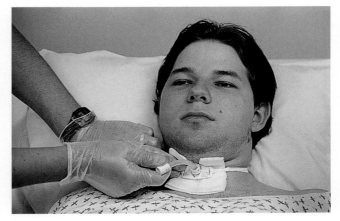

Step 3h(5)   Reinserting the inner cannula.

Steps	Rationale

i. If a disposable inner cannula is used:
   (1) Remove cannula from manufacturer's packaging.
   (2) While touching only the outer aspect of the tube, withdraw inner cannula and replace with new cannula. Lock into position.
   (3) Dispose of contaminated cannula in appropriate receptacle.
j. Using hydrogen peroxide–prepared cotton-tipped swabs and 4 × 4 gauze, clean exposed outer cannula surfaces and stoma under faceplate, extending 5 to 10 cm (2 to 4 inches) in all directions from stoma (see illustration). Clean in circular motion from stoma site outward, using dominant hand to handle sterile supplies.
k. Using NS–prepared cotton-tipped swabs and 4 × 4 gauze, rinse hydrogen peroxide from tracheostomy tube and skin surfaces.
l. Using dry 4 × 4 gauze, pat lightly at skin and exposed outer cannula surfaces.
	Maintains sterility of the inner aspect of the new cannula.
	
	Aseptically removes secretions from stoma site.
	
	Rinses hydrogen peroxide from surfaces, preventing possible irritation.
	
	Dry surfaces prohibit formation of moist environment from growth of microorganisms and skin excoriation.

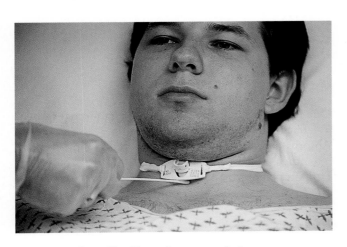

Step 3j   Cleansing around stoma.

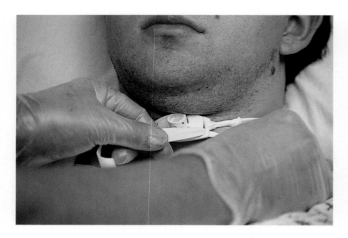

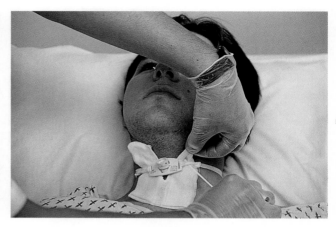

Step 3m(2)   Replacing tracheostomy ties when an assistant is not available. Do not remove old tracheostomy ties until new ones are secure.

Step 3n   Applying tracheostomy dressing.

Steps	Rationale
m. Instruct assistant, if available, to hold tracheostomy tube securely in place while ties are cut.	Promotes hygiene, reduces transmission of microorganisms, and secures tracheostomy tube.

NURSE ALERT   *Assistant must not release hold on tracheostomy tube until new ties are firmly tied to reduce risk of accidental extubation. If no assistant is present, do not cut old ties until new ties are in place and securely tied. (Follow manufacturer's guidelines for Velcro ties.)*

(1) Cut length of twill tape long enough to go around client's neck 2 times, about 60 to 75 cm (24 to 30 inches) for an adult. Cut ends on a diagonal.	Cutting ends of tie on a diagonal aids in inserting tie through eyelet.

NURSE ALERT   *Secure tracheostomy ties with one-finger slack. For accidental extubation, call for assistance and manually ventilate client with Ambu-bag, if necessary. Tracheostomy obturator should be kept at bedside with a fresh tracheostomy to facilitate reinsertion of the outer cannula, if dislodged. An additional tracheostomy tube of the same size and shape should be kept on hand for emergency replacement.*

(2) Insert one end of tie through faceplate eyelet, and pull ends even (see illustration).	
(3) Slide both ends of tie behind head and around neck to other eyelet, and insert one tie through second eyelet.	
(4) Pull snugly.	
(5) Tie ends securely in double square knot, allowing space for only one finger in tie.	One-finger slack prevents ties from being too tight when tracheostomy dressing is in place.
n. Insert fresh tracheostomy dressing under clean ties and faceplate (see illustration).	Absorbs drainage. Dressing prevents pressure on clavicle heads.
o. Position client comfortably, and assess respiratory status.	Promotes comfort. Some clients may require post–tracheostomy care suctioning.

4. See Completion Protocol (inside front cover).

· · · · · · · · · · ·

EVALUATION

1. Auscultate lungs and observe that airway is in proper position with tape/ties secure and comfortable for client. ET tube should be at the same depth as before care (as per physician order), with the same centimeter marking at lips and equal bilateral breath sounds.
2. Measure client's temperature; observe stoma for signs of infection.
3. Compare oral mucosa and airway assessments before and after artificial airway care. Observe for signs of tissue breakdown or persistent dried secretions.
4. Observe client's actions to determine compliance with the procedure.
5. Have client indicate when tracheostomy care is required, and independently demonstrate the technique for tracheostomy tube care.

Unexpected Outcomes and Related Interventions

1. Tube is not secure, and artificial airway moves in or out or is coughed out by client.
   a. Adjust or apply new ties.
2. Breath sounds not equal bilaterally with an ET tube in place.
   a. Evaluate ET tube for proper depth. If incorrect, arrange for ET tube to be repositioned as allowed by institution.
   b. Obtain order for chest x-ray study to verify placement if applicable.
   c. Assess client's respiratory status, and observe for the presence of mucus plugs.
3. Breakdown, pressure areas, or stomatitis (tracheostomy tube) are observed.
   a. Increase frequency of tube care.
   b. Make sure skin areas are clean and dry.
4. Hard, reddened areas with or without excessive or foul-smelling secretions are observed.
   a. Indicates infection. Notify physician.
   b. Increase frequency of tube care.
   c. Remove inner cannula, if applicable, for cleaning and suctioning.

5. Accidental extubation
   a. Call for assistance
   b. Maintain patent airway: Replace old tracheostomy tube with new tube.
   c. Observe vital signs and signs of respiratory distress.

Recording and Reporting

- Record respiratory assessments before and after care.
- Record ET tube care: depth of ET tube, frequency and extent of care, client tolerance, and any complications related to presence of the tube.
- Record tracheostomy care: type and size of tracheostomy tube, frequency and extent of care, client tolerance, and any complications related to presence of the tube.

Sample Documentation

0800 Routine ET tube care done. Size 7.5-cm tube remains with 22-cm marking at lips. No irritation or skin breakdown noted. Mouth care given. Respirations even and easy at a rate of 16 breaths per minute. Clear breath sounds bilaterally.

⊛ SPECIAL CONSIDERATIONS ⊛

Pediatric Considerations
Children who have recently undergone a tracheostomy must be closely monitored for hemorrhage, edema, aspiration, accidental decannulation, tube obstruction, or the entrance of free air into the pleural cavity (Wong and others, 1999).

Geriatric Considerations
Older adult skin may be more fragile and prone to breakdown from secretions or pressure or to tearing when tape is removed.

Home Care Considerations
Caregivers in the home must know signs and symptoms of respiratory and stomal infections (see Chapter 40).

Skill 31.5

Managing Closed Chest Drainage Systems (Including Managing Postoperative Autotransfusions)

Trauma, disease, or surgery can interrupt the closed negative-pressure system of the lungs, causing lung collapse. Air (pneumothorax) or fluid (hemothorax) may leak into the pleural cavity. A chest tube is inserted, and a closed chest drainage system is attached to promote drainage of air and fluid (Figure 31-8). Suction may be added to assist gravity in draining the lung. Lung reexpansion and improved oxygenation occur as the fluid or air is removed.

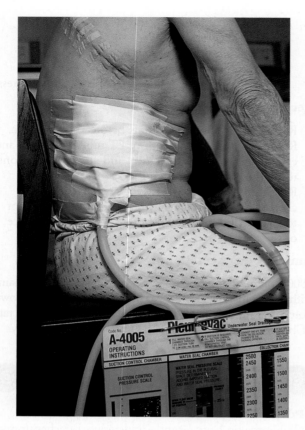

Figure 31-8 Pleural chest tube in place following open heart surgery.

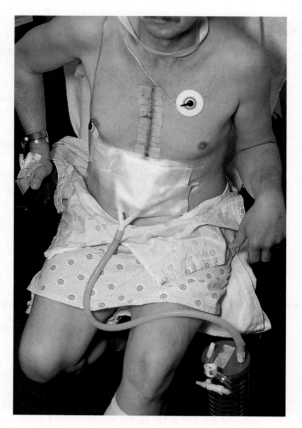

Figure 31-10 Mediastinal chest tube.

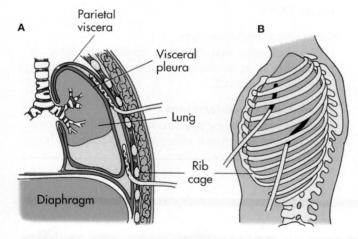

Figure 31-9 Diagram of sites for chest tube placement.

The location of the chest tube indicates the type of drainage expected. Because air rises, apical and anterior chest tube placement (Figure 31-9, *A*) promotes removal of air. Chest tubes are placed low and posterior or lateral (Figure 31-9, *B*) to drain fluid. A mediastinal chest tube is placed just below the sternum (Figure 31-10) and drains

blood or fluid, preventing its accumulation around the heart (e.g., after open heart surgery).

Although single-bottle systems are available, single-unit water-seal or waterless systems are most often used. The water-seal system is composed of two or three compartments or chambers (Figure 31-11). Fluid is drained into the first chamber. The second chamber contains the water seal, which allows air to escape because of the force of expiration but not to reenter on inspiration. If suction is to be used, a third chamber is used. The amount of suction depends on the amount of sterile water in the suction chamber.

The waterless system (Figure 31-12) follows the same principles, except sterile water is not required for setup. The water seal is replaced by a one-way valve located near the top of the system. Most of the single unit is the drainage chamber. The suction chamber contains a suction control float ball that is set by a suction control dial after the suction source is turned on.

Autotransfusion can be linked with chest drainage after open heart surgery or thoracic surgery to replace mediastinal blood lost and allow lung reexpansion (Figure 31-13). Autotransfusion enables the client to avoid other donor blood transfusion. The client's own blood is drained from the chest and re-infused.

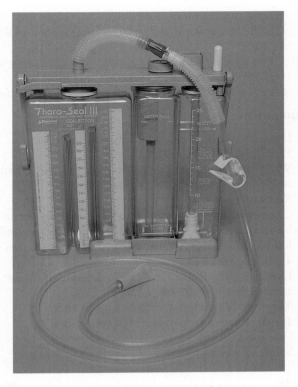

Figure 31-11   Disposable chest drainage system.

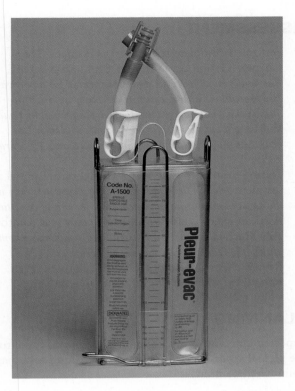

Figure 31-13   Example of reinfusion replacement bag.

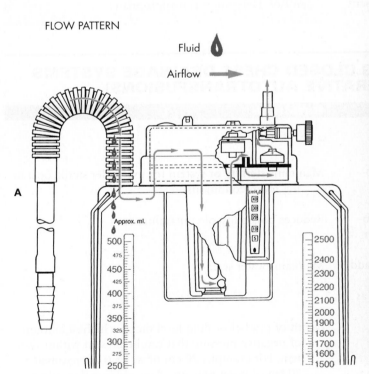

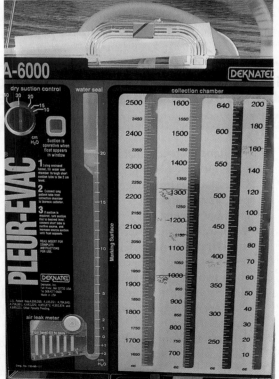

Figure 31-12   A, Suction-regulating device. **B,** Collection chamber is marked at specified intervals to monitor amount of drainage.

ASSESSMENT

1. Perform a complete respiratory assessment (see Chapter 13) and baseline vital signs and oximetry. *Rationale: Baseline vitals signs are essential for any invasive procedure. Clients requiring chest tube insertion frequently have respiratory distress. Sharp stabbing chest pain with or without decreased blood pressure and increased heart rate may indicate a tension pneumothorax (Woodruff, 1999).*
2. During procedure observe for changes from initial assessment. *Rationale: Changes in these parameters may indicate worsening or improvement from the initial condition.*
3. Assess if client is able to breathe deeply and comfortably. *Rationale: Detects early signs and symptoms of complications. Promotes reexpansion of the lung.*
4. Review client's hemoglobin and hematocrit levels. *Rationale: Parameters reflect if blood loss is occurring.*

PLANNING

Expected outcomes focus on removal of air and fluid from the pleural space and re-expansion of the lung with maximum client comfort.

Expected Outcomes

1. Client's respirations are nonlabored.
2. Client's breath sounds are present in all lobes, and lung expansion is symmetrical.
3. Client's vital signs, hemoglobin level, and hematocrit are within normal ranges by discharge.

4. Client uses breathing exercises.
5. Client reports improved comfort using a scale of 0 to 10.
6. Chest tube remains in place, and chest drainage system remains airtight and functioning properly.
7. Client's oxygen saturation is within client's normal range.

Equipment

- Local anesthetic, if not an emergent procedure
- Prescribed drainage system
- Water-seal system versus waterless system: sterile water or NS as per manufacturer's directions
- Suction, if used
- Chest tube tray (all items are sterile), typically: knife handle, chest tube clamp, small sponge forceps, needle holder, knife blade, suture, sterile drape, two clamps, 4 × 4 sponges, suture scissors
- Dressings: petroleum gauze, large dressing of choice, additional 4 × 4 dressings, tape
- Two shodded hemostats for each chest tube
- 1-inch adhesive tape for taping connections
- Face mask/shield
- Sterile gloves

Delegation Considerations

The skill of chest tube management requires the critical thinking and knowledge application unique to an RN. Delegation is inappropriate.

IMPLEMENTATION FOR MANAGING CLOSED CHEST DRAINAGE SYSTEMS (INCLUDING MANAGING POSTOPERATIVE AUTOTRANSFUSIONS)

Steps	Rationale
1. See Standard Protocol (inside front cover).	
2. **Set up water-seal system.**	
a. Obtain a chest drainage system. Remove wrappers, and prepare to set up as a two- or three-chamber system.	Maintains sterility of system for use under sterile operating room conditions.
b. While maintaining sterility of the drainage tubing, stand system upright and add sterile water or NS to appropriate compartments.	Reduces possibility of contamination.
c. For a two-chamber system (without suction), add sterile solution to water-seal chamber (second chamber), bringing fluid to the required level as indicated.	Maintains water seal.
d. For a three-chamber system (without suction), add sterile solution to the water-seal chamber (second chamber). Add amount of sterile solution prescribed by physician to the suction control (third) chamber, usually 20 cm (8 inches). Connect tubing from suction control chamber to suction source.	Depth of rod below fluid level dictates highest amount of negative pressure that can be present within system. For example, 20 cm of water is approximately 20 cm of water pressure. Any additional negative pressure applied to system is vented into atmosphere through suction control vent. This safety device prevents damage to pleural tissues from an unexpected surge of negative pressure from suction source.

Steps	Rationale
3. Set up waterless system.	
a. Remove sterile wrappers, and prepare to set up.	Maintains sterility of system for use under sterile operating room conditions.
b. For a two-chamber system (without suction), nothing is added or needs to be done to system.	Waterless two-chamber system is ready for connecting to client's chest tube after opening wrappers.
c. For a three-chamber waterless system with suction, connect tubing from suction control chamber to suction source.	Suction source provides additional negative pressure to system.
d. Instill 15 ml sterile water or normal saline into diagnostic indicator injection port located on top of system.	This is not necessary for mediastinal drainage because there will be no tidaling. Also, in an emergency, this is not necessary because system does not require water for setup.
4. Tape all connections in a spiral fashion using 1-inch adhesive tape. Then check both systems for patency by:	Prevents atmospheric air from leaking into system and client's intrapleural space. Provides chance to ensure airtight system before connecting it to client. Allows correction or replacement of system if it is defective before connecting it to the client.
a. Clamping the drainage tubing that will connect client to system	
b. Connecting tubing from the float ball chamber to suction source	

NURSE ALERT   *Bubbling will be seen at first because there is air in tubing and system initially. This should stop after a few minutes unless other sources of air are entering system. If bubbling continues, check connections and locate source of air leak as described in Table 31-3.*

Steps	Rationale
c. Turning on suction to prescribed level.	
5. Turn off suction source, and unclamp drainage tubing before connecting client to system.	Having client connected to suction when it is initiated could damage pleural tissues from sudden increase in negative pressure. Suction source is turned on again after client is connected to three-chamber system.
6. Position the client. During tube insertion, position client so the side in which the tube will be placed is accessible to physician. After tube placement client is positioned:	
a. Using semi-Fowler's to high-Fowler's position to evacuate air (pneumothorax)	Permits optimum drainage of fluid and/or air. Air rises to highest point in the chest.
b. Using high-Fowler's position to drain fluid (hemothorax)	Permits optimum drainage of fluid.
7. Assist physician with chest tube insertion by providing needed equipment, analgesic, and offering support and instruction to the client.	
8. Help physician attach drainage tube to chest tube.	Connects drainage system and suction (if ordered) to chest tube.
9. Tape tube connection between chest and drainage tubes. One method: One long strip of tape on each side with an overlapping tape wrapped spirally enables connections to be observed and remain secure.	Secures chest tube to drainage system and reduces risk of air leaks causing breaks in airtight system.
10. Check patency of air vents in system.	
a. Water-seal vent must have no occlusion.	Permits displaced air to pass into atmosphere.
b. Suction control chamber vent must have no occlusion when using suction.	Provides safety factor of releasing excess negative pressure into atmosphere.
c. Waterless systems have relief valves without caps.	
11. Coil excess tubing on mattress next to client. Secure with a rubber band and safety pin or system's clamp.	Prevents excess tubing from hanging over edge of mattress in a dependent loop. Drainage could collect in loop and occlude drainage system (Gordon and others, 1997).

Table 31-3

Problem Solving With Chest Tubes

Assessment	Intervention
1. Air leak can occur at insertion site, connection between tube and drainage, or within drainage device itself. Continuous bubbling is noted in water-seal chamber and water seal.	Locate leak by clamping tube at different intervals along the tube. Leaks are corrected when constant bubbling stops.
2. Assess for location of leak by clamping chest tube with two rubber shod or toothless clamps close to the chest wall. If bubbling stops, air leak is inside client's thorax or at chest insertion site.	**NURSE ALERT** *Unclamp tube, reinforce chest dressing, and notify physician immediately. Rationale: Leaving chest tube clamped can cause collapse of lung, mediastinal shift, and eventual collapse of other lung from buildup of air pressure within the pleural cavity.*
3. If bubbling continues with the clamps near the chest wall, gradually move one clamp at a time down drainage tubing away from client and toward suction control chamber. When bubbling stops, leak is in section of tubing or connection between the clamps.	Replace tubing, or secure connection and release clamps.
4. If bubbling still continues, this indicates the leak is in the drainage system.	Change the drainage system.
5. Assess for tension pneumothorax: • Severe respiratory distress • Low oxygen saturation • Chest pain • Absence of breath sounds on affected side • Tracheal shift to unaffected side • Hypotension and signs of shock • Tachycardia	Make sure chest tubes are patent: remove clamps, eliminate kinks, or eliminate occlusion. *Rationale: Obstructed chest tubes trap air in intrapleural space when air leak originates within the thorax.* Notify physician immediately, and prepare for another chest tube insertion. A flutter (Heimlich) valve or large-gauge needle may be used for short-term emergency release of pressure in the intrapleural space. Have emergency equipment, oxygen, and code card available because condition is life threatening.
6. Water seal tube is no longer submerged in sterile fluid because of evaporation.	Add sterile water to water-seal chamber until distal tip is 2 cm under surface level.

Steps	Rationale
12. Adjust tubing to hang in a straight line from top of mattress to drainage chamber.	Promotes drainage.
13. Provide two shodded hemostats for each chest tube. Shodded hemostats are usually attached to top of client's bed with adhesive tape or clamped to client's clothing during ambulation.	Chest tubes are double-clamped under specific circumstances: (1) to assess for an air leak (see Table 31-3) and (2) to empty or change collection bottle or chamber or disposable systems. Have new system ready to be connected before clamping tube so that transfer can be rapid and drainage system reestablished.
14. **Care for client with chest tubes** a. Assess vital signs; oxygen saturation; skin color; breath sounds; and rate, depth, and ease of respirations.	Provides baseline and information about procedure-related complications.
b. Monitor color, consistency, and amount of drainage every 15 minutes for the first 2 hours, indicating level of drainage fluid, date, and time on chamber's write-on surface.	Provides baseline for continuous assessment of type and quantity of drainage. Ensures early detection of complications.

Steps	Rationale
(1) From mediastinal tube less than 100 ml/hr is expected and a total of approximately 500 ml in first 24 hours.	Sudden gush of drainage may result from coughing or changing client's position; releasing blood rather than indicating active bleeding.
(2) From a posterior chest tube between 100 and 300 ml is expected during first 2 hours after insertion, which decreases, and a total of 500 to 1000 ml can be expected in first 24 hours.	
(3) From an anterior chest tube that primarily removes air, much less drainage is expected.	

COMMUNICATION TIP *Discuss client's continued participation in care, as appropriate. Medicate as needed.*

c. Observe chest dressing for drainage.	Increase in drainage may indicate blockage in chest tube.
d. Palpate around the tube for swelling and crepitus as evidenced by crackling.	Indicates presence of air trapping in subcutaneous tissues. Large area that travels to neck or face can result in respiratory distress (O'Hanlon-Nichols, 1996).
e. Check tubing to ensure it is free of kinks and dependent loops. Excess tubing should be coiled on bed or chair.	Promotes drainage.
f. Observe for fluctuation of drainage in the tubing during inspiration and expiration. Observe for clots or debris in tubing.	If fluctuation or tidaling stops, it means either the lung is fully expanded or the system is obstructed.
g. Keep drainage system upright and below level of the client's chest.	Promotes gravity drainage and prevents backflow of fluid and air into the pleural space.
h. Check for air leaks by monitoring the bubbling in the water seal chamber: Intermittent bubbling is normal during expiration when air is being evacuated from the pleural cavity, but continuous bubbling during both inspiration and expiration indicates a leak in the system.	Absence of bubbling may indicate that the lung has expanded, sealing the opening.
15. Obtain specimen.	
a. Cleanse resealing diaphragm or tubing with an antiseptic.	Reduces transmission of microorganisms.
b. Insert needle with bevel in the fresh drainage.	
c. Gently aspirate appropriate amount of fluid, and place into properly labeled container.	
d. Recleanse diaphragm with antiseptic swab.	
16. Assist in chest tube removal.	
a. Administer prescribed medication for pain relief about 30 minutes before procedure.	Reduces discomfort and relaxes client.
b. Assist client with sitting on edge of bed or lying on side without chest tubes.	Physician prescribes client's position to facilitate tube removal.
c. Physician prepares an occlusive dressing of petroleum gauze on a pressure dressing and sets it aside on a sterile field.	Essential to prepare in advance for quick application to wound during tube withdrawal.
d. Physician asks client to take a deep breath and hold it or exhale completely and hold it.	Prevents air from being sucked into chest as tube is removed.

COMMUNICATION TIP *Support client physically and emotionally while physician removes dressing and clips sutures.*

e. Physician holds prepared dressing at point of tube insertion and quickly pulls out chest tube.	Prevents entry of air through chest wound.

Steps	Rationale
f. Physician quickly and firmly secures it in position with elastic bandage (Elastoplast) or wide tape. Physician sometimes uses skin clips or draws purse-string sutures together before applying dressing.	Keeps wound aseptic. Prevents entry of air into chest. Wound closure occurs spontaneously. Clips or sutures aid in skin closure.

17. Perform postoperative autotransfusion.

Steps	Rationale
a. Set up the Pleur-evac autotransfusion system (ATS) using technique that maintains the sterility of unit and following three steps printed on front of unit (Deknatel, Inc) (see Figure 31-13, p. 777).	Contamination of unit provides a ready source of infection to client.
b. Make sure all connections are tight and all clamps are open.	Tight connections ensure an airtight system, and open clamps allow chest drainage to enter the ATS bag.
c. A mesh filter is located in the ATS bag to filter drainage.	Filtering drainage removes extraneous materials and microemboli.
d. ATS collection bag has a capacity of 1000 ml, marked in increments of 25 ml, and an area for marking times and amounts.	
e. Continue collection.	
(1) Open Pleur-evac A-1500 replacement bag using proper technique, and close two white clamps.	Contamination of unit provides a ready source of contamination to client. Closed clamps maintain a closed system during replacement.
(2) Use high-negativity relief valve to reduce excessive negativity.	Eases removal of initial collection bag from metal support stand.
(3) Perform bag transfer.	
(a) Close clamp on chest drainage tubing.	Prevents air from entering chest cavity through tube and collapsing lung.
(b) Close two white clamps on top of initial ATS collection bag.	Maintains a closed system for reinfusion, preventing contamination of blood.
(c) Connect chest drainage tube to new ATS bag using red containers. Make certain that all connections are tight.	
(d) Open all clamps on chest drainage tube and replacement bag.	Reestablishes an autotransfusion collection system.
f. Connect red and blue connectors on top of initial collection bag, and remove it by lifting it from side hook and then from foot hook.	Maintains a closed system within bag and removes it for use in autotransfusion.
g. Secure replacement bag by connecting foot hook, replacing metal frame into side hook of Pleur-evac unit, and pushing down to secure frame into hook.	Secures collection device and reduces risk of unit tipping over.
h. Replacement bag is removed by placing the thumbs on top of metal frame and pushing up with fingers to slide bag out.	
i. Initiate Pleur-evac autotransfusion re-infusion.	
(1) Use a new microaggregate filter to reinfuse each autotransfusion bag.	Prevents infusion of microemboli and provides maximum filtration for each bag.
(2) Access bag by inverting it, spiking it through spike port with microaggregate filter, and twisting.	Connects autotransfusion bag to transfusion tubing.
(3) With bag upside down, gently squeeze it to remove the air and prime the filter with blood.	Gentle pressure is used to prevent hemolysis.

Steps	Rationale
(4) Hang bag on an intravenous (IV) pole, and continue to prime tubing until all air is gone. Clamp tubing, attach it to client's IV access, and adjust clamp to deliver the reinfusion at the appropriate rate.	Removes all air from transfusion tubing and establishes the reinfusion. Gravity, a blood cuff (not to exceed 150 mm Hg pressure), or a blood-compatible IV pump may be used.
(5) If ordered, anticoagulants (i.e., heparin) can be added to the reinfusion through self-sealing port in autotransfusion connector.	Prevents clotting in the autotransfusion.

NURSE ALERT   *Stripping or milking the chest tube is controversial and should be performed according to hospital policy. Stripping creates a high degree of negative pressure and potentially may pull lung tissue or pleura into drainage holes of chest tube.*

---

    j. Discontinue autotransfusion.

(1) Clamp chest drainage tube, and connect it directly to Pleur-evac unit using red and blue connectors.	Prevents air from entering chest cavity through tube and collapsing lung.
(2) Open chest drainage tube clamp.	All drainage will be collected directly in Pleur-evac unit and must be appropriately discarded.

18. See Completion Protocol (inside front cover).

• • • • • • • • • •

EVALUATION

1. Assess client for decreased respiratory distress and chest pain.
2. Auscultate client's lungs, and observe chest expansion.
3. Monitor vital signs, hematocrit, and hemoglobin level.
4. Evaluate client's ability to use deep-breathing exercises while maintaining comfort.
5. Reassess client level of comfort (on a scale of 0-10) comparing level with comfort prior to chest tube insertion.
6. Monitor continued functioning of system, as indicated by reduction in the amount of drainage, resolution of the air leak, and complete reexpansion of the lung.
7. Monitor client's oxygen saturation.

Unexpected Outcomes and Related Interventions

1. Air leak is unrelated to client's respiration.
   a. See Table 31-3 on p. 780 for determining the source of an air leak and problem solving.
2. Chest tubes become obstructed by a clot or kinked tube.
   a. Observe client for mediastinal shift or respiratory distress, which may constitute a medical emergency.
   b. Determine source of obstruction, as noted by lack of flow through tube or clot detected in system. If kinked, straighten tubing and adjust to prevent continued problems.
   c. If clot is identified, notify physician.

3. Chest tube becomes dislodged.
   a. Immediately apply pressure over chest tube site with anything that is within immediate reach (e.g., several layers of client's hospital gown, bed-sheet, towel, gauze dressings).
   b. Have assistant obtain a sterile petroleum dressing. Apply as client exhales. Secure dressing with a tight seal.
   c. Notify physician.
4. Substantial increase in bright-red drainage is observed.
   a. Observe for tachycardia and hypotension.
   b. Report to physician, because this may indicate that client is actively bleeding.
5. Drainage system is knocked on side or damaged.
   a. Observe for signs of increasing pneumothorax, which would indicate that water seal is not being maintained. Notify physician.
   b. Obtain a second unit, and change system after following setup guidelines.

Recording and Reporting

- Record respiratory assessment; amount of suction, if used; amount of drainage since the previous assessment; type of drainage in chest tubing; presence or absence of an air leak, including amount if present.
- Record integrity of dressing and presence of drainage.
- Record client comfort and tolerance.

Sample Documentation

0800 Client resting comfortably, denies complaint. Respirations even and easy. Lungs clear with breath sounds heard over all lung fields. Posterior chest tube and dressing remain intact with oscillation present in water-seal chamber. No air leak noted. 50 ml serous drainage collected in past 8 hours. Continues to take deep breaths as instructed without complaints of discomfort.

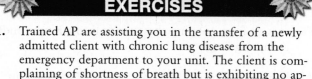
CRITICAL THINKING EXERCISES

1. Trained AP are assisting you in the transfer of a newly admitted client with chronic lung disease from the emergency department to your unit. The client is complaining of shortness of breath but is exhibiting no apparent respiratory distress. Vital signs are blood pressure 160/88 mm Hg, heart rate 92 beats per minute, respirations 20 breaths per minute, and temperature 99.4° F, with an oximetry reading of 86%. Supplemental oxygen per nasal cannula has been ordered at 2 liters but has not been started. What interventions would you as the RN perform, and what might you delegate to AP?
2. Your client has a permanent tracheostomy tube. Can you delegate suctioning? What would you tell the AP about this procedure?
3. Assessment of a client with a chest tube reveals a "new" air leak. What further assessment should be performed? What are possible interventions for your findings?

REFERENCES

Brooks D and others: Clinical practice guidelines for suctioning the airway of the intubated and non-intubated patient, *Can Respir J* 8(3):163, 2001.

Gordon PA and others: Positioning of chest tubes: effects on pressure and drainage, *Am J Crit Care* 6(1):33, 1997.

Kryger M, Roth T, Dement W: *Principles and practice of sleep medicine*, Philadelphia, 1994, Saunders.

Lueckenotte AG: *Gerontologic nursing*, ed 2, St Louis, 2000, Mosby.

McKelvie S: Endotracheal suctioning, *Nurs Crit Care* 3(5):244, 1998.

National Asthma Education and Prevention Program: *Expert panel report II: guidelines for the diagnosis and management of asthma*, Bethesda, Md, 1997, National Heart Lung and Blood Institute, National Institutes of Health.

O'Hanlon-Nichols T: Commonly asked questions about chest tubes, *Am J Nurs* 96(5):60, 1996.

Perry AG, Potter PA: *Clinical nursing skills and techniques*, ed 5, St Louis, 2002, Mosby.

St. John RE: Airway management, *Crit Care Nurse* 19(4):79, 1999.

Wong DL and others: *Whaley and Wong's nursing care of infants and children*, ed 6, St Louis, 1999, Mosby.

Woodruff DW: Pneumothorax, *RN* 62(9):62, 1999.

Intubation of the stomach with a flexible tube passed through the client's nares, nasopharynx, and esophagus and into the stomach (Figure 32-1) is sometimes performed after surgical procedures, when vomiting and gastric distention occur, and for irrigation of the stomach. In addition, there are times following major surgery, trauma, or as a result of conditions affecting the gastrointestinal tract when normal peristalsis temporarily becomes altered. Because peristalsis is slowed or absent, a client cannot eat or drink fluids without causing abdominal distention. When these conditions occur, temporary insertion of a nasogasrtric (NG) tube serves to decompress the stomach, keeping it empty until peristalsis returns.

Decompression of the stomach with removal of fluids and gas promotes abdominal comfort, decreases the risk of aspiration, and allows surgical anastomoses to heal without distention. When used for decompression, the tube is usually attached to low intermittent suction to facilitate the removal of secretions. For clients who are unable to swallow, the NG tube is frequently used for the administration of medications and may be used as a temporary feeding tube. The tube can also be used to irrigate the stomach and to remove toxic substances, such as in poisoning.

NG tubes are typically of a larger diameter (12 to 18 Fr) than feeding tubes (see Chapter 33) to enhance the removal of thick secretions or to instill fluids rapidly. Their stiffer composition and larger diameter make these tubes more uncomfortable for the client, and these tubes cause more irritation of the sensitive nasopharyngeal mucosa. NG tubes are constructed of a single lumen (Levin tube) or a central lumen and a separate air vent lumen (Salem sump tube). Important nursing measures for the client with an NG tube include measures to maintain patency of the tube, such as irrigation, and measures to promote comfort, such as positioning the tube to prevent pressure on the nares, cleansing around the nares, and lubrication of the oral and nasal membranes (Viall, 1996).

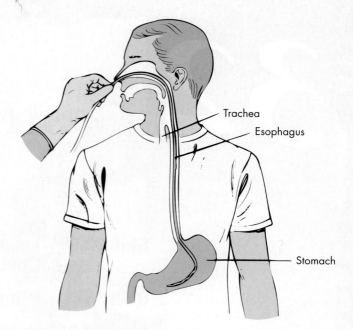

Figure 32-1   Placement of nasogastric tube.

NURSING DIAGNOSES

Nursing diagnoses for clients who may undergo NG intubation include **Risk for Aspiration,** in which clients are at risk of aspiration related to nausea and vomiting or delayed gastric emptying, and this risk is a primary reason for placement of the tube. The presence of an NG tube can lead to the diagnosis of **Impaired Oral Mucous Membrane** because NG tubes typically cause irritation, drying, and crusting of secretions. Removal of gastric secretions can produce **Deficient Fluid Volume** associated with altered electrolyte imbalance (see Chapter 30).

Skill 32.1

Inserting Nasogastric Tube (Includes Checking Placement of Nasal Tube)

This skill includes insertion of a large-bore flexible tube into the client's nares, nasopharynx, esophagus, and stomach. Placement of an NG tube requires a physician's order. The tube can be accidentally displaced into the pulmonary system, lie in the distal esophagus or gastric antrum rather than well into the stomach, or kink on itself in the stomach. In addition to displacement, other complications of NG tubes include impaired skin integrity of nares and nasal mucosa, sinusitis, earache, esophagitis, gastric or esophageal ulceration and bleeding, and pulmonary aspiration.

Clean technique is adequate for NG tube insertion. The procedure is, however, uncomfortable. Clients complain of a sensation of burning as the tube passes through the nasal mucosa. In addition, clients may also have dry, irritated nasal mucosa; the nares may be excoriated; frequent oral hygiene is also needed because clients with NG tubes frequently breathe through their mouth.

ASSESSMENT

1. Ask client about past history of nasal surgery or trauma. Inspect client's nares and oral cavity for deviated nasal septum, nasal surgery, inability to breathe well when either nasal opening is occluded, and nasal or oral irritation or bleeding. *Rationale: This information determines which naris the tube should be inserted through, provides baseline data about the condition of nasal and oral cavity, and determines the need for special measures for oral hygiene or comfort after the tube is inserted.*

2. Palpate client's abdomen for distention or pain, and auscultate for bowel sounds. *Rationale: Provides baseline information about the client's level of comfort, level of abdominal distention, and presence of abdominal sounds.*

3. Determine if client has had an NG tube insertion in the past. *Rationale: Procedure is uncomfortable; client's previous experience will complement any explanation.*

4. Assess client's level of consciousness and ability to cooperate or assist with the procedure and the need for special positioning during insertion.

5. Check medical record for physician's order, type of NG tube to be placed, and whether tube is to attach to suction or drainage bag. *Rationale: Procedure requires a physician's order. Adequate stomach decompression depends on NG suction.*

PLANNING

Expected outcomes focus on decompression of the stomach, comfort, adequacy of fluid volume, adequacy of nutrition, and prevention of complications related to NG intubation.

Expected Outcomes

1. Client's stomach remains soft without distention.
2. Client's level of comfort improves or remains the same.
3. Client's NG tube remains patent.
4. Client's nasal mucosa remains moist and intact.

Equipment (Figure 32-2)

- 14 to 15 Fr NG tube (smaller-lumen catheters are not used for compression in adults because they are not able to remove thick secretions)
- Water-soluble lubricating jelly

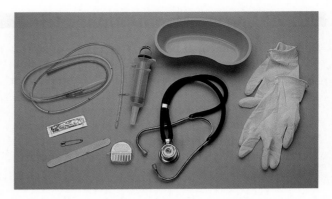

Figure 32-2 NG tube insertion equipment.

- pH test strips (measure gastric aspirate acidity)
- Tongue blade
- Flashlight
- 60-ml catheter tip syringe
- 1-inch (2.5 cm) wide hypoallergenic tape (3 to 4 inches long) or commercial fixation device
- Safety pin and rubber band
- Clamp, drainage bag, or suction machine or pressure gauge if wall suction is to be used
- Emesis basin
- Towel
- Glass of water with straw
- Facial tissues
- Tincture of benzoin (optional)
- Suction equipment
- Clean disposable gloves

 Delegation Considerations

This skill requires the critical thinking and knowledge application unique to a nurse. Assistive personnel (AP) may measure and record the drainage from the NG tube and provide oral and nasal hygiene. AP should also be taught how to properly secure the NG tube.

IMPLEMENTATION FOR INSERTING NASOGASTRIC TUBE (INCLUDES CHECKING PLACEMENT OF NASAL TUBE)

Steps	Rationale

1. See Standard Protocol (inside front cover).

NURSE ALERT *Have suction equipment and emesis basin within reach in case of vomiting.*

Steps	Rationale
2. Prepare equipment at bedside. Cut a piece of tape about 4 inches (10 cm) long, and split one half of it into two pieces to form a Y, or have NG tube fixator device available.	Ensures well-organized procedure. Tape or fixator device will be used to hold the tube in place after insertion.
3. Place client in high-Fowler's position with pillows behind head and shoulders. Raise bed to a horizontal level comfortable for the nurse.	Promotes client's ability to swallow during procedure. Good body mechanics prevents injury to nurse or client.
4. Place towel over client's chest; give facial tissues to client.	Prevents soiling of client's gown. Tube insertion through nasal passages may cause tearing and coughing with increased salivation.
5. Instruct client to relax and breathe normally while occluding one naris. Then repeat with other naris. Select nostril with greater airflow.	Tube passes more easily through naris that is more patent.
6. Stand on client's right side if right-handed, left side if left-handed.	
7. Measure distance to insert tube:	Approximates distance from naris to stomach. Tube should extend from naris to stomach; distance varied with each client.
a. Measure distance from tip of nose to earlobe to xiphoid process (see illustration).	
b. Mark a 50-cm point on the tube, then do traditional measurement. Tube insertion should be midway point between 50 cm (20 inches) and previous method.	
8. Mark this distance on tube with a removable piece of tape or an indelible marker.	
9. Curve 10 to 15 cm (4 to 6 inches) of end of tube tightly around index finger and then release.	Curving tube tip aids insertion and decreases tube stiffness.
10. Lubricate about 7.5 to 10 cm (3 to 4 inches of the distal end of the tube with a water-soluble lubricant.	Minimizes friction against nasal mucosa and aids in tube insertion.
11. Tell client that insertion is about to begin, and ask client to extend neck back against pillow (see illustration).	Promotes comfort and reduces friction during insertion. Position facilitates initial passage of tube through naris and maintains clear airway for open naris.
12. Insert tube slowly through naris with curved end pointing downward. Continue to insert tube along floor of nasal passage aiming down toward ear. If resistance is met, apply gentle downward pressure to advance tube. (Do not force past resistance.)	Minimizes discomfort of tube rubbing against upper nasal turbinates. Resistance is caused by posterior nasopharynx. Downward pressure helps tube curl around corner of nasopharynx.

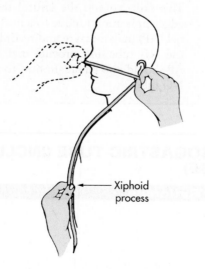

Xiphoid process

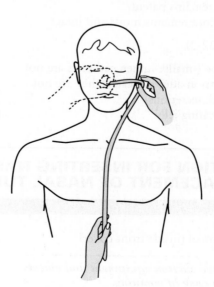

Step 7a Technique for measuring distance to insert NG tube.

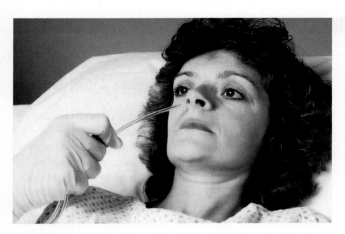

Step 11   Insert NG tube with curved end pointing downward.

Steps	Rationale
13. If resistance is met, try to rotate the tube and see if it advances. If still resistant, withdraw tube, allow client to rest, relubricate tube, and insert into other naris.	Forcing against resistance can cause trauma to mucosa.

NURSE ALERT   *If unable to insert tube in either nares, stop procedure and notify physician.*

Steps	Rationale
14. Continue insertion of tube until just past nasopharynx by gently rotating it toward the opposite nostril, then pass the tube just above oropharynx.	Helps prevent coiling of tube in oropharynx.
a. Stop tube advancement, allow client to relax, and provide tissues.	Relieves anxiety; tearing is a natural response to mucosal irritation, and excessive salivation may occur because of oral stimulation.
b. Explain to client that next step requires that client swallow. Give client glass of water, unless contraindicated.	Sipping of water aids passage of NG tube into esophagus.
15. With tube just above oropharynx, instruct client to flex head forward and swallow small sips of water. Advance tube 2.5 to 5 cm (1 to 2 inches) with each swallow.	Flexed position closes off upper airway to trachea and opens esophagus. Swallowing closes epiglottis over trachea and helps move the tube into the esophagus.
16. If client begins to cough, gag, or choke, withdraw slightly and stop tube advancement. Instruct client to breathe easily and take sips of water.	Tube may be displaced into larynx and produce coughing. Swallowing water eases gagging or choking. Risk for aspiration increases if vomiting occurs.

NURSE ALERT   *If vomiting occurs, assist client in clearing airway; oral suctioning may be needed. Do not proceed until airway is cleared.*

Steps	Rationale
17. If client continues to gag and cough or complains that tube feels as though it is coiling in back of throat, check back of oropharynx using tongue blade to compress client's tongue. If tube has coiled, withdraw it until the tip is back in the oropharynx. Then reinsert with client swallowing.	Tube may coil around itself in the back of throat and stimulate gag reflex.
18. Continue to advance tube with swallowing until tape or mark is reached. Temporarily anchor tube to cheek with a piece of tape until placement is checked.	Tip of tube must be well within stomach for adequate decompression. Tube should be anchored before placement is verified.

Steps	Rationale

19. Verify tube placement: Check agency policy for preferred methods for checking NG tube placement.

a. Ask client to speak.

Inability to speak can indicate that tube is through vocal cords into the lungs.

b. Inspect posterior pharynx for presence of coiled tube.

Tube is pliable and can coil up in back of pharynx instead of advancing into esophagus.

c. Draw up 30 ml of air into syringe. Attach the catheter-tipped syringe to end of tube, flush tube with the 30 ml of air before aspirating. Then aspirate gently back on syringe to obtain gastric contents, observing color.

Gastric contents are usually cloudy and green, but may be off-white, tan, bloody, or brown. Aspiration of contents provides a means to measure fluid pH and determine tube tip placement in gastrointestinal tract (Metheny and others, 1998a).

d. Measure pH of aspirate with color-coded pH paper with range of whole numbers at least 1 to 11 (see illustration).

Gastric secretions are usually highly acidic, preferably 4 or less, compared with intestinal aspirates, which are usually greater than 4, or respiratory secretions, which are usually greater than 5.5 (Metheny and others, 1998a, 1998b; Metheny and Titler, 2001).

NURSE ALERT   *Be sure to use gastric (Gastrocult) pH and not Hemoccult test.*

e. If tube is not in stomach, advance tube by about 2.5 to 5 cm (1 to 2 inches) and repeat Steps a through d to verify tube placement.

Tube must be in stomach to provide decompression.

20. Anchor tube.

a. After tube is properly inserted and position verified, either clamp distal end or connect tube to drainage bag or suction source.

Drainage bag is used if gravity drainage is ordered. Intermittent suction is most effective for gastric decompression. If the client is going to the operating room, the tube may be clamped.

b. Tape tube to nose; avoid putting pressure on nares.

Prevents tissue necrosis.

(1) Before taping tube to nose, apply small amount of tincture of benzoin to lower end of nose and allow it to become "tacky."

Benzoin secures tape by preventing loosening of tape if client perspires.

(2) Carefully wrap two split ends of tape around tube (see illustration).

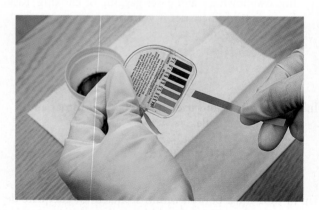

Step 19d   Checking pH of gastric aspirate.

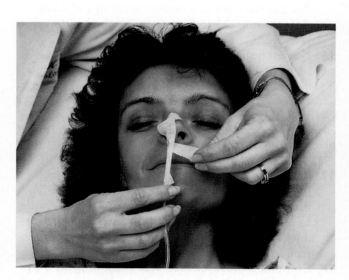

Step 20b(2)   Tape is crossed over and around NG tube.

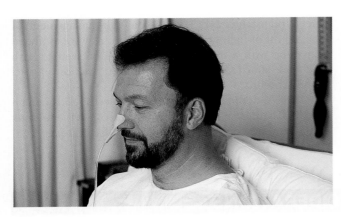

Step 20b(3)   Client with tube fixation device.

Steps	Rationale
(3) *Alternative:* Apply tube fixation device using shaped adhesive patch (see illustration).	
c. Fasten rubber band to end of NG tube in a slip knot, and pin rubber band to client's gown, allowing enough slack for movement of head.	The weight of the tube can irritate nasal mucosa with increased movement or activity. Pinning the tube to the gown stabilizes the tube and decreases friction and pressure.
d. Keep head of bed elevated at least 30 degrees unless physician orders otherwise.	Helps prevent esophageal reflux and minimizes irritation of tube against posterior pharynx.
e. Explain to client that sensation of tube should decrease somewhat with time.	
f. Remove gloves, and perform hand hygiene.	Reduces transmission of microorganisms.
21. Once placement of tube is confirmed:	
a. Place a mark, either a red mark or tape, on the tube to indicate where the tube exits the nares or	Mark provides a visual guide to indicate whether tube displacement may have occurred.
b. Measure tube length from nares to connecter	
c. Document findings from a or b in client's record	
22. Provide regular oral hygiene (see Chapter 7) every 2 to 3 hours.	
23. See Completion Protocol (inside front cover).	

• • • • • • • • • •

EVALUATION

1. Palpate client's abdomen for distention and pain. Auscultate for bowel sounds.
2. Ask client to rate comfort
3. Observe color of gastric secretions and patency of NG tube.
4. Observe client's oral and nasal mucosa.

Unexpected Outcomes and Related Interventions

1. Client develops abdominal distention, vomiting, or absence of drainage from tube.
    a. Assess patency of tube, and irrigate tube as needed.
2. Client complains of sore throat from dry, irritated mucous membranes.
    a. Perform oral hygiene more frequently.
    b. Ask physician whether client can suck on ice chips or throat lozenges or chew gum.
3. Client develops chronic inflammation and erosion of nasal mucosa.
    a. Consider removal or tube and reinsertion into opposite naris (physician's order necessary).
4. Client develops signs and symptoms of pulmonary aspiration: fever, shortness of breath, pulmonary congestion.
    a. Contact physician to report symptoms.
    b. Prepare for chest x-ray examination.

Recording and Reporting

• Record length, size, and type of gastric tube inserted and through which nostril it was inserted.
• Record the client's response to tube insertion, any symptoms that could indicate tube malposition, the client's status after the tube was inserted, and level of client comfort.

- Record the pH readings that were obtained to indicate correct placement and the amount and color of secretions withdrawn from the tube.
- Record insertion distance.

Sample Documentation

1000 Inserted 16 Fr nasogastric tube into left nares and advanced it to 50-cm mark. Client assisted with insertion by swallowing and states he is comfortable following procedure. Understands NPO status and self-management of tube. 50 ml of light-green gastric secretions were aspirated from tube with a measured pH of 3. Tube secured with tape and attached to low intermittent suction. Bowel sounds absent.

1200 Abdomen soft, nontender. Bowel sounds remain absent. Client given oral hygiene; mucosa remains pink and moist. No complaints of increased discomfort.

SPECIAL CONSIDERATIONS

Pediatric Considerations

- In some cases it may be necessary to have the parent with the child to assist in a timely completion of the procedure.
- The amount of preprocedure preparation is dependent on the child's developmental level, as well as the health care needs; when possible, prepare the child. Never surprise the child with this procedure (Wong and others, 2001).

Geriatric Considerations

- Geriatric clients may have sensory deficits that affect their ability to assist with NG tube insertion. If the client has hearing impairment, make sure that the client's hearing aid is in place and adjusted appropriately so that the client will be able to hear instructions.

- Check for ill-fitting dentures, and remove them for the client's safety and comfort during the insertion.
- Oral and nasal mucosal drying may be present. Be sure that the tube is adequately lubricated for insertion.

Home Care Considerations

Clients are seldom sent home with NG suction. If long-term decompression of the stomach is required, such as when the bowel is obstructed, a permanent decompression tube, such as a gastrostomy tube, is surgically inserted. Clients and caregivers should be taught how to take care of the gastrostomy tube and suction device. A portable, intermittent suction device is usually used in the home.

Skill 32.2

Irrigating Nasogastric Tube

This skill involves irrigation of the NG tube with an isotonic saline solution (normal saline) to maintain patency of the tube. Irrigation should be performed when the tube's patency is in question, such as when the volume of gastric secretions has decreased or the client is experiencing symptoms such as abdominal pain or nausea, or if the client's abdomen is distended. The NG tube should also be irrigated before and after its use for the administration of medications. Before irrigating the NG tube, the nurse must always verify tube placement.

ASSESSMENT

1. Assess the volume, color, and character of gastric secretions. *Rationale: Thick secretions and a reduced volume of secretions may indicate the need to irrigate the NG tube.*

Color can also be an indicator of tube placement (Figure 32-3).

2. Assess client's abdomen for distention or pain. *Rationale: Abdominal distention indicates that NG tube may not be patent.*
3. Turn off gastric suction, and auscultate for bowel sounds and note any passage of flatus. *Rationale: Determines presence of peristalsis. Gastric suction noise will obliterate bowel sounds.*

PLANNING

Expected outcomes focus on maintenance of tube patency to ensure adequate decompression of the stomach.

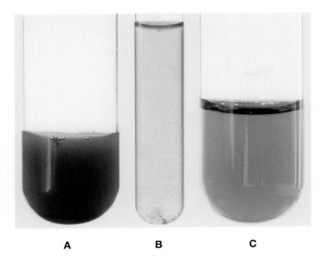

Figure 32-3 Gastric contents. **A,** Stomach. **B,** Stomach. **C,** Intestinal. (Courtesy Dr. Norma Metheny, St Louis University School of Nursing.)

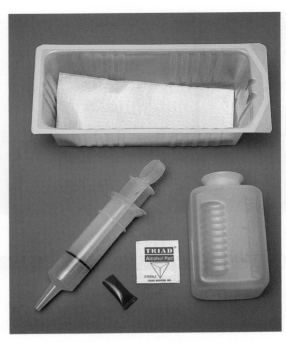

Figure 32-4 NG tube irrigation equipment.

Expected Outcomes

1. Client's NG tube remains patent.
2. Tube remains in proper position
3. Client denies abdominal discomfort or nausea.

Equipment (Figure 32-4)

- 60-ml catheter tip syringe
- Normal saline solution for irrigation
- Towel
- Disposable gloves

Delegation Considerations

The skill of irrigating an NG tube requires the critical thinking and knowledge application unique to a nurse and should not be delegated to assistive personnel (AP).

IMPLEMENTATION FOR IRRIGATING NASOGASTRIC TUBE

Steps	Rationale

1. See Standard Protocol (inside front cover).
2. Verify that NG tube is properly placed (see Skill 32.1, Steps 19 a-d). Once tube position is verified, proceed with irrigation.

    Reduces risk of pulmonary aspiration of irrigating solution.

3. Draw up 30 ml of normal saline solution into large syringe.

    Use of normal saline minimizes loss of electrolytes from stomach fluids.

4. Pinch or clamp NG tube, and disconnect from connection tubing. Lay end of connection tubing on towel.

    Prevents soiling of client's gown and bed by drainage of gastric secretions.

5. Insert tip of irrigation syringe into end of NG tube, and unclamp tubing (see illustration, p. 794). Hold syringe with top pointed at floor, and inject saline slowly and evenly. Do not force solution.

    Position of syringe prevents introduction of air into vent tubing, which could cause gastric distention.
    Solution introduced under pressure can cause gastric irritation or gastric trauma.

NURSE ALERT *Do not introduce saline through blue "pigtail" air vent on Salem sump tube.*

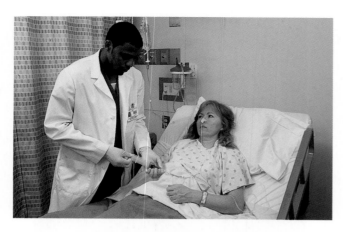

Step 5 Irrigating NG tube.

Steps	Rationale
6. If resistance occurs, check for kinks in tubing. Reposition client on left side, and try again. Repeated resistance should be reported to physician.	Tip of tube may be against stomach wall. Repositioning may dislodge tube away from stomach lining. Buildup of gastric secretions will cause abdominal distention and nausea and vomiting.
7. After instilling saline, immediately aspirate fluid by pulling back gently on syringe to withdraw fluid. If amount aspirated is greater than amount instilled, record the difference as output. If amount aspirated is less than amount instilled, record the difference as intake.	Irrigation clears tubing, so stomach should remain empty. Fluid remaining in stomach is considered intake and must be recorded.
8. Reconnect NG tube to suction. Remove and discard gloves, and perform hand hygiene.	Reestablishes gastric drainage system; irrigation may need to be repeated until NG tube drains properly.
9. See Completion Protocol (inside front cover).	

• • • • • • • • • •

EVALUATION

1. Palpate client's abdomen for distention, pain, and rigidity.
2. Auscultate bowel sounds.
3. Inspect the color, volume, and character of NG secretions.
4. Verify correct position of tube.
5. Determine client's level of comfort.

Unexpected Outcomes and Related Interventions

1. Client's NG tube cannot be irrigated and is no longer patent.
   a. Contact physician. The buildup of secretions poses a risk for aspiration.
2. Client's NG tube can be irrigated, but irrigation fluid cannot be withdrawn and the tube continues to drain poorly.
   a. Contact physician.
   b. Position of tube may need to be confirmed.

Recording and Reporting

- Record volume and color of drainage from the NG tube before irrigation of the tube and any symptoms of discomfort that the client is having.
- Record difference in volume instilled and volume withdrawn. If equal, no documentation is required.
- Record the amount and type of irrigation solution.
- Record whether there was any difficulty irrigating the tube and the volume of secretions withdrawn after irrigation.
- Record the client's response to irrigation, including any discomfort or relief of symptoms.

Sample Documentation (See Skill 9.1, p. 200)

0800 NG tube draining scant amounts. Position of tube verified, pH 3.0. Irrigated with 30 ml normal saline. Initially NG tube irrigated sluggishly but became easier to irrigate. Withdrew 20 ml light green fluid at end of irrigation. Client stated he had been feeling mild nausea.

1000 Increased volume of light-green gastric secretions draining from NG tube at low suction. Client states he no longer feels nauseated. Abdomen remains soft and nontender.

Skill 32.3

Removing Nasogastric Tube

This skill involves removal of the NG tube when it is no longer needed for decompression of the stomach. A physician's order is required for this procedure. Generally, an NG tube is no longer required when gastric secretions empty normally into the duodenum through the pyloric sphincter and when intestinal motility returns. The client's ability to handle gastric secretions is sometimes evaluated by removing the NG tube from suction and putting it to gravity drainage or by clamping the NG tube for a specified number of hours per day. If the client has not had a return of gastric or intestinal motility, the symptoms of abdominal distention, discomfort, or nausea will return.

ASSESSMENT

1. Palpate for pain or abdominal distention. *Rationale: Abdominal distention and pain may contraindicate tube removal; contact physician before proceeding.*
2. Ask client about nausea or abdominal pain.
3. Turn off gastric suction, and auscultate abdomen for such presence of bowel sounds. Also note if client has had bowel movements or is passing flatus. *Rationale: Return of flatus, bowel sounds, and bowel movements confirms the presence of peristalsis and bowel functioning. Gastric suction noise will obliterate bowel sounds.*

PLANNING

The expected outcome focuses on minimizing the discomfort caused by removal of the tube.

Expected Outcome

1. Client remains comfortable after removal of the tube.
2. Client's abdomen remains soft and nontender, and bowel sounds are normal.

Equipment

- Tissues
- Towel
- Disposable gloves
- 60-ml catheter tip syringe

 Delegation Considerations

The skill of removing an NG tube requires the critical thinking and knowledge application unique to a nurse and should not be delegated to assistive personnel (AP).

IMPLEMENTATION FOR REMOVING NASOGASTRIC TUBE

Steps	Rationale
1. See Standard Protocol (inside front cover).	
2. Verify physician's order.	Physician's order is required.

COMMUNICATION TIP *Tell client that removal of tube is less distressing than the insertion.*

Steps	Rationale
3. Place towel over client's chest to protect gown and cover tube.	Towel will protect client's gown and bed linens.
4. Turn off suction, and disconnect NG tube from drainage bag or suction. Remove tape or NG tube fixation device from bridge of client's nose, and unpin tube from client's gown.	Tube is free of connections before removal.
5. Stand on client's right side if right-handed, left side if left-handed.	Allows for easy manipulation of tube.
6. Attach large syringe to tube, and flush with 30 ml of air.	Clears gastric fluids from tube that could irritate esophagus and mouth during tube removal.
7. Hand the client facial tissue, and ask client to take a deep breath and hold it as tube is removed.	Client may wish to blow nose after tube is removed. Airway is partially occluded during removal of tube.
8. Tell client that removal of tube is about to begin.	Reduces anxiety and enhances cooperation.

Steps	Rationale
9. Clamp or kink tube securely, and pull tube out steadily and smoothly onto towel while client holds breath.	Kinked tube is less likely to expel gastric contents (if present) into throat or trachea. Breath holding minimizes risk of aspirating gastric contents if spilled from tube during removal.
10. Measure volume of drainage, and note character of content. Record on Intake and Output Summary (see Chapter 9). Dispose of NG tube, remove and discard gloves, and perform hand hygiene.	Maintains accurate intake and output.
11. Clean nares, and provide mouth care.	Promotes comfort.
12. See Completion Protocol (inside front cover).	

• • • • • • • • • • •

EVALUATION

1. Ask client about level of comfort after removal of the tube and after provision of mouth care.
2. Palpate client's abdomen and auscultate for bowel sounds.

Unexpected Outcomes and Related Interventions

1. Client complains of nares or throat pain after removal of the NG tube.
   a. Consult with physician about the use of topical anesthetics to reduce pain from irritated nasal mucosa.
   b. Encourage client to ingest warm, soothing liquids if able. Be alert for any swallowing problems that may indicate erosion of the esophagus.
2. Abdominal distention and pain occur.
   a. Notify physician
   b. Prepare to reinsert NG tube and/or obtain abdominal x-ray examination.

Recording and Reporting

- Record whether there was any difficulty removing the NG tube.
- Record abdominal assessment findings (e.g., absence of distention, presence of bowel sounds)
- Record the client's level of comfort and any symptoms after removal of the tube.
- Record any nursing interventions for client's discomfort or relief of other symptoms.

Sample Documentation

1300 Removed NG tube without difficulty. Mouth care provided after the removal. Client stated throat was sore but mouth care provided some relief. Abdomen remains soft, nontender. Bowel sounds auscultated in all four quadrants. Skin at left naris red and intact.

CRITICAL THINKING EXERCISES

1. While the nurse is inserting an NG tube, the client initially complains of burning and then begins to gag repeatedly as the tube reaches the back of the throat. When requested to swallow, the client requires some effort to swallow and has difficulty swallowing to assist in tube passage. What actions should the nurse take?
2. The nurse irrigates Mrs. Alvera's NG tube with 20 ml of saline solution and senses a sudden release of pressure. When withdrawing the fluid, the nurse obtains 150 ml of light green fluid. Is this normal? What could explain these findings?
3. Ms. Olivera has an NG tube placed during surgery to prevent fluid buildup around her surgical anastomosis. On the first postoperative day Ms. Olivera complains of stomach distention, and the nurse notices that her abdomen appears distended. The drainage from her tube has decreased over the last 4 hours, and Ms. Olivera states that she accidentally pulled on the tube when trying to reach for her glasses. The tube appears to be the same length as before. What actions should the nurse consider?

REFERENCES

Metheny NA, Titler MG: Assessing placement of feedings tubes, *Am J Nurs* 101(5):36, 2001.

Metheny NA and others: Detection of improperly positioned feeding tubes, *J Healthcare Risk Manage* 98:37, 1998a.

Metheny NA and others: pH, color and feeding tubes, *RN* 61(1):25, 1998b.

Viall C: When your patient has an NG tube, what's the most important thing?—location, location, location, *Nursing* 26(9):43, 1996.

Wong DL and others: *Wong's essentials of pediatrics*, ed 6, St Louis, 2001, Mosby.

CHAPTER
33

Enteral Nutrition

Enteral nutrition is the administration of nutrients directly into the gastrointestinal (GI) tract by way of a feeding tube. The most desirable and appropriate method of providing nutrition is the oral route; however, there are clients with a functional GI tract who are unable or unwilling to ingest oral nutrients. In this case enteral tube feedings are an alternative. Enteral feedings are most commonly given via small-bore (diameter) tubes (8 Fr to 12 Fr), inserted through the nose and advanced to either the stomach or proximal small intestine (Metheny and Titler, 2001) (Figure 33-1).

Nasogastric (NG) and nasointestinal (NI) feedings are typically used for short-term management of nutritional problems during acute illness and recovery. Clients may also require tube feeding because of ineffective swallowing or a weakened gag reflex causing aspiration. Some clients have an increased metabolism as a result of sepsis or burns and are unable to ingest enough calories to meet their bod-

ies' metabolic needs. After a feeding tube is placed, all clients remain at risk for aspiration and need careful nursing management to avoid this complication. For short-term nutritional support, 4 weeks or less, soft, small-bore enteral feeding tubes placed nasally into the stomach, duodenum, or jejunum are preferred (Eisenberg, 1994).

Tube feedings may also be used to provide long-term nutritional support for clients who cannot swallow safely or those who are unable to eat enough to sustain daily function. These groups may include clients with brain injury or an altered or reduced level of consciousness and clients with neuromuscular diseases who have a high incidence of aspiration, such as those with amyotrophic lateral sclerosis (ALS) and muscular dystrophy (MD). In these clients, tubes may be placed endoscopically or surgically through the abdominal wall gastrostomy (into the stomach) or jejunostomy (into the small intestine) (see Figure 33-1).

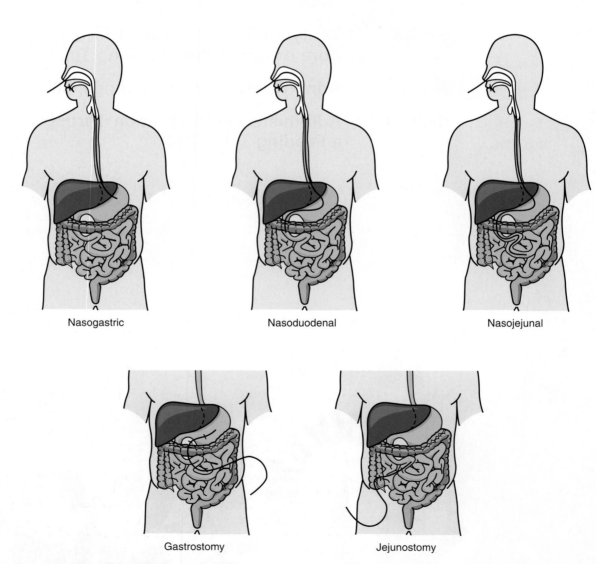

Nasogastric   Nasoduodenal   Nasojejunal

Gastrostomy   Jejunostomy

Figure 33-1 Tube feeding routes. (From Beare PG, Myers JL: *Principles and practice of adult health nursing,* ed 3, St Louis, 1998, Mosby.)

A variety of enteral feeding formulas are available in whole protein or partially digested form. Special enteral formulas for renal disease, hepatic disease, pulmonary disease, or diabetes are also available. Adult and pediatric formulas can be chosen.

Tube feedings may be administered in several ways. They can be given as a bolus amount via gravity, several times a day through a large-bore syringe; as an intermittent gravity drip administered for $1/2$ to 1 hour several times per day using a pouch to hang the feeding; or as a continuous drip per infusion pump, administered over 24 hours or whatever time interval best meets the client's needs.

Checking for placement of a feeding tube before administering medication or tube feeding is critical to safe client care. A feeding tube is improperly positioned when it is accidentally placed in the lung, esophagus, or even the stomach when it should be in the small bowel (Metheny and others, 1998a, 1998b). Tubes can easily be misplaced as a result of either normal movements or those of a confused or agitated client. In addition, a tube's distal tip can migrate upward or downward from its original correct position, even when the external portion of the tube is taped in place (Metheny and Titler, 2001). When a tube migrates to the lung, complications such as aspiration, pneumonia, pneumothorax, and peritonitis can develop if feedings are subsequently administered.

Placing an NG or NI feeding tube needs to be verified by x-ray examination to determine that the tube is in the stomach or intestine rather than in the airways (Levy, 1998; Metheny and others, 1990a, 1990b). Chest x-ray films are considered the standard of care. Unfortunately, not all institutions have policies mandating this method. X-ray examinations are also not usually performed for large-diameter NG tubes, because clinicians usually believe the tubes are less likely to enter the lung undetected (Metheny and others, 1998a). pH measurement is the next best method for confirming feeding tube placement. By testing the pH of fluid aspirated from a newly inserted feeding tube, it is possible to make reliable assumptions about the tube's location (Metheny and others, 1998b). Research is being conducted to test the efficacy of capnography and bilirubin testing in determining tube placement (Metheny and Titler, 2001).

Traditionally the auscultatory method was used to determine NG tube placement. The use of a syringe to insufflate air through a tube and then using a stethoscope to listen for a gurgling sound over the epigastric region was long thought to indicate proper tube placement. Studies have shown that the reliability of this method is highly questionable, and it should not be used to rule out inadvertent respiratory positioning of feeding tubes (Metheny and others, 1990b; 1998a).

Many potential complications may arise from prolonged intubation, including nasal erosion, sinusitis, esophagitis, gastric ulceration, and pulmonary aspiration. The cost of managing the ensuing complications and infections is expensive. Complications may be related to the tube itself, such as placement in the lung, frequent tube clogging, or the tube being inadvertently pulled out. Complications may also occur when the administered feeding causes delayed gastric emptying, bloating, or diarrhea (Bowers, 1996).

NURSING DIAGNOSES

Imbalanced Nutrition: Less Than Body Requirements related to inability to ingest or digest food or absorb nutrients is appropriate when there is evidence of weight loss, a reduction in food intake, and physical signs of malnutrition. **Impaired Swallowing** related to neuromuscular impairment makes a client a likely candidate for feeding tube placement. **Risk for Aspiration** is another indication for use of tube feedings, but it is also a condition that a client receiving tube feedings is predisposed to. Clients may experience **Diarrhea** or be at **Risk for Constipation** related to altered intake associated with tube feedings. If enteral feeding tubes are not managed correctly, **Impaired Oral Mucous Membrane** can be a common complication.

Skill 33.1

Intubating the Client With a Small-Bore Nasogastric or Nasointestinal Feeding Tube

Large-bore NG tubes are contraindicated when used primarily for enteral feedings because they carry an increased risk of aspiration and are more irritating to the nasopharyngeal and esophageal mucosa (Lehmann, 1992). Occasionally, large-bore GI tubes inserted for gastric decompression will be used to initiate enteral feeding because they are already in place. If the feeding continues for more than a few days, the nurse should consult with the physician about placement of a small-bore enteral feeding tube. Small-bore feeding tubes are available in weighted (tungsten) or unweighted designs (Figure 33-2). Weighted tubes were thought to pass more easily into the duodenum or jejunum via peristalsis; however, research has not demonstrated an advantage of the weight in promoting intestinal passage (Lord and others, 1993). Nonetheless, weighted tubes are used more frequently than non-

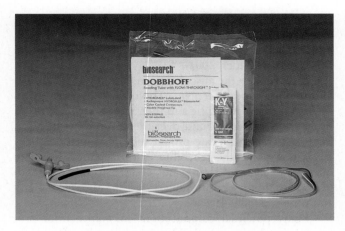

Figure 33-2 Small-bore feeding tubes.

weighted tubes for nasoduodenal and nasojejunal feedings because they are believed to remain in correct position longer than nonweighted tubes; however, research data regarding this belief are conflicting. Because the tubes are flexible, a guide wire or stylet is used to provide rigidity and to facilitate positioning, and then removed once correct placement is verified. Small-bore tubes can be left in place for an extended period with less irritation to the nasopharyngeal, esophageal, and gastric mucosa. Placing an NG or NI feeding tube requires a physician's order.

ASSESSMENT

1. Assess client's need for enteral tube feedings and intubation: impaired swallowing, head or neck surgery, decreased level of consciousness, surgeries involving upper alimentary tract, or facial trauma. Obtain order after consultation with physician. *Rationale: Recent head or neck surgery, esophageal surgery, or facial trauma may necessitate tube placement by a physician.*
2. Assess weight for client's height, hydration status, electrolyte balance, and organ function. *Rationale: Enteral feeding preserves function and mass of the gut, promotes wound healing, and may decrease the incidence of infection in the critically ill (Zaloga, 1994).*
3. Have client close each nostril alternately and breathe. Examine each naris for patency and skin breakdown. *Rationale: Assessment determines most patent naris for tube insertion.*
4. Assess medical history: nosebleeds, nasal surgery, deviated septum, anticoagulant therapy, and coagulopathy. *Rationale: Factors may require nurse to seek physician's order to change route of nutritional support.*
5. Assess client for gag reflex. Place tongue blade in client's mouth, touching uvula. *Rationale: Identifies client's ability to swallow and determines if risk for aspiration exists.*
6. Assess client's mental status. *Rationale: An alert client is better able to cooperate with procedure.*
7. Assess for bowel sounds (notify physician if sounds are absent). *Rationale: Absence of bowel sounds may indicate decreased or absent peristalsis and increased risk of aspiration or abdominal distention.*

PLANNING

Expected outcomes focus on safe insertion of feeding tube with placement in stomach, duodenum, or jejunum.

Expected Outcomes

1. Tube is placed in stomach or intestine.
2. Client does not develop aspiration
3. Client has no complaints or signs of discomfort or nasal trauma.

Equipment

- NG or NI tube (8 to 12 Fr) with guide wire or stylet
- 60-ml or larger Luer-Lok or catheter-tipped syringe
- Stethoscope
- Hypoallergenic tape and tincture of benzoin with cotton-tipped applicator or tube fixation device
- pH indicator strip (scale 0.0 to 14.0)
- Glass of water and straw
- Emesis basin
- Safety pin
- Rubber band
- Towel
- Facial tissues
- Clean gloves
- Suction equipment in case of aspiration
- Penlight
- Tongue blade

Delegation Considerations

This skill requires the critical thinking and knowledge application unique to a nurse. For this skill, delegation to assistive personnel (AP) is inappropriate.

IMPLEMENTATION FOR INTUBATING THE CLIENT WITH A SMALL-BORE NASOGASTRIC OR NASOINTESTINAL FEEDING TUBE

Steps	Rationale

1. See Standard Protocol (inside front cover).
2. Position client in sitting or high-Fowler's position. If client is comatose, place in semi-Fowler's position. — Reduces risk of pulmonary aspiration in event client should vomit.
3. Explain procedure to client.

COMMUNICATION TIP *To help the client have a chance to participate and feel a sense of control, explain how to try to relax and communicate during tube insertion. "Now I will explain each step as we go along. The tube will cause a slight burning pain as it passes through your nose. I want you to raise one finger to tell me if it's too uncomfortable so that I can be gentle and at the same time get this done as quickly as possible."*

---

4. Check feeding tube for flaws: rough or sharp edges on distal end and closed or clogged outlet holes. — Flaws in feeding tube hamper tube intubation and can injure client.
5. Determine length of tube to be inserted, and mark with tape or indelible ink (see illustration). — Determines approximate depth of insertion.

NURSE ALERT *Tip of tube must reach stomach. Measure distance from tip of nose to earlobe to xyphoid process of sternum (see illustration). Add additional 20 to 30 cm (8 to 12 inches) for NI tube (Hanson, 1979; Lord and others, 1993; Welch, 1996).*

---

6. Prepare NG or NI tube for intubation:
   a. Plastic tubes should *not* be iced. — Tubes will become stiff and inflexible, causing trauma to mucous membranes.
   b. Inject 10 ml of water from 30-ml or larger Luer-Lok or catheter-tipped syringe into the tube. — Aids in guide wire or stylet insertion.
   c. Make certain that guide wire is securely positioned against weighted tip and that both Luer-Lok connections are snugly fitted together. — Promotes smooth passage of tube into GI tract. Improperly positioned stylet can induce serious trauma.

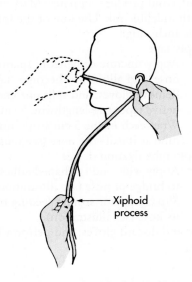

Xiphoid process

Step 5 Determining length of feeding tube.

Steps	Rationale
7. Cut tape 10 cm (4 inches) long.	
8. [hand icon] Inspect nares for any irritation or obstruction.	Determines naris to use for tube insertion.
9. Dip tube with surface lubricant into a glass of water.	Activates lubricant to facilitate passage of tube into naris to GI tract.

COMMUNICATION TIP *Explain that you are now about to insert the feeding tube. Let client know how he or she can assist. "I will insert the tube through your nose toward the back of your throat. Once the tip is in the back of your throat, I will ask you to begin to swallow. The water (ice chips) are something we may use if you find it hard to swallow. I will tell you when to stop swallowing"*

Steps	Rationale
10. Hand client a glass of water with straw or glass with crushed ice (if able to swallow).	Client is asked to swallow to facilitate tube passage.
11. Gently insert tube through nostril to back of throat (posterior nasopharynx). This may cause client to gag. Aim back and down toward ear.	Natural contour facilitates passage of tube into GI tract.
12. Have client flex head toward chest after tube has passed through nasopharynx.	Closes off glottis and reduces risk of tube entering trachea.
13. Have client mouth breathe and swallow. Give small sips of water or ice chips when possible. Advance tube as client swallows. Rotate tube 180 degrees while inserting.	Swallowing facilitates passage of tube past oropharynx. Rotating tube decreases friction.

NURSE ALERT *Do not force tube. If resistance is met or client starts to cough, choke, or become cyanotic, stop advancing the tube and pull tube back.*

Steps	Rationale
14. When tip of tube reaches the carina (about 25 cm, or 10 inches, in an adult), stop and listen for air exchange from the distal portion of the tube.	If air can be heard, tube could be in the respiratory tract; remove tube and start over (Metheny, 2000).
15. Continue to advance tube until desired length has been passed.	Ensures correct tube placement.
16. Check for position of tube in back of throat with penlight and tongue blade.	Tube may be coiled, kinked, or entering trachea.
17. Check placement of tube (see Skill 33.2, p. 805).	Proper position is essential before starting feedings.
18. After gastric aspirates are obtained, anchor tube to nose and avoid pressure on nares. Mark exit site on tube with indelible ink. Use one of the following options for anchoring:	A properly secured tube allows client more mobility and prevents trauma to nasal mucosa.
a. Apply tape	
(1) Apply tincture of benzoin sparingly to nose, and allow it to become "tacky."	
(2) Remove gloves, and split one end of the adhesive tape strip lengthwise 5 cm (2 inches).	
(3) Wrap each of the 5-cm strips around the tube as it exits the nose (see illustration).	
b. Apply tube fixation device	
(1) Apply wide end of shaped adhesive patch to bridge of nose (see illustration).	
(2) Slip connector around feeding tube as it exits nose (see illustration).	
19. Remove and discard gloves, and perform hand hygiene.	Reduces transmission of microorganisms.

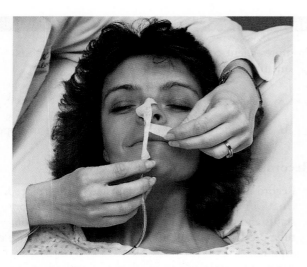

Step 18a(3) Applying tape to secure feeding tube.

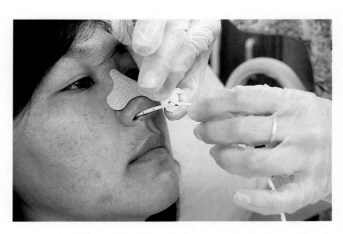

Step 18b(2) Slip connector around feeding tube.

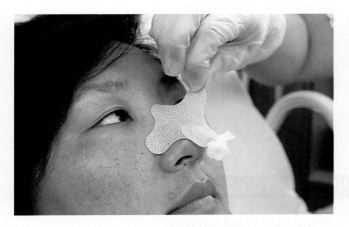

Step 18b(1) Applying fixation device patch to bridge of nose.

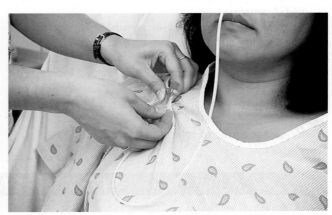

Step 20 Fasten feeding tube to client's gown.

Steps	Rationale
20. Fasten end of tube to client's gown by looping rubber band around tube in slip knot. Pin rubber band to gown (see illustration). Allow slack for movement of head.	Reduces traction on naris when tube is moved.
21. For intestinal placement, position client on right side when possible until radiological confirmation of correct placement has been verified. Otherwise, assist client to a comfortable position.	Promotes passage of the tube into the small intestine (duodenum or jejunum).

NURSE ALERT *Leave guide wire or stylet in place until correct position is ensured by x-ray film. Never attempt to reinsert partially or fully removed guide wire or stylet while feeding tube is in place. Guide wire or stylet may perforate GI tract, especially esophagus or nearby tissue, and seriously injure the client.*

22. Obtain x-ray film of abdomen.	Placement of tube is verified by x-ray examination (Metheny, 1988).

Steps	Rationale

23. Apply gloves, and administer oral hygiene. Cleanse tubing at nostril.

Promotes client comfort and integrity of oral mucous membranes.

24. See Completion Protocol (inside front cover).

• • • • • • • • • •

EVALUATION

1. Observe client to determine response to NG or NI tube intubation:
   a. Persistent gagging
   b. Paroxysms of coughing
2. Confirm x-ray results, and auscultate lung sounds.
3. Inspect condition of nasal mucosa, and ask client if experiencing pain or soreness. Reinspect mucosa at least every 8 hours.

Unexpected Outcomes and Related Interventions

1. Persistent gagging leads to vomiting with aspiration of GI contents.
   a. Position client on side, remove feeding tube if gagging continues, and suction airway as needed (see Skill 31.1, p. 748).
   b. Contact physician, and consider need for immediate chest x-ray film.
2. Nasal mucosa becomes inflamed, tender, and/or eroded.
   a. Retape tube to relieve pressure on mucosa.

   b. Consider removal of tube, and reinsert in opposite naris (physician order required).

Recording and Reporting

- Record in nurse's notes type and size of tube placed, length of tube insertion, client's baseline respiratory status and tolerance of procedure, confirmation of tube position by x-ray film, and pH and appearance of aspirate.
- Report to physician any incidence of aspiration or suspected change in tube position.

Sample Documentation

1000 Number 10 Fr small-bore feeding tube inserted into right naris, advanced approximately 60 cm. Client experienced slight discomfort without gagging or vomiting. Chest x-ray film confirmed duodenal placement. Intestinal aspirate tested at pH 7.0, bile colored in appearance.

SPECIAL CONSIDERATIONS

Pediatric Considerations

- Premature infant and neonate: measure length of tube from bridge of nose to just beyond tip of sternum. Older child: Measure from tip of nose to earlobe to tip of sternum.
- In infant, assess for vagal stimulation during insertion, evidenced by decreased heart rate.

Geriatric Considerations

Ensure adequate lubrication of tube to decrease discomfort for the older adult, who may have decreased oral or nasopharyngeal secretions.

Home Care Considerations

- Assess client or primary caregiver's ability to maintain tube and feeding program.
- Assess environmental safety and sanitation of client's home to determine potential for infection or injury if tube is to be inserted for ongoing nutritional support.
- See Home Care Considerations for Skill 33.2, on facing page.

Verifying Tube Placement for a Large-Bore or Small-Bore Feeding Tube

Testing placement of a small-bore or a large-bore feeding tube is a responsibility of the nurse. First, nurses must assess for GI versus respiratory placement when tubes are initially blindly inserted. Failure to detect pulmonary placement of a feeding tube can lead to serious complications, especially if formula or medications are instilled through the tube. Documentation of nonrespiratory placement by x-ray examination is standard practice when a small-bore tube is initially inserted because such a tube can enter the airway without causing obvious respiratory symptoms. Even a large-bore tube may not produce obvious respiratory symptoms when accidentally inserted into the airway of a semiconscious or unconscious client.

Following verification that a tube is positioned in the desired site (either stomach or small intestine), the nurse is responsible for ensuring that the tube has remained in the intended position before administering formula or medications through the tube. Therefore verification of correct tube placement is performed before each intermittent feeding, at least once every 12 hours when continuous feedings are given, and before medications are administered through the tube.

The risk for aspiration of regurgitated gastric contents into the respiratory tract is increased when the tip of an NI tube accidentally dislocates upward into the stomach or when the tip of either an NG or NI tube dislocates upward into the esophagus.

ASSESSMENT

1. Identify signs and symptoms of accidental respiratory migration of feeding tube: coughing, choking, or cyanosis. *Rationale: Signs and symptoms indicate accidental insertion of tube into airway. However, absence of signs and symptoms does not ensure nonrespiratory placement, especially in clients with decreased level of consciousness or altered cough and gag reflex.*
2. Identify conditions that increase risk of spontaneous tube dislocation from intended position: retching/vomiting, nasotracheal suctioning, severe bouts of coughing. *Rationale: Tube may move from stomach to esophagus or intestine to stomach.*
3. Observe for the external portion of the tube marked in ink to indicate tube placement. Observe if the

mark has moved away from the naris. *Rationale: Increased external length of tube may indicate distal tip is no longer in correct position.*
4. Review client's medication record: gastric acid inhibitors and proton pump inhibitors. *Rationale: H_2 receptor antagonists reduce volume of gastric acid secretion and the concentration (acid content) of secretions (McKenry and Salerno, 1998).*
5. Review client's history for previous tube displacement. *Rationale: History places client at increased risk.*
6. Auscultate client's bowel sounds. *Rationale: Determines if normal peristalsis is present.*

PLANNING

Expected outcome focuses on correct placement of feeding tube tip.

Expected Outcomes

1. Gastric fluid aspirated from point of tip insertion tests at a pH of 1 to 4.
2. Intestinal fluid aspirated from point of tip insertion tests at a pH greater than 6.
3. Tube feeding formula infuses smoothly into client's GI tract.
4. Client does not experience respiratory distress (e.g., coughing, dyspnea, increased respirations, reduced SpO_2).

Equipment

- 30-ml or larger Luer-Lok or catheter-tip syringe
- Medicine cup
- Stethoscope
- Clean gloves
- pH indicator strip (scale of 0.0 to 14.0 preferred)

Delegation Considerations

The verification of feeding tube placement requires the critical thinking and knowledge application unique to a nurse. For this skill, delegation to assistive personnel (AP) is inappropriate.

IMPLEMENTATION FOR VERIFYING TUBE PLACEMENT FOR A LARGE-BORE OR SMALL-BORE FEEDING TUBE

Steps	Rationale
1. See Standard Protocol (inside front cover)	
2. Perform measures to verify tube placement: a. When tube is initially inserted.	Establishes placement with initiation of treatment.
b. For intermittently fed clients, test placement immediately before feeding (usually a period of at least 4 hours will have elapsed since previous feeding).	More frequent checking has been associated with increased clogging of small-bore tubes (Powell and others, 1993). To avoid this problem flush tube with water after checking residual volume (Edwards and Metheny, 2000).
c. For continuously tube-fed clients, test at least once every 12 hours.	Confirms placement with reduced risk of clogging.
d. Wait at least 1 hour after medication administration.	Premature aspiration of gastric fluid will remove medication, reducing dose delivered to client. Medication may also interfere with pH testing.
3. Draw up 30 ml of air into syringe, then attach to end of feeding tube. Flush tube with 30 ml of air before attempting to aspirate fluid. More than one bolus of air may be needed in some cases.	Burst of air aids in aspirating fluid more easily (Metheny, 1993).

NURSE ALERT *It will likely be more difficult to aspirate fluid from the small intestine than from the stomach. Repositioning client from side to side may help.*

Steps	Rationale
4. Draw back on syringe, and obtain 5 to 10 ml of gastric aspirate (see illustration). Observe appearance of aspirate.	Aspirates of continuously tube-fed clients often have appearance of curdled formula. Aspirates from NI tubes are often bile stained. Gastric fluid may be grassy green with sediment, brown (if blood is present), or clear and colorless (often with shreds of tan mucus). Tracheobronchial secretions primarily consist of off-white to tan mucus. Pleural fluid usually looks watery and straw colored. Intestinal aspirate is generally more transparent than gastric aspirate and may appear bile stained, ranging in color from light to dark golden yellow or brownish-green (Metheny and Titler, 2001).
5. Gently mix aspirate in syringe, and expel into medicine cup. (*Option:* Apply few drops directly to pH test strip.) Measure pH of aspirate by dipping the pH strip into the fluid. Compare the color of the strip with the color on the chart provided by the manufacturer (see illustration) (Metheny and others, 1998a).	Quantity is sufficient for pH testing. Mixing ensures equal distribution of contents for testing. pH paper covering a range from 0 to 14 provides most accurate readings of gastric pH levels (Metheny and others, 1994).
a. Gastric fluid from client who has fasted for at least 4 hours usually has PH range of 1 to 4.	Range of 1 to 4 is reliable indicator of stomach placement, especially when gastric acid inhibitor is not being used.
b. Fluid from NI tube of fasting client usually has pH greater than 6.	Intestinal contents are less acidic than stomach.
c. Client with continuous tube feeding may have pH of 5 or higher.	Formulas contain solutions that are basic.
d. pH of pleural fluid from tracheobronchial tree is generally greater than 6.	The pH of pleural fluid makes it difficult to differentiate between respiratory and intestinal placement (Metheny and others, 1999).

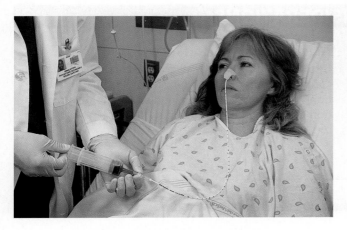

Step 4   Aspirate gastric contents.

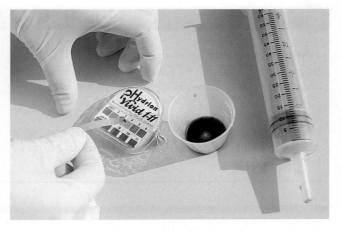

Step 5   Compare color on test strip with color on pH chart.

Steps	Rationale

NURSE ALERT *Auscultation is no longer considered a reliable method for verification of tube placement because a tube inadvertently placed in the lungs, pharynx, or esophagus can transmit a sound similar to that of air entering the stomach (Ghahremani and Gould, 1986; El-Gamel and Watson, 1993; Metheny and others, 1998b; Metheny and others, 1998c).*

6. If after repeated attempts, it is not possible to aspirate fluid from a tube that was originally established by x-ray examination to be in desired position, and (a) there are no risk factors for tube dislocation, (b) tube has remained in original taped position, and (c) client is not experiencing difficulty, assume tube is correctly placed (Metheny and others, 1993).	It is reasonable to assume tube is correctly placed. When abdominal x-ray films are obtained for clinical reasons, the nurse can take advantage of reports to monitor tube location.
7. See Completion Protocol (inside front cover).	

• • • • • • • • • •

EVALUATION

1. Obtain pH reading.
2. Observe flow rate of enteral formula.
3. Observe client for respiratory distress: persistent gagging, paroxysms of coughing, respiratory patterns (e.g., rate) inconsistent with baseline.

Unexpected Outcomes and Related Interventions

1. Client develops respiratory distress evidenced by dyspnea and changes in arterial blood gas or oxygen saturation values.
   a. Contact physician immediately.
   b. Be prepared to obtain chest x-ray examination, initiate oxygen therapy.
   c. Turn off feeding pump or withhold intermittent feedings.
2. Unable to aspirate fluid or the pH is greater than or equal to 6.

   a. Determine the client's risk of dislodgment (retching, vomiting, severe coughing, or frequent nasotracheal suctioning). If risk is low and the tube has remained taped in original position, start next feeding. If risk is high and tube has moved, consider need to verify placement with an x-ray film (Metheny and Titler, 2001).

Recording and Reporting

• Record type of tube, pH, appearance of aspirate, condition of naris, and client's tolerance to tube feeding.

Sample Documentation

1430 Feeding tube placement confirmed, aspirant pH of 3.0., dark green bile colored. Skin of naris clear and intact. Bowel sounds normoactive.

SPECIAL CONSIDERATIONS

Pediatric Considerations

In an infant, inject 0.5 to 1.0 ml of air before aspiration of gastric secretions for pH measurement.

Geriatric Considerations

Older adults frequently take medications that may affect pH, including H_2 receptor antagonists, proton pump inhibitors, or antacids.

Home Care Considerations

Instruct client or family caregiver to check that tube is in correct position before administering feedings or medications, why this is important, and to withhold administration of any fluid if placement is in doubt.

Skill 33.3

Administering Tube Feedings

Enteral tube feeding is preferred over parenteral nutrition (see Chapter 38) because it improves utilization of nutrients, is generally safer for clients, maintains structure and function of the gut, and is less expensive. Enteral feedings are most commonly given via small-bore tubes, inserted through the nose and advanced to either the stomach or small intestine. NG feedings are the most common, allowing tube-feeding formulas to enter the stomach and then pass more gradually through the intestinal tract to ensure absorption. NI tubes allow for successful postpyloric feeding, in which formula is placed directly into the small intestine beyond the pyloric sphincter of the stomach (Kudsk, 1994). The advantage of NI feedings is decreased gastric reflux, which reduces the risk of aspiration. However, gastric ileus (decreased or absent peristalsis affecting the stomach but not the intestines), delayed gastric emptying, or gastric resections contraindicate NG feedings.

This skill includes the administration of tube feeding via bolus, intermittent and continuous drip via gravity, and continuous via infusion pump. It is very important to check placement of NG and NI tubes before initiating feedings. Using good hand hygiene technique and clean equipment and hanging formula only for the recommended time (8 hours in open system, 24 hours in closed system) to prevent spoiling are critically important for avoiding contamination of the system and subsequent infection in the client.

ASSESSMENT

1. Assess client's need for enteral tube feedings: unable to eat, unwilling to eat, has increased energy requirements, requires bowel rest.
2. Identify signs and symptoms of malnutrition, including baseline weight and laboratory values (albumin, protein, lymphocyte, etc.). *Rationale: Conditions such as GI diseases, cancer, metabolic diseases make clients candidates for enteral nutrition.*
3. Verify physician orders for tube feeding formula, rate, and frequency. Laboratory data and bedside assessments, such as finger-stick blood glucose measurements, are also ordered by the physician.
4. Assess for food allergies. *Rationale: Prevents client from developing localized or systemic allergic reactions.*
5. Assess abdomen for distention or tenderness. Auscultate over left upper quadrant for bowel sounds before each feeding. *Rationale: Abdominal distention may indicate increased gastric residual. Absent bowel sounds indicate inability of the GI tract to digest or absorb nutrients.*

PLANNING

Expected outcomes focus on safe administration of tube feeding formula, client tolerance of the formula, and avoidance of complications related to tube feeding administration.

Expected Outcomes

1. Client's nutritional status improves (laboratory values, weight status, wound healing, intake and output) by discharge.
2. Client verbalizes no complaints of abdominal discomfort.
3. Client experiences no aspiration or signs of respiratory distress.
4. Client has residual volume less than 100 ml before each tube feeding or per institution's protocol (check agency's protocol).

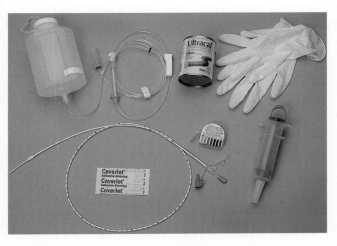

Figure 33-3 Graduate feeding container with tubing, 50 to 60-ml syringe with catheter tip, pH test strip, formula, gloves, feeding tube with guide wire, and fixation device.

Equipment (Figure 33-3)

- Prescribed enteral formula
- 30-ml or larger Luer-Lok or catheter-tip syringe (catheter tip for large-bore tubes, Luer-Lok tip for small-bore tubes)
- pH test strip (range 0.0 to 14.0)

- Stethoscope
- Tap water
- Administration set:

  Bolus syringe: 60-ml bulb or plunger syringe
  Gavage/intermittent infusion: plastic feeding bag with drip chamber and tubing, *or*
  Continuous infusion: infusion pump with plastic feeding bag and appropriate drip chamber and tubing for pumps; use pump designed for tube feedings

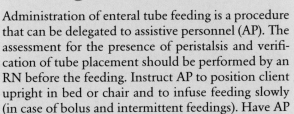

Delegation Considerations

Administration of enteral tube feeding is a procedure that can be delegated to assistive personnel (AP). The assessment for the presence of peristalsis and verification of tube placement should be performed by an RN before the feeding. Instruct AP to position client upright in bed or chair and to infuse feeding slowly (in case of bolus and intermittent feedings). Have AP report any difficulty infusing the feeding or any distress experienced by client immediately.

IMPLEMENTATION FOR ADMINISTERING TUBE FEEDINGS

Steps	Rationale
1. See Standard Protocol (inside front cover).	
2. Prepare administration set to administer formula intermittently or continuously:	
a. Check expiration date on formula and integrity of feeding bag container.	Ensures GI tolerance of formula. Prevents leakage of tube feeding.
b. Have tube feeding at room temperature.	Cold formula causes gastric cramping.
c. Connect infusion tubing to feeding bag container. (NOTE: Tubing may be part of feeding bag system.)	
d. Shake formula container well, and fill feeding bag with formula (see illustration). Open stopcock of infusion tubing, and fill tubing with formula to remove air. Hang bag on intravenous (IV) pole.	Filling tube with formula prevents excess air from entering GI tract once infusion begins.
3. For bolus syringe feeding, have syringe ready and be sure formula is at room temperature.	
4. Elevate head of bed to high-Fowler's, at least 30 degrees, or reverse Trendelenburg if spinal injury present.	Reduces risk of aspiration during feeding with head higher than stomach.

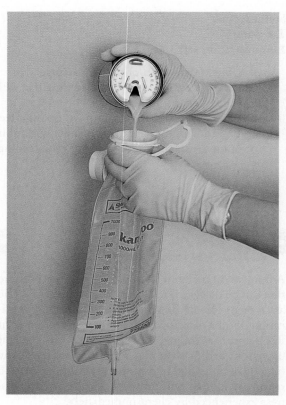

Step 2d Fill feeding bag with formula.

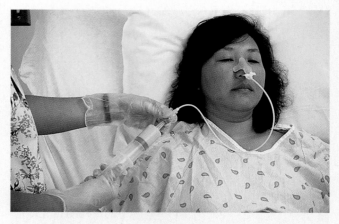

Step 6a Check for gastric residual (small-bore tube).

Steps	Rationale
5. Check placement of feeding tube (see Skill 33.2, p. 805). Consider together the results from pH testing and the aspirate's appearance.	Ensures proper tube placement. Sometimes color alone may differentiate gastric from intestinal placement. Because most intestinal aspirates are stained by bile to a distinct yellow color, and most gastric aspirates are not, the difference can often distinguish sites (Metheny and others, 1999). Pleural fluid is a clear light yellow or off white and often contains mucus.
6. Check for gastric residual.	
a. Connect syringe to end of feeding tube; pull back evenly to aspirate gastric contents (see illustration).	Residual volume indicates if gastric emptying is delayed. Delayed gastric emptying may be reflected by 100 ml or more remaining in the client's stomach (McClave and others, 1992).
b. Return aspirated contents to stomach unless the volume exceeds 100 ml or as defined by agency policy.	Return of aspirate prevents fluid and electrolyte imbalance.

NURSE ALERT *If residual amount is greater than last hour's infusion or greater than 100 ml, hold feeding 1 hour and recheck residual (Bockus, 1993) or refer to agency policy. It may be necessary to notify physician.*

7. Flush tubing. Prepare 30-ml syringe with 30 ml of tap water or normal saline. Pinch proximal end of feeding tube, and insert tip of catheter into end of tube. Release tube, and slowly instill irrigating solution. If unable to instill fluid, reposition client on left side and try again.	Irrigation clears tubing. Tip of tube may lie against stomach wall. Changing client's position may move tip away from stomach wall. Notify physician if unable to irrigate.

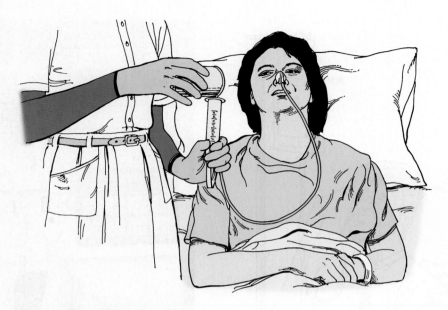

Step 8a(3) Fill syringe with measured amount of formula.

Steps	Rationale

8. Initiate feeding:

a. Bolus syringe or intermittent feeding

(1) Pinch proximal end of feeding tube.

(2) Remove plunger from syringe, and attach barrel of syringe to end of tube.

(3) Fill syringe with measured amount of formula (see illustration). Release tube, and elevate syringe to no more than 18 inches (45 cm) above insertion site and allow it to empty gradually by gravity over several minutes. Refill syringe until prescribed amount has been delivered to client.

Gradual emptying of tube feeding by gravity from syringe reduces risk of abdominal discomfort, vomiting, or diarrhea induced by bolus or too rapid infusion of tube feedings.

b. Intermittent gavage infusion

(1) Take prepared administration set, and attach infusion tubing to end of feeding tube. Set rate by adjusting roller clamp on infusion tubing. Allow bag to empty gradually over 30 to 60 minutes (see illustration, p. 812). Label bag with tube-feeding type, strength, and amount. Include date, time, and initials.

Gradual emptying of tube feeding by gravity from feeding bag reduces risk of abdominal discomfort, vomiting, or diarrhea induced by too rapid infusion of tube feedings.

c. Continuous drip method

(1) Hang feeding bag and tubing on IV pole.

(2) Connect distal end of tubing to proximal end of feeding tube.

(3) Connect tubing through infusion pump, and set rate (see manufacturer's directions) (see illustration, p. 812).

Continuous feeding delivers prescribed hourly rate of feeding, thus reducing abdominal discomfort. Clients who receive continuous drip feedings should have residuals checked every 8 to 12 hours and tube placement verified.

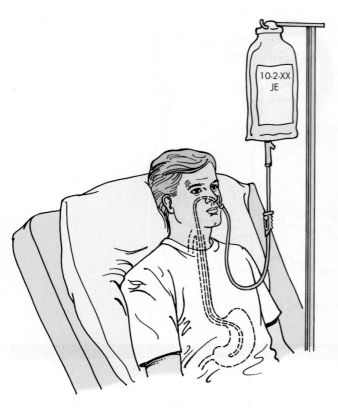

Step 8b(1)   Gravity intermittent feeding.

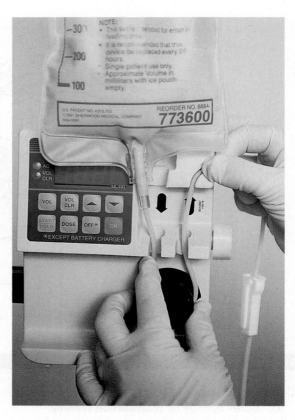

Step 8c(3)   Place infusion tubing in tube feeding pump.

Box 33-1

Advancing the Rate of Tube Feeding

INTERMITTENT

1. Start formula at full strength for isotonic formulas (300 to 400 mOsm) or at ordered concentration.
2. Infuse formula over at least 20 to 30 minutes via syringe or feeding container.
3. Begin feedings with no more than 150 to 250 ml at one time. Increase by 50 ml per feeding per day to achieve needed volume and calories in six to eight feedings. (NOTE: Concentrated formulas at full strength may be infused at slower rate until tolerance is achieved.)

CONTINUOUS

1. Start formula at full strength for isotonic formulas (300 to 400 mOsm) or at ordered concentration. Usually hypertonic formulas are also started at full strength but at a slower rate.
2. Begin infusion rate at designated rate.
3. Advance rate slowly (e.g., 10 to 20 ml/hr) per day to target rate if tolerated (tolerance indicated by absence of nausea and diarrhea, and low gastric residuals).

Steps	Rationale

NURSE ALERT *Maximum hang time for formula is 8 hours in an open system, 24 hours in closed, ready-to-hang system.*

9. Ask if client is comfortable while the infusion is continuing. Assess for presence of fullness, cramping, nausea, vomiting, and diarrhea.

10. Advance rate of concentration of tube feeding gradually (Box 33-1).

Complaints of cramping may indicate tube feeding is too cold or is infusing too fast. Symptoms indicate rapid distention of the intestine (McKenry and Salerno, 1998). Diarrhea should be reported to the physician.

Prevents diarrhea and gastric intolerance to formula.

Steps	Rationale
11. Following intermittent or bolus infusion or at end of continuous infusion, flush feeding tube with 30 ml water, using irrigating syringe. Repeat every 4 to 6 hours around the clock (Simon and Fink, 1999). Clamp or plug end of tube when no feedings are infusing. Have registered dietitian recommend total free water requirement per day.	Provides client with source of water to help maintain fluid and electrolyte balance. Clears tubing of formula. Clamp or plug prevents air from entering stomach between feedings.
12. Rinse syringe or bag and tubing with warm water whenever feedings are completed. Remove and discard gloves, and perform hand hygiene.	Rinsing removes formula left in equipment, reduces potential for bacterial growth, and allows for reuse of equipment. Most institutions require replacement with new equipment every 24 hours.
13. See Completion Protocol (inside front cover).	

● ● ● ● ● ● ● ● ● ●

EVALUATION

1. Weigh client daily until maximum administration rate is reached and maintained for 24 hours, then weigh client 3 times per week. Observe for return of normal laboratory values.
2. Monitor finger-stick blood glucose level every 6 hours until maximum administration rate is reached and maintained for 24 hours.
3. Monitor intake and output every 8 hours (Metheny, 2000).
4. Ask client if abdominal cramping, nausea, or discomfort is noted during or following feedings.
5. Auscultate client's lungs and observe respiratory rate and character.
6. Monitor and record residual volume (tube-feeding aspirate) on an ongoing basis.

Unexpected Outcomes and Related Interventions

1. Gastric residual exceeds 100 ml (use agency policy).
   a. Hold feeding, and notify physician.
   b. Maintain client in semi-Fowler's or at least have head of bed elevated 30 degrees.
   c. Recheck residual in 1 hour.
2. Client aspirates formula. Respirations are rapid and shallow, color is ashen. Breath sounds full of rhonchi. Client coughs up secretions that are similar to tube feeding.
   a. Turn off tube feeding immediately.
   b. Position client in Fowler's position, suction, and notify physician immediately.
   c. Prepare for chest x-ray examination.
3. Client's feeding tube cannot be aspirated or injected with air or water.
   a. For a newly inserted tube, notify physician and obtain x-ray confirmation of placement (Metheny and others, 1998a).

   b. Attempt to flush tubing with large-bore syringe and warm water. (Avoid using a small-bore syringe because this exerts large amount of pressure and may rupture tube.)
   c. Notify physician if unable to clear feeding tube.
   d. If tube cleared, keep patent by flushing every 4 hours, before clamping off each time, and before and after each feeding and medication infusion.
4. Client develops diarrhea 3 or more times in 24 hours, indicating intolerance.
   a. Notify physician, and confer with dietitian to determine need to modify type of formula, concentration, or rate of infusion.
   b. Determine if receiving antibiotics and medications containing sorbital, which can induce diarrhea (Guenther and others, 1991).
5. Client develops nausea and vomiting.
   a. May indicate gastric ileus. Withhold tube feeding and notify physician.
   b. Be sure tubing is patent; aspirate for residual.

Recording and Reporting

- Record amount and type of feeding, client's response to tube feeding, patency of tube, and any adverse effects.
- Record volume of formula and any additional water on intake and output (I&O) form.
- Report type of feeding, status of infusion and feeding tube, client's tolerance, and any adverse effects.

Sample Documentation

0900 NG feeding tube placement confirmed, aspirant pH 3.0. Bowel sounds normoactive over all four quadrants. Abdomen soft and nondistended. Full-strength Osmolyte hung per infusion pump at 60 ml/hr. Head of bed elevated 45 degrees. Lungs clear to auscultation. Denies abdominal discomfort.

SPECIAL CONSIDERATIONS

Pediatric Considerations

Short-term intermittent feeding is preferred in infants because of possible perforation of the stomach, nasal airway obstruction, ulceration, and irritation to mucous membranes with continuous feedings.

Geriatric Considerations

- Assess client regularly for hyperglycemia, because older adults may be more susceptible to high glucose concentration in enteral formulas.
- Assess routinely for gastric residual, because older adults may have decreased transit time so that formula remains in the stomach longer.
- Use of intestinal feeding tubes may reduce the risk of aspiration of feedings for the older adult.

Home Care Considerations

- Teach client or primary caregiver to check placement of tube and method of measurement before administering any formula.
- Instruct client or primary caregiver not to administer a feeding if there is any doubt concerning tube placement.
- Reinforce importance of giving feeding at room temperature.

Long-Term Care Considerations

It is desirable to transition a client to an oral diet as soon as possible. Enteral nutrition can usually be discontinued once a client is able to consume about 50% to 75% of nutrient and fluid needs over 24 to 48 hours without GI upset (American Society for Parenteral and Enteral Nutrition, 1998).

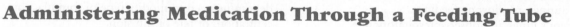

Skill 33.4

Administering Medication Through a Feeding Tube

This skill involves the safe administration of oral medications through a feeding tube. Specific attention must be paid to proper placement of the tube and whether the medication can be crushed for administration through the tube (Box 33-2). Liquid medication and elixirs are the best choice to administer through a feeding tube, but some medicines only come in tablet form. Most tablets may be crushed; however, those that are sublingual, enteric coated, or sustained release should not be given by tube, because their absorption, metabolism, and effectiveness will be unpredictable. Capsules (except sustained-release preparations) may be opened and contents emptied of powder, dissolved, and given through the feeding tube (McKenry and Salerno, 1998). A pharmacist should be consulted before pills are crushed or before capsules are opened and dissolved for tube feeding administration.

Medications should not be mixed in with tube feedings because of potential interruptions in tube feeding flow (e.g., turning feeding off while client is in radiology department), spillage, delayed absorption of the medication, or possible drug precipitation. It is always best to consult with a pharmacist before administering medications through a feeding tube.

ASSESSMENT

1. Assess for any contraindications to client receiving oral medication: Has the client been diagnosed as having bowel inflammation or reduced peristalsis? Has client had recent GI surgery? Does client have gastric suction? *Rationale: Alterations in GI function interfere with drug distribution, absorption, and excretion. Clients with GI suction might not receive benefit from the medication because it may be suctioned from GI tract before it can be absorbed.*

2. Assess medical history: history of allergies, type of medications, and diet history. *Rationale: These factors can influence how certain drugs act. Information also reflects client's need for medications.*

3. Gather and review assessment (e.g., bowel sounds, abdominal distention or pain, laboratory data that may influence drug administration.) *Rationale: Physical examination or laboratory data may contraindicate drug administration.*

4. Assess for potential drug-food interactions if you must administer drugs with a feeding (e.g., penicillin G and most tetracyclines).

Box 33-2

Medications That Should Not Be Crushed

The following is a partial list only.

Afrinol Repetabs	Feosol Spansule
Allerest Capsule	Feosol tablet
Aminodur Duratab	Ferro-Grad 500 tablet
Artane Sequel	Kaon tablet
ASA Enseals	Nitrospan capsule
Azulfadine EN-Tab	Nitroglycerin tablet
Betaphen-VK	Ornade Spansule
Compazine Spansule	Quinaglute Dura-Tab
Diamox Sequel	Quinidex Extentab
Donnatal Extentab	Slow-K tablet
Drixoral tablet	Sudafed SA capsule
Ecotrin tablet	Teldrin capsule
E-Mycin tablet	Theo-Dur tablet
Entozyme tablet	Trental

Expected Outcomes

1. Client experiences desired medication effect within period of onset of medication.
2. Client's feeding tube remains patent after medication administration.

Equipment

- 50- to 60-ml syringe, catheter tip for large-bore tubes, Luer-Lok tip for small-bore tubes
- pH test strip (scale 0.0 to 14.0)
- Graduate container
- Medication to be administered
- Pill crusher if medication in tablet form
- Syringe with needle if medication in gelatin form
- Warm water (to dissolve dry/gelatin medication)
- Tap water
- Tongue blade or straw to stir dissolved medication
- Disposable gloves (required if handling medications)

5. Check with the pharmacy for availability of liquid preparations for client's medications. *Rationale: Liquid preparations are always preferable to crushing tablets.*

PLANNING

Expected outcomes focus on administration of appropriate medication via the tube feeding route and avoidance of tube clogging from medication administration.

Delegation Considerations

The skill of administering medication through a feeding tube requires the critical thinking and knowledge application unique to a nurse. Delegation is inappropriate.

IMPLEMENTATION FOR ADMINISTERING MEDICATION THROUGH A FEEDING TUBE

Steps	Rationale
1. See Standard Protocol (inside front cover).	
2. Prepare medication for instillation in feeding tube.	

NURSE ALERT *Verify that medications to be administered do not include any sublingual, enteric-coated, or sustained-release medications.*

Steps	Rationale
a. Review six rights for administration of medication (see Chapter 16).	Essential to reduce medication errors.

NURSE ALERT *Do not mix medications and tube feedings; give at separate intervals to avoid potential drug-food interactions (McKenry and Salerno, 1998).*

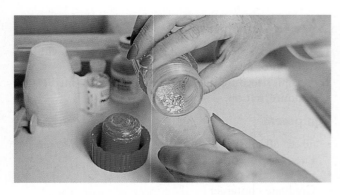

Step 2b   Crush tablets to fine powder.

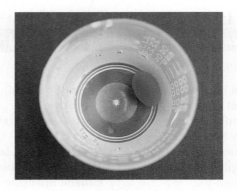

Step 2d   Capsule dissolving in water.

Steps	**Rationale**

b. *Tablets:* Crush pill (in its package if possible) with pill crusher (see illustration). Dissolve the powder in 15 to 30 ml warm water.

Crushing medication in its package prevents some from being lost.

c. *Capsules:* Open and dissolve the powder in 15 to 30 ml warm water.

d. *Gelatin capsules:* Aspirate with a syringe, or capsule may be dissolved in warm water (see illustration) over several minutes. After capsule dissolves, remove its gelatin outer layer.

Less medication is wasted if capsule is dissolved in warm water, but this may require 15 to 20 minutes before administration.

3. Elevate head of bed to high-Fowler's, at least 30 degrees, or in reverse Trendelenburg if spinal injury present.

Reduces risk of aspiration, keeping head above stomach.

4. Check placement of feeding tube (see Skill 33.2, p. 805).

5. Aspirate stomach contents for residual volume (see Skill 33.3, p. 808), determine volume with graduate container if necessary, and reinstill to client (see illustration).

If residual remains greater than 100 ml, hold medication and contact physician for further orders or follow agency protocol.

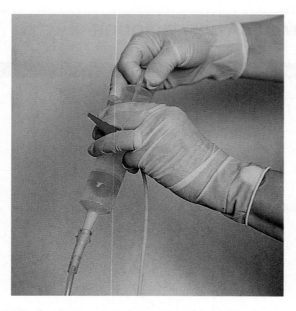

Step 5   Aspirate stomach contents for residual volume.

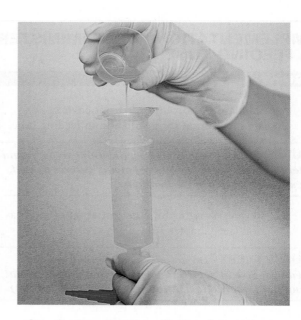

Step 6   Pour liquid medication into syringe.

Steps	Rationale
6. Pour dissolved medication into syringe, and allow to flow by gravity into feeding tube (see illustration). Flush with 10 ml water after each medication.	If a problem develops during medication administration (e.g., spillage, coughing, tube clogging), nurse can tell which medications have been lost and which are still available for later administration.
7. Follow last medication with 30 to 60 ml of water.	Avoids tube clogging with medication and ensures medication enters stomach, where it can be absorbed.
8. After instillation of medications, position client upright and turned slightly to the left if the medication is for local effect in the stomach (e.g., antacid), and have client remain there for several minutes.	Promotes drug absorption and delivery.
9. See Completion Protocol (inside front cover).	

• • • • • • • • • • •

EVALUATION

1. Observe for desired effects within appropriate time frame depending on medication administered.
2. Observe tube patency before and after medication administration.

Unexpected Outcomes and Related Interventions

1. Client is unable to receive medication because of blockage in tube.
   a. For newly inserted tube, notify physician and obtain x-ray confirmation of positioning.
   b. Attempt to flush tube with large-bore syringe and warm water to clear clog. (Avoid using a small-bore syringe because this exerts large amounts of pressure and may rupture tube.)
   c. If unable to flush clog, contact physician for replacement of tube and potential need to reroute medication if dose cannot be skipped or delayed until a new feeding tube is placed.

Recording and Reporting

• Record in nurses' notes placement of NG tube, volume of stomach aspirate, pH and appearance of stomach aspirate.
• Record time each drug was administered on the medication administration record (MAR) or computer printout. Include initials and signature (check agency policy).
• If drug is withheld, record reason in nurses' notes. Circle time the drug normally would have been given on the MAR or computer printout.
• Report adverse effects/client response to nurse in charge or physician.

Sample Documentation

NOTE: Documentation for medications via feeding tube is usually done on the medication sheet, the same as for any other medication. Other documentation occurs only if a problem is noted.

1300 Unable to administer medication because of clogged NG tube, despite efforts to irrigate. Physician notified, medications held pending placement of new tube.

✸ SPECIAL CONSIDERATIONS ✸

Geriatric Considerations

Assess the client for use of medications that may affect the pH of gastric secretions, such as H_2 receptor antagonists or antacids.

Home Care Considerations

• Teach the client or primary caregiver to check placement of tube before administering any medication.
• Instruct the client or primary caregiver not to administer medication if there is any doubt concerning the placement of the tube.
• Instruct the client or primary caregiver on the types of medications that can be safely given via a feeding tube. Stress that elixirs may clog feeding tubes. Be sure to administer water before and after giving the medications.
• Instruct the client or primary caregiver that sublingual, enteric-coated, or sustained-release pills *cannot* be given through the tube.

CRITICAL THINKING EXERCISES

1. Your client has a small-bore feeding tube in place. You need to administer two medications via the tube. One medication is an elixir; the other is a gelatin capsule. Describe your nursing actions related to the medication administration.

2. You have been caring for Mrs. Ellis, who has a feeding tube because of her nutritional deficiency related to cancer. She has been receiving continuous tube feedings at 50 ml/hr. Your assessment at the beginning of the shift finds that the tube feeding is 2 hours behind. You disconnect the feeding tube from the infusion and attempt to aspirate stomach contents. You get no return. What should you assess about the condition of Mrs. Ellis's feeding tube? What action should you then take?

3. You have just checked the placement of your client's NG tube. You obtain a pH reading of 7.0. Discuss the implications of this value and what nursing actions you would take.

REFERENCES

American Society for Parenteral and Enteral Nutrition, Board of Directors: *Clinical pathways and algorithms for delivery of parenteral and enteral nutrition support in adults,* Silver Spring, Md, 1998.

Bockus S: When your patient needs tube feedings: making the right decision, *Nursing* 23(7):34, 1993.

Bowers S: Tubes: a nurse's guide to enteral feeding devices, *Medsurg Nurs* 5(5):315, 1996.

Edwards S, Metheny N: Measurement of gastric residual volume: state of the science, *Medsurg Nurs* 9(3):125, 2000.

Eisenberg PG: Nasoenteral tubes: a nurse's guide to tube feeding, *RN* 57(10):62, 1994.

El-Gamel A, Watson D: Transbronchial intubation of the right pleural space: a rare complication of nasogastric intubation with a polyvinylchloride tube—a case study, *Heart Lung* 22:223, 1993.

Ghahremani GG, Gould RJ: Nasoenteric feeding tubes: radiographic detection of complications, *Dig Dis Sci* 31: 574, 1986.

Guenther P and others: Tube feeding related diarrhea in acutely ill patients, *JPEN J Parenter Enteral Nutr* 15(3): 277, 1991.

Hanson RL: Predictive criteria for length of nasogastric tube insertion for tube feeding, *JPEN J Parenter Enteral Nutr* 3(3):160, 1979.

Kudsk K: Clinical applications of enteral nutrition, *Nutr Clin Pract* 12(1):20, 1994.

Lehmann S: Parenteral and enteral access devices. In Teasley-Strausberg KM, editor: *Nutrition support handbook,* Cincinnati, 1992, Harvey Whitney Books.

Levy H: Nasogastric and nasoenteric feeding tubes, *Gastrointest Endosc Clin N Am* 8(3):529, 1998.

Lord L and others: Comparison of weighted vs unweighted enteral feeding tubes for efficacy of transpyloric intubation, *JPEN J Parenter Enteral Nutr* 17(3):271, 1993.

McClave SA and others: Use of residual volume as a marker for enteral feeding intolerance: prospective blinded comparison with physical examination and radiographic findings, *JPEN J Parenter Enteral Nutr* 16(2):99, 1992.

McKenry LM, Salerno E: *Mosby's pharmacology in nursing,* ed 20, St Louis, 1998, Mosby.

Metheny N: Measures to test placement of nasogastric and enteral feeding tubes: a review, *Nurs Res* 37(6):323, 1988.

Metheny N: Minimizing respiratory complications of nasoenteric tube feedings: state of the science, *Heart Lung* 22:213, 1993.

Metheny N: Personal correspondence, 2000.

Metheny N, Titler M: Assessing placement of feeding tubes, *Am J Nurs* 101(5):36, 2001.

Metheny N and others: Detection of inadvertent respiratory placement of small bore feeding tubes: a report of 10 cases, *Heart Lung* 19(6):631, 1990a.

Metheny N and others: Effectiveness of the auscultatory method in predicting feeding tube location, *Nurs Res* 39(5):262, 1990b.

Metheny N and others: Effectiveness of pH measurements in predicting feeding tube placement: an update, *Nurs Res* 42(6):323, 1993.

Metheny N and others: Characteristics of aspirates from feeding tubes as a method for predicting tube location, *Nur Res* 43(5):282, 1994.

Metheny N and others: Detection of improperly positioned feeding tubes, *J Healthc Risk Manage* 18(3):37, 1998a.

Metheny N and others: pH, color, and feeding tubes, *RN* 61(1):25, 1998b.

Metheny N and others: Testing feeding tube placement: auscultation vs pH method, *Am J Nurs* 98(5):37, 1998c.

Metheny N and others: Indicators of feeding tube placement in neonates, *Nurs Clin Pract* 14(6):307, 1999.

Powell KS and others: Aspirating gastric residuals causes occlusion of small bore feeding tubes, *JPEN J Parenter Enteral Nutr* 17:243, 1993.

Simon T, Fink AS: Current management of endoscopic feeding tube dysfunction, *Surg Endosc* 13:403, 1999.

Welch SK: Certification of staff nurses to insert enteral feeding tubes using a research-based procedure, *Nutr Clin Pract* 11(1):21, 1996.

Zaloga G: Timing and route of nutritional support. In Zaloga G, editor: *Nutrition in critical care,* St Louis, 1994, Mosby.

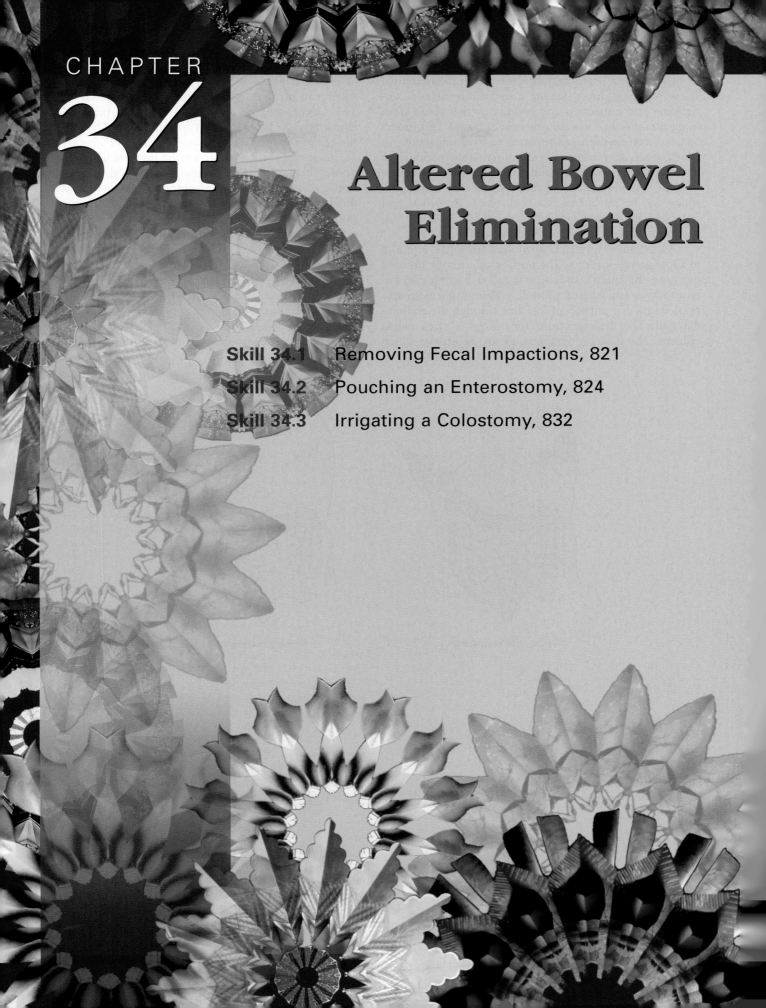

CHAPTER 34

Altered Bowel Elimination

Disorders of the bowel may be caused by various factors. Those requiring direct nursing intervention include constipation and impaction and conditions that result from surgical removal of various portions of bowel. Left unrecognized, constipation can progress to fecal impaction, in which stool may block the intestinal lumen. Stasis of bowel contents produces abdominal distention and pain. In some cases, liquid stool passes around the obstruction, which can be misinterpreted as diarrhea. If enemas and suppositories do not facilitate passage of stool, the impaction may need to be removed manually.

An ostomy is a surgical opening made in the intestine to allow passage of feces. The portion of intestine brought out onto the client's abdomen is called a stoma. An enterostomy is any surgical procedure that produces an artificial stoma in a portion of intestine through the abdominal wall. The drainage from the stoma is often called effluent. The forms of enterostomy are ileostomy, which involves the ileum of the small intestine, and colostomy, which can involve various segments of the colon (Figure 34-1). Depending on the reason for the surgery, an enterostomy can be permanent or temporary. Ostomies of the genitourinary (GU) tract are addressed in Chapter 35.

Care of a client with an ostomy involves many dimensions. These include providing the physical care of the stoma, containing the ostomy output or effluent, protecting the skin around the stoma (peristomal skin), preventing peristomal irritation, and preventing fecal contamination of the surgical wound (Hampton and Bryant, 1992). Teaching the client ostomy self care is critical. This includes pouch change techniques, colostomy irrigation, and diet management.

Regardless of the type of ostomy, a threat to body image may be perceived (Quayle, 1994; Walsh and others, 1995; Kluka and Kristijanson, 1996; Piper and Mikols, 1996; Piper, Mikols, and Grant, 1996). Clients with ostomies have concerns about stool leakage and odor, body

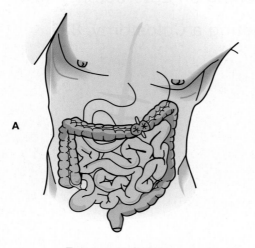

Transverse colostomy

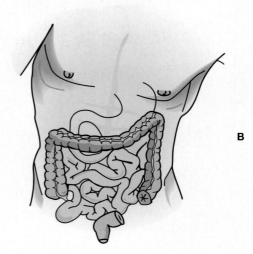

Sigmoid colostomy

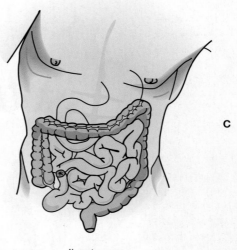

Ileostomy

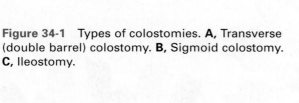

Figure 34-1   Types of colostomies. **A,** Transverse (double barrel) colostomy. **B,** Sigmoid colostomy. **C,** Ileostomy.

image changes, social support, self-care, health and life expectations, and surgical complication management. Some other concerns the client may have are fears of mutilation, rejection by friends or family, embarrassment with intimacy, and even a loss of normal sexual functioning (Golis, 1996).

NURSING DIAGNOSES

Nursing diagnoses associated with clients who have an impaction include **Constipation** related to dehydration, decreased activity, postsurgical ileus, or inadequate dietary fiber; and **Acute Pain** and/or **Chronic Pain** related to bowel distention. Those common diagnoses associated with clients who have ostomies may include **Deficient Knowledge** related to ostomy management, **Disturbed Body Image** related to presence of the ostomy, **Risk for Impaired Skin Integrity** related to irritation of peristomal skin, and **Anxiety** related to altered bowel function or rejection by friends. Foul-smelling odors, spillage or leakage of liquid stools, and the inability to regulate bowel movements give the client a sense of **Powerlessness** and **Situational Low Self-Esteem.** **Ineffective Sexuality Patterns** may occur related to perceived negative body image.

Skill 34.1

Removing Fecal Impactions

This skill is usually performed when the administration of enemas (see Skill 9-4, p. 213) or suppositories has been unsuccessful at removing impacted stools. Fecal impaction, the inability to pass a hard collection of stool, occurs in all age groups. Physically and mentally incapacitated persons and institutionalized older adult clients are at greatest risk (Prather and Ortiz-Camacho, 1998). Digital removal of an impaction may be embarrassing and uncomfortable for the client. Excessive rectal manipulation may cause irritation to the mucosa and subsequent bleeding or vagus nerve stimulation, which can produce a reflex slowing of the heart rate.

ASSESSMENT

1. Assess client's normal and current bowel elimination pattern as to frequency, characteristics of stool, use of laxatives, enemas, and other medications; urge to defecate but inability to do so; and abdominal discomfort, especially when attempting to defecate. *Rationale: This information is valuable in determining contributing factors and preventing recurrence of this problem.*
2. Palpate client's abdomen for distention, discomfort, or masses. *Rationale: Distention may contribute to pain, constipation, or diarrhea. When severe constipation occurs, a palpable mass may be felt.*
3. Auscultate all four quadrants for the presence of bowel sounds. *Rationale: Hypoactive bowel sounds may result from partial obstruction of the gastrointestinal (GI) tract as with constipation or masses. Hyperactive bowel sounds may be present due to intestinal irritation, as with diarrhea, or partial obstruction of GI tract or before defecation.*
4. Observe consistency of stool, seepage of liquid stool, or continual passage of small amounts of hard stool. *Rationale: Seepage of stool is symptomatic of an impaction high in colon. Client may be able to pass small pieces of hard stool or have episodes of passing small amounts of liquid stool (Prather and Ortiz-Camacho, 1998).*
5. Measure client's current vital signs and level of pain to establish a baseline. *Rationale: Vagus nerve stimulation during digital stimulation may result in reflex slowing of heart rate.*
6. Determine if client is receiving anticoagulant therapy. *Rationale: Procedure may be contraindicated because irritation and manipulation of the rectum may cause bleeding of rectal mucosa.*
7. Check client's record for physician's order for digital removal of impaction. *Rationale: A physician's order is necessary because of possible vagus nerve stimulation.*

PLANNING

Expected outcomes focus on removal of the impaction and prevention of further occurrences.

Expected Outcomes

1. Client's rectum is free of stool.
2. Client's vital signs remain normal after procedure.
3. Bowel sounds return to normal.
4. Client resumes normal defecation within 2 to 3 days.
5. Client experiences minimal discomfort.
6. Client/family verbalizes ways to prevent constipation.

Equipment

- Clean, disposable gloves
- Water-soluble local anesthetic lubricant (NOTE: Some institutions may require use of water-soluble lubricant without anesthetic when a nurse performs the procedure.)

- Waterproof, absorbent pads
- Bedpan
- Bedpan cover
- Bath blanket
- Basin, washcloth, towel, and soap
- Tissue

Delegation Considerations

The skill of removing an impaction requires the critical thinking and knowledge appplication unique to a nurse and should not be delegated. Instruct assistive personnel (AP) to inform the nurse if client is able to pass normal stool after procedure is completed.

IMPLEMENTATION FOR REMOVING FECAL IMPACTIONS

Steps	Rationale
1. See Standard Protocol (inside front cover).	
2. Assist client to a left side-lying position with knees flexed.	Relaxes abdominal muscles and provides access to the rectum.
3. Drape client's trunk and lower extremities with bath blanket, and place waterproof pad under buttocks.	Prevents unnecessary exposure of body parts.
4. Place bedpan next to client.	

COMMUNICATION TIP *At this time, instruct client to take slow, deep breaths during procedure. Breathe slowly with client.*

5. Lubricate gloved index finger of dominant hand with lubricant.	Lessens discomfort and permits smooth insertion of finger into anus and rectum.

NURSE ALERT *Observe for the presence of irritation to perianal skin, which would indicate the need for postprocedure skin care to area.*

6. Gradually insert index finger, and feel the anus relax around the finger. Then insert the middle finger.	Maneuver helps to dilate the anal sphincter (Prather and Ortiz-Camacho, 1998).
7. Gradually advance fingers slowly along rectal wall toward umbilicus.	Allows nurse to reach impacted stool high in rectum.
8. Gently loosen fecal mass by moving fingers in a scissors motion to fragment the fecal mass. Work fingers into hardened mass.	Loosening and penetrating mass allows nurse to remove it in small pieces, resulting in less discomfort to client.
9. Work stool downward toward end of rectum. Remove small sections of feces.	Prevents need to force finger up into rectum and minimizes trauma to mucosa.
10. Periodically assess heart rate, and look for signs of fatigue.	Vagal stimulation slows heart rate and may cause dysrhythmias. Procedure may exhaust client.

NURSE ALERT *Stop procedure if heart rate drops or rhythm changes or if rectal bleeding occurs.*

11. Continue to clear rectum of feces, and allow client to rest at intervals. If needed, use tissue.	Rest improves client's tolerance of procedure.
12. After removal of impaction, provide washcloth and towel to wash buttocks and anal area.	
13. Remove bedpan, and dispose of feces. Remove gloves by turning inside out and discarding in proper receptacle.	Reduces transmission of microorganisms.

Steps	Rationale
14. Assist client to toilet or clean bedpan. (Procedure may be followed by enema or cathartic.)	Disimpaction may stimulate defecation reflex.
15. See Completion Protocol (inside front cover).	

• • • • • • • • •

EVALUATION

1. Perform rectal examination for presence of retained stool or bleeding.
2. Obtain vital signs and assess level of pain, and compare to baseline values.
3. Auscultate bowel sounds.
4. Palpate abdomen to determine if it is soft and nontender.
5. Monitor bowel elimination patterns.

Unexpected Outcomes and Related Interventions

1. Client has seepage of liquid fecal material after removal of impaction.
   a. Contact physician. An enema may be needed to remove hardened feces higher in the rectum.
   b. Increasing fluids, fiber in the diet, and activity level may aid peristaltic activity.
2. Client experiences bradycardia, decrease in blood pressure, and decrease in level of consciousness as a result of vagus nerve stimulation.
   a. Stop procedure.
   b. Notify physician immediately.
   c. Monitor the client's vital signs and level of consciousness.
   d. Be prepared for potential emergency intervention.
3. Client has trauma to the rectal mucosa, as evidenced by blood on the gloved finger.
   a. Stop procedure if bleeding is excessive.
   b. If bleeding continues, notify physician for further treatment measures.

Recording and Reporting

- Record and report any changes in vital signs, character of pain, presence of bleeding, client's tolerance of procedure, amount and consistency of stool removed, and adverse effects.

Sample Documentation

1600 Moderate amount of hard, dark brown stool removed from rectum. Pulse ranged 86 to 94 beats per minute. Procedure tolerated without rectal bleeding, pain, or fatigue. Bowels sounds auscultated in all four quadrants. No abdominal distention or complaints of pain.

  ## SPECIAL CONSIDERATIONS

Geriatric Considerations

- Many older adult clients are especially prone to dysrhythmias and other problems related to vagal stimulation; monitor heart rate and rhythm closely.
- At least 28% of older adults are constipated as a result of insufficient dietary bulk, inadequate fluid intake, laxative abuse, diminished muscle tone and motor function, decreased defecation reflex, mental or physical illness, and presence of tumors or structures (Ebersole and Hess, 1998).
- For older adults, instituting a diet adequate in dietary fiber (6 to 10 g/day) adds bulk, weight, and form to stool and improves defecation (Ebersole and Hess, 1998).
- Consider development of a regular toileting routine that includes responding to the urge to defecate (Lueckenotte, 2000).

Home Care Considerations

- Consider having client or family member keep a week's diary of meals and fluid intake. Determine if dietary pattern contributes to constipation. Recommend a diet adequate in fiber.
- Have client or family member maintain a weekly bowel diary.

Long-Term Care Considerations

In long-term care, maintenance of activity can be very important in maintaining peristalsis.

Skill 34.2

Pouching an Enterostomy

Immediately after surgical diversion or removal of a portion of bowel, it is necessary to place a pouch (also called an appliance) over the newly created stoma because in noncontinent ostomies effluent (drainage) may begin immediately. The initial postoperative drainage is usually gas and old blood. Once the bowel starts functioning, fecal effluent is present.

The ostomy pouch collects all effluent and protects the skin from irritating drainage. A pouch with its skin barrier must fit comfortably, cover the skin surface around the stoma, not cut the stoma, and create a good seal. The postoperative pouch should allow visibility of the stoma (Black, 2000).

Pouching a newly formed stoma differs from techniques used to pouch a stoma several days or weeks old. The new stoma is edematous during the postoperative healing process. An incision line from the bowel resection may lie close to the stoma. The stoma itself often has a series of small stitches around its perimeter. A pouch and its skin barrier must be applied so that they do not constrict the stoma or traumatize healing tissues (Thompson, 2000). Initially the pouch over a postoperative colostomy may not need to be emptied frequently because drainage is diminished or lacking. Several days may pass before a client's normal elimination pattern returns. In the case of an ileostomy, the client will have frequent loose or watery stools when peristalsis returns (Black, 2000).

Many types of pouches and skin barriers are available. Some pouches are one piece and have skin barriers directly preattached and are called one-piece pouching systems (Bradley and Pupiales, 1997). The manufacturer already precuts some to size, and others must be custom cut to fit the client's stoma. Other systems are two separate pieces. The pouch can be applied to the skin barrier by attaching it to the flange (a plastic ring) on the barrier. Often the skin barrier must be custom cut to the client's specific stoma size. For two-piece systems, the skin barrier with flange must be used with the corresponding size pouch that fits that *flange from the same manufacturer.*

Nurses should understand how to use each of these different pouching systems. An ostomy nurse specialist, who has advanced education and experience in ostomy care, is a valuable resource to both client and nursing staff to assist in selecting proper equipment, fit, and application of an ostomy pouch.

ASSESSMENT

1. Identify the type of ostomy (e.g., colostomy or ileostomy) the client has (see Figure 34-1, p. 820). *Rationale: Client preference and type of ostomy are impor-*

tant when deciding on type of pouching system to use. Pouch type will vary as to amount and consistency of drainage and client's stoma characteristics.

2. Auscultate for bowel sounds. *Rationale: Documents presence of peristalsis.*

3. Observe skin barrier and pouch for leakage and length of time in place. Depending on type of pouching system used (such as an opaque pouch), the nurse may have to remove the pouch (with gloves) to fully observe the stoma. *Rationale: Extended exposure of the skin to effluent can cause maceration.*

4. Observe peristomal skin for blistering, redness, irritation, rash, or skin breakdown. *Rationale: Improper ostomy fit may cause pressure on the skin, ostomy adhesives may cause skin irritation, and moisture can further increase the risk of skin breakdown.*

NURSE ALERT *Intact skin barriers with no evidence of leakage do not need to be changed daily and can remain in place for 3 to 5 days (Ayello, 2000).*

---

5. Assess client's stoma for the following characteristics:
   a. *Size:* Use a measuring card to determine the correct size of the client's stoma (Figure 34-2). *Rationale: Accurate stoma size is critical for planning and selecting ostomy pouch size. Stoma opening needs to be $1/8$ to $1/16$ inch larger than the client's stoma. During the 6- to 8-week postoperative phase the client's ostomy will change size and shape. Thus the new stoma needs to be remeasured with each change in pouch.*
   b. *Shape:* If the stoma is round, use the precut, presized pouches as an option. *Rationale: Irregularly*

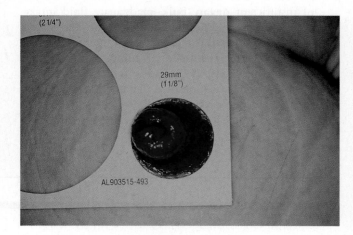

Figure 34-2 Measuring an ostomy using a measuring grid.

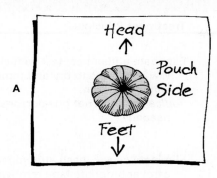

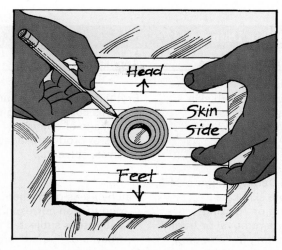

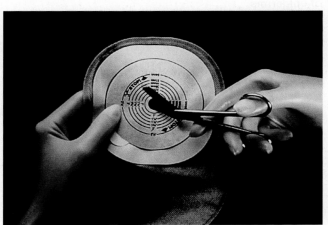

Figure 34-3   Steps for preparing skin barrier and pouch. (Permission to use and/or reproduce this copyrighted photo has been granted by the owner, Hollister Incorporated.)

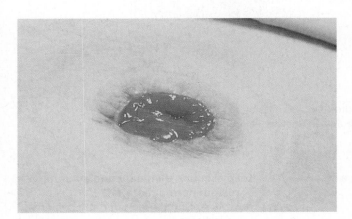

Figure 34-4   Flush stoma. (Permission to use and/or reproduce this copyrighted photo has been granted by the owner, Hollister Incorporated.)

shaped stomas require a custom-cut shape made on the skin barrier to match the shape of the stoma (Figure 34-3).

c. *Type:* Determine whether the stoma is flush to the skin or protruding (Figure 34-4). *Rationale: Type of stoma is important when selecting skin barrier, pouch, and accessories such as paste, strips, or binders.*

d. *Color:* Stoma should be pink-red in color. Peristomal skin is assessed for redness and trauma, such as ulceration, cuts, or necrosis (Table 34-1). *Rationale: Dark-colored stoma can indicate stoma necrosis, which is most common in the first 3 to 5 postoperative days.*

e. *Effluent:* Determine amount and consistency of the fecal drainage from the stoma (Table 34-2). *Rationale: Differences in drainage in the type of ostomies should be considered when selecting the ostomy pouch. Pouches are available in different sizes and closed or open ended. Only a pouch designed for stool should be used.*

PLANNING

Expected outcomes focus on helping client adjust to life with an ostomy emotionally and physically when performing ostomy self care, preventing peristomal skin breakdown, and containing effluent.

Expected Outcomes

1. Client denies discomfort.
2. Stoma is moist and reddish pink.

Table 34-1

Peristomal Skin Damage

Type or Cause of Damage	Appearance	Treatment Principles
Chemical Damage Effluent in contact with skin Incorrect use of adhesives or solvents	Erythematous and denuded areas corresponding to leakage of effluent *or* areas of product use (adhesives, solvents)	Eliminate effluent contact with skin; allow adhesives to dry and remove solvents from skin. *Topical:* Skin barrier powder; sealants if needed
Mechanical Damage (Figure 34-5, *A*) Inappropriate skin care (scrubbing or "picking") Incorrect tape removal or fragile skin, resulting in "stripping" of epidermis	Patchy areas of erythema or denudation corresponding with areas subjected to trauma or "taped" areas	Eliminate cause; teach atraumatic skin care, appropriate tape removal, and use of sealants when indicated. *Topical:* Skin barrier powder; sealant as indicated

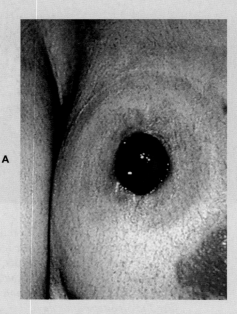
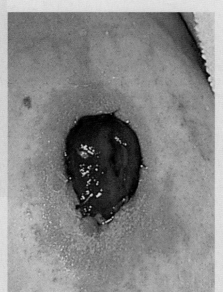

Figure 34-5 **A,** Mechanical injury. **B,** Candidiasis. (Permission to use and/or reproduce this copyrighted photo has been granted by the owner, Hollister Incorporated.)

Type or Cause of Damage	Appearance	Treatment Principles
Fungal Rash *(Candida)* (Figure 34-5, *B*) Antibiotics resulting in fungal overgrowth Persistent skin moisture	Maculopapular rash with satellite lesions	Keep skin dry; eliminate pooled urine; restore normal flora. *Topical:* Antifungal powder and sealant as indicated
Allergic Reaction Can be caused by any product	Areas of erythema or pruritus corresponding to area of skin exposed to allergen	Use patch test if needed to determine allergen; eliminate contact with allergen. *Topical:* Corticosteroid agent if needed for control of pruritus (cream or spray, not ointment, which would interfere with pouch adherence)

Modified from Hampton BG, Bryant RA: *Ostomies and continent diversions: nursing management,* St Louis, 1992, Mosby.

Table 34-2

Characteristic Output of GI Stomas

Type	Amount (ml)	Consistency	pH
Esophagostomy	1000-1500	Saliva	Slightly alkaline
Gastrostomy	2000-2500	Liquid	0.5-1.5
Jejunostomy	1000-3000	Liquid	Slightly acid
Ileostomy	750-1000	Toothpaste	Alkaline
Cecostomy and ascending colostomy	500-750	Toothpaste	Alkaline
Transverse colostomy*		Mushy to semiformed	Alkaline
Descending and sigmoid colostomy*		Semiformed to formed	Alkaline

*Unable to estimate volume.

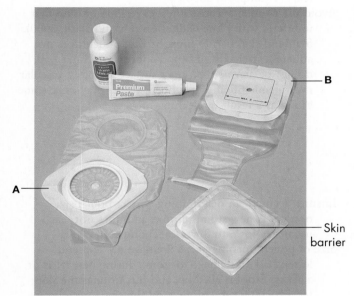

A

 B

Skin barrier

Figure 34-6 Ostomy pouches and skin barriers.
A, Two-piece detachable system. (NOTE: Skin barrier would need to be custom cut according to stoma size.) The pouch opening is already precut by the manufacturer to fit the size of the flange on the skin barrier.
B, One-piece pouch with skin barrier attached.

Equipment

- Pouch, clear drainable colostomy/ileostomy in correct size for two-piece system or custom cut-to-fit one-piece type with attached skin barrier (Figure 34-6)
- Pouch closure device, such as a clamp
- Ostomy measuring guide
- Adhesive remover (optional)
- Clean disposable gloves
- Ostomy deodorant
- Gauze pads or washcloth
- Towel or disposable waterproof barrier
- Basin with warm tap water
- Scissors
- Skin barrier such as sealant wipes or wafer (Figure 34-6)
- Stoma paste or stomahesive (optional)
- Tape or ostomy belt

3. Stoma is functioning with moderate amount of liquid or soft stool and flatus in pouch. Bowel sounds are present. (Flatus is noted by bulging of pouch in absence of drainage; flatus initially indicates return of peristalsis after surgery.)
4. Skin is intact and free of irritation; sutures are intact.
5. Client observes stoma and steps of procedure carefully.
6. Client indicates readiness to learn and to begin self-care.

 Delegation Considerations

The skill of pouching a stoma requires the critical thinking and knowledge application unique to a nurse. In some agencies the pouching of an established ostomy may be delegated. In this case the care provider should be instructed in the expected amount, color, and consistency of drainage from the ostomy. In addition the care provider should report changes in the stoma and surrounding skin integrity.

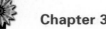

IMPLEMENTATION FOR POUCHING AN ENTEROSTOMY

Steps	Rationale
1. See Standard Protocol (inside front cover).	
2. 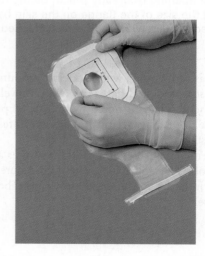 Inspect pouch periodically to see if it has to be emptied or empty ostomy pouch when pouch is one-third to one-half full of stool or gas. Remove gloves.	Minimizing leaking fosters a positive body image (Baxter, 2000). A full, heavy ostomy pouch will break the seal and cause leakage.
3. Place towel or disposable waterproof barrier under client.	Protects bed linens.
4. Remove used pouch and skin barrier gently by pushing down on the skin and lifting up on the barrier. An adhesive remover may be needed.	Reduces skin trauma. Improper removal of pouch and barrier can irritate client's skin and can cause skin tears (Thompson, 2000).
5. Cleanse peristomal skin gently with warm tap water using gauze pads or clean washcloth. Do not scrub skin; dry completely by patting skin with gauze or towel.	Avoid use of soap because it leaves residue on skin that interferes with pouch adhesion to skin (Black, 2000). Skin and skin barrier must be dry; pouch does not adhere to wet skin. If blood appears on gauze pad, do not be alarmed. Stoma's surface is highly vascular mucous membrane. If rubbed, stoma may ooze some blood as a result of cleaning process.

NURSE ALERT *Bleeding into pouch is abnormal.*

COMMUNICATION TIP *While caring for the stoma, talk in a pleasant tone and use normal facial gestures to convey acceptance. Encourage the client by saying "the stoma appears to be healing well," for example.*

6. Measure stoma for correct size of pouching system needed (see Figure 34-2, p. 824).	Ensures accuracy in determining correct pouch size needed. A new stoma shrinks and does not reach usual size for 6 to 8 weeks (Thompson, 2000).
7. Select appropriate pouch for client based on assessment. With a custom cut-to-fit pouch, use an ostomy guide to cut opening on the pouch $\frac{1}{16}$ to $\frac{1}{8}$ inch larger than stoma before removing backing. Barrier of flange of two-piece appliance should be at least $\frac{1}{4}$ inch bigger than the stoma. Prepare pouch by removing backing from barrier and adhesive (see illustration).	Size of pouch opening keeps drainage off skin and lessens risk of damage to stoma during peristalsis or activity. Stool is alkaline, and this irritates the skin; fecal bacteria can colonize on the skin and increase risk of infection.

NURSE ALERT *The stoma should be measured at each pouching system change to determine the correct size of equipment needed (Thompson, 2000). Follow each ostomy pouch manufacturer's directions and measuring guide as to which size ostomy pouch to use based on the client's actual stoma measurement size.*

Step 7 Removal of backing from barrier and pouch.

Steps	Rationale
8. Apply thin circle of barrier paste around opening of pouch; allow to dry.	Paste facilitates seal and protects skin. Paste is used for flush or poorly located stoma sites to fill in abdominal creases or folds.

NURSE ALERT *When applying a skin barrier to a stoma that is close to a client's abdominal incision, the skin barrier may have to be trimmed for it to fit.*

Steps	Rationale
9. Apply skin barrier and pouch. If creases exist next to stoma, use barrier paste to fill in; let dry 1 to 2 minutes.	Prevents leakage of fecal material onto the client's skin.
a. **For one-piece system**	
(1) Use skin sealant wipes on skin around stoma; allow to dry. Starting from the bottom and working up and around sides, press adhesive backing of pouch and/or skin barrier smoothly against skin.	Ensures smooth, wrinkle-free seal.
(2) Hold pouch by barrier, center over stoma, and press down gently on barrier. For ambulatory clients, the bottom of the pouch should point toward client's knees.	Attaches pouch to barrier already present on client's skin.
(3) Maintain gentle finger pressure around barrier and pouch for 1 to 2 minutes.	Excessive pressure may cause the client pain.
b. **For two-piece system**	
(1) Apply barrier-paste flange (barrier with adhesive wafer) as in steps for one-piece system. Then snap on pouch, and maintain finger pressure.	Creates wrinkle-free, secure seal; decreases irritation from adhesive on skin. Some two-piece pouching systems may have a snapping or clicking sound that occurs when attaching pouch to skin barrier (Black, 2000).
10. For both pouching systems gently tug on pouch in a downward direction	Determines that pouch is securely attached.
11. Apply nonallergenic paper tape around the skin barrier in a "picture frame" method. Half of the tape should be on the skin barrier and half on the client's skin. Some clients may prefer a belt attached to the pouch for extra security rather than tape.	"Picture framing" the pectin skin barrier keeps the pouch system attached securely.
12. Make sure a client who chooses to wear an ostomy belt can position two fingers between belt and skin.	An ostomy belt that is too tight can cause damage to the underlying stoma, discomfort to the client, and damage to the seal between skin barrier and pouching system (O'Brien, 1999).
13. Although many ostomy pouches are odor-proof, some nurses and clients like to add a small amount of ostomy deodorant into the pouch. Do not use "home remedies" to control ostomy odor.	Home remedies may cause damage to pouch and defeat purpose of an odor-proof pouch. In addition, these remedies may damage the stoma or peristomal skin surface.

NURSE ALERT *Aspirin should never be added to the ostomy pouch. It can cause stomal bleeding.*

Steps	Rationale
14. Fold bottom of drainable open-ended pouches up once, and close using a closure device such as a clamp (or follow manufacturer's instructions for closure).	Maintains secure seal to prevent leaking.
15. Properly dispose of old pouch and soiled equipment. Remove and discard gloves, and perform hand hygiene. Consider using room deodorant if needed.	
16. Change pouch every 3 to 7 days unless leaking; pouch can remain in place for tub bath or shower; after bath, pat adhesive dry.	Avoids unnecessary trauma to skin from too frequent changes. Dryness ensures adhesion of pouch.
17. See Completion Protocol (inside front cover).	

• • • • • • • • •

EVALUATION

1. Ask client to rate level of comfort around stoma and peristomal area. If an incision is present, as is the case with a new ostomy, ask about client's incisional discomfort using a scale of 0 to 10.
2. Observe appearance of stoma for color, swelling, trauma, and healing.
3. Auscultate bowel sounds, and observe amount, color, consistency, and frequency of fecal elimination (effluent) from the stoma.
4. Observe peristomal skin and existing incision (if present) for signs of skin breakdown.
5. Observe integrity of skin barrier and pouching system. Check bag for leakage. Check for odor and seepage under the skin barrier.
6. Observe client's behavior when looking at stoma and handling equipment. Note whether client talks about stoma.

Unexpected Outcomes and Related Interventions

1. Client's peristomal skin is irritated, and/or client complains of a burning sensation.
   a. Assess for causes of the skin breakdown.
   b. Remeasure the stoma size.
   c. Check if the selected pouch is correct for client's stoma size.
   d. Obtain referral for enterostomal therapy.
   e. Use a skin barrier for subsequent pouch changes. Determine that there is no undermining of pouching system by fecal contents.

2. Client's stoma develops a prolapse.
   a. Prolapse may be seen in clients with a temporary loop colostomy, commonly seen in surgery for colon cancer (Black, 2000).
   b. Notify physician because bowel is not properly sutured to the abdominal surface (Black, 2000).
3. Client's skin barrier and pouch leak.
   a. Assess if client is waiting too long (e.g., if pouch more than half full of stool) to empty pouch.
   b. Remeasure stoma, and reevaluate pouch and skin barrier size (Thompson, 2000).
   c. Determine if client is cutting out the correct size on the skin barrier.
   d. Evaluate if stoma is in a skinfold or whether other irregularities exist (Figure 34-7).
   e. Assess for peristomal hernia (Figure 34-8).
   f. Determine whether a convex disk, skin barrier paste, or other measures are needed to prevent leakage (Young, 1992).
4. Client cannot perform ostomy pouching change.
   a. Determine if client lacks the physical or mental ability to do ostomy self-care.
   b. Eliminate distractions and other factors (e.g., pain) that might interfere with client's performance of ostomy self care (Ball, 2000).
   c. Reevaluate client's understanding of ostomy self-care (Ball, 2000).
   d. Reevaluate client's problems with self-image, coping skills, and support systems (Baxter, 2000).

Recording and Reporting

- Chart type of pouch and skin barrier applied.
- Record size, color, and shape of stoma, and condition of peristomal skin and sutures.
- Record amount and appearance of stool or drainage in pouch.

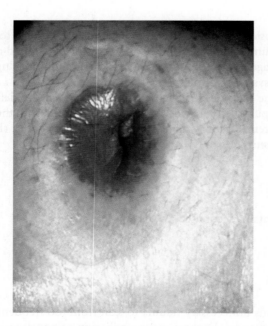

Figure 34-7 Irregular stoma (flush on right side, raised on left with skin irritation.)

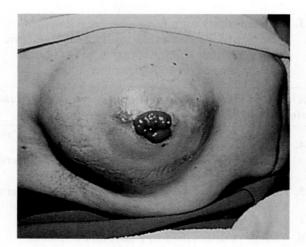

Figure 34-8 Peristomal hernia. (Permission to use and/or reproduce this copyrighted photo has been granted by the owner, Hollister Incorporated.)

- Report any of the following to the charge nurse and/or physician:

  Abnormal appearance of stoma, suture line, peristomal skin, character of output, absence of bowel sounds.

  No flatus in 24 to 36 hours and no stool by third day.
- Document abdominal distention and excessive tenderness, nature of bowel sounds.
- Record client's level of participation and need for teaching.

Sample Documentation

1600 Colostomy stoma is ½ in diameter, round, slightly swollen, and red in color. Peristomal skin is intact. Stoma is functioning, 3300 ml of dark brownish liquid stool. Normal bowel sounds present. Two-piece ostomy pouching system with hydrocolloid skin barrier in place without odor or other signs of leaks. Client has not yet looked at stoma. ET nurse began instruction of client's ostomy self-care technique.

SPECIAL CONSIDERATIONS

Pediatric Considerations

- Because babies swallow large amounts of air while sucking, a considerable amount of flatus is normal. Be sure pouch can accommodate increased flatus, or be prepared to release flatus frequently (Brown and Ricketts, 1994).
- Stoma prolapse occurs more often in pediatric clients because of the increase in intraabdominal pressure that occurs with crying (Brown and Ricketts, 1994).
- Use pouching system designed for pediatric clients that (Brown and Ricketts, 1994):

  Is flexible to cover infant, toddler's stomach contours

  Is thin enough to avoid undermining of fecal contents under skin barrier

  Can accommodate more that one stoma

- Whenever possible, adolescents requiring an ostomy benefit from presurgical contact with other adolescents who have an ostomy (Erwin-Toth, 1999; O'Brien, 1999).

Geriatric Considerations

- Evaluate the older adult's cognitive status for understanding ostomy self-care instructions.
- Evaluate the older adult's motor and visual ability to prepare ostomy equipment. For clients who are unable to custom cut the size of their skin barriers, consider having barriers precut by the ostomy equipment supplier or using a precut two-piece system.

- Teach older clients about the change in the number of eliminations (from an incontinent ostomy) that would be normal on a daily status.
- Financial concerns about the cost of ostomy supplies and reimbursement may be an important issue for clients on Medicare (Halvorson and Kertz, 1996).

Home Care Considerations

- Evaluate the client's home toileting facilities. This includes:

  The presence of adequate functioning and accessible toileting facilities

  Number and location of toileting facilities

  Number of other people living with the client who must share the toileting facilities

  Identification of the toileting facilities pattern of use as to time of day and amount of time spent in bathroom by the other people living with the client

- Evaluate the client's ostomy routine in relationship to usual lifestyle after discharge.
- Caution the client that most ostomy pouches and barriers cannot be flushed down the toilet; they clog the system. Dispose of used ostomy pouch according to local sanitation regulations.
- Provide client/family with education material regarding diet and activities (e.g., drinking with straws, chewing gum, and smoking) that increase intestinal gas (Thompson, 2000).

Skill 34.3

Irrigating a Colostomy

The purpose of a colostomy irrigation is to establish a pattern of regular bowel elimination after ostomy surgery, to cleanse the bowel of feces before tests or surgical procedures, and to relieve constipation. Irrigation of a colostomy is a simple procedure that clients can learn. The muscular quality of the colon allows it to be safely irrigated with a relatively large amount of fluid. Some clients who perform irrigations at home learn to establish an irrigation routine so that regular evacuation of the bowel occurs without stomal discharge between irrigations. Irrigations for achieving regular bowel evacuation can be achieved only with descending and sigmoid end colostomies and are not usually done for pediatric clients. Clients who successfully irrigate their colostomies have improved continence, reduced equipment costs, and fewer problems with sleeping, sexual activities, and skin complications (Leong and Yunos, 1999).

Irrigating an ileostomy is rarely necessary, except in cases of food blockage near the stomal outlet. Only a qualified person such as an enterostomal therapy (ET) nurse may perform a gentle lavage. An ileostomy produces liquid drainage containing a high concentration of electrolytes such as sodium, chloride, potassium, magnesium, and bicarbonate. Because excessive lavage could lead to a serious fluid and electrolyte imbalance, normal saline solution is used. Smaller amounts of solution are used on pediatric clients. The physician determines volume.

ASSESSMENT

1. Assess frequency of defecation, character of stool, and placement of stoma, as well as client's regular nutritional pattern. *Rationale: May indicate a need to irrigate to stimulate elimination function; consistency of stool varies along length of GI tract.*

2. Assess time when client normally irrigates colostomy. In the case of a new ostomy, confer with physician about whether and when irrigations can begin. Obtain written order. *Rationale: Irrigation helps to establish regular bowel emptying. Bowel must be totally healed so irrigation fluid will not cause perforation. This usually occurs 3 to 7 days after surgery.*

3. Confer with client for best time to irrigate. *Rationale: Irrigation can be planned to coincide with other hygiene activities.*

4. Assess client's understanding of procedure and ability to perform techniques. *Rationale: Determines level of participation to expect from client, level of explanations nurse should provide, and if client/caregiver is able to perform irrigation.*

PLANNING

Expected outcomes focus on regular bowel evacuation and client learning to perform the colostomy irrigation.

Expected Outcomes

1. Large amount of flatus, formed stools, and fluid is expelled.
2. Client achieves regular bowel movements from the stoma with little or no spillage of stool between irrigations.
3. Client denies abdominal pain or cramping.
4. Client independently performs the colostomy irrigation procedure.

Equipment

- Ostomy irrigation set that consists of an irrigation solution bag and tubing with a fluid control clamp and cone tip (Figures 34-9 and 34-10)
- Irrigation sleeve (with belt tabs or stick-on ring and end-closure device)
- Water-soluble lubricant
- Ostomy pouch and skin barrier or stoma cap cover
- Ostomy deodorant
- Clean disposable gloves

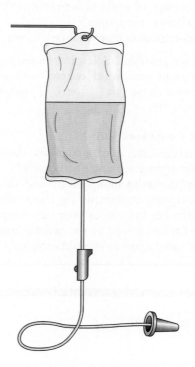

Figure 34-9 Irrigation bag with tubing and control clamp.

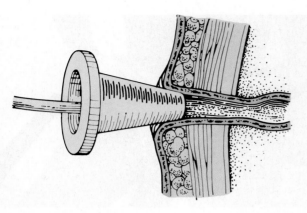

Figure 34-10 Cone tip: Irrigation cone against stoma opening.

- Toilet facilities that include a flushable toilet, a hook or some device to hold the irrigation container, toilet tissue, running water (that is suitable for use)

For Clients Who Are Bedridden

- Bedpan
- Towels
- Waterproof pad

Delegation Considerations

The skill of irrigating a newly established colostomy requires the critical thinking and knowledge application unique to a nurse. However, in some settings assistive personnel (AP) may be trained to perform irrigations on established ostomies. Review agency policy.

IMPLEMENTATION FOR IRRIGATING A COLOSTOMY

Steps	Rationale
1. See Standard Protocol (inside front cover).	
2. Summarize for client how procedure will be performed. Encourage questions as you proceed.	Helps client anticipate steps in procedure. Active dialogue during procedure can enhance learning (Black, 2000; Thompson, 2000).
3. Position client. (NOTE: Gloves are optional for client who is doing self-care.) a. On toilet or in chair in front of toilet, if ambulatory. b. On side, with head slightly elevated, if unable to be out of bed. Place bedpan nearby.	Allows for placement of irrigation sleeve into toilet or bedpan.
4. For adult clients, close clamp on irrigation bag, then fill bag with 500 to 1000 ml warm irrigation solution (tap water or saline solution) (see illustration). Open clamp to clear tubing of air. Close clamp.	Volume will adequately distend colon and cause evacuation. Cold solution can cause cramping and/or syncope; hot solution could injure mucosa. Air entering colon can cause cramping.

NURSE ALERT *Do not use tap water for irrigation if tap water in region is not suitable for drinking. Replace with bottled water.*

Steps	Rationale
5. Hang the irrigation bag on a hook so that the lower end of the bag is no higher than client's shoulder height when sitting or 18 to 20 inches (45 to 50 cm) above stoma.	This position prevents too high water pressure and reduces possibility of bowel damage.
6. Remove client's pouch by gently pushing skin from adhesive and barrier; dispose of according to hospital policy for standard precautions (save clamp if attached to pouch).	Prevents skin irritation, controls odor in room.

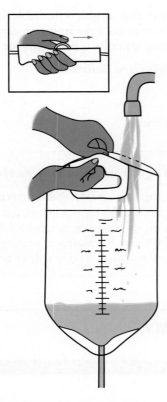

Step 4   Filling irrigation bag.

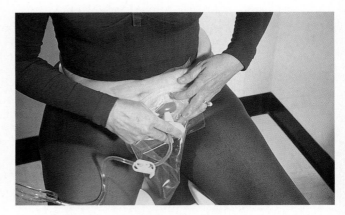

Step 8   Client placing irrigation cone into stoma.

Steps	Rationale
7. Place irrigation sleeve over client's stoma. Angle sleeve for appropriate flow of fecal returns (e.g., if client is using bedpan, place the irrigation sleeve at a 45-degree angle). Know particular use of the selected irrigation equipment. Some irrigation sleeves attach to flange of the two-piece skin barrier. Some sleeves require use of a belt. If so, adjust belt so it fits comfortably and is not too tight or too loose.	Make sure irrigation sleeve is correctly attached. Angle of irrigation sleeve facilitates flow of fecal returns. End of sleeve must be in toilet or bedpan to prevent spillage of feces.
8. Lubricate tip of irrigating cone. Reach through the top of the irrigation sleeve and, using gentle pressure, hold cone tip snugly against stomal opening (see Figure 34-10, p. 833). Do not force cone into stoma (see illustration).	Prevents trauma, tearing, bleeding, and rupturing of stoma. Cone tip avoids perforation of bowel.

NURSE ALERT   *Only use a cone tip to do irrigations. (Do not use a tube without a cone tip because it carries a higher risk for perforation of colon.) Insert cone securely into stoma, using just enough pressure to create a seal; do not insert entire length of irrigation cone into stoma. Too little pressure will cause the irrigation to flow around the side of cone rather than into the client. Too much pressure can block flow of irrigation solution into client.*

9. While client is holding cone, open flow control clamp and allow solution to flow. Start with 500 ml; this should take 5 to 10 minutes. Adjust the direction of the cone to facilitate inflow of solution as needed.

Too rapid instillation of irrigation solution can cause cramping and risk bowel perforation. Cone aids in retaining solution during inflow. Aiming flow of solution toward direction of bowel aids inflow.

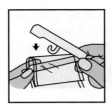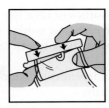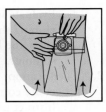

Step 13   Closing ostomy pouch.

Steps	Rationale
10. If cramping occurs, reduce or stop flow of irrigation fluid.	Client's complaint of abdominal cramps indicates need to stop irrigating and wait until cramps subside.
11. When all the irrigation fluid has been instilled into client's stoma, close flow control clamp and wait 15 seconds before removing irrigation cone from stoma. Close top of irrigation sleeve using appropriate closure method (e.g., Ziploc top). Discard gloves.	Avoids backflow of solution from stoma.
12. Allow 15 to 20 minutes for initial evacuation of stool. Keep end of sleeve in toilet or bedpan.	Keeps the device balanced and prevents injury from bumping against objects.

COMMUNICATION TIP   *Now is a good time to review with client importance of instilling fluid slowly. Reinforce positive performance. "You did very well. Remember, it helps to hold the cone so that fluid runs easily. Next time, you can show me how you would insert it."*

---

13. After initial evacuation of stool is over, dry tip of irrigation sleeve and close end with the clip or closure device (see illustration). Leave in place 30 to 45 minutes while waiting for the secondary evacuation. Client may get off toilet and may walk around, shower, or shave.	Exercise stimulates bowel.
14. Unclamp sleeve, and empty any fecal contents into toilet or bedpan. Rinse sleeve by pouring a small amount of water through the top, then remove sleeve. Rinse with liquid cleanser and cool water. Hang sleeve to dry.	Maintains sleeve in clean condition for future use.
15. Wipe stoma with toilet tissue to remove any stool. Put an appropriate colostomy pouch over stoma. If client is using a two-piece pouching system, place a new flange cap or closed-end pouch onto skin barrier (see Skill 34.2 , p. 824).	An appropriate pouch or cap may be worn to contain feces in case of elimination between irrigations.
16. See Completion Protocol (inside front cover).	

• • • • • • • • • •

EVALUATION

1. Observe amount and character of fecal material and fluid that is returned after the irrigation.
2. Evaluate degree to which regularity of bowel movements is being achieved.
3. Observe client's comfort and response to the irrigation procedure.
4. Observe client's ability to do the irrigation procedure correctly, and determine if client has fecal drainage between irrigations.

Unexpected Outcomes and Related Interventions

1. Client has feces from the colostomy stoma between irrigations.
    a. Reassess if client is an appropriate candidate for this management option.
    b. Evaluate whether anything has changed in client's treatment plan or lifestyle that could account for this finding.
    c. Evaluate whether client understands to follow the schedule for irrigation at the same time each day.

d. Evaluate if sufficient time has occurred since beginning the irrigation routine (6 to 8 weeks) to allow the bowel time to react to the irrigation stimulus.

2. Client cannot independently perform the irrigation procedure correctly.
   a. Instruct primary caregivers in this technique.
   b. Reassess client's self-irrigation technique for accuracy.
   c. Observe client perform the irrigation technique, and monitor for errors in technique that could account for this finding.

3. Client has no fecal returns after the irrigation.
   a. Evaluate client for possible absence of bowel sounds, abdominal pain, or distention. More often, lack of fecal returns may indicate that client is dehydrated.
   b. Encourage client to increase fluid intake, to alter diet intake if constipated, and to wear a pouch that can contain the expected fecal output until the next scheduled irrigation.

Recording and Reporting

- Record procedure, time of irrigation, volume and type of solution, amount and type of return, and client's tolerance.
- Record reapplication of skin barrier and pouch and condition of stoma and skin.
- Report symptoms of extreme discomfort, onset of severe diarrhea, inadequate results, or excessive bleeding to nurse in charge or physician.

Sample Documentation

0800 Second colostomy irrigation done in bathroom by client with minimal nurse assistance. 500 ml lukewarm water instilled easily into stoma using cone applicator. Passed large amount of brownish fluid and semisoft stool. Tolerated procedure without cramping or complaints. Correctly replaced ostomy pouch onto ostomy skin barrier at end of irrigation procedure. States, "Feels like I'm beginning to do this right."

 SPECIAL CONSIDERATIONS

Pediatric Considerations

Irrigations are not routinely done on pediatric clients. Irrigations in this population may be done before diagnostic procedures.

Geriatric Considerations

- Assess the client's physical ability to do ostomy self-irrigations. Motor and/or visual limitations may make it difficult but not impossible for client to do the procedure. Some adaptations in the irrigation technique may need to be made to enable older clients with motor and/or visual limitations to successfully do self-irrigation.
- Some older adults become upset if they do not have a daily bowel movement. With some irrigation routines, irrigation is not done daily; therefore the client will not have a daily bowel movement. Client needs to understand and accept this.

Home Care Considerations

- Evaluate the client's home toileting facilities (see Skill 34-2, p. 831).
- Establish scheduled time (approximately 1 hour) for uninterrupted ostomy care.
- Irrigation sleeve may be attached by a belt, by a stick-on, or by snapping directly onto the flange of the skin barrier. For home care, two-piece system is easier to use and more cost-effective; it allows client to remove pouch from flange and then attach irrigation sleeve, then snap on a clean pouch or stoma cap when evacuation is completed.

CRITICAL THINKING EXERCISES

1. An 80-year-old client was admitted yesterday with a diagnosis of weakness and dehydration. The history indicates no bowel movement for the past 6 days, and the client is having small liquid stools today. Because suppositories and enema did not result in bowel evacuation, you have determined that your client needs to have impacted stool removed digitally. What assessments are needed before this? What would you delegate to assistive personnel following the procedure?
2. You just started irrigating your client's colostomy, and the client begins to complain of cramping. What should you do and why?
3. You have a client using a two-piece pouching system who tells you she is having difficulty maintaining the seal on the pouch, and stool leaks. What nursing assessments are important to make at this time?

REFERENCES

Ayello E: ABCD's of stoma assessment and pouching. Personal correspondence, 2000.

Ball EM: A teaching guide for continent ileostomy, *RN* 63(12):35, 2000.

Baxter A: Stoma care nursing, *Nurs Stand* 14(19):59, 2000.

Black P: Practical stoma care, *Nurs Stand* 14(41):47, 2000.

Bradley M, Pupiales M: Essential elements of ostomy care, *Am J Nurs* 97(7):38, 1997.

Brown KC, Ricketts RR: Current management of the neonatal patient with an ostomy, *Progressions* 6(3):28, 1994.

Ebersole P, Hess P: *Toward healthy aging: human needs and nursing response,* ed 4, St Louis, 1998, Mosby.

Erwin-Toth P: The effect of ostomy surgery between the ages of 6 and 12 years on psychosocial development during childhood, adolescence, and young adulthood, *J Wound Ostomy Continence Nurs* 26(2):77, 1999.

Golis AM: Sexual issues for the person with an ostomy, *J Wound Ostomy Continence Nurs* 23(1):1, 1996.

Halvorson ML, Kertz JM: Changes in Medicare reimbursement for ostomy supplies: an overview, *J Wound Ostomy Continence Nurs* 23(1):26, 1996.

Hampton BG, Bryant RA: *Ostomies and continent diversions: nursing management,* St Louis, 1992, Mosby.

Kluka S, Kristijanson LJ: Development and testing of the ostomy concerns scale: measuring ostomy-related concerns of cancer patients and their partners, *J Wound Ostomy Continence Nurs* 23(3):166, 1996.

Leong AFPK, Yunos ABM: Stoma management in a tropical country: ostomy irrigation versus natural evacuation, *Ostomy Wound Manage* 45(11):52, 1999.

Lueckenotte AG: *Gerontologic nursing,* ed 2, St Louis, 2000, Mosby.

O'Brien B: Coming of age with an ostomy, *Am J Nurs* 99(8):71, 1999.

Piper B, Mikols C: Predischarge and postdischarge concerns of persons with an ostomy, *J Wound Ostomy Continence Nurs* 23(2):105, 1996.

Piper B, Mikols C, Grant TRD: Comparing adjustment to an ostomy for three groups, *J Wound Ostomy Continence Nurs* 23(4):197, 1996.

Prather CM, Ortiz-Camacho CP: Evaluation and treatment of constipation and fecal impaction in adults, *Mayo Clin Proc* 73(9):881, 1998.

Quayle BK: Making positive choices: body image and the new ostomy patient, *Ostomy Wound Manage* 40(4):16, 1994.

Thompson J: A practical ostomy guide, part I, *RN* 63(11):61, 2000.

Walsh BA and others: Multidisciplinary management of altered body image in the patient with an ostomy, *J Wound Ostomy Continence Nurs* 22(5):227, 1995.

Young MJ: Convexity in the management of problem stomas, *Ostomy Wound Manage* 38(4):53, 1992.

Altered Urinary Elimination

Catheterization is the placement of a tube into the bladder to remove urine from the bladder. Catheterization requires a physician's order and strict sterile technique. The steps for inserting an indwelling and a single-use straight catheter are the same. The difference lies in the inflation of a balloon to keep the indwelling catheter in place and in providing a closed drainage system. Urinary catheters are made with either latex or Silastic material and are available in a variety of sizes. In general, it is recommended that the narrowest, softest tube that will suffice should be selected. Assessment for latex allergy is essential before insertion of a latex catheter. Silastic catheters have been recommended for short-term use after surgery because of a decreased incidence or urethritis. Because of its lower cost and similar long-term outcomes, latex is the catheter of choice for long-term use (Cravens and Zweig, 2000).

Usually a size 14 to 16 Fr is adequate for adult clients, and rarely is a size greater than 18 appropriate. A size 12 Fr catheter was found appropriate in men with acute urinary retention (Cravens and Zweig, 2000). Factors that influence the size of the urethra include the age and size of the client, history of previous catheterization, and length of time the catheter is in place. Special circumstances may alter the location and appearance of the urethra. For example, during labor, immediately following childbirth, and after a vaginal hysterectomy women may have extensive perineal swelling and tenderness. Altered appearance of the urinary meatus may exist many years later.

There are three types of catheters: single-, double- and triple-lumen catheters (Figure 35-1). Catheterization done using a single-lumen catheter (see Figure 35-1, *A*) involves removal of the catheter as soon as the bladder is empty (see Skill 35.3, p. 850). When catheterization is done with an indwelling catheter with two lumens, one lumen allows urine to drain while the other lumen is used to inflate a balloon that keeps the tip of the catheter in the bladder (see Figure 35-1). Catheterization with a triple-lumen catheter (see Figure 35-1, *C*) may be done postoperatively to irrigate the bladder continuously, which prevents obstruction of urine outflow with blood clots (see Skill 35.4, p. 854). It can also be used to irrigate the bladder with medications. The triple-lumen catheter has one lumen to drain the bladder. The second lumen is used to inflate the balloon. The third lumen carries fluid from the irrigation

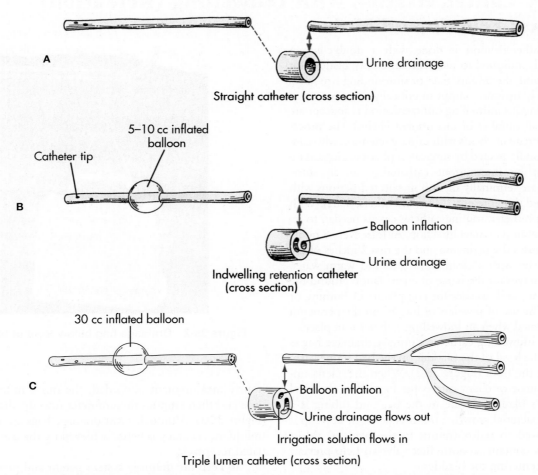

Figure 35-1   A, Straight catheter (cross section). **B,** Indwelling retention catheter (cross section). **C,** Triple-lumen catheter (cross section).

bag into the bladder. Indwelling (Foley) catheters are actually approximately one size larger than the equivalent straight catheter because of the circumference of the balloon (Wong, 1999). The size of the balloon for indwelling catheters varies from 3 ml (for a child), to 30 ml for continuous bladder irrigation (CBI). The size of the balloon is usually printed on the catheter port.

Urinary diversions are needed with partial or complete removal of the bladder because of cancer, neurogenic bladder, congenital anomalies, strictures, or trauma or chronic infections with altered renal function (Lewis and others, 2000). Urinary diversions may be continent or incontinent (see Skill 35.6, p. 860). A continent urinary diversion is constructed so that urine does not leak involuntarily. A catheter is used periodically to empty the bladder. An incontinent diversion uses a pouch over the opening to collect urine. Initially a temporary appliance is used. Seven to 10 days postoperatively a permanent appliance is fitted.

These have a faceplate that adheres to the skin and a collecting pouch with an opening to drain the pouch. An enterostomal therapist can provide information on where to purchase supplies, location of ostomy clubs, and follow-up support and assistance (Lewis and others, 2000).

NURSING DIAGNOSES

Urinary Retention may result from obstructions, trauma, paralysis, or inadequate muscle tone of the bladder. There are five types of urinary incontinence. **Total Urinary Incontinence** is the constant flow of urine with lack of awareness of bladder filling or incontinence. When a client has a urinary diversion, **Risk for Impaired Skin Integrity** related to irritation from incontinence or adhesive around the stoma may also apply. **Sexual Dysfunction** or **Disturbed Body Image** may be related to presence of a catheter for a prolonged time or presence of a urinary diversion.

Skill 35.1

Urinary Catheterization With Indwelling (Retention) Catheter: Female and Male

Indwelling catheterization is done with a double-lumen catheter and is indicated to maintain an empty bladder for surgery involving the urinary tract or surrounding structures or to accurately measure output in critically ill or comatose clients. Continuous indwelling catheterization is appropriate only in a small number of incontinent clients. The procedure is appropriate in clients with urinary retention who cannot be successfully treated by surgical or pharmacological intervention or by intermittent catheterization, in some persons who are terminally ill, and in selected persons with severe impaired skin integrity (Maas and others, 2001). With an indwelling catheter, routine catheter care is needed to reduce the risk of urinary tract infection. At least every 8 hours the nurse cleanses the perineum and the first 2 inches of the exposed catheter with a clean washcloth and warm water. The nurse observes for discharge or encrustation around the urethral meatus, and assesses for complaints of burning or discomfort. The use of powders or lotions on the perineum is contraindicated when an indwelling catheter is in place.

With an indwelling catheter a urinary drainage bag is hung below the level of the bladder on the bed frame without touching the floor (Figure 35-2). When the client ambulates, the nurse or client carries the bag below the level of the client's bladder. Urine in the bag and tubing is a medium for bacterial growth, and infection can develop if urine is allowed to reflux (return to the bladder). Most drainage bags contain an antireflux valve to help prevent urine from reentering the bladder.

A spigot at the base of the bag provides a means for emptying the bag. Some urinary drainage bags have special urometers for measuring small volumes of urine. When

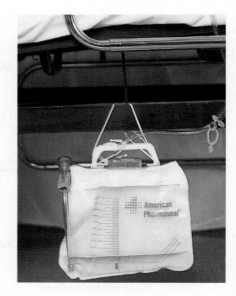

Figure 35-2 Drainage bag below level of bladder.

hourly measurement is needed, the nurse notes the volume and then empties the urometer into the drainage bag (Figure 35-3). Although most drainage bags are marked in milliliters, accuracy is better achieved by the use of a graduated receptacle.

To keep the drainage system patent and prevent stasis of urine in the tubing, the nurse checks for kinks in the tubing, avoids pressure on the drainage tubing, and observes for clots or sediment that may occlude the tubing.

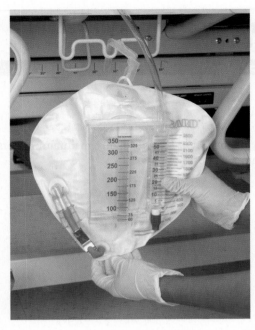

Figure 35-3   Urine collection bag with urometer for hourly output measurement.

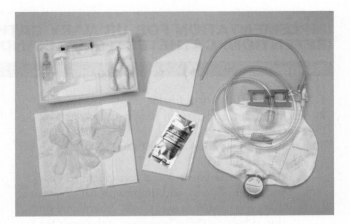

Figure 35-4   Kit for indwelling catheterization (includes drainage device, specimen cup, sterile drapes, sterile gloves, indwelling catheter, cleansing solution, sterile saline, sterile cotton balls, forceps, and lubricant).

ASSESSMENT

1. Assess client's knowledge and prior experience with catheterization. *Rationale: Reveals need for client instruction and likelihood of client cooperation (Evans, 1999).*
2. Assess client's weight, age, level of consciousness, ability to cooperate, and mobility of lower extremities. *Rationale: Determines catheter size and how much assistance is needed to properly position the client.*
3. Ask client the time of last voiding and to describe urine (if nurse did not observe). *Rationale: This determines if urinary retention is likely.*
4. Palpate for bladder over symphysis pubis. *Rationale: Distended bladder is palpable.*
5. Inspect perineal region, observing for perineal landmarks, erythema, drainage, or discharge. *Rationale: Determines the visibility of the urethra and need for cleansing the perineum.*
6. Ask client and check chart for allergies. *Rationale: Identifies allergy to antiseptic, tape, latex, and lubricant. Povidone-iodine allergies are common; if client is unaware of allergy, ask instead if allergic to shellfish.*
7. Assess any pathological condition that may impair passage of catheter (e.g., enlarged prostate gland in men).
8. Review client's medical record, including physician's order and nurses' notes. Note previous catheterization, including catheter size, response of client, and time of last catheterization. *Rationale: Identifies purpose of inserting catheter and can indicate potential difficulty with catheter insertion.*

PLANNING

Expected outcomes focus on emptying the bladder and on client comfort.

Expected Outcomes

1. Client's bladder drains freely.
2. Client verbalizes absence of discomfort or bladder fullness.
3. Client has a urine output of at least 30 ml/hr.

Equipment

- Catheter kit (Figure 35-4) and the appropriate-size catheter (Catheter kits vary. Check list of contents on the package. Some contain everything needed, some do not contain the catheter or drainage bag.)
- Nonallergenic tape or catheter strap (to secure catheter)
- Extra sterile gloves and catheter
- Clean gloves
- Washcloth, towel, soap, and basin for water
- Flashlight or lamp
- Flat sheet or bath blanket
- Measuring container for urine

 Delegation Considerations

The skill of urinary catheterization may be delegated to assistive personnel (AP) in some settings (see agency policy). First-time catheterizations or catheterization of clients in an acute care setting or with urethral trauma requires the critical thinking and knowledge application unique to a nurse, and delegation is inappropriate.

IMPLEMENTATION FOR URINARY CATHETERIZATION WITH INDWELLING (RETENTION) CATHETER: FEMALE AND MALE

Steps	Rationale
1. See Standard Protocol (inside front cover).	
2. Tell client you will explain the procedure step by step as you proceed.	
3. Arrange for extra nursing personnel to assist with positioning as needed.	Female clients often have difficulty maintaining dorsal recumbent position.
a. *Position female* client dorsal recumbent (on back with knees flexed), and drape with bath blanket so that only perineum is exposed. Alternately position side-lying (Sims') position with upper leg flexed at knee and hip and rectal area covered with the drape to reduce risk of contamination. Alternate position is more comfortable if client cannot abduct leg at the hip joint (e.g., if client has arthritic joints or contractures). Support client with pillows if necessary to maintain position.	
b. *Position male* client supine with legs extended and thighs slightly abducted. Cover upper body with small sheet or towel. Cover legs with separate sheet so that only genitals are exposed.	
4. ✥ Cleanse client's perineal area with soap and water, rinse, and dry. Place a waterproof pad under the client. Remove and discard gloves.	

COMMUNICATION TIP   *Encourage client to lie still to avoid accidental contamination of the sterile equipment. Tell client each step as you proceed and before actually beginning to insert the catheter.*

---

5. Position light to illuminate perineum, or have assistant available to hold the flashlight to visualize the urinary meatus	
6. While standing on the left side of the bed (if right-handed) or the right side of the bed (if left-handed), place catheter kit on clean surface and open outer wrap using sterile technique (see Chapter 4) (see illustration). If packaged separately, open drainage system, close clamp, and place drainage bag over edge of bottom bed frame and drainage tube up between mattress and side rail.	Outer wrap serves as sterile work field. Closed systems have catheter preattached to the drainage tubing and bag, which helps maintain a sterile system.
7. **Put on sterile gloves (see Chapter 4).**	

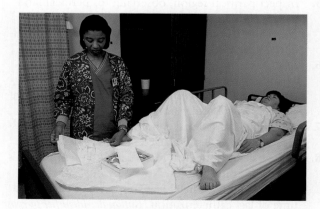

Step 6 Position doral recumbent with drapes for comfort and privacy.

Steps	**Rationale**

8. **Drape the perineum (see illustrations).**
   a. *Drape female:* With a cuff over both hands, ask client to lift hips and slip drape between client's thighs under buttocks.
   b. Place a second sterile drape with center opening so that perineum is covered and only the labia are exposed *(optional)* (see illustration).
   c. *Drape male:* Apply drape over thighs, just below penis. Place fenestrated drape with opening centered over penis (see illustration).
9. Arrange supplies on sterile field, maintaining sterility of gloves:
   a. Place closed-system outer container with drainage bag, catheter, and attached syringe toward the foot of the bed. If using a closed system, secure bag clamp at this time.
   b. Place top tray with cotton balls, lubricant, forceps, and drapes on the sterile drape between client's legs.

Technique keeps upper surface of drape sterile.

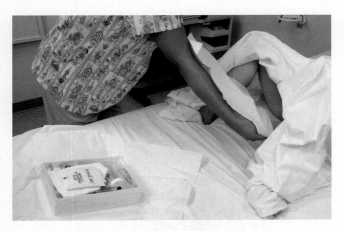

Step 8a   Place sterile drape under buttocks as client lifts hips slightly off the bed.

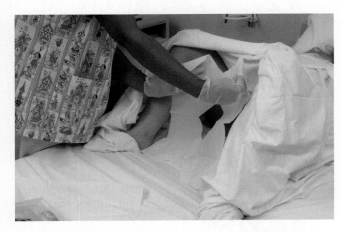

Step 8b   Place sterile fenestrated drape (with opening in center) over perineum with labia exposed.

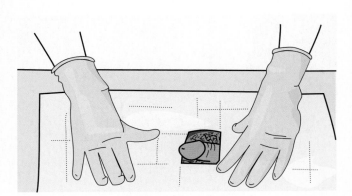

Step 8c   Draping male.

Steps	Rationale
10. If present, remove the plastic sleeve from the catheter, being careful not to contaminate the catheter. Inject saline solution into balloon port (see illustration). Withdraw if no leakage.	Tests the integrity of the balloon. If leakage is present, a different catheter will be needed.
11. Lubricate catheter with water-soluble gel 2.5 cm to 5 cm (1 to 2 inches) for women and 12.5 to 17.5 cm (5 to 7 inches) for men (see illustration).	Facilitates insertion of the catheter with minimal tissue irritation. Female urethra is shorter.
12. Pour antiseptic solution over all but one cotton ball (see illustration).	Dry cotton ball is used to remove excess antiseptic solution from meatus.

13. Cleanse the urinary meatus with antiseptic solution, holding the cotton ball with forceps and making a single stroke with each of the three cotton balls (see illustrations).

    a. *Cleansing female:* Separate labia with fingers of nondominant hand (now contaminated), and retain this position until catheter has been inserted. Using forceps to hold cotton balls, cleanse labia and urinary meatus with three strokes: (1) anterior to posterior along farthest side from nurse near meatus, (2) along side of meatus near nurse, and (3) down the center of the meatus.

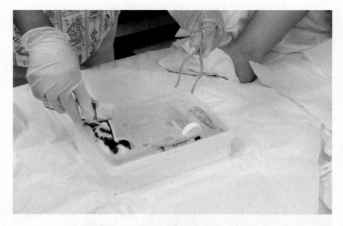

Step 12 Pouring antiseptic solution over cotton balls.

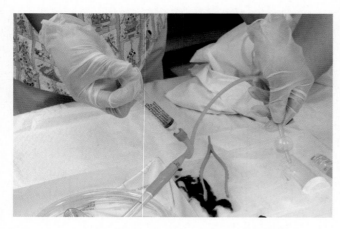

Step 10 Inflating balloon on double-lumen catheter to test integrity.

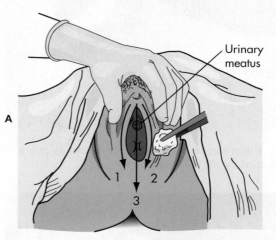

Step 13a Cleansing female perineum.

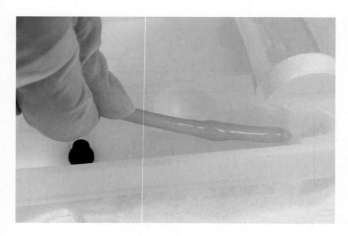

Step 11 Lubricating catheter.

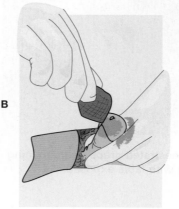

Step 13b Cleansing male urinary meatus.

Steps	Rationale

b. *Cleansing male:* Hold shaft of penis at right angle to body with nondominant hand (now contaminated) while retracting foreskin (if present). This hand remains in this position for remainder of the procedure. Using forceps to hold cotton ball and using circular strokes, cleanse from meatus outward and downward with three cotton balls (see illustration).

COMMUNICATION TIP   *As you prepare to cleanse the area, tell the client "This will feel cold and wet." Before you insert the catheter ask her to bear down gently as if passing urine. Explain that catheter insertion will not hurt, but pressure is usually felt and may be uncomfortable.*

14. Hold catheter 7.5 cm to 10 cm (3 to 4 inches) from the tip. Ask client to bear down gently and insert catheter.

  a. *Inserting catheter (female):* Insert catheter 2 to 3 inches (see illustrations Step 14a, *A* and *B*) or until urine flows, then advance another 1 to 2 inches (2.5 to 5 cm). Insert for a total of 2 to 3 inches (5 to 7.5 cm) (see illustration *C*).

Appearance of urine indicates that catheter tip is in bladder or lower urethra. Advancement ensures bladder placement and passage of balloon in bladder.

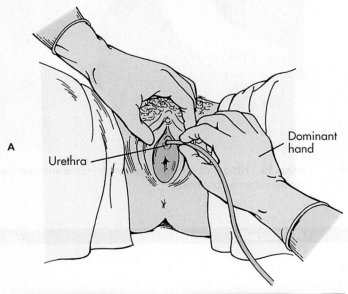

A

Urethra

Dominant hand

Step 14a   A, Inserting catheter into female urinary meatus. **B,** Catheter in place with balloon inflated (female side view). **C,** Catheter tip placed in bladder.

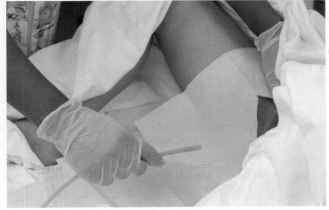

B

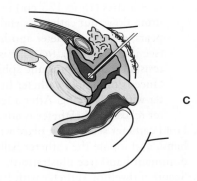

C

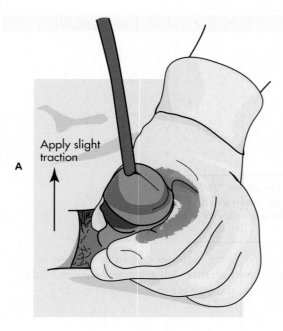

Apply slight
traction

A

B

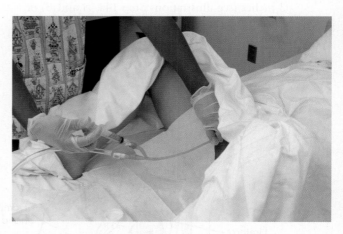

Step 14b   A, Inserting catheter into male urinary meatus.
B, Catheter inserted 6 to 7 inches and balloon inflated in
urinary bladder (male side view).

Step 15   Hold catheter in place with nondominant hand
while inflating balloon.

Steps	Rationale

    b. *Inserting catheter (male):* Gently apply traction to
penis (see illustration *A*), and insert catheter 7
to 9 inches (15 to 17.5 cm) in adult or until
urine flows out catheter's end. When urine appears, advance catheter another 1 to 2 inches
(see illustration *B*). NOTE: It is normal to meet
resistance at the prostatic sphincter. When resistance is met, hold catheter firmly against sphincter without forcing. After a few seconds, sphincter relaxes and catheter is advanced.

15. Hold catheter securely in place with nondominant
hand, and inflate the catheter balloon using the
dominant hand (see illustration).

Bladder or sphincter contraction may cause expulsion of
    catheter if it is not held in place.

16. Secure indwelling catheter with hypoallergenic tape
or catheter strap.

Minimal tension on catheter prevents trauma to urethra.

    a. *Female:* Secure catheter to inner thigh with tape
or a catheter strap, allowing enough slack to prevent tension (see illustration).

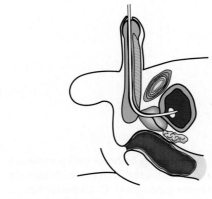

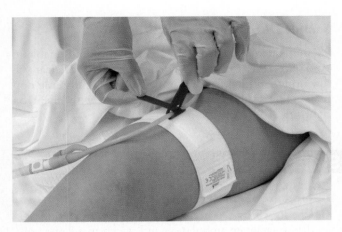

Step 16a   Secure catheter with tape (female).

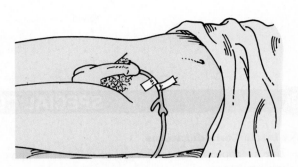

Step 16b   Securing catheter to top of thigh or to abdomen with tape (male).

Steps	Rationale
b. *Male:* Secure to top of thigh or lower abdomen with tape or catheter strap (see illustration). Replace foreskin if present. NOTE: If not previously connected, attach catheter to the drainage bag.	
17. Position drainage bag lower than bladder, and coil tubing on bed.	Facilitates drainage of urine by gravity.
18. Cleanse and dry perineal area. Position client for comfort.	Povidone-iodine is irritating to skin.
19. Measure urine.	Monitors output as baseline assessment.

NURSE ALERT   *Agency policy may restrict maximum volume of urine drained at one time to about 800 to 1000 ml. Rapid emptying of an extremely distended bladder can alter hemodynamics, resulting in shock.*

20. See Completion Protocol (inside front cover).

· · · · · · · · · ·

EVALUATION

1. Palpate bladder and observe amount, color, and clarity of urine.
2. Ask client if comfortable.
3. Measure intake and output (I&O) (see Skill 9.1, p. 200).

Unexpected Outcomes and Related Interventions

1. Client complains of discomfort during inflation of balloon.
   a. Stop inflation immediately.
   b. Advance another 1 inch (2.5 cm), and reattempt inflation.
   c. If client sill complains of pain, remove catheter and report to physician.
2. Catheter does not insert easily into urethra.
   a. Have client take deep breaths to relax, and attempt reinsertion.
   b. If still unable to advance, do not force it. Remove, and report to physician.

3. Catheter goes into vagina.
   a. Leave catheter in vagina.
   b. Recleanse urinary meatus. With another sterile catheter, insert catheter into meatus.
   c. Remove catheter in vagina after inserting second catheter in bladder.
4. Sterility is broken during catheterization by nurse or client.
   a. Replace gloves if contaminated, and start over.
   b. If client sterile field is touched, but equipment remains sterile, avoid touching that part of the sterile field.
   c. If equipment is contaminated, replace it with sterile items or start over again with new kit.

Recording and Reporting

· Record the following:
  Reason for catheterization.
  Type and size of catheter inserted.

Amount of fluid used to inflate balloon.
Client's response to procedure.
• Initiate I&O records.

Sample Documentation

0800 Bladder distended. C/O full sensation but unable to void. No. 18 Fr catheter inserted, and 700 ml of clear yellow urine returned. Balloon inflated with 5 ml sterile normal saline. Catheter to bedside drainage with client on right side.

SPECIAL CONSIDERATIONS

Pediatric Considerations
• Use an appropriate size/length of catheter to prevent urethral trauma. Up to age 3 years size 5 to 8 Fr is used. Ages 4 to 8 years may need size 8 to 10 Fr, and ages 8 to 12 years may need size 12 to 14 (Wong, 1999).
• Lubrication of the urethra before catheterization with a lubricant containing 2% lidocaine may eliminate burning and discomfort. The use of lidocaine jelly can slow the drainage of urine; therefore allow additional time for urine to flow (Wong, 1999).
• Preparation for catheterization includes instruction on pelvic muscle relaxation. Toddler, preschooler, or younger child may blow a pinwheel, sing a song, or simply breathe deeply and slowly while pressing the hips against the bed during catheterization. These actions help relax the pelvic and periurethral muscles.

Geriatric Considerations
• The frail older adult client who is physically compromised is at high risk of developing septicemia, a life-threatening infection that has spread to the blood. The client who is incontinent should not be routinely catheterized.
• An adequate oral fluid intake of 2000 ml/day and assisting the older adult to toilet on a regular timed basis will help bladder retraining and minimize the need for catheterization.

Home Care Considerations
• Clients who are at home may use a leg bag during the day to facilitate ambulation and switch to a larger volume bag at night.
• Clients may catheterize themselves at home on an intermittent basis using clean technique (see Skill 35.2). Self-catheterization has been shown to be successful in maintaining continence and results in fewer infections than with the use of indwelling catheters.

Long-Term Care Considerations
• Unfortunately, indwelling catheters are used in 10% to 30% of incontinent individuals living in long-term care institutions and are a major cause of urinary tract infections (Maas and others, 2001).
• An alternative to indwelling catheters is the use of clean intermittent catheterization at regular intervals.
• If indwelling catheters are used, the balloon should be inflated with 10 ml of fluid to avoid slippage and risk of obstruction.

Skill 35.2

Removal of an Indwelling Catheter

Indwelling catheters should be removed as soon as possible because the presence of the catheter increases the risk for urinary tract infection. Following surgery, catheters may be removed after 8 to 24 hours depending on the type of surgery. In some situations the catheter will have been in place for days or even weeks. The longer the catheter has been in place, the greater the risk that the client will have difficulty voiding after it has been removed. Clients are expected to void adequately no more than 8 hours after removal. Clients who have had an overdistended bladder or who have altered sensory perception because of regional anesthesia, such as a spinal or epidural block, may also have difficulty voiding following removal of the catheter.

The presence of a urinary catheter increases the risk of urinary tract infection, which is one of the most common types of iatrogenic infections and often develops 2 to 3 or more days after catheter removal. With early discharge from the acute care setting, clients often are at home by this time. Before discharge clients need to be informed of the risk for infection, prevention measures, and signs and symptoms that need to be reported to the physician.

ASSESSMENT

1. Check physician's order.
2. Note length of time catheter was in place. *Rationale: The longer a catheter has been in place, the greater the risk for decreased bladder muscle tone and inflammation of the urethra.*
3. Assess client's knowledge of what to expect. *Rationale: Many clients anticipate discomfort or fear inability to void successfully after removal of the catheter.*

PLANNING

Expected outcomes focus on comfort and teaching to promote successful voiding as well as prevention and early detection of infection.

Equipment

- 10-ml syringe without a needle or larger depending upon volume of solution used to inflate the balloon (Figure 35-5)
- Waterproof pad
- Clean disposable gloves
- Urine "hat"

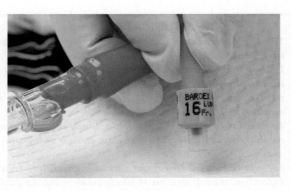

Figure 35-5   Note size of balloon printed on catheter.

Expected Outcomes

1. Client will void at least 250 ml within 8 hours of catheter removal.
2. Client will drink 1000 ml of fluid within 6 hours of catheter removal.
3. Client will verbalize the signs and symptoms of urinary tract infection.

Delegation Considerations

The skill of removing a retention catheter can be delegated to assistive personnel (AP); however, assessment and teaching require the critical thinking and knowledge application unique to a nurse. Instruct AP to measure first voiding and to report time and amount to the nurse.

REMOVAL OF INDWELLING CATHETER

Steps	Rationale

1. See Standard Protocol (inside front cover).
2. Position the client supine, and place a water-proof pad under the catheter. Females will need to abduct the legs with the drape between thighs. Drape can lay on male's thighs.
3. Insert hub of syringe into inflation valve (balloon port). Aspirate until tubing collapses, indicating that entire contents of balloon has been removed.
4. Remove catheter steadily and smoothly.
5. Wrap catheter in waterproof pad. Unhook collection bag and drainage tubing from bed.
6. Measure urine, and empty the drainage bag. Record output.
7. Cleanse the perineum with soap and water, and dry area thoroughly.

NURSE ALERT   *Catheter should slide out very easily. Do not use force. If any resistance is noted, repeat Step 3 to remove remaining water.*

COMMUNICATION TIPS

- *Tell the patient it is important to have fluid intake of 1.5 to 2 L/day (unless contraindicated).*
- *Instruct the client of need to void within 8 hours and that each voiding will be into the "hat" and measured to ensure ability to empty the bladder adequately.*
- *Explain that many clients experience mild burning or discomfort with first voiding, which soon subsides.*
- *Inform the client to report any signs urinary tract infection, which are most likely to develop in 2 to 3 days.*

---

8. Place the urine "hat" on the toilet seat.
9. See Completion Protocol (inside front cover).

• • • • • • • • • •

EVALUATION

1. Observe time and amount of first voided specimen.
2. Monitor I&O.
3. Ask client to list the signs and symptoms of urinary tract infection.

Unexpected Outcomes and Related Interventions

1. Client is unable to void 8 hours after catheter removal, having had adequate fluid intake. Bladder is distended.
   a. Provide pain medication if tension and discomfort is being experienced.
   b. Assist to normal position for voiding.
   c. Provide privacy.
   d. If all else fails, catheter may need to be reinserted to prevent overdistention.
2. Client voids small amounts frequently and states that bladder does not feel empty.
   a. Consider possible urinary retention with overflow.
   b. Secure physician's order for catheterization for residual urine.

   c. Catheterize immediately after the next voiding. If more than 150 ml is present in the bladder, catheter may be left in place.

Recording and Reporting

- Record and report time catheter was removed.
- Record teaching relating to increasing fluid intake and signs and symptoms of urinary tract infection.
- Record and report time, amount, and characteristics of first voiding.
- Record I&O.

Sample Documentation

1600 Foley catheter removed without difficulty. Client encouraged to drink 8 to 10 ounces per hour and told that first void will be measured. Informed that first void may be uncomfortable and voiding within 6 to 8 hours is to be expected. Client has had urinary tract infections before. Signs and symptoms reviewed.
　1930 Voided 350 ml with mild burning discomfort.

Skill 35.3

Inserting Straight Catheter for Specimen Collection or Residual Urine

Straight catheterization is done to empty a distended bladder when a client cannot void, to collect a specimen, or to determine if residual urine is in the bladder after voiding. Because as many as 20% of older clients have bacterial infection from a single catheterization, a urine sample should be obtained from a voided specimen if possible (Yoshikawa, Nicolle, and Normal, 1996). Straight catheterization is also done intermittently for clients with paralysis following spinal cord injury or with complications involving peripheral nerve damage (Gray, 2000). Although catheteriztion is frequently used for older clients in the management of incontinence, it is no longer recommended. Clean intermittent catheterization, when practical, is preferable to long-term catheterization (Cravens and Zweig, 2000).

A client's ability to void depends on feeling the urge to urinate, on being able to control the urethral sphincter, and on being able to relax. If a client is unable to void, every effort is made to promote urinary elimination before catheterization is performed. This involves assisting the client in assuming the normal voiding position. Females usually assume a sitting or a squatting position. Males usually void more easily in the standing position. Other measures to promote voiding include having the client listen to running water, putting a client's hand in warm water, or stroking a female client's inner thigh. Clients should be given privacy and not be rushed. Comfort and adequate fluid intake are also important factors in facilitating voiding.

Urinary retention is the inability of the bladder to fully empty. Residual urine is the volume of urine in the bladder after voiding. Clients at risk for large residual volumes include those receiving bladder training exercises, including clients with spinal cord injuries, who have suffered a cerebrovascular accident, or who have had bladder surgery resulting in swelling and partial obstruction of the urethra. Intermittent catheterization has become the standard of care for clients with spinal cord injuries (Warren, 1997).

ASSESSMENT

1. Review I&O record for frequency and amount of each voiding over previous 8 to 24 hours. *Rationale: May indicate likelihood of bladder fullness.*
2. Ask client to describe any discomfort experienced while voiding. *Rationale: Pain is associated with bladder spasms that can alter voiding pattern.*
3. Review physician's orders, which may specify parameters for catheterization for residual (e.g., "Check residual urine bid until amount obtained is less than 100 ml").
4. Identify time client voids. *Rationale: Residual urine determinations need to be performed immediately after voiding to obtain accurate data.*
5. Assess client's knowledge and experience with urinary retention and catheterization. *Rationale: Reveals level of knowledge and teaching needed.*

PLANNING

Expected outcomes focus on monitoring quantity of residual urine, promoting comfort, and preventing urinary tract infection.

Expected Outcomes

1. Quantity of residual urine trends toward 100 ml or less.
2. Urine remains clear, straw colored, and without foul odor.

3. Client reports voiding without difficulty or discomfort.
4. Client explains the purpose of the procedure and what is expected.

Equipment

- Disposable gloves
- Bed protector
- Bath blanket
- Flashlight or appropriate additional lighting
- Basin with warm water, soap, washcloth, and towel
- Catheterization kit for straight catheterization: contains collection chamber, single-lumen catheter, cotton balls, antiseptic solution, forceps, drapes (one is fenestrated with center hole), gloves, lubricant, and specimen container (Figure 35-6). (NOTE: Contents vary. Read contents on outer package and add necessary items.)

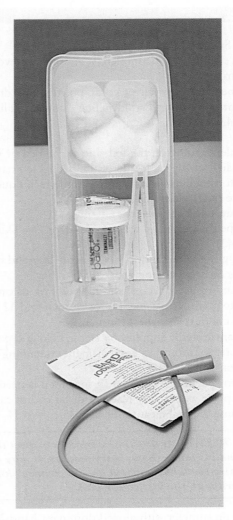

Figure 35-6 Kit for straight catheterization for specimen or residual (outer collection container with cotton balls, antiseptic solution, drape with center opening, specimen container, lubricant, rectangular drape, disposable sterile gloves, straight catheter, and forceps).

Delegation Considerations

The skill of obtaining catheterized specimens for residual urine may be delegated to assistive personnel (AP) in some settings (see agency policy). Initial client assessment and coordination of repeated catheterizations requires the critical thinking and knowledge application unique to a nurse and delegation is inappropriate.

IMPLEMENTATION FOR INSERTING STRAIGHT CATHETER FOR SPECIMEN COLLECTION OR RESIDUAL URINE

Steps	Rationale
1. See Standard Protocol (inside front cover).	
2. Ask client to void completely, and measure volume of urine.	Helps determine how effectively client is emptying bladder.
3. Immediately after client voids, position and drape client as for inserting indwelling catheter (Skill 35-1, p. 843).	Urine is being produced and collected in the bladder continuously. A delay in the procedure would give inaccurate information about the client's ability to empty the bladder.
4. While standing on the left side of the bed (if right-handed) or the right side of the bed (if left-handed), open catheterization kit using sterile technique and place outer plastic bag within reach.	Provides a container for disposal of used supplies.
5. **Apply sterile gloves (see Chapter 4).**	
6. Drape the perineum with sterile drape (see Skill 35.1, p. 843)	
7. Using sterile technique, place sterile tray and contents on sterile drape between legs.	
8. Open lubricant packet, and lubricate tip of catheter; 2.5 to 5 cm (1 to 2 inches) for women and 12.5 to 17.5 cm (5 to 7 inches) for men.	Eases insertion of catheter through the urethra with minimal discomfort.
9. Organize sterile supplies on sterile field and pour antiseptic solution into compartment containing sterile cotton balls.	
10. Open specimen container (if specimen is needed), and place within easy reach of distal end of catheter.	
11. Cleanse urethral meatus (see Skill 35.1, Step 14, p. 844).	

NURSE ALERT *At this time carefully inspect the perineum and visualize the urinary meatus. It may help to gently raise the labia upward as you cleanse slowly downward with the last cotton ball.*

---

12. Pick up catheter with gloved dominant hand 2.5 to 5 cm (1 to 2 inches) from catheter tip. Hold catheter loosely coiled in palm of dominant hand.
13. Insert catheter gently until urine flows.

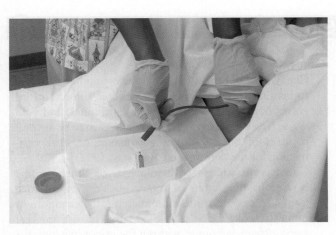

Step 14 Collecting urine for specimen with straight catheter.

Steps	Rationale
14. Collect 10 to 30 ml of urine in specimen container, then allow remaining urine to collect in outer container (see illustration).	Sterile specimen is obtained for culture.
15. Allow bladder to empty fully unless institution policy restricts maximal volume of urine drained (see agency policy).	Retained urine may serve as reservoir for growth of microorganisms.
16. Steadily and smoothly remove straight catheter.	
17. Assist client to a comfortable position. Wash and dry perineal area.	Promotes comfort.
18. See Completion Protocol (inside front cover).	

• • • • • • • • • •

EVALUATION

1. Accurately measure urine obtained.
2. Note if urine appears clear, straw colored, and without foul odor.
3. Ask client to describe level of discomfort using a scale of 0 to 10, 10 being the worst.
4. Ask client to explain the purpose of the procedure and what is expected.

Unexpected Outcomes and Related Interventions

1. Residual volume is greater than 100 ml of urine.
   a. Continue to catheterize after each voiding for residual urine according to physician's orders. If amounts exceed a prescribed volume, it may be necessary to insert an indwelling catheter. If this is anticipated, the nurse may perform residual catheterization with a Foley catheter.
2. Urinary incontinence of small amounts of urine occurs from overflow incontinence with bladder distention.
   a. Physician should be notified.
3. Client has evidence of bladder infection, which may include fever and chills; dysuria; frequent voiding in small amounts; dull or aching pain localized in the flank, back, lower abdomen, or groin; and cloudy, bloody, or foul-smelling urine.
   a. Physician may order urinalysis for culture and sensitivity.
   b. Encourage increased fluid intake.
   c. Antibiotics may need to be prescribed.

Recording and Reporting

• Record the following:
  Amount of urine voided.
  Amount and characteristics of urine obtained from catheterization.
  Client's response to procedure.

Sample Documentation

1300 Voided 200 ml clear urine without discomfort. Catheterized for a residual of 125 ml of clear yellow urine. Reported minimal discomfort during the procedure; however, expresses concern about how many more times this procedure needs to be done.

SPECIAL CONSIDERATIONS

Pediatric Considerations

- Bladder catheterization is used to obtain a specimen that is urgently needed or when the child is unable to void. Catheterization is used to obtain a sterile urine specimen in the presence of urethral obstruction or anuria caused by renal failure.
- Suprapubic aspiration may be used when the bladder cannot be accessed through the urethra, such as with some birth defects; however, access to the bladder via the urethra is preferred whenever possible because it has a much higher success rate and is less painful.
- It is important to insert an appropriate length of tubing to prevent knotting of the catheter in the bladder. The extra length coils in the bladder and becomes knotted as the bladder decompresses.
- Also see Pediatric Considerations for Skill 35.1, p. 840.

Geriatric Considerations

A urinary tract infection in an older adult can develop into septicemia, infection in the circulation, which can be life threatening. Prevention, early detection, and treatment are crucial in this age group.

Home Care Considerations

- Clients may be taught to use a double-voiding technique to help decrease the amount of residual urine. This involves having the client void, wait 5 minutes, and void again. The relaxation between voidings may be helpful in cases of bladder outlet obstruction or weak contractility of the detrusor muscle (Gray, 1992).
- Clients with paraplegia, hemiplegia, or other chronic conditions that limit voluntary bladder control may learn to perform intermittent self-catheterization at home (see Skill 35.2, p. 848). Many can use medical asepsis (clean technique) without the risk of infection because the body's natural resistance to microorganisms normally found in their home makes risk for infection minimal. Some clients who are prone to infection choose to use sterile technique. *If the procedure is performed by the nurse, sterile technique is indicated.*

Long-Term Care Considerations

Equipment in the long-term care setting may include a kit that has the outer container, drape, and lubricant. The catheter and specimen container may need to be obtained separately.

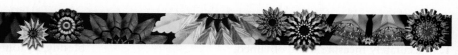

Skill 35.4

Continuous Bladder Irrigation

CBI is a continuous infusion of a sterile solution into the bladder, usually using a three-way irrigation closed system with a triple-lumen catheter (see Figure 35-1, *C*, p. 839). One lumen goes to the client to drain urine, one goes to the irrigation solution, and one is used to inflate the catheter balloon (Figure 35-7). The primary use of CBI is following genitourinary surgery to use an indwelling catheter to keep the bladder clear and free of blood clots or sediment. CBI is frequently ordered after bladder surgeries.

The physician must order the solution, strength, and flow rate. If the physician only specifies solution, check your agency's protocol for strength and rate. The irrigation solution infuses continuously through one lumen while the second lumen drains the urine and irrigation solution.

ASSESSMENT

1. Assess client's level of consciousness and ability to cooperate.

2. Palpate bladder for distention and tenderness. *Rationale: Bladder distention indicates flow of urine may be blocked from draining.*

3. Ask client to describe bladder pain or spasms. *Rationale: Serves as baseline. Accumulation of blood clots can increase bladder spasms.*

4. Observe urine for color, amount, clarity, and presence of mucus, clots, or sediment. *Rationale: This indicates if client is bleeding or sloughing tissue and determines necessity for increasing irrigation rate.*

5. Review I&O record to verify that the hourly output into the drainage bag is in appropriate proportion to the irrigating solution entering the bladder. *Rationale: Determines if system is obstructed. Expect more output than fluid instilled because of urine production.*

6. Assess client's knowledge regarding purpose of performing catheter irrigation.

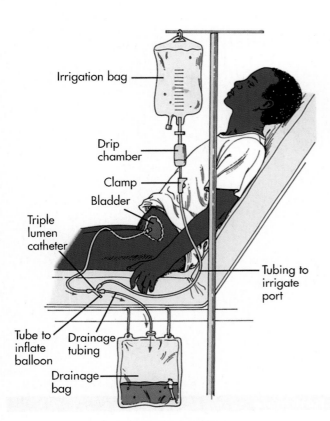

Irrigation bag

Drip chamber

Clamp

Bladder

Triple lumen catheter

Tubing to irrigate port

Tube to inflate balloon

Drainage tubing

Drainage bag

Figure 35-7   CBI setup.

2. Client's urine output has decreased blood clots and sediment. (NOTE: Urine will be bloody following bladder/urethral surgery, gradually becoming lighter and blood tinged in 2 to 3 days.)
3. Client does not complain of bladder pain or spasms.

Equipment

- Clean gloves
- Irrigation solution at room temperature as prescribed
- Irrigation tubing with clamp to regulate irrigation flow rate
- Y connector (optional) to connect irrigation tubing to double-lumen catheter
- Intravenous (IV) pole
- Antiseptic swab

PLANNING

Expected outcomes focus on continuous urine flow and client comfort.

Expected Outcomes

1. Output is greater than volume of irrigating solution instilled.

Delegation Considerations

The skill of catheter irrigations requires the critical thinking and knowledge application unique to a nurse. Delegation to assistive personnel (AP) is inappropriate.

IMPLEMENTATION FOR CONTINUOUS BLADDER IRRIGATION

Steps	Rationale
1. See Standard Protocol (inside front cover).	
2. Place label on irrigation solution bag with client's name, room number, date and time, type of solution, and any additives. Clearly mark bag for GU IRRIGATION ONLY.	Indicates fluid is not to be infused intravenously.
3. Hang bag on IV pole.	
4. Using aseptic technique, insert (spike) tip of sterile irrigation tubing into bag containing irrigation solution (see illustration).	
5. Close clamp on tubing, and fill the drip chamber one-half full by squeezing the chamber. Open the clamp to completely fill tubing and remove air. Close the clamp.	Air in the tubing may cause bladder fullness and spasms.

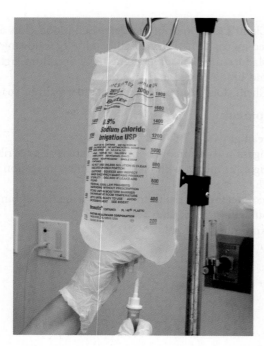

Step 4 Spiking bag of sterile irrigation solution for CBI.

Steps	Rationale

6. Using aseptic technique, wipe off irrigation port of triple-lumen catheter with antiseptic swab and connect to irrigation tubing.

NURSE ALERT *Be sure the drainage tubing from indwelling catheter is patent (not clamped or obstructed). If irrigation solution continues to infuse rapidly and drainage from the bladder is blocked by a blood clot, overdistention can result in extreme discomfort and bladder damage or rupture.*

---

7. Calculate drip rate, and adjust rate at roller clamp (according to physician's orders or agency protocol).

8. If urine is bright red or has clots, increase irrigation rate until drainage appears pink.

Continuous drainage is expected and assists with prevention of clotting in the presence of active bleeding in bladder and flushes clots out of bladder.

9. Replace bag of irrigation solution as needed.

10. Empty catheter drainage bag as needed.

Bag will fill rapidly and may need to be emptied every 1 to 2 hours.

11. Compare urine output with infusion of irrigation solution every hour.

12. See Completion Protocol (inside front cover).

• • • • • • • • • •

EVALUATION

1. To determine actual urine output, subtract total amount of fluid infused from the total volume drained.
2. Observe client's urine for blood clots and sediment.
3. Ask if client is experiencing pain and assess for fever.

Unexpected Outcomes and Related Interventions

1. Irrigation solution will not infuse or is slower than previously set.
   a. Check for kinks in the tubing.
   b. Examine drainage tubing for clots, sediment, or kinks.

c. Notify physician if irrigant is retained, client complains of severe pain, or bladder is distended.

2. Drainage output is less than amount of irrigation solution infused.
   a. Assess for clots. With a physician's order, manual irrigation with 50 ml sterile normal saline (NS) "using gentle pressure" may be done.
   b. Assess client for bladder spasms and distended bladder (may need antispasmodics).
   c. Notify physician.

3. Bright-red bleeding occurs even with irrigation drip wide open.
   a. Assess for hypovolemic shock (vital signs, skin color and moisture, anxiety level).
   b. Leave irrigation drip wide open, and notify physician.

4. Client has bladder spasms.
   a. Try nonpharmacological methods of pain relief (e.g., apply warmth to lower abdomen, repositioning with knees flexed to 45 degrees).

b. Administer ordered urinary antispasmodics.
c. If unrelieved, call physician.

Recording and Reporting

- Record amount and type of solution used as irrigant, amount influenced, amount returned as drainage, and characteristics of output.
- Record I & O.
- Report catheter occlusion, sudden bleeding, infection, or increased pain to physician.

Sample Documentation

0800 Lower abdomen soft and flat. Catheter drainage of 225 ml of bright-red urine with moderate-size dark bloody clots. 3000 ml of NS infusing at 60 gtt per minute. Client rates bladder spasms at 5 on a 0 to 10 scale (with 10 the worst). Lying on left side, knees flexed.

Skill 35.5

Suprapubic Catheters

A suprapubic catheter is a very small tube inserted surgically into the bladder through the abdominal wall above the symphysis pubis (Figure 35-8). This type of catheter may be used following gynecological and bladder surgery when there is likely to be excessive swelling and pain in the perineal area that could interfere with voiding, to promote bladder healing after trauma, and to empty the bladder in the presence of spinal cord injuries. A suprapubic catheter drains urine until the client is able to void naturally after the swelling has subsided and the suprapubic catheter is clamped. It is generally more comfortable than an indwelling catheter and the incidence of urinary tract infection may be lower than with an indwelling catheter. Numerous suprapubic catheters and appliances are available.

Suprapubic catheters may be sutured to the skin or secured with an adhesive material. In some cases clients are discharged home with the suprapubic catheter and must learn to maintain patency, empty the drainage bag, clean the site, and observe for infection.

ASSESSMENT

1. Assess catheter insertion site for inflammation including erythema, edema, and drainage. *Rationale: If insertion site is new, slight inflammation may be expected as part of normal wound healing.*
2. Assess urine in catheter or bag for amount, color, clarity, and sediment. *Rationale: Abnormal findings may indicate potential complications such as blockage or urinary tract infection.*
3. Assess for fever and chills. *Rationale: These are signs of urinary tract infection or infection at the catheter site.*
4. Assess tape site for signs of irritation. *Rationale: Repeated taping may lead to skin irritation and breakdown.*

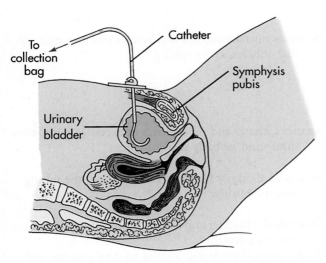

Figure 35-8   Suprapubic catheter in female client.

5. Identify allergies. *Rationale: Client may be sensitive to tape or antiseptic solution.*
6. Assess level of discomfort on scale of 0 to 10.

PLANNING

Expected outcomes focus on maintaining the patency of the catheter, maintaining comfort, and prevention of infection.

Expected Outcomes

1. Client's catheter is patent, and output is 30 ml or greater per hour.
2. Client's catheter site is free of erythema, edema, discharge, or tenderness.
3. Client remains afebrile, and urine is clear, free from odor, sediment, and bacteria.
4. Client's level of discomfort is less than baseline assessment.
5. Client correctly demonstrates care for insertion site and drainage bag by discharge.

6. Client verbalizes signs and symptoms of urinary tract infection and insertion site infection by discharge.

Equipment

- Gloves: sterile and clean
- Sterile gauze for cleaning site
- Antiseptic solution
- Drain (split) gauze
- Tape
- Biohazardous waste bag (for soiled dressing)

Delegation Considerations

The skill of caring for a newly established suprapubic catheter requires the critical thinking and knowledge application unique to a nurse. Delegation to assistive personnel (AP) is inappropriate.

IMPLEMENTATION FOR SUPRAPUBIC CATHETERS

Steps	Rationale
1. See Standard Protocol (inside front cover).	
2. Remove dressing; discard gloves (see Skill 24.1, p. 573).	
3. **Put on sterile gloves.**	
4. Inspect insertion site and patency of catheter.	
5. Without creating tension, hold catheter erect with nondominant hand while cleaning. Cleanse in circular motion starting near the catheter insertion site and continuing in outward widening circles for approximately 2 inches (5 cm) (see illustration).	Follows principle of sterile technique to move from area of least contamination to area of most contamination. Tension on the catheter may cause discomfort or cause the catheter to slip out of place.
6. With a fresh moistened gauze, gently cleanse the base of the catheter, moving up and away from site of insertion (proximal to distal).	Removes microorganisms that resides and any drainage that adheres to the tubing.
7. With sterile gloved hand, apply drain dressing (split gauze) around catheter and tape in place (see illustration).	
8. Secure catheter to abdomen with tape or Velcro multipurpose tube holder to reduce tension on insertion site.	Secures catheter and reduces risk of excessive tension on suture and/or body seal.
9. Coil excess tubing on bed, and secure it to the dressing. Keep drainage bag below level of bladder at all times.	Prevents kinking or backflow of urine from the tubing into the bladder.
10. With a physician's order the suprapubic catheter may be clamped for several hours.	Distends the bladder and allows the client to initiate voiding normally.
11. If the client is unable to void and feels uncomfortably full, unclamp the catheter, and reclamp it according to physician's orders.	As the surgical site heals, normal voiding patterns will return.

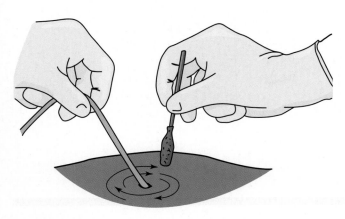

Step 5 Cleansing around suprapubic catheter, avoiding tension on catheter.

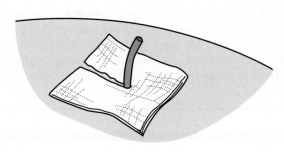

Step 7 Split drain dressing for suprapubic catheter.

Steps	Rationale
12. Once the client has voided normally while the suprapubic tube is clamped, residual urine can be evaluated by releasing the clamp and measuring remaining urine volume.	Residual urine amounts of less than 100 ml indicate that normal bladder function has returned. The physician may order the removal of the suprapubic catheter.
13. See Completion Protocol (inside front cover).	

• • • • • • • • • •

EVALUATION

1. Monitor suprapubic catheter output.
2. Monitor body temperature, complete blood count for elevated white blood cell count, and observe client's urine for clarity, sediment, or unusual odor.
3. Observe catheter insertion site for erythema, edema, discharge, or tenderness.
4. Ask client to rate discomfort using a scale of 0 to 10.
5. Observe client demonstrate care of insertion site and drainage bag.
6. Ask client to state signs and symptoms of urinary tract infection and insertion site infection.

Unexpected Outcomes and Related Interventions

1. Urine through catheter is obstructed with blood clots, catheter tip against wall of bladder, or sediment collection.
   a. Irrigate catheter to achieve patency.
   b. If unable to irrigate, notify physician.
   c. Increase fluids (if not contraindicated) to at least 1500 ml/day.
2. Client has urinary tract infection or catheter site infection.
   a. Increase fluids to at least 1500 ml/day (if not contraindicated).
   b. Increase protein, cereal, and grain foods to increase acidity of urine, and increase intake of cranberry juice.
   c. Monitor body temperature, and notify physician for temperatures greater than 101° F (38.3° C).

   d. Follow agency or Centers for Disease Control and Prevention protocol, and culture drainage at site of catheter.
   e. Administer antibiotics as ordered.
3. Catheter becomes dislodged.
   a. Apply sterile gauze to site.
   b. Apply pressure if bleeding.
   c. Reassure client.
   d. Notify physician.
4. When catheter is clamped, client complains of distended bladder before time to release clamp.
   a. Release clamp, and drain no more than 800 to 1000 ml of urine at one time depending on agency policy.
   b. Recalculate time for clamping, if off schedule.

Recording and Reporting

• Record the following:
   Urine output, color, and characteristics.
   Dressing changes, including assessments of wound.
   Tolerance of client.

Sample Documentation

0800 Catheter draining 100 ml of clear yellow urine in 2 hours. Dressing removed from suprapubic catheter site. Small amount of dark-brown drainage on gauze. No redness, edema, or drainage at the site. Cleansed with povidone-iodine and dressed with drain dressing. Describes discomfort at 3 (scale of 0 to 10) during dressing change.

SPECIAL CONSIDERATIONS

Home Care Considerations
Before discharge from the hospital with a suprapubic catheter the client must be able to clean and dress the suprapubic site; list signs of catheter obstruction, urinary tract infection, and wound infection; empty the catheter drainage bag; and observe characteristics of the urine.

Skill 35.6

Urinary Diversions (Continent and Incontinent)

A urinary diversion is a surgical opening on the abdomen or ostomy through which urine is eliminated. This is performed on clients who have partial or complete excision of the bladder (cystectomy) because of malignancy or trauma. There are two types of urinary diversions: (1) continent and (2) incontinent. Continent diversion consists of an internal pouch or reservoir for urine, surgically created from a segment of the small bowel (Figure 35-9, *A*.) The stoma has a muscular closure or valve similar to the sphincter at the urinary meatus so urine does not leak involuntarily. The client regularly performs self-catheterization every 4 to 6 hours and does not need to wear an external appliance. Periodic irrigation of the reservoir is also necessary because mucus is secreted from pouches constructed from the bowel. When the catheter is not in use, a small gauze pad covers the stoma to protect the client's clothes from mucus drainage. For continent diversions use of pouch varies with recovery phase, postoperative care as long as 3 weeks.

The second type of urinary diversion is an incontinent urinary diversion, such as the ileal conduit, in which the ureter is transplanted into a closed-off portion of the ileum of the small bowel, which has an opening going to the outer wall of the abdomen (Figure 35-9, *B*). With a ureterostomy there is an opening from one or both ureters to the abdomen's outer wall (Figure 35-9, *C* and *D*). The stoma of a urinary diversion is normally red or pink and protrudes slightly above the skin. These diversions require a pouch to collect urine that drains continuously. The pouch must be emptied frequently, and the adhesive holding the pouch may cause skin irritation. Numerous products on the market are available for pouching and skin barrier protection.

ASSESSMENT

1. Inspect pouch for amount of urine, leakage, and length of time in place. *Rationale: Expect output of at*

least *30 ml/hr. Pouches are emptied when one-third to one-half full because weight of urine in pouch can weaken the seal, resulting in leaking. To prevent skin irritation one-piece pouch or skin barrier from two-piece system should be changed, if not leaking, every 3 to 7 days.*

2. Inspect stoma and all external suture lines for healing progress. Stoma should be moist and reddish pink; immediately after surgery it is edematous and usually

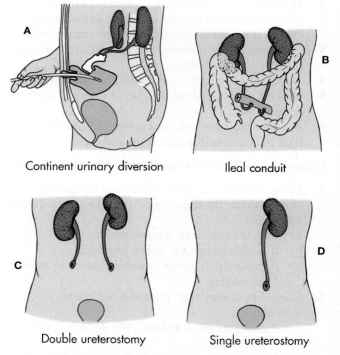

Figure 35-9   Types of urinary diversions. **A,** Continent urinary diversion. **B,** Ileal loop. **C,** Double ureterostomy (stoma from each ureter). **D,** Single ureterostomy (stoma from one ureter).

has urinary stents in place. *Rationale: Ureteral stents are sutured in place with dissolvable sutures and are used to maintain patency of ureters. Stents remain in place 10 to 14 days and are removed by the physician (Black and Matassarin-Jacobs, 1997).*

3. Observe and palpate skin around stoma for erythema, excoriation, edema, and drainage. *Rationale: Determines need for skin barrier.*
4. Assess level of comfort on a scale of 0 to 10.
5. Observe abdomen for abdominal contours, folds, and suture line. *Rationale: Helps to determine proper pouch type and size.*
6. Assess client's emotional response, knowledge, and understanding of ostomy. *Rationale: Helps to determine the extent client is able to participate in care and facilitates discharge planning.*

PLANNING

Expected outcomes focus on maintaining urine output, a healthy stoma, skin integrity, and promoting self-care.

Expected Outcomes

1. Urine drains freely from stents or stoma at least 30 ml/hr.
2. Stoma remains red, shiny, and moist.
3. Peristomal skin is free of irritation. Sutures are intact, and incision is well approximated.
4. Client rates discomfort at less than baseline assessment (scale of 0 to 10).
5. Client and/or primary caregiver are willing to view stoma and correctly care for stoma, skin, and pouch by discharge.

Equipment (Figure 35-10)

- Clean gloves
- Underpad, washcloth, towel, and warm water
- Scissors with pointed end

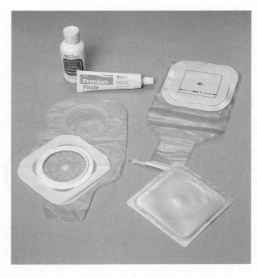

Figure 35-10   Ostomy pouches and skin barriers.

- Measuring guide
- Tissue or toilet paper
- Gauze pad or tampon
- New pouch, skin barrier, and adhesive if required
- Urinary drainage bag

Delegation Considerations

Pouching an incontinent urinary diversion requires the critical thinking and knowledge application unique to a nurse. In some agencies a stoma nurse specialist is available to provide this care. Assistive personnel (AP) who provide personal care are instructed to report any leakage of urine and/or breakdown of skin integrity to the nurse.

IMPLEMENTATION FOR URINARY DIVERSIONS (CONTINENT ANDINCONTINENT)

Steps	Rationale
1. See Standard Protocol (inside front cover).	
2. Position client supine to allow for easy access to stoma so that abdomen is as smooth or flat as possible. Be sure client can view procedure.	When client is sitting, more skin wrinkles on the abdomen complicate pouch application and increase the tendency for leaking.
3. Prepare pouch by removing backing from barrier and adhesive; if using cutting to fit; cut opening $1/16$ to $1/8$ inch larger than stoma before removing backing (see illustration). Some pouches have standard opening that attaches to plastic ring. Some urinary pouches have special skin barrier that melts and forms secure seal around base of stoma.	Barrier facilitates seal and protects skin. Correct size of opening keeps urine off skin and reduces risk of maceration and skin irritation. New stoma will shrink and does not reach optimal size for 6 to 8 weeks.
4. Place a towel or disposable waterproof barrier under client. Tightly roll several gauze pads separately to form "wicks" (or use tampons).	Rolled gauze pads are used to absorb urine during pouch change. Urine drains almost continuously.

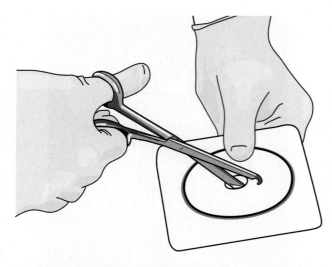

Step 3   Cutting opening of pouch to fit stoma.

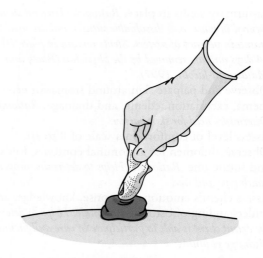

Step 5   Holding wick in place to prevent leaking.

Steps	Rationale
5. Remove used pouch gently by pushing skin away from barrier, avoiding any tension on stents (if present). Immediately place a wick, tampon, or sterile gauze pad over stoma (see illustration). If stents are present, place sterile gauze pad underneath tips.	Gauze or tampon wick keeps urine from leaking onto the skin.

NURSE ALERT   ***If stents are present, avoid tension on them. Stents are usually sutured in place with dissolvable sutures.***

6. Cleanse skin around the stoma gently with warm tap water using gauze pads. Do not scrub skin. Wick stoma continuously.	Avoid soap, which leaves a residue on skin that interferes with pouch adhesion. Using a wick at stoma tip prevents peristomal skin from becoming wet with urine. Pouch does not adhere to wet skin.
7. If uric acid crystals are present, saturate a washcloth with a solution of one-third vinegar and two-thirds warm water. Soak the involved area for several minutes. Rinse with warm tap water, and dry completely with dry gauze or towel. Remove copious mucus from the surface of the stoma if present.	Vinegar solution helps remove uric acid crystals.
8. If creases form next to stoma, use barrier paste or seal to fill in; let dry 1 to 2 minutes.	Creates smooth surface for pouch placement and inhibits leaking.
9. Apply skin sealant in circular area around base of stoma to skin not protected by barrier; let dry.	
10. *Apply one-piece pouch.* Hold pouch by barrier, center over stoma and stents, and press down gently. Bottom of pouch is angled slightly to attach to bedside urinary drainage bag.	Angling pouch minimizes trauma to the skin and avoids uneven twisting, which can disrupt seal.
a. Use another skin sealant on skin in contact with adhesive; allow to dry. Press adhesive backing smoothly against skin starting from the bottom and working up and around sides (see illustration).	
b. Maintain gentle finger pressure around barrier for 1 to 2 minutes.	Ensures molding and adherence of skin barrier.
11. *Apply two-piece pouch.* Apply flange (barrier with adhesive) as above (see illustration), then snap on pouch. If client is mostly ambulatory and upright, apply pouch vertically.	Weight of urine in the bag is pulled down by gravity. Pulling at an angle can disrupt the seal and create leakage.

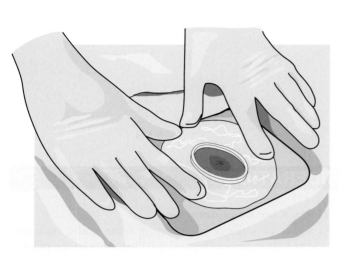

Step 10a   Press pouch firmly to secure in place.

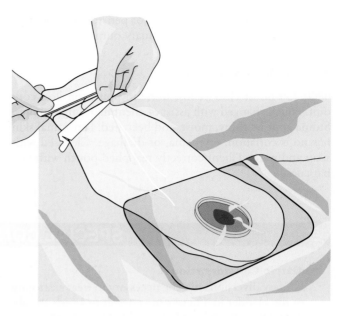

Step 13   Clamping pouch after emptying.

12. Dispose of used pouch and soiled equipment in a plastic bag, and place it in the appropriate trash receptacle (see agency policy).

Avoids odor in the room.

13. Empty bag when one-half to two-thirds full of urine. Measure and record urine output. Secure clamp on end of bag opening for repeated emptying (see illustration).

Prevents tension on the bag that can irritate the skin and disrupt the seal.

14. See Completion Protocol (inside front cover).

• • • • • • • • • •

EVALUATION

1. Observe urine output through stoma: urine is free flowing and greater than 240 ml every 8 hours.
2. Inspect and palpate stoma for color, shine, moistness, edema, or tenderness.
3. Observe peristomal skin for excoriation or erythema. If suture line is present, inspect for approximation and signs of inflammation.
4. Ask client to rate discomfort using a scale of 0 to 10.
5. Ask client to view stoma, and observe client demonstrating pouch care.

Unexpected Outcomes and Related Interventions

1. Output from pouch is less than 30 ml/hr or 240 ml per 8 hours.
   a. Assess for pressure or fullness in stoma region.
   b. Observe for leakage around stent.
   c. Determine if stents or stoma could be blocked by blood clot or debris.
   d. Irrigation may be indicated. Notify physician.
2. Skin irritation around stoma: itching and burning.
   a. Remove pouch immediately.
   b. Apply new pouch.

3. Odors are coming from pouch.
   a. If pouch is leaking, change complete pouch.
   b. Increase intake of cranberry juice, ascorbic acid, protein, grains, and cereals. (This will acidify the urine and decrease odor and potential for infection.)
4. Client will not participate in care of stoma.
   a. Listen to client's feelings with empathy.
   b. Contact local support group with physician's approval.
   c. Guard against displaying disapproval or disgust while caring for client.

Recording and Reporting

• Record type of pouch, time of change, condition and appearance of stoma and peristomal skin, character of urine, time of irrigation, and client response.
• Record actual urinary output and characteristics of urine.
• Document client's, family's, or significant other's verbal and nonverbal reaction to stoma and level of participation.

- Report abnormalities in stoma or peristomal structures and absence or decrease in urinary output to nurse in charge or physician.

Sample Documentation

0800 250 ml of clear yellow urine in pouch on ileal conduit. Pouch changed with assist of client handling supplies. Stoma appears shiny, moist, and beefy red. Peristomal skin has no excoriation, erythema, or drainage. Cleansed with soap and water. Client correctly reapplied pouch with verbal cues.

 SPECIAL CONSIDERATIONS

Pediatric Considerations

- Urinary diversions may be necessary to treat exstrophy of the bladder in a newborn, a defect in which the abdominal wall and underlying bladder structures are exposed.
- It is helpful to discuss the advantages of a permanent urinary diversion with a well-fitted ileostomy bag, which allows the child almost unrestricted freedom in activities enjoyed by other children (Wong, 1999).
- There are no major alterations in toileting, except emptying the bag at periodic intervals. This is extremely important to older children and adolescents, who want to be accepted as one of the group.
- Substantial psychological support and guidance are needed to help with the adjustment and fears related to appearance of the genitalia, and potential rejection by peers, especially the opposite gender.

Geriatric Considerations

- Some older clients may try to cope with the continuous flow of urine from the stoma by decreasing the amount of fluid they drink so they will have less output. This can be very dangerous because older adults are more susceptible to dehydration. Client needs appropriate teaching to prevent this misconception.
- Limitations in physical and visual ability may require adaptation and assistance in self-ostomy routine.

Home Care Considerations

- Stress importance of reporting fever, chills, back or flank pain, or cloudy, foul-smelling urine to the physician as soon as possible.
- At home, pouch spout should be opened and connected to larger drainage bag at night.
- Many different types of one-piece and two-piece pouching systems are available. All disposable pouches are odor proof. Clients should be encouraged to find a pouch that they can apply easily and that is comfortable for them.
- Clients should avoid replacing pouches in an extremely hot or cold environment, because temperature may affect the barrier and adhesive materials.
- Pouch covers are available or can be easily made. Special underwear and sleep garments are also available.
- Advise clients when they travel to always keep spare ostomy supplies with them in case luggage gets lost.
- While swimming, clients may find that applying waterproof tape to the skin barrier and/or wearing an ostomy belt prevents the pouch and skin barrier from becoming dislodged.
- Client needs to wear medical alert bracelet or necklace.

CRITICAL THINKING EXERCISES

1. A client had a vaginal hysterectomy 2 days ago. The Foley catheter has been removed, and now she is having difficulty emptying her bladder. She feels the urge to void frequently but is only able to void 75 to 100 ml each time. The orders include the following: "Catheterize for residual volume. If greater than 150 ml, leave catheter in place."
   a. What assessments would you make to determine the client's bladder status?
   b. What equipment would you gather to perform catheterization for this client?
   c. How would you collect a specimen for urinalysis if the Foley catheter is left in place?

2. A client has a suprapubic catheter in place. She has decreased urine output, the urine is cloudy, and she is experiencing fever and chills. The physician orders urinalysis for culture and sensitivity.
   a. How could you collect a urine specimen for culture and sensitivity?
   b. What teaching is appropriate for this client?

3. A client has had prostate surgery and returns from the recovery room with a CBI. You note that the urine output is bright red and there are several clots in the drainage tubing. The client is complaining of excruciating bladder pains, 10 (scale of 0 to 10), that come and go. The vital signs are within normal limits except that the blood pressure is slightly elevated. The amount of irrigation solution instilled is 250 ml greater than the amount of drainage in the past hour.
   a. What are the possible reasons for these developments to occur?
   b. What is your first priority in this situation?

REFERENCES

Black I, Matassarin-Jacobs E: *Medical-surgical nursing: clinical management for continuity of care,* ed 3, Philadelphia, 1997, WB Saunders.

Cravens DD, Zweig S: Urinary catheter management, *Am Fam Physician* 61(1):369, 2000.

Evans E: Indwelling catheter care: dispelling the misconceptions, *Geriatr Nurs* 20(2):85, 1999.

Fiers S: Indwelling catheters and devices: avoiding the problems, *Urol Nurs* 14(3):141, 1994.

Gray M: Urinary retention: management in the acute care setting, part II, *Am J Nurs* 100(8):36, 2000.

Hiser V: Nursing interventions for urinary incontinence in home health, *J Wound Ostomy Continence Nurs* 26(3):142, 1999.

Lewis S and others: *Medical-surgical nursing: assessment and management of clinical problems,* ed 5, St Louis, 2000, Mosby.

Maas M and others: *Nursing care of older adults: diagnoses, outcomes, and interventions,* St Louis, 2001, Mosby.

Warren JW: Catheter-associated urinary tract infections, *Infect Dis Clin North Am* (11):609, 1997.

Wong D: *Nursing care of infants and children,* ed 6, St Louis, 1999, Mosby.

Yoshikawa TT, Nicolle LE, Normal DC: Management of complicated urinary tract infection in older patients, *J Am Geriatr Soc* 44:1235, 1996.

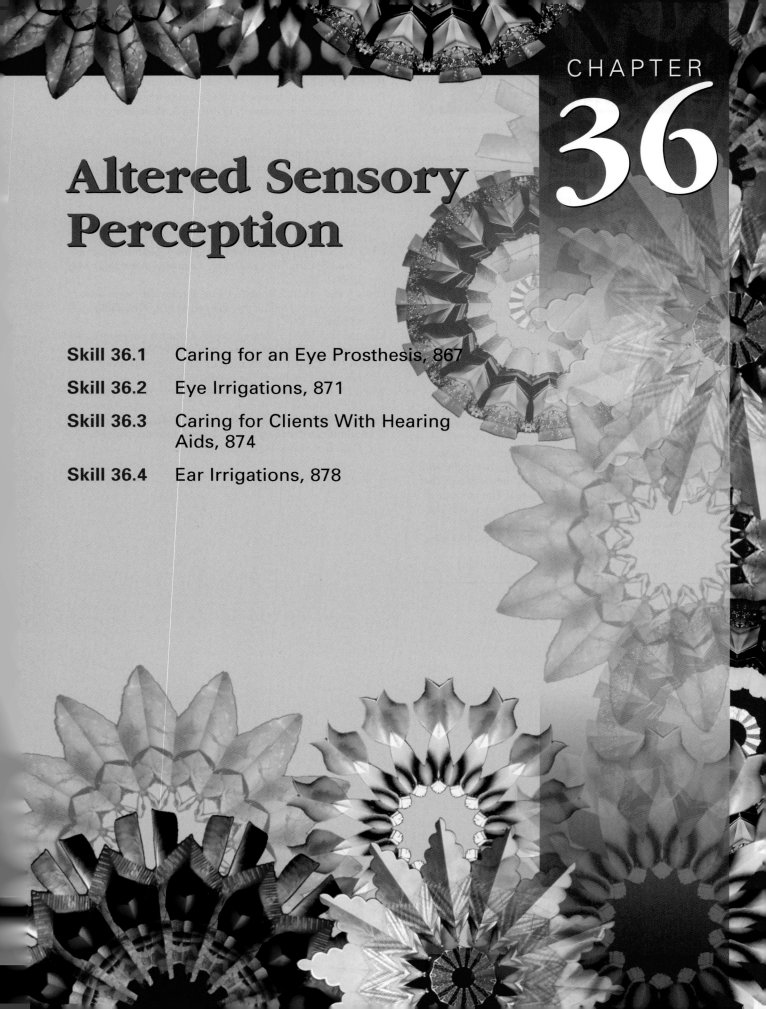

Altered Sensory Perception

Meaningful sensory stimuli allow a person to learn about the environment and are necessary for healthy functioning and normal development. Many clients seeking health care have preexisting sensory alterations, whereas others might develop alterations after medical treatment. The nurse plays an important role in helping clients care for sensory aids such as eye prosthetics and hearing aids. In addition, the nurse provides care, such as eye or ear irrigations, that promotes the integrity of sensory organs.

Whenever you care for clients with sensory alterations, safety is a priority. The nurse must be able to anticipate how the client's sensory alteration places the client at risk for injury. Orientation to any new environment, arranging an existing living environment to minimize safety hazards, and educating family and friends about ways to help clients adapt to sensory loss are just some of the interventions nurses may use.

In an acute care environment the nurse may need to provide clients more direct supervision. When assisting with ambulation for a visually impaired client, the nurse should stand on the client's nondominant side approximately one step ahead, with the client lightly holding the nurse's arm. Items such as the call light, over-bed table, and telephone should be placed within the client's reach and their locations described to the client. If a client has a hearing deficit, the nurse may need to ensure the client can understand the caregivers' communication. The nurse faces the client before beginning to speak and makes sure there is enough light for the client to see the nurse's lips. By eliminating external noises, speaking in a slow, clear, normal tone of voice, and accentuating facial gestures, the nurse helps the client to hear correctly. Sign language, lipreading, writing with pad and pencil, or use of communication boards may be necessary for hearing-impaired clients. Family or friends should be taught these same techniques so that they can become a source of support.

Clients may be very sensitive about lens or prosthetic care. Accidental breakage or malfunction of the client's sensory aids may seriously impair sensory function and threaten self-esteem if the client becomes dependent on others for assistance. Most clients have established routines for cleaning contact lenses or eye prostheses. Nurses should adapt to these routines as much as possible when administering care to clients. Likewise, clients should be encouraged to participate in care of sensory aids as much as possible. Careful handling of these devices is vital to avoid damage or injury.

A visual or hearing impairment may be caused by the presence of foreign bodies, irritants, or secretions. In the older adult or in clients who wear hearing aids, cerumen impaction can cause discomfort and further hearing loss. Inflammation or infection of the eyes may produce drainage or secretions that reduce vision. Irrigation of the eye or ear may help restore or maintain existing function. The presence of a foreign body or irritant in the eye or ear requires immediate intervention to restore function and prevent possible permanent sensory loss.

NURSING DIAGNOSES

An appropriate nursing diagnosis associated with a visual or hearing impairment is **Disturbed Sensory Perception (Visual/Auditory),** in which clients experience a change in how they perceive and respond to environmental stimuli. Clients with a hearing loss may also have **Impaired Verbal Communication,** depending on their ability to use and understand language. Clients requiring irrigations of the eye or assistance with eye prostheses may be at **Risk for Infection** if the client does not use the proper technique. A client with a sensory impairment in an unfamiliar environment, such as a hospital room, is especially at **Risk for Injury.** A nursing diagnosis of **Pain (Acute** or **Chronic)** may also apply when injury or infection involves the eye or ear. Clients who are unable to demonstrate proper care techniques may have **Deficient Knowledge.** Visual or hearing impairments can also affect psychosocial status, resulting in **Impaired Social Interaction** or **Social Isolation.**

Skill 36.1

Caring for an Eye Prosthesis

As a result of tumor, infection, congenital blindness, or severe trauma to the eye, clients may have to undergo an enucleation, a procedure involving the complete removal of the eyeball. All that remains is the socket and eyelids. For obvious cosmetic purposes, clients who have had an enucleation are often fitted with an artificial eye, or prosthesis.

Artificial eyes are made of glass and plastic and fit just behind the client's eyelids. Each prosthesis is designed to take on the appearance of the client's natural iris, pupil, and sclera. Prostheses are relatively easy to remove and insert and can be worn day and night. Cleansing with soap and water can be done daily or any time up to several months based on client preference.

ASSESSMENT

1. Determine which eye is artificial (no movement or pupillary reaction to light).
2. Inspect surrounding tissues of eyelid and eye socket for inflammation, tenderness, swelling, or drainage

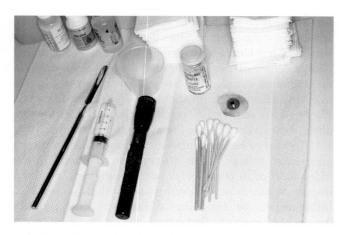

Figure 36-1 Equipment for eye prosthetic care.

3. Client demonstrates no signs of infection, such as redness, tenderness, swelling, or discharge of socket or eyelid margins.
4. Client verbalizes that prosthetic eye fits comfortably.
5. Client demonstrates the proper technique for removing, cleaning, and reinserting prosthesis.

Equipment (Figure 36-1)

- Soft washcloth or cotton gauze square
- Washbasin with warm water or saline
- 4 × 4 gauze pads
- Mild soap
- Facial tissues
- Bath towel
- Suction device (e.g., rubber bulb syringe, medicine dropper bulb) (Optional: Bulb syringe removes prosthesis by suction if manual removal is not successful.)
- Disposable gloves
- Covered plastic storage case

after prosthesis removal. Wear gloves if drainage is suspected or present. *Rationale: Infections can spread easily to neighboring eye, underlying sinuses, or brain tissue.*

3. Assess client's routines for prosthetic care: frequency and methods of cleaning. *Rationale: Determines compliance with and knowledge of self-care.*
4. Assess client's ability to remove, clean, and reinsert prosthesis.

PLANNING

Expected outcomes focus on client's comfort and prevention of infection.

Expected Outcomes

1. Client verbalizes feelings regarding prosthesis removal.
2. Client's eyelid margins and eye socket are clean and of normal pink color, with lashes turned away from prosthesis.

Delegation Considerations

The skills of removal, cleansing, and insertion of an eye prosthesis can be delegated to assistive personnel (AP).
- Stress importance of careful handling of the device.
- Stress the importance of maintaining client's privacy during procedure.
- Inform care provider of types of findings to report (e.g., inflammation, drainage).

IMPLEMENTATION FOR CARING FOR AN EYE PROSTHESIS

Steps	Rationale
1. See Standard Protocol (inside front cover).	
2. With thumb, gently retract lower eyelid against lower orbital ridge (see illustration).	Exposes lower edge of eye prosthesis.
3. Exert slight pressure below eyelid (see illustration). If prosthesis does not slide out, use bulb syringe or medicine dropper bulb to apply direct suction to prosthesis.	Maneuver breaks suction, causing prosthesis to rise and slide out of socket (Bocking and others, 1990).
4. Place prosthesis in palm of hand, and clean with mild soap and water or plain saline by rubbing between thumb and index finger.	Tears and secretions containing microorganisms may collect on surface of prosthesis. Soap is less irritating than detergents.

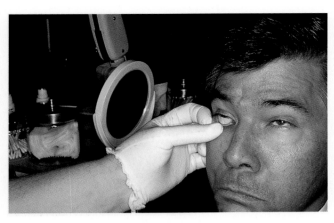

Step 2 Retraction of lower lid to aid removal of eye prosthesis.

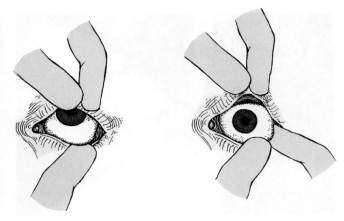

Step 3 Exertion of pressure below eyelid and removal of prosthesis.

Steps	Rationale

COMMUNICATION TIP *During this time make client feel at ease by using a calm, gentle approach. Now is a good time to ask, "Tell me how often you find it necessary to clean your artificial eye. Have you ever had difficulty with that?"*

5. Rinse well under running tap water, and dry with soft washcloth or facial tissue (see illustration, p. 87).

Soft cloth or tissue maintains shinny appearance of prosthesis. Paper towel may dull finish.

6. If client is not to have prosthesis reinserted, store in sterile saline or water in plastic storage case. Label with client's name and room number.

7. Clean eyelid margins and socket.
    a. Retract upper and lower eyelids with thumb and index finger. (Inspection can be done at this time.)

Exposes eye socket.

    b. Wash socket with washcloth or gauze square moistened in warm water or saline.

Removes secretions that may contain microorganisms.

    c. Remove excess moisture with gauze pads.

Removes moisture that can harbor microorganisms.

    d. Wash eyelid margins with mild soap and water. Wipe from inner to outer canthus, using a clean part of cloth with each wipe. Dry eyelids using the same method.

Prevents secretions from entering tear duct in inner canthus.

NURSE ALERT *If crusts are difficult to remove, place moistened cloth over eyelids for several minutes during cleaning. This will help to remove crusts.*

8. Moisten prosthesis with water or saline.

Makes insertion easier because dry plastic would rub against tissue surfaces.

9. Retract client's upper eyelid with index finger or thumb of nondominant hand (see illustration, p. 87).

Eases prosthesis insertion.

10. With dominant hand, hold prosthesis so that notched or pointed edge is positioned toward nose. Iris faces outward.

Correct positioning of prosthesis ensures proper fit (Bocking and others, 1990).

11. Slide prosthesis up under upper eyelid as far as possible. Then push down lower lid to allow prosthesis to slip into place.

Prosthesis will fit evenly into socket.

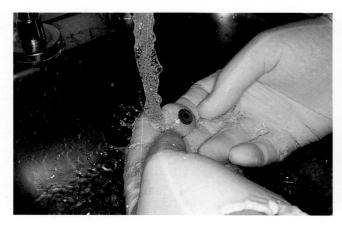

Step 5 Rinsing of eye prosthesis.

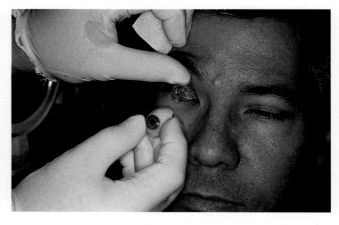

Step 9 Replacement of eye prosthesis into eye socket.

Steps	Rationale

NURSE ALERT *Do not force prosthesis into socket.*

12. Gently wipe away excess fluid if necessary. Remove and discard gloves, and perform hand hygiene.

Wipe toward nose to prevent dislodgement.

13. See Completion Protocol (inside front cover).

• • • • • • • • • •

EVALUATION

1. Ask client about feelings regarding prosthesis removal.
2. Inspect eyelids and eye socket for cleanliness, color, and position of eyelashes. Wear gloves if drainage is suspected or visible.
3. Inspect eyelids and socket for signs of infection.
4. Ask client if prosthesis fits comfortably.
5. Observe client demonstrating technique for prosthesis care.

Unexpected Outcomes and Related Interventions

1. Client states prosthesis feels uncomfortable.
   a. Reposition prosthesis.
   b. Remove prosthesis. Inspect for any rough areas.
2. Inflammation develops in tissues of socket or lid margins.
   a. Remove prosthesis for a few days if necessary. Clean eyelid and socket.
   b. Provide client with comfortable eye patch until inflammation subsides.
3. Client develops excessive, purulent, or foul-smelling drainage.
   a. Wearing clean gloves, remove prosthesis and clean area. Inspect socket and surrounding tissue.
   b. Place prosthesis in appropriate cleaning and storage solution.
   c. Provide eye patch if desired and perform hand hygiene.
   d. Instruct client on proper handwashing and procedures to use to help reduce infection.
   e. Notify physician of assessment findings.

4. Client is unable to perform prosthesis care correctly.
   a. Teach and demonstrate prosthetic care to client and significant other.
   b. Provide literature regarding prosthetic eye care.
   c. Observe return demonstration until correctly performed.

Recording and Reporting

• Record appearance and condition of eye socket in nurses' notes.
• Record and report any signs and symptoms of infection involving eye socket.

Sample Documentation

1400 Client complaining of tenderness around left artificial eye. Prosthesis removed. No scratches or rough edges noted on prosthesis. Slight redness and edema noted at outer canthus. Socket and eyelids cleaned with normal saline. Client agrees not to wear prosthesis until symptoms improve. Prosthesis cleaned and stored. Eye patch provided.

SPECIAL CONSIDERATIONS

Pediatric Considerations

- Young children, even infants and toddlers, are able to be fitted with eye prostheses.
- Prostheses are easily removed; the child may accidentally dislodge this during play. Parents need to be encouraged to explain to the child that this "special eye" may fall out but can be easily put back in place after it has been properly cleaned (Wong and others, 1999).

Geriatric Considerations

- Older adults normally experience a reduction in visual function. With only one eye, the older adult may require greater assistance with respect to safety precautions.

- If an older adult has underlying thyroid disease and has some exophthalmos, it is necessary to have an oculist determine that the prosthesis fits appropriately (Salvi and others, 1999).

Home Care Considerations

- For clients receiving new prostheses, instruct in prosthetic care and have client perform return demonstration.
- If a client becomes disabled and suffers an inability to perform self-care measures on a regular basis, be sure the prosthesis is cleaned regularly to prevent possible infection.
- Assess client's home, and determine need for special precautions.
- Determine if client is able to use available equipment in the home to care for prosthesis.

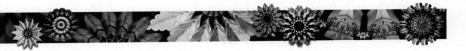

Skill 36.2

Eye Irrigations

Eye irrigation is performed to flush out exudates or irritating solutions. It is a procedure typically used in emergency situations when a foreign object or some other substance has entered the eye. When a chemical or irritating substance contaminates the eyes, irrigate immediately with copious amounts of water for at least 15 minutes to prevent corneal burning (McConnell, 1991). In addition, contact lenses wearers may need eye irrigation to wash out particles of dust causing eye irritation.

ASSESSMENT

1. Assess reason for eye irrigation. *Rationale: This information determines the amount and type of solution and the immediacy of treatment.*
2. Assess the eye for redness, excessive tearing, and discharge. Assess the eyelids and lacrimal glands for edema. Ask client about itching, burning, pain, blurred vision, or photophobia (McConnell, 1991). *Rationale: Provides baseline for condition of eye.*
3. Assess client's ability to cooperate. *Rationale: Extra assistance may be needed.*

PLANNING

Expected outcomes focus on client's physical and psychological comfort and improving vision.

Expected Outcomes

1. Client verbalizes reduced burning/itching after eye irrigation.
2. Client demonstrates minimal anxiety during irrigation.
3. Client verbalizes improved visual acuity after eye irrigation.
4. Client maintains normal pupillary reaction and eye movement after irrigation.

Equipment

- Prescribed irrigating solution: volume usually varies from 30 to 180 ml at 98.6° F (37° C). (For chemical flushing, use tap water or prescribed intravenous [IV] fluid in volume to provide continuous irrigation over 15 minutes.)
- Sterile basin for solution
- Curved emesis basin
- Waterproof pad or towel
- Cotton balls
- Soft bulb syringe, eyedropper, or IV tubing
- Disposable gloves

Delegation Considerations

This skill requires the critical thinking skills and knowledge application unique to a nurse. Delegation is inappropriate.

IMPLEMENTATION FOR EYE IRRIGATIONS

Steps	Rationale
1. See Standard Protocol (inside front cover).	
2. Remove contact lenses (if possible) before beginning irrigation (Box 36-1).	Prompt removal of lenses is needed to safely and completely irrigate foreign substances from client's eyes.
3. Assist client to side-lying position on the same side as the affected eye. Turn head toward affected eye.	Irrigation solution will flow from inner to outer canthus, preventing contamination of unaffected eye and nasolacrimal duct (see illustration for Step 9).

COMMUNICATION TIP *Reassure client that eye can be closed periodically and that no object will touch eye.*

Steps	Rationale
4. Place waterproof pad under client's face.	
5. With cotton ball moistened in prescribed solution (or normal saline), gently clean eyelid margins and eyelashes from inner to outer canthus.	Minimizes transfer of debris from lids or lashes into eye during irrigation.
6. Place curved emesis basin just below client's cheek on side of affected eye.	

Box 36-1

Removal of Contact Lenses

SOFT LENSES (WEAR GLOVES IF DRAINAGE IS SUSPECTED OR PRESENT)

- If possible, have client look straight ahead. Retract lower eyelid, and expose lower edge of lens.
- Using pad of index finger, slide lens off cornea to white of eye.
- Pull upper eyelid down gently with thumb of other hand, and compress lens slightly between thumb and index finger.
- Gently pinch lens, and lift out without allowing edges to stick together.
- If lens edges stick together, place lens in palm and soak thoroughly with sterile saline.
- Place lens in storage case.
- Follow procedure for cleansing and disinfecting.

RIGID LENSES (WEAR GLOVES IF DRAINAGE IS SUSPECTED OR PRESENT)

- Be sure lens is positioned directly over cornea. If it is not, have client close eyelids. Place index and middle fingers of one hand beside the lens, and gently but firmly massage lens back over cornea.

- Place index finger on outer corner of client's eye, and draw skin gently back toward ear.
- Ask client to blink. Do not release pressure on lids until blink is completed.
- If lens fails to pop out, gently retract eyelid beyond edges of lens. Press lower eyelid gently against lower edge of lens.
- If client is unable to assist, use a specially designed suction cup. Place cup on center of lens and while applying suction, gently remove lens off client's cornea.
- Place lens in storage case.
- Follow procedure for cleansing and disinfecting.

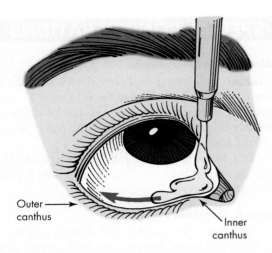

Outer canthus

Inner canthus

Step 9 Irrigation of eye from inner to outer canthus.

Steps	Rationale
7. With gloved finger, gently retract upper and lower eyelids to expose the conjunctival sacs. To hold lids open, apply pressure to lower bony orbit and bony prominence beneath eyebrow. Do not apply pressure over eye.	Retraction minimizes blinking and allows irrigation of conjunctiva.
8. Hold irrigating syringe, dropper, or IV tubing approximately 1 inch (2.5 cm) from the inner canthus.	If irrigator touches the eye, there is risk of injury.

COMMUNICATION TIP *Use a calm, confident, soft voice when talking with client and reinforcing the importance of the procedure. For example, "You are doing great; just relax; that's it, we need to flush this out of your eye as completely as possible to lessen the chance of an eye injury."*

9. Ask client to look up. Gently irrigate with a steady stream toward the lower conjunctival sac, moving from the inner to the outer canthus (see illustration).	Allows irrigation solution to flow freely, washing out the irritant from the eye.
10. Allow client to close the eye periodically.	Lid closure moves secretions from upper to lower conjunctival sac.
11. Continue irrigation until all solution is used or secretions have been cleared. (NOTE: An irrigation of 15 minutes or more is needed to flush chemicals.)	
12. Dry eyelids and facial area with sterile cotton ball.	
13. See Completion Protocol (inside front cover).	

• • • • • • • • • •

EVALUATION

1. Assess client's comfort level after eye irrigation.
2. Observe for verbal and nonverbal signs of anxiety during irrigation.
3. Ask client if vision is blurred after irrigation.
4. Observe pupillary reaction (to light and accommodation) and extraocular eye movement.

Unexpected Outcomes and Related Interventions

1. Client demonstrates extreme anxiety during irrigation.
   a. Reinforce the rationale for irrigation.
   b. Allow client to close eye periodically during irrigation.
   c. Instruct client to take slow, deep breaths.
   d. Seek extra assistance if needed to prevent injury.

2. Client complains of pain and foreign body sensation in the eye after irrigation. Excessive tearing and photophobia noted.
   a. Advise client to close the eye and to avoid eye movement.
   b. Notify physician or eye care practitioner of findings.

Recording and Reporting

- Record in nurses' notes condition of eye, type and amount of solution used for irrigation, length of time for irrigation, and client's report of pain and visual status.
- Report continued symptoms of pain and visual blurring to physician.

Sample Documentation

0800 Client complaining of blurred vision and tenderness in left eye. Yellow, crusty drainage noted on eyelids with slight edema and redness of conjunctiva. Eyelids cleaned and eye irrigated with 30 ml warm, sterile, normal saline for 10 minutes. Neosporin ophthalmic ointment applied. Client had no complaint of discomfort.

0900 Client states that eye "feels better." Vision clearer. Pupils equal, round, reactive to light, accommodation. Normal eye movements noted. Conjunctiva remains red with slight edema.

🌸 SPECIAL CONSIDERATIONS 🌸

Pediatric Considerations
- Children with foreign bodies or chemicals in the eye are quite panicked. It may be necessary to use a mummy restraint so that the eye can be safely and quickly irrigated and thus reduce the risk of damage (Wong and others, 1999).
- Parents need education and demonstration when having to continue eye irrigations at home (Wong and others, 1999).

Geriatric Considerations
Due to changes in fine motor coordination or mobility, an older adult who needs eye irrigations in the home setting may need the assistance of a family member or friend. Therefore this significant other must be present for client teaching (Lueckenotte, 2000).

Home Care Considerations
- If client suffered injury in the home, instruct in ways to minimize chemical injuries in the future. Have client wear eye goggles when working with chemicals or in a dusty environment.
- Instruct client and family in how to perform emergency irrigation of the eye.

Skill 36.3

Caring for Clients With Hearing Aids

Hearing is vital for normal communication and orientation to sounds in the environment. Sensorineural hearing loss is a major disabling condition in the United States, affecting 20 to 26 million people (Larson and others, 2000). For people with hearing loss, a proper hearing aid improves the ability to hear and understand spoken words. Hearing aids amplify so that sound is heard at a more effective level. All aids have four basic components:

1. A microphone, which receives and converts sound into electrical signals
2. An amplifier, which increases the strength of the electrical signal
3. A receiver, which converts the strengthened signal back into sound
4. A power source (batteries)

In addition, programmable hearing aids are now available. The programmable hearing aids are in analog and digital formats. Clients seeking these aids need to be evaluated by a licensed audiologist to determine the type of aid and which frequencies are needed for the individual client (National Institute on Deafness and Other Communication Disorders [NIDCD], 2002). These aids input signals rather than just amplifying the sounds. They are programmed by an audiologist with the use of a computer specific to a client's hearing impairment. These aids are adjusted to accommodate the range of the client's residual hearing. Programmable aids independently amplify high-frequency (soft-spoken consonants) from low-frequency (loudly spoken vowels) sounds; this process occurs rapidly and continuously (ReSound Corporation, 1994, 1995). Several styles of hearing aids are available to clients today (Figure 36-2).

1. *In-the-Ear (ITE)* hearing aids fit completely in the outer ear and are used for mild to severe hearing loss. The case, which holds the components, is made of hard plastic. ITE aids can accommodate added technical mechanisms such as a telecoil, a small magnetic

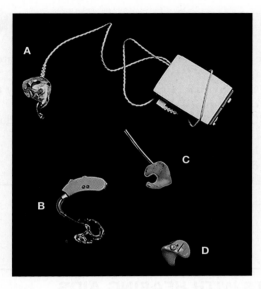

Figure 36-2 Types of hearing aids. **A,** Older aid with a battery pack worn on the body and a wire connected to the ear mold. **B,** Behind-the-ear (BTE) battery with ear mold. **C,** In-the-ear (ITE) mold with battery. **D,** Small in-the-canal (ITC) mold. (Courtesy CLG Photographics, Inc.)

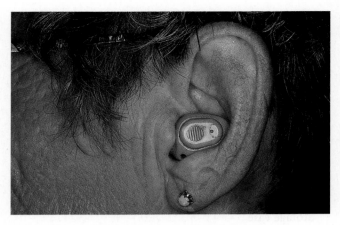

Figure 36-3   Small canal type, hearing aid.

coil contained in the hearing aid that improves sound transmission during telephone calls. ITE aids can be damaged by earwax and ear drainage, and their small size can cause adjustment problems and feedback. They are not usually worn by children because the casings need to be replaced as the ear grows.

2. *Behind-the-Ear (BTE)* hearing aids are worn behind the ear and are connected to a plastic earmold that fits inside the outer ear. The components are held in a case behind the ear. Sound travels through the earmold into the ear. BTE aids are used by people of all ages for mild to profound hearing loss. Poorly fitting BTE earmolds may cause feedback, a whistle sound caused by the fit of the hearing aid, or by buildup of earwax or fluid.

3. *Canal Aids* fit into the ear canal and are available in two sizes. The *In-the-Canal (ITC)* hearing aid is customized to fit the size and shape of the ear canal and is used for mild or moderately severe hearing loss (Figure 36-3). A *Completely-in-Canal (CIC)* hearing aid is largely concealed in the ear canal and is used for mild to moderately severe hearing loss. Because of their small size, canal aids may be difficult for the user to adjust and remove, and may not be able to hold additional devices, such as a telecoil. Canal aids can also be damaged by earwax and ear drainage. They are not typically recommended for children.

4. *Body Aids* are used by people with profound hearing loss. The aid is attached to a belt or a pocket and connected to the ear by a wire. Because of its large size, it is able to incorporate many signal processing options, but it is usually used only when other types of aids cannot be used. (http://www.nidcd.nih.gov/health/hearing/the basicshearingaid.asp. Last updated December 2, 2002.)

ASSESSMENT

1. Assess client's knowledge of and routines for cleansing and caring for hearing aid. *Rationale: Determines compliance with and knowledge of self-care.*

2. Observe whether client can hear clearly with use of aid by talking slowly and clearly in normal tone of voice. *Rationale: Inability to hear may indicate faulty function of the hearing aid or may indicate that aid is no longer effective for client's auditory loss.*

3. Assess if hearing aid is working by removing from client's ear. Close battery case, and turn volume slowly to high. Cup hand over hearing aid. If squealing sound (feedback) is heard, it is working. If no sound is heard, replace batteries and test again.

4. Inspect ear mold for cracked or rough edges. *Rationale: Poorly fitting hearing aids cause irritation to external ear canal.*

5. Inspect for accumulation of cerumen around aid and plugging of opening in aid. *Rationale: Cerumen can block sound reception.*

PLANNING

Expected outcomes focus on facilitating communication and promoting comfort and appropriate self-care.

Expected Outcomes

1. Client hears conversation spoken in normal tone of voice and responds appropriately.
2. Client responds appropriately to environmental sounds.
3. Client demonstrates proper care of the hearing aid.
4. Client verbalizes that the aid fits comfortably.

Equipment

- Over-bed table
- Soft towel and washcloth
- Brush or wax loop
- Storage case
- Disposable gloves (if drainage is present)

Delegation Considerations

The skill of caring for a hearing aid can be delegated to assistive personnel (AP).
- Confirm that care provider knows proper way to care for prosthetic device.
- Clarify communication tips to use for individual client while aid is being cleaned.
- Have care provider report presence of any drainage to RN.

IMPLEMENTATION FOR CARING FOR CLIENTS WITH HEARING AIDS

Steps	Rationale
1. See Standard Protocol (inside front cover).	
2. Have equipment at bedside for client to see.	
3. **Cleaning hearing aid**	
a. Wipe aid with soft washcloth. Use wax loop or brush (supplied with aid) or tip of syringe needle to clean the holes in the aid. Hold hearing aid so that canal faces sink or waste can.	Impaction of wax blocks normal sound transmission (Meador, 1995). Holding hearing aid canal toward sink or waste can allows wax particles to fall out the openings of the device (McConnell, 1996).

NURSE ALERT *Caring for a hearing aid should protect the device from moisture, heat, breakage, and loss.*

COMMUNICATION TIP *Ask client to share at this time any tips for care of the aid. Use the time to discuss whether the client is having any difficulty hearing or using the aid at home, at work, or in social situations. When clients are children, involve parents.*

Steps	Rationale
b. Open battery door, and allow it to air dry.	Increases battery life and allows moisture to evaporate (Olson, 1995).
c. Wash ear canal with washcloth moistened in soap and water. Rinse and dry.	Removes cerumen from ear canal.
d. If hearing aid is to be stored, place in dry storage case with desiccant material. Label case with client's name and room number. If more than one aid, note right or left. Turn off hearing aid when not in use.	Protects hearing aid against damage, moisture, and breakage.
4. **Inserting hearing aid**	
a. Check batteries (see Assessment).	
b. Turn aid off and volume control down.	Protects client from sudden exposure to feedback sounds.
c. Hold aid so that the canal—the long portion with the hole(s)—is at the bottom. Guiding the aid along client's cheek, bring it to the ear.	Proper orientation is important for hearing aid insertion.

Steps	Rationale
d. Insert canal portion of the aid into the ear first. Use other hand to pull up and back on outer ear. Gently push aid into ear until it is in place and fits snugly in the midline.	
e. Adjust volume gradually to comfortable level for talking to client in regular voice 3 to 4 feet away. Rotate volume control toward nose to increase volume and away from nose to decrease volume.	Gradual adjustment prevents exposing client to harsh squeal or feedback. Client should hear nurse comfortably.

NURSE ALERT   *Programmable aids have the volume control located on the remote. For most clients, hearing aids work best at lower volume settings.*

---

5. See Completion Protocol (inside front cover).

• • • • • • • • • •

EVALUATION

1. Converse with client in a normal tone of voice, and observe response.
2. Observe client's response to environmental sounds.
3. Observe client perform hearing aid care.
4. Ask client about comfort after hearing aid insertion.

Unexpected Outcomes and Related Interventions

1. Client is unable to hear conversations or environmental sounds clearly. Client's verbal responses are inappropriate.
   a. Remove hearing aid, and check battery for power and correct placement.
   b. Inspect ear mold and ear canal for cerumen blockage.
   c. Change volume setting as needed.
   d. If problems persist, contact audiologist or hearing aid specialist.
2. Client is unable to perform care of hearing aid.
   a. Demonstrate correct aid care.
   b. Observe return demonstration until correctly performed.

3. Client complains of ear discomfort and may complain of whistling sound.
   a. Remove aid and reinsert.
   b. Assess external ear for signs of inflammation.
   c. If problems persist, contact audiologist or hearing aid specialist.

Recording and Reporting

- Record that hearing aid is removed and stored if client is going for surgery or special procedure.
- Report to nursing staff and document on plan of care tips that promote communication with client.

Sample Documentation

1000 Client responding inappropriately to questions. Unable to hear normal conversation tone. Complains of hearing an "echo." Volume turned down on ITE aid in right ear. Daughter states that client frequently turns the volume up so he can "hear better." Reviewed proper volume settings and improved listening techniques with client and daughter.

SPECIAL CONSIDERATIONS

Pediatric Considerations

- As children grow older, they can become self-conscious of a hearing aid. Changes in hair style may assist some children in overcoming self-consciousness (Wong and others, 1999).
- Changes in style and size occur as child gets bigger.

Geriatric Considerations

- The small size of hearing aids may make it difficult for older adults to handle and manipulate the devices. Clients who have this difficulty should contact their hearing aid specialist for assistance. Family members may be able to assist with care of device.

- High-pitched signals associated with consonants *f, p, t, k, ch, sh,* and *st* are more difficult to hear clearly as people age (Lueckenotte, 2000).
- Inappropriate responses to questions or situations, inattentiveness, difficulty following instructions, monopolization of conversation should alert the nurse or family members that the client may have some hearing loss that needs to be evaluated. People incorrectly may assume the client is confused (Cavendish, 1998).
- Be alert for client assessment findings that may indicate some depression. Hearing loss and depression are common, and correction of hearing loss may actually resolve depression in some clients (Jupiter and Spivey, 1997).

Continued

SPECIAL CONSIDERATIONS—*Cont'd*

- Age-related hearing loss, presbycusis, is common. Clients and their families can overcome this auditory change by speaking slowly and clearly. Not all clients with this type of hearing loss require a hearing aid (Meecham, 1999).

Home Care Considerations
- Initial use of a hearing aid should be restricted to quiet situations in the home. Clients need to adjust gradually to voices and household sounds (Lewis, Collier, and Heitkemper, 2000).
- Avoid exposure of aid to extreme heat or cold. Do not leave in case near stove, heater, or sunny window. Do not use with hair dryer on hot settings or with sunlamp.

- Remove aid for bathing and when at hair stylist.
- Hair spray tends to clog hearing aid.

Long-Term Care Considerations
- Because of the potential high number of hearing aids in long-term care facilities, clients and their families need to clearly mark the hearing aid.
- The hearing aid must always be stored in the client's bedside table
- When possible, instruct family to buy an extra battery to keep in client's bedside table.
- Instruct clients not to remove their aids in common rooms (e.g., sunroom, recreation areas).

Skill 36.4

Ear Irrigations

The common indications for irrigation of the external ear are presence of certain foreign bodies and accumulation of cerumen. The procedure is not without potential hazards. Damage to the external auditory meatus may occur by scratching the lining of the canal if the client suddenly moves or if there is inadequate control of the irrigating syringe (Meador, 1995). Improperly drying the ear may lead to an episode of acute otitis externa. If the client moves suddenly during irrigation, the tympanic membrane can be perforated. Water pressure can also cause perforation. Never irrigate the ear if vegetable matter is occluded in the canal, the tympanic membrane is ruptured, or the client has otitis externa, myringotomy tubes, or a mastoid cavity (McConnell, 1992; Zivic and King, 1993). Irrigations should be done with liquid warmed to body temperature to avoid vertigo or nausea in clients (McKenry and Salerno, 1998).

In addition to irrigation, cerumen can be removed by use of a curette, which is performed by a physician or advanced nurse practitioner. Instillation of ceruminolytic agents that soften and loosen the matter for cleaning is another alternative.

ASSESSMENT

1. Review prescriber's medication order, including solution to be instilled and the affected ear(s)—right (AD), left (AS), or both (AU)—to receive irrigation. *Rationale: Ensures safe and correct administration of medication.*

2. Review medical history for ruptured tympanic membrane, myringotomy tubes, or surgery of auditory canal. *Rationale: These factors contraindicate ear irrigation.*
3. Inspect the pinna and external auditory meatus for redness, swelling, drainage, abrasions, and presence of cerumen or foreign objects. *Rationale: Provides baseline information to monitor effects of irrigation.*
   a. Attempt to remove foreign object in ear by straightening ear canal. *Rationale: Straightening of canal may cause object to fall out and negate need for irrigation.*
   b. If vegetable matter (e.g., dried bean or pea) is occluding canal, do not perform irrigation. *Rationale: Irrigant may cause object to absorb solution and swell, causing further damage.*
4. Use an otoscope to inspect deeper portions of the auditory canal. *Rationale: If client's tympanic membrane (eardrum) is not intact, irrigation is contraindicated.*
5. Assess client's comfort level using a scale of 0 to 10. *Rationale: Provides baseline to evaluate changes in client's condition. Presence of pain is symptomatic of ear infection or inflammation.*
6. Assess client's hearing ability in the affected ear. *Rationale: Occlusion of canal by cerumen or foreign object can impair hearing.*
7. Assess client's knowledge of proper ear care.

PLANNING

Expected outcomes focus on client comfort and improved auditory perception.

Expected Outcomes

1. Client denies increased pain, using a scale of 0 to 10, during instillation.
2. Client verbalizes increased comfort, using a scale of 0 to 10, after irrigation.
3. Client demonstrates minimal anxiety during irrigation.
4. Client's ear canal is clear of discharge, cerumen, or foreign material after irrigation.
5. Client demonstrates improved hearing acuity in the affected ear after irrigation.

Equipment

- Clean disposable gloves
- Otoscope
- Irrigation syringe
- Basin
- Towel
- Cotton balls
- Prescribed sterile irrigating solution warmed to body temperature or mineral oil, over-the-counter softener
- Medication administration record (MAR) or computer printout

Delegation Considerations

The skill of irrigating the external ear requires the critical thinking and knowledge application unique to a nurse. Delegation is inappropriate.

IMPLEMENTATION FOR EAR IRRIGATIONS

Steps	Rationale
1. See Standard Protocol (inside front cover).	
2. Assist client to a sitting or lying position with head turned toward the affected ear. Place towel or waterproof pad under client's head and shoulder. Have client help hold basin under affected ear (see illustration).	Position minimizes leakage of fluids around neck and facial area. Solution will flow from ear canal to basin.
3. Pour prescribed irrigating solution into sterile basin. Check the temperature of the solution (98.6° F, or 37° C) by pouring a small drop on your inner forearm.	Solution that is too hot or too cold can cause nausea, vertigo, and vomiting.
4. Gently clean auricle and outer ear canal with moistened cotton applicator. Do not force drainage or cerumen into ear canal.	

NURSE ALERT *Advise client to not make any sudden moves, to prevent trauma to the ear.*

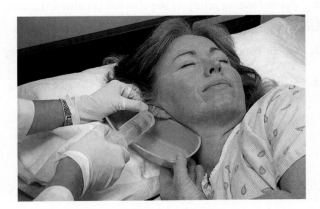

Step 2 Irrigation of affected ear.

Steps	Rationale
5. Fill irrigating syringe, and expel air. *If using dental irrigating device, use low setting.*	Prevents sudden expulsion of fluid.
6. For adults and children over age 3 years, gently pull pinna up and back. In children 3 years or younger, pinna should be pulled down and back (Lilley and Aucker, 1999). Place the tip of the irrigating device just inside the external meatus. Leave a space around the irrigating tip and canal.	Pulling of pinna straightens external ear canal. Prevents obstruction of canal with device, which can lead to increased pressure on tympanic membrane.
7. Direct the fluid slowly and gently toward the superior aspect of the ear canal. Do not occlude canal with syringe.	Fluid is directed back behind impacted cerumen.

COMMUNICATION TIP *Talk in a confident, calm voice to help the client relax. As you begin the irrigation, say, "Now you are going to feel the warm water. I am going to be sure to do this gently. If you feel any discomfort at all, let me know."*

Steps	Rationale
8. Maintain the flow of the irrigation in a steady stream until you see small to large pieces of cerumen flow from the canal.	
9. Periodically ask if the client is experiencing pain, nausea, or vertigo.	Symptoms indicate irrigating solution is too hot or too cold.
10. Drain excessive fluid from the ear by having client tilt the head toward the affected side.	
11. Dry the canal gently with a cotton-tipped applicator, and then chemically dry with an antiseptic otic solution such as VoSol HC Otic Solution or 70% isopropyl alcohol (Meador, 1995). Remove and discard gloves, and perform hand hygiene.	Drying prevents buildup of moisture that can lead to otitis externa.
12. See Completion Protocol (inside front cover).	

· · · · · · · · · ·

EVALUATION

1. Ask client about pain level during irrigation.
2. Ask client about pain level after irrigation.
3. Observe for verbal and nonverbal signs of anxiety during irrigation.
4. Inspect condition of external meatus and ear canal.
5. Assess hearing acuity in the affected ear after irrigation.

Unexpected Outcomes and Related Interventions

1. Client complains of increased ear pain during irrigation.
   a. Discontinue irrigation, and notify physician.
2. Client's ear canal remains occluded. Client's hearing acuity has not improved in the affected ear.
   a. Repeat irrigation if prescribed.
   b. If condition persists, notify physician.

Recording and Reporting

- Record type of solution and amount, ear irrigated, appearance of irrigant, and condition of external ear canal.
- Report if client complains of sudden pain or if irrigation results in drainage of purulent-looking fluid.

Sample Documentation

1000 Client complaining of difficulty hearing in right ear. Cerumen plug noted in canal. Irrigated right ear with 50 ml warm normal saline. Return fluid clear with brown particles. No complaints of pain or discomfort. States that hearing "is fine." Responding appropriately to normal conversation tone. Right ear canal clear.

SPECIAL CONSIDERATIONS

Pediatric Considerations
- Be certain that child's head is immobilized to prevent puncturing eardrum.
- It may be helpful to have parent help calm the child during procedure.

Geriatric Considerations
- Older adults often require ongoing ear care for cerumen removal. Use of a softening agent, such as slightly warmed mineral oil (0.5 to 1 ml), twice daily for several days before irrigation is helpful.
- Older adults with higher risk of cerumen impaction include those with large amounts of ear canal hair, those with benign growths that narrow the ear canal, and those who habitually wear hearing aids (Lueckenotte, 2000).

Home Care Considerations
- Instruct client to clean ears with a damp washcloth wrapped around a finger. Do not use a cotton-tipped applicator.
- If client uses a ceruminolytic agent, instruct that these are softening products and that they will not remove the impaction (Meador, 1995).
- Severe cerumen impactions may cause a decrease in hearing, pain, ringing, or a crackling noise in the ear. This requires referral to a physician.

 CRITICAL THINKING EXERCISES

1. Ms. Sorenstam comes to the clinic with a complaint of eye pain during the past 24 hours. She appears to have inflammation of the conjunctiva. Your assessment reveals that she wears soft contact lenses. Ms. Sorenstam reports that she cleans her lenses daily, using a prescribed disinfectant from her ophthalmologist and tap water for rinsing. What might be the source of Ms. Sorenstam's eye discomfort? What are your nursing interventions?
2. Cathy Janes has a prosthetic eye. She has had the device for 6 years and does not have any problems with its care. At present she is in the hospital for bilateral broken collar bones and has limited arm movement. Can you delegate care of her eye prosthesis to AP? What information would you want reported back to you?
3. Mr. Zisk is a 74-year-old client who wears a programmable hearing aid. He has noted a decrease in hearing over the past 2 weeks despite use of the hearing aid. What nursing assessment is appropriate and what intervention might Mr. Zisk require, and why?

REFERENCES
Bocking H and others: Artificial eyes, *Nurs Times* 86(18):40, 1990.
Cavendish R: Clinical snapshot: adult hearing loss, *Am J Nurs* 98(8):50, 1998.
Jupiter T, Spivey V: Perception of hearing loss and hearing handicap on hearing aid use by nursing home residents, *Geriatr Nurs* 18(5):201, 1997.
Larson V and others: Efficacy of 3 commonly used hearing aid circuits: a crossover trial, *JAMA* 284(14):1806, 2000.
Lewis SM and others: *Medical-surgical nursing: assessment and management of clinical problems*, ed. 5, St Louis, 2000, Mosby.
Lilley LL, Aucker RS: *Pharmacology and the nursing process*, ed 3, St Louis, 1999, Mosby.
Lueckenotte AG: *Gerontologic nursing*, ed 2, St Louis, 2000, Mosby.
McConnell E: How to irrigate the eye, *Nursing* 21(3):28, 1991.
McConnell E: How to irrigate the ear, *Nursing* 22(1):66, 1992.
McConnell E: Handling your patient's hearing aid, *Nursing* 26(7):22, 1996.
McKenry LM, Salerno E: *Pharmacology in nursing*, ed 20, St Louis, 1998, Mosby.
Meador JA: Cerumen impaction in the elderly, *J Gerontol Nurs* 21(12):43, 1995.
Meecham E. Audiology and healing impairment: improving the quality of care, *Nurs Stand* 13(43):42, 1999.
National Institute on Deafness and Other Communication Disorders: Health information: hearing aids, http://www.nided.nih.gov/health/hearing/thebasics_hearingaid.asp. Last updated December 2, 2002.
Olson R: Now hear this! *RN* 58(8):43, 1995.
ReSound Corporation: *Hear what you've been missing*, Redwood City, Calif, 1994, ReSound Corporation.
ReSound Corporation: ReSound hearing health care, *Hearing J* 48(7):53, 1995.
Salvi M and others: Expulsion of an artificial eye in a patient with thyroid-associated ophthalmopathy and surgical anophthalmos, *Am J Med* 107(2):191, 1999.
Wong DL and others: *Whaley and Wong's nursing care of infants and children*, ed, 6, St Louis, 1999, Mosby.
Zivic RC, King S: Cerumen impaction management for clients of all ages, *Nurse Pract* 18(3):29, 1993.

Emergency Measures for Life Support in the Hospital Setting

The cardiovascular and pulmonary systems work together to transport oxygen to the tissues and remove carbon dioxide and other waste products of metabolism. The amount of oxygen delivered to the tissues depends on several physiological components including the amount of oxygen entering the blood and carbon dioxide leaving the lungs (ventilation), blood flow to the lungs and tissues (perfusion), and the movement of oxygen to the red blood cells (diffusion). Diffusion occurs at the alveolar level. Critical to the transport of oxygen to the tissues is the ability of the heart to pump blood between the lungs and the periphery. Other components to be considered are the oxygen-carrying capacity of the blood and oxygen requirements of the tissues. The oxygen-carrying capacity of blood depends on the presence of adequate numbers of hemoglobin molecules and an environment conducive to the attachment of oxygen and carbon dioxide to the hemoglobin molecule.

Respiratory arrest and cardiac arrest are emergency situations that the nurse must be prepared to handle at any time. Respiratory arrest, or cessation of breathing, results in the absence of oxygen delivery to the alveoli. This in turns leads to no oxygen or carbon dioxide exchange, which creates a buildup of waste products in the tissues. Cardiac arrest is the cessation of circulating blood, which in turn eliminates oxygen transport.

Predisposing factors to a cardiac or pulmonary arrest may include illnesses involving the cardiopulmonary system, presence of an airway obstruction, fluid and electrolyte imbalances, and ingestion of toxic substances. Unless otherwise indicated, such as a client having a do not resuscitate (DNR) status, all clients receive cardiopulmonary resuscitation (CPR) in the event of arrest. Individual hospital policy and procedures define methods of identification of a client's resuscitation status.

Advance directives offer valuable information concerning resuscitation status and individual client decisions regarding resuscitation efforts. Although advance directives may be addressed before or during the client's hospital admission, the nurse can play an important role in encouraging clients to complete the document. Nurses, because of their unique relationship with clients and the associated high level of trust, are the ideal facilitators for the initiation of advance directives. The American Nurses Association (ANA) *Position Statement on Nursing and the Patient Self-Determination Acts* state that it is the nurse's responsibility to facilitate informed decision making for patients making choices about end-of-life care. Clients want to discuss end-of-life care, and they expect providers to initiate these conversations. Though further research is required on the degree of improvement of end-of-life care, there is some evidence that advance directives give clients a means of controlling treatment decisions about the end of their life. (Ditto and others, 2001). An advance directive may be used as a tool to minimize disagreements among family members regarding resuscitation status determination when the client is physically unable to make decisions. Many hospitals have a mechanism to assist the client/family regarding this issue. Social services and an ethics committee may be of assistance to the client and family.

NURSING DIAGNOSES

Nursing diagnoses that apply to clients who receive CPR include **Ineffective Breathing Pattern,** in which a client who is not breathing (respiratory arrest) is unable to achieve adequate gas exchange of oxygen and carbon dioxide. This may be related to injury, paralysis affecting the diaphragm or phrenic nerve, a collapsed lung (pneumothorax), chest trauma with blood accumulation in the chest (hemothorax), or drug overdose. **Ineffective Airway Clearance** related to copious secretions associated with pneumonia or airway obstruction can also result in respiratory distress. **Impaired Gas Exchange** can be associated with cardiac and pulmonary disorders that interfere with the body's ability to exchange carbon dioxide and oxygen at the cellular level. **Decreased Cardiac Output** occurs when there is a cardiac arrest and/or cardiac disorders such as dysrhythmias, blockage of coronary arteries, or congestive heart failure (CHF). Finally, **Ineffective Tissue Perfusion** of vital organs (e.g., brain, kidney, heart) occurs if cardiopulmonary function is not maintained or restored.

Skill 37.1

Resuscitation

Cardiopulmonary arrest is identified by the absence of pulse and respiration. Once this is assessed, the nurse must immediately begin CPR. CPR is an emergency procedure that combines artificial breathing techniques with external cardiac massage. This is labeled by the American Heart Association as basic cardiac life support (BCLS) and is accomplished in an established and orderly pattern known as the ABCs of resuscitation. Resuscitation efforts include ABCD, establishing the airway *(A)*, initiating breathing *(B)*, and maintaining circulation *(C)*. This has been expanded to include defibrillation *(D)* (see Skill 37-2, p. 891). Defibrillation involves delivery of a direct electrical current, through the heart, that is sufficient to depolarize cells of the myocardium. The intent of defibrillation is that subsequent repolarization of the heart will allow the sinoatrial (SA) node to resume the role of pacemaker. The heart will then resume more normal conduction. Early CPR followed by electrical defibrillation of the heart within 5 minutes (when indicated) and advanced cardiac life support (ACLS) can improve the survival of cardiopulmonary arrest victims to as high as 49%, twice the rate of those previously reported. (AHA, 2000).

ACLS training and certification combines cognitive and psychomotor skills with systematic critical-thinking skills in the management of the client experiencing cardiopulmonary arrest. ACLS teaches how to establish an endotracheal airway and other advanced skills in support of ventilation, establishment of intravenous (IV) access, recognition of dysrhythmias, administration of drugs, and delivery of electrical shock. Early ABCD is crucial for a favorable client outcome. Without oxygen delivery, brain damage can begin within 4 minutes of arrest, brain damage almost always occurs at 6 minutes, and brain death is certain at 10 minutes (AHA, 2000).

Being prepared for a cardiopulmonary arrest is important. The ability of non–ACLS-trained nurses to initiate resuscitative efforts can prevent lethal dysrhythmias such as ventricular fibrillation from deteriorating to a systole (absence of cardiac electrical activity) and improve the chance of the heart returning to a normal rhythm. This improves the heart and brain's ability to function and improves sur-

vivability. Equipment may be readily available at the bedside or in a designated area of the hospital unit. It is the nurse's responsibility to know the location and use of emergency equipment, including the resuscitation cart. It is also the nurse's responsibility to know the contents of the resuscitation cart (Figure 37-1).

ASSESSMENT

1. Determine if client is unconscious by shaking the client and shouting, "Are you OK?" *Rationale: Assists the nurse in determining if the client is unconscious rather than intoxicated, sleeping, or hearing impaired.*
2. Activate the emergency system immediately according to agency policy and procedure (e.g., call a code blue). *Rationale: The majority of adult victims are in ventricular fibrillation and need defibrillation and antidysrhythmic drugs as soon as possible. Early access to emergency cardiac care systems improves client outcome.*

PLANNING

Expected outcomes focus on the establishment and maintenance of artificial breathing and circulation.

Expected Outcomes

1. Adequate oxygenation and tissue perfusion are maintained during artificial resuscitation.
2. Client regains spontaneous respirations during resuscitation.
3. Client regains adequate cardiac output as a result of resuscitation.

Equipment

- Air-mask-bag unit (Ambu-bag)
- CPR pocket mask or barrier device (Figure 37-2)
- Clean gloves, face shield, and gown if available
- Suction apparatus

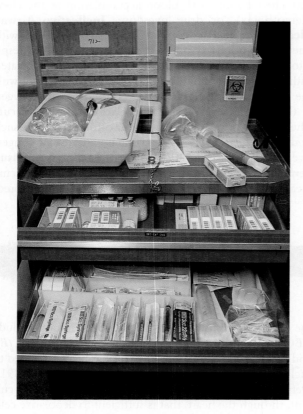

Figure 37-1   Emergency resuscitation cart.

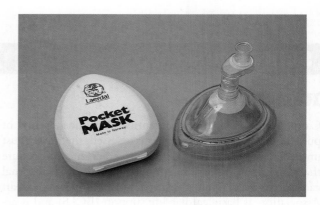

Figure 37-2   Pocket mask.

* Resuscitation cart with

> Cardiac monitor with defibrillator and pads
> Emergency medications
> Endotracheal intubation equipment
> IV catheters (sizes 16 and 18), tubing, and fluids
> (0.9% normal saline [NS])
> Pulse oxymetry monitoring equipment

Delegation Considerations

The skill of CPR can be performed by assistive personnel (AP) who are certified in basic life support (BCLS) techniques.
* Caution the care provider to make certain the client is indeed pulseless, or lacks signs of circulation, before initiating chest compressions.
* The procedures for opening the airway should be reviewed with care provider if the client has any risk for cervical neck trauma.

IMPLEMENTATION FOR RESUSCITATION

Steps	Rationale
1. Assess responsiveness, and call for help.	Determines initial client status and activates emergency response system.
2. Observe for signs of circulation and chest movement; open airway; look, listen and feel for breaths. This should take no longer than 10 seconds.	Determine if client has spontaneous respirations. The tongue is the most common cause of blocked airway in an unresponsive victim.

NURSE ALERT *The nurse must be aware if the client has a DNR status.*

3. **Open the airway**
   a. If no head or neck trauma is suspected, use the head-tilt, chin-lift method (see illustration). Place the heel of the hand on the client's forehead; apply firm backward pressure with the palm of the hand tilting the head back. Place the fingers of the other hand under the bony part of the lower jaw near the chin, lifting the jaw upward, bringing it forward.

   The head-tilt, chin-lift maneuver prevents the tongue from obstructing the airway of the unconscious client, while avoiding unnecessary neck trauma. The tongue is the most common obstruction.

   b. If head or neck trauma is suspected, use the jaw-thrust maneuver only. Grasp angles of client's lower jaw and lift with both hands, displacing the mandible forward (see illustration).

   This maneuver allows opening of airway without disrupting head and neck alignment, therefore preventing any further damage.

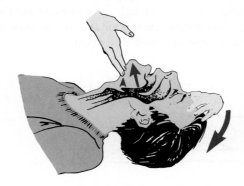

Step 3a Heat tilt, chin lift.

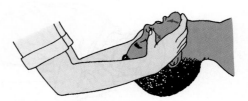

Step 3b Jaw thrust.

Steps	Rationale

4. If client is breathing and no trauma is present, place client in the modified lateral recovery position (see illustration).

In the recovery position, the airway is more likely to remain open, and unrecognized airway obstruction (the tongue) is less likely to occur. A true lateral position is unstable and involves excessive lateral flexion of the cervical spine, resulting in less free drainage from the mouth (AHA, 2000).

5. If no respirations are detected, or inadequate respirations (agonal) are assessed, call for assistance. Rapid intervention of rescue breathing is required.

One person cannot maintain effective CPR indefinitely. The helper can also obtain the resuscitation cart or equipment.

6. 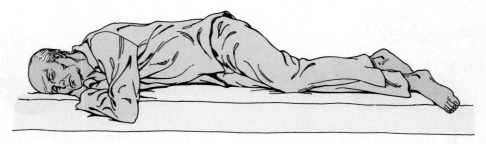 Place victim in a supine position on a firm, flat surface, such as floor or ground, or use the backboard found on the resuscitation cart or the headboard of the hospital bed. If the client must be moved to the supine position, use the logrolling technique to maintain spinal integrity.

Places client in proper position for CPR. External cardiac compressions are most effective when the heart is compressed between the sternum and a hard surface (AHA, 2000).

7. Correctly position for resuscitative efforts

   a. *One-person rescue:* Face client while kneeling parallel to the client's sternum with knees shoulder width apart and shoulders directly over sternum.

Allows rescuer to move quickly between head and sternum.

   b. *Two-person rescue:* One person faces client while kneeling parallel to the client's head. Second person is on the opposite side parallel to the client's sternum. When third person is available, the person should be at the head looking from head to toe.

Allows one rescuer to perform artificial respirations while the second rescuer performs chest compressions. Third person would be available to assist with ventilations.

8. Mouth-to-mouth artificial respirations

   a. *Adult*

     (1) Pinch client's nose with thumb and index finger, and occlude mouth with rescuer's mouth or use face shield or CPR pocket mask. Attempt two slow breaths, $1\frac{1}{2}$ to 2 seconds per breath.

Forms an airtight seal around the client's mouth and prevents air from escaping through the nose. Give breaths with only enough force to make the chest rise. Slow breaths deliver air at a low pressure to reduce the risk of gastric distention. If using pocket mask, position hands to ensure a tight seal.

     (2) The rescuer should take a breath after each ventilation.

Taking a breath ensures the client is receiving an adequate volume of oxygenated air with each ventilation.

     (3) Allow the client to exhale between breaths.

An excess of air may result in gastric distention.

     (4) Continue with 12 breaths per minute, 1 breath every 5 seconds.

   b. *Child (1 to 8 years of age)*

     (1) Pinch the victim's nose tightly with thumb and forefinger. Place rescuer's mouth, face shield, or CPR pocket mask over client's mouth, forming an airtight seal. Give two slow breaths, 1 to $1\frac{1}{2}$ seconds per breath.

Forms an airtight seal around the client's mouth and prevents air from escaping through the nose. Give breaths with only enough force to make the chest rise. Slow breaths deliver air at a low pressure to reduce the risk of gastric distention.

Step 4 Recovery position.

Steps	Rationale
(2) Pause after the first breath to take a breath and to allow the victim to exhale.	Taking a breath ensures the client is receiving an adequate volume of oxygenated air with each ventilation. An excess of air may result in gastric distention
(3) Continue with 20 breaths per minute, 1 breath every 3 seconds.	
c. *Infant (less than 1 year of age)*	
(1) Place the rescuer's mouth, face shield, or pocket mask over the infant's nose and mouth, forming an airtight seal.	Rescue breaths are the single most important maneuver in assisting a nonbreathing infant or child. Ensure mask is proper size so as not to occlude eyes and result in poor seal.
(2) Give two breaths slowly at 1 to $1\frac{1}{2}$ seconds per breath.	Infants and children have small airways that provide high resistance to airflow. To minimize the resistance and to prevent gastric distention, give breaths slowly. The correct volume for each breath is the volume that makes the chest rise (Guidelines, 2000).
(3) Continue with 20 breaths per minute, 1 breath every 3 seconds.	
9. Bag-valve-mask artificial respirations	
a. *All ages*	
(1) Connect oxygen supply tubing to bag-valve-mask and oxygen flowmeter. Adjust oxygen to 100% fractional inspired oxygen concentration (FiO_2) or ordered rate.	Provides supplemental oxygen.
(2) Insert oropharyngeal airway if available.	Prevents tongue from obstructing the airway and provides patent airway.
(3) Position the face mask of the bag-valve-mask over the client's mouth and nose. When a bag-valve-mask is available, ensure the mask does not occlude the eyes.	Selection of the proper size face mask is essential to achieving an airtight seal. If using pocket mask or bag-valve-mask, be sure a tight seal is maintained.
(4) Give slow breaths by squeezing the bag over 1 to 2 seconds. If a bag-valve-mask is used without oxygen, provide breath over 2 seconds. Observe for chest to rise.	As the bag is compressed, oxygen enters the client. When supplemental oxygen is used, a decreased volume is necessary because of the oxygen-rich air provided.
(5) Allow time for client to exhale.	Exhalation prevents overinflation of the lungs and gastric distention.
10. If ventilation attempt is unsuccessful, reposition the client's head and reattempt rescue breathing. If ventilation attempt remains unsuccessful, the airway may be obstructed by a foreign body that will need to be removed.	Patent airway and oxygen delivery must be ensured before beginning compressions.
a. *Adult:* Foreign body removal may be facilitated by abdominal thrusts (see illustration) and blind finger sweeps. Begin with five abdominal thrusts, below the xiphoid process and above the naval, while straddling the client. If unsuccessful, open client's mouth and observe for foreign body in throat. Grasp both the tongue and lower jaw between the thumb and fingers and lift. Finger sweep, using the index finger of the opposite hand to sweep the back of the mouth and throat (see illustration). If this is unsuccessful, give two breaths, reposition the head, give two more breaths, and repeat the process until foreign body is cleared or advanced procedures are available to establish an airway.	Abdominal thrusts result in a rapid pressure change that may dislodge an obstruction from the airway. Opening the airway in this manner draws the tongue from the back of the throat and away from foreign body. Finger sweep to remove loosened objects from the airway. It is necessary to establish an airway and oxygenate the client before proceeding to cardiac compressions.

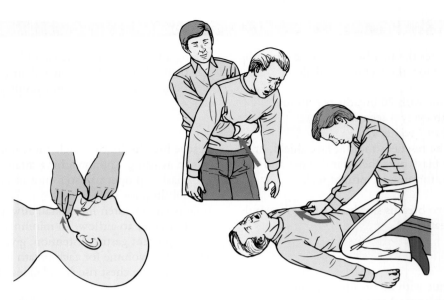

Step 10a Finger sweep and abdominal thrusts. (From Lewis SM, Collier I, Heitkemper MM: *Medical-surgical nursing: assessment and management of clinical problems,* ed 5, St Louis, 2000, Mosby.)

Steps	Rationale
b. *Child:* Abdominal thrusts are recommended in the same sequence as described in Step 9a, with the exception of finger sweeps. Finger sweep only when an object is visualized in the back of the throat.	Finger sweep may push foreign body back into the airway or damage the airway.
c. *Infant:* Back blows and chest thrusts are recommended. After establishing an inability to ventilate the infant, perform five back blows between the shoulder blades in an upward glancing method, followed by five chest thrusts on the breast bone between the nipples. Check the mouth to see if an object can be visualized; do not perform a blind finger sweep. Repeat until infant can be ventilated.	Serious complications and damage to the internal organs are associated with the use of abdominal thrusts in infants, including rupture of the stomach, diaphragm, esophagus, and jejunum (Stapleton and others, 2001).
	Finger sweep may push foreign body back into the airway or damage the airway.
11. Suction secretions as needed, or turn client's head to the side and clear the airway if no trauma is suspected.	Suctioning secretions assists in preventing airway obstruction. Turning the head to one side allows the secretions to drain to gravity.
12. Check for the presence of carotid pulse in adult and child or brachial pulse in infant. Feel for 3 to 5 seconds on the side you are on.	Carotid pulse is present when other peripheral pulses are not. The neck of an infant is usually fat and chubby, so the carotid pulse is difficult to locate. Delivering cardiac compressions in the presence of a pulse is contraindicated.
13. If no pulse, initiate chest compressions.	

NURSE ALERT *Ensure fingers are off the ribs and the lowermost part of the xiphoid process. This minimizes the chance of rib fracture that could result in punctured lung or liver laceration.*

a. *Adult:* Place heel of hands, one atop the other, on lower half of the sternum. Lock elbows and maintain shoulders directly above sternum (see illustrations). Avoid compressing on xiphoid process.	Correct positioning of the hands decreases chance of injury.

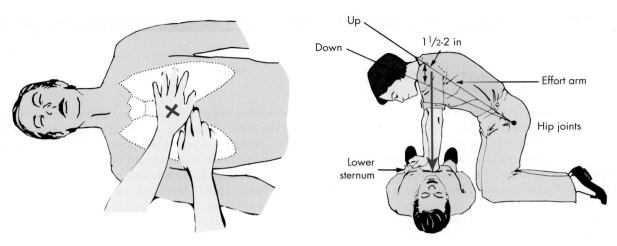

Step 13a   Positioning for CPR adult.

Steps	Rationale
b. *Child:* Place the heel of one hand on the lower half of the sternum. If possible, maintain open airway with the other hand (see illustration).	The one-hand chest compression technique for the child is used to minimize delays is restoring circulation if no trauma is present, and it will allow the rescuer to maintain airway patency during compressions (Guidelines, 2000).
c. *Infant:* Place two fingers one fingerwidth below the level of the infant's nipples (see illustration).	
14. Compress chest downward to proper depth, and then release. Maintain constant contact with skin. If contact is lost, landmarks must be reestablished a. *Adult:* 1½ to 2 inches (4 to 5 cm) b. *Child:* 1 to 1½ inches (2.5 to 4 cm) c. *Infant:* ½ to 1 inch (1 to 2.5 cm)	Compression of the sternum provides circulation as a result of direct compression of the heart and increase in intrathoracic pressure (Stapleton and others, 2001).
15. Maintain correct ratio proportionate to number of rescuers: a. *Adult:*	Number of effective compressions per minute determines the cardiac output.

One rescuer: 15 compressions, 2 breaths
Two rescuers: 5 compressions, 1 breath
Minimum of 80 to 100 compressions per minute

   b.   *Child:* One and two rescuers:

5 compressions to 1 breath
Minimum of 100 compressions per minute

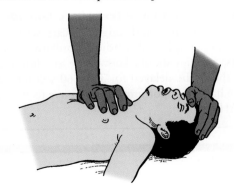

Step 13b   Positioning for CPR child.

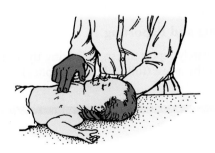

Step 13c   Positioning for CPR infant.

Steps	Rationale

c. *Infant:* One and two rescuers:

5 compressions to 1 breath
Greater than 100 compressions per minute

16. Continue artificial respiration.

17. Monitor the adequacy of the compressions during two-rescuer CPR with palpation of the carotid (adult, child) or brachial (infant) pulse during compressions. Have the rescuer performing the breathing palpate the pulse during compression. Do not delay compression.

18. Continue CPR until the rescuer is relieved, client regains cardiopulmonary function independently, or physician directs that CPR be discontinued.

19. See Completion Protocol (inside front cover).

Maintains oxygen concentration during compressions.
If the pulse is not palpable, compressions may not be strong enough or hand position on the sternum may be incorrect. CPR should not be interrupted for more than 5 seconds. Interruption of CPR for intubation should be closely monitored to avoid prolonged cessation of life-support measures.
Artificial respiration and cardiac function are provided as long as necessary.

• • • • • • • • • • •

EVALUATION

1. Inspect client's chest wall for rise and fall during administration of artificial breathing. Monitor for adequate seal over client's mouth.

2. Palpate for presence of pulse after the initial four cycles of compressions and breaths. Assess every few minutes thereafter.

3. Observe for return of respirations and pulse.

Unexpected Outcomes and Related Interventions

1. Client develops a fractured rib or sternum or a laceration of an internal organ such as a lung or the liver.
   a. Monitor correct hand placement during the administration of CPR, and continue compressions.
   b. Assess client for predisposing factors that make the client susceptible to injury during CPR.
   NOTE: CPR takes precedence over predisposing factors for injury and must be performed.

2. Patient aspirates because of reflux that results from increased gastric distention and reduced lung volume.
   a. Ensure correct volume of air is provided with each breath.
   b. Avoid overventilation by providing just enough for chest to rise.
   c. Rescuer should remove mouth and take a breath to allow patient to exhale between breaths.
   d. If client regurgitates, turn head to side and clear airway.

Recording and Reporting

• Immediately report arrest, indicating the exact location of the arrest (follow hospital policy).

• Record in nurses' notes onset of arrest; actions taken, including all medications and treatments, and client's response. A special resuscitation sheet is available in most acute care settings.

Sample Documentation

2230 Client found lying in bed and unresponsive. No breathing noted. Code blue called, CPR begun.

2342 Client resuscitated by code blue team and transferred to the medical intensive care unit with team in attendance.

☸ SPECIAL CONSIDERATIONS ☸

Geriatric Considerations

• In the older adult, compressions often result in rib and cartilage fractures. Cardiopulmonary resuscitation should be continued.

• Loose-fitting dentures should be removed to avoid obstructing the airway. If dentures fit securely, leave them in to assure a tight seal when providing ventilations.

• If dentures are removed, place them in a soft, secure location.

Home Care and Long-Term Care Considerations

In the community and long-term care settings, clients may have implanted cardiodefibrillators. For these clients, families should know how to administer CPR. CPR should be delayed for 30 to 60 seconds, until the device has the opportunity to complete its treatment cycle (AHA, 2000).

Skill 37.2

Code Management

This skill includes the initial response and management of cardiopulmonary arrest. Care must be taken to perform the basic skills of CPR immediately after discovery of an unresponsive client. In many hospital settings a code team or cardiac arrest team is available to respond and assist in resuscitation of a client with cardiac arrest.

The team usually includes a physician, intensive care nurse, respiratory therapy personnel, radiology and laboratory technologists, and other personnel. A representative from pastoral care may be available to be with the family. Family and visitors are usually asked to wait in a nearby area. If the client is in a two-bed room and the roommate can be assisted to leave, this is appropriate. If the roommate cannot leave, it is appropriate for AP to remain with the person. Excess furniture is moved out of the way, and resuscitation equipment is brought into the room.

CPR is initiated and maintained by the discovering staff until the code team arrives. As soon as possible, the client's cardiac rhythm is determined and the client is defibrillated if warranted. The client may also be intubated, and a bag-valve-mask is used for ventilatory support. Usually specially trained staff from the code team initiates defibrillation. When code teams are not used, nurses should be proficient with defibrillation and individual hospital policy should be followed. A code team should have access to a defibrillator immediately or within 1 to 2 minutes of cardiac arrest. Statistics show that defibrillation within 1 minute can result in a successful rescue as high as 90%; however, statistics drop off rapidly to 50% after 5 minutes, 30% after 7 minutes, and 10% after 9 to 11 minutes (AHA, 2000).

Automatic external defibrillators (AEDs) are available. The advantage of the AED is that BCLS personnel, who have less training than ACLS personnel, can defibrillate. AEDs eliminate the training in rhythm interpretation and make early defibrillation practical and achievable. The AED is an external defibrillator that incorporates a rhythm analysis system. The device attaches to a client by two adhesive pads and connecting cables. The pads can relay the rhythm for interpretation and deliver the electric shock. A fully automatic defibrillator requires only that the operator attach the pads and turn on the device.

A cardiopulmonary arrest is approached in a systematic and organized fashion to ensure the most expedient care. The goal is to restore cardiopulmonary function as soon as possible and decrease the likelihood of an adverse outcome. The Committee on Emergency Cardiac Care (AHA, 2000) continues to research cardiac arrest treatment and outcomes and has created guidelines for the initial care of these situations. Special specific recommendations for emergency cardiac drugs, electrical defibrillation, and supportive measures are included in the ACLS guidelines (Cummins, 2001).

ASSESSMENT

1. Assess client's unresponsiveness. *Rationale: This information assists the nurse in determining if the client is unconscious rather than asleep, intoxicated, or hearing impaired.*
2. Activate the emergency medical service in accordance with hospital policy and procedure (e.g., call a code blue or 99). *Rationale: The majority of adult victims are in ventricular fibrillation and need defibrillation and antidysrhythmic drugs as soon as possible. Early access to emergency cardiac care systems improves client outcomes (AHA, 2000).*
3. Begin CPR efforts (see Skill 37.1, p. 883). *Rationale: Without oxygen delivery, brain damage begins within 4 minutes. Brain damage almost always occurs at 6 minutes, and brain death is certain at 10 minutes (Stapleton and others, 2001).*

PLANNING

Expected outcomes focus on the goals of care, which are restoration of cardiac and pulmonary function before irreversible organ damage occurs.

Expected Outcome

1. Client regains cardiopulmonary function without adverse effects.

Equipment

*   Crash cart: Most crash carts have the following equipment:

    Gloves, gown, protective eyewear
    Oxygen source
    Bag-valve-mask
    Laryngoscope, handle, straight and curved blades
    Endotracheal tube, various sizes (6 to 8 Fr)
    Tape
    Cardiac board
    Defibrillator
    IV needles (14 to 18 gauge), tubing, fluids (9% NS, D_5W)
    Syringes
    Lab specimen tubes
    Arterial blood gas kit
    Code medications

*   Suction machine and suction equipment if not with crash cart

Delegation Considerations

The skill of CPR can be performed by assisitve personnel (AP) who are certified in BCLS procedures. The administration of emergency drugs and treatment is the responsibility of the RN and physician. An ACLS-certified RN is preferred for coordinating nursing and some ancillary department activities in a code situation.

IMPLEMENTATION FOR CODE MANAGEMENT

Steps	Rationale

COMMUNICATION TIP *When assisting a client sharing a room with the victim, remain calm and assist the client to another location. Use words that convey a sense of urgency and also portray a sense of competency and assurance. "There will be many people in the room soon to help your roommate. I will help you to a less busy area/room." If the client must stay in the room because it is impossible to leave, stay with the client. "A team of professionals is going to help your roommate. It will be a very busy area and may be noisy. I will be with you to answer questions." Remember the issue of confidentiality when answering questions. If the family is at the bedside, assist them away from the area. "Your brother is in an emergency situation. We need to give the emergency team time and space to work to help your brother. I will keep you informed of his condition frequently."*

1. Follow Skill 37.1, p. 883. Establish absence of respirations, begin artificial respirations, establish absence of pulse, and begin compressions (ABC).

NURSE ALERT *This skill requires that you know the client's code status, that CPR be performed immediately after discovery of the client with cardiopulmonary arrest, and that electrical defibrillation equipment be obtained as soon as possible.*

2. First available person brings the resuscitation cart with emergency drugs, intubation equipment, IV access supplies, and other equipment.

   Positive client outcome is directly related to the timeliness of administration of ACLS.

3. If an AED is available:

   Survival rates after ventricular fibrillation arrest decrease approximately 7% to 10% with every minute that defibrillation is delayed (AHA, 2000).

   a. Turn on the power.

   Turning on the power allows the machine to warm up while the defibrillator pads are being applied.

   b. Attach the device. Stop CPR before attaching the pads. Place the first electrode pad on the upper right sternal border directly below the clavicle. Place the second electrode pad lateral to the left nipple with the top of the pad a few inches below the axilla. Ensure that the cables are connected to the AED. Do not attach pads to a wet surface, over a medication patch, or over a pacemaker or implanted defibrillator.

   Stopping CPR ensures proper placement and adhesiveness of the electrode pads. This placement of the electrodes maximizes current flow through the cardiac chambers (Cummins, 2001).

   Wet surface, implanted defibrillator, and medication patch may reduce the effectiveness of the defibrillation attempt and result in complications.

Steps	Rationale
c. Initiate analysis of the rhythm. Each brand of AED is different, so familiarity with the model is important. Some devices will require an analysis button be pressed. Clear rescuers and bystanders from the victim, and ensure that no one is touching the victim.	The AED automatically interprets the rhythm upon operator's command. Clearing the victim prevents artifact errors and avoids all movement during analysis (Cummins, 2001) and prevents shock from being delivered to bystanders.
d. Deliver the shock in a series of three as indicated by the AED. The AED has a pause time of 5 to 15 seconds for rhythm analysis. Before pressing shock button, announce loudly to clear the victim and perform a visual check to ensure that no one is in contact with the victim. Do not resume CPR until directed to do so.	Series of three repeated shocks decreases intrathoracic pressure to the electrical current (Cummins, 1997). This pause time is the exception to American Heart Association (AHA) guidelines, which recommend that CPR not be stopped for more than 5 seconds. Clearing the client ensures safety for those involved in rescue efforts.
e. After three shocks, check for signs of circulation: pulse, respirations, movement. If no pulse, resume CPR for 1 minute, then begin the shock sequence again.	The AED may not automatically deliver another shock. The purpose of defibrillation is to return the heart to a rhythm that produces a pulse.
4. If time did not allow this to be done previously, have someone assist the victim's roommate away from the code scene.	The victim's privacy must be protected. The code scene is intense and has the potential to create emotional distress for the roommate.
5. Have client's chart available, and be prepared to relay information about the client to the team. This information includes events occurring immediately before the arrest, vital signs, laboratory results, radiology findings, and medications. The code leader may want information about the location of family members.	This information is critical in the selection of appropriate treatment for the client.
6. If respirations are absent but pulse is present, assist the code team:	
a. Administer oxygen at high flow rate by mask or bag-valve-mask (see illustration).	Increases the oxygen concentration in the blood circulating to the tissues.
b. Monitor vital signs, including cardiac rhythm, via resuscitation monitor (see illustration).	A cardiac dysrhythmia resulting in hypotension requires immediate intervention.
c. Prepare for endotracheal intubation. Have available laryngoscope, handle, curved and straight blades, and endotracheal tubes (6 to 8 Fr).	Intubation provides a patent airway and increases pulmonary ventilation (Cummins, 2001).
d. Establish IV access with large-bore needle (14 to 18 gauge), and begin infusion of 0.9% NS.	Provides a route for rapid drug administration, access for blood samples, and fluid administration. Physiological saline is isotonic.

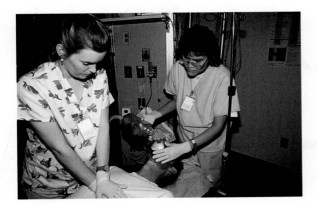

Step 6a   Administer oxygen using bag-valve mask.

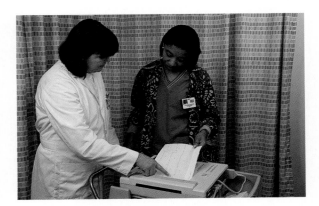

Step 6b   Monitor cardiac rhythm.

Steps	Rationale
e. Assist ancillary team in obtaining blood samples, including arterial blood gases (ABGs).	Provides valuable information regarding electrolytes, oxygenation, and ventilation.
f. Review history for suspected causes of cardiac arrest.	Hypotension, shock, pulmonary edema, and dysrhythmias are possible causes of a respiratory arrest. Treatment depends on the cause.

7. If respirations and pulse are absent and no AED is available, assist the code team:

a. Team prepares for defibrillation and defibrillates. NOTE: Defibrillation is performed only by personnel trained and certified to do so.

b. Defibrillator is turned on, and proper energy level is selected.

Output delivered in joules or watts per second. Shock may be delivered at 200 J and increased as necessary to 200 to 300 J, then 360 J, following the recommendations of the American Heart Association (Hazinski, Cummins, and Field, 2000).

c. Conductive materials (electrode gel or defibrillator gel pads) are applied to client's chest where defibrillator paddles will be placed.

Decreases electrical opposition and helps minimize burns to skin (Cummins, 2001).

d. Paddles are charged and placed on the client's chest wall by trained personnel with one to the right of the sternum just below the clavicle and the other to the left of the precordium as previously described in Step 3b (see illustration).

Placement ensures appropriate discharge of current throughout.

e. Operator applies a firm pressure to the paddles, announces to clear the client and intent to shock the client, and does a visual scan to make sure no personnel are directly or indirectly in contact with the client.

Firm pressure lowers transthoracic impedance of the electrical current (Cummins, 2001).

Anyone in direct or indirect contact with the client during the shock will also receive the shock.

NURSE ALERT *Verify that no one is in physical contact with the client, bed, or any item contacting the client during defibrillation. A warning must be called out before initiating the charge.*

---

f. Operator depresses the buttons on the defibrillator paddles at the same time to discharge the electrical current.

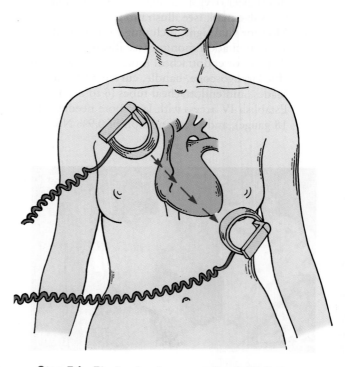

Step 7d Electrode placement for defibrillation.

Table 37-1

Common Medications Used in a Code

Medication	Dosage	Administration Frequency
Epinephrine	1 mg, IV	Every 3-5 minutes
Vasopressin	40 U IV	1 time only
Atropine	1 mg IV	Repeat every 3-5 minutes up to a total of 0.04 mg/kg
Amiodarone	150 mg IV over 10 minutes	Maximum: 2.2 g IV in 24 hours
Lidocaine	0.5 to 0.75 mg/kg IV	May repeat in 5 to 10 minutes
		Maximum dose: 3 mg/kg
Procainamide	20 mg/kg IV infusion	Maximum total dose: 17 mg/kg
Sodium bicarbonate	1 mEq/kg IV bolus	Repeat half this dose every 10 minutes thereafter

Reproduced with permission from: *Handbook of emergency cardiovascular care for healthcare providers,* © 2000, copyright American Heart Association.

Steps	Rationale
g. The first defibrillation activity is performed as a rapidly repeated series of three if the monitor displays persistent ventricular fibrillation or ventricular tachycardia without a pulse.	The series of three repeated shocks decreases the intrathoracic impedance to the electrical current. Shock for defibrillation are currently recommended at 200 J, 200 to 300 J, and 360 J (Hazinski, Cummins, and Field, 2000).
8. If three shocks fail or a different dysrhythmia is present: a. Continue CPR.	The code team is trained to interpret dysrhythmias and intervene with appropriate treatment.
b. Establish IV access with large bore needle if not previously completed.	
c. Prepare to administer medications through established IV access or endotracheal tube as directed by ACLS-trained personnel (Table 37-1).	Timely drug administration can be life saving.
d. Establish ventilation (intubation) as described in Step 6c. This is performed by ACLS personnel.	Airway necessary for oxygen delivery.
e. Repeat shocks if warranted.	
9. If not involved in the performance of CPR, nurse should obtain supplies and drugs as requested and keep family informed as directed. Another nurse may also be the designated recorder and is responsible to chart all activity, CPR, delivery of medication, AED shocking, intubation, and so on (see illustration).	The code team is specially trained in advanced life support techniques. Rapid location of supplies assists the team in providing care to clients.

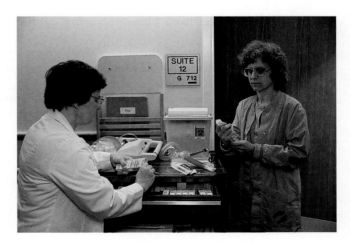

Step 9 Obtain supplies as needed.

Steps	Rationale
10. Anticipate the types of vasoactive medications that will likely be used. Double-check dosages to be given.	Ensures prompt and accurate administration of medications.
11. Remain in the room during the resuscitative phase.	Nurse caring for the client is the person most familiar with the client's medical history, which aids in diagnosis and treatment by the code team.
12. Keep unnecessary personnel out of the room during the resuscitative phase.	Cardiopulmonary arrest situations attract many hospital personnel. Too many people may interfere with the expeditious delivery of care.
13. Ensure all interventions, medication administration, and client responses are being recorded.	At the onset of a code, designation of a recorder is important. Several medical personnel are performing different interventions in a rapid sequence. Accurate recording of the events assists the code team in planning the next intervention.
14. Continue resuscitative efforts until the client regains pulse or until the physician determines cessation of efforts.	Maintains oxygenation and circulation.
15. See Completion Protocol (inside front cover).	

• • • • • • • • • •

EVALUATION

1. Inspect the client's chest wall for rise and fall during administration of artificial respiration.
2. When available, observe client's pulse oximetry levels to determine adequacy of oxygenation.
3. Assess pulse during compressions to determine the adequacy of compressions. NOTE: CPR is not interrupted for more than 5 seconds. CPR is resumed between all interventions.
4. If client has osteoporosis or chest trauma from motor vehicle injury, observe for rib fractures that might have occurred during chest compressions.

Unexpected Outcomes and Related Interventions

1. Client experiences injury as a result of cardiac compressions, such as rib or sternum fracture or lacerated lung or liver.
   a. Monitor correct hand placement before cardiac compressions.
2. Client converts back to life-threatening dysrhythmia of ventricular fibrillation or pulseless ventricular tachycardia.
   a. Continuously monitor cardiac rhythm and vital signs after resuscitation phase.
   b. Reinitiate or continue CPR.
3. Client is pronounced dead by physician member of the code team after all emergency life-support interventions are unsuccessful.
   a. Support family/significant others during initiation of grieving process.
   b. Perform postmortem care (see Skill 39.2, p. 934).
   c. Review resuscitation efforts with team members, and evaluate effectiveness of interventions.
   d. Discuss personal feeling regarding client's death and resuscitative efforts with team members, supervisor, or other professional as needed.

Recording and Reporting

- Cardiopulmonary arrest requires precise documentation. Most hospitals use a form designed specifically for in-hospital arrests. These forms are reviewed by a committee to ensure the code was performed according to ACLS recommendations.
- Information included in the form are time of the arrest; initiation, continuation, and cessation of CPR; cardiac rhythm; pulse; defibrillation attempts; medication administration; procedures performed; and the client's response.

Sample Documentation (Without Code Sheet)

0734 Client found unresponsive in bed. Code blue called. Compression board under client. CPR begun.

0736 Code blue team arrives. Cardiac monitor shows ventricular fibrillation. CPR continues.

0738 Client defibrillated at 200, 300, and 360 J with monitor showing continued ventricular fibrillation. No pulse. Continue CPR.

0740 18-gauge IV inserted in right and left antecubital site. Blood sent to lab for electrolytes and complete blood count. NS wide open via right antecubital site. ABG drawn via right femoral site by physician.

0741 Intubated with #8 endotracheal tube, left side of mouth at 26 cm. Securely taped. CPR continues. Epinephrine 1 mg IV given left antecubital site.

0742 Repeat defibrillation at 360 J. Monitor shows sinus tachycardia. Carotid pulse felt. Blood pressure 96/46 mm Hg.

0745 Prepare for transport to cardiac care unit with physician, RN, and respiratory therapist. Client remains intubated with monitor showing sinus tachycardia. Client is nonresponsive.

 ## CRITICAL THINKING EXERCISES

1. A code blue is called in Room 211, bed 2. Your client is in Room 211, bed 1. Upon entering the room, what should you assess? What would you do after making your assessment?

2. You find your client on the floor without respirations or pulse. You know the client has terminal illness but has been unable to make a resuscitation decision. What do you do?

3. The nurse discovers the client, a nursing home resident with severe Alzheimer's disease and contractures, unresponsive in bed. The nurse calls a code 99 and begins cardiac compressions. AP arrive to assume CPR, and the nurse leaves the room to get the client's chart. Critique this nurse's critical thinking and activities.

REFERENCES

American Heart Association: Guidelines 2000 for cardiopulmonary resuscitation and emergency cardiovascular care: international consensus on science, *Circulation*: I-371, 2000.

Cummins RO, editor: *ACLS provider manual,* Dallas, 2001, American Heart Association.

Ditto PH and others: Advance directives as acts of communication: a randomized control trial, *Arch Intern Med* 161(3):421, 2001.

Hazinski MF, Cummins RO, Field JM: *2000 Handbook of emergency cardiovascular care for healthcare providers,* Dallas, 2000, American Heart Association.

Keen JH, Baird MS, Allen JH: *Mosby's critical care and emergency drug reference,* St Louis, 1994, Mosby.

Stapleton ER and others, editors: *Basic life support for healthcare providers,* Dallas, 2001, American Heart Association.

CHAPTER 28

Care of the Client With Special Needs

Clients with special needs include the population with complex medical and nursing diagnoses, who require nursing interventions that are more elaborate than those of basic nursing care. These interventions require a higher level of problem solving and coordination. Many of the interventions required by these clients are performed in cooperation with physicians or allied health professionals, which means that communication skills are also a part of these processes. It is common for facilities to have in-service or certification programs that are required before implementation of these skills; the nurse should be familiar with the facility's expectations and standards of performance in the clinical area.

The role of assessment on the part of the nurse takes on special importance in these skills. Because of more frequent and more prolonged contact with the client in most instances, the nurse has a unique perspective on the progress toward goals and outcomes that affect that progress. This includes positive factors such as family support and adequate resources, as well as factors that might have a negative impact on the outcome, such as the development of complications or the presence of family stressors. The observation and interpretation of all data will be critical in the ongoing process of client care, and the foundation of this must be assessment. Systematic and objective assessments on the part of the nurse ensure the highest-quality, individualized client care.

NURSING DIAGNOSES

The following nursing diagnoses apply to multiple skills in this chapter. **Disturbed Body Image** is related to physical changes brought on by illness or side effects of treatment. Clients may also exhibit **Anxiety** related to possible outcomes of both treatment and disease process and ongoing reliance on therapies. These skills are highly technical and can be complex; therefore clients will often demonstrate **Deficient Knowledge** related to inexperience with procedures. In addition, because of the complex nature of these skills and the need for the client's understanding of these skills, **Noncompliance** and/or **Ineffective Coping** related to possible side effects of treatment, knowledge deficit, or poor relationships with the health care team may also be appropriate.

Clients are at **Risk for Injury** and/or **Risk for Impaired Skin Integrity** related to the disease process, invasive treatment procedures, and altered fluid/nutritional balance. Clients requiring any of the skills may present with **Deficient Fluid Volume, Excess Fluid Volume,** and/or **Risk for Imbalanced Fluid Volume** related to disease process and/or side effects of medication or treatment. Lastly, **Risk for Infection** related to disease process and/or invasive treatment procedures should be considered.

Additional nursing diagnoses may be applicable as a result of the unique implications for each skill. The nurse must use critical thinking in selecting nursing diagnoses that are appropriate.

Skill 38.1

Managing Central Venous Lines

Long-term central venous access devices are indicated for some clients who will receive intravenous (IV) therapy or hemodialysis for longer than 7 days and up to several years. The lines are used to administer IV fluids, medications, blood products, and parenteral nutrition fluids or for hemodialysis procedures. They may be single-lumen or multilumen catheters. The use of intravascular devices is frequently complicated, including instances of septic thrombophlebitis, endocarditis, bloodstream infection, and metastatic infection (e.g., osteomyelitis or arthritis). Catheter-related infections are associated with increased morbidity and mortality rates, prolonged hospitalization, and increased medical costs.

Central venous catheters are inserted by physicians through the subclavian or jugular veins and in emergencies through the femoral veins. The former sites are preferred in providing a flat, relatively immobile area on the chest and blood flows at a high rate, but the risk of infection is higher with internal jugular veins than subclavian (Mermel

and others, 2001). Double-, triple-, or quadruple-lumen catheters are used when the client requires several different infusions. Each port is labeled with the gauge size and position (e.g., 16-gauge distal). The largest gauge is used for blood therapy and colloid administration. If total parenteral nutrition (TPN) is administered, it should be infused through the most distal unused port available. The TPN port remains designated for TPN only throughout the life of the catheter. The middle port is used for central venous pressure (CVP) monitoring or IV infusions, and the proximal port is used for IV infusions. The proximal lumen should be used for obtaining blood specimens (Infusion Nursing Society, 2000).

Peripherally inserted central catheters (PICCs) are inserted by specially trained nurses or physicians, with the insertion from the antecubital site and the distal end of the catheter resting in the central circulation. These catheters may be inserted at the client's hospital bedside, in the outpatient department, or in the client's home. Other long-term devices may be divided into two categories: surgically tunneled catheters, which are designed to have a portion lie within a subcutaneous (SQ) passage before exiting the body (e.g., Broviac, Hickman, or Groshong); and surgically implanted infusion ports, which are placed in a vessel, body cavity, or organ and are attached to a reservoir placed under the skin (e.g., Port-A-Cath).

ASSESSMENT

1. Assess client for indications for long-term device:
   a. IV therapy anticipated for longer than 7 days, including transfusions, TPN administration, long-term antibiotics, or continuous infusions such as narcotics
   b. Infusion of vesicants or irritants, such as in chemotherapy
   c. Poor peripheral venous circulation
   d. Frequent long-term phlebotomy
2. Assess vital signs and intake and output (I&O). *Rationale: Provides a baseline to determine client's response to fluid therapy.*
3. Assess catheter patency by testing for blood return in catheter and free infusion of IV fluid or a manual flush. *Rationale: A patent line is necessary for the safe infusion of fluids, blood products, and TPN.*
4. Assess insertion site for integrity of catheter and skin. *Rationale: Development of phlebitis or infiltration requires prompt removal of catheter.*

PLANNING

Expected outcomes focus on maintaining a patent channel of venous access, maintaining fluid and electrolyte balance, and preventing complications related to maintenance of access devices.

Expected Outcomes

1. Intake and output remains in balance with electrolytes within normal limits.
2. IV infusion setup is intact and functioning properly with infusion flowing freely.

3. Client has no evidence of complications: clotting, local inflammation or phlebitis, systemic infection, venous thrombosis, air embolus, extravasation (leaking of medication into the tissues around the site), or migration of catheter.

Equipment

Site Care and Dressing Change

- Gloves (sterile and nonsterile)
- Alcohol and povidone-iodine swabs or combination swabs (chlorhexidine if client is allergic to povidone-iodine)
- Transparent or gauze dressing
- Label

Blood Drawing Through Central Venous Catheter

- Nonsterile gloves
- Povidone-iodine swabs (chlorhexidine or alcohol if client is allergic to povidone-iodine)
- 5-ml Luer-Lok syringes
- 10-ml Luer-Lok syringes
- Vacutainer system
- Saline flush
- Heparin flush (10 to 100 μ/ml)
- Blood tubes, including waste tube
- Needleless injection cap

Removal of Central Venous Catheter

- Nonsterile gloves
- Povidone-iodine swabs (or chlorhexidine if client is allergic to povidone-iodine)
- Suture removal set
- 4 × 4 gauze
- Tape

 Delegation Considerations

The skill of maintenance of central venous access devices requires critical thinking and knowledge application unique to an RN. Delegation is inappropriate for this skill.

IMPLEMENTATION FOR MANAGING CENTRAL VENOUS LINES

Steps	Rationale
1. See Standard Protocol (inside front cover).	
2. **Insertion site care**	
a. Provide insertion site care every 24 to 48 hours and as needed (prn) for gauze dressings, every 7 days and prn for transparent dressings.	Allows visual inspection of site for rapid detection of infection or other complications. Transparent dressing has been shown to remain intact longer without development of infection at site.

Steps	Rationale
b. Provide client education with respect to maintenance of catheter.	Decreases client's fears and anxieties and enables client to make choices.
c. Don mask.	Prevents aerosolization of microorganisms over IV site.
d. Remove old dressing and tape. Discard in receptacle.	
e. Inspect the catheter, insertion site, suture, and surrounding skin.	Provides baseline for condition of catheter site.
f. **Remove and discard nonsterile gloves; apply sterile gloves.**	Sterile technique required to apply new dressing.
g. Using combination antiseptic swab, cleanse catheter and site, working outward in a circular motion, or follow Steps 2h and 2i if combination swab not available.	Removes microorganisms resident on skin.
h. Using alcohol swab, cleanse catheter and site, working outward in a circular motion. Repeat × 2; allow to dry completely. Use chlorhexidine if client is allergic to alcohol.	Alcohol swabs defat the skin. Circular cleansing motions move bacteria on the skin away from the insertion site.
i. Using povidone-iodine swab, cleanse catheter and site, working outward in a circular motion (see illustration). Use chlorhexidine if client is allergic to povidone-iodine. Repeat with new swab. Allow povidone-iodine to dry completely.	Povidone-iodine reduces the skin surface bacteria. Allowing to dry completely promotes maximum bactericidal effectiveness.
j. Apply sterile clear occlusive dressing or gauze dressing (see illustration).	
k. Tape gauze dressing so that it is occlusive. Tape outer perimeter of transparent dressing	Reduces entrance of microorganisms. Permits visual inspection while securing dressing.
l. For PICC lines, coil extension tubing, and tape securely to client's arm.	Prevents accidental dislodgement and catheter breakage.
m. Write the date, time, and your initials on the label.	Provides means to determine when next dressing change is due.
n. Clamp lumens to catheter one at a time, and remove injection caps.	
o. Cleanse ports with povidone-iodine and allow to dry completely.	
p. Put new caps in place then open clamps for infusion.	To decrease the risk of catheter-related infection, routine cap changes should be done (Ray, 1999).
q. See Completion Protocol (inside front cover).	

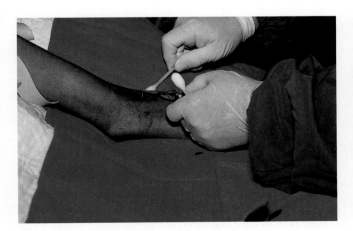

Step 2i Cleanse catheter site.

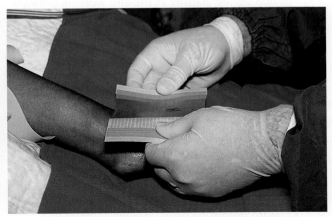

Step 2j Application of transparent dressing to PICC site.

Steps	Rationale

3. Blood drawing through injection cap

a. See Standard Protocol (inside front cover).

b. Explain procedure to client.

c. Cleanse injection cap with povidone-iodine, and allow to dry completely.

> If solution is not allowed to dry, new cap may be difficult to remove with next change.

d. Stop IV infusion. NOTE: If infusion is critical for client's well-being, draw blood instead through a different peripheral vein.

> Prevents interruption of critical fluid therapy.

e. Flush catheter port with 5 ml normal saline (NS).

> Clears IV catheter.

f. Aspirate 3 to 5 ml blood and discard, or attach Vacutainer device and draw a red-top blood tube for discard.

> Initial specimen is diluted with saline solution. Amount of discard will vary with catheter size and length; check manufacturer's guidelines. Vacutainer system reduces risk of blood exposure.

g. Aspirate the appropriate amount of blood required for ordered specimen and place in appropriate laboratory tube(s), or obtain specimens with Vacutainer system.

> Multiple specimens can be removed at one time and placed in various different tubes.

h. Flush catheter with 10 ml NS solution.

> Reduces risk of clotting in tube after procedure.

i. Flush catheter port with 3 ml heparin solution.

> Flush volumes will vary with type of catheter used. Heparin flush is believed to reduce incidence of clot formation at tip of catheter.

j. Clamp lumen, and remove cap.

k. Cleanse port with povidone-iodine, and allow to dry completely.

l. Put on new cap. Open clamps for infusion, and resume IV infusion.

m. See Completion Protocol (inside front cover).

4. Removal of central venous catheter

a. See Standard Protocol (inside front cover).

b. Explain procedure to client.

c. Place client in Trendelenburg's or supine position.

> Trendelenburg's position reduces the risk of an air embolism entering the cerebral circulation.

d. Place moisture-proof underpad beneath site.

e. Remove old dressing and tape. Discard in receptacle. Inspect catheter and insertion site.

> Provides baseline for condition of catheter site.

f. Cleanse site using combination antiseptic or povidone-iodine swabs, or according to institution policy, starting at site and working outward in a circular motion. Allow to air dry.

> Removes microorganisms on surrounding skin.

NURSE ALERT *Avoid pulling exposed part of suture through skin.*

---

g. If sutures present, open suture removal set.

h. With nondominant hand, grasp suture with forceps. Using dominant hand, cut suture carefully with sterile scissors, making sure to avoid damage to skin or catheter. Lift suture out and discard.

i. Using nondominant hand, apply sterile 4 × 4 gauze to site. Instruct client to take deep breath and hold it as catheter is withdrawn.

> Holding breath involves a Valsalva maneuver that reduces the risk of air embolus by decreasing negative pressure in respiratory system.

j. With dominant hand, remove catheter in a smooth, continuous motion. Apply pressure to site immediately, and continue for 5 to 10 minutes. Observe for bleeding.

> Client is at risk for bleeding and needs direct pressure on site to prevent hematoma or hemorrhage.

Steps	Rationale

k. Apply betadine ointment and sterile gauze dressing to site. Write the date and time and initials on the dressing.

> Antibiotic ointment reduces chance of bacterial growth at old insertion site.

l. Inspect catheter integrity, and discard.

NURSE ALERT   *If catheter is removed because of suspected infection, send tip to laboratory for culturing per facility policy and procedure. In addition, two sets of blood samples should be drawn for culture (Mermel and others, 2001). If catheter tip is broken or compromised in some way, place catheter in container, apply label with client's name and date. Risk management of facility may need catheter for investigation.*

---

m. See Completion Protocol (inside front cover).

• • • • • • • • • •

EVALUATION

1. Monitor I&O every 8 hours for fluid balance, and monitor laboratory values for electrolyte balance as ordered.
2. Inspect IV setup and catheter or port every 8 hours and prn for leaks or tears, secure connections, integrity of dressing, tubing free of obstruction or kinks, correct solution, tubing labeled, and electronic infusion pump functioning properly.
3. Evaluate for complications:
   a. Evaluate for signs of clot formation in catheter, including difficulty flushing, sluggish infusion, and absent or sluggish blood return.
   b. Inspect insertion site every 4 hours for the first 48 hours, then every 8 hours for warmth, tenderness, swelling, drainage, or bruising or bleeding. Observe skin around the site for cellulitis. Check institution policies; more frequent inspection may be delineated.
   c. Monitor for systemic infection every 12 hours, including fever, hypotension, tachycardia, increased white blood cell (WBC) count, confusion or change in level of consciousness, and decreased urinary output.
   d. Observe for thrombosis every 8 hours, including pain, tenderness, or numbness in the neck, shoulder, or arm on affected side of the body.
   e. Observe for air embolism every 8 hours, including dyspnea, respiratory distress, or cyanosis.
   f. Observe for extravasation during infusions, including burning or swelling around insertion site or port (Port-A-Cath).
   g. Observe for migration of catheter or port every 12 hours:
      (1) *All catheters:* irregular heart rate or dysrhythmia
      (2) *PICC:* frequent nausea and emesis; frequent, severe episodes of coughing.
      (3) *Hickman/Groshong:* swelling, burning sensation

Unexpected Outcomes and Related Interventions

1. Client has broken or leaking catheter.
   a. *Hickman/Broviac:*
      (1) Cease use of catheter.
      (2) Clamp with nonserrated instrument between the broken area and the exit site.
      (3) Cover the broken part with sterile gauze, and tape securely.
   b. *PICC:*
      (1) Cease use of catheter.
      (2) Cover the broken part with sterile gauze, and tape securely.
2. Client has extravasation.
   a. Stop infusion immediately.
   b. Consult clinical pharmacist for antidote.
3. Client has air embolus.
   a. Close off open end of catheter.
   b. Place client in Trendelenburg's position on left side.
   c. Obtain immediate emergency assistance.
4. Client has bright-red blood filling syringe or tracheal compression with respiratory distress, indicating arterial laceration.
   a. Notify physician.
   b. Apply direct pressure to artery for 15 minutes.

Recording and Reporting

- Notify physician immediately for signs/symptoms of the following: local or systemic infection; thrombosis/thrombophlebitis; air embolus; extravasation; suspected catheter or port occlusion or migration; dysrhythmias; or leaks, tears, or breaks in catheter.
- Notify physician or nurse who inserted PICC immediately for phlebitis/cellulitis of affected arm; suspected catheter occlusion/migration; or leaks, tears, or breaks in catheter.
- Document for catheter removal: client position (Trendelenburg's or supine), appearance of site, integrity of catheter on removal, client's tolerance of procedure, and presence/absence of bleeding every 15 minutes × 4.

- Document for site care and changing injection caps: appearance of site, catheter, and suture; date and time of dressing change; injection caps changed.
- Document for drawing blood via injection cap: date, time, sample drawn.
- Document unexpected outcomes, physician notification, and interventions in nurses' notes.

Sample Documentation

1400 Central line dressing change to right subclavian triple-lumen catheter per protocol. No redness, drainage, or swelling to site. Sutures intact. All ports with good blood return and flush without difficulty. IV fluids infusing per distal port without difficulty. Middle port attached to CVP monitoring. Injection cap to proximal port changed.

SPECIAL CONSIDERATIONS

Pediatric Considerations

Flush volumes and discard volumes will be less due to smaller catheter length and circumference; check manufacturers' guidelines. Discard volumes are also less because pediatric clients have a smaller amount of total circulating blood volume.

Geriatric Considerations

The older adult client is at greater risk for alterations in skin integrity, nutritional imbalance, and fluid and electrolyte imbalance.

Home Care Considerations

- Ongoing assessment by the home care provider is critical in the early detection of infection and the possible salvage of long-term–use catheters (Ray, 1999).
- Instruct client/significant other to notify the nurse/physician immediately for pain, swelling, burning, or numbness at site, affected arm, or side of body; bleeding or leaking; difficulty breathing; any perceived change in well-being; or pump alarming.
- Instruct client/significant other in flushing technique, site care and dressing change, and emergency interventions.

Long-Term Care Considerations

- Long-term care facilities have varying levels of health care providers (e.g., licensed practical nurses [LPNs], RNs, IV therapy provider, durable medical equipment provider); therefore a care coordination form is helpful in designating central line responsibilities in writing (Fitzpatrick, 1999).
- The acute care facility should discharge the client to the long-term care facility with the instructions taught to the client so that consistent care is provided.

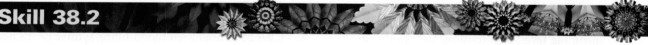

Skill 38.2

Administration of Total Parenteral Nutrition

TPN is the administration through a central vein of a nutritionally complete formula including amino acids, glucose, lipids, electrolytes, vitamins, and trace elements in clients with a nonfunctioning gastrointestinal (GI) tract. The purpose of the administration of TPN is to promote wound healing and avoid malnutrition. Hyperalimentation solutions that have very high osmolarities (i.e., containing 15% to 30% dextrose) are infused into a wide-diameter, high-flow central vein to reduce the risk of chemical phlebitis. The commonly accepted sites for vascular access of the central venous system are the subclavian and internal jugular veins. The catheter tip location is usually the superior vena cava (Figure 38-1), although other sites may be the innominate vein, the intrathoracic subclavian vein, and the right atrium (for silastic catheters only).

TPN is typically used for clients with critical illness such as pancreatitis, sepsis, cardiac conditions, trauma, liver failure, GI conditions impairing absorption, or anorexia nervosa. The regimen is individually designed for a client; the prescription is ordered by the physician and reviewed daily, with special consideration given to the electrolyte, fluid, and nitrogen balance. Collaboration with the dietitian is also important. The choice of solution varies with the client's condition and nutritional needs. Many facilities use a three-in-one solution, a mixture of dextrose, amino acids, and lipids in one bag (Perry and Potter, 2002).

ASSESSMENT

1. Assess indications of and risks for protein-calorie malnutrition: weight loss from baseline or ideal, muscle atrophy/wasting/weakness, edema, lethargy, failure to wean from ventilatory support, chronic ill-

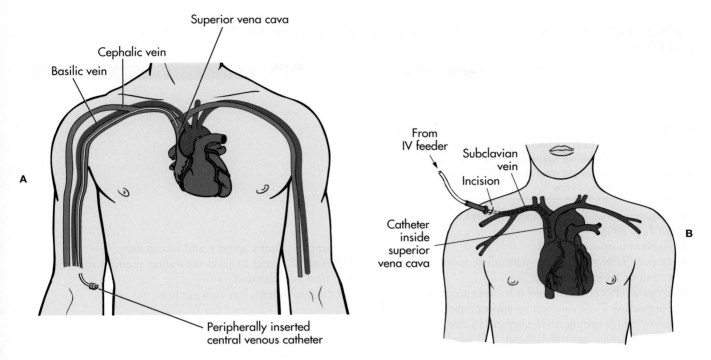

Figure 38-1   A, Placement of PICC through antecubital fossa. (Modified from Lewis SM and others: *Medical-surgical nursing: assessment and management of clinical problems,* ed 5, St Louis, 2000, Mosby.) **B,** Placement of central venous catheter inserted into subclavian vein.

ness, allergy to foods (especially eggs), and nothing by mouth (NPO) more than 6 days. *Rationale: Clinical indications for parenteral nutrition.*

2. Assess levels of serum albumin, total protein, transferrin, prealbumin, triglycerides, glucose, and urine nitrogen balance as ordered by physician. *Rationale: Provides baseline measure of nutritional status and blood glucose level.*

3. Consult with physician and dietitian on calculation of calorie, protein, and fluid requirements for client. *Rationale: Provides multidisciplinary plan for client's nutritional support.*

4. Assess baseline vital signs and weight. *Rationale: Subsequent measures will evaluate effectiveness of nutritional support.*

5. Verify physician's order for nutrients, vitamins, minerals, trace elements, electrolytes, and flow rate. *Rationale: Ensures safe and accurate TPN administration.*

PLANNING

Expected outcomes focus on adequacy of nutrition, adequacy of fluid volume, and prevention of complications related to TPN therapy.

Expected Outcomes

1. Client will achieve/maintain ideal body weight.
2. Client will achieve/maintain fluid and electrolyte balance.
3. Client will maintain serum glucose levels at less than 200 mg/dl.
4. Client will remain free of local and systemic infection.

Equipment

- Glucometer kit
- IV tubing
- IV solution of TPN
- IV infusion pump
- IV filter (optional: 0.22 μ for dextrose/amino acids, 1.2 μ for three-in-one solutions)
- Alcohol swabs
- Sterile needles

 Delegation Considerations

The skill of TPN management requires the critical thinking skills and knowledge application unique to an RN. Delegation of all skills except blood glucose monitoring is inappropriate.

IMPLEMENTATION FOR ADMINISTRATION OF TOTAL PARENTERAL NUTRITION

Steps	Rationale

1. See Standard Protocol (inside front cover).

COMMUNICATION TIP *Describe for client the nutrients contained in the solution. Also explain, "We will be checking your blood often to be sure your blood sugar level is just right and that other blood values are where we want them."*

---

2. Initiate central line management protocol (see Skill 38.1, p. 899).

3. Explain purpose of TPN. — Minimizes client's anxiety and uncertainty.

4. Inspect TPN solution for particulate matter or separation of fat into a layer. — Presence of matter or lipid separation requires that solution be discarded.

5. Prepare TPN solution and infusion tubing. Before connecting TPN solution to appropriate IV tubing, prime or fill tubing, then connect to dedicated port of multilumen central catheter, and label port. — Establishes patent, free-flowing line.

6. Use IV pump or volume controller (see illustration) to infuse solution at ordered rate. — Pump reliably delivers prescribed volume at ordered rate.

7. Assess appearance of central line site routinely (see agency policy).

8. Change tubing every 24 hours. — Client is at increased risk of infection because of impaired nutritional status. High concentration of glucose in infusion also increases risk of infection.

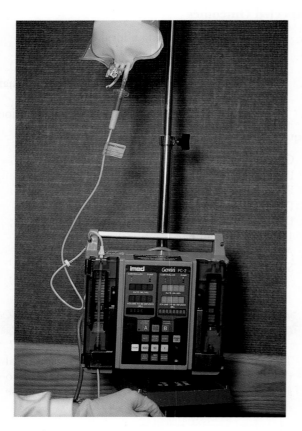

Step 6   IV pump in use to infuse TPN.

Steps	Rationale

9. If bag or tubing contamination is suspected or integrity of product may have been compromised, discard bag and tubing.

10. Do not add medications to parenteral nutrition solution.

In rare circumstances, medications may be administered via the Y-site below the TPN filter if verified as compatible by pharmacy or nutrition support service and no other ports are available.

11. Make sure additional bag of solution is available to ensure continuous infusion if ordered.

Blood glucose levels must be monitored and maintained to avoid complications of hypoglycemia. Patency of line must be maintained to ensure continued use.

NURSE ALERT *Have backup fluids ($D_{10}W$) available if new TPN solution cannot be obtained on time.*

---

12. See Completion Protocol (inside front cover).

• • • • • • • • • •

EVALUATION

1. Monitor daily or biweekly weights for trend toward normal.

2. Monitor I&O, and evaluate for fluid overload or dehydration (see Chapter 9).

3. Monitor finger-stick blood glucose level every 6 hours or as ordered (see Chapter 14).

4. Monitor for signs and symptoms of infection at infusion site, including redness, swelling, tenderness or drainage; monitor for systemic signs of infection, including fever, elevated WBC count, and malaise.

Unexpected Outcomes and Related Interventions

1. Client develops hypoglycemia or hyperglycemia.
   a. Client may need gradual adjustment of concentration of glucose in TPN solution.
   b. Insulin may be necessary to maintain proper blood glucose level.

2. Client has sharp chest pain, dyspnea, decreased breath sounds on one side, crepitus, cyanosis, or resonance to percussion. These indicate pneumothorax, hydrothorax, or hemothorax.
   a. Stop infusion.
   b. Obtain chest x-ray examination as ordered by physician.
   c. Monitor vital signs.

   d. Provide emotional support.
   e. Assist with insertion of chest tube if necessary.
   f. Assist with removal of catheter and insertion of replacement.

Recording and Reporting

• Report to physician deviation from baseline assessment or laboratory parameters and signs/symptoms of dehydration or fluid overload.

• Document assessment of physical condition, capillary blood glucose values, and IV solution on applicable flow sheet.

• Document I&O and weight on graphic sheet.

• Document unexpected outcomes, notification of physician, and interventions on nurses' notes/plan of care.

Sample Documentation

0700 Weight maintained at 58 kg for 1 week. Central line insertion site free of infection. Vital signs stable. Client denies discomfort from catheter. Daily infusions continued with 2000 ml/day as ordered. 150 g dextrose, 42.5 ml amino acids, 200 ml fat emulsion, 50 mEq Na, 30 mEq K, 4.5 mEq Ca, 5 mEq Mg, 50 mEq Cl, 12 mEq PO_4, 10 ml multivitamins, 1 ml trace minerals, and 100 units heparin.

SPECIAL CONSIDERATIONS

Geriatric Considerations

- TPN is appropriate treatment for older adults with the following conditions:

  Cachexia (chronic protein-calorie malnutrition), which is more common in older adults with cancer, hepatic disease, or chronic neurological disease. Manifestations of cachexia include emaciation, loss of subcutaneous fat and lean body mass, brittle hair, and banded nails.

  Older adults may also have protein malnutrition. Malnutrition is primarily the result of protein losses (not reduced intake), as with burns, pemphigus, or albuminuria.

- Older adults are at higher risk for complications related to TPN therapy.

Home Care Considerations

- Assess client's/family member's ability to manage parenteral feedings. Also assess environmental conditions: sanitation, equipment storage, power source. Make referral to home IV agency.
- For long-term management of TPN administration, the client and significant others must be taught to monitor the results as outlined above and should be instructed to report the following immediately: perceived change in physical condition, weight change, altered glucose values, or change in skin turgor or integrity; pain, redness, or swelling at infusion site; infusion pump alarm that cannot be corrected.
- Instruct client/family member in proper steps used to obtain capillary blood sample and measure glucose level.

Long-Term Care Considerations

As with central line care, the use of a care coordination form is helpful in designating responsibilities in writing.

Skill 38.3

Mechanical Ventilation

Mechanical ventilation controls or assists the client's respirations when the client is unable to maintain adequate gas exchange because of respiratory or ventilatory failure (Table 38-1). The treatment takes over the physical work of moving air in and out of the lungs, but it does not replace or alter the physiological function of the lung. Mechanical ventilation is used to maintain or improve ventilation, oxygenation, and breathing pattern. It corrects profoundly impaired ventilation that may be evidenced by hypercapnia and symptoms of breathing difficulty. Invasive mechanical ventilation typically requires the use of an endotracheal or tracheostomy tube (see Chapter 31) and delivers room air under positive pressure or oxygen-enriched air in concentrations of up to 100%. Noninvasive mechanical ventilation uses a special face or nasal mask (see Chapter 31).

The ultimate goal of timely and successful discontinuation of mechanical ventilation is achieved differently with every client. In general, clients will remain on mechanical ventilation only as long as necessary and will not require reintubation within 24 to 48 hours of discontinuation of treatment. Management of the client receiving mechanical ventilation is a continual challenge. Strong inter-disciplinary collaboration among physicians, nurses, respiratory therapists, pharmacists, nutritionists, pastoral care personnel, and rehabilitation services is essential to manage and eventually terminate mechanical ventilatory assistance. Nursing care for the client requiring mechanical ventilation includes provision of emotional support, prevention of equipment failure, prevention of complications (e.g., pneumothorax, atelectasis, decreased cardiac output, pulmonary barotrauma, stress ulcer, or infection), and promotion of optimum gas exchange.

ASSESSMENT

1. Assess the client's level of consciousness and ability to cooperate with the procedure and the need for special positioning and sedation during the intubation procedure. *Rationale: Combative behavior on the part of the client not only makes the procedure more difficult but also requires greater respiratory effort for the client.*

2. Assess the client's ability (e.g., use of notepad or alphabet board or hand signals) and willingness to communicate, and establish an appropriate means to do so. *Rationale: Decreasing apprehension and facilitating*

Table 38-1

Overview of Mechanical Ventilation Types

Types	Description	Nursing Considerations
Positive Pressure		
Continuous positive-airway pressure (CPAP)	Applies positive pressure during entire respiratory cycle.	Used for clients who breathe spontaneously but have hypoxemic respiratory failure; also useful during weaning.
Positive end-expiratory pressure (PEEP)	Applies positive pressure during expiration.	Used for treating hypoxemic respiratory failure.
Volume-cycled	Delivers a preset volume to client; peak inspiratory pressure will vary.	Used in short-term ventilation and with ventilator weaning.
Pressure-cycled reached.	Delivers volume to client until a preset pressure is reached; tidal volume will vary.	Useful when excessive inspiratory pressure could damage lungs, as in neonates; tidal volume varies with airway resistance and lung compliance.
High Frequency		
High-frequency jet ventilation (HFJV)	Delivers gas rapidly under low pressure via special injector cannula. Delivers 100-200 breaths per minute with tidal volume of 50-400 ml.	Clients on any mode of high-frequency ventilation require continuous sedation and neuromuscular blocking agent administration.
High-frequency oscillatory ventilation (HFOV)	Delivers over 200 breaths per minute or 900-3000 vibrations, with tidal volume of 50-80 ml, airway pressures controlled.	Most common of high-frequency types; maintains alveolar ventilation with low airway pressure; useful for treating esophageal or bronchopleural fistulas or pneumothorax; may avert barotrauma in high-risk clients if used early in treatment.
High-frequency positive-pressure ventilation (HFPPV)	Delivers 60-100 breaths per minute, with tidal volume of 3-6 ml/kg.	Tidal volume is less than the normal 5-7 ml/kg.
Mode of Use		
Control	Fully regulates ventilation in client with paralysis or in arrest. Delivers set tidal volume at prescribed rate, using predetermined inspiratory/expiratory times.	Client may require sedation to reduce competition with ventilator.
Assist	Client initiates inspiration and receives preset tidal volume that augments ventilatory effort.	
Assist-control	Client initiates breathing, but backup control delivers a preset number of breaths at a set volume.	
Synchronized intermittent mandatory ventilation (SIMV)	Ventilator delivers set number of breaths at specified volume; client may breathe spontaneously between SIMV breaths at volumes differing from those set on machine; used for weaning.	Requires frequent monitoring during weaning process.

communication will allow the client to remain calmer and more cooperative during mechanical ventilation.

3. Assess the client's need for specialized nutritional support. *Rationale: Client will not be able to have any oral intake and will have increased nutritional needs from the stress related to the condition.*

4. Assess the client's baseline vital signs and laboratory values (e.g., electrolytes, arterial blood gases [ABGs], hemoglobin [Hg]/hematocrit [Hct]) ordered by the physician. After initiation of mechanical ventilation, monitor and evaluate client's arterial hemoglobin saturation (SpO_2) per pulse oximetry and end-tidal carbon dioxide concentration ($EtCO_2$) continuously, and monitor ABGs as ordered and prn with respiratory distress. *Rationale: Provides means to monitor client's response and tolerance to mechanical ventilation.*

PLANNING

Expected outcomes focus on establishing and maintaining a patent airway, facilitating effective gas exchange, maintaining adequate fluid volume and nutrition, and preventing complications related to intubation and mechanical ventilation.

Expected Outcomes

1. Client's airway remains clear of secretions.
2. Client's partial pressure of oxygen in arterial blood (PaO_2), respiratory pattern, and SpO_2 remain within desired parameters.
3. Client's oral and nasal mucous membranes and lips remain moist and clear of abrasions, excoriations, or erosions.

4. Client maintains fluid and electrolyte balance.
5. Client maintains mental status and level of consciousness.
6. Client remains free of lung infection.

Equipment

- In-line suction catheter
- Suction unit
- Nonsterile latex gloves
- 10-ml syringe
- Stethoscope
- Manual resuscitation bag with oxygen tubing
- 1-inch adhesive tape
- Scissors
- Bite block
- Oral airway
- Pulse oximeter (SpO_2) probe and monitor
- Capnography ($EtCO_2$) window and monitor

 Delegation Considerations

The skill of maintenance of mechanical ventilation requires the critical thinking and knowledge application unique to an RN. Delegation is inappropriate.

IMPLEMENTATION FOR MECHANICAL VENTILATION

Steps	Rationale
1. See Standard Protocol (inside front cover).	
2. Explain the ventilator system to the client, using descriptions of anticipated experiences and benefits. Include family in discussion, especially when client is not responsive.	Allays anxiety when ventilator alarms sound and when staff become attentive in providing routine ventilator care.
3. Set up a communication system, and reassure the client that assistance will always be nearby.	Presence of endotracheal tube prevents client from being able to talk.

NURSE ALERT *Be sure that communication device/system is always within reach and available to client.*

4. If client does not have an endotracheal or tracheostomy tube, assist physician with insertion; verify placement with $EtCO_2$, then order chest x-ray examination.	$EtCO_2$ verifies placement of tube in trachea and not esophagus (Ahrens, Wijeweera, and Ray, 1999). X-ray examination evaluates correct tube level placement in trachea.

Steps	Rationale
5. Implement safety and infection-control measures:	
a. Check ventilator, EtCO₂, SpO₂, and cardiac alarms at beginning of each shift and after visits to bedside by others and after examinations or treatments.	Determines client's cardiopulmonary status.
b. Check for endotracheal tube position in centimeters every shift, and secure stabilization of artificial airway with every client contact (see Skill 31.4, p. 768).	Prevents accidental migration of tube into right or left bronchus or extubation of tube.
c. Keep airway, face mask, and manual resuscitation bag at bedside.	Necessary to ventilate client if endotracheal tube is inadvertently removed.
d. Ensure availability of emergency supplies on unit (e.g., extra endotracheal tubes, tracheostomy tube, chest tubes).	
e. Check endotracheal tube cuff using minimal leak technique every shift and after any change in tube position.	Ensures stable position of tube.
f. Verify tube position after every chest x-ray examination.	Physician will note correct position of tube in trachea to ensure not too close to carina, not in the right mainstem bronchus, or position is not proximal.
g. Using inline catheter, suction prn; suction oropharynx/nasopharynx after endotracheal suctioning and before any cuff manipulation.	Maintains patency of airway.
h. Use swivel adapter between endotracheal tube and ventilator.	Minimizes movement of endotracheal tube.
i. Move oral endotracheal tube from one side of mouth to the other every 24 hours; retape endotracheal tube every 24 hours when repositioned and prn, using skin prep pads.	Helps to minimize oral mucosa irritation and erosion.
j. Perform oral hygiene every 2 hours with oral suction close at hand.	Suction of secretions during oral care prevents risk of aspiration.
k. Monitor in-line temperature and humidity continuously.	Overheating can cause increase in client's body temperature.
l. Keep ventilator tubing clear of condensation and secretions. Always drain tubing away from client into fluid traps in ventilator tubing system before repositioning of client.	Prevents accidental spillage into client's airway.
m. Place bite block or insert oral airway if client is biting tube.	Prevents obstruction to air flow
n. Administer sedatives or neuromuscular blocking agents as ordered if client is fighting ventilator and ineffective ventilation occurs; observe carefully after administration.	Establishes more relaxed breathing pattern.
o. Troubleshoot high-pressure and low-pressure alarms within 15 seconds. Intervene as necessary to correct cause.	Some causes for high-pressure alarms include tube obstruction from secretions, kinked tubing or airway, increased airway resistance from bronchospasm or worsening lung disease (pneumothorax, decreased compliance). Possible causes for low-pressure alarms include accidental extubation, disconnection of tubing, or inadequate tracheal tube cuff inflation.
6. When possible, place client in semi-Fowler's position.	Promotes lung expansion and prevents aspiration if client is on enteral feedings.
7. If client becomes confused or combative, consult physician on use of soft restraints to prevent the client from extubating self. A time-limited physician's order is required.	

Steps	Rationale

COMMUNICATION TIP *Reassure the client, "This is a way of helping you remember not to pull out the tube that you need to help you breathe."*

---

8. Monitor $EtCO_2$ continuously and ABGs intermittently to detect possible overventilation or inadequate alveolar ventilation.

Overventilation causes respiratory alkalosis from decreased carbon dioxide. Inadequate ventilation may cause respiratory acidosis from increased carbon dioxide (Ahrens, Wijeweera, and Ray, 1999).

  a. Monitor oxygen saturation continuously (see Skill 12.2, p. 289).

Provides ability to continuously assess pulmonary function (Ahrens and Tucker, 1999).

  b. Assess $EtCO_2$ and SpO_2 whenever ventilator settings are changed.

Confirms endotracheal tube placement and cardiopulmonary status.

  c. Pulse oximetry and capnography may be used for continuous monitoring with the addition of periodic laboratory analysis of ABG specimens.

  d. Check ABGs whenever a sudden change in client condition occurs.

Provides more accurate measure of O_2 saturation and partial pressure of oxygen.

9. Perform the following at least hourly:

  a. Make sure that the client can reach the call light if able to use it.

Ensures mode of communication for client.

  b. Check all connections between the client and the ventilator, making sure that the alarms are turned on, including both high- and low-pressure alarms and volume alarms.

Maintains pressure within system.

  c. Verify that the ventilator settings are correct and that the ventilator is operating at those settings. Compare the client's respiratory rate with the setting. Make sure that the spirometer reaches the correct volume for volume-cycled mode; for pressure-cycled modes, assess exhaled tidal volume.

Maintains integrity of system and ensures that settings are consistent with current physician's orders.

NURSE ALERT *Do not assume that ventilator settings are correct, because they may be altered accidentally or intentionally by other personnel such as respiratory therapists or physicians. Do not assume that the machine is operating correctly, because loose connections or obstructions in tubing can cause altered function despite ventilator settings.*

---

  d. Check the humidifier, and refill if necessary. Check the corrugated tubing for condensation, and drain any accumulation to be discarded.

Do not return condensation to humidifier because of possible bacterial contamination. Responsibilities for ventilator management will vary from facility to facility, check your facility's policy.

  e. Check temperature gauges, and make sure that gas is being delivered at the correct temperature. The desired range of temperatures is between 89.6° F (32° C) and 98.6° F (37° C).

Maintain client's body temperature.

10. At least every 4 hours, assess client for:

  a. Confusion, anxiety/restlessness, agitation/lethargy, headache

Sign of inadequate ventilation/gas exchange.

  b. Adventitious breath sounds, dyspnea, tachypnea, inability to move secretions

Signs of inadequate gas exchange.

  c. Decreased urine

Sign of inadequate renal perfusion.

  d. Nasal flaring, tracheal tug, intractable cough, fremitus, use of accessory muscles

Signs of ineffective breathing patterns, possibly related to problem with equipment.

Steps	Rationale
e. Changes in respiratory depth, prolonged expiratory phase, or altered chest excursion during spontaneous breaths	Signs of inadequate ventilation.
11. Auscultate for decreased breath sounds on the left side. Arrange for chest x-ray films as ordered.	Determines whether the tube has slipped into the right mainstem bronchus.
12. Auscultate over trachea for presence of air leaks.	
a. Using minimal occlusive pressure, inflate cuff with 10-ml syringe.	Excessive cuff pressure causes tissue necrosis.
b. Leave syringe attached to cuff of tubing, or place on ventilator for easy access.	Cuff deflation destroys seal and results in inadequate ventilation.
13. Monitor fluid I&O and electrolyte balance. Weigh client as ordered.	Fluid retention can signal early pulmonary edema.
14. Using aseptic technique, change the tubing only when needed, including the humidifier, the nebulizer, and the ventilator. During the tubing change the client should be manually ventilated.	Changing the ventilator circuit only with a mechanical failure or when visibly soiled rather than routine changing does not increase the risk of ventilator-associated pneumonia (Kollef and others, 1995).
15. Change the client's position frequently.	Avoids impaired circulation of both air and blood flow.
16. Perform chest physiotherapy (see Chapter 31) as necessary, including percussion and postural drainage as appropriate.	Promotes clearing of secretions from alveoli and tracheobronchial tree.
17. Monitor GI function to prevent complications:	Inactivity and stress can produce decreased bowel function.
a. Administer H_2 blockers and other medications as ordered.	Reduces gastric acid production to prevent stress ulcer.
b. Auscultate for decreased bowel sounds, and check for abdominal distention, which may signal paralytic ileus.	Nasogastric tube may be needed to provide decompression.
c. Check nasogastric secretions for blood using Gastroccult or other agency-approved reagent.	Stress ulcer is a common complication of mechanical ventilation.
18. Provide emotional support to minimize stress.	Apprehension and anxiety can increase client's respiratory rate and respiratory effort.
a. Ensure that means of communication is intact.	

COMMUNICATION TIP   *Explain procedures even to clients who are unresponsive, because they may still be able to hear and understand. "I am going to suction you now so that you can breathe better."*

---

b. Explain procedures and events to client.	
19. Develop plan for activity: turning, repositioning, up to chair or ambulation as tolerated.	During night hours allow 2-hour interval of uninterrupted sleep with activity during day and evening hours.
a. Do passive/active range-of-motion (ROM) exercises.	Maintains joint mobility and venous return.
b. Change position every 2 hours and prn.	Reduces incidence of skin breakdown.
c. Evaluate for rotational therapy.	Rotational therapy is a special form of positioning on a rotating bed that will turn in a constant cycle to reduce incidence of atelectasis and pneumonia
d. Assist client to chair 2 to 3 times daily if tolerated.	
e. Assist client to stand and walk in place at bedside if tolerated.	Builds tolerance to exercise.
20. Initiate interdisciplinary consults as indicated.	Potential needs for nutritional support, spiritual support, physical therapy, speech therapy, or other support.
21. See Completion Protocol (inside front cover).	

• • • • • • • • • •

EVALUATION

1. Assess client for secretions, and suction as needed to maintain airway patency.
2. Continuously assess SpO_2 and $EtCO_2$, and assess respiratory pattern and vital signs at least every 2 hours for acutely ill clients and at least every 4 hours in stable chronically ill clients.
3. Inspect oral/nasal mucosa and lips for integrity and adequate moisture.
4. Monitor daily weights, I&O, and related laboratory values.
5. Use Glasgow Coma Scale to evaluate mental status and level of consciousness.
6. Monitor for signs and symptoms of infection including fever, elevated WBC count, and sputum characteristics.
7. Evaluate for signs and symptoms of sleep deprivation: irritability, increased sensitivity to pain and discomfort, stupor, confusion, and/or decreased level of consciousness.

Unexpected Outcomes and Related Interventions

1. Client develops signs/symptoms of inadequate ventilation/gas exchange/ineffective breathing pattern:
   a. Remove from ventilator, and ventilate with bag/mask device at 100% oxygen.
   b. Search for reversible cause.
   c. Have assistant call code blue or agency's cardiac/respiratory emergency system if indicated.
2. Client develops signs of inadvertent extubation/malposition of endotracheal tube or leak in cuff, characterized by vocalization/gurgling sounds, activated low-pressure alarm, decreased/absent breath sounds, gastric distention, asymmetrical chest expansion, increased/decreased peak inspiratory pressure (PIP), air leak around mouth/nose, loss of tidal volume, radiographic evidence of malposition.
   a. Manually ventilate client with manual resuscitation bag until reintubation or repositioning of tube is achieved.
   b. Have assistant notify physician.
3. Client develops extubation/malposition of endotracheal tube.
   a. Deflate cuff if still in airway, and remove endotracheal tube.
   b. Ventilate with manual resuscitation bag/mask device at 100% fraction of inspired oxygen (FiO_2).
   c. Prepare for reintubation.
4. Client develops signs/symptoms of pneumothorax: absent/diminished breath sounds on the affected side, acute chest pain, and possibly tracheal deviation or submucosal or mediastinal emphysema.
   a. Remove from ventilator, and ventilate with manual resuscitation bag/mask device at 100% FiO_2.

   b. Prepare for chest tube insertion (see Chapter 31).
5. Client develops signs of atelectasis, characterized by decreased or bronchial breath sounds, increased breathing effort, tracheal deviation toward side of normal findings, increased PIP, decreased lung compliance, decreased PaO_2, SpO_2 in the presence of constant ventilator parameters, or localized consolidation on chest x-ray film.
   a. Notify physician.
6. Client develops oxygen toxicity (clients receiving high concentrations of oxygen are especially at risk), characterized by substernal chest pain, increased coughing, tachypnea, decreased lung compliance and vital capacity, and decreased PaO_2 without a change in oxygen concentration.
   a. Notify physician, and prepare to reduce oxygen concentration.
7. Client develops signs of ventilator-associated pneumonia, characterized by purulent secretions or change in consistency/color of secretions, decreased bronchial breath sounds, coarse rales/rhonchi/wheezes, positive sputum Gram stain, positive sputum and/or blood cultures, progressive/persistent infiltrate on chest x-ray film.
   a. Notify physician.
   b. Administer antibiotics as prescribed.
   c. Suction prn, and obtain cultures as ordered.
8. Client develops signs of nutritional deficiencies as characterized by progressive weight loss, decreased serum plasma protein levels (albumin, prealbumin, transferrin), decreased lymphocyte count, slow wound healing, lethargy.
   a. Notify physician.
   b. Initiate dietary consult as ordered.

Recording and Reporting

- Document the following on appropriate forms in client record:
  Date/time ventilatory support initiated, size of endotracheal tube, insertion depth in centimeters
  Ventilator settings and client mechanics, including FiO_2 delivered/exhaled tidal volume, minute ventilation, mode of ventilation, breaths per minute, positive end-expiratory pressure (PEEP), inspiration/expiration ratio or inspiratory time, PIP, compliance, date/time of changes in ventilator parameters
  Physical assessment findings, weight, vital signs, lung sounds, and hemodynamic parameters and waveforms
  SpO_2 and $EtCO_2$ values
  ABG results and other laboratory work
  Interventions/comfort measures and client's response

Sample Documentation

0930 Intubated with 7 Fr endotracheal tube; insertion depth marked at 24 cm. $EtCO_2$ level 39 with good waveform upon intubation. Cuff inflated to minimal occlusive pressure as verified by auscultation for air leaks. 10-ml syringe at bedside. FiO$_2$ at 100%; will titrate down to maintain SpO$_2$ at or above 92%. Ventilator set on assist control, with respiratory rate at 12 and tidal volume at 700 ml. Client was sedated with 2 mg midazolam IV push; will sedate per sedation protocol if client is combative or fighting ventilator. Tube placement verified with chest x-ray film; no epigastric gurgling noted; bilateral breath sounds auscultated. Client tolerated procedure without adverse effects.

SPECIAL CONSIDERATIONS

Pediatric Considerations
Endotracheal tubes used in neonates and small children are cuffless. Strict vigilance to placement is imperative.

Geriatric Considerations
- Older adult clients are at risk for complications with greater frequency and intensity than younger clients.
- Because of alterations in sensory capabilities, the older adult client has special considerations in communication techniques and emotional support.
- Alterations in electrolyte balance, nutritional status, or cardiovascular function can produce sudden changes in the client's cognitive and physical condition.
- Underlying medical conditions and the presence of multiple medications can have significant negative effects on the client's progress.
- The older adult client is at greater risk for infection because of diminished immune function.
- The nurse must exercise diligence in monitoring the older adult client's condition on an ongoing basis and perform interventions to limit or control complications quickly and aggressively.

Home Care Considerations
- Determine if family/significant others are able to accept responsibility for performing all procedures related to mechanical ventilation support, as allowed by available equipment. If not, client will require long-term care management
- Backup supplies must be present, including airways, oxygen supply, Ambu-bags, and tracheostomy tubes.
- The preparation for transition to the home must begin as soon as possible to allow maximum time to instruct family members and evaluate their return demonstrations.
- Emergency interventions should be clearly outlined to prevent life-threatening complications of treatment.

Long-Term Care Considerations
- Long-term care facilities accepting clients on mechanical ventilation require the placement of a tracheostomy for long-term airway management.
- These facilities have respiratory therapists and often a pulmonary medical specialist on staff to assist with ventilator management and weaning.

Skill 38.4

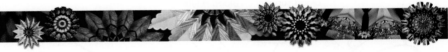

Care of Client Receiving Hemodialysis

The purpose of hemodialysis is to remove toxic wastes and other impurities from the blood in a client with renal failure. The blood is removed from the body through a surgically created access site, pumped though a dialyzing unit to filter out toxins, and returned to the body (Figure 38-2). The procedure may be performed in an emergency in acute renal failure, or it may be performed as a long-term therapy in end-stage renal disease. The frequency and duration of dialysis are determined by the client's condition; a client in chronic renal failure may need treatments up to 3 to 4 hours in length, 3 times a week. The goals of hemodialysis are to help restore or maintain acid-base balance, restore or maintain electrolyte balance, prevent complications associated with uremia, and help restore or maintain fluid balance. These goals are accomplished by extracting by-products of protein metabolism (especially urea and uric acid), creatinine, excess water, and other unmeasured toxins. This is done by allowing the client's blood to flow between surfaces of semipermeable membranes. At the same time, the dialysis solution (called dialysate) is pumped around the other side of the apparatus using hydrostatic pressure. The dialysate is an aqueous fluid usually containing isotonic concentrations of sodium and chloride ions; low concentrations of potassium, calcium, and magnesium ions; and high concentrations of bicarbonate and glucose. The toxic wastes and excess water are removed as a result of the differing pressure and concentration gradients between the blood and the dialysate.

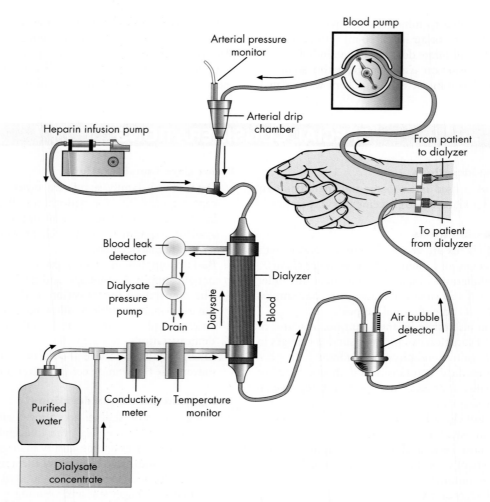

Figure 38-2 Components of a hemodialysis system. (Redrawn from Thelan LA, Davie JK, Urden LD: *Textbook of critical care nursing: diangosis and management,* ed 3, St Louis, 1998, Mosby.)

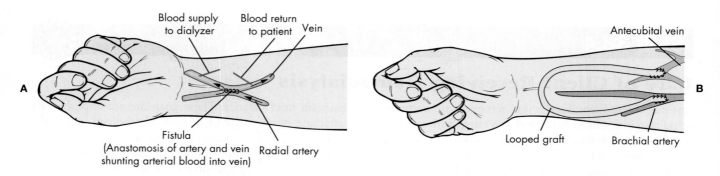

Figure 38-3 Methods of vascular access for hemodialysis. **A,** Internal arteriovenous fistula. **B,** Looped graft in forearm. (From Lewis SM, Collier JC, Heitkemper MM: *Medical-surgical nursing: assessment and management of clinical problems,* ed 5, St Louis, 2000, Mosby.)

Because the blood has greater concentrations of hydrogen ions and other electrolytes than the dialysate, the solutes diffuse across the semipermeable membrane into the solution. In the other direction, glucose and acetate are more highly concentrated in the dialysate, so they diffuse across the semipermeable membrane into the blood.

Vascular access with high blood flow is required for hemodialysis. For chronic, long-term dialysis an arteriovenous fistula or graft is created. Internal arteriovenous fistulas and vein or synthetic grafts (Figure 38-3, *A* and *B*) are created in the forearm or thigh. The increased pressure of the arterial blood flow through the vein causes the vein to dilate and toughen, allowing easy access for venipuncture. The fistula or graft is accessed using two large-gauge steel needles. For temporary dialysis, dual-lumen or triple-lumen dialysis catheters can be placed in the subclavian, internal jugular, or femoral veins.

Additional procedures using temporary dialysis catheters include hemofiltration and ultrafiltration. These therapies are termed continuous renal replacement therapies. Continuous arteriovenous hemofiltration (CAVH) and continuous venovenous hemofiltration (CVVH) are used to treat hemodynamically unstable clients with fluid overload who do not need dialysis. Continuous arteriovenous hemofiltration dialysis (CAVHD) and continuous venovenous hemofiltration dialysis are used to dialyze clients who are hemodynamically unstable and require both fluid removal and dialysis. These procedures mechanically filter toxic wastes and infuse a replacement fluid such as Ringer's lactate. Ultrafiltration is similar to CAVH but is slower.

Nurses who work in outpatient dialysis centers receive specialized training to administer dialysis. Clients visit these centers usually 3 times per week with treatment lasting 3 to 4 hours. When these clients become acutely ill and hospitalized, nursing staff must know how to monitor their status and provide appropriate supportive care.

ASSESSMENT

1. Assess client's weight, and compare to weight from end of previous dialysis and dry weight. *Rationale: Fluid retention can be quickly assessed by weight gain.*
2. Assess client's vital signs with blood pressure taken in both supine and standing positions if able. *Rationale: Provides baseline to evaluate response to dialysis.*
3. Assess client for changes in mentation, speech, and thought processes. *Rationale: Change in cognition can reveal fluid and electrolyte imbalance.*
4. Assess client's peripheral pulses with special attention to extremity where dialysis access is located. *Rationale: Determines adequacy of peripheral circulation.*
5. Assess client's heart rate and rhythm. *Rationale: Determines adequacy of systemic circulation and establishes*

baseline for assessments after dialysis. Also assesses myocardial irritability secondary to possible hyperkalemia and increased blood toxins.
6. Assess client's respiratory rate, rhythm, and quality and character of lung sounds. *Rationale: Determines baseline for assessing client's respiratory status after dialysis, because of potential changes related to fluid overload.*
7. Inspect condition of skin around vascular access. If external device is present, inspect insertion site.

PLANNING

Expected outcomes focus on relieving client's anxiety; maintaining comfort; maintaining adequacy of fluid volume, electrolyte balance, and nutrition; and preventing complications related to the dialysis process.

Expected Outcomes

1. Excess fluid and solute wastes are removed from the blood and lymph as evidenced by decreased weight, blood pressure within normal limits (WNL), and electrolyte balance.
2. Client relates a feeling of improved well-being.
3. Client has no complications as evidenced by absence of nausea, vomiting, cardiovascular complications, or alteration in mental status.
4. Vascular access is patent and intact.
5. Client verbalizes understanding of dialysis purpose and procedure.

Equipment

- Stethoscope
- Antiseptic swabs
- 4 × 4 gauze squares or 2-inch gauze roll
- Nonallergenic tape (optional)

Delegation Considerations

The skill of providing care to the client receiving hemodialysis treatment requires the critical thinking and knowledge application unique to an RN. Delegation is inappropriate.

IMPLEMENTATION FOR CARE OF CLIENT RECEIVING HEMODIALYSIS

Steps	Rationale
1. See Standard Protocol (inside front cover).	
2. Thoroughly review steps of procedure with client and family member if new to procedure. If client has received dialysis in the past, ask if there are any questions or if client wants to discuss the experience.	Relieves anxiety and promotes client's cooperation.

Steps	Rationale
3. Restrict fluids to 1 to 1.5 L/day.	Reduced renal function limits volume of fluid that can be filtered by body.
4. Develop adequate diet plan in collaboration with dietitian and client. Encourage adherence on the part of the client.	Reduced renal function limits type and quantity of nutrients that can be metabolized/excreted by the body.

COMMUNICATION TIP   *Review with client the role diet plays in disease management by asking questions such as, "Have you noticed a difference in the way you feel when you go off your prescribed diet?"*

5. Before dialysis, provide light meals.	Large meals cause shunting of blood to gut. Hemodynamics are altered during dialysis. Hypotension and vomiting may develop.
6. Routine administration of medications must be altered to avoid complications of dialysis.	Hemodialysis may remove some medications if given before dialysis.
a. Antihypertensives must be withheld in vast majority of clients until after treatment.	If client is normotensive before dialysis and medication is given, the client might become hypotensive.
b. For IV fluids, lactated Ringer's solution must not be used because of potassium load.	Hyperkalemia is a serious risk for client in renal failure.
c. Calcium for use as a phosphate binder must be given with meal, not just "around mealtime."	Calcium must be given with meal to act as a phosphate binder rather than a calcium supplement.
7. For care of access	
a. Palpate fistula or graft for thrill, and auscultate for bruit. Client should learn to assess bruit/thrill daily.	A thrill on palpation or bruit on auscultation indicates patency of fistula or graft.

COMMUNICATION TIP   *Be sure that client knows how to properly assess patency of access site by asking for return demonstration. "Please show me where you feel your shunt to be sure that it is not clotted."*

b. If clotting is suspected or confirmed, declotting is usually performed in radiology department.	Risk of damage to access site; risk of clotting. Goal is to avoid stagnation of flow to decrease clotting and reduce risk of infection.
c. Use dual-lumen catheters for blood draws and IV fluids only with approval of nephrologist. Catheter must be flushed with correct amount of heparin flush after blood draw.	Repeated access of catheters may result in clotting or catheter damage.
d. Post a warning sign in prominent location, and instruct client to refuse to allow others to perform venipuncture or blood pressure measurements on affected extremity.	

NURSE ALERT   *No blood pressures, needle sticks, or any constricting procedure should be performed on access arm.*

e. If access device is external and newly placed, clean around insertion site with antiseptic swab. **Using sterile gloves, apply sterile gauze squares or gauze roll, or transparent dressing (see agency policy).**	Some agencies only allow dialysis staff to care for access sites.
8. See Completion Protocol (inside front cover).	

• • • • • • • • • •

EVALUATION

1. Compare weight and blood pressure to preprocedure parameters. A weight change of 1 kg is equivalent to 1 L of fluid.
2. Ask client to describe general feeling of well-being.
3. Observe for nausea, vomiting, change in vital signs, or altered level of consciousness. NOTE: Temperature may rise because blood urea nitrogen (BUN) is an antipyretic and is decreased with dialysis. Hypotension may indicate hypovolemia or a drop in hematocrit. Rapid respirations may indicate hypoxemia.
4. Palpate arteriovenous shunt for thrill, and auscultate for bruit.
5. Ask client to describe the purpose and process of hemodialysis.

Unexpected Outcomes and Related Interventions

1. Client develops internal bleeding, which may be manifested by apprehension; restlessness; pale, cold, clammy skin; excessive thirst; hypotension; rapid, weak, thready pulse; increased respirations; or decreased body temperature.
   a. Report to physician immediately.
   b. Prepare to transfuse if ordered.
2. Client develops excessive site bleeding.
   a. Maintain pressure on site, and notify physician.
3. Client develops fever.
   a. Assess for sources and signs of infection.
   b. Culture blood as ordered.
   c. Administer antipyretics and antibiotics as ordered.
4. Client develops hypotension, which may be related to antihypertensive medications, inadequate sodium in diet, unstable cardiovascular disease, hypoalbuminemia, or hypovolemia from excessive fluid and sodium removal during dialysis.
   a. Elevate client's feet.
   b. Administer 100 to 500 ml NS boluses as ordered by physician.
   c. Measure blood pressure frequently during episode.
   d. Administer colloid osmotic agent as ordered.

Recording and Reporting

- After dialysis, record the following in the client's record:
  Client education given and client's ability to discuss
  All vital signs measured, all laboratory data, and client's weight before and after treatment
  All food and fluid intake before treatment
  Assessment of vascular access before treatment, including site inspection and assessment of thrill and bruit

Sample Documentation

1045 Client scheduled for hemodialysis. Discussed wife's concerns about patency of fistula. Arteriovenous fistula in left forearm has palpable thrill; able to auscultate bruit. Dry weight before treatment 91.2 kg. Blood pressure (BP) 170/102 mm Hg (sitting); 155/97 mm Hg (standing).

 # SPECIAL CONSIDERATIONS

Geriatric Considerations

Older adults are at greater risk for complications, including systemic or peripheral circulatory problems such as hypotension and hypoxia that can be life threatening.

Home Care Considerations

- The client must be taught to care for the vascular access site, which includes keeping incision clean and dry to prevent infections and cleaning site with soap and water daily until healing is complete and sutures are removed; notifying health care team of pain, swelling, redness, or drainage in accessed arm; palpation technique to assess thrill daily; free use of arm after site has healed, with care not to exert excessive pressure on it; avoiding any treatments or procedures on the access arm; and use of exercises for access arm to promote vascular dilation and enhance blood flow.

- The client who will be performing hemodialysis at home must thoroughly understand all aspects of the procedure. A specialized home care dialysis team referral is needed to assist the client with the transition to home. The client should be given the phone number for contacting the health care team for any questions or to report any problems. The client should be encouraged to have another person present during the home dialysis sessions in case problems develop.

Long-Term Care Considerations

- Long-term care facilities providing hemodialysis often have specialized RNs similar to those in acute care settings to administer hemodialysis.
- Nocturnal hemodialysis is another alternative in the long-term care setting.

Skill 38.5

Peritoneal Dialysis

Peritoneal dialysis removes toxins from the blood of a client with acute or chronic renal failure who does not respond to or tolerate other treatments. In addition, lifestyle and client choice may dictate the use of peritoneal dialysis. Peritoneal dialysis is a procedure that infuses a hypertonic solution into the peritoneal cavity. The solution is left for a specified period of time and then drained. The semipermeable peritoneal membrane filters excess water, electrolytes, and toxins from the blood. Peritoneal dialysis catheters that may be used include the Missouri swan neck and the Moncrief and Toronto Western devices (Figure 38-4). Presternal catheters

tunneled from the chest with the exit site approximately at the third to fourth intercostal space may also be used. A hypertonic dialysate is instilled through a catheter inserted into the peritoneal cavity; then diffusion moves the excessive concentrations of electrolytes and uremic toxins across the membrane into the dialysate. Excessive water is removed in the same way by osmosis. After an appropriate dwell time, the dialysate solution is removed, to be replaced by fresh solution. The procedure may be performed manually or by a cycler machine (Figure 38-5). Table 38-2 summarizes the types of peritoneal dialysis.

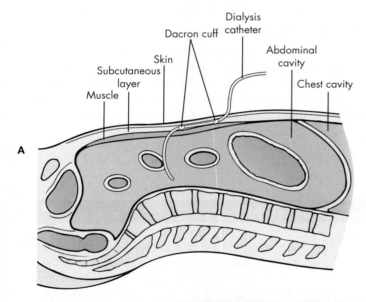

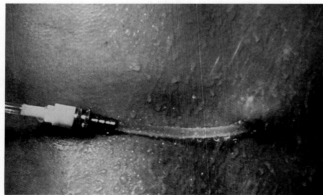

Figure 38-4 **A,** Tenckhoff catheter used in peritoneal dialysis. (From Lewis SM, Collier IC, Heitkemper MM: *Medical-surgical nursing: assessment and management of clinical problems,* ed 5, St Louis, 2000, Mosby.) **B,** Placement of peritoneal catheter. (Courtesy Baxter Healthcare.)

Table 38-2

Methods of Peritoneal Dialysis

Type	Description
Continuous ambulatory peritoneal dialysis (CAPD)	Manual; three to five exchanges daily; last bag of solution remains in abdomen overnight.
Continuous cycling peritoneal dialysis (CCPD)	Cycler machine changes solution 3-5 times or more overnight; last bag of solution remains in abdomen during daytime.
Intermittent peritoneal dialysis (IPD)	Manual or automated; connected for about 10 hours, with cycle changing every 30-60 minutes; abdomen left "dry" between sessions.

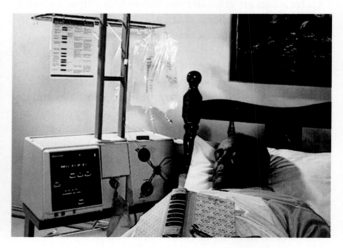

Figure 38-5 Automated peritoneal dialysis cycler, which is used while the client is sleeping at night. (Courtesy Baxter Healthcare.)

ASSESSMENT

1. Assess client's weight and vital signs before treatment. Blood pressure should be measured with the client standing and supine. *Rationale: Provides predialysis baseline.*
2. Assess client's serum electrolyte levels, especially potassium. *Rationale: Determines amount of potassium to be added to dialysate, ordered by physician.*
3. Assess client's knowledge and compliance with diet plan. Review sources of high sodium, potassium, and phosphorous that often require restriction.

PLANNING

Expected outcomes focus on successful filtering of toxic wastes from the client's blood, adequacy of fluid volume and of nutrition, and prevention of complications related to the dialysis treatment.

Expected Outcomes

1. Excess fluid and solute wastes are removed from the blood and lymph as evidenced by decreased weight, blood pressure within normal limits, and electrolyte balance (especially potassium).

2. Client relates a feeling of improved well-being.
3. Client has no complications as evidenced by absence of nausea, vomiting, cardiovascular complications, respiratory distress, or alteration in sensorium.
4. Client's catheter remains patent and intact.
5. Client verbalizes understanding of peritoneal dialysis purpose and procedure.

Equipment

* Peritoneal dialysis administration set
* Mask
* Graduated containers for measuring I&O or scale for weighing dialysate drained
* Stethoscope

 Delegation Considerations

The skill of performing peritoneal dialysis requires the critical thinking and knowledge application unique to an RN. Supportive comfort or assistive measures may be performed by other members of the health care team or by family members.

IMPLEMENTATION FOR PERITONEAL DIALYSIS

Steps	Rationale
1. See Standard Protocol (inside front cover).	
2. Review client's understanding of treatment (Jassal and Oreopoulos, 1999), and provide emotional support.	

COMMUNICATION TIP *Client often is fatigued and may experience other symptoms because of blood toxins. Keep discussion simple and focused on client needs.*

Steps	Rationale
3. Warm dialysate solution to body temperature according to agency procedure.	Avoids hypothermia and shock during procedure.
4. Add any prescribed medications to dialysate aseptically.	Some agencies require medications to be added in pharmacy.
5. Apply mask, and then prepare dialysis administration set. Have client wear mask during connection and disconnection of administration set.	Avoids introducing pathogens into peritoneal cavity.
a. Place drainage bag below client.	Facilitates drainage by gravity.
b. Connect outflow tubing to drainage bag (Figure 38-6).	Provides route for removal of dialysate solution.
6. Connect dialysis infusion lines to the bags/bottles of dialysate, and hang at client's bedside.	
7. Place client in supine position when the equipment and solutions are ready.	Promotes comfort and relaxation. Abdominal distention from fluid instillation may make breathing difficult in Fowler's or semi-Fowler's position. If the tube is new, supine position helps prevent hernias.

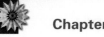

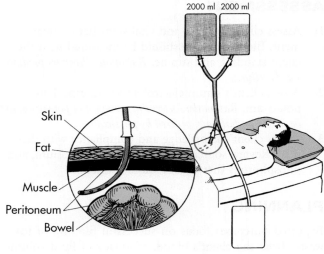

Figure 38-6 Patient receiving peritoneal dialysis. Dialysis fluid being inserted into peritoneal cavity. (From Phipps WJ and others: *Medical-surgical nursing,* ed 6, St. Louis, 1999, Mosby.)

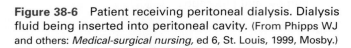

Steps	Rationale
8. Prime infusion tubing by allowing solution to fill tubes. Keeping clamps closed, connect one infusion line to the abdominal catheter.	Maintains integrity of system and prevents air from entering line.

NURSE ALERT *Avoid introducing air into peritoneal cavity.*

Steps	Rationale

9. Check patency of catheter:
  a. Rapidly instill 500 ml of dialysate into client's peritoneal cavity.
  b. Immediately unclamp the outflow line, and let fluid drain into the collection bag.
	Ensures that catheter is ready for use and that client will tolerate initiation of treatment.

10. Open the clamps on the infusion lines, and infuse the prescribed amount of dialysate over 5 to 10 minutes; allow solution to dwell for prescribed interval (10 minutes to 4 hours). Remove and discard gloves, and perform hand hygiene.	Fluid dwell time varies, dependent on concentration of electrolytes to be removed.
11. When dwell time is completed, open the outflow clamps and allow the solution to drain into the collection bag. Client may need to change position, roll from side to side.	Position helps to eliminate all of dialysate.
12. Repeat the cycles of infusion-dwell-drainage (using new batches of solution each cycle) until the prescribed amount of dialysate and the prescribed number of cycles have been achieved.	Prescribed cycling is necessary to achieve desired fluid and electrolyte balance.
13. **When the dialysis treatment is completed, mask the client and put on mask and sterile gloves, then clamp the catheter.**	Sterile technique needed.
14. After carefully disconnecting the inflow line from the catheter, place a sterile cap over the catheter end. Then discard gloves.	Avoid introducing pathogens into the peritoneal cavity.
15. Monitor vital signs every 10 minutes until stable, then every 2 to 4 hours as ordered.	Client is at risk for respiratory distress from fluid overload.
16. During treatment, have client change positions frequently, do ROM exercises, and do deep breathing.	Improves client comfort, reduces risk of skin integrity impairment, reduces risk of respiratory complications, and enhances dialysate drainage.
17. Maintain adequate nutrition, adhering to any prescribed diet.	Protein needed to replace that lost during dialysis.

18. Maintain standard precautions when emptying collection bag and measuring solution.
19. Change dressing every day and prn.
    a. See Standard Protocol (inside front cover).
    b. Cleanse insertion site with wound cleanser.
    c. Apply two split-drain sponges around the site, and tape securely in place.
20. See Completion Protocol (inside front cover).

Fluid is contaminated and may carry transferable diseases such as hepatitis.
Reduces development of infection at catheter insertion site.

• • • • • • • • • •

EVALUATION

1. Compare weight and blood pressure to preprocedure parameters. A weight change of 1 kg is equivalent to 1 L of fluid. Monitor electrolytes (especially potassium).
2. Ask client to describe general feeling of comfort.
3. Observe for respiratory distress indicating fluid overload or leakage of dialysate into pleural cavity. Watch for abdominal pain, cloudiness of effluent, and fever, which can indicate peritonitis.
4. Observe catheter for kinks, and observe outflow for cloudiness, blood, or blood clots. Clear fluid drainage should be present after a few fluid changes. Observe the site for signs of infection.
5. Ask client to describe the purpose and process of peritoneal dialysis.

Unexpected Outcomes and Related Interventions

1. Client develops peritonitis, which may be manifested by abdominal pain and elevated temperature.
   a. Notify physician.
   b. Culture all sites to determine portal of entry: transluminal, periluminal, hematogenous, or through bowel wall.
   c. Administer prescribed antibiotics.
   d. Consult with physician for possible removal of catheter.
2. Client develops exit site infection, which may be manifested by redness, swelling, heat, and pain.
   a. Notify physician.
   b. Assess response to cleansing agents.
   c. Continue thorough daily site care.
   d. Administer antibiotics as ordered.
3. Client develops abdominal pain.
   a. If pain is related to rapid inflow, decrease rate of infusion during initial exchanges.
4. Client develops shoulder pain, which may be related to abdominal distention secondary to air in the peritoneal cavity.
   a. Prime new tubing carefully, and do not use vented systems.
5. Client develops increased body temperature, abdominal pain, or cardiac dysrhythmias related to receiving overheated dialysate.
   a. Drain solution.
   b. Treat for hyperthermia.
   c. Evaluate warming procedure.

6. Client develops hypothermia, which may be related to receiving inadequately warmed dialysate.
   a. Drain solution.
   b. Treat hypothermia.
   c. Evaluate warming procedure.
7. Client develops fluid overload, which may be manifested by dyspnea, altered mental status, and alteration in breath sounds.
   a. Calculate fluid balance accurately.
   b. Use a more hypertonic dialysate as ordered by physician.
   c. Limit fluid intake.
   d. Shorten dwell time.
   e. Correct any catheter malfunction.
   f. Monitor weight, vital signs, and cardiorespiratory status frequently.
8. Client develops fluid deficit, which may be manifested by alteration in fluid and electrolyte balances.
   a. Calculate fluid balance accurately.
   b. Discontinue use of hypertonic solution.
   c. Replace fluid and sodium losses.
   d. Monitor vital signs and weight closely.
   e. Lengthen dwell time.
9. Client develops hypokalemia, which is manifested by decreased levels of serum potassium.
   a. Monitor serum potassium.
   b. Add potassium to dialysate for clients with normal levels.
   c. Instruct clients with chronic problems to increase dietary intake of potassium.

Recording and Reporting

• Document the client's vital signs, weight, laboratory results, type of solution, number of cycles, and volume of infusion and return.
• Document any unexpected outcomes and interventions performed.
• Report any significant changes to physician.

Sample Documentation

1015 Weight after peritoneal dialysis is 70 kg. Electrolytes are WNL. Vital signs: BP 159/82 mm Hg, pulse 94 beats per minute, respirations 20 breaths per minute. Temperature 37° C. Inflow 2 L in 10 minutes, dwell time 4 hours, drained 2300 ml in 15 minutes. Effluent clear pale yellow. Site nontender without redness or drainage. Client reports feeling much better. Denies questions or concerns about the procedure.

SPECIAL CONSIDERATIONS

Geriatric Considerations

- The older adult client is at risk for complications related to metabolic and nutritional changes and difficulty in following through with instructions because of alterations in sensory perceptions and judgment.
- The client must be monitored carefully to ensure that complications are prevented or minimized.

Home Care Considerations

- The client who will perform continuous ambulatory peritoneal dialysis (CAPD) or continuous cycling peritoneal dialysis (CCPD) at home will usually undergo a 2-week training program before performing the treatment independently.
- The client must be able to understand and perform all the necessary steps of the procedure, in addition to verbalizing when to report any untoward effects of treatment such as infection and fluid imbalance.
- A support group can be helpful in facilitating adjustment to the client's new regimen.
- Home care nursing can provide periodic supervision and assessment of the client's performance of the treatment.
- The client should be able to verbalize the following items related to care of the insertion site and catheter: no shower until exit site has healed; once site has healed, showering only; no bathing in tub or swimming in unchlorinated pools or in lakes or rivers; no running through fountains; no sports in which trauma to the abdomen is probable; and no heavy weight lifting.
- The client should carry emergency medical information and identification at all times, including the phone number of the dialysis center.
- The client should record vital signs, weight, and response to each treatment.
- The nurse stresses the importance of follow-up visits with the dialysis team to evaluate the effectiveness of the treatment and detect any problems that may arise.

Long-Term Care Considerations

- Staff of long-term care facilities may be trained in the use of either the Y-bag system or cycler system with support from a continuous peritoneal dialysis unit (Carey and others, 2001).
- The transition from acute care to home care will be improved by consistent use of one system as selected by the client and physician.

 ## CRITICAL THINKING EXERCISES

1. Your client Mr. H is intubated and on mechanical ventilation for pneumonia. He has a history of chronic obstructive pulmonary disease (COPD). He has been having large amounts of secretions and requires suctioning every 30 to 60 minutes. The ventilator alarms high pressure. What are your nursing interventions for this client?

2. Mrs. J has just completed hemodialysis. She has a history of hypertension, peripheral vascular disease, coronary artery disease, and now acute renal failure secondary to an aortic aneurysm repair. During dialysis a total of 3 L is removed. It is time for her antihypertensive medication. Her vital signs are BP, 88/46 mm Hg; pulse, 125; respirations, 24; and temperature, 36.8° C. What are your priorities for this client?

3. A client receiving TPN via a long-term implanted catheter (Broviac) feels moisture on his gown and calls for assistance. The catheter is leaking. What should you do?

4. Your client's central line transparent dressing has been in place for 4 days; however, it is loose on the edge. What should you assess, and what intervention would you do?

REFERENCES

Ahrens T, Tucker K: Pulse oximetry, *Crit Care Nurs Clin North Am* 11(1):87, 1999.

Ahrens T, Wijeweera H, Ray S: Capnography: a key under-utilized technology, *Crit Care Nurs Clin North Am* 11(1):49, 1999.

Carey HB and others: Continuous peritoneal dialysis and the extended care facility, *Am J Kidney Dis* 37(3):580, 2001.

Fitzpatrick LM: Care and management issues regarding central venous access devices in the home and long-term care setting, *J Intraven Nurs* 22(suppl 6):S40, 1999.

Infusion Nurses Society: *Policies and procedures for infusion nursing,* 2000, The Society.

Jassal SV, Oreopoulos DG: *Techniques in peritoneal dialysis in therapy in nephrology and hypertension,* Philadelphia, 1999, WB Saunders.

Kollef MH and others: Mechanical ventilation with or without 7-day circuit changes, *Ann Intern Med* 123(3):168, 1995.

Lewis SL, Collier IC, Heitkemper MM: *Medical-surgical nursing: assessment and management of clinical problems,* ed 4, St Louis, 1996, Mosby.

Macklin D: How to manage PICCs, *Am J Nurs* 97(9):21, 1997.

Mermel LA and others: Guidelines for the management of intravascular catheter-related infections, *Clin Infect Dis* 32:1249, 2001.

Perry A, Potter P: *Clinical nursing skills and techniques,* ed 5, St Louis, 2002, Mosby.

Ray CE Jr: Infection control principles and practices in the care and management of central venous access devices, *J Intraven Nurs* 22(suppl 6):S18, 1999.

Thelan LA, Davie JK, Urden LD: *Textbook of critical care nursing: diagnosis and management,* ed 3, 1998, Mosby.

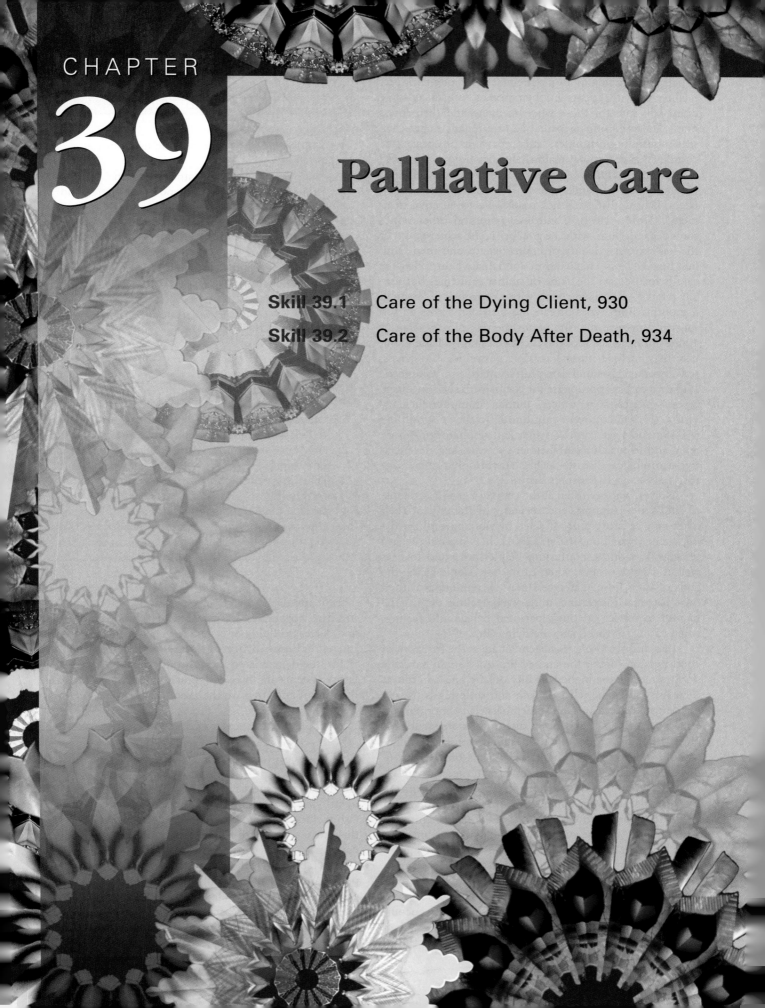

39

Palliative Care

Whether practicing in an inpatient setting, long-term care facility, or with clients in their homes, nurses at some point will care for those who are dying and their loved ones. The provision of palliative care entails many challenges and opportunities, encompassing physical, psychosocial, and spiritual realms, and has unique legal and ethical implications. According to the World Health Organization, palliative care is "the active total care of clients whose disease is not responsive to curative treatment" (Storey, 1994). Control of pain and other symptoms is paramount, with the goal being the achievement of the best possible quality of life for clients and their families. Box 39-1 lists characteristics of palliative care. Hospice care is focused on the same or similar principles but usually refers to care given clients with a prognosis of less than 6 months. Both types of care are provided across all settings and involve the care of an interdisciplinary team to address holistic needs of the client and family. Team members may include nurses, assistive personnel, physicians, social workers, pastoral care professionals, and volunteers. Palliative care is appropriate for clients with such end-stage disease processes as cancer, human immunodeficiency virus (HIV)/acquired immunodeficiency syndrome (AIDS), end-stage cardiovascular and respiratory diseases, renal and liver failure, Alzheimer's disease, and degenerative neurological diseases such as amyotrophic lateral sclerosis (ALS) and Parkinson's disease.

Nurses, who are often at the center of enabling people to find relief, support, and meaning at the end of their lives, may be profoundly affected by working with the dying client (Ferrell and Coyle, 2001). It is natural to have feelings of sadness, confusion, helplessness, and loss, as well as a sense of awe, when caring for people facing the ends of their lives. Caregivers may be reminded of their own personal losses and unresolved feelings. It can be helpful to reflect on one's personal beliefs and feelings when caring for those who are dying (Box 39-2).

Pain and symptom management are at the forefront of good nursing care at the end of life. All people have the right to receive the highest quality of care and comfort as their lives end. The relief of pain and suffering is usually of utmost concern to family members. It is important to remember that pain and other discomforts are what people say they are and require thorough, ongoing assessment without judgment (see Chapter 11). Fears on the part of the client and/or family about using pain medications, especially narcotics, can be barriers to effective pain control. It is essential to give accurate and complete information.

One challenge in end-of-life care involves incorporating norms for disease progression and symptom management different from those applied in a curative model. Symptoms considered abnormal in a curative approach may be normal for a person who is dying (Ferrel and Coyle, 2001). One example is the change in focus in regard to nutrition. For a curative approach, it is appropriate to encourage food and fluids to increase strength and healing. When

---

a client approaches death, however, body systems are slowing. This slowing results in a decreased caloric requirement and decreased fluid perfusion. The client generally has less interest in eating. By forcing intake or providing parenteral fluids, the demands on the gastrointestinal (GI) and circulatory systems are increased, potentially creating increased discomfort and stress on the client.

PSYCHOSOCIAL/SPIRITUAL CARE

An important aspect of nursing care of a dying person is identifying and meeting emotional needs. It is crucial to also include the needs and concerns of family members in this process. Elisabeth Kübler-Ross identified five stages of coming to terms with the dying process (Kübler-Ross, 1969) (Table 39-1). It is important to be aware that each person does not pass through all these stages, nor is progression in an orderly, sequential manner. Clients may jump stages or move back and forth between stages. A strong, therapeutic, trusting relationship between client,

Table 39-1

Behaviors and Responses Related to Stages of Grieving

Stage	Reasons for Client/Family Behaviors	Caregiver Response
Denial	A normal reaction, usually temporary. May be unable to absorb the news. Allows time for a terrifying idea to be digested.	Patience and willingness to talk are important; understand why the person is grasping at straws, without reinforcing nonreality.
Anger	Helps to relieve the anguish of dying. A sense of helplessness may turn to rage and may seem unreasonable. Anger may come unexpectedly and be hard to control; may cause guilt feelings. A difficult but necessary stage.	Treat with understanding and respect, not by returning anger. Consider that anger comes from feelings of loss and powerlessness. Do not take the anger as directed at you personally.
Bargaining	Usually involves a change in behavior or a specific promise in exchange for more time to live and/or freedom from pain. Person may want to wait for a specific milestone, such as an anniversary or birthday, and/or wish to complete some unfinished business. Bargaining is a part of hope and stems from a willingness to do anything to change prognosis or fate. This may be mostly an internal process.	If the person's bargain is revealed, listen with respect, reinforce feelings of hope, normalcy of feelings.
Depression	May occur when a dying person or family member faces the losses that dying brings and/or mourns what has already been lost. This is a normal stage, often starting when symptoms of terminal illness become impossible to ignore. Dying person may also feel guilt and shame for causing sadness to family and friends or for being a burden.	Attempts to cheer and reassure are counterproductive. Person needs to express sorrow fully and without hindrance. Active listening is essential.
Acceptance (Resolution)	The dying person is often tired and weak, wanting fewer visitors. It may be a time of emotional calm without great fear, joy, or sadness. The person is coming to terms with reality and beginning the process of separation.	Being fully present is important. Help family accept expressions of client's awareness of approaching death. Can be a painful time for the family.

Stages from Kübler-Ross E: *On death and dying.* New York, 1969, Macmillan.

family, and nurse is essential, as is the need for competence and compassion in the provision of care. Nurses' fundamental beliefs about humankind and caring have a profound influence on the quality of the care provided and the response of the client to the practitioner. Compassion and attentiveness may be conveyed in many ways, including the therapeutic use of touch (Figure 39-1), active listening, and sometimes simply sitting and being present with the client.

The concepts of fear and hope take on great significance at this time, and it is important to address both when concerned with a client's psychosocial well-being. Those with terminal illness may fear pain, isolation and loneliness, loss of control, or being a burden. The greatest fear of many people is the possibility of dying alone. Fear intensifies pain, and pain intensifies fear. Encouraging the expression of fears may help the client find ways to alleviate them. At the same time the nurse may support the client's ability to hope. A sense of hope can lend meaning to a person's existence, whether it is hoping for another day, for relief from suffering, for a "good" death, not to die, to see someone, or to heal a relationship.

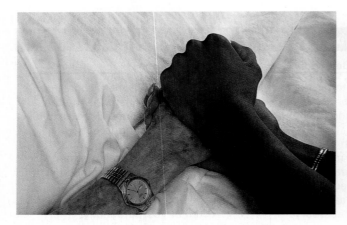

Figure 39-1 Touch can communicate caring and compassion.

Another important element of palliative care is promoting a client's spirituality, which is defined in many ways. It may be seen as the life of one's spirit, soul, or being, the very essence of each, and unique to each human being (Macrae, 1997). Crisis situations, such as serious illness and impending death, bring one face-to-face with the ultimate issues of life, the limitations of one's humanness, the loss of personal and environmental control, and the meaning of pain and suffering in the overall purpose of life (Stoll, 1979). A spiritual assessment helps to identify ways a person finds a sense of purpose and meaning in life as his or her life draws to a close (Box 39-3). Addressing such concerns may arouse feelings of discomfort or uncertainty on the part of the nurse and the client; it is best to limit data collection to that which is deemed essential in assisting the client and family. To enhance the person's comfort, select appropriate timing of questions relating to spirituality within the nursing history. Use sensitivity to discern when rapport has been established, and explain that these issues are being discussed in order to provide the client and family with the best, most holistic care possible.

A major part of many people's spiritual life is their faith or religion. Religious practice relates to a person's beliefs and behaviors associated with a specific religious tradition or denomination (O'Brien, 1999). Knowing about faith traditions is important in the provision of spiritual care (Box 39-4). Involvement of a priest, rabbi, pastor, or hospital chaplain can be very helpful in providing supportive care (Figure 39-2).

Cultural sensitivity is crucial in end-of-life care. Social and demographic trends in the United States have resulted in enormous changes in ethnic, racial, and cultural characteristics of populations served by health care providers (Kemp, 2000). Client and family health care beliefs and practices, communication patterns, family structures, and other factors may be challenging for caregivers to understand. Staff members' health care beliefs and practices,

Box 39-3
Spiritual Assessment Guide

CONCEPT OF GOD OR DEITY
- What gives your life meaning and purpose?
- Is religion or God significant to you? If yes, can you describe how?
- What values or beliefs are central to your life?

SOURCES OF HOPE AND STRENGTH
- Who are the people most supportive to you?
- Where do you get your strength during difficult times?
- What helps you the most when you feel afraid?

RELIGIOUS/SPIRITUAL PRACTICES
- What does spiritual support mean to you?
- Are there certain practices or rituals that are meaningful to you?
- What do you do when you want to find peace and serenity?

RELATIONSHIP BETWEEN SPIRITUAL BELIEFS AND HEALTH
- What is the most difficult thing you are facing?
- Has being sick or what you are facing now made a difference in your spiritual beliefs?
- What are your goals, things you still want to achieve?

Modified from Stoll R: Guidelines for spiritual assessment, *Am J Nurs* 79(9):1574, 1979.

communication patterns, organizational structures, and other factors may be even more challenging for clients and families to understand (Kemp, 2000). To provide appropriate care, nurses must look beyond personal assumptions and preconceived ideas to understand the needs of those in their care.

The death of a loved one ushers in a period of grieving for the survivor(s). Grief refers to the emotional and behavioral response to loss. Survivors experience Elizabeth Kübler-Ross's (1969) stages of grieving. Initial manifestations of a survivor's grief may include sadness, relief, denial, shock, or inertia. There may also be guilt and/or anger. The process of grieving is a journey that is experienced and expressed uniquely but ideally leads to the bereaved person adjusting to and reorganizing life without the deceased (Kemp, 1999). Multiple losses compound the experience of grief, whereas those who are marginalized in society or do not have sufficient social supports may experience what is referred to as disenfranchised grief. These examples of complicated grief often require ongoing bereavement support and/or referral for professional help (Kemp, 1999).

Box 39-4

Some Religious Practices Related to Dying and Death

Judaism: Some branches do not subscribe to the concept of eternal life, believing that one's good deeds in this life live on in memories of loved ones (O'Brien, 1999). Because life is valued as a gift of God, all efforts to continue a productive life are supported. After death there should be no preparation of the body until it is known whether members from the Jewish Burial Society are coming. A family member may stay with the body until burial. It is customary to be buried within 24 hours, but not on the Sabbath. There is a prescribed mourning period during which grief is expressed openly and in keeping with ritual (Kemp, 1998). Often cremation, autopsy, and embalming are avoided.

Christianity: Virtually all denominations believe in eternal life. Some may request Sacrament of the Sick, confession, Holy Eucharist, Holy Communion. Prayer and reading from the Bible may be appropriate forms of spiritual care. There may be a period of viewing or wake before burial. A funeral or memorial service is the norm. Usually there is no prohibition of cremation, autopsy, or embalming.

Islam: There is belief in eternal life and the will of God (Allah). Clients may wish to face Mecca, in the East, as they are dying (O'Brien, 1999). Cleanliness and modesty are very important. Regular 5-times-daily prayer should continue as long as possible; honoring that schedule shows respect to the client, family, and faith (Kemp, 1998). Loved ones usually remain with the sick person 24 hours a day; they may wish to prepare the body through ritual washing and wrapping in a white cloth. Burial is usually in a Muslim cemetery within 24 hours.

Hinduism: Hindus believe in one supreme deity, also in lesser gods with power and interest in specific areas of one's life. Beliefs include reincarnation, karma (how one has lived in this world affects how one might return in the next one). Client may want the presence of Brahmin priest; prayers are chanted by the priest. The family is responsible for washing and preparing the body. Cremation is traditional.

Buddhism: There is no supreme deity. The "eight-fold path" consists of right belief, right intent, right speech, right conduct, right endeavor, right mindfulness, right effort, and right meditation. The goal is to reach the eternal state of nirvana, or inner peace and happiness. Death is a transition and part of life. There is belief in rebirth and cremation. The client may want to remain conscious in order to be able to think right and wholesome thoughts during the dying process.

Confucianism: In Confucianism there is respect for the memories and contributions of ancestors, elaborate death and burial rituals, and belief in continuity of life after death.

Secular/Humanist: Often the focus is on values, relationships, and life accomplishments; the person may be remembered and honored at a nonreligious service.

Pagan/Indigenous spiritual traditions: Nature is sacred. From nature come teachings, inspiration, deepest sense of connection. These traditions acknowledge the mystery of life and death (Starhawk, 1997).

 ## LEGAL/ETHICAL ISSUES

An advance directive is a document that may include a living will, a person's directions about future medical care, or a health care power of attorney, which designates another person to make medical decisions if the individual is unable to do so (Perry and Potter, 2002). Advance directives generally express the desire to avoid or limit the use of life-sustaining devices and extraordinary medical procedures when there is no chance of recovery or death is imminent. Often the nurse can facilitate discussion between the client and family members about their wishes at the end of life. Issues such as the desire for fluid and nutrition, comfort measures, life support measures, and other wishes unique to the individual can be addressed. Laws relating to advance directives vary state by state, so it is imperative to

know those that apply. Institutions usually have written policies regarding advance directives. Copies should be given to the physician and responsible family members and filed in the medical record. The physician writes "Do not resuscitate" orders when the decision is made by the client and family not to initiate cardiopulmonary resuscitation when the client's heart fails. The discussion of these issues requires sensitivity, because they may be emotionally laden for the client and family.

Some clients may raise questions about or express the desire for physician-assisted suicide. This topic has received a great deal of attention in recent years, is very controversial, and arouses strong feelings. The appropriate, consistent delivery of palliative care can alleviate client concerns (Bloomer, 1998). For example, open, nonjudgmental discussions with the client may clarify concerns and fears and lead to the implementation of suitable sup-

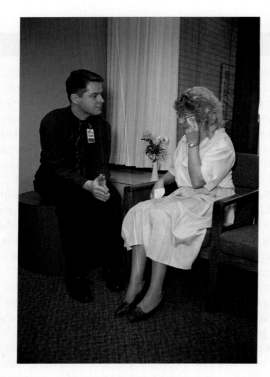

Figure 39-2 Referral to a chaplain can be a helpful nursing intervention for a client and/or family member experiencing loss and grief.

port measures such as more aggressive and consistent pain control. Depression and spiritual distress are common issues for clients facing death. The selection of appropriate interventions requires input from all members of the interdisciplinary team.

NURSING DIAGNOSES

While appropriate nursing diagnoses will vary according to the disease process and individual client/family needs, the following are commonly addressed when providing palliative care. The diagnosis of **Acute Pain** and/or **Chronic Pain** will apply when pain is unrelieved and/or requires ongoing evaluation. **Risk for Constipation** is often related to use of narcotic analgesia and immobility. **Risk of Impaired Skin Integrity** is related to immobility, poor nutrition, and muscle wasting. **Anxiety** may be diagnosed by self-report; the client may have difficulty sleeping; agitation or restlessness may be observed. A client who is having difficulty using his or her belief system as a source of strength, hope, or meaning may be at risk for **Spiritual Distress. Anticipatory Grieving** occurs before the actual loss, often leading to a greater ability to cope with the situation (Kemp, 1998). **Dysfunctional Grieving** (increasingly referred to as complicated grief) applies when clients and families are unsuccessful in working through the process of grieving. This is not a matter of making a value judgment but may indicate the need for further intervention (Kemp, 1999).

Skill 39.1

Care of the Dying Client

Promoting comfort is of the utmost importance as the client moves towards death. There is often a need for an increase in opioid dose in the final days and weeks of life, whether for pain control or the alleviation of respiratory distress (Morita, 1998). The client may have impairment of any body system, depending on disease process; there is, however, a typical pattern of progression apparent in the dying process and imminent death, as well as appropriate interventions (Table 39-2). It is helpful for the family to know what to expect so they may be as involved as possible, emotionally prepared for the death, and present at the time of death if desired.

ASSESSMENT

1. Assess each symptom in terms of onset, precipitating factors, quality, severity, and what has helped to relieve symptoms in the past. If client is nonverbal, use such cues as facial grimacing and restlessness to determine discomfort or distress. *Rationale: Thorough individualized assessment helps in determining level of distress and appropriate interventions.*

2. Listen for information that indicates spiritual distress on the part of client/family, such as "Why has God done this to me," "I haven't accomplished what I wanted to in life," or "If only I had more time."
3. Determine barriers to expression of feelings. *Rationale: Lack of privacy, pain, stress, or fatigue may create barriers to self-expression.*
4. Elicit information from client/family that may determine stage of grieving process and strength of coping abilities.

PLANNING

Expected outcomes focus on promoting comfort, autonomy, family involvement, and dignity throughout the dying experience.

Expected Outcomes

1. Client demonstrates relief from pain and other distressful symptoms.
2. Client/family make decisions regarding end-of-life care.

Table 39-2

Physical Changes Indicating Impending Death

Signs and Symptoms	Interventions
Coolness and color changes in extremities.	Place socks on feet, cover person with light blankets.
Increased periods of sleeping/unresponsiveness.	Sit with the client, perhaps holding a hand and talking quietly; encourage family/friends to speak to the client even though there may be a lack of response.
Incontinence of urine or bowel.	Change bedding as appropriate, use bed pads, good skin care. Foley catheter may be indicated.
Congestion/increased secretions.	Elevate the head, gently turn the head to drain secretions. Consider a medication such as atropine to help decrease secretions.
Restlessness.	Speak calmly to the client, reduce light. Gentle touch or massage, soothing music.
Decreased intake of food or fluids.	Do not force client to eat or drink. Offer ice chips, popsicles, sips of fluid, apply lip balm. Use sponge mouth swabs.
Decreased urine output.	None.
Altered breathing pattern (apnea, labored respirations).	Elevate the head, hold hand, speak gently to client, administer anxiolytics, opioids as ordered to relieve pain and apprehension.

Perry A, Potter P: *Clinical nursing skills and techniques,* ed 5, St Louis, 2002, Mosby.

3. Client/family are involved in provision of care according to their desires.
4. Client/family demonstrate satisfaction with emotional/spiritual support.

Equipment

- Personal care items most preferred by client

Delegation Considerations

Personal care may be delegated to assistive personnel (AP), but in-depth psychosocial/spiritual care requires the critical thinking and knowledge application unique to a nurse.

IMPLEMENTATION FOR CARE OF THE DYING CLIENT

Steps	Rationale
1. See Standard Protocol (inside front cover).	
2. Promote relief from pain (see Chapter 11).	
a. Administer appropriate analgesics on an around-the-clock (ATC) schedule, including medication for breakthrough pain, as ordered.	ATC is the most effective method for maintaining adequate pain control (Jacox and others, 1994). The goal of treating breakthrough pain is to minimize episodes of pain without overmedicating.
b. Consider the use of adjuvant medication (in collaboration with physician).	Adjuvant medications are those that either enhance opioid effectiveness or treat certain kinds of pain not relieved by opioid use (Jacox and others, 1994). Those commonly used in palliative care are antidepressants and anticonvulsants for neuropathic pain and antiinflammatory drugs for bone pain.
c. Choose the most effective route for analgesics.	Chosen route is based on client's level of consciousness, GI and circulatory status, and type of medication.
d. Monitor effectiveness of medication regimen and adverse side effects at regular intervals (Ferrell and Coyle, 2001).	Allows for modification of analgesic treatment as needed.

Steps	Rationale
e. Monitor for major side effects of narcotic analgesics.	Major side effects of narcotic analgesia include constipation, usually necessitating ongoing use of laxatives, and sedation, which is usually transitory but may necessitate a decrease in dose. Nausea, vomiting, or dry mouth is not uncommon.
f. Consider nonpharmacological methods of pain control such as relaxation, repositioning, heat/cold, massage, and diversion (see Chapter 11).	These adjuvant therapies may enhance the effectiveness of pain medication and/or allow clients to develop an ability to control themselves and their situation (Kemp, 1999).
3. Promote emotional well-being.	The process of dying creates unfamiliar psychosocial problems and brings old ones into focus (Kemp, 1999).
a. Talk with client/family about stressors, anxieties, and fears.	Helps identify sources of emotional distress and measures to alleviate the distress.
b. If client is unable to verbalize, observe for signs and symptoms of agitation and emotional distress. It may be difficult to differentiate pain from emotional distress.	Accurate assessment ensures more timely and appropriate therapies.
c. Administer antianxiety medications as indicated and ordered. Observe for signs of depression and possible need for pharmacological treatment.	Severe anxiety and/or depression require a multidisciplinary approach and may respond to appropriate medication.
d. Use members of interdisciplinary team to aid in support.	Consulting with members of team may help in determining best approaches. Client/family may benefit from counseling.
e. Facilitate communication between client and significant others. A social work referral may be helpful.	Intervention may be helpful if client and significant others are in conflicting stages of grieving or there is unresolved conflict (Kemp, 1998).
f. Involve family in providing care as desired and appropriate, such as assisting with bathing, feeding, repositioning (see illustration).	This is important to the client-family relationship before death and helps in the grieving process after death (Kemp, 1998).
g. Teach family what changes to expect as client's condition worsens.	Family members cope better if they are prepared and involved.
4. Promote spiritual well-being.	
a. Facilitate spiritually meaningful activities, such as saying a prayer with the client, reading the Bible or Koran.	Helps client move toward peace and reconciliation near the end of life.
b. Identify sources of spiritual pain and support. Encourage visits by clergy, chaplain, or religious leaders who are a source of support to client/family.	Spiritual pain can be most distressful and may negatively influence symptoms during the dying process (Kemp, 1999).

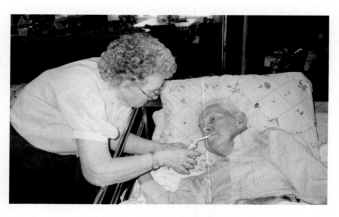

Step 3f Involve family in care.

Steps	Rationale
c. Encourage discussion of goals, life review, values, and sense of meaning/hope.	
d. Clarify who is handling client's affairs and what funeral arrangements are to be made.	Best done in context of conversation when client/family are able to express feelings and wishes (Perry and Potter, 2002).
5. Promote skin integrity and personal hygiene.	Skin integrity is compromised because of immobility, poor nutrition, and weight loss. It is best to prevent pressure areas, because they can be a major source of discomfort.
a. Reposition frequently.	Skin may become sore and irritated.
b. Use pressure-reducing devices.	
c. Aggressively treat pressure sores.	
d. Apply lotion as needed and desired.	
e. Provide personal care that is important to the client, such as nail and hair care.	Personal care individualized according to client preferences and level of comfort facilitates a sense of autonomy, dignity, and well-being.
f. Bathe frequently if incontinent.	
6. Promote nutrition as tolerated.	It is most effective to prevent nausea from occurring.
a. Medicate for nausea and vomiting on a regular schedule.	Anorexia is common near the end of life, as is difficulty swallowing.
b. Provide good oral hygiene, using sponge swabs as necessary.	
c. Offer small amounts of food and fluids in a relaxed manner, encouraging client to identify what is most appealing.	Gradual dehydration may be a natural way for the body to prevent distressing symptoms such as congestion, excess secretions, shortness of breath, vomiting, and edema (Smith and Andrews, 2000).
d. Avoid foods with strong odors.	Strong smells tend to intensify nausea. Offering food and fluid symbolizes love and nurturing, so this can be a difficult adjustment for family members (Smith and Andrews, 2000).
e. As their loved one's desire to eat decreases, give information and support to family members. Keep expectations low.	
7. Maintain adequate elimination.	Narcotic use causes constipation. Other factors that may contribute are inactivity and decreased intake.
a. Ensure regular use of stool softeners and laxatives, especially if taking narcotic analgesia.	Natural position for defecation promotes elimination; helps maintain client's autonomy.
b. Encourage use of bedside commode as long as possible.	
8. Promote oxygenation.	Alleviating respiratory distress is a comfort measure that facilitates ease of breathing.
a. Elevate head of bed.	
b. Administer oxygen as ordered.	
c. Promote measures to conserve energy.	
d. Consider opioid use for severe dyspnea and atropine to decrease secretions.	
9. See Completion Protocol (inside front cover).	

• • • • • • • • • •

EVALUATION

1. Evaluate client's degree of relief from pain and other symptoms, such as nausea, fatigue, and anxiety.
2. Ask about progress in decision making identified by client and family as essential at this time.
3. Observe level of participation in care of client, based on wishes of client/family.
4. Ask if client/family are satisfied with emotional/spiritual support.

Unexpected Outcomes and Related Interventions

1. Pain and/or other symptoms are not under control with prescribed treatment plan.
   a. Collaborate with physician for alternative medications.
   b. Talk with client/family about what other measures may be helpful.

c. Assess whether there are other factors (e.g., emotional/spiritual) that may be interfering with symptom control.
2. Client/family in conflict over decision making.
   a. Offer self or other member of interdisciplinary team to intervene if desired.
   b. Encourage communication by active listening, reflecting feelings, and clarifying issues.
3. Family members not present or not participating in care.
   a. Determine cause of nonparticipation; reinforce any teaching if appropriate.
   b. Be nonjudgmental. The client and family need support for what is working for them.
4. Client and/or family members appear to be in emotional/spiritual distress.
   a. Seek to elicit cause through assessment skills.
   b. Refer to supportive agencies as appropriate.

Recording and Reporting

- Record:
  Interventions for pain and symptom management, including client response.
  Any changes in mental, emotional, spiritual status.
  Family presence and involvement.
  Unresolved issues and concerns.
- Report when a previously alert client becomes unresponsive.

Sample Documentation

15:00 Client less responsive to verbal stimuli. No oral intake this shift. Mouth care given every 2 hours. Unable to rate pain, having occasional periods of restlessness. Appears calmer when family members are present. Hospital chaplain and grandchildren in to visit. Family members tearful and verbalizing awareness that client is nearing death. A family member plans to remain with client at all times.

SPECIAL CONSIDERATIONS

Pediatric Considerations

- The family and child are treated as a unit. Parents should be encouraged to stay with the child and participate in care as much as possible.
- Many people are affected by the death of a child, including grandparents, friends, neighbors, school personnel, and staff caring for the child.
- Decisions to end treatment can be more difficult when children are involved.
- The age and developmental level of the child must be considered in assessment and intervention strategies.
- Key points include information, support, and teaching of parents, support for siblings, and cultural sensitivity (Ferrell and Coyle, 2001).

Geriatric Considerations

- There may be more than one disease process (comorbidity) and increased disability in members of this population.

- Many chronic illnesses have an uncertain prognosis.
- Knowledge of interactions of multiple medications and geriatric pharmacology is essential.
- Pain, respiratory distress, and delirium are the most common symptoms in the dying older adult (Ferrell and Colye, 2001).
- Older adults may have experienced multiple losses in their lives, which may affect reactions to subsequent losses.

Home Care Considerations

- The primary responsibility for care rests on the family, necessitating ongoing teaching and support.
- Volunteers may be needed to give the family respite time.
- Educate family about approaches to use for symptom management.

Skill 39.2

Care of the Body After Death

When a client's death is pronounced, the physician certifies the death in the medical record and records the time of death and a description of therapies or actions taken. The physician may request permission from the family for an autopsy, although this is unusual when the death is an-ticipated. An autopsy, or postmortem examination, may be performed to confirm or determine the cause of death, gather data regarding the nature and progress of a disease, study the effects of therapies on body tissue, and provide statistical data for epidemiology and research purposes. A consent form must be signed by the appropriate family member and the physician or designated requestor. Autopsies normally do not delay burial.

It is the responsibility of the nurse to prepare and care for the client's body with dignity. Often the family members wish to view the body before final preparations are made and/or they may wish to help with preparations. The nurse should give the family the time it needs to say good-bye before the body is prepared for transfer to the morgue.

ASSESSMENT

1. Assess for presence of family members or significant others and whether they have been informed of the client's death. Determine who is legally defined as next of kin. *Rationale: Physician usually informs the family of client's death, depending on the circumstances.*
2. Assess the family's grief response. *Rationale: Nurse assumes role of providing emotional support and guidance such as active listening, acknowledgment of feelings.*
3. Approach next of kin for tissue donation or call organ/tissue request team (check agency policy). *Rationale: Trained requestors are sensitive to approaches needed to make request. Successful recovery of tissues or organs depends on a timely process.*
4. Assess client's religious preference and/or cultural heritage. *Rationale: May influence family's preferences for viewing or preparation of the body.*
5. Determine if autopsy is planned. *Rationale: If autopsy is planned, some procedures such as removal of tubes and lines may be altered or prohibited.*

PLANNING

Expected outcomes focus on preventing injury to the deceased's body tissue and facilitating grieving of family and friends.

Expected Outcomes

1. Significant others will express grief.
2. Client's body is prepared with involvement of family as desired.
3. Deceased's body will be free of skin damage.

Equipment

- Disposable gloves, gown, and other protective clothing
- Plastic bag for hazardous waste disposal
- Washbasin, washcloth, warm water, and bath towel
- Clean gown or disposable gown for body (consult agency policy)
- Absorbent pads
- Body bag or shroud kit (consult agency policy)
- Paper tape and gauze dressing
- Paper bag, plastic bag, or other suitable receptacle for client's clothing, belongings, and other items to be returned to family
- Valuables envelope
- Identification tags as specified by agency policy

 Delegation Considerations

Care of the body after death can be delegated to assistive personnel (AP). However, the critical thinking knowledge application unique to a nurse will be needed in providing support to grieving loved ones.

IMPLEMENTATION FOR CARE OF THE BODY AFTER DEATH

Steps	Rationale
1. See Standard Protocol (inside front cover).	
2. There is no need to hurry at this time. Help the family do what they need to at this time according to cultural, spiritual, personal preferences.	The sense of being in a hurry may be caused by the family's pain and staff's discomfort (Kemp, 1999). Slowing things down allows time for the family to begin understanding the reality of what has happened and to say good-bye.
3. Have body placed in a private room, or have roommate moved to another area as body is being prepared.	Provides staff with an area to make the body presentable for family to visit in private.
4. Check with significant others about notifying other family members/friends of the death. Request the name of the funeral home.	Following a death, significant others may have difficulty remembering details.
5. Discuss procedure of caring for the body with significant others. Inquire if there are particular cultural or spiritual practices that are important to know.	Discussing these aspects increases the appropriateness of care and conveys caring and concern.

Steps	Rationale
6. Determine if family wants to be involved in final preparation of the body.	The family may value being able to participate in this final aspect of care, which can facilitate grieving and acknowledgment of the death.
7. If tissue donation has been made, consult agency policy for specific guidelines on care of the body.	Retrieval of tissues (e.g., eye, skin) may require special preparation measures.
8. 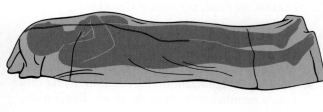 Apply gown or protective barriers as applicable.	Body excretions may harbor infectious microorganisms. Withdrawal of IV tubing or other tubing may cause temporary bleeding.
9. Identify the body according to agency policy. Leave identification in place as directed in agency policy.	Ensures proper identification of the body for delivery to morgue, autopsy room, and funeral home.
10. If in keeping with agency policy, remove all indwelling catheters, intravenous (IV), oxygen, and other tubes. (If an autopsy is to be performed, policy may direct to leave these devices in place.) Dress puncture wounds with a small dressing.	Creates a normal appearance.
11. Remove soiled dressings, and replace with clean gauze dressings using paper tape.	Changing dressings helps to control odors caused by microorganisms and to creates a more acceptable appearance. Paper tape minimizes skin trauma.
12. If the person wore dentures, insert them. If mouth fails to close, place a rolled-up towel under the chin.	It is difficult to insert dentures after rigor mortis occurs. Dentures maintain natural facial expression.
13. Position client as outlined in agency procedures. In general, do not place one hand on top of the other.	Client appears natural and comfortable. Placing one hand on top of another can lead to skin discoloration.
14. Place small pillow or folded towel under the head, or elevate head of bed 10 to 15 degrees.	Prevents pooling of blood in the face and subsequent discoloration.
15. Close eyes gently by grasping the eyelashes and pulling lids over corneas of eyes.	Closed eyes present a more natural appearance. Pressure on the lids can lead to discoloration.
16. Wash body parts soiled by blood, urine, feces, or other drainage (a mortician will provide a complete bath). Place an absorbent pad under the client's buttocks.	Prepares body for viewing and reduces odors. Relaxation of sphincter muscles after death may cause release of urine or feces.
17. Place a clean gown on the client (agency policy may require removal before body is wrapped).	Prepares body for viewing.
18. Brush and comb client's hair. Remove any clips, hairpins, or rubber bands.	The client should appear well-groomed for viewing by family. Hard objects such as pins can damage or discolor the face and scalp.
19. Remove all jewelry, and give to designated family member. Exception: If family requests that wedding band be left in place, place a small strip of tape around client's finger over the ring.	Prevents loss of client's valuables.

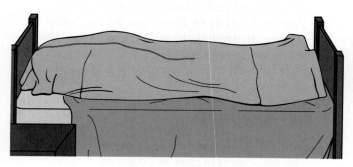

Step 21   Body in body bag and shroud.

Steps	Rationale
20. If significant others request viewing, place a sheet or light blanket over the body with only the head and upper shoulders exposed. Remove unneeded equipment from the room. Provide soft lighting, and offer chairs. Determine whether significant others would like to be alone or to have a staff person in the room.	Maintains dignity and respect for the client and significant others. Prevents exposure of body parts.
21. After the significant others have left the room, remove all linen and the client's gown (refer to agency policy). Place body in body bag or apply the shroud as required by the agency (see illustration).	
22. Label the body as directed by agency policy.	
23. Arrange transportation of the body to the morgue or mortuary.	Ensures proper identification of the body. If delay is anticipated before the mortician arrives, the body should be cooled in the morgue to prevent further tissue damage.
24. Be sure family/loved ones have no questions or concerns before they leave.	

• • • • • • • • • •

EVALUATION

1. Observe significant others' response to the loss.
2. Determine if family has received appropriate emotional/spiritual support after the death.
3. Note appearance and condition of client's skin during preparation of the body.

Unexpected Outcomes and Related Interventions

1. Significant others may become immobilized by their grief and have difficulty functioning.
   a. Do not rush family. Give them time to ask questions and express their grief.
   b. Consider pastoral care or social work consultation.
2. Lacerations, bruises, or abrasions are noted on skin surfaces of deceased.
   a. Cleanse areas thoroughly before family viewing.
   b. Inform family of any bruises or lacerations that they may see.
   c. Document any skin tears or breakdown.

Recording and Reporting

• Record date and time of death, time physician notified, name of physician pronouncing death, delivery of postmortem care, identification of body, consent form signed by significant other, disposition of the body, and information provided to significant others.
• Document any marks, bruises, wounds on body before death or those observed during care of the body.
• Document how valuables and personal belongings were handled and who received them. Secure signatures as required by agency policy.

Sample Documentation

0245 David Knight pronounced dead by Dr. J White at 0213. Wife and other family members present at time of death and assisted with preparation of the body. Hospital chaplain provided support. Two bruises, approximately 1 cm in diameter each, on left forearm noted. Allen and Son Funeral Home notified of death. Teeth, glasses, hearing aid, and clothes sent with body to morgue with security personnel.

✹ SPECIAL CONSIDERATIONS ✹

Home Care Considerations

• The trend is toward more people choosing to die at home.
• The family needs to know whom to call for help if symptom control is needed, and what to do at the time of death, who must be notified, and how the body is to be transported.
• Knowledge of types of home care reimbursement is essential, including Medicare and Medicaid hospice benefits.

Long-Term Care Considerations

• Less physician involvement means nurses have an important role in assessing and managing pain and symptom control.
• Challenges include providing privacy and autonomy for the client and family, involving the family as much as possible or desired, individualizing care, keeping family members informed of changes, and making the environment as homelike as possible.

CRITICAL THINKING EXERCISES

1. James J. is a 58-year-old man dying of cancer. He is short of breath at rest and rates his pain as 4 (scale of 0 to 10) 1 hour after receiving his analgesic medication. His daughter is flying in to see him tonight, and he asks frequently when she will arrive. Identify three nursing diagnoses in order of priority and an appropriate intervention for each.

2. You are taking care of an Islamic client of Saudi-Arabian descent. What would you need to assess in order to provide adequate psychosocial/spiritual care?

REFERENCES

Bloomer B: Palliative care, *J Assoc Nurses AIDS Care* 9(2):45, 1998.

Ferrell B, Coyle N: *Textbook of palliative nursing*, New York, 2001, Oxford University Press.

Jacox A and others: *Management of cancer pain*, Clinical practice guideline No. 9, Rockville Md, 1994, Agency for Health Care Policy and Research, Public Health Service, U.S. Department of Health and Human Services.

Kemp C: *Terminal illness: a guide to nursing care*, ed 2, Philadelphia, 1999, Lippincott.

Kemp C: Culture and the end of life, *J Hosp Palliat Nurs* 2(3):109, 2000.

Kübler-Ross E: *On death and dying*, New York, 1969, Macmillan.

Macrae J: Nursing spiritual healing practices with emphasis on Florence Nightingale. Paper presented at Spirituality and Healing in Medicine-II, Los Angeles, March 20-22, 1999 (cited in Sheldon, 2000), Chicago.

Morita T: A prospective study on the dying process in terminally cancer patients, *Am J Hosp Palliat Care* 15(4):217, 1998.

O'Brien M: *Spirituality in nursing: standing on holy ground*, 1999, Boston, Jones and Bartlett Publishers.

Perry A, Potter P: *Clinical nursing skills and techniques*, ed 5, St Louis, 2002, Mosby.

Smith S, Andrews M: Artificial nutrition and hydration at the end of life, *Medsurg Nurs* 9(5):233, 2000.

Starhawk: *The pagan book of living and dying*, San Francisco, 1997, Harper.

Stoll R: Guidelines for spiritual assessment, *Am J Nurs* 79(9):1574, 1979.

Storey P: *Primer of palliative care*, Gainesville, Fla, 1994, Kendell Hunt.

CHAPTER
40

Client Teaching and Home Health Management

The goals of client and family teaching and home health management are to promote healthy behaviors, encourage the client's involvement in health care decisions, and to improve outcomes (Joint Commission on Accreditation of Healthcare Organizations [JCAHO], 2000). The JCAHO's standard for client education include standards that promote healthy behaviors, support recovery and rapid return to function, and enable clients to be involved in decisions about their own care. These standards require that assessment consider cultural and religious practices, emotional barriers, desire and motivation to learn, physical and cognitive limitations, language barriers and financial implications. The goals of client and family education include assessing client educaton progams available, formulating individualized client health education goals, and determining and prioritizing specific client education needs. In addition these standards require that client education continuously elicits feedback to ensure that the information is understood, appropriate and useful. Evidence of successful client education must be documented in the client's medical record. Comprehensive client education includes three important purposes, (See Box 40-1, Topics for Health Education). Teaching needs to be based on assessment of the client's knowledge level and learning need, psychosocial, spiritual, and cultural values, as well as physical and emotional readiness to learn (Redman, 2001). Teaching begins at the time of admission to the health care facility, integrated throughout the client's stay in the health care facility and continued in the home setting.

Discharge planning is an organized, coordinated, interdisciplinary process that provides a plan of care for the client leaving the health care setting. The teaching and support provided needs to include the promotion of healthy behaviors, support recovery, and facilitate an effective return to normal function.

Client teaching is currently considered an essential part of practice in state practice acts for most health professionals, in various federal and state regulations, and in accreditation criteria. Practice guidelines, which define the standard of practice based on research, are now widely used in health care settings to improve the quality of care (Redman, 2001).

Nurses have an ethical responsibility to teach their clients. In the *Patient Care Partnership* the American Hospital Association (2003) indicates that clients have the right to make informed decisions about their care. The information required to make informed decisions must be relevant, current, and presented clearly. The nurse often clarifies information provided by physicians and other health care providers and may become the primary source of information for adjusting to health problems.

The nurse's role in discharge planning follows the nursing process. The nurse must assess the learning needs, abilities, preferences, and readiness to learn. The assessment considers cultural and religious practices, emotional barriers, desire to learn, physical and cognitive limitations,

---

Box 40-1

Topics for Health Education

HEALTH PROMOTION AND ILLNESS PREVENTION
- Avoidance of risks (e.g., smoking, alcohol)
- Relaxation
- Growth and development
- Immunizations
- Prenatal care
- Childbirth education
- Nutrition
- Exercise
- Safety
- Screening (e.g., blood pressure, vision, cholesterol)

COPING WITH IMPAIRED FUNCTION
- Long-term care
- Rehabilitation
- Environmental modifications
- Physical therapy
- Occupational therapy
- Speech therapy
- Prevention of complications
- Implications of noncompliance with therapy

RESTORATION OF HEALTH RELATED TO DISEASE PROCESS
- Body system affected
- Cause of disease
- Origin of symptoms
- Diagnostic tests
- Prognosis
- Limitation of function
- Treatment plan
- Dietary modifications
- Medication
- Surgical intervention (if appropriate)
- Client participation in care
- Adaptations in ADLs (bathing, toileting, eating, etc.)
- Activity modifications
- Self-help devices
- Home care

---

language barriers, and the financial implications of care choices (JCAHO, 2000). The discharge needs are determined from the analysis of the total assessment, and nursing diagnoses are then identified.

In the planning phase the nurse and client jointly identify goals and expected outcomes. Achievement of these goals involves support and coordination of activities and resources using a collaborative and interdisciplinary approach. The nurse identifies family and community resources available and facilitates the referral process.

Because of shortened length of stays and complexity of client needs, many agencies have an interdisciplinary discharge planning team that includes nurses, physicians, social workers, and respiratory, physical, and occupational therapists to assist in preparing the client for discharge. Clear, concise, accurate documentation of the client's needs and abilities on the discharge plan improves the continuity of care. The nurse also documents the client's and family's knowledge of and ability to follow through with discharge instructions.

When clients become actively engaged in the learning process, teaching/learning effectiveness is enhanced. The best way for the nurse to evaluate a client's understanding of self-care behaviors is to observe the client in relation to the treatment regimen and to have the client or family demonstrate the specific knowledge and skills they need to meet ongoing health care needs. Guidelines for client education include safe and effective use of medication and medical equipment, diet and nutrition, rehabilitation, educational resources in the community, and follow-up care (JCAHO, 2000). Finally, the discharge plan is confirmed with the client and family after discharge. Telephone follow-up several days after discharge provides the opportunity to answer questions or facilitate continued follow-up with a referral of the client to a home health agency of the client's choice.

NURSING DIAGNOSES

Health-Seeking Behaviors is appropriate when the client is in stable health and is actively seeking to alter personal habits to achieve better health.

Ineffective Health Maintenance is appropriate when a client or family is unable to identify, manage, or seek help to maintain health. **Noncompliance** may be used when lack of support, health beliefs, cultural influences, spiritual values, financial constraints, and the client-provider relationship result in difficulty with self-care therapies. **Ineffective Therapeutic Regimen Management** may apply when clients have a complex treatment regimen, little or no previous experience with the plan of care, or no perceived susceptibility to complications, resulting in failure to integrate treatments into their daily lives. For these nursing diagnoses, referral to a home health agency can offer continued support to help the client identify and remove or minimize barriers that interfere with recovery.

Deficient Knowledge is appropriate when the client is exposed to a new procedure, lacks recall, or verbalizes misinterpretation of information. **Anxiety** results from the client's concern about how illness may change lifestyle or about adapting to a new behavior and performing it correctly in the home environment.

Disturbed Sensory Perception influences the teaching/learning process and may apply when sensory acuity is decreased as a result of the aging process and chronic illnesses such as diabetes mellitus and cataracts and adaptations to the home environment may be needed. **Impaired Physical Mobility** from perceptual or cognitive impairment, disabilities, or age-related changes may limit the client's ability to take medications or perform self-care skills. **Risk for Injury** and **Risk for Falls** can apply in the presence of potentially unsafe environmental conditions (e.g., physical setup of the home) and when sensory, cognitive, or motor disabilities are present.

Risk for Impaired Home Maintenance may be associated with client's disease or disability, motor skills, inadequate support systems, decreased knowledge of available resources and ways to initiate contact, communication skills, and impaired cognitive or emotional functioning. Finally, **Caregiver Role Strain** may be appropriate whenever a client requires extensive or continuous complex care resulting in disruption of the family routines and roles.

Skill 40.1

Client Teaching

Health teaching is an important role of the professional nurse. One of the most important goals in health care today is to engage clients and families in maintaining health and managing health problems. The purposes of health teaching include conveying knowledge and skills, dispelling myths, and assisting clients in dealing with the fears that can interfere with the learning process. Nurses provide information to clients that will promote self-care and independence and help prevent complications (Edelman and Mandle, 2002). For example, a client whose ability to move one side of the body is impaired after a stroke must learn new ways of bathing, walking, and eating. The client with a draining surgical wound needs to learn to how to complete dressing changes. A newly diagnosed diabetic must learn about diet, exercise, monitoring blood glucose levels, and insulin administration. During each interaction with every client, the nurse also has an opportunity to provide information and promote attitudes needed for healthy living. For example, the nurse can encourage maintaining a healthy weight, stress reduction, and developing a regular exercise program. Much health teaching is informal and integrated into daily routines. Teaching takes place in a variety of settings, including hospitals, clinics, classrooms, and the community.

Teaching uses basic principles while following the same steps as the nursing process (i.e., assessment, analysis, planning, implementation, and evaluation). To be effective, teaching priorities are established based on the client's needs. The content and teaching methods are individualized for the client, and the client's cultural beliefs about health information are taken into account. Health teaching includes active involvement of the client and family within the client's support network.

ASSESSMENT

1. Assess clients' learning needs and readiness to learn by asking what they know about their disease and treatment, how they are coping with symptoms, how they prefer to learn new information, and what is of concern to them at this time. *Rationale: Clients are more ready to learn when (1) they believe that they are able to take action that will make a difference, (2) the benefits of learning outweigh the barriers, (3) anxiety is at a manageable level, and (4) they are physically and mentally capable of taking in new information.*

2. Assess attention span, short-term memory, pain, fatigue, high anxiety level, sensory deficits, language limitations, and distractions. *Rationale: These factors and others may interfere with learning (Redman, 2001).*

3. Assess client's attitudes toward learning and willingness to follow health care provider recommendations. Determine the client's perceived benefit of action, perceived barrier to action, interpersonal influences such as family and peers, and commitment to a plan of action. *Rationale: These variables are major sources of motivation for changing behavior, and nursing interventions should be targeted toward these variables (Pender, 1996).*

4. Review risk factors from nursing history in relation to lifestyle patterns: smoking, stress, seat belt use, drug use, alcohol use, exercise routines, and personal hygiene. *Rationale: Unhealthy lifestyle habits or choices frequently increase the risk for developing illnesses or disabilities.*

5. Review client's employment history to determine risks within the work setting. *Rationale: Occupational inhalants such as asbestos, plastics, dusts, and gases have potential for causing chronic lung diseases or cancer.*

6. Assess client's and family's understanding of therapies, restrictions resulting from health alterations, and possible complications. *Rationale: Determines level and extent of health education needed by client.*

7. Determine client's actual or potential limitations resulting from sensory, motor, cognitive, or physical changes. *Rationale: This identifies the need for special teaching methods and family assistance.*

8. Consult other health care team members about ongoing needs (e.g., dietitian, social worker, home care nurse). Facilitate appropriate referrals. *Rationale: Members of all health care disciplines collaborate to determine client's needs and functional abilities.*

PLANNING

Expected outcomes focus on increasing the client's knowledge level, motivation to learn, and identification of risk factors and on a change in client behavior related to health issues.

Expected Outcomes

1. The client identifies unhealthy choices and implements a plan to change these behaviors.
2. The client identifies strategies for illness prevention or early detection of disease.

Delegation Considerations

The skill of client teaching requires the critical thinking and knowledge application unique to a nurse. Delegation is inappropriate.

IMPLEMENTATION FOR CLIENT TEACHING

Steps	Rationale
1. See Standard Protocol (inside front cover).	
2. Use every contact with the client as an opportunity to teach (use time when giving a bath, passing medications, ambulating, or feeding client). Identify who is responsible for follow-up care in the home, and incorporate them in the teaching/learning process (see illustration).	Gives client opportunity to practice new skills, ask questions, and obtain necessary feedback to facilitate learning. Incorporating teaching during care activities maximizes use of available time.

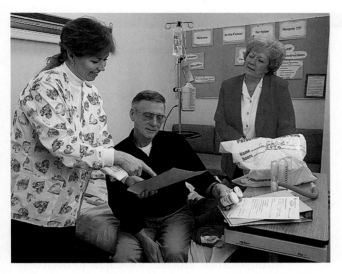

Step 2 Select appropriate setting for client teaching.

Steps	Rationale
3. Together with the client and family, identify what the learner needs to accomplish and how achievement will be measured.	Clients learn best when they set their own goals and priorities (Redman, 2001). Objectives are client oriented and reflect what the learner will be able to do after completion of the instruction (Redman, 2001).
4. Select media, methods of teaching, and aids (e.g., hands-on equipment, pamphlets, audiovisual materials) appropriate to client's needs.	One of the most effective teaching methods is to verbally deliver information, leave written information, and ask the client for follow-up questions after the client hears and reads the information. Videos work well with clients who cannot read. Effective learning often requires repetition (Murphy and Davis, 1997).
5. Establish an environment that encourages clients and families to ask questions and participate in decision making and care.	
6. When presenting information, vary the tone of voice, use simple, clear language, and if possible reinforce with pictures or demonstrations. Repeat and highlight key points.	
7. Set up equipment, and demonstrate self-care to the client using supplies and equipment that client will use at home.	Clients learn most easily in the "real" setting. Most clients learn best by doing.
8. Employ teaching techniques of repetition, rephrasing, and summarizing.	Repetition enhances learning.
9. Have client demonstrate skill. Provide client with positive feedback. Have client/family member become as independent as possible with skill while direct support and assistance are available.	Application of newly learned material in practical situations increases memory retention (Redman, 2001).
10. Elicit feedback from the client/family frequently.	Feedback can determine that the information is understood and that it is appropriate, useful, and usable in practical terms (JCAHO, 2000).
11. Teach health promotional activities as appropriate, including avoidance of risks (smoking, alcohol), safety, screening (e.g., blood pressure, vision, cholesterol, cancer), nutrition, and exercise.	Some clients may not have major learning needs related to current illness but could benefit from learning how to reduce risks of certain diseases (e.g., cardiopulmonary disease, cancer, obesity). There is supportive evidence that with certain disorders, exercise and nutrition enable wellness (Zernike and Henderson, 1998).

Steps	Rationale

12. As appropriate, teach client how to recognize stress and measures to deal effectively with psychophysiological effects (see Skill 10.2).

Prolonged stress response can increase client's risk of stress-related illnesses.

13. Review material repeatedly as care is provided, asking questions to encourage the client to think through implications for self-care.

Teaching small amounts of information over time is most effective, and repetition leads to compliance (Katz, 1997).

14. Give clients praise for return demonstrations that are done correctly and for behavior changes resulting from information given.

Learners tend to be motivated by clear feedback about what they did right.

15. See Completion Protocol (inside front cover).

• • • • • • • • • • •

EVALUATION

1. Observe ability to demonstrate skills needed for self-care and compliance with therapeutic regimen.

2. Ask client to describe strategies for illness prevention or early detection of disease.

Unexpected Outcomes and Related Interventions

1. Client demonstrates self-care skill(s) incorrectly or needs verbal prompting throughout.
   a. Provide opportunities for the client/family to repeat the skill several times with assistance until they are able to do it independently.
   b. Encourage the client and family to ask questions and identify areas difficult for them.
   c. Identify the need for adaptations if possible. When adaptations are not recommended, the client and family need to understand the consequences of failing to follow the treatment plan (Redman, 2001).
   d. Provide additional educational materials such as pamphlets and videotapes. Consider adaptations needed. For example, if a client is visually impaired, audiotape or large-print handouts may be more appropriate.
   e. Provide repetition, adequate time, and praise as appropriate throughout learning sessions.

2. Client is able to correctly verbalize or demonstrates desired skills or behaviors, but evidence suggests there may be difficulty with compliance.

   a. Identify factors that interfere with desired behavior, such as expense of equipment or time/place inconvenience. Problem solve how to overcome this barrier.
   b. A written chart may be helpful if client is forgetful, rather than intentionally neglecting desired behaviors.
   c. Encourage client and/or family support system to develop additional strategies to enhance compliance.
   d. Consider need for referral for home health follow-up visits.

Recording and Reporting

• Record:
   What is being taught
   Methods used
   Client response to teaching/learning
• Report inability to verbalize or demonstrate desired behaviors or anticipated or actual non-compliance.

Sample Documentation

0830 Client reviewed the procedure for measuring blood glucose level, including viewing a videotape and reading a pamphlet with step-by-step instructions. Procedure demonstrated to client and husband using the equipment that will be used following discharge. Plans to complete the procedure herself with assistance at 1100 today.

SPECIAL CONSIDERATIONS

Pediatric Considerations
• Education provided to children should be based on their developmental level. Use age-appropriate language and teaching methods. Infants need attention to promoting oral-motor development and trust; toddlers need encouraged mobility, exploration, and language development; preschoolers need to learn self-care; school-age children need opportunity for socialization; and adolescents need increased independence and opportunity for privacy (Wong and others, 1999).
• Children younger than 5 years need to know how procedures will affect them. For example, during a chest x-ray examination they have to stand still, hold their breath for a few seconds, and will not feel anything (Redman, 2001).

SPECIAL CONSIDERATIONS—*Cont'd*

- Include family/caregiver when doing teaching whenever possible.
- When school-age children or adolescent clients are hospitalized for long periods of time, hospitals must comply with state and local laws that may specify the requirements for meeting the child's schooling needs. Although not responsible for providing schoolteachers directly, hospitals are required to provide access to schooling (JCAHO, 2000).

Geriatric Considerations
- Older adults may have reduced visual and hearing acuity and difficulty understanding language because high-frequency tones are less perceptible. Therefore speak in a slow, low-pitched voice when teaching the older adult. Also, provide written teaching materials in at least 14-point type. This is printed in 14-point type.
- In the absence of mental changes such as dementia or delirium, the capacity for learning new information remains as we age (Lueckenotte, 2000). Allow adequate time and number of teaching sessions to support successful learning.

Procedural Guideline 40-1

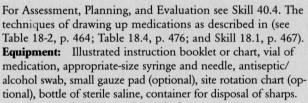

Teaching Clients Self-Injections

For Assessment, Planning, and Evaluation see Skill 40.4. The techniques of drawing up medications as described in (see Table 18-2, p. 464; Table 18.4, p. 476; and Skill 18.1, p. 467).
Equipment: Illustrated instruction booklet or chart, vial of medication, appropriate-size syringe and needle, antiseptic/alcohol swab, small gauze pad (optional), site rotation chart (optional), bottle of sterile saline, container for disposal of sharps.
1. See Standard Protocol (inside front cover).
2. Have client hold and manipulate a syringe and medication vial. If client cannot manipulate syringe, an alternative plan must be developed (e.g., have significant other prepare medication).
3. Explain which parts of the syringe must remain sterile (free of germs) and which can be touched.
4. Discuss medication dosage, and show client how much medication should be drawn into syringe. Show client where to find the types of the medication on the vials. Concentration of insulin in units and number of units marked on syringe must match; for example, 100-unit syringe is used only with U-100 insulin.
5. Have client examine medication for color change or clumping. If appropriate, mix solution by gently rotating bottle or rolling it. If medication has been refrigerated, allow it to warm to room temperature to minimize discomfort and regulate absorption.
6. Often the easiest site to learn self-injections is the anterior thigh (see illustration *A*). Many clients learn to self-administer subcutaneous injections into the abdomen (see illustration *B*), which has approximately 100 sites. The posterior upper arm can also be used; however, it is less easily accessible. For the arm the client presses back of arm against wall or back of chair and "rolls" arm down to push up the skin. Different anatomical locations for injections provide different absorption rates. It is often recommended that one area is consistently used for a month at a time to promote regulation of effectiveness.

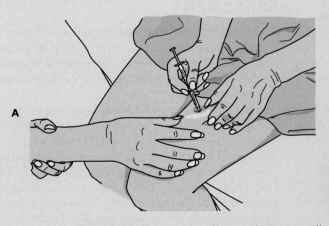

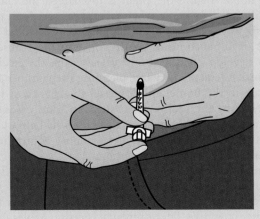

Step 6   **A,** Encourage client to insert needle quickly. **B,** Insert needle to the hub.

Continued

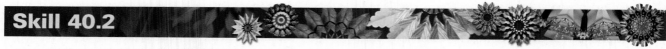

Teaching Clients Self-Injections—cont'd

7. Encourage client to insert needle quickly into prepared site all the way to the hub. Some clients may need you to gently push on their hand at first.

COMMUNICATION TIP *Tell the client to inject on the count of 3, then count slowly and rhythmically, and say "Go."*

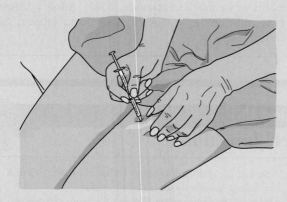

Step 7 Syringe is inserted all the way to the hub.

8. Once needle is inserted, instruct client to slowly let go of skin and transfer free hand to barrel of syringe.

9. Have client push plunger all the way in at a slow and steady rate to administer the medication.

10. Once medication has been administered, have client quickly remove needle at same angle at which it was inserted and exert gentle pressure on the site with a small gauze pad.

11. Teach client to dispose of uncapped needle or needle enclosed in safety shield in a sharps container or, at home, a hard plastic bottle. The legal regulations vary depending on local ordinances. Clients need to be aware of the laws that apply where they live. Some hospitals provide containers and offer to dispose of full containers regularly.

12. Discuss rotation of sites, and have client indicate on a chart where injection was given.

13. Encourage client to practice preparing prescribed dose using a bottle of sterile saline.

14. Discuss where medication and syringes will be secured at home so that children will not have access to them.

15. See Completion Protocol (inside front cover).

Skill 40.2

Risk Assessment and Accident Prevention

This skill focuses on preparing the client to go home to a safe environment. Discharge from an agency can be stressful if a client and family are not ready to resume normal activities or are unable to adapt therapeutic regimens to living at home. Before the client is discharged the client and family need to know what to expect regarding any continuing physical challenges. Inability to understand restrictions or implications of health concerns may cause a client to develop complications after leaving the health care setting. Adequate discharge planning prepares for adequate care in the home and decreases the chance of the client reentering the health care system. In some cases referral to a physical or occupational therapist is helpful. A home visit before discharge can help identify appropriate modifications for accident prevention.

Unintentional injuries can occur at all ages of the life span. Many of these injuries result from hazards that are easily overlooked and easily fixed. Knowledge of specific motor and cognitive developmental needs enables the nurse to assess the potential for injury for each client. After the area of risk is identified, the nurse designs interventions to eliminate or reduce the threat to the client's safety.

ASSESSMENT

1. Assess client's physical and mental status before discharge, and determine the type of adaptations necessary in the home. *Rationale: The nature of physical and cognitive limitations determines the type of adjustments to be made in the home.*

2. Assess client's attitudes toward returning home and following health care provider recommendations. Determine the client's perceived benefit of action, perceived barrier to action, interpersonal influences such as family and peers, and commitment to a plan of action. *Rationale: These variables are major sources of motivation for changing behavior, and nursing interventions are targeted toward these variables (Pender, 1996).*

3. Determine client's actual or potential limitations resulting from sensory, motor, cognitive, or physical changes. *Rationale: These factors increase client's risk of injury.*
4. Consult other health care team members about needs after discharge (e.g., physical therapist, occupational therapist, respiratory therapist, dietitian, social worker, home care nurse). Make appropriate referrals. *Rationale: Members of all health care disciplines collaborate to determine client's needs and functional abilities.*

PLANNING

Expected outcomes focus on identification of risk factors, provision of a safe environment, and ability to safely perform self-care in the home environment.

Expected Outcomes

1. Client/family identifies safety risks in the home.
2. Client/family identifies community resources available and how to initiate contact.

Equipment

- Assessment form(s)
- Home safety checklist

Delegation Considerations

An RN, a physical therapist, or an occupational therapist is best qualified to determine what alterations or revisions are needed based on the client's physical and/or cognitive limitations and to conduct a thorough home safety assessment. Delegation to assistive personnel (AP) is not appropriate. The nurse may elicit practical suggestions that have a commonsense approach from AP such as home health aides, who spend significantly more time with clients.

IMPLEMENTATION FOR RISK ASSESSMENT AND ACCIDENT PREVENTION

Steps	Rationale
1. See Standard Protocol (inside front cover).	
2. Before discharge involve the client and family as active participants in a home safety assessment using a checklist (Table 40-1). NOTE: The assessment may need to be validated later with the client in the home.	
3. With the client and family, identify ways to make home environment safe.	Client's level of independence and ability to retain function can be maintained within safe environment.
4. Reduce the number of different pain medications used.	Prevents oversedation.
5. Schedule diuretics early in the day.	Minimizes interruption in sleep and trips to the bathroom at night because of urinary elimination.
6. Explore benefits and challenges of all recommendations.	
7. Consider changing physical environment to reduce predisposition to falls.	
8. Provide for safe disposal of in-home medical supplies:	Prevents injury to self or others and prevents pollution.
a. Instruct client to place needles, syringes, lancets, or other sharp objects in a hard plastic or metal container such as a soda bottle or laundry detergent container with screw-on or tightly secured lid.	
b. Soiled bandages, disposable sheets, and medical gloves are placed in securely fastened plastic bag before being placed in garbage can.	

Table 40-1

Home Safety Checklist

Criteria	Yes	No
Front and Back Entrances/Walkways		
1. Walkways and steps are smooth and well lighted. Sturdy handrail is on both sides of stairs to entrance.	☐	☐
2. Nonskid strips/safety treads or bright paint is used on outdoor steps. Steps are of uniform depth and risers.	☐	☐
3. A shelf or bench is located by front/back doors to place grocery bags or packages if needed.	☐	☐
Kitchen		
1. Client wears clothes with short or close-fitting sleeves when cooking.	☐	☐
2. Stove control dials are easy to see and use, and stove top and oven are clean and grease free.	☐	☐
3. Items in kitchen cabinets and shelves are easily to reach without climbing.	☐	☐
4. There is adequate lighting over sink, stove, and work areas.	☐	☐
Floors		
1. All carpeting and mats are secure. Skid backing is present under area rugs, or throw rugs are removed.	☐	☐
2. Walkways are kept free of clutter.	☐	☐
Bathrooms		
1. Door lock can be unlocked from both sides.	☐	☐
2. Tub or shower is equipped with nonskid mats, abrasive strips.	☐	☐
3. Tub/shower has at least one grab bar kept free of towels or other items.	☐	☐
4. Shower has a stable stool or chair and handheld sprayer.	☐	☐
5. Cold and hot water faucets are clearly marked, and temperature on water heater is 120° F or less.	☐	☐
6. A night-light is available.	☐	☐
Bedroom		
1. Client can turn on light without having to get out of bed in the dark.	☐	☐
2. Furniture is arranged to provide clear path from bed to bathroom.	☐	☐
3. Phone with emergency numbers is within easy reach of bed.	☐	☐
4. Alarm systems are available. There are listening devices for invalid clients.	☐	☐
Living Room/Family Room		
1. Light can be turned on without having to walk into dark room.	☐	☐
2. Lamp, extension, or phone cords are kept out of traffic ways.	☐	☐
3. Furniture is arranged so that it can be walked around easily.	☐	☐
Fire Safety		
1. Sufficient numbers of functional smoke detectors are in appropriate locations.	☐	☐
2. Emergency exit plans are in place in case of fire.	☐	☐
3. Family has determined a meeting place outside the house.	☐	☐
4. Portable space heaters are used and kept 3 ft away from flammable items.	☐	☐
5. Furnace area is free of things that can catch on fire.	☐	☐
6. Furnace and chimney are checked annually by a qualified professional.	☐	☐
7. Emergency numbers for police, fire, and poison control are posted near phone.	☐	☐
8. Fire extinguisher is available and easy to handle and manipulate.	☐	☐
Electrical Safety		
1. Electrical cords are in good condition, not frayed, spliced, or cracked.	☐	☐
2. Electrical cords are kept away from water.	☐	☐
3. Extension cord/outlet extenders have built-in circuit breaker or fuse.	☐	☐
4. Wall outlets and switches have cover plates.	☐	☐
5. Light bulbs are of correct wattage for each fixture.	☐	☐
6. Fuse box is easily accessible and clearly labeled.	☐	☐
7. Lamp switches are easy to turn to avoid burns from hot light bulbs.	☐	☐
Carbon Monoxide Prevention		
1. Furnace flues are checked regularly for patency.	☐	☐
2. Carbon monoxide detector is in home.	☐	☐

9. Offer client and family appropriate information about community health care resources, including homemakers, transportation, Meals on Wheels, retirement communities, home care, adult day care, respite care, rehabilitation, and long-term care.

10. See Completion Protocol (inside front cover).

· · · · · · · · · ·

EVALUATION

1. Client implements a successful plan that eliminates safety risks and leads to safe health behavior choices.

2. Ask client to identify safety risks.

3. Ask client and family to identify resources available for a particular problem and how to initiate contact with that resource.

Unexpected Outcomes and Related Interventions

1. Client is unable to identify safety risks.
   a. Reevaluate home environment with client and family members.
   b. Teach client the rationale for preventing and removing potential hazards from home environment.

Recording and Reporting

· Retain copy of the home safety assessment in the client's home health record.

The emphasis is to keep the client in the home for as long as it is safe and desirable to do so. During the decision-making period regarding the need for care outside the home, the role of the nurse is to support the older adult and the family and to provide information about options available (Potter and Perry, 2001).

· Record assessment of the client's cognitive and mental status, recommended interventions, and client's and caregiver's response in progress notes.

· Record any instruction provided, client's response, and changes made to the environment in progress notes.

Sample Documentation

0900 Safety checklist completed with client and family members before discharge. Plans made for family to remove throw rugs and to install handrails in bathroom. Heartland Home Health Care Agency referral made with physician's order and discussed with client and family members.

 ## SPECIAL CONSIDERATIONS

Pediatric Considerations

· Measures to ensure the safety of children in the home are based on the child's developmental level. Families are instructed to use safety devices (e.g., safety gates on staircases and cabinet locks) as applicable.

· All medications, cleaning products, and other potentially poisonous materials must be placed where children cannot reach them and should be locked up when possible.

· To identify dangers present in the home to young children, suggest that families get down on the floor to survey the environment from the child's view (Wong and others, 1999).

· Children are imitators and copy what they see and hear. Practicing safety teaches safety, which applies to parents and their children and to nurses and their clients. Saying one thing and doing another confuses children (Wong and others, 1999).

· If there are guns in the house, they should be stored unloaded and kept under lock and key.

· Families should also be taught car safety based on the child's age, developmental level, and size. Children should be restrained in the appropriate restraint system, and if the car has airbags, children under 12 years of age should ride in the back seat.

Geriatric Considerations

· Physiological changes and mental status alterations that accompany aging, such as a slower reaction time, muscular weakness, reduced pain and temperature perception, reduced depth perception and color discrimination, reduced visual acuity, confusion, memory loss, and poor orientation, place older adults at risk for injury in the home environment.

Continued

SPECIAL CONSIDERATIONS—*Cont'd*

- Older adults learn to negotiate their environments relatively well and are usually more aware of potential dangers.
- Frail older adults should not ride in the passenger side of the car if the car has airbags. They should be taught to sit in the back seat or sit at least 10 inches away from the airbag.

Home Care and Long-Term Care Considerations
- Any changes in the client's home environment should be made to retain as much of the client's independence as possible.

- Before making any revisions to a client's home, know the client's financial resources and wherever possible let the client be the final decision maker in the types of alterations to be made.
- Caregivers must learn the importance of preserving client autonomy, and any modifications to the home environment should consider the client's physical strengths and remaining functional abilities, not just the client's disabilities.

Skill 40.3

Adapting the Home Setting for Clients With Cognitive Deficits

An important aspect of safety is a person's ability to perform routine activities of daily living (ADLs) and to make the correct decisions for home management activities. This includes the use of the telephone, cleaning, shopping, money management, meal preparation, and taking medications. When there are cognitive limitations, a person's autonomy is clearly threatened. Family members may misunderstand mental changes and need assistance to determine whether a client is competent to remain at home safely.

It is a myth that all older adults experience cognitive dysfunction. However, it is the older adult who is most likely to develop cognitive dysfunction. Accurate assessment includes mental health, physical health, social and economic status, functional status, and the environment (Ebersole and Hess, 1998). A person may have certain mental processes intact (e.g., orientation to name, time, and place), while at the same time other processes are compromised (e.g., short-term memory of life events).

To further complicate the issue of differentiating mental status and cognitive changes, it is important to recognize that many older adults suffer from depression, which also can result in cognitive impairment (Lueckenotte, 2000). Depression can occur alone or in combination with cognitive disorders such as dementia. Depression can also occur secondary to isolation when the older adult is homebound and has few social visitors.

This skill attempts to provide guidelines for helping clients with varying degrees of cognitive impairment and for making adaptations to preserve their ability to function safely within the home.

ASSESSMENT

1. Ask client to describe own level of health and how it affects ability to provide self-care skills, including bathing, dressing, eating, and toileting. Ask family members to confirm description. *Rationale: Question requires client to describe abilities and health challenges. This allows assessment of the client's attention, concentration, and perceptions of health limitations.*

2. Listen carefully to the client. Provide a quiet, well-lit space, and avoid interruptions or distractions. Accommodate as necessary for sensory disabilities, and avoid a lengthy assessment that results in fatigue. *Rationale: Improves likelihood of gathering accurate relevant data.*

PLANNING

Expected outcomes focus on adaptation of the home environment and the client's ability to perform ADLs.

Expected Outcomes

1. Client is able to complete as many home management responsibilities as possible within existing limitations.
2. Family caregiver(s) use techniques that help client perform home management activities as needed.

Equipment

- Mini-Mental State Examination (see Chapter 13)
- Calendar
- Paper for making lists
- Bulletin board or poster board (optional)

Delegation Considerations

This skill requires the critical thinking and knowledge application unique to a nurse and cannot be delegated.

IMPLEMENTATION FOR ADAPTING THE HOME SETTING FOR CLIENTS WITH COGNITIVE DEFICITS

Steps	Rationale
1. See Standard Protocol (inside front cover).	
2. If client has difficulty remembering when to perform self-care routines, create a list or use a calendar. A wristwatch with an alarm may be used to signal time of scheduled activity.	Memory function in older adults tends to be preserved for relevant, well-known material (Lueckenotte, 2000). Lists will help client complete required tasks.
3. Schedule medications likely to cause confusion at bedtime.	Maintains mental status during the day at the maximum level possible.
4. Space antihypertensives and antiarrhythmics at different times to minimize side effects.	These drugs can cause hypotension and dizziness, increasing the risk of falls.
5. When client has difficulty completing tasks with multiple steps, reduce steps it takes to complete the task or simplify the task.	Prevents frustration and/or forgetting one or more steps that lead to task being unfinished.
6. Help client and family develop a schedule for routine daily activities such as eating, bathing, and exercise. Post a large calendar for appointments or special events.	Consistency creates a sense of security and keeps client more easily oriented to daily activities.
7. Have caregiver(s) set up activities so that client can complete them (e.g., lay out clothes to wear for the day, place food for simple meals for the day out on the counter).	Helps client complete tasks even though unable to plan and perform all the steps.
8. Encourage simple and direct communication using a calm and relaxed approach. Use eye contact and touch. Speak in simple words and short sentences. Use nonverbal gestures that complement verbal messages.	Facilitates effective communication and minimizes anxiety.
9. Keep clocks, calendars, and personal items (pictures, scrapbooks, personal gifts from loved ones) throughout rooms where easily seen.	Reinforces reality orientation.
10. Routinely remind client of who caregiver is and what the next step is to be.	Improves productivity and responses (Lueckenotte, 2000).
11. Facilitate regular naps or rest periods.	Fatigue adds to mental status changes.
12. Encourage and support frequent visits by family and friends. Encourage use of humor and reminiscing of favorite stories.	Prevents boredom and reduces restlessness.
13. See Completion Protocol (inside front cover).	

• • • • • • • • • •

EVALUATION

1. To determine ability to recall events ask client to review the home management activities completed the morning of that day and the previous day.
2. Ask caregiver to review schedules of daily routines and review approaches used.

Unexpected Outcomes and Related Interventions

1. Client is unable to complete daily activities as planned.
   a. Review what occurred, and identify barriers.
   b. Identify strategies for maintaining adequate support.
2. Caregiver is unable to implement techniques that improve orientation and ability to complete activities.
   a. Support for caregiver may be necessary before caregiver can learn how to help the client.
   b. Consider that the caregiver may not be able to provide necessary support. Consider other living arrangements or support services.

Recording and Reporting

- Record cognitive abilities and mental status, recommended interventions, and client's and caregiver's response.
- Report significant decline in cognitive or mental status to physician.

Sample Documentation

2100 Oriented to person and place, but not to time. Reported that she is waiting for breakfast. Reoriented by having client look outside to see it is dark and telling her it will soon be bedtime. Acknowledged awareness without difficulty.

◉ SPECIAL CONSIDERATIONS ◉

Pediatric Considerations

Children with cognitive impairment are often not aware of inherent dangers during play and daily activities. Adult supervision is critical.

Geriatric Considerations

- Many clients experience progressive loss of function, requiring continuous adaptations and adjustments.
- Stress created for caregiver by older adult demonstrating problematic behaviors may be reduced by increased understanding of the behaviors and practice with management techniques.

Skill 40.4

Helping Clients With Self-Medication and Medical Device Safety

Clients who are taking medications or doing routine procedures frequently have difficulty managing to follow through consistently at home. Difficulty with prescribed medications often exists for several reasons: clients stop taking medications once symptoms subside, regimens involving multiple drugs are confusing, the consequences of not taking medications are not understood, prescriptions are costly, and clients may fear addiction. Procedural Guideline 40-1 describes teaching clients self-injections. The assessment, planning, and evaluation are similar regardless of the techniques and equipment used.

Medical device safety includes the administration of medications and the use of medical devices such as syringes, blood glucose monitoring equipment, dressings, and in some cases even intravenous devices. This includes administration, storage, and waste disposal. Safety involves correct techniques and prevention of infection.

Clients who have special needs include those with acute sensory or neurological impairment, chronic illnesses such as diabetes or arthritis, and physical limitations that make manipulation of medical devices and handling medications difficult. In some cases a family member or other caregiver must learn to provide this care (Figure 40-1).

ASSESSMENT

1. Assess client's and family caregiver's visual, cognitive, musculoskeletal, and neurological function, level of consciousness or sedation, vision, hearing, literacy, swallowing ability, and willingness to cooperate (see Chapter 13). *Rationale: Helps to identify appropriate assistive devices needed.*
2. Assess client's medication regimen and length of time client has been receiving each drug.

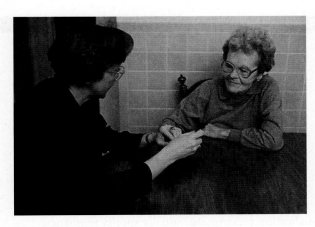

Figure 40-1 A family member or other caregiver may need to learn about prescribed medications.

Rationale: Determines complexity of medication regimen and degree of familiarity of client with each drug.

3. Identify where medications are stored in the home and the type of storage containers used.
4. Assess resources (transportation and financial) for obtaining medications when needed. *Rationale: Lack of financial resources or transportation are two major factors that interfere with self-medication at home.*

PLANNING

Expected outcomes focus on the client's ability to manage medications and medical devices safely.

Expected Outcomes

1. Client will state purpose of each medication, common side effects, and when to notify physician about drug problems.

2. Client is able to reach each label and explain when each drug is to be taken.
3. Client/caregiver will be able to prepare and administer prescribed nonparenteral medications and/or injections independently.
4. Client/caregiver will store items properly and dispose of items safely.

Equipment

- Written instructions or charts
- Medication
- Liquid to take with medication
- Container for daily or weekly preparation
- Measuring devices (e.g., medicine cup, teaspoon, syringe)
- Colored marking pens
- Labels
- Puncture-resistant sharps container or 2-L soda bottle with cap
- Duct or adhesive tape

Delegation Considerations

Assessment of client risks in using medical devices and administering medication requires the critical thinking and knowledge application unique to a nurse and cannot be delegated. Assistive personnel (AP), such as home health aides, may observe how clients use these adaptations and need to know to report deviations that may be unsafe.

IMPLEMENTATION FOR HELPING CLIENTS WITH SELF-MEDICATION AND MEDICAL DEVICE SAFETY

Steps	Rationale

1. See Standard Protocol (inside front cover).
2. For prescribed medications and over-the-counter (OTC) medications scheduled and prn review with clients:
   a. Purpose of medications and their expected effects
   b. How medications work
   c. Dosage schedules and rationale
   d. Common side effects, what to do to relieve side effects
   e. What to do if dose is missed
   f. When to call the physician

Steps	Rationale

3. Plan for use of appropriate devices to monitor medications taken as scheduled:

a. Calendars may be made for each week with plastic bags of medications to take at specific times.

b. Egg cartons may be divided into color-coded sections with medications for the day, using color coding for drug types (e.g., blue for sedative, red for pain pill).

c. Use pillboxes that are set up daily or weekly to separate pills into slots for each day of the week and appropriate time of day (see illustration).

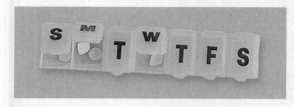

Step 3c Pill organizer for each day of the week.

4. Medicine prescribed must only be used as prescribed and by the person for whom it was prescribed.

Medication prescriptions usually specify frequency, dosage, and special instructions, (e.g., before meals, at bedtime). Other members of the household with similar symptoms may be tempted to take medications prescribed for another, which is an unsafe practice.

5. Monitor expiration dates.

It is unsafe to take medication more than a year past the expiration date on the container.

6. Keep medications in the container they came in, and make sure the label is clearly legible. Have pharmacy provide large print labels if appropriate. If client is legally blind, Braille labels may be used.

Some clients like to put several different kinds of medications in the same container for convenience. This is an unsafe practice, because they can mix up dosage or schedule of administration.

7. Finish prescribed medications, and if ordered, get refills before the container is empty.

Some medications need to be taken until they are gone. Clients may be tempted to keep some medication when the symptoms are gone, planning to use them later. This is an unsafe practice. It is essential to order refills so that there is no interruption in the medication routine.

8. Identify appropriate adaptations to facilitate ease and accuracy in administration of nonparenteral medications:

a. Have medications dispensed by the pharmacist in a container client can open easily if manual dexterity is limited.

Most pharmacies dispense medications in childproof containers, which may be difficult to open if client has limited mobility of fingers/hands.

NURSE ALERT *If there are small children in the home or children who frequently visit, help establish a safe place for medications to reduce risk of accidental ingestion.*

---

b. When many medications are prescribed, a color-coding system may be useful. For example, tops of containers may be marked with the same color when they are taken at the same time.

9. For teaching self-injection techniques see Procedural Guideline 40-1, p. 945.

10. See Completion Protocol (inside front cover).

• • • • • • • • • •

EVALUATION

1. Ask client to state purpose of each medication, common side effects, and when to notify physician about drug problems.

2. Observe client reading each label, and ask to explain when each drug is to be taken.

3. Observe client/caregiver preparing and administering medications independently.

4. Ask to see where client/caregiver stores items, and observe disposal of medical supplies, including sharps and contaminated supplies.

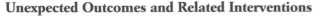

Unexpected Outcomes and Related Interventions

1. Client makes errors in preparing medications or is unable to recall and explain related drug information.
   a. Provide written instructions at client's/caregiver's level of understanding. Often pictures are very helpful. Some commercially prepared booklets may contain instructions that are too complex or are difficult to understand.
   b. Repeat and reinforce elements of the information. Give positive feedback for accurate recall of information.
   c. Provide repeated supervised practice until a system is working in which client can self-administer medications safely.
2. Self-medication is not possible due to client's self-care deficits.
   a. Develop alternate plan, which may rely on family, friends, or home health agency.
   b. Consider the need for alternative living arrangements.
3. Excess or insufficient pills are found in pill container during pill count.
   a. Incorrect dosage is being taken.
   b. Reevaluate use of dosage reminders.
   c. Establish additional monitoring system until client is able to self-medicate accurately.
4. Medications and medical devices/supplies are not stored in a secure or appropriate location.
   a. Client may choose to store items conveniently rather than safely.
   b. Identify barriers, and identify appropriate alternatives.
   c. Implement plans to maintain client safety.

Recording and Reporting

- Document instruction given, including details of medications included. Often a discharge instruction sheet lists details about prescribed medications. Pharmacy may also provide helpful teaching sheets for each prescribed medication.
- Describe system planned for ensuring all prescribed medications are being taken in a timely fashion.

Sample Documentation

Client instructed on self-administration of both Digoxin and Lasix. Able to state purpose of each medication and common side effects, when to notify physician about drug-related concerns. Able to read each label and state when each drug is to be taken. Demonstrated how to take her own pulse correctly. Demonstrated understanding of appropriate storage of blood glucose monitor and disposal of sharps and contaminated supplies in the home.

SPECIAL CONSIDERATIONS

Pediatric Considerations

- All medications, medical supplies, and equipment must be kept safely out of reach of children.
- Caregivers should not compare medications to treats, even artificially sweetened varieties, because this could add to risk of child overdosing by mistaking medicine for candy.

Geriatric Considerations

- Capacity for learning new information remains as we age (in the absence of dementia). However, additional time is needed to accomplish learning. Allow adequate time and number of teaching sessions to support successful learning.
- It may be necessary for a home health nurse to fill weekly pillbox if client/family cannot reliably complete this task.

Skill 40.5

Using Home Oxygen Therapy

Clients with alterations in oxygenation often require continuous oxygen therapy. The duration of therapy may be several weeks or months as clients recover from an acute lung injury or continuously for the remainder of their lives for chronic conditions. Oxygen is a drug and is administered and monitored with the same care as any other medication. Box 40-2 lists oxygen safety measures to be followed.

Medicare and other third-party payers usually cover a portion of oxygen therapy. Medicare has specific guidelines for reimbursement of oxygen therapy in the home (e.g., serious reduction in oxygenation during sleep or following exercise). Medicare requires a written physician's order for home oxygen (Rice, 2001).

Three types of oxygen are available for home use: liquid oxygen, oxygen concentrators, and compressed oxygen. Liquid oxygen systems have smaller portable units that are filled from a larger stationary unit in the home. When at home the client uses the stationary unit. The

Box 40-2
Oxygen Safety Guidelines

- Oxygen is a medication and should not be adjusted without a physician's order.
- No smoking should be allowed in the client's room.
- A "No Smoking" sign is placed in a spot visible to visitors.
- Oxygen delivery systems must be kept 10 feet from any open flames.
- Oxygen supports combustion; however, it will not explode.
- When oxygen cylinders are used, they must be secured so that they will not fall over. Oxygen cylinders are stored upright and chained or in appropriate holders.
- When oxygen tanks are transported in a car, they should be secured in a seat, not placed in the trunk.
- Never store oxygen tanks in a car.

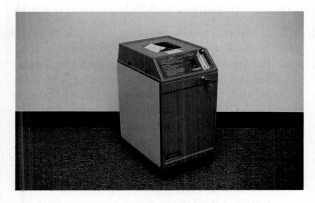

Figure 40-2   Oxygen concentrator. (From Sorrentino SA: *Assisting with patient care,* St Louis, 1999, Mosby.)

Table 40-2
Time in Hours of Oxygen Availability Depending on Liter Flow per Minute and Tank Size/Type

L/min	STATIONARY RESERVOIRS		PORTABLE UNITS	
	17,000 L	25,000 L	800 L	1000 L
1	248	396	7	14
2	124	196	3	7
3	83	134	2	4½
4	61	99	1½	3½
5	40	80	—	—
6	—	—	1	2

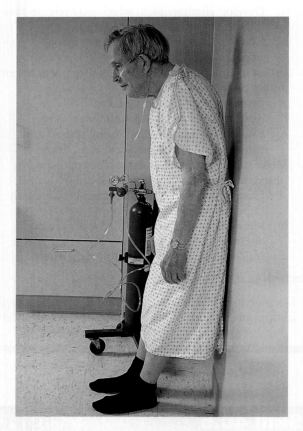

Figure 40-3   Portable compressed oxygen.

reservoir unit is refilled weekly or more often depending on the client's use. Liquid oxygen is the most portable and the most expensive. Table 40-2 lists the length of time a liquid oxygen system will last depending on the liter flow. Oxygen concentrators are moderate-size units that extract oxygen from the room air, concentrate it, and deliver the prescribed liter flow to the client. Oxygen concentrators (Figure 40-2) are the most economical but do not provide portability. Clients with an oxygen concentrator usually have small E cylinder tanks available for trips outside the home (Figure 40-3). Compressed oxygen is usually available in large H cylinders and in the small E cylinder tanks on carts, which are easily pulled along as the client walks. The large H cylinder tank will last approximately 50 hours at 2 L/min.

The type of oxygen delivery is based on a thorough assessment of the client's needs. Criteria for determining the right oxygen delivery for the client include the client's activity level, the amount of oxygen prescribed for the client, the client's physical ability, the availability of assistance for activities such as refilling a liquid tank, and where the client lives. A client who is very mobile and active would benefit from a liquid oxygen system to encourage continuation of activities. A client who is homebound is best served with an oxygen concentrator and smaller E cylinder for infrequent trips outside the home. The nurse, physi-

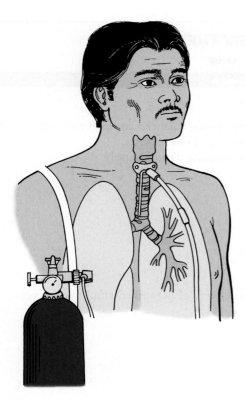

Figure 40-4 Transtrachael oxygen delivery via a catheter placed directly into the trachea.

cian, client, and home health company can determine the right system to meet a client's needs.

The client at home who needs oxygen therapy usually receives oxygen via nasal cannula. Occasionally oxygen is administered through a reservoir nasal cannula, which stores oxygen in a chamber during the expiratory phase of respirations (Rice, 2001), or through a Venturi mask. Transtracheal oxygen is delivered directly into the trachea via a catheter (Figure 40-4). A T tube with reservoir or tracheostomy collar is used for clients with a permanent tracheostomy.

Nasal cannulas are replaced weekly or cleaned with mild soap and water. Face masks, T tubes, and tracheostomy collars are cleaned daily with mild soap and water and allowed to air dry. Clients should have more than one delivery device so they can clean one and hang it to air dry while using the other.

This skill involves setting up and administering oxygen therapy to the client requiring oxygen administration in the home.

ASSESSMENT

1. Assess client and family's ability to apply and manipulate oxygen equipment while in the hospital or in the home. *Rationale: Physical or mental impairment may indicate a need for assistance in the home.*

2. Assess client and family's ability to determine the signs and symptoms of hypoxia. *Rationale: Hypoxia can occur at home when client uses oxygen and can be caused by worsening of the client's physical problem or an underlying change in respiratory status.*

3. Assess the availability of community resources for home oxygen therapy. *Rationale: Durable medical equipment company (DME) usually responsible for repair service.*

4. Assess client and family's ability to recognize signs and symptoms of carbon dioxide narcosis. *Rationale: Carbon dioxide narcosis can result from inappropriate oxygen flow rate and result in respiratory arrest.*

5. Determine appropriate backup system, if compressor or concentrator is used, in event of power failure.

PLANNING

Expected outcomes focus on correct and safe use of the home oxygen equipment.

Expected Outcomes

1. Client receives oxygen at prescribed rate.
2. Client and family verbalize the purpose and correct use of home oxygen by discharge.
3. Client and family demonstrate how to set up the oxygen system.
4. Client and family are able to verbalize safety guidelines for oxygen use and troubleshoot problems (i.e., broken tubing, tubing disconnected, or not in nostrils correctly).
5. Client and family are able to verbalize emergency plan of care.

Equipment

- Oxygen delivery device
- Nasal cannula
- Simple mask
- Tracheostomy collar
- Oxygen tubing
- Oxygen source
- Oxygen cylinders
- Liquid system
- Concentrator

Delegation Considerations

This skill requires the critical thinking and knowledge application unique to the nurse. The nurse assumes accountability for appropriate assessment and implementation of home oxygen therapy by the client or appropriate caregiver after the teaching has occurred.

IMPLEMENTATION FOR USING HOME OXYGEN THERAPY

Steps	Rationale
1. See Standard Protocol (inside front cover).	
2. Place oxygen system in a clutter-free environment.	Keeps the device balanced and prevents injury from bumping against objects.
3. Check oxygen level remaining. Maintain a backup supply.	Ensures adequate oxygen supply.
a. Check liquid system by depressing button at lower right corner and reading the dial on the Liberator or Stroller (see illustration).	
b. Check cylinders by reading amount on pressure gauge.	
4. Connect oxygen delivery device (e.g., nasal cannula) to oxygen system.	
5. Determine and set correct liter flow rate.	Ensures delivery of prescribed amount of oxygen.

NURSE ALERT   *Equipment vendor and nurse instruct client how frequently Liberator and Stroller must be filled. Small Liberator (Sprint) has 4-hour capacity, whereas 9½-pound Stroller has 8-hour capacity. Refilling occurs automatically and takes a few seconds to a minute, depending on amount of oxygen required to fill Stroller.*

---

6. Review the safety guidelines (see Box 40-2, p. 956).
7. Place oxygen delivery device on client (see illustration).
8. When client is leaving the home and needs portability, the following steps are needed to prepare the portable units:
   a. Verify adequate supply of oxygen in tank by reading gauge on regulator. If necessary, replace with a full tank.

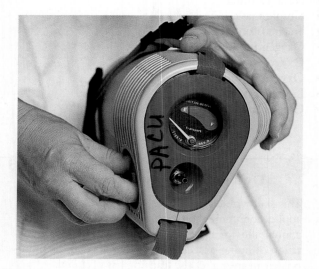

Step 3a   Depress button and read dial to check liquid oxygen system.

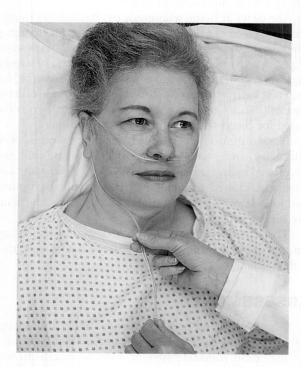

Step 7   Placing oxygen delivery system on client.

b. Connect appropriate oxygen delivery device and oxygen tubing to oxygen source.

   c. Place Stroller on cart.

   d. Set prescribed flow rate, and lock flow meter (if appropriate).

9. See Completion Protocol (inside front cover).

· · · · · · · · · ·

EVALUATION

1. Observe client's respiratory pattern, and ask client if feeling short of breath to determine if oxygen therapy is effective as prescribed.
2. Ask client and family to describe reasons for and correct setup for home oxygen use.
3. Observe client and family use of home oxygen system to determine ability to set up equipment correctly.
4. Ask client and family to describe safety guidelines for home oxygen use.

Unexpected Outcomes and Related Interventions

1. Client develops signs and symptoms associated with hypoxemia.
   a. Determine if oxygen delivery device and source are delivering oxygen properly.
   b. Determine if prescribed oxygen flow rate is set correctly.
   c. Assess client for change in respiratory status, such as airway plugging, respiratory infection, or bronchospasm.

2. Client uses unsafe practices with oxygen therapy, such as using oxygen near fire or cigarette smoking or setting incorrect flow rate.
   a. Discuss with client risks created through unsafe behavior.
   b. Attempt to identify reason client is unable to use oxygen correctly (e.g., health beliefs, incorrect information).

Recording and Reporting

- Record teaching plan for instructing client and family to use home oxygen.
- Record information given to client and family and any validation of learning on progress notes.
- Communicate client or family's learning progress to other health care providers involved.

Sample Documentation

1600 Client and family able to return demonstrate appropriate use of liquid oxygen system, including safety guidelines. Correctly stated signs and symptoms of hypoxemia.

 ## SPECIAL CONSIDERATIONS

Pediatric Considerations

- Plastic hoods are the best method to use to deliver oxygen therapy to infants (Wong and others, 1999).
- Nasal cannula or prongs can be used with older infants and children. Children generally do not tolerate oxygen administration given by mask (Wong and others, 1999).

Geriatric Considerations

- Older adults have less efficient respiratory systems and less surface area for gas exchange, so their response to decreased oxygen and infection may cause cerebral anoxia and lead to confusion. They may be unable to recognize respiratory problems or problems with the delivery system; therefore they must have frequent contact with a designated caregiver.
- Older adults are prone to skin breakdown; therefore it is important to keep skin dry under the mask and wash with mild soap and water. Cotton balls or foam pads provided by vendor can be used to prevent skin breakdown from the cannula on the ears.

Home Care and Long-Term Care Considerations

- Oxygen desaturation and decreased oxygen delivery to the brain can impair the client's ability to remember previous learning. Thus written or pictorial instructions should be provided for the home setting.
- Some clients are able to manage portable oxygen system but are unable to fill portable system.
- Assess the home for availability of a three-pronged (grounded) outlet for the compressor/concentrator to prevent electric shock.
- Equipment must be kept out of reach of children in the home, because manipulation of dials or flow meters could have disastrous effects on the oxygen-delivery process.

CRITICAL THINKING EXERCISES

1. Mr. Davis, age 65, is being discharged from the hospital after an acute exacerbation of his chronic obstructive pulmonary disease (COPD). The physician has ordered home oxygen therapy for Mr. Davis. What teaching needs to be done for Mr. Davis and his wife before sending him home with his oxygen?

2. Mrs. Taylor, age 80, is returning to her home following bilateral cataract surgery. In spite of the corrective surgery, she continues to have difficulty seeing well enough to read the labels on her medication bottles. She expresses concern to you about correctly taking her heart and blood pressure medication. As the nurse, how might you help Mrs. Taylor take her medications safely?

REFERENCES

American Hospital Association, *Patient Care Partnership: understanding expectations, rights, and responsibilities*, 2003, The Association.

Ebersole P, Hess P: *Toward healthy aging: human needs and nursing response*, ed 5, St Louis, 1998, Mosby.

Edelman CL, Mandle CL: *Health promotion throughout the lifespan*, ed 5, St Louis, 2002, Mosby.

Joint Commission on Accreditation of Healthcare Organizations: *Hospital Accreditation Standards*, Oakbrook Terrace, Ill, 2000, The Association.

Katz JR: Back to basics: providing effective patient teaching, *Am J Nurs* 5:33, 1997.

Lueckenotte A: *Gerontologic nursing*, ed 2, St Louis, 2000, Mosby.

Murphy PW, Davis TC: When low literacy blocks compliance, *RN* 60(10):58, 1997

Pender NJ: *Health promotion in nursing practice*, ed 3, Stamford, Conn, 1996, Appleton & Lange.

Potter P, Perry A: *Clinical nursing skills and techniques*, ed 5, St Louis, 2001, Mosby.

Redman B: *The practice of patient education*, ed 9, St Louis, 2001, Mosby.

Rice R: *Home care nursing practice*, ed 3, St Louis, 2001, Mosby.

Sorrentino SA: *Assisting with patient care*, St Louis, 1999, Mosby.

Wong DL and others: *Whaley & Wong's nursing care of infants and children*, ed 6, St Louis, 1999, Mosby.

Zernike W, Henderson A: Evaluating the effectiveness of two teaching strategies for patients diagnosed with hypertension, *J Clin Nurs* 7(1):37, 1998.

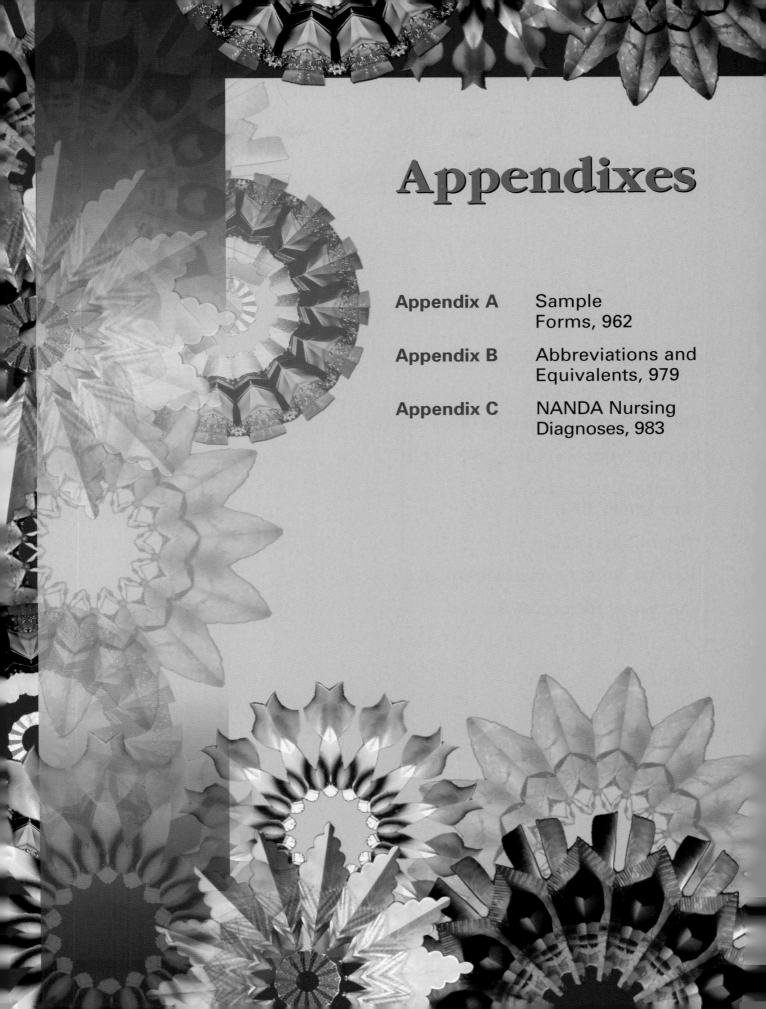

Appendixes

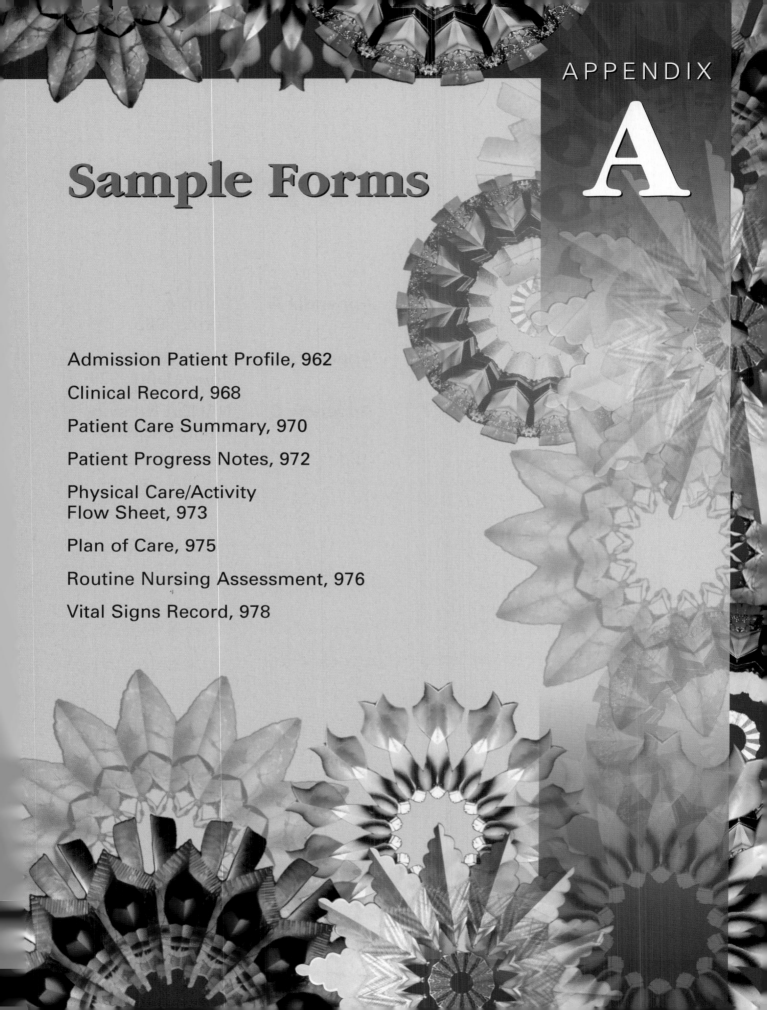

Sample Forms

ST. JOHN'S HOSPITAL
800 E. Carpenter St.
Springfield, Illinois 62769

ADMISSION PATIENT PROFILE

Known Allergies: (List)   **Describe reaction:**

Food: _____   ☐ N/V ☐ Rash ☐ Other:_____

_____   ☐ N/V ☐ Rash ☐ Other:_____

Drug: _____   ☐ N/V ☐ Rash ☐ Other:_____

_____   ☐ N/V ☐ Rash ☐ Other:_____

_____   ☐ N/V ☐ Rash ☐ Other:_____

_____   ☐ N/V ☐ Rash ☐ Other:_____

Contact allergies: _____

Latex allergy: ☐ No ☐ Yes   (If yes, initiate Latex precautions) _____

X-ray dye allergy: ☐ No ☐ Yes   _____

CURRENT MEDICATIONS: (Include over-the-counter medications, i.e., ASA™, Tylenol™, vitamins, herbals, etc.)

Name of medication	Dose	Dosing time	Day/Time of last dose	Brought to hospital (If yes, indicate disposition of the medication)
				☐ No ☐ Yes
				☐ No ☐ Yes
				☐ No ☐ Yes
				☐ No ☐ Yes
				☐ No ☐ Yes
				☐ No ☐ Yes
				☐ No ☐ Yes
				☐ No ☐ Yes
				☐ No ☐ Yes
				☐ No ☐ Yes
				☐ No ☐ Yes
				☐ No ☐ Yes
				☐ No ☐ Yes
				☐ No ☐ Yes
				☐ No ☐ Yes
				☐ No ☐ Yes
				☐ No ☐ Yes
				☐ No ☐ Yes
				☐ No ☐ Yes
				☐ No ☐ Yes
				☐ No ☐ Yes

#4678 (R 04/01)
(1 of 6)

ADMISSION PATIENT PROFILE
(Nurses Notes)

(Courtesy St. John's Hospital, Springfield, Ill.)

HEALTH HISTORY

Information obtained from: ☐ Patient ☐ Family ☐ Friend ☐ Old Chart ☐ Transfer Sheet ☐ ED Record

Reason for admission (as stated by patient): _____

Previous surgery(ies)/hospitalizations: _____

_____

_____

_____

_____

Previous blood transfusion(s)? ☐ No ☐ Yes Date _____

COGNITIVE / NEURO / SENSORY

History:

☐ CVA ☐ Seizures
☐ Head injury ☐ Headache
☐ Syncope ☐ Stiff neck
☐ Vertigo

Associated signs/symptoms:

☐ Oriented to: ☐ Time ☐ Place ☐ Person
☐ Cooperative ☐ Anxious
*☐ Memory problem: ☐ Short term ☐ Long term
*☐ Confused ☐ Withdrawn ☐ Comatose

Additional Comments

☐ * Asterisk denotes potential barriers to learning

***Vision problems:**

☐ Blind: ☐ Rt. ☐ Lt.
☐ Cataracts: ☐ Rt. ☐ Lt.
☐ Implants: ☐ Rt. ☐ Lt.
☐ Glaucoma: ☐ Rt. ☐ Lt.
☐ Eye prosthesis: ☐ Rt. ☐ Lt.

Associated signs/symptoms:

☐ PERLA
☐ Pupil asymmetry; describe:_____
*☐ Blurry or double vision
*Difficulty reading small print? ☐ Yes ☐ No
Wears glasses? ☐ Yes ☐ No
Wears contacts? ☐ Yes ☐ No

***Communication problems:**

☐ Deaf:
☐ Uses hearing aid: ☐ Rt. ☐ Lt.
☐ Hearing difficulty:(with appliance if used) ☐ Mild ☐ Moderate ☐ Severe
☐ Aphasia ☐ Dysphasia
☐ Language barrier; describe:_____

☐ All above areas addressed

CARDIAC / PERIPHERAL VASCULAR

History:

☐ Angina
☐ Heart attack, date:_____
☐ Arrhythmia
☐ CHF
☐ Heart murmur
☐ Rheumatic Fever
☐ Peripheral Vascular Disease
☐ DVT
☐ Pulmonary Embolus
☐ Hypertension
☐ High cholesterol
☐ Family history of heart disease

Procedures: **Date:**

☐ Cardiac Catheterization _____
☐ Balloon Angioplasty _____
☐ Stent _____
☐ Bypass surgery _____
☐ Valve surgery _____
☐ Pacemaker _____
(Obtain copy of ID card.)
☐ Internal Cardiac Defibrillator_____
(Obtain copy of ID card.)

Use Additional Comments section as necessary to indicate surgeon, cardiologist or other pertinent information.

Pulses:

Apical Pulse: ☐ Reg. ☐ Irreg.
Radial: _____ Rt. _____ Lt.
Posterior Tibial: _____ Rt. _____ Lt.
Pedal: _____ Rt. _____ Lt.
(P = Pulse present by palpation,
D = Pulse audible with doppler,
A = Absent)

Additional Comments

Associated signs/symptoms:

☐ Dizziness on standing
☐ SOB w/ activity
☐ Awakening from sleep w/ SOB
☐ Swelling of ankles
☐ Sleeps w/ greater than 2 pillows

☐ Palpitations
☐ Passing out spells
☐ Pain in legs when walking (intermittent claudication)
☐ Leg cramps
☐ Chest pain (describe:)_____

☐ All above areas addressed

OXYGENATION

History:

☐ Asthma
☐ COPD
☐ Pneumonia
☐ TB
☐ Recent URI
☐ Sinus problems
☐ Cigarette smoking: Packs/day: _____ # of years_____
☐ Pipe ☐ Cigar ☐ Chew

Associated signs / symptoms:
Breath Sounds:
☐ Clear bilaterally
☐ Abnormal, describe: _____
_____

☐ SOB: ☐ @ rest; ☐ w/ exertion
☐ Cough
☐ Sputum, describe: _____
_____

☐ Apnea
☐ Sleep apnea: ☐ BiPAP or ☐ CPAP
O₂ / Resp. Therapy at home? _____

Pulse Ox _____ (if indicated)
☐ room air ☐ on O₂_____ lpm

☐ Quit; date:_____

Additional Comments

☐ All above areas addressed

#4678 (R 04/01)
(2 of 6)

ADMISSION PATIENT PROFILE
(Nurses Notes)

ST. JOHN'S HOSPITAL
800 E. Carpenter St.
Springfield, Illinois 62769

ADMISSION PATIENT PROFILE

SKIN CONDITION / WOUND ASSESSMENT

Indicate locations of any of the following by number:

1. Abrasion   6. Laceration
2. Burn   7. Rash
3. Contusion   8. Scars
4. Bruise   9. Sutures
                   10. Lower extremity ulcers
5. Decubitus*

* Complete Pressure Ulcer Therapy Form

☐ **Wound, Ostomy, Continence Nurse Referral**
Date:_____

Skin color: _____
Skin temp.: _____
Skin moisture: _____

Edema: ☐ Yes   ☐ No
    Location: _____
    Describe: _____

Wound location/description:
_____
_____

Body piercing: Date: _____
          Site: _____

☐ **All above areas addressed**

PAIN ASSESSMENT (INITIAL)

1. **Indicate all areas of pain on the body drawing.**   ☐ **Denies pain**
   [Mark as external (E) or internal (I).]

2. Current pain meds: _____
   _____

3. How long since last dose of pain medication? _____

4. Intensity: (Rate pain on a 0 - 10 scale)   Present: _____
                                              Most severe: _____
                                              Least pain: _____

5. What level of pain is acceptable to you? _____ (0-10 scale)

6. Quality:(Use patient's own words, e.g. ache, burn, throb, pull, sharp.)
   _____
   _____

7. What relieves your pain(s)? _____
   _____

8. What makes your pain(s) worse? _____
   _____

9. How does your pain affect your activities of daily living? (Appetite, physical activity, concentration, etc.)
   _____
   _____

10. Other comments: _____

FUNCTIONAL ASSESSMENT

SELF-CARE ABILITY:	Independent	Assistive device +/or assistance from one person	Dependent	Change in last week Yes	Change in last week No
	(Place ✔ in appropriate column)			Yes	No
Eating/drinking					
Bathing					
Dressing/grooming					
Toileting					
Bed mobility*					
Transferring					
Walking					
Stair climbing					
Household chores					

* If bedbound or chairbound complete Pressure Ulcer Therapy Form

Is it anticipated that function would improve with rehabilitation? If so, Registered Nurse to obtain an M.D. order regarding a referral for Rehabilitation Services based on this functional assessment.

Referral made: ☐ Yes   ☐ No
          Date: _____
          Time: _____

Additional comments: _____
_____
_____
_____
_____
_____

ASSISTIVE DEVICES

☐ None   ☐ Cane   ☐ Wheelchair   ☐ Walker   ☐ Crutches

☐ Splint/Brace/Immobilizer   ☐ Trapeze   ☐ Bedside commode   ☐ Stool riser

☐ Other _____

☐ **All above areas addressed**

HISTORY:

☐ Arthritis   Gait: ☐ Steady   ☐ Muscle weakness
☐ Gout   ☐ Unsteady   ☐ Paralysis
☐ Fracture: Location: _____   Time frame: _____
☐ Amputation: _____
☐ Prosthesis: _____
☐ Contractures: _____

ADMISSION PATIENT PROFILE
(Nurses Notes)

IMMUNE FUNCTION   Additional Comments

☐ Fever in last 48°   Transplant history: _____   _____

☐ Radiation Therapy (date)_____ Malignancy history: _____   _____

☐ Chemotherapy (date)_____   _____

Implanted port: ☐ Yes ☐ No Site: _____ Type: _____ Date: _____   _____

Tunneled catheter: ☐ Yes ☐ No Site: _____ Type: _____ Date: _____   _____

PICC: ☐ Yes ☐ No Site: _____ Type: _____ Date: _____   _____

Single lumen: ☐ Yes ☐ No Site: _____ Type: _____ Date: _____   _____

Multi lumen: ☐ Yes ☐ No Site: _____ Type: _____ Date: _____   _____

Peripheral IV access: ☐ Yes ☐ No Site: _____ Type: _____ Date: _____   _____

Other:_____   ☐ Yes ☐ No Site: _____ Type: _____ Date: _____   _____

History of autoimmune diseases: ☐ Yes   ☐ No   _____
    (e.g. lupus; scleroderma)   _____

History of MRSA: ☐ Yes   ☐ No   ┌─────────────────────────────┐   _____
                                       │   Vaccinations: │
History of VRE: ☐ Yes   ☐ No   │ ☐ Flu (date:_____)   │   _____
                                       │ ☐ Pneumonia (date:_____) │
☐ All above areas addressed   │ ☐ Tetanus (date:_____) │   _____
                                       └─────────────────────────────┘   _____

ENDOCRINE / METABOLIC   Additional Comments

History: _____

☐ Diabetes: ☐ Insulin controlled*   ☐ Diet controlled   ☐ Oral meds   _____

  Do you check your blood sugar at home? ☐ Yes ☐ No If yes, how often?:_____   _____

*Do you give your own insulin? ☐ Yes ☐ No If no, who does administer your insulin?:_____   _____

☐ Hepatitis: Type:_____   Thyroid problems ☐ Yes ☐ No   _____

☐ Alcohol use: Average # of drinks per day _____; or per week _____   _____

Other: _____   _____

☐ All above areas addressed   _____

NUTRITION   Additional Comments

Home Diet: _____   Recent appetite: ☐ Good ☐ Fair ☐ Poor   _____

Using supplements: ☐ No ☐ Yes Type:_____   _____

Recent weight changes? ☐ No ☐ Yes ☐ Increase ☐ Decrease Amount _____   _____

    ☐ Intentional   ☐ Unintentional   _____

☐ Nausea ☐ Vomiting   _____

☐ Swallowing difficulty   _____

☐ Tube feedings: _____ ☐ G-tube(Date inserted/changed:_____) ☐ J-tube(Date inserted/changed:_____)

☐ All above areas addressed.   ┌──────────────────────────┐
                                                       │ ☐ Clinical Dietitian referral │
                                                       │ Date:_____   │
                                                       └──────────────────────────┘

ADMISSION PATIENT PROFILE
(Nurses Notes)

ST. JOHN'S HOSPITAL
800 E. Carpenter St.
Springfield, Illinois 62769

ADMISSION PATIENT PROFILE

ELIMINATION   Additional Comments

Bowel History: Typical bowel pattern: (describe) _____
☐ GI Bleed   Last B.M.? _____
☐ Ulcerative Colitis   ☐ Abdominal distention   Bowel sounds: ☐ Present ☐ Absent
☐ Diverticulitis   ☐ Constipation
☐ Irritable bowel   ☐ Diarrhea freq. _____
☐ Hemorrhoids   ☐ Involuntary stools
☐ Colostomy   ☐ Stool changes: (describe)_____
☐ Ileostomy   Laxative use on a regular basis: ☐ No ☐ Yes Med:_____

Urinary History:
☐ Renal disease:_____   ☐ Burning   ☐ Nocturia
☐ Renal stent   ☐ Urgency   ☐ Hematuria
☐ Ureteral stent   ☐ Retention   ☐ Dysuria
☐ Kidney stones   ☐ Incontinence   ☐ Ileo-Conduit
☐ Stream initiation difficulty   ☐ Suprapubic catheter   ☐ Nephrostomy
                                    ☐ Foley in place: date inserted/changed _____
☐ **All above areas addressed**

SEXUAL FUNCTION / REPRODUCTIVE   Additional Comments

Female: (Staff reminder: For females over 20, unless pap smear has been performed
Date of last pap smear: _____   within the previous year, add pap smear label to MD order sheet.)

LMP: _____   ☐ Breast changes/problems: _____
☐ Menstrual changes/problems:
                                            _____
_____   ☐ Mammogram   Date: _____
☐ History of sexually transmitted disease: Pregnant: ☐ No
                                            ☐ Yes EDC: _____
_____
Male:
☐ Prostate problems   ☐ Testicular changes/problems: _____
☐ History of sexually transmitted disease: _____
☐ **All above areas addressed**

PSYCHO-SOCIAL / SPIRITUAL / CULTURAL   Additional Comments

☐ Lives with spouse   Do you plan to return to the same living arrangement?: ☐ Yes ☐ No
☐ Lives alone   Do you have a family member or someone else that could help you at home?:
☐ Lives with family   ☐ Yes ☐ No   Name:_____
☐ Lives with friend   Relationship:_____
☐ Lives in a nursing home Do you want your family or significant other to be included in your treatment
☐ Other:_____   decisions and care planning? ☐ Yes ☐ No

                           Are you the primary caregiver for someone at home?: ☐ Yes ☐ No | ☐ **Pastoral Care referral**
Do you have special religious, spiritual, or cultural requests during this hospitalization? ☐ Yes ☐ No | Date:_____
   Describe: _____ | ☐ **Social Service referral**
☐ **All above areas addressed** | Date:_____

COPING / INDEPENDENCE

Significant losses: Major life changes or stressors (e.g. divorce, death, job change, retirement, victim of traumatic event) Note time frame.
_____
_____

Do you anticipate changes due to this illness? (job, housing, family) _____
Due to an increase in awareness regarding abuse and domestic violence, we ask all patients:
Are you being hurt, hit or frightened by anyone at home or in your life? ☐ No ☐ Yes
If yes, explain _____
☐ **All above areas addressed**   ☐ **Social Service referral   Date:_____**

#4678 (R 04/01)   **ADMISSION PATIENT PROFILE**
(5 of 6)   (Nurses Notes)

ADVANCE DIRECTIVES

Has the patient received a copy of the Patient Services Directory? ☐ Yes ☐ No

Does the patient have an advance directive (Living Will or Power of Attorney for Health Care) ☐ Yes ☐ No

☐ Patient is a minor; does not apply.

Patient HAS an advance directive:

Do we have a current copy? ☐ Yes ☐ No

☐ With patient or ☐ In a record from a previous admission

If in a record from a previous admission, Nursing to proceed with the following steps:

(Nursing): _____ Obtain copy from Medical Records Dept.

(Nursing): _____ Patient and RN/LPN to initial and date document if information is correct.

(Nursing): _____ Place document in patient's chart, affix a Notice Sticker to front of the chart, update the FIN sheet and place a new FIN on chart.

The patient indicated that,

name: _____

telephone#: _____

was named as Power of Attorney for Health Care.

Patient DOES NOT HAVE an advance directive:

Do you want to see a short video (15 min.) which would provide you with information? ☐ Yes ☐ No

[Available on Patient Education Channel. Consult the directory]

Do you want to complete an advance directive on this admission? ☐ Yes ☐ No

If yes,

(Nursing): Send an Infogram to Pastoral Care Department.

Inform the patient that they will be contacted during this admission by hospital staff who will assist them in the completion of an advance directive.

If the request is urgent, page Pastoral Care Chaplain on duty (Pager 1140).

Signature of data collector _____ **Date** _____ **Time:** _____

INITIAL TEACHING NEEDS / DISCHARGE PLANNING / REFERRALS (*MUST* be completed by RN)

1. Patient/family teaching needs identified at this time:

☐ Medication _____ ☐ Pre-op _____ ☐ Diagnosis/illness _____

☐ Dietary _____ ☐ Pre-Procedure _____

☐ Diabetic _____

☐ Other (specify) _____

2. Current utilization of community resources: ☐ None ☐ Church group ☐ Hospice Home Care ☐ Adult Day

☐ Meals on Wheels ☐ Homemaker AideCare ☐ Home Health Care (notify Home Health of pt's admission)

☐ Community group _____ ☐ Other _____

3. Based on this Admission Patient Profile do you anticipate the patient needing any assistance when they are discharged from the hospital? ☐ Yes ☐ No

If yes, specify _____

Signature of Pre-Admission nurse: _____ **Date** _____

Profile completed/verified by unit staff nurse admitting the patient _____ **Date** _____

Time _____

ADMISSION PATIENT PROFILE
(Nurses Notes)

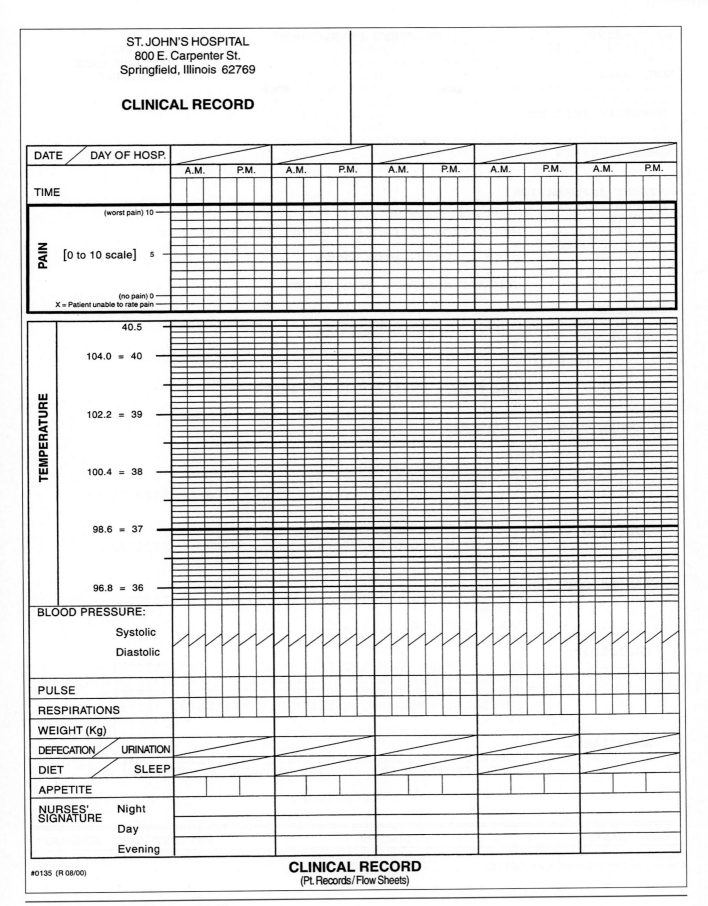

ST. JOHN'S HOSPITAL
800 E. Carpenter St.
Springfield, Illinois 62769

CLINICAL RECORD

DATE / DAY OF HOSP.											
	A.M.	P.M.	A.M.	P.M.	A.M.	P.M.	A.M.	P.M.	A.M.	P.M.	
TIME											

PAIN [0 to 10 scale]
(worst pain) 10
5
(no pain) 0
X = Patient unable to rate pain

TEMPERATURE
40.5
104.0 = 40
102.2 = 39
100.4 = 38
98.6 = 37
96.8 = 36

BLOOD PRESSURE:
    Systolic
    Diastolic

PULSE

RESPIRATIONS

WEIGHT (Kg)

DEFECATION / URINATION

DIET / SLEEP

APPETITE

NURSES' SIGNATURE   Night
    Day
    Evening

CLINICAL RECORD
(Pt. Records / Flow Sheets)

#0135 (R 08/00)

(Courtesy St. John's Hospital, Springfield, Ill.)

```
4S    -2196              ST.JOHNS DEVELOPMENT
01/13/03  15:44              (QAB$$P)                        PAGE 001
===================================================    PATIENT CARE
DOE, JANE                      M U S  63                    SUMMARY
ACCT#: 020027891000            MR#: 02002789
SERV: MEDICAL                  4S      00426A           PT TYPE: IP
 NONSTAFF,TEST MD              ADM: 01/10/03
DR:                            DOB: 01/01/40
===================================================
SUMMARY: 01/14 07:00    TO 15:15


PATIENT INFORMATION:
 NO PUBLICITY
MEDICATION ALLERGIES:
     01/10         MEDICATION ALLERGY: CODEINE, REACTION--N/V
DIET ALLERGIES:
     01/10         DIET ALLERGY: NONE KNOWN
CONTACT ALLERGIES:
     01/10         CONTACT ALLERGY: NONE KNOWN

 CHECKLIST:
___ CARE PLAN    ___ PT ED      ___ PRN FOLLOW-UP    ___ PAIN ASSESS
___ MD ORDERS    ___ TELE       ___ PT CHARGES

NURSING INFORMATION:
     01/10         ADMISSION WEIGHT:WT: 73.5 KG
     01/10         ADMIT DX:  TRIGEMINAL NEURITIS
     01/10         AD: N

ALL CURRENT MEDICAL ORDERS:

  MD TO NURSE ORDERS:
     01/10      1. ACTIVITY BRP, (0060)
     01/10      2. BLOOD: ACCUCHECK DAILY, (0060)
     01/10      3. 0700 AND 1700 CALL IF LESS THAN 60 OR GREATER THAN
                    250, (0060)

  DIET/I&O:
     01/10      4. DIET STANDARD DIABETIC/NO CONC. SWEETS, <01/10/03>,
                    (0060)

  LABORATORY:
     01/10      5. ANTI-NEUTROPHIL CYTOPLASM AB, TODAY, (01/10/03),
                    (0060)
     01/10      6. ANA, TOMORROW, (01/11/03), (0060)

  RADIOLOGY:
     01/10      7. X-RAY: CHEST PA & LATERAL (ROUTINE), INDICATION:--
                    HYPERTENSION, SCHEDULE: TOMORROW, (01/11/03), (0060)
     01/10      8. X-RAY: MRA HEAD W/WO CONTRAST TRIGEMINAL NEURITIS,
                    SCHEDULE: TOMORROW, HANDLING: WHEELCHAIR, (01/11/03),
                    (0060)

  ANCILLARY:
     01/10      9. ELECTROENCEPHALOGRAM, NO PREP, INDICATION: CVA, LT
                    SIDE, SEDATION OK: CHLORAL HYDRATE, SCHEDULE: ASAP,

                         CONTINUED

===================================================================
DOE, JANE                  02002789              PATIENT CARE SUMMARY
```

(Courtesy St. John's Hospital, Springfield, Ill.)

```
01/13/03  15:44              (QAB$$P)                    PAGE 003
=====================================================   PATIENT CARE
DOE, JANE                    M U S  63                      SUMMARY
ACCT#: 020027891000          MR#: 02002789
SERV: MEDICAL                4S      00426A              PT TYPE: IP
 NONSTAFF,TEST MD            ADM: 01/10/03
DR:                          DOB: 01/01/40
=====================================================
SUMMARY: 01/14 07:00     TO 15:15
```

MEDICATION ALLERGIES:
      01/10   *MEDICATION ALLERGY: CODEINE, REACTION--N/V*

ALL CURRENT PHARMACY/INFUSION ORDERS:

  SCHEDULED MEDICATIONS:
```
  01/10     11. LASIX FUROSEMIDE 40MG TAB, #1, PO, DAILY 09,
                 (01/11/03 09:00-..), (02 OF 02), (0060) 09
  01/10     13. PLAVIX CLOPIDOGREL 75MG TAB, #1, PO, DAILY 09,
                 (01/11/03 09:00-..), (02 OF 02), (0060) 09
  01/10     14. ZANTAC RANITIDINE 150MG TAB, #1, PO, BID, (01/10/03
                 21:00-..), (0060) 09
  01/10     15. LOTREL NONFORMULARY AMLODIPINE 5MG/ BENAZEPRIL 10MG
                 CAP, #1, PO, DAILY AT, 1200, (01/11/03 12:00-..),
                 (0060) 12
  01/10     16. GLUCOPHAGE METFORMIN 500MG TAB, #1, PO, DAILY AT, 0800
                 , (01/11/03 08:00-..), (0060) 08
  01/10     17. AMARYL NONFORMULARY GLIMEPIRIDE 4MG TAB, #1, PO,
                 DAILY AT, 0800, (01/11/03 08:00-..), (0060) 08
  01/10     18. LESCOL FLUVASTATIN 20MG CAP, #1, PO, DAILY 21,
                 (01/10/03 21:00-..), (0060)
  01/10     19. CATAPRES TTS CLONIDINE 7.5MG TRANSDERMAL DISK
                 (0.3MG/24HR), TO SKIN, START ON 11/10/03 WEEKLY, 0900,
                 (11/10/03 09:00-..), (0060)
  01/10     20. NORVASC AMLODIPINE 5MG TAB, #1, PO, DAILY AT, 2200,
                 (01/10/03 22:00-..), (0060)
  01/10     21. NORMODYNE LABETALOL 100MG TAB, #1, PO, DAILY AT, 2000,
                 (01/10/03 20:00-..), (0060)
  01/10     23. LOPRESSOR METOPROLOL 100MG TAB, #1, PO, DAILY 09,
                 (01/11/03 09:00-..), (02 OF 02), (0060) 09
```

  PRN MEDICATIONS:
```
  01/10     24. TYLENOL ACETAMINOPHEN 500MG CAP, #1, PO, Q3H, PRN,
                 <01/10/03 15:20-..>, (0060)
  01/10     25. VIOXX ROFECOXIB 25MG TAB, #1, PO, DAILY 09, PRN,
                 <01/10/03 15:20-..>, (0060)
  01/10     26. AMBIEN ZOLPIDEM 5MG TAB, #1, PO, HS-PRN, <01/10/03
                 15:20-..>, (0060)
```

                                      LAST PAGE

```
=====================================================================
DOE, JANE                    02002789              PATIENT CARE SUMMARY
-*-
```

ST. JOHN'S HOSPITAL
Springfield, Illinois

PATIENT PROGRESS NOTES

DATE	TIME	PROGRESS NOTES	SIGNATURE

#299 (02/96)

PATIENT PROGRESS NOTES

(Courtesy St. John's Hospital, Springfield, Ill.)

ST. JOHN'S HOSPITAL
800 E. Carpenter St.
Springfield, Illinois
PHYSICAL CARE / ACTIVITY

KEY:

BRN	=	brown	AMB	=	ambulate	RS	=	right side
CL	=	clear	C	=	chair	LS	=	left side
GR	=	green	D	=	dangle	B	=	back
PT	=	pink tinged	BR	=	bathroom	JT	=	jejunostomy tube
R	=	red	BED	=	bedrest	GT	=	gastrostomy tube
T	=	tan	G	=	good	FT	=	feeding tube
W	=	white	WL	=	well	N/G	=	nasogastric tube
Y	=	yellow	F	=	fair	RM	=	right mouth
LG	=	large	P	=	poor	LM	=	left mouth
MOD	=	moderate	AB	=	absent	RN	=	right nare
SM	=	small	PR	=	present	LN	=	left nare
Ø	=	No/None	*	=	see nurses notes			
SP	=	see care plan	Blank	=	non applicable			
			✓	=	performed			

CIRCULATORY AID CODES:

KEN	=	kendall boots
TED	=	Ted Hose
ACE	=	Ace wraps
JOB	=	Jobst stockings

LOCATION:

RA	=	right arm
LA	=	left arm
BA	=	both arms
RL	=	right leg
LL	=	left leg
BL	=	both legs

Date:

Time:

HYGIENE / ELIMINATION

- Bed bath / Assist bath
- Self bath
- Bony areas inspected
- Oral care / Skin care
- Foley catheter care
- Incontinence Care   Urine / Stool
- HS care

ACTIVITY

- Turn and reposition / # of assists
- Activity: Type
- Tolerance / # of assists

SAFETY

- Top rails up / All rails up
- Bed in low position / Awake or asleep
- Call bell in reach / Armband in place
- Camera on / Visitors present
- Reoriented to surroundings
- Bedside commode used
- Patient monitored while in BR
- Reminded to call for assist to BR
- Toilet before bedtime
- Items left within reach for patient

PHYSICAL CARE / ACTIVITY
(Patient Records/Flow Sheets)

#5003 (R 08/99)
(1 of 2)

(Courtesy St. John's Hospital, Springfield, Ill.)

			Date:													
			Time:													
RESPIRATION			Deep Breathe & Cough / Incentive Spirometry													
			Pulse Oximetry													
			Trach Care / Size													
	SUCTIONING		Tracheostomy Color / Amt.													
			Oral Color / Amt.													
			Pharyngeal Color / Amt.													
			ETT Color / Amt.													
	ETT		Site / Care													
			Chest Tube CM suction / Tidaling													
NUTRITION			NPO													
			Eats with Assist / Total Feed													
			Nourishment													
			NG or Feeding Tube													
			Placement Verified / Irrigated													
			Residual													
			Enteral feeding type													
			Bag & Tubing Change													
			Route / Rate													
OTHER ASSESSMENTS/ TREATMENTS			Isolation (type)													
			Circulatory Aide / Pressure Reduction Device													
			K-Pad / Ice Bag (location)													
			EKG patches dated & off Pectoral Sites													
			EKG monitor alarms on Upper limit / Lower limit													
SIGNATURE																

#5003 (R 08/99)
(2 of 2)

```
4S    -2197              ST.JOHNS DEVELOPMENT                        PAGE 001
01/13/03  15:47              (QAY$$P)                       \\\\\ \\\\\ \\\\\
=================================================          \  \   \   \   \
DOE, JANE                     M U S  63                    \\\\\ \   \   \ \
ACCT#: 020027891000           MR#: 02002789               \\\\\ \   \   \ \
SERV: MEDICAL                 4S      00426A               \    \   \   \ \
DR:NONSTAFF,TEST MD           ADM: 01/10/03                \     \\\\\ \\\\\
DR:                           DOB: 01/01/40
=================================================          PLAN OF CARE


    ADMIT DX:    TRIGEMINAL NEURITIS

   CURRENT PROBLEMS/ISSUES:


01/13 15:30    PAIN                                                      ARYA

01/13 15:30    HIGH RISK FOR INJURY: SAFETY
               R/T: UNSTEADY GAIT                                        ARYA
   EXPECTED OUTCOMES:                           DATE:
01/13 15:30    PT REMAINS FREE OF INJURY        PRIOR TO DC    ARYA
01/13 15:30    PT/FAMILY/S.O. VERBALIZE KNOWLEDGE OF
               SAFETY PRECAUTIONS AT ALL TIMES  PRIOR TO DC    ARYA
   APPROACHES:
01/13 15:30    PLACE BELONGINGS WITHIN REACH
01/13 15:30    CALL LIGHT WITHIN REACH
01/13 15:30    INSTRUCT IN CORRECT USE OF ASSISTIVE
               DEVICES. SPECIFY--WALKER


01/13 15:30    PAIN: CHRONIC
               R/T: COMPRESSION OF NERVES                                ARYA
   EXPECTED OUTCOMES:                           DATE:
01/13 15:30    PT WILL MAINTAIN OPTIMAL MOBILITY PRIOR TO DC   ARYA
01/13 15:30    PT WILL USE ADEQUATE COPING
               MECHANISMS FOR CHRONIC PAIN MGMT  BY:01/15/03   ARYA
   APPROACHES:
01/13 15:30    ASK PT TO RATE PAIN USING APPROPRIATE
               SCALE --WHENEVER VITAL SIGNS ASSESSED
01/13 15:30    ASSESS LEVEL OF SEDATION
01/13 15:30    IDENTIFY FACTORS THAT AGGRAVATE PAIN
               QSHIFT
01/13 15:30    EVALUATE EFFECTIVENESS OF PAIN CONTROL
01/13 15:30    DISCUSS PREVENTION OF CONSTIPATION:
               ENCOURAGE FLUIDS, INCREASE ACTIVITY,
               INCREASE IN BULK, & STOOL SOFTENERS


KEY: YEATES,AMY RN




                              LAST PAGE






    ===================================================================
    DOE, JANE                   02002789                  PLAN OF CARE
    -*-
```

(Courtesy St. John's Hospital, Springfield, Ill.)

ST. JOHN'S HOSPITAL
800 E. Carpenter St.
Springfield, Illinois 62769

ROUTINE NURSING ASSESSMENT
MEDICAL/SURGICAL

Edema: +1 = 0" - ¼"
+2 = ¼" - ½"
+3 = ½" - 1"

Key:

	Ø = negative / no	OTA = open to air		G = green	
	✓ = observed or positive response	PU = purulent		P = pink	
Blank = no assessment at this time		SS = serosanguinous		A = amber	
NN = see nurses notes		B = brown		C = Clear	
LE = lower extremity		R = red		CL = cloudy	
UE = upper extremity		Y = yellow			

Date									
Time									
MENTAL STATUS	Alert								
	Oriented / disoriented								
	Lethargic								
	Unresponsive								
BEHAVIOR	Agitated								
	Anxious								
	Restless								
MOTOR / SENSORY FUNCTION	Moves all extremities								
	Weakness UE LT / RT								
	LE LT / RT								
	Paralysis UE LT / RT								
	LE LT / RT								
	Numbness / tingling								
	Location								
SKIN / MUCOUS MEMBRANE	Temperature: warm / cool								
	Moisture: dry / moist								
	Skin: pink / pale								
	flushed / cyanotic								
	jaundiced								
	Mucous membrane pink / pale								
	flushed / cyanotic								
	Edema:								
	location								
CARDIO-VASCULAR	Apical rate: reg. / irreg.								
	Dorsalis pedis LT / RT								
	Posterior tibial LT / RT								

#4747 (R 01/02)
(1 of 2)

ROUTINE NURSING ASSESSMENT - MEDICAL/SURGICAL
(Patient Records/Flow Sheets)

(Courtesy St. John's Hospital, Springfield, Ill.)

Date										
Time										
RESPIRATORY	Quality: unlabored/labored									
	deep / shallow									
	O_2 therapy:									
	Sounds: clear LT / RT									
	diminished LT / RT									
	rales (crackles) LT / RT									
	rhonchi LT / RT									
	wheeze LT / RT									
	Cough: productive/nonproductive									
	Sputum: color									
GASTROINTESTINAL/ ABDOMEN	Nondistended / distended									
	Sounds: present / absent									
	Firm / soft									
	Hyperactive / hypoactive									
	Expelling flatus / nausea									
	Date of last bowel movement									
WOUND	Location (✓ = no redness or edema)									
	#1									
	#2									
	#3									
DRESSING	Location (✓ = clean and dry)									
	#1									
	#2									
	#3									
DRAINAGE	Device and location	description	description	description	description	description	description	description	description
	#1									
	#2									
	#3									
PAIN	Absent / present									
	Location									
	#1									
	#2									
	Severity scale (0 - 10) #1 / #2									
	Intervention									
PATIENT TEACHING	Description									
	#1 Pain management									
	#2									
	#3									
Signature										

#4747 (R 01/02)
(2 of 2)

ST. JOHN'S HOSPITAL
800 E. Carpenter St.
Springfield, Illinois 62769

VITAL SIGNS RECORD

KEY:

V	=	systolic	•	=	temperature	RA =	right arm
∧	=	diastolic	A	=	axillary	LA =	left arm
LY	=	lying	O	=	oral	RL =	right leg
ST	=	standing	R	=	rectal	LL =	left leg
SIT	=	sitting	S	=	skin	NN =	Nurses Notes
D	=	doppler	P	=	temperature probe		

Date																				Date
Time																				Time
Weight (kg)																				Weight (kg)
Temp site																				Temp site
B/P site																				B/P site
Pulse Oximetry																				Pulse Oximetry

Left scale		Right scale
43.0 - 240		240 43.0
42.5 - 230		230 42.5
42.0 - 220		220 42.0
41.5 - 210		210 41.5
41.0 - 200		200 41.0
40.5 - 190		190 40.5
40.0 - 180		180 40.0
39.5 - 170		170 39.5
39.0 - 160		160 39.0
38.5 - 150		150 38.5
38.0 - 140		140 38.0
37.5 - 130		130 37.5
37.0 - 120		120 37.0
36.5 - 110		110 36.5
36.0 - 100		100 36.0
35.5 - 90		90 35.5
35.0 - 80		80 35.0
34.5 - 70		70 34.5
34.0 - 60		60 34.0
33.5 - 50		50 33.5
33.0 - 40		40 33.0

Pain (0-10)																				Pain (0-10)
Pulse																				Pulse
Respiration																				Respiration

VITAL SIGNS RECORD
(Pt. Records / Flow Sheets)

#284 (R 09/99)

Abbreviations and Equivalents

ABBREVIATIONS AND CONVERSION FROM APOTHECARY TO METRIC

grain (gr) = 60 milligrams (mg)
15 gr = 1 gram (g, gm)
15 minims = 1 milliliter (ml, mL)
1 dram (dr) = 4 ml
1 ounce (oz) = 30 cubic centimeters (cc, ml)

ABBREVIATIONS FOR CONVERSION USING HOUSEHOLD MEASURES

1 drop (gtt) = 1 minim
1 teaspoon (1 tsp) = 5 ml
3 tsp = 1 tablespoon (tbsp)
1 cup = 8 oz
16 oz = 1 pound (lb)

STANDARD EQUIVALENTS, ABBREVIATIONS, AND CONVERSIONS

1000 mg = 1 g
1000 ml = 1 liter (L)
2.2 lb = 1 kilogram (kg) = 1000 g
1 tsp = 5 ml (cc)
1 dr = 4 ml (cc)
mEq: milliequivalent
mcg (μg): microgram

SYMBOLS

/	Per
<	Less than
>	More than
≤	Equal to or less than
≥	Equal to or more than
≅	Approximately equal to
+/−, ±	Plus or minus
♂	Male
♀	Female
1°	Primary; first degree
2°	Secondary; second degree
3°	Tertiary; third degree
↑	Up; increase
↓	Down; decrease
μ	Micron

ABBREVIATIONS RELATED TO TYPES OF INTRAVENOUS (IV) FLUIDS

D5W, D_5W: 5% dextrose and water
NS: normal saline
LR: lactated Ringer's solution
D5NS, D_5NS: 5% dextrose in 0.9% (normal) saline
D5 ½ NS, D_5½ NS: 5% dextrose in 0.45% saline
D5 ⅓ NS, D_5⅓ NS: 5% dextrose in 0.33% saline

ABBREVIATIONS

$\bar{a}$: before
abd: abdomen
ABGs: arterial blood gases
ac: before meals
ad lib: as desired
ADH: antidiuretic hormone
ADLs: activities of daily living
AFB: acid-fast bacillus (related to tuberculosis)
AIDS: acquired immunodeficiency syndrome
ALL: acute lymphoblastic leukemia
AMB: ambulatory
AP (and lateral chest): anterior and posterior
ASA: aspirin
ASHD: arteriosclerotic heart disease
ax: axillary
BE: barium enema
bid: twice a day
BM: bowel movement
BP: blood pressure
BPH: benign prostatic hypertrophy
BR: bed rest
BRP: bathroom privileges
BSE: breast self-examination
BSI: body substance isolation
BUN: blood urea nitrogen
bx: biopsy
$\bar{c}$: with
C&S: culture and sensitivity
CA: cancer
CABG: coronary artery bypass graft
CAD: coronary artery disease
cap: capsule
CBC: complete blood count
CBI: continuous bladder irrigation
CBR: complete bed rest
CC: chief complaint
CDC: Centers for Disease Control and Prevention
CHF: congestive heart failure
Cl: chloride
CN: cranial nerve
CNS: central nervous system
c/o: complains of
CO_2: carbon dioxide

COPD: chronic obstructive pulmonary disease
CPM: continuous passive motion
CPR: cardiopulmonary resuscitation
CSF: cerebrospinal fluid
CT: computed tomography
CVA: cerebrovascular accident (stroke)
CVP: central venous pressure
DAT: diet as tolerated
D/C: discontinue
DM: diabetes mellitus
DNR: do not resuscitate
DSD: dry sterile dressing
DTR: deep tendon reflex
DVT: deep venous thrombosis
dx: diagnosis
EC: enteric coated
ECG, EKG: electrocardiogram
elix: elixir
ER: extended release
ESR: erythrocyte sedimentation rate
ESRD: end-stage renal disease
ET: enterostomal therapist
FUO: fever of unknown origin
fx: fracture
g: gram
GI: gastrointestinal
gtt: drops
GU: genitourinary
Hb, Hgb: hemoglobin
HBV: hepatitis B virus
HCO_3^-:   bicarbonate
Hct: hematocrit
HCV: hepatitis C virus
HEPA: high-efficiency particulate air
HIV: human immunodeficiency virus
h/o: history of
HOB: head of bed
HR: heart rate
hs: at bedtime
HTN: hypertension
I&O: intake and output
ICP: intracranial pressure
ICU: intensive care unit
IDDM: insulin-dependent diabetes mellitus
IM: intramuscular
IPPB: intermittent positive-pressure breathing
IV: intravenous
JVD: jugular vein distention
K: potassium
KUB: kidney, ureter, bladder
KVO: keep vein open (run IV very slowly)
LLQ: left lower quadrant
LMP: last menstrual period
LOC: level of consciousness
lytes: electrolytes
MAP: mean arterial pressure

MCHC: mean corpuscular hemoglobin
          concentration
MCV: mean corpuscular volume
MI: myocardial infarction
MRI: magnetic resonance imaging
N: nitrogen
Na: sodium
NaCl: sodium chloride
neg: negative
NG: nasogastric
NPO: nothing by mouth
NSAIDs: nonsteroidal antiinflammatory drugs
O_2:   oxygen
O.D.:   right eye
OOB: out of bed
OR: operating room
O.S.:   left eye
OT: occupational therapy
OTC: over the counter (medicine without
          prescription)
O.U.:   both eyes
P: pulse
PACU: postanesthesia care unit
pc: after meals
PCA: patient-controlled analgesia
PE: pulmonary embolism
PID: pelvic inflammatory disease
PMH: past medical history
PMI: point of maximal impulse
PO: by mouth
postop: after surgery
preop: before surgery
prep: preparation
prn: as needed
pt: patient
PT: physical therapy
PT: prothrombin time
PTT: partial thromboplastin time
PVD: peripheral vascular disease
q: each
qd: daily
q__h (fill in number of hours), e.g., q3h: every
                                        3 hours
qid: four times a day
qod: every other day
qs: sufficient quantity
R: respirations
RA: rheumatoid arthritis
RBC: red blood cell
R/O: rule out (eliminate possibility of a condition)
ROM: range of motion
ROS: review of systems
r/t: related to
RUQ: right upper quadrant
Rx: treatment
$\bar{s}$:   without

SC (SQ):   subcutaneous
sl (SL):   sublingual
SOB: shortness of breath
sp gr: specific gravity
SR: sustained release
STAT: immediately
STD: sexually transmitted disease
supp: suppository
susp: suspension
sx: symptoms, signs
T: temperature
T&C: type and crossmatch
tab: tablet
TB: tuberculosis
TCDB: turn, cough, deep breathe
tid: three times a day

TPN: total parenteral nutrition
TPR: temperature, pulse, respirations
TURP: transurethral resection of prostate
UA: urinalysis
up ad lib: up as desired
URI: upper respiratory infection
US: ultrasound
UTI: urinary tract infection
VS: vital signs
VTBI: volume to be infused
WBC: white blood cell
WC: wheelchair
WNL: within normal limits
wt: weight

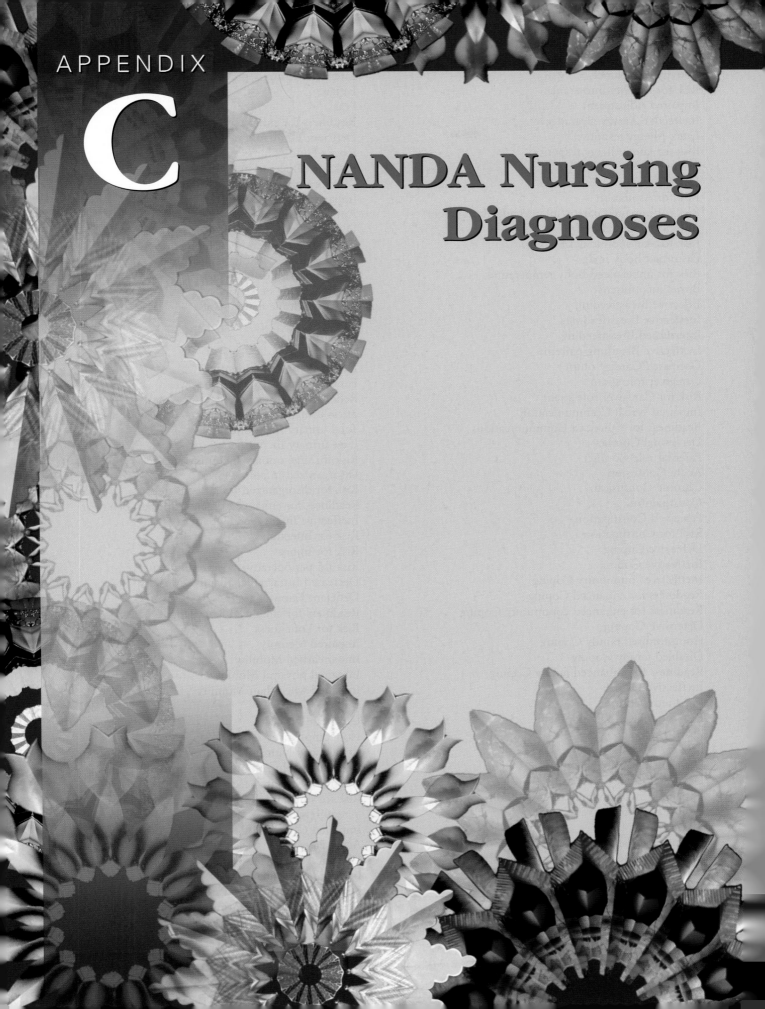

APPENDIX

C

NANDA Nursing Diagnoses

Activity intolerance
Risk for Activity intolerance
Impaired Adjustment
Ineffective Airway clearance
Latex Allergy response
Risk for latex Allergy response
Anxiety
Death Anxiety
Risk for Aspiration
Risk for impaired parent/infant/child Attachment
Autonomic dysreflexia
Risk for Autonomic dysreflexia
Disturbed Body image
Risk for imbalanced Body temperature
Bowel incontinence
Effective Breastfeeding
Ineffective Breastfeeding
Interrupted Breastfeeding
Ineffective Breathing pattern
Decreased Cardiac output
Caregiver role strain
Risk for Caregiver role strain
Impaired verbal Communication
Readiness for enhanced Communication
Decisional Conflict
Parental role Conflict
Acute Confusion
Chronic Confusion
Constipation
Perceived Constipation
Risk for Constipation
Defensive Coping
Ineffective Coping
Ineffective community Coping
Readiness for enhanced Coping
Readiness for enhanced community Coping
Defensive Coping
Compromised family Coping
Disabled family Coping
Readiness for enhanced family Coping
Ineffective Denial
Impaired Dentition
Risk for delayed Development
Diarrhea
Risk for Disuse syndrome
Deficient Diversional activity
Disturbed Energy field
Impaired Environmental interpretation syndrome
Adult Failure to thrive
Risk for Falls
Dysfunctional Family processes: alcoholism
Family processes
Readiness for enhanced Family processes

Interrupted Family processes
Fatigue
Fear
Readiness for enhanced Fluid balance
Deficient Fluid volume
Excess Fluid volume
Risk for deficient Fluid volume
Risk for imbalanced Fluid volume
Impaired Gas exchange
Anticipatory Grieving
Dysfunctional Grieving
Delayed Growth and development
Risk for disproportionate Growth
Ineffective Health maintenance
Health-seeking behaviors
Impaired Home maintenance
Hopelessness
Hyperthermia
Hypothermia
Disturbed personal Identity
Functional urinary Incontinence
Reflex urinary Incontinence
Stress urinary Incontinence
Total urinary Incontinence
Urge urinary Incontinence
Risk for urge urinary Incontinence
Disorganized Infant behavior
Risk for disorganized Infant behavior
Readiness for enhanced organized Infant behavior
Ineffective Infant feeding pattern
Risk for Infection
Risk for Injury
Risk for perioperative-positioning Injury
Decreased Intracranial adaptive capacity
Deficient Knowledge
Readiness for enhanced Knowledge
Risk for Loneliness
Impaired Memory
Impaired bed Mobility
Impaired physical Mobility
Impaired wheelchair Mobility
Nausea
Unilateral Neglect
Noncompliance
Imbalanced Nutrition: less than body requirements
Imbalanced Nutrition: more than body requirements
Readiness for enhanced Nutrition
Risk for imbalanced Nutrition: more than body requirements
Impaired Oral mucous membrane
Acute Pain
Chronic Pain
Impaired Parenting
Readiness for enhanced Parenting
Risk for impaired Parenting
Risk for Peripheral neurovascular dysfunction

NANDA International: *NANDA Nursing Diagnoses: Definitions and Classification 2003-2004.* Philadelphia, 2002, NANDA.

Risk for Poisoning
Post-trauma syndrome
Risk for Post-trauma syndrome
Powerlessness
Risk for Powerlessness
Ineffective Protection
Rape-trauma syndrome
Rape-trauma syndrome: compound reaction
Rape-trauma syndrome: silent reaction
Relocation stress syndrome
Risk for Relocation stress syndrome
Ineffective Role performance
Bathing/hygiene Self-care deficit
Dressing/grooming Self-care deficit
Feeding Self-care deficit
Toileting Self-care deficit
Readiness for enhanced Self-Concept
Chronic low Self-esteem
Situational low Self-esteem
Risk for situational low Self-esteem
Self-mutilation
Risk for Self-mutilation
Disturbed Sensory perception (specify)
Sexual dysfunction
Ineffective Sexuality patterns
Impaired Skin integrity
Risk for impaired Skin integrity
Sleep deprivation
Disturbed Sleep pattern
Readiness for enhanced Sleep
Impaired Social interaction

Social isolation
Chronic Sorrow
Spiritual distress
Risk for Spiritual distress
Readiness for enhanced Spiritual well-being
Risk for Suffocation
Risk for Suicide
Delayed Surgical recovery
Impaired Swallowing
Effective Therapeutic regimen management
Ineffective Therapeutic regimen management
Readiness for enhanced Therapeutic regimen
    management
Ineffective community Therapeutic regimen management
Ineffective family Therapeutic regimen management
Ineffective Thermoregulation
Disturbed Thought processes
Impaired Tissue integrity
Ineffective Tissue perfusion (specify)
Impaired Transfer ability
Risk for Trauma
Impaired Urinary elimination
Readiness for enhanced Urinary elimination
Urinary retention
Impaired spontaneous Ventilation
Dysfunctional Ventilatory weaning response
Risk for other-directed Violence
Risk for self-directed Violence
Impaired Walking
Wandering

Index

---

*f indicates figure; t indicates table.

INDEX OF SKILLS*

*Page numbers given indicate the beginning of Skill.